OXFORD MEDICAL PUBLICATIONS

Oxford Desk Reference

Clinical genetics and genomics

Oxford Desk Reference: Acute Medicine
Edited by Richard Leach, Derek Bell, and Kevin Moore

Oxford Desk Reference: Cardiology
Edited by Hung-Fat Tse, Gregory Y. Lip, and
Andrew J. Stewart Coats

Oxford Desk Reference: Clinical Genetics 2e
Helen V. Firth and Jane A. Hurst

Oxford Desk Reference: Critical Care
Carl Waldmann, Neil Soni, and Andrew Rhodes

Oxford Desk Reference: Geriatric Medicine
Edited by Margot Gosney, Adam Harper, and
Simon Conroy

Oxford Desk Reference: Major Trauma
Edited by Jason Smith, Ian Greaves, and Keith Porter

Oxford Desk Reference: Nephrology
Jonathan Barratt, Kevin Harris, and Peter Topham

**Oxford Desk Reference: Obstetrics and
Gynaecology**
Edited by Sabaratnam Arulkumaran, Lesley Regan,
Aris Papageorghiou, Ash Monga, and David Farquharson

Oxford Desk Reference: Oncology
Edited by Thankamma V. Ajithkumar, Ann Barrett,
Helen Hatcher, and Natalie Cook

Oxford Desk Reference: Respiratory Medicine
Edited by Nick Maskell and Ann Millar

Oxford Desk Reference: Rheumatology
Edited by Richard Watts, Gavin Clunie, Frances Hall, and
Tarnya Marshall

Oxford Desk Reference: Toxicology
Edited by D. Nicholas Bateman, Robert D. Jefferson,
Simon H. L. Thomas, John P. Thompson, and
J. Allister Vale

Oxford Desk Reference
Clinical genetics and genomics

Second Edition

Helen V. Firth

Consultant in Clinical Genetics, Cambridge University Hospitals, Cambridge, UK
and Hon Faculty Member, Wellcome Trust Sanger Institute, Hinxton, UK

Jane A. Hurst

Consultant in Clinical Genetics, Great Ormond Street Hospital, London, UK

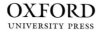

OXFORD
UNIVERSITY PRESS

OXFORD

UNIVERSITY PRESS

Great Clarendon Street, Oxford, OX2 6DP,
United Kingdom

Oxford University Press is a department of the University of Oxford.
It furthers the University's objective of excellence in research, scholarship,
and education by publishing worldwide. Oxford is a registered trade mark of
Oxford University Press in the UK and in certain other countries

First Edition published in 2005
Second Edition published in 2017

Impression: 1

Published in the United States of America by Oxford University Press
198 Madison Avenue, New York, NY 10016, United States of America

British Library Cataloguing in Publication Data
Data available

Library of Congress Control Number: 2016958194

ISBN 978–0–19–955750–9

Printed and bound by
CPI Group (UK) Ltd, Croydon, CR0 4YY

Preface to the second edition

Welcome to the second edition of *Oxford Desk Reference: Clinical Genetics and Genomics*. We were surprised and delighted by the amazingly positive response to the first edition and apologize to readers who have been eagerly awaiting the second edition that it has taken so long to reach publication. Since sending the first edition to press, Helen has become Clinical Lead for DECIPHER (http://decipher.sanger.ac.uk) and the Deciphering Developmental Disorders (DDD) study (http://www.ddduk.org), and Jane became Clinical Lead for Genetics at Great Ormond Street Hospital, London. While these roles have kept us both very busy, they have expanded our network of Expert Advisers and clinical practice and we hope you will see the benefits of that in this new edition.

Like many of our readers, we are learning how to navigate the opportunities and challenges of the new sequencing technologies that have led to an explosion in knowledge and potential for diagnosis. Establishing safe models of practice that reap the diagnostic benefits, while minimizing the potential harms of misdiagnosis and overdiagnosis, is a challenge for all working in clinical genetics. Addressing that challenge is essential if we are to offer up-to-date and accurate advice to patients and their families. We hope that this new edition, revised throughout from a genomic perspective, will help in that endeavour.

Helen Firth and Jane Hurst

Preface to the first edition

When Helen and Jane asked me whether a desk reference in clinical genetics would be useful, I enthusiastically replied 'yes'. Who has not been asked to see a child on the ward and not been able to remember the approach to a relatively common, but recently forgotten, disorder? During an outreach clinic, you are scheduled to see a family with a common disorder and they turn out to have two or three rare complications, and you do not have access to 'real' textbooks. You get a call from a good colleague who asks you 'simple' questions about the workings of a well-known syndrome and you do not want to appear stupid to your friend. This book can be your 'lifesaver' in many situations.

The book includes many common-sense approaches, useful standards and definitions, suggestions for appropriate testing, and excellent references. It is meant to be 'first line' and a way to jog your memory. Certainly, you will need to consult other texts and data sources. However, this book can be carried around in your briefcase or handbag—so to speak a peripheral brain. Blank pages are distributed throughout the book to enable you to update and personalize your copy with notes from current journals, guidelines, seminars, and lectures.

If it turns out to be useful, and I certainly expect that it will, there will surely be additional editions. The authors would therefore like feedback and suggestions. Genetic information is changing so quickly that a 2-year half-life can be expected.

Medical genetics registrars, residents, and fellows should particularly find this book useful, but I would anticipate that the mature and experienced clinical geneticist would also find it useful and thoughtfully constructed.

If you are the lucky new purchaser of *Oxford Desk Reference: Clinical Genetics*—'congratulations'. If you are considering buying it—'do it'. If you need an easy-to-use, handy reference that can be carried around so you appear more competent and well informed—'don't hesitate'.

Enjoy this new approach.

Judith G. Hall, OC, MD, FRCP(C), FAAP, FCCMG, FABMG
Emeritus Professor of Pediatrics and Medical Genetics,
University of British Columbia, Vancouver, Canada

Acknowledgements

In writing this book, we are indebted to the many colleagues and friends who have kindly given of their time and expertise to review each section of the book. Their wide experience of particular clinical areas has enhanced the book in many ways, improving accuracy and clarity and ensuring that the entries are as up-to-date as we can make them. We owe special thanks to our Cancer chapter expert advisers Marc Tischkowitz and Ian Frayling. We would also like to thank Rebecca Firth and Hannah Firth for their work as editorial assistants. Thanks also to Fiona Richardson at Oxford University Press for her commitment to this project over several years and special thanks to Fiona Chippendale for overseeing the production of the book.

We also owe a debt of gratitude to Judy Hall for her sustained encouragement and enthusiasm and enormous thanks to our husbands and children for their love and forbearance.

Reviews

Published reviews of the first edition

'... a comprehensive and highly focussed guide to clinical genetics that should certainly rank as an indispensable handbook for consultants in clinical genetics, genetic counsellors and paediatricians. However, it should also be extremely useful for PhD students in nearly all disciplines within medical and/or human genetics. Its major strength is the well-conceived and clearly laid out format which enables the reader to obtain a rapid yet quite substantial overview of a plethora of difficult topics ...'

Human Genetics

'The authors of [this book] deserve to be congratulated for achieving the impossible... Overall this book is a winner and is a must for every clinical genetics department. This is arguably the most important book ever published for trainees in genetics...[but] can be considered as an extremely useful reference source to any genetics physician...this book is a 'peripheral brain' and 'lifesaver' for geneticists in many situations!'

Ulster Medical Journal Vol 75, no 3

'If there was a Booker Prize for new texts on clinical genetics, then the winner this year would be a foregone conclusion. No one else could possibly come up with an entry as good as this.... the definitive hands-on guide to clinical genetics.... The breadth and depth of information provided is remarkable.... As a practical guide to the specialty of clinical genetics this book has no match, and overall it represents an awesome achievement. How did the authors manage to acquire and collate all this knowledge? Where did they find all this information? ... If your department can only afford one book this year, make it this one. Better still, buy your own copy and keep it hidden because it is going to be much in demand.'

BMJ

'This is an amazing compilation of genetic knowledge. It provides a fantastic tool for clinical geneticists who require a fast review of specific genetic subjects while performing clinical consultations.... Condensation of the amount of information included in this wonderful book could not be done any better.... This is a most-have tool for all clinical geneticists who require quick and specific reviews in clinical practice.... Dr Firth and Hurst have achieved a tremendous goal. They have been able to summarize a tremendous amount of information in clinical genetics and convert it to an excellent tool for the practice of the specialty. It could not be done any better. The magnificent work done suggests that as the field of clinical genetics expands, further editions will be needed. This is a must have book, and a second edition would be expected.'

Doody's Journal

Pre-publication reviews of the first edition

'It is very refreshing to review a book written for clinicians by clinicians, which is in a format that reflects situations actually encountered in practice. Information provided by the referring doctor to a clinical geneticist or other specialist before a clinic or ward consultation is usually limited. This new text takes common referral indications and, in a standardized format that manages to be brief and clear without skimping on detail, reminds the clinician of diagnostic possibilities and strategies for investigation and management. This will allow the best possible use to be made of an individual consultation by both the patient and the doctor.'

Dian Donnai, Professor of Medical Genetics, University of Manchester,
Consultant Clinical Geneticist, Regional Genetics Service,
St Mary's Hospital, Manchester, UK.

'I have been impressed with the thoughtfulness of the topics. This should be a great help to many people who are part of the clinical genetics team.... There are up-to-date summaries for the staff member who needs a refresher, as well as the glossary and the headings on fundamental topics, like AD inheritance, for those just starting out.'

Lewis B. Holmes, Professor of Pediatrics, Harvard Medical School and Chief,
Genetics and Teratology Unit, Massachusetts General
Hospital for Children, Boston, Massachusetts, USA.

Brief contents

Detailed contents

Appendix 805

System-based contents

Cardiac disorders

Cranial imaging abnormalities

Cranial size and shape abnormal

Developmental delay/ intellectual disability and neurodevelopmental disorders

Skin disorders

Teratogens

Glossary of terms used in dysmorphology

Accessory nipple Additional nipple arising on the 'milk line' that runs caudally from the normally sited nipple and cranially towards the axilla

Agenesis A condition in which a body part is absent or does not develop completely

Ala nasi The flaring cartilaginous area forming the outer side of each nostril

Alopecia Absence, loss, or deficiency of hair; may be patchy or total

Amelia Complete absence of one or more limbs from the shoulder or pelvic girdle

Aniridia Absence of the iris

Anisocoria Unequal pupil size

Ankyloblepharon Adhesion of the eyelids by synechiae or fibrous bands

Ankyloglossia A short or tight lingual frenulum attaching the anterior half of the inferior aspect of the tongue to the floor of the mouth, just beneath or directly onto the posterior alveolar ridge, which restricts tongue movement

Anodontia Absence of teeth

Anonychia Absence of nails

Anophthalmia Congenital absence of one or both eyes. Genetically, anophthalmia may represent an extreme form of microphthalmia and both forms may coexist in the same patient or in different family members

Antimongoloid slant Downward slant of the palpebral fissure of the eye, with the outer canthus (outer corner) lying below the level of the inner canthus

Aphakia Absence of the ocular lens

Arachnodactyly Long, slender hands, feet, fingers, and toes. Literally 'spider digits'

Areola Pigmented skin surrounding the nipple

Arrhinia Congenital absence of the nose

Atresia A condition in which an opening or passage for the tracts of the body is absent or closed, e.g. anal atresia, duodenal atresia

Bathing trunk naevus A congenital giant pigmented naevus over the area of the body covered by swimming trunks. The naevus can be hairy, deeply pigmented, and very large. It may undergo malignant transformation, so expert advice from a paediatric dermatologist is essential

Birthmark An area of altered skin colour present from birth or arising in early infancy and caused by vascular or pigment distribution anomalies

Blaschko line Streak of abnormally pigmented skin following the line of a dermatome. Linear distribution along limbs; hemicircumferential on the trunk

Body mass index (BMI) BMI = weight (kg)/height^2 (m^2). See 'Obesity with and without developmental delay' in Chapter 2, 'Clinical approach' for table

Bone age Radiological assessment of skeletal maturity based on ossification of the carpal and hand bone epiphyses. By convention, a radiograph of the left wrist is taken. The skeletal age is compared with the chronological age. Normal values and standard deviations are defined and thus an assessment can be made as to whether skeletal maturation is delayed, normal, or advanced. A more accurate assessment can be made under the age of 2 years by evaluation of the epiphyses at the knees by comparison with an atlas of normal knees at different ages

Blepharophimosis Decrease in the palpebral fissure aperture; the distance between the inner and outer canthi of each eye is reduced

Brachycephaly Flattening of the back of the head

Brachydactyly Short fingers

Brushfield spot Mottle, marbled, or speckled elevation of the iris due to increased density of the anterior border layer of the iris. Present in 85% of individuals with Down's syndrome—similar appearances may also be seen in normal individuals

Buphthalmos Congenital enlargement of the eye, usually secondary to congenital glaucoma

Café-au lait-spot Macular area of coffee-coloured pigmentation >0.5 cm in diameter

Calvarium Upper, dome-like portion of the skull

Campomelia Literally 'bent limb', as seen in campomelic dysplasia or oto-palato-digital syndrome type II

Camptodactyly Literally 'bent fingers'; usually involving contractures of the fingers

Canthal distance, inner Distance between the inner canthi (inner corners) of the two eyes

Canthal distance, outer Distance between the outer canthi (outer corners) of the two eyes

Carrying angle With the arms hanging by the sides and palms facing forwards, the deviation of the forearm relative to the humerus

Cavernous haemangioma Elevated vascular naevus or 'strawberry mark'; usually a dense red colour. Often not apparent or minimal at birth and growing rapidly during infancy; usually involuting spontaneously from the first birthday

Cebocephaly Severe form of holoprosencephaly with ocular hypotelorism and a centrally placed nose with a single blind-ended nostril

Cheilion Most lateral point of the corner of the mouth

Chordee Abnormal position of the penis caused by a band of tissue that holds the penis in a ventral or lateral curve

Clinodactyly Lateral or medial curve of one or more fingers or toes away from the third finger. Mild fifth finger clinodactyly is a common autosomal dominant (AD) trait

Club-foot Abnormal resting position of the foot. May be positional or structural. The two most common types are talipes equinovarus (the forefoot is plantar-flexed and medially rotated) and talipes calcaneovalgus (the forefoot is dorsiflexed and everted)

Coloboma Congenital fissure of the eye. May involve the iris and/or retina or eyelid. Inferior colobomas arise early in embryonic life due to incomplete fusion of the optic cup. Colobomas of the lower eyelid may be found in Treacher–Collins syndrome

Columella nasi Fleshy inferior border of the nasal septum, between the nostrils

Craniorachischisis Congenital failure of closure of the skull and spinal column

Crown–rump length (CRL) Distance from the top of the head to the bottom of the buttock. The most accurate measure of gestational age in the embryo between 6 and 11+ weeks' gestation

Cryptophthalmos Complete congenital adhesion of the eyelids; fused eyelid

Cryptorchidism Failure of the testis to descend into the scrotum; undescended testes

Cubitus valgus Increased carrying angle at the elbow

Cupid's bow The upper edge of the upper lip; shaped like the double-curved bow carried by Cupid

Cutis aplasia Absence of skin in a specific area—commonly on the scalp over the vertex

Cystic hygroma Accumulation of lymphatic fluid found usually at the back of the neck

Depigmentation Area of absent or reduced pigment due to lack of functional melanocytes

Dermatoglyphics Pattern of ridges and grooves over the fingertips, palms, and soles

Dermatome Segmental area of skin supplied by nerves from a single spinal nerve root

Dermis Inner layer of the skin; the outer layer is the epidermis. Thickness of the dermis varies from <0.5 mm over the eyelid to 2–3 mm over the back

Developmental delay Delayed acquisition of developmental milestones (e.g. smiling, sitting independently, walking, first words) in comparison with the normal range for chronological age

Developmental quotient Ratio of developmental age/chronological age

Dimple Indentation or depression of the skin where the subcutaneous tissues are deficient and the skin may be tethered to underlying structures, e.g. bone

Distichiasis A second row of eyelashes arising from the meibomian glands, as seen in the lymphoedema–distichiasis syndrome caused by mutations in *FOXC2*

Dolicocephaly Elongation of the skull. The skull is long in its anteroposterior dimension and narrow in its bitemporal dimension

Drusen Drusen are deposits on the optic nerve head present in 0.3% of the population, of which 70% occur bilaterally. An irregular knobbly disc margin, anomalous branching of the vessels, and autofluorescence help the differentiation from papilloedema

Dystopia canthorum Lateral displacement of the inner canthi of the eye (e.g. Waardenburg type 1)

Eclabion Eversion of the lips, as seen in congenital Harlequin ichthyosis

Ectopia lentis Displacement of the ocular lens, as seen in Marfan's syndrome and homocystinuria

Ectopic Abnormally sited

Ectrodactyly Commonly used to describe a 'split hand' or 'split foot' where there is deficiency of the middle ray(s) of the hand/foot

Ectropion Eversion of the eyelid

Encephalocele Congenital herniation of the brain through a bony deficiency of the skull. May be frontal or occipital (e.g. Meckel syndrome)

Enophthalmos Abnormal retraction of the eye into the orbit, producing deeply set eyes

Entropion Inversion of the eyelid

Epicanthic fold Congenital fold of the skin medial to the eye, sometimes covering the inner canthus. It is commonly seen in association with a hypoplastic nasal bridge

Epicanthus inversus Congenital fold of the skin medial to the eye, sometimes covering the inner canthus, with the fold broader inferiorly than superiorly. May occur in association with blepharophimosis and ptosis in BPES (blepharophimosis–ptosis–epicanthus inversus) syndrome due to mutations in *FOXL2*

Epidermis Superficial keratinized layer of the skin

Epiphora Flow of tears down the cheek due to blockage or stenosis of the nasolacrimal duct

Epispadias Abnormal location of the urethral meatus on the dorsal surface of the penis

Esotropia Inward deviation of an eye when both eyes are open and uncovered; convergent strabismus (squint)

Exophthalmos Abnormal protrusion of the eyes (as seen in Crouzon or Apert syndromes)

Exotropia Outward deviation of an eye when both eyes are opened and uncovered; divergent strabismus (squint)

Flexion crease Crease in the skin on the ventral surface of a joint, secondary to movement at that joint

Fontanelle Membrane-covered space remaining in the incompletely ossified skull of a fetus or infant in the line of the sutures. The anterior fontanelle at the junction of the sagittal, coronal, and metopic sutures is patent in the first 6–12 months of life and usually closes by the end of the first year

Frenulum Small fold of mucous membrane, e.g. arising between the upper central incisors and extending to the upper lip, or beneath the tongue. Additional frenulae may be found in oral–facial–digital (OFD) syndrome

Frontal bossing Prominence of the anterior portion of the frontal bone of the skull

Gastroschisis Congenital fissure of the anterior abdominal wall, adjacent to, but not involving, the insertion of the umbilical cord. Part of the intestine may herniate through the defect

Genu valgum Outward bowing of the knee; bow-leg

Genu varum Inward deviation of the knee; knock-knee

Gibbus Extreme kyphosis or hump; deformity of the spine in which there is a sharply angulated segment, the apex of the angle being posterior

Glabella The most prominent midline point between the eyebrows

Glossoptosis Downward displacement or retraction of the tongue; sometimes held by a frenulum (tongue-tie)

Gnathion The lowest median point on the inferior border of the mandible

Gonion The most lateral point of the posteroinferior angle of the mandible

Height Distance from the top of the head to the sole of the foot in a standing position

Heterochromia iridis Unequal colour of the irises where the entire iris of one eye is of a distinctly different colour, as seen in Waardenburg syndrome. A wedge-shaped segment of anomalous eye colour is called heterochromia iridum

Hirsutism Excessive body and facial hair

Holoprosencephaly Failure of midline cleavage of the embryonic forebrain

Hydrocephalus Abnormal increase in the amount of cerebrospinal fluid, accompanied by dilatation of the cerebral ventricles

Hyperextensibility Excessive stretch of the skin or excessive range of movement of a joint

Hypertelorism Increased distance between two paired structures such as the nipples or eyes. Ocular hypertelorism is used to describe the appearance of wide-set eyes due to an increased interpupillary distance

Hypertrichosis Excessive body hair that is long and often involves the face

Hypodontia Reduced number and/or size of teeth due to disturbance of tooth bud development/patterning

Hyponychia Small dysplastic nails

Hypospadias Abnormal location of the urethral meatus on the ventral surface of the penis: may be glandular (1°), penile (2°), scrotal (3°), or perineal (4°)

Hypotelorism Decreased interpupillary distance; eyes unusually close together

Imperforate anus Absence of the normal anal opening. Usually results from abnormal development of the urorectal septum, resulting in incomplete separation of the cloaca into urogenital and anorectal portions

Intelligence quotient (IQ) Measure of intellectual functioning, as assessed by standardized tests; usually measures verbal and non-verbal reasoning and expresses results as a quotient standardized for age, with 100 being the mean

Interpupillary distance Distance between the centres of the pupils of the eyes

Iridodonesis Tremor of the iris on movement, usually secondary to dislocation of the lens

Keratoconus Conical protrusion of the cornea, usually associated with thinning of the cornea

Koilonychia Spoon-shaped nails

Kyphoscoliosis Abnormal curvature of the spinal column, both anteroposteriorly and laterally

Kyphosis Curvature of the spine in the anteroposterior plane. A normal kyphosis exists in the shoulder area

Lagophthalmos Condition in which the eyelid cannot be completely closed

Lanugo Embryonic or fetal hair: fine, soft, unmedullated

Length Distance between the top of the head and the sole of the foot when the individual is lying down—used as a surrogate for height in the first year of life

Lentigo Round or oval, flat, brown, pigmented skin spot due to deposition of melanin by an increased number of melanocytes at the epidermodermal junction

Leukocoria White pupillary reflex. The pupillary reflex is usually red

Leukonychia White spots or stripes on the nails; may involve the whole nail

Lingua plicata Fissured tongue

Lisch nodule Hamartomatous iris structure seen in neurofibromatosis type 1 (NF1). Lisch nodules are iris freckles that project above the surface of the iris (unlike normal iris pigmentation) and thus are detectable by slit-lamp examination

Lordosis Curvature of the spinal column with a forward (ventral) convexity. A normal lordosis exists in the lumbar area

Lower segment Distance from the top of the pubic bone to the sole of the foot

Macrocephaly Abnormally large skull. Occipital–frontal circumference >3 standard deviations

Macrodactyly Abnormally large digit

Macroglossia Abnormally large or hypertrophic tongue (as seen in Beckwith–Wiedemann syndrome)

Madelung deformity A developmental abnormality of the wrist characterized by anatomical changes in the radius, ulna, and carpal bones, leading to palmar and ulnar wrist subluxation ('dinner-fork deformity'). It is seen in individuals with deletions or mutations of the *SHOX* gene on Xp22.3 (e.g. Leri–Weill syndrome) and sometimes in Turner's syndrome. The deformity usually becomes evident clinically between the ages of 6 and 13 years. Madelung deformity can result in wrist pain and restriction of forearm rotation (pronation/supination)

Male pattern baldness Loss of hair at the temples and on the top of the head

Manubrium Cranial portion of the sternum that articulates with the clavicles and the first two pairs of ribs

Melanocyte Pigment cell in the skin

Meromelia Partial absence of a limb

Mesomelic Referring to the middle segment of the limb

Microcephaly Abnormally small head. Occipital–frontal circumference <3 standard deviations

Micrognathia Abnormally small mandible giving a small chin

Microphallus Abnormally small penis: micropenis. If the genitalia are ambiguous, it may be difficult to distinguish a micropenis from an enlarged clitoris

Microphthalmia Abnormally small eye

Microstomia Abnormally small opening of the mouth

Mid-parental height Sum of parents' heights divided by two

Miosis Small contracted pupil

Mole Circumscribed area of darkly pigmented skin, which is often raised

Mongolian blue spot Bluish area of skin, mostly over the sacrum. The discoloured area of skin is not raised. More frequent in black, Hispanic, and Asian people

Müllerian duct Embryonic precursor of the female reproductive tract (Fallopian tubes, uterus, and upper one-third of the vagina)

Mydriasis Large, dilated pupil. Mydriatics are used to facilitate fundoscopy

Naevus sebaceous Raised, waxy patch with a mostly linear distribution

Nyctalopia Poor night vision due to loss or dysfunction of rod photoreceptors in the retina, e.g. in retinitis pigmentosa

Nystagmus Involuntary rapid movement of the eyeball that may be horizontal, vertical, rotatory, or mixed

Occipital–frontal circumference (OFC) Distance around the head. The largest measurement with the tape measure passing across the forehead, over the ears, and over the occiput

Oligodontia Less than the normal number of teeth (see also 'Hypodontia', this glossary)

Omphalocele Failure of embryonic herniation of the intestines to return inside the abdominal cavity. The intestines (and sometimes parts of the liver) protrude through a defect in the abdominal wall at the umbilicus and are covered by a thin membrane composed of the amnion and peritoneum

Ophthalmoplegia Paralysis of the eye muscles (may occur in some mitochondrial disorders)

Pachyonychia Thickened nails

Palpebral fissure length Distance between the inner and outer canthi of one eye

Patterning Process whereby embryonic cells acquire their spatial identities

Pectus carinatum Undue prominence of the sternum, often referred to as a pigeon chest

Pectus excavatum Undue depression of the sternum, often referred to as a funnel chest

Pes cavus High arched foot

Philtrum Vertical groove in the midline extending from beneath the nose to the Cupid's bow in the vermilion border of the upper lip

Pili torti Hair twisted by 180° angle

Plagiocephaly Asymmetric head shape

Poland anomaly Hypoplastic pectoral muscle often found in association with ipsilateral breast hypoplasia. Often found in association with a terminal transverse limb defect

Polydactyly Extra digit(s)—may be preaxial or post-axial or insertional

Polysyndactyly Extra digit(s) with fused digit(s)

Polythelia Occurrence of an extra nipple(s)—usually found in the milk line that runs caudally from the normal position of the nipples and cranially towards the axilla

Portwine naevus Dark angioma that can be purple in colour (as seen in Sturge–Weber syndrome)

Post-axial Posterior or lateral to the axis (e.g. post-axial polydactyly where the extra digit is lateral to the fifth finger or fifth toe)

Preaxial Anterior or medial to the axis (e.g. preaxial polydactyly where the extra digit is medial to the thumb or hallux)

Prognathism Prominence of the jaw leading to an unusually prominent chin

Pterygium A wing-shaped web, e.g. a skin web across a joint

Ptosis Drooping of the upper eyelid

Range of movement Range of place or position through which a particular joint can move

Rhizomelic Referring to the proximal portion of a limb

Scaphocephaly Abnormally long and narrow skull as a result of premature closure of the sagittal suture

Scoliosis Appreciable lateral deviation from the normally straight vertical line of the spine

Shawl scrotum Congenital ventral insertion of the scrotum

Sidney crease Proximal flexion crease of the palm that extends all the way across the palm; the distal flexion crease is still present

Simian crease Single palmar crease

Sitting height Distance from the top of the head to the buttocks when in the sitting position

Skinfold thickness Thickness of skin in designated areas (e.g. triceps, subscapular, suprailiac) used to assess subcutaneous fat and nutrition

Span Distance between the tips of the middle fingers of each hand when the arms are stretched out horizontally from the body with the palms facing forwards

Sprengel deformity Congenital upward displacement of the scapula

Stadiometer Upright measuring device for accurate assessment of height

Stellate iris A lacy, 'star-like' reticulate pattern radiating out from the pupil

Stork mark Pink vascular mark localized over the middle of the forehead, or the nape of the neck in the newborn. It represents the fetal circulatory pattern in the skin and those on the face resolve spontaneously

Strabismus Deviation of the eye (squint); the visual axes assume a position relative to each other different from that required by physiological conditions

Symblepharon Adhesion of the eyelid to the eyeball

Symphalangism Bony fusion of interdigital spaces resulting in fixed extension of joints

Syndactyly Webbing or fusion of fingers or toes

Synechia Adhesion of parts, especially adhesion of the iris to the cornea or to the lens

Syngnathia Intraoral bands, possibly remnants of the buccopharyngeal membrane extending between the jaws

Synophyrys Confluent eyebrow growth across the glabella

Tanner stages Grading system to establish standards for the stages of puberty

Telangiectasia Prominence of blood vessels on the surface of the skin

Telecanthus Increased distance between the inner canthi of the eyes

Teratogenic effect Any harmful fetal effect arising from an exposure during pregnancy

Torticollis 'Wry neck'—contracted state of the cervical muscles, resulting in twisting of the neck and restriction of movement, especially rotation. The most common causes are trauma, inflammation, or a congenital malformation involving the cervical vertebrae and/or the sternocleidomastoid muscle on one side

Trichorrhexis Nodular swelling of the hair. The hair is light-coloured and breaks easily

Trigonocephaly Triangular-shaped head and skull resulting from premature synostosis of the portions of the frontal bone with prominence of the metopic suture

Triphalangeal thumb Thumb with three phalanges (as in the fingers)

Triradii Dermatoglyphic pattern where three sets of ridges converge

Turricephaly Tall or high skull; the top of the head is pointed—may be caused by premature closure of the lamboid and coronal sutures

Vermilion border Red-coloured edge to the lip where it meets the normal skin of the face

Vertex Highest point of the head in the mid-sagittal plane, when the head is held erect

Widow's peak Pointed frontal hairline in the midline

Wolffian duct Embryonic precursor of the male reproductive tract (vas deferens, seminal vesicles, and prostate)

Woolly hair Tightly curled, kinky hair with a reduced shaft diameter

Wormian bone Small irregular bone in the suture between the bones of the skull

Expert adviser: Judith G. Hall, Emeritus Professor of Pediatrics and Medical Genetics, University of British Columbia, Vancouver, Canada.

Reference

Hall JG, Froster-Iskenius UG, Allanson JE. *Handbook of normal physical measurements*. Oxford University Press, Oxford, 1995.

Glossary of genetic and genomic terms

Acrocentric A chromosome where the centromere is near one end. The gene-coding material is usually located only on the long arm. The human acrocentric chromosomes are 13, 14, 15, 21, and 22

Activating mutation These mutations are site-specific and usually result in constitutive activation of a specific protein function

Allele One of several alternative forms of a gene occupying a given locus on a chromosome

Allele dropout (ADO) The failure, for technical reasons, to detect an allele that is present in a sample; the failure to amplify an allele during a polymerase chain reaction

Allele frequency The frequency in a population of each allele at a polymorphic locus

Alternative splicing A mechanism by which different forms of mature mRNAs are generated from the same gene. Different exons from a single gene are used to produce isoforms of a protein

Aneuploidy In *full aneuploidy*, there is an abnormal chromosome number differing from the usual diploid or haploid set by loss or addition of one or a small number of chromosomes, e.g. 45,X or 47,XY + 21. It can be the result of non-disjunction in (i) a premeiotic mitotic division in the germline of either parent, (ii) a first or second meiotic division in either parent, or (iii) an early embryonic mitotic (post-zygotic) division in an affected individual. In *partial aneuploidy*, the imbalance involves the gain or loss of part of a chromosome

Anticipation Worsening of disease severity in successive generations. Characteristically occurs in triplet repeat disorders where there is expansion of the triplet repeat in the maternal or paternal line, e.g. myotonic dystrophy

Antisense mRNA mRNA transcript that is complementary to endogenous mRNA. Introducing a transgene coding for antisense mRNA is a strategy used experimentally, but not currently in clinical practice, to block expression of an endogenous gene of interest

Apoptosis Programmed cell death

ARMS (amplification refractory mutation system) A specific robust polymerase chain reaction system for routine genetic testing that can be readily multiplexed, e.g. 29-mutation kit for cystic fibrosis (CF) testing

Array-CGH Microarray-based comparative genomic hybridization (see 'Microarray' and 'Comparative genomic hybridization (CGH)', this glossary)

ART (assisted reproductive technology) Assisted reproductive technology, e.g. *in vitro* fertilization (IVF) and intracytoplasmic sperm injection (ICSI), has revolutionized the treatment of infertility. In conjunction with single-cell genetic analysis based on polymerase chain reaction (PCR) or fluorescent *in situ* hybridization (FISH), it has also made pre-implantation genetic diagnosis (PGD) possible for some genetic disorders. See 'Assisted reproductive technologies: *in vitro* fertilization (IVF), intracytoplasmic sperm injection (ICSI), and pre-implantation genetic diagnosis (PGD)' in Chapter 6, 'Pregnancy and fertility', p. 706

Ascertainment bias A tendency for a study to be non-representative of the true population, because individuals of a particular type are more likely to be sampled

Associated* Significantly enriched in disease cases, compared to matched controls

Autosome A chromosome that is not an X or Y chromosome. There are 22 pairs of autosomes in the human chromosome complement

BAC (bacteria artificial chromosome) A cloning vector derived from an *Escherichia coli* plasmid. BACs can be used in the cloning of large DNA fragments, on average ~200 kb long, and are ideal as cloning vectors for the sequencing of whole genomes. BACs are convenient for use as FISH probes

BAM file The Binary Alighment Map (BAM) file is a binary format for storing sequence data

Band/banding Differential staining of a chromosome leading to distinction of chromosomal segments. A Giemsa-stained (G-banded) karyotype has 850 bands visible at prometaphase (Mitelman 1995)

Bioinformatics Bioinformatics is a broad discipline related to the fields of computational biology and biostatistics. Bioinformatics can be categorized into three domains:

- analytical method development;

- construction and curation of computational tools and databases;

- data mining, interpretation, and analysis.

Birth prevalence The number of cases of disorder/condition per number of live births (usually per 1000)

Bivalent Describes a pair of homologous chromosomes that align and undergo synapsis and recombination. The double structure is termed a bivalent

bp (base pair) In DNA, a purine and pyrimidine base on each strand that interact with each other through hydrogen bonding

cDNA DNA complementary to, and copied from, an RNA molecule. cDNA libraries of living cells therefore represent the RNA content of those cells, and thereby represent expressed gene sequences

Centimorgan (cM) Unit of genetic map distance corresponding to a recombination fraction of 0.01

Centromere The constricted region of a chromosome that includes the site of attachment to the mitotic or meiotic spindle

Chimerism The presence in an organism of two or more cell lines that are derived from different zygotes. Such an organism is termed a chimera. Chimerism is extremely rare in humans

Chip See 'Microarray', this glossary

Chromatid A chromosome that has undergone replication has two identical sister chromatids that are joined at the centromere before they separate into two distinct chromosomes during cell division

Chromatin The DNA helix is wrapped around core histones to form a simple 'beads on a string' configuration where the beads represent nucleosomes. This is then folded into higher-order chromatin. Chromatin can be modified by processes such as DNA methylation and histone modification (acetylation, phosphorylation, methylation, and ubiquitylation). The regulation of higher-order chromatin structures is crucial for genome reprogramming during early embryogenesis and gametogenesis and for tissue-specific gene expression and global gene silencing

Chromosome A thread-like structure composed mainly of chromatin that carries a highly ordered sequence of linked genes and resides in the nucleus of eukaryotic cells

Chromosome walking The method of moving from a linked marker to a gene

Clinical genome The portion of the genome within which genetic variation can substantially influence disease risk or response to therapy

Cloning Production of genetically identical cells (or organisms from a single ancestral cell (or nucleus)). Also a technique used in molecular biology to propagate single or discrete DNA fragments of interest. See also 'Reproductive cloning', this glossary

CNV (copy number variant) A structural variant that alters the copy number of a segment of the genome. CNVs are typically deletions or duplications (though larger amplifications, e.g. triplications, occur) and range in size from ~100 bases to several Mb

Coding strand The coding strand of DNA has a complementary sequence to mRNA since it serves as the template for mRNA synthesis

Comparative genomic hybridization (CGH) Reference and test DNA samples are fluorescently labelled, e.g. one with green probes, the other with red probes. After hybridization of labelled probe mixes to metaphase chromosome spreads, the ratio of green to red fluorescence along each chromosome is compared in an attempt to identify genomic imbalance in the test DNA

Compound heterozygote An individual that has altered gene function because each copy of the gene is altered by different mutations, e.g. an individual with cystic fibrosis may have the *CFTR* genotype deltaF508/G542X, i.e. there are two mutations in both alleles at the same locus. (NB. A double heterozygote is an individual who is heterozygous at two different loci.)

Concordance Presence of the same trait in both members of a pair (as in twins) or in all members of a set of similar individuals

Confidence interval (CI) The CI provides a means of quantifying the range of uncertainty around a result (e.g. for a relative risk (RR) = 0.7 with a 95% CI, the range is 0.5–0.8). The smaller the range of the CI, the more precise the estimate is likely to be. Where a CI spans 1.0, this indicates no significant observed effect

Consanguinity Parents are related (i.e. have a recent common ancestor) and share a proportion of their genetic material. In practice, a consanguineous relationship is often considered as one between individuals who are second cousins or closer

Consultand An individual seeking advice about a genetic disorder

Contig A set of overlapping sequences or clones from which a sequence can be obtained

Copy number The number of copies of a given chromosomal locus which are present. For an autosomal locus with a heterozygous deletion, e.g. Smith–Magenis syndrome on 17p11.2, the copy number for the deleted region is 1, compared with 2 for normal individuals and 3 for individuals carrying a 17p11.2 duplication. For a male with an AZFa deletion on his Y chromosome, the copy number will be 0, compared with 1 for a normal male

CRAM file CRAM files are sequence alignment files similar to BAM files, but requiring less data storage space. CRAM files are a more compressed version of the alignment where nucleotides identical to the reference sequence are not individually represented, e.g. for a reference sequence of ACTGGGC, an individual sequence of AC**C**GGGC in a BAM file format would be represented as --C---- in a CRAM file

CRISPR/Cas9 A powerful technology that can be used to create a targeted modification in the genome of a living cell (see entry on Genome editing). The CRISPR/Cas9 complex is an RNA-guided nuclease (the guide RNA is 20 nucleotides in length) that can be used to efficiently cleave DNA; it is often referred to as 'molecular scissors'. The cleavage process induces the cell's own DNA repair machinery to repair the break. This strategy can be used to create a null allele or to revert a variant on one allele to that of its homologue by triggering homology directed DNA repair at the break site. An alternative strategy is to co-introduce a DNA fragment containing the intended replacement bespoke DNA sequence along with the CRISPR/Cas9 complex, to study its functional impact. In this instance, the DNA repair machinery can use this introduced DNA template to change the targeted variant to this intended sequence

Cumulative risk Cumulative risk of a disease by age *n* is the probability of an individual being diagnosed with that disease by their *n*th birthday

Damaging A damaging variant alters the normal levels or biochemical function of a gene or gene product

Deleterious A deleterious variant reduces the reproductive fitness of carriers and would thus be targeted by purifying natural selection

Deletion Loss of part of a chromosome, or part or all of a gene or DNA sequence

Differentially methylated region (DMR) DNA segments in imprinted genes that show different methylation patterns between paternal and maternal alleles, e.g. SNRP (small nuclear ribonuclear protein). Some DMRs acquire DNA methylation in the germ cells, whereas others acquire DNA methylation during embryogenesis

Digenic inheritance Two genes are involved, with at least one mutation at both loci needed, in order to produce the phenotype, e.g. Connexin 26 and 30 in sensorineural deafness, and *HFE* and *HAMP* in juvenile haemochromatosis and *BBS2* and *BBS4* in Bardet–Biedl syndrome

Diploid (2n) A paired set of chromosomes comprising two of each autosome and two sex chromosomes. Diploid chromosome sets occur in somatic cells, e.g. 46,XX and 46,XY. Often used as a diploid cell or a diploid organism

Discordance A twin pair or set of individuals in which the members differ in whether they exhibit a certain trait

Dizygotic twins (DZ) Two individuals born together derived from two separate eggs fertilized by two separate sperms

Domain A discrete portion of a gene or protein with its own function

Dominant A trait in which the mutant allele is dominant to the wild-type allele, i.e. the disease or disorder is manifest when one copy of the mutant allele is inherited, e.g. achondroplasia

Dominant negative mutation A mutation in one copy of a gene, resulting in a mutant protein that has not only lost its own function, but also prevents the wild-type protein of the same gene from functioning normally. Commonly acts by producing an altered polypeptide (subunit) that prevents the assembly of a multimeric protein

Double heterozygote An individual who is heterozygous at two *different* loci. (NB. An individual who is a compound heterozygote has two different mutations at the same locus.)

Downstream A region of DNA that lies 3′ to the point of reference

Duplicon A duplicated segment of the genome. Pericentromeric regions of human chromosomes are preferential sites for the integration of duplicated DNA, or 'duplicons', which often contain gene fragments. Duplicons appear to mediate genomic fluidity in both disease and evolutionary processes. Duplicons are implicated in the recurring 15q11–q13 deletion seen in PWS/AS (Prader–Willi syndrome/Angelman syndrome) and also in 22q11 deletion syndrome

Dynamic mutation A trinucleotide repeat expansion that can change in size during meiosis or, in some instances, mitosis

Embryonic stem cell Cell derived from the inner cell mass of an early embryo that can replicate indefinitely and differentiate into many cell types

Empiric risk Risk of recurrence that has been observed based on family studies—often used for complex multifactorial disorders

Epigenetic Any heritable influence (in the progeny of cells or of individuals) on chromosome or gene function that is not accompanied by a change in DNA sequence, e.g. X-chromosome inactivation, imprinting, centromere inactivation, and position effect variegation

ESAC (extrastructurally abnormal chromosome) Term synonymous with 'marker chromosome'. Some are composed entirely of heterochromatin and do not influence phenotype; others contain euchromatin and may adversely affect phenotype

EST (expressed sequence tag) A small segment of DNA with a characteristic (or perhaps unique) sequence derived from a cDNA clone. Used to map the positions of expressed sequences

Euchromatin The lightly staining regions of the nucleus that generally contain decondensed, transcriptionally active regions of the genome; gene-rich areas of chromatin that are typically decondensed and therefore lightstaining in nuclei and chromosomes

Exome The protein-coding portion of the genome, typically 1–2% of the entire genome. The total length of coding and splicing regions is estimated to be ~35 Mb

Exon A segment of an interrupted gene that is represented in the mature RNA product

Expressivity Variation in the severity of a disorder in individuals who have inherited the same disease alleles. Note the difference from penetrance, which is the percentage of individuals expressing the disorder to any degree, from the most trivial to the most severe

FISH (fluorescent *in situ* hybridization) *In situ* hybridization in which the DNA probe is labelled with a fluorophore. Using fluorescence microscopy, the probe can be visualized binding to a specific chromosomal region. The efficacy of FISH is limited in some applications by low-resolution sensitivity

Founder effect A high prevalence of a genetic disorder in an isolated or inbred population due to the fact that many members of the population are derived from a common ancestor who harboured a disease-causing mutation. Founder effects are seen both for dominant and recessive disorders and, if the disorder is due to a founder effect, the affected individuals in a given population carry the same mutation (founder mutation). Examples include the recessive disorders Meckel syndrome, hydrolethalus syndrome, Cohen syndrome, and congenital Finnish nephropathy, which all occur with disproportionately high incidence in Finland, compared with other European populations

Founder mutation A disease-causing mutation that is found repeatedly in a given population and is derived from a common ancestor who harboured that mutation

Frameshift mutation Deletion or insertion of a number of bases that is not a multiple of three, leading to alteration of the reading frame

Gain-of-function mutation These mutations are site-specific and usually result in constitutive activation of a specific protein function

Gene The fundamental unit of heredity. A sequence of DNA involved in producing a polypeptide chain—it includes coding segments (exons) and intervening sequences (introns), together with regulatory elements, e.g. promoter. A gene is functionally defined by its product

Gene conversion A non-reciprocal recombination process between alleles or loci that results in an alteration of the sequence of a gene to that of its homologue. Gene conversion occurs as a consequence of mismatch repair after heteroduplex formation. Gene conversion events are common between the telomeric and centromeric *SMN* genes (spinal muscular atrophy (SMA)) and between the *NEMO* gene and its pseudogene in incontinentia pigmenti (IP)

Gene panel This term has two meanings: (i) a pull-down technology to isolate a subset of genes (e.g. cancer predisposition genes) for sequencing or (ii) a virtual panel against which a whole exome or whole genome is analysed

Genetic counselling The process by which individuals or relatives at risk of a disorder that may be hereditary are advised of the consequences of the disorder, the probability of developing or transmitting it, and the ways in which this may be prevented, avoided, or ameliorated (Harper 2004)

Genome The entire genetic complement of a prokaryote, virus, mitochondria, or chloroplast, or the haploid nuclear genetic complement of a eukaryotic species. The human genome contains ~20 000 genes

Genome architecture The structure, content, and organization of a genome, including the location and order of genes

Genome editing A protein (eg. Cas9) is combined with a specific 'guide RNA' (typically 20 nucleotides long) to create a complex to target a specific DNA sequence in the genome and create a break. This break can then be used to engineer in a mutation or edit out a section of DNA that harbours a mutation. The former approach can be used to study the functional significance of DNA elements; the latter approach has the potential to 'correct' pathogenic mutations in order to develop mutation targeted therapy for some genetic disorders. CRISP/Cas9 is one of the most widely-used systems (see entry on CRISP/Cas9).

Genome-wide scan A systematic survey to discover if a phenotypic trait or genetic disease is linked to a genetic mapping marker(s) used to try and identify the gene(s) responsible for a given disease

Genome-wide significance A statistical measure of the confidence with which a gene or variant is associated to a phenotype/disease that incorporates correction for multiple testing

Genotype The genetic constitution of an individual, at one or more gene loci

Germline mosaicism The presence in a gonad of genetically distinct populations of cells, usually implying that the mosaicism is confined to the ovary/testis. If both parents appear unaffected, but one parent is a germline mosaic, this can result in recurrence of affected children, e.g. TSC

Haploid (n) A set of chromosomes comprising one of each autosome and one sex chromosome. Haploid chromosome sets (n) occur in the gametes, e.g. 23,X and 23,Y

Haploinsufficiency Situation in which the product of only one allele is produced and is insufficient for normal function. It arises when the normal phenotype requires the protein product of two alleles, and reduction of 50% of the gene product results in an abnormal phenotype

Haplotype A set of closely linked alleles on a single chromosome that tend to be inherited en bloc, i.e. not separated by recombination at meiosis

Hedgehog genes A highly conserved family of genes that encode signalling molecules. Sonic hedgehog (*SHH*) plays a major part in the growth and patterning of many tissues and organ systems. Indian hedgehog (*IHH*) is important in endochondral bone formation, and desert hedgehog (*DHH*) regulates male germline development

Helicases Enzymes that unwind double-stranded DNA into two single strands

Hemizygous The presence of only one copy of a gene. Males are hemizygous for most genes on the X chromosome (with the exception of the pseudoautosomal regions, which are also represented on Y)

Heritability The proportion of variation in a given characteristic or state within a particular population that can be attributed to genetic factors

Heterochromatin Regions of the genome that are permanently in a highly condensed condition, are not transcribed, and are late-replicating. Heterochromatin includes both repetitive DNA (e.g. highly repetitive satellite DNA and ribosomal DNA gene clusters) and some protein-coding genes

Heterodisomy See 'Uniparental disomy (UPD)', this glossary

Heteroduplex Double-stranded DNA fragment that has a mismatch between the two strands due to a mutation. The mismatched bases cannot pair as normal and so destabilize the DNA molecule

Heteroplasmy The existence of more than one mitochondrial DNA (mtDNA) type in the same cell, tissue, or individual, e.g. mitochondria containing a mixture of mtDNA carrying the MELAS 3243 point mutation and mtDNA with the wild-type sequence. In mitochondrial disorders, because of the thousands of mitochondria in each cell, there are often a variable percentage of mutant and wild-type mtDNAs between different cells and especially between different tissues. See 'Homoplasmy', this glossary

Heterozygous The presence of two different alleles at a specified locus

Histones Small, highly conserved basic proteins that associate with DNA to form a nucleosome (the basic structural subunit of chromatin)

Homeobox The conserved 60-amino acid DNA-binding homeodomain in a *HOX* gene

Homeobox (HOX) genes A family of genes that encode proteins with a conserved DNA-binding homeobox domain that are involved in regulating patterning events of early embryonic development. The *HOX* genes provide a remarkably conserved system for providing regional identity to the primary body axis of developing embryos. They encode transcription factors with a conserved 60-amino acid DNA-binding homeodomain (homeobox) and are organized in four clusters on the chromosomes (*HOXA, HOXB, HOXC,* and *HOXD*). In *Drosophila*, they specify segment identity along the rostrocaudal axis. To date, only two *HOX* genes *HOXD13* (synpolydactyly) and *HOXA13* (hand–foot–genital syndrome) have been found to be mutated in human malformation syndromes. Both genes are located at the 5′ end of their respective clusters and play a role in the specification of the most caudal structures, i.e. the most distal parts of the limb and the genital tubercle

Homeotic genes A class of genes that are crucial for controlling the early development and differentiation of embryonic tissues, e.g. homeobox (*HOX*) genes and paired box (*PAX*) genes

Homoplasmy The existence of only one mitochondrial DNA (mtDNA) type in the same cell, tissue, or individual, e.g. mitochondria containing only mtDNA carrying the A1555G sensorineural deafness sequence. See 'Heteroplasmy', this glossary

Homozygosity by descent Seen in consanguineous families where both copies of an allele or haplotype arise from a common ancestor. Can be a useful mapping strategy for autosomal recessive (AR) disorders

Homozygous The presence of two identical alleles at a specified locus

Housekeeping gene A gene that is ubiquitously expressed and encodes a protein performing a basic function common to most cells

HOX **genes** See 'Homeobox (*HOX*) genes', this glossary

Hybridization The artificial pairing of two complementary strands of DNA (or one strand of DNA and one of RNA) to form a double-stranded molecule. One strand is often labelled and used as a probe to detect the presence of the other

Hypomorphic mutation/allele A mutation which leads to impaired function of the gene product, in contrast to a null mutation which leads to absence or complete loss of function of the gene product

ICSI (intracytoplasmic sperm injection) Used as an adjunct to IVF to overcome infertility due to oligospermia and/or immotile sperm and for polymerase chain reaction (PCR)-based pre-implantation genetic diagnosis (PGD) techniques, to avoid the risk of extra sperm buried in the zona pellucida contaminating the assay

Implicated An implicated variant or gene possesses evidence consistent with a pathogenic role, with a defined level of confidence

Imprinting A genetic mechanism by which genes are selectively expressed from the maternal or paternal homologue of a chromosome. This expression may be time-specific and even tissue-specific. For a small number of genes, epigenetic mechanisms can determine expression from one generation of an organism to the next. Imprinting invokes a variety of mechanisms that distinguish the maternal and paternal homologue and affect the chromatin structures that determine transcriptionally silent and active states. The inactive allele is epigenetically marked by histone modification, cytosine methylation, or both. Imprints once established are erased during the early development of the male and female germ cells and then reset prior to germ cell maturation. In humans, about 50 genes are imprinted, i.e. differentially expressed according to their origin in either the oocyte or spermatozoa. These imprinted genes have roles in growth and development, as well as in tumour suppression

Imprinting centre Controls resetting of a cluster of closely linked imprinted genes during transmission through the opposite sex, e.g. *UBE3A* in Angelman syndrome

Incest Incest is defined as sexual intercourse between close relatives. In English law, it is the crime of sexual intercourse between parent and child or grandchild, or between siblings or half-siblings (*Shorter Oxford English Dictionary*)

Incidence The number of new cases arising in a specified population over a given period of time

Indel An insertion or deletion, typically <100 bp. Currently, the distinction between indels and CNVs is largely determined by the technology by which they are ascertained, with 'indel' primarily used for variants identified by sequencing and 'CNV' for variants identified by genomic array. Biologically, there is a continuum in size from deletion or duplication of a single nucleotide, to deletion or duplication of many megabases, or even an entire chromosome

Informed choice 'An informed choice is one that is based on relevant knowledge consistent with the decision maker's values and behaviourally implemented' (O'Connor and O'Brien-Pallas 1989)

In-frame mutation Deletion or insertion of multiples of three bases that lead to a deletion or insertion to the encoded protein, but not to early termination

In situ Refers to carrying out experiments with intact tissue

Interphase The period between mitotic cell divisions; divided into G1, S, and G2

Intron A segment of DNA that is transcribed, but removed from within the transcript by splicing together the coding sequences (exons) on either side of it

Inverse PCR (iPCR) iPCR is a technique to amplify genomic DNA flanking the insertion site of a transposon. The flanking genomic DNA obtained can be sequenced to determine the position of insertion of the transposon

Isodisomy See 'Uniparental disomy (UPD)', this glossary

Isoelectric focusing gels Thin-layer acrylamide gels that separate proteins by mass and charge, e.g. the different mutants of alpha-1 antitrypsin have characteristic migration profiles

IVF (*in vitro* fertilization) An assisted reproductive technology (ART) procedure that involves collecting eggs from a woman's ovaries (egg retrieval) and fertilizing them in the laboratory. The resulting embryos are then transferred back into the uterus through the cervix. Hormone therapy is administered to stimulate ovulation prior to egg collection and to prepare the endometrium to facilitate implantation of the embryo(s). Usually a maximum of two embryos are implanted to minimize the risk of triplets and higher-order multiple births

Karyotype The chromosome complement of a cell or species. In humans, the karyotype of a normal male is 46,XY and that of a normal female is 46,XX

kb (kilobase) 10³ base pairs of DNA

Knockout Usually refers to a genetically engineered organism (e.g. a mouse) carrying a targeted mutation (in all of their somatic and germline cells) that inactivates the gene of interest. Interbreeding of heterozygous knockout mice can generate homozygous knockouts

Lambda (λ) The ratio of the frequency of a multifactorial disease in the relative of an affected person, compared with its rate in the general population, e.g. in sib pair studies, lambda is the ratio of the frequency of the disease in siblings, compared with the general population. Lambda is a measure of relative risk and hence of disease heritability

LCR (low-copy repeat element) LCRs have been found to mediate the recurrent interstitial deletions on 7q (Williams), 15q11–q13 (PWS/AS (Prader–Willi syndrome/Angelman syndrome)), and 22q11. LCRs are either chromosome-specific, e.g. LCR-22, or specific to a particular chromosomal region(s). Three large region-specific LCRs, composed of different blocks (A, B, and C), flank the Williams syndrome deletion interval and are thought to predispose to misalignment and unequal crossing-over, causing the deletions

Linkage disequilibrium Linkage disequilibrium occurs when the probability of the occurrence of particular DNA variants at two sites physically close to one another on the chromosome is significantly greater than that expected from the product of the observed allelic frequencies at each site independently, i.e. the DNA variants occur together more frequently on individual chromosomes in the population than expected by chance

Locus A unique chromosomal region that corresponds to a gene or some other DNA sequence

Locus heterogeneity The disease phenotype caused by mutation in one gene can also be caused by mutations in another gene at a different location in the genome, e.g. tuberous sclerosis can be caused by a mutation in *TSC1* on 9q or by a mutation in *TSC2* on 16p

LOD (logarithm of the odds ratio) score A measure of genetic linkage, defined as the log10 ratio of the probability that the data would have arisen if the loci are linked to the probability that the data could have arisen from unlinked loci. The conventional threshold for declaring linkage is an LOD score of 3.0, i.e. a 1000:1 ratio (which must be compared with the 50:1 probability that any random pair of loci will be linked)

LOF (loss of function) Referring to a type of mutation resulting in inactivation of the gene product

LOH (loss of heterozygosity) When a region of a chromosome becomes homozygous for alleles that were expected to be heterozygous (usually due to a deletional event or loss of chromosomal material, often seen in the evolution of tumours)

LOI (loss of imprinting) Loss of imprinting is a phenomenon seen in many cancers

Marker chromosome Term synonymous with ESAC (extrastructurally abnormal chromosome)

Mb (megabase) 10⁶ base pairs of DNA

Meiosis The process by which haploid (*n*) germ cells are produced by two successive cell divisions without an intervening round of DNA replication. The first meiotic division (MI) is called the reduction division because it reduces the chromosome number from 2*n* to *n*. Sister chromatids separate from each other only at the second

meiotic division (MII). This yields haploid cells that differentiate into ova or sperm. Recombination occurs in the prophase of MI

Microarray (chip) A high-density miniaturized array of oligonucleotides spotted onto a glass slide. Expression arrays hybridize mRNA to quantify gene expression. Genomic arrays hybridize DNA to identify cryptic deletions and duplications

Microsatellite A stretch of DNA in which a short motif (usually 1–5 nucleotides long) is repeated several times, e.g. a poly A tract (A)13. The most common microsatellite in humans is a (CA)*n* repeat which occurs in tens of thousands of places in the genome. Microsatellites are often polymorphic, e.g. (CA)11, (CA)14, (CA)15, and (CA)20

Microsatellite instability (MSI) The situation in which germline microsatellite alleles (see 'Microsatellite', this glossary) gain or lose repeat units during mitosis. This generates a variety of repeat lengths for specific microsatellites in different somatic cells of the same individual. Microsatellite instability is a feature of hereditary non-polyposis colorectal cancer (HNPCC)

Minisatellite See 'VNTR (variable number tandem repeat)', this glossary

Minor allele frequency (MAF) When there are more than two alleles, MAF refers to the second most frequent

Mismatch repair Nucleotide mismatches occur normally when two strands of DNA replicate, but almost all such errors are quickly corrected by a molecular proofreading mechanism (encoded by the mismatch repair genes, e.g. *MSH2* and *MLH1*). Defective mismatch repair facilitates malignant transformation by allowing the rapid accumulation of mutations that inactivate genes that ordinarily have key functions in the cell

Missense mutation Nucleotide substitution that results in an altered amino acid residue in the encoded protein

Mitosis The process by which the genetic material in a cell is duplicated and divided equally between two daughter cells. Each chromosome undergoes duplication to produce two closely adjacent sister chromatids that separate from each other to become two daughter chromosomes

MNV (multinucleotide variant) A combination of two or three single nucleotide polymorphisms (SNPs) that, when found in the same codon/haplotype in a given individual, change the interpretation of protein-coding variants

Modifier gene A gene whose expression can influence a phenotype resulting from a mutation at another locus

Monogenic A trait or disease governed by the individual action of a single gene (as in classical Mendelian disorders)

Monosomy One copy of a chromosome. Usually two copies are present in a somatic cell (2*n*). Autosomal monosomy is invariably lethal in early pregnancy. Females with Turner's syndrome are typically monosomic for X, i.e. 45,X

Monozygotic twins (MZ) Two individuals born together derived from one sperm and one egg

Mosaicism The presence of two or more cell populations derived from the same conceptus, but in which one has subsequently acquired a genetic difference, either by mitotic non-disjunction, trisomy rescue, or occurrence of a somatic new mutation. Examples include trisomy 21 mosaicism arising either from a normal conceptus with mitotic non-disjunction in the early zygote or from a trisomy 21 conceptus with subsequent trisomy rescue establishing a euploid cell line 47XY + 21/46XY, or segmental neurofibromatosis type 1 (NF1) in which cells in just a few dermatomes have acquired a neurofibromin mutation

Multifactorial disease A disease caused by the interaction of several genes and the environment

Multiplex ligation-dependent probe amplification (MLPA) A new method for the relative quantification of up to 40 different DNA sequences. Each MLPA probe consists of two oligonucleotides that are ligated by a thermostable ligase if they bind to the target sequence. Target sequences are small (50–70 nucleotides). The ligated probe is then amplified by polymerase chain reaction (PCR), rather than the target sequence as in conventional assays. Each MLPA probe is designed to have a specific size so that, when the amplification products of the PCR are run on a gel, the product of each probe can be identified by its size. This technique can be used to identify exon deletions and duplications and, potentially, the copy number of any unique sequence

Multiplex polymerase chain reaction (PCR) In this test, PCR is used with a mixture of different primer pairs. Each primer pair is designed to amplify a single region of interest (e.g. an exon of dystrophin) using genomic DNA as a template

Mutation A permanent change in the genetic material that can be transmitted to offspring. A pathogenic mutation results in an alteration in the function of the gene product

Nested polymerase chain reaction (PCR) A technique for improving the sensitivity and specificity of PCR by the sequential use of two sets of oligonucleotide primers in two rounds of PCR. The second pair (known as 'nested primers') are located within the segment of DNA that is amplified by the first pair

Next-generation sequencing (NGS) Describes a group of high-throughput technologies that use massively parallel DNA sequencing to substantially increase capacity and reduce costs. NGS technologies usually sequence DNA in short fragments many times over, then longer sequences or whole genomes are subsequently reconstructed computationally

Non-disjunction The failure of homologous chromosomes to segregate at meiosis, resulting in one daughter cell with two copies, and one daughter cell with no copies of the chromosome in question. Trisomy 21 usually arises by non-disjunction in maternal meiosis

Nonsense-mediated decay (NMD) A pathway ensuring that mRNAs that bear premature stop codons are eliminated as templates for translation

Nonsense mutation A mutation resulting in the introduction of a stop codon that causes the premature truncation of a protein

Non-synonymous variant A sequence variant that results in a change in the amino acid sequence of the protein

Northern blotting Technique for transferring RNA from an agarose gel to a nitrocellulose filter on which it can be hybridized to complementary DNA

Nucleosome The basic structural subunit of chromatin, consisting of 200 bp of double-helical DNA and an octamer of histone proteins comprising two of each core histone (H2A, H2B, H3, and H4)

Nucleotide A purine or pyrimidine base to which a sugar and phosphate groups are attached

Null mutation/allele A mutation which leads to absence or complete loss of function of the gene product, in contrast to a hypomorphic mutation which leads to impaired function of the gene product

Odds ratio (OR) The association of an exposure and an outcome measure can be estimated by the calculation of an odds ratio, which is the ratio of the odds of exposure among cases to the odds of exposure among controls. An OR greater than one (>1) means the exposure is estimated to increase the odds of an event; conversely, an OR <1 will decrease the odds. If the OR = 1, then the exposure is estimated to have no effect on the outcome

Offspring risk The risk that an affected parent will have an offspring with the same genetic condition. For a fully penetrant autosomal dominant condition, this risk will be 50%. See relevant sections of Chapter 1, 'Introduction'

Oligogenic A trait or disease governed by the simultaneous action of a few (2–3) gene loci

Oligonucleotide (oligo) A short fragment of single-stranded DNA that is typically 5–50 nucleotides long

Oncogene A gene normally involved in promoting cell proliferation or differentiation, whose overactivity contributes to carcinogenesis. Oncogenes usually act dominantly at the cellular level, i.e. an activating mutation in just one copy of the gene is sufficient to drive carcinogenesis

Open reading frame (ORF) A sequence of DNA following an initiation codon that does not contain a stop codon. Implies the presence of a gene that codes for a protein or functional RNA

Panel See 'Gene panel', this glossary

Paracentric inversion A structural alteration to a chromosome that results from breakage, inversion, and reinsertion at the sites of breakage of the fragment at the same breakpoints where both breakpoints lie on the same arm of the chromosome, i.e. the inversion does not span the centromere

Paralogues Homologous genes that are related by a duplication event

Parent of origin (PoO) When inheritance expression differs, depending on from which parent (mother or father) a gene or trait is inherited (see 'Imprinting', this glossary) and allelic expansion

Pathogenic* A pathogenic variant contributes mechanistically to disease but is not necessarily fully penetrant (i.e. may not be sufficient in isolation to cause disease)

PAX (paired box) genes Genes that encode transcription factors involved in early embryological development of many tissues. Their DNA-binding domain resembles that of paired genes of *Drosophila*

PCR (polymerase chain reaction) A technique in which cycles of denaturation, annealing with primer, and extension with DNA polymerase are used to amplify the number of copies of a target DNA sequence by >106 times (Lewin 2000)

Penetrance The probability of the carrier of a germline mutation showing signs of the disease, from the most trivial to the most severe. If all individuals who have a disease genotype show the disease phenotype, then the disease is said to be 'fully penetrant' or to have a penetrance of 100%

Pericentric inversion A structural alteration to a chromosome that results from breakage, inversion, and reinsertion of the fragment at the same breakpoints where one breakpoint lies on the p arm and the other on the q arm, i.e. the inversion spans the centromere

PGD (pre-implantation genetic diagnosis) IVF (*in vitro* fertilization) techniques are used (ovarian hyperstimulation, oocyte retrieval, and *in vitro* fertilization) to obtain fertilized embryos. One to two cells are removed for genetic analysis from several cleavage-stage embryos at the 8- to 16-cell stage (day 3). Only embryos in which genetic testing predicts that the developing embryo will not develop the genetic disorder under test are then implanted in the mother

Phase Describes whether particular alleles at adjacent loci are on the same (*cis*) or different (*trans*) chromosomes

Phenocopy The mimicking of a disorder usually caused by mutations in a given gene, by mutations in a different gene, or by environmental factors

Phenotype The appearance or other characteristics of an organism, resulting from the interaction of its genetic constitution with the environment

Pleiotropy The production by a single gene of two or more apparently unrelated diseases, e.g. limb-girdle dystrophy, partial lipodystrophy, and Charcot–Marie–Tooth disease can all be caused by different mutations in the lamin A/C (*LMNA*) gene on 1q21. Conversely, the term may refer to the pleiotropic effects (e.g. multiple system involvement) of a single gene (e.g. eye, bone, and heart involvement in Marfan's syndrome due to mutations in *FBN1*)

pLI score A measure of the probability of loss of function intolerance

Polygenic A trait or disease governed by the simultaneous action of many (>3) gene loci

Polymorphism The existence of two or more variants (alleles, sequence variants, chromosomal variants) that are non-pathogenic, the less common occurring at a frequency of >1% in a normal population

Polyploid (3n or 4n) Multiple sets of chromosomes, e.g. triploid 69,XXX or 69,XXY, or 69,XYY or tetraploid 92,XXXX or 92,XXYY, sometimes found in spontaneous abortions

Predictive testing Determining the genotype of an individual at risk for an inherited disorder who, at the time of testing, has no symptoms or features of the disorder. Usually contemplated in the context of adult-onset degenerative disorders, e.g. Huntington's disease, or disorders for which burdensome screening will be undertaken in at-risk individuals, e.g. familial amyloid polyneuropathy, retinoblastoma

Premutation A mutation that has no phenotypic effect but that predisposes to a pathogenic mutation in subsequent generations, e.g. triplet repeat expansions in fragile X syndrome

Primers Oligonucleotides that anneal to template DNA to prime synthesis mediated by DNA polymerase

Private mutation A mutation unique to a given individual or family

Proband The first person in a pedigree to be identified clinically as being affected by a genetic disorder

Promoter A region of DNA involved in the binding of RNA polymerase to initiate transcription of a gene

Proteome The set of all expressed proteins for a given organism

Proto-oncogene A normal cellular gene that, by activating mutations, can be converted into an oncogene

Pseudogene A DNA sequence that was derived originally from a functional protein-coding gene that has lost its function, owing to the presence of one or more inactivating mutations

PSV (paralogous sequence variant) Sequence variants observed between duplicated segments of the genome

Quantitative real-time polymerase chain reaction (PCR) A procedure in which the PCR reaction is tracked as it progresses, by monitoring the accumulating signal that is provided by a fluorescent dye released during each PCR cycle

QTL (quantitative trait locus) A genetic locus or chromosomal region that contributes to variability in complex quantitative traits (e.g. height, weight, IQ). Quantitative traits are typically affected by several genes and by the environment

Read depth The number of sequencing calls generated for a given nucleotide or targeted region or across the exome/genome. The confidence with which heterozygous variants or mosaicism can be called is dependent upon the read depth. Typically, a read depth of ~30× enables high confidence in identifying heterozygous sites in WGS. Due to the greater variability in read depth in WES, sequencing is usually done to a higher average depth, typically 70–80×

Recessive A trait in which the mutant allele is recessive to the wild-type allele, i.e. the disease is manifest only when two mutant alleles are inherited, e.g. cystic fibrosis

Recurrence risk The chance of an event happening again. In genetic counselling, this term is usually used when advising parents who have experienced the birth of a child with a specific problem about the chance of that problem occurring again in a subsequent pregnancy. For a Mendelian condition following autosomal recessive inheritance, the recurrence risk will be 25% for each pregnancy (see relevant sections in Chapter 1, 'Introduction')

Relative risk (RR; or risk ratio) The ratio of the risk of developing a disease in individuals who have been exposed to (or inherited) a risk factor to that in individuals who have not been exposed to (or not inherited) the risk factor. An RR >1 means a person is estimated to be at an increased risk, while an RR <1 represents a decrease in risk. An RR of 1.0 means there is no apparent effect on risk

Repeat sequences Roughly half of the human genome is composed of repeat sequences. The majority of repeated sequences are transposable 'parasitic' elements such as long interspersed elements (LINEs) and short interspersed elements (SINEs) (e.g. Alu elements). Together, LINE1 and Alu account for >60% of all repeated sequences in our genome. About 5% of the genome is made up of large duplicated regions, e.g. chromosome-specific low-copy repeats (LCRs)

Reporter gene Easily detected gene/gene product used to report the expression of a gene of interest, e.g. β-galactosidase (enzyme encoded by the bacterial *LacZ* gene that converts a substrate to fluorescent compounds), green fluorescent protein (a protein derived from jellyfish that fluoresces spontaneously when excited by light of an appropriate wavelength)

Reproductive cloning The use of cloning technology to create a new organism. A reproductive clone is an organism that develops from the genetic information contained in one somatic cell of its parent and is genetically identical to that parent

Restriction fragment length polymorphism (RFLP) A genetic marker based on the presence or absence of a target for a restriction enzyme due to a polymorphism at a single base pair

Reverse phenotyping The use of genetic data to improve the phenotypic definition of a disorder

RNA interference (RNAi) RNA interference is a natural process through which small interfering RNAs (siRNAs)—small stretches of double-stranded RNA—act as guides for an enzyme complex that uses the sequence of the siRNAs to identify and destroy complementary messenger RNA, thus silencing gene expression in a sequence-specific manner

RT-PCR (reverse transcriptase polymerase chain reaction) A form of PCR that amplifies RNA by first converting it to cDNA using reverse transcriptase

Satellite DNA Consists of many tandem repeats (identical or related) of a short basic repeating unit

Screening The systematic application of a test or enquiry in order to identify individuals at sufficient risk of a specific disorder to warrant further investigation or direct preventive action among persons who have not sought medical attention on account of symptoms of that disorder (UK National Screening Committee)

Segmental aneusomy An unbalanced karyotype arising from a deletion or duplication, such that a segment of the genome is represented in additional or fewer copies than normal, e.g. 46,XY del 7q11.2 (Williams syndrome)

Segregation analysis A means to trace a DNA change through a family to test whether the change is co-inherited with the disease state

Sensitivity The frequency with which a test result is positive when the disorder/disease is present

Silent substitution (synonymous change) A nucleotide substitution that does not result in an amino acid substitution in the encoded protein because of redundancy of the genetic code

Small interfering RNAs (siRNAs) See 'RNA interference (RNAi)', this glossary

SNP (single nucleotide polymorphism, 'Snip') The occurrence in a population of different nucleotides at particular sites in the genome. Assuming a tight definition of polymorphism, SNPs are not typically disease-causing (though SNP and SNV are often used interchangeably in the literature, so caution is advised). SNPs are present at an appreciable frequency in the population (typically 1% or greater). They can be used in association studies and several adjacent SNPs can be combined into a haplotype

SNV (sincle nucleotide variant) A variant that differs from the reference sequence at a single nucleotide

Somatic mosaicism The presence in a given individual of genetically distinct populations of somatic cells that have derived from one zygote, usually implying the germline is not affected by the genetic change

Somatic recombination Pairing of homologous chromosomes, followed by recombination (crossing-over), is a central feature of meiosis. In contrast, chromosomes do not generally pair during mitotic cell division and recombination (homologous or heterologous) is a rare event. Occasional cells do, however, undergo recombination events and this can be an important mechanism in disease. For example, mosaicism for paternal uniparental isodisomy (UPD) occurring as a result of somatic recombination may underlie some cases of Beckwith–Wiedemann syndrome (BWS). Somatic recombination can cause loss of heterozygosity (LOH), which is often an important step in tumour development

Southern blotting Procedure for transferring denatured DNA that has been cut with restriction enzymes from an agarose gel to a nitrocellulose filter where it can be hybridized with a radioactively labelled probe (complementary nucleic acid sequence). Used to size high-copy repeats, e.g. in Huntington's disease, myotonic dystrophy, fragile X

SOX genes Group of genes that encode transcription factors that influence embryonic development of many tissues. Sox refers to Sry-like high mobility group box transcription factor

Specificity The frequency with which a test result is negative when the disorder/disease is absent

Splice acceptor site Junction between the dinucleotide AG at the end of an intron and the start of the next exon

Splice donor site Junction between the end of an exon and the dinucleotide GT at the start of the next intron

Splicing The process by which introns are removed from the primary transcript and the exons are joined together. Some genes have alternative splice variants where a single gene gives rise to more than one mRNA sequence that may have different tissue distributions

Stem cell A cell of a multicellular organism that is pluripotent and capable of giving rise to indefinitely more cells of the same type, and that retains the potential to undergo terminal differentiation, e.g. into a neuron or an oligodendrocyte or into a red blood cell or a white blood cell

Structural variant (SV) A region of DNA of ≥1 kb that may be an inversion, a balanced translocation, an insertion, or a deletion. Insertion or deletion SVs are commonly referred to as copy number variants (CNVs)

Stutter bands The signals that indicate the presence of DNA fragments that are one or two repeats shorter than the true allele, owing to a 'slippage' artefact that arises from the polymerase chain reaction (PCR)

STR (short tandem repeat) An array of short sequences, each normally 2- to 4-bp nucleotides in length. Often used in DNA profiling

STS (sequence-tagged sites) Short segments of genomic DNA for which the base sequence is known; they serve as physical landmarks for mapping

Synapsis Side-by-side pairing and union of homologous chromosomes

Synonymous variant A sequence variant that, due to redundancy of the genetic code, does not result in a change in the amino acid sequence in a protein. Synonymous variants can still be pathogenic, e.g. if they affect splicing

TaqMan A propietary system that allows the progression of a polymerase chain reaction (PCR) to be monitored in real time

Targeting vector DNA fragment usually derived from a virus or plasmid that carries the mutation to be introduced during gene targeting (genetic engineering). It contains the mutation and is flanked by long stretches of homologous DNA sequences to ensure proper exchange with the targeted endogenous gene

T-box genes A highly conserved family of genes, found in vertebrates and invertebrates, encoding transcription factors that bind DNA through a motif called the T-box and are important in the development of many organ systems

Telomere The tip of a chromosome. In humans, it consists of a tandem repeat of the sequence TTAGGG and ends in a 3′ extension that may be bent over like a hairpin. All ends of human chromosomes must have a telomeric cap to be stable. If a telomere is lost in a terminal deletion, at least three mechanisms exist to maintain the chromosome end: stabilization of a terminal deletion through a process of telomere regeneration ('telomere healing'); retention of the original telomere producing an interstitial deletion; and formation of a derivative chromosome by obtaining a different telomeric sequence through cytogenetic rearrangement ('telomere capture')

Tiling path The set of clones that represents the sequence of a region or an entire chromosome with the minimum overlap

Transcription factor A protein that regulates the expression of one or more genes (its target genes). To do so, it must enter the nucleus and bind to a specific sequence in its target gene's DNA

Transgene A foreign gene, typically a gene produced by recombinant DNA techniques. In reference to mice, transgenic refers to mice whose genetic make-up has been changed by the introduction of a transgene (see 'Transgenic', this glossary)

Transgenerational When effects occur across more than one generation, e.g. from grandparent to grandchild

Transgenic An organism (often a mouse) whose genome has been modified by introducing a new DNA sequence (e.g. a human gene) into the germline (by manipulation of the egg)

Transition A DNA substitution mutation between two-ring purines, e.g. A<->G, or one-ring pyrimidines, e.g. C<->T

Transposon (transposable element) A DNA sequence that can move from one chromosomal location to another

Transversion A DNA substitution mutation resulting in the substitution of a two-ring purine for a one-ring pyrimidine, or vice versa, e.g. A<->C or A <->T, or G<->C or G<->T

Trisomy Three copies of a chromosome. Usually two copies are present in a somatic cell ($2n$). The most common human trisomy surviving to live birth is Down's syndrome, e.g. 47,XY + 21

Truncating mutation A deletion or insertion of one or more bases (but not multiples of three) that disrupt the open reading frame, or a substitution leading to the creation of a stop codon. All result in premature termination of translation

Tumour suppressor gene A gene normally involved in inhibition of cell proliferation or differentiation, whose inactivation contributes to carcinogenesis. Tumour suppressor genes usually act recessively at the cellular level, i.e. inactivating mutations in both copies of the gene are necessary to drive carcinogenesis

Two-dimensional gel electrophoresis A method by which proteins are separated by charge in the first dimension and by size in the second

Uniparental disomy (UPD) A euploid cell in which one of the chromosome pairs has been inherited exclusively from one parent. If two identical homologues are inherited, this is called *isodisomy*; if non-identical homologues are inherited, the term *heterodisomy* is used. This occurs when non-disjunction during meiosis in one parent leads to formation of a disomic gamete. A trisomic zygote is formed and trisomic rescue with loss of the chromosome from the other parent occurs. UPD is of particular importance in imprinted regions of the genome

Upstream A region of DNA that lies 5′ to the point of reference

VCF (variant call file) VCF is a text file format (most likely stored in a compressed manner). It contains meta-information lines, a header line, and then data lines, each containing information about a position in the genome. VCF records use a single general system for representing genetic variation data composed of:

- allele: representing single genetic haplotypes (A, T, ATC);
- genotype: an assignment of alleles

for each chromosome of a single named sample at a particular locus.

VCF record A record holding all segregating alleles at a locus (as well as genotypes, if appropriate, for multiple individuals containing alleles at that locus). VCF records use a simple haplotype representation for REF and ALT alleles to describe variant haplotypes at a locus

VNTR (variable number tandem repeat) Also known as minisatellites, these are a class of highly repetitive sequences that consist of a sequence 10–100 bp long, repeated in tandem arrays which vary in size from 0.5 to 40 kb. They tend to occur near telomeres

Western blot Detection of specific proteins by transfer to a membrane and reaction with labelled antibodies

Wild-type The term used to indicate the normal allele (often symbolized as +) or the normal phenotype

X-inactivation The process by which most of the genes on one of the X chromosomes in female somatic cells are inactivated or turned off during embryonic development. Also termed lyonization

YAC (yeast artificial chromosome) Cloning vector system able to accommodate large genomic fragments. YACs are grown in yeast

Zygote A diploid cell resulting from the fusion of two haploid gametes; a fertilized ovum

Expert advisers (first edition): Martin Bobrow, Professor of Medical Genetics, University of Cambridge, Cambridge, England and Judith G. Hall, Emeritus Professor of Pediatrics and Medical Genetics, University of British Columbia, Vancouver, Canada.

References

Gardner RJM, Sutherland GR. *Chromosome abnormalities and genetic counseling, Oxford monographs on medical genetics No. 31*, 3rd edn. Oxford University Press, New York, 2004.

Goodman FR. Congenital abnormalities of body patterning: embryology revisited. *Lancet* 2003; **362**: 651–62.

Harper PS. *Practical genetic counselling*. 6th edn. Hodder Headline Group, London, 2004.

Lewin B. *Genes VII*. Oxford University Press, Oxford, 2000.

MacArthur DG, Manolio TA, Dimmock DP, *et al*. Guidelines for investigating causality of sequence variants in human disease. *Nature* 2014; **508**: 469–76.

Mitelman F (ed.). *ISCN (1995): an international system for human cytogenetic nomenclature*. Karger, Basel, 1995.

O'Connor A, O'Brien-Pallas LL. Decisional conflict. In: Mcfarlane GK, Mcfarlane EA (eds). *Nursing Diagnosis and Intervention*, pp. 486–96. Mosby, Toronto, 1989.

Strachan T, Read AP. *Human molecular genetics*, 3rd edn. Garland Science, Philadelphia, 2003.

Sudbery P. *Human molecular genetics*. Longman, Essex, 1998.

Abbreviations

3β-HSD	3-beta-hydroxysteroid dehydrogenase
17β-HSD	17-beta-hydroxysteroid dehydrogenase
11β-OHase	11-beta-hydroxylase
21-OHase	21-hydroxylase (deficiency)
17-OHP	17-OH-progesterone
3C	craniocerebellocardiac (dysplasia)
3D	three-dimensional
AAA	achalasia–addisonianism–alacrima (syndrome)
AAIDD	American Association on Intellectual and Developmental Disabilities
AASA	amino adipic semialdehyde
AC	abdominal circumference
AC	Amsterdam criteria
ACALD	adult cerebral adrenoleukodystrophy
ACC	agenesis of the corpus callosum
ACE	angiotensin-converting enzyme
aCGH	array comparative genomic hybridization
AChR	acetylcholine receptor
ACMG	American College of Medical Genetics
ACS	acrocallosal syndrome
ACTH	adrenocorticotrophic hormone
AD	autosomal dominant
ADA	adenosine deaminase
ADCA	autosomal dominant cerebellar ataxia
ADHD	attention-deficit/hyperactivity disorder
ADNFLE	autosomal dominant nocturnal frontal lobe epilepsy
ADO	allele dropout
AdolCALD	adolescent cerebral adrenoleukodystrophy
ADOS	autosomal dominant Opitz syndrome
ADPKD	autosomal dominant polycystic kidney disease (adult PKD)
ADRP	autosomal dominant retinitis pigmentosa
ADULT	acro-dermato-ungual-lacrimal-tooth (syndrome)
AEC	ankyloblepharon–ectodermal dysplasia–clefting (syndrome)
AEG	anophthalmia–(o)esophageal atresia–genital anomalies (syndrome)
aEEG	amplitude integrated electroencephalography
AF	amniotic fluid
AFAP	attenuated familial adenomatous polyposis
AFP	alpha-fetoprotein
AFO	ankle–foot orthosis
AGS	Aicardi–Goutières syndrome
AHO	Albright hereditary osteodystrophy
AID	artificial insemination by donor
AIDS	acquired immune deficiency syndrome
AIS	androgen insensitivity syndrome
ALD	adrenoleukodystrophy
ALK	activin-like receptor kinase
ALL	acute lymphocytic leukaemia
ALT	alanine aminotransferase
AMH	anti-Müllerian hormone
AML	acute myeloid leukaemia
AML	angiomyolipoma
AMN	adrenomyeloneuropathy
ANCL	adult neuronal ceroid lipofuscinosis
ANF	antinuclear factor
AOA	ataxia with oculomotor apraxia (AOA-1, AOA-2)
AOS	Adams–Oliver syndrome
AP	anteroposterior
APA	American Psychiatric Association
APC	activated protein C
APECED	autoimmune polyendocrinopathy–candidiasis– ectodermal dystrophy
APOB	apolipoprotein B
APOE	apolipoprotein E
APTT	activated partial thromboplastin time
AR	autosomal recessive
A2RA	angiotensin II receptor antagonist
ARAS	autosomal recessive Alport syndrome
ARB	angiotensin receptor blocker
ARC	arthrogryposis multiplex congenita, renal dysfunction, and neonatal cholestasis (syndrome)
ARCA	autosomal recessive cerebellar ataxia
ARH	autosomal recessive hypercholesterolaemia
ARMS	amplification refractory mutation system
ARND	alcohol-related neurodevelopmental disorder
ARPKD	autosomal recessive polycystic kidney disease (infantile PKD)
ARSACS	autosomal recessive spastic ataxia of Charlevoix–Saguenay
ART	assisted/artificial reproductive technology
ARVC	arrythmogenic right ventricular cardiomyopathy

ARVD	arrythmogenic right ventricular dysplasia
ARX	Aristaless-related homeobox (gene)
AS	Alport syndrome
AS	Alström syndrome
AS	Angelman syndrome
ASD	atrial septal defect
ASD	autism spectrum disorders
ASH	asymmetric septal hypertrophy
ASHG	American Society of Human Genetics
ASO	antisense oligonucleotide
ASPA	aspartoacylase (gene)
ASSA	aminopterin syndrome sine amniopterin
AST	aspartate transaminase
AT	ataxia telangiectasia
ATLD	ataxia telangiectasia-like disorder
ATM	A-T mutated
ATP	adenosine triphosphate
ATRX	X-linked alpha-thalassaemia/mental retardation syndrome
AV	atrioventricular
AVM	arteriovenous malformation
AVR	aortic valve replacement
AVSD	atrioventricular septal defect
AZF	azoospermia factor (e.g. AZFa, AZFb)
BAC	bacteria artificial chromosome
BAER	brainstem auditory evoked response
BAV	bicuspid aortic valve
BAVM	brain arteriovenous malformation
BBS	Bardet–Biedl syndrome
BCC	basal cell carcinoma
BCECTS	benign childhood epilepsy with centrotemporal spikes
BCG	bacille Calmette–Guérin (immunization)
BCS	brittle cornea syndrome
BDNF	brain-derived neurotrophic factor
BFNIS	benign familial neonatal–infantile seizures
BHD	Birt–Hogg–Dubé (syndrome)
BMD	Becker muscular dystrophy
BMI	body mass index
BMP	bone morphogenetic protein
BMPR2	bone morphogenetic protein receptor II
BMT	bone marrow transplantation
BOADICEA	Breast and Ovarian Analysis of Disease Incidence and Carrier Estimation Algorithm
BOCA	brown oculocutaneous albinism
BOF	branchio-oculo-facial (syndrome)
BOR	branchio-oto-renal (syndrome)
bp	base pair
BP	blood pressure

BPD	biparietal diameter
BPES	blepharophimosis–ptosis–epicanthus inversus syndrome
BPNH	bilateral periventricular nodular heterotopia
BRR	Banayan–Riley–Ruvalcaba (syndrome)
BRR–PHTS	Banayan–Riley–Ruvalcaba/Cowden syndrome
BRRS	Bannayan–Riley–Ruvalcaba syndrome
BS	Bruck syndrome (BS1, BS2)
BSA	body surface area
BSER	brainstem evoked response
BSO	bilateral salpingo-oophorectomy
BTD	biotinidase
BWS	Beckwith–Wiedemann syndrome
CA	chronological age
CA125	cancer antigen 125
CADASIL	cerebral autosomal dominant arteriopathy with subcortical infarcts and leukoencephalopathy
CAH	congenital adrenal hyperplasia
CAIS	complete androgen insensitivity syndrome
CAKUT	congenital abnormalities of the kidney and urinary tract
CAL	café-au-lait (spot)
CAL M	café-au-lait macule
cAMP	cyclic adenosine monophosphate
CaSR	calcium-sensing receptor
CAUV	congenital absence of the uterus and vagina
CAVM	cerebral arteriovenous malformation
CBAVD	congenital bilateral absence of the vas deferens
CBS	cystathionine beta-synthase
CCA	congenital contractural arachnodactyly
CCALD	childhood cerebral adrenoleukodystrophy
CCAM	congenital cystic adenomatoid malformation
CCD	central-core disease
CCHS	congenital central hypoventilation syndrome
CCMS	cerebrocostomandibular syndrome
CD	Canavan disease
CDG	congenital disorders of glycosylation
CDH	congenital dislocation of the hip
CdLS	Cornelia de Lange syndrome
cDNA	complementary DNA
CDP	chondrodysplasia punctata
CEDNIK	cerebral dysgenesis, neuropathy, ichthyosis, and palmoplantar keratoderma (syndrome)

CEMRI	contrast-enhanced magnetic resonance imaging
CES	cat-eye syndrome
CF	cystic fibrosis
CFC	cardiofaciocutaneous (syndrome)
cffDNA	cell-free fetal DNA
cffRNA	cell-free fetal RNA
CFNS	craniofrontonasal dysplasia
CFTR	cystic fibrosis transmembrane conductance regulator (gene)
CGD	chronic granulomatous disease
CGH	comparative genomic hybridization
CGHT	congenital generalized hypertrichosis terminalis
CGRP	calcitonin-gene related peptide
CH	congenital hypothyroidism
CHARGE	coloboma–heart defects–atresia choanae–retardation of growth and/or development–genital defect–ear anomalies and/or deafness
CHD	congenital heart disease
CHED	congenital endothelial dystrophy
CHI	congenital hyperinsulinism of infancy
CHILD	congenital hemidysplasia–ichythiosiform erythroderma–limb defects (syndrome)
CHL	congenital hypertrichosis lanugosa
CHRPE	congenital hypertrophy of the retinal pigment epithelium
CHS	Chediak–Higashi syndrome
CHSP	complex hereditary spastic paraplegia
CHT	congenital hypothyroidism
CI	confidence interval
CINCA	chronic infantile neurologic cutaneous and articular (syndrome)
CIPA	congenital insensitivity to pain with anhidrosis
CJD	Creutzfeldt–Jakob disease
CK	creatine kinase
CLE	congenital lobar emphysema
CLOVE	congenital lipomatous overgrowth, vascular malformation, and epidermal naevi (syndrome)
CL/P	cleft lip and palate
CLS	Coffin–Lowry syndrome
CLS	cholestasis–lymphoedema syndrome
cm	centimetre
cM	centimorgan
CM	cardiomyopathy
CM	complete hydatidiform mole
CMA	chromosomal microarray analysis
CMD	congenital muscular dystrophy
CMG2	capillary morphogenesis protein 2

CML	chronic myelogenous leukaemia
CMMRD	constitutional mismatch repair disorder
CMN	congenital melanocytic naevus
CMR	cardiac magnetic resonance imaging
CMS	congenital myasthenic syndromes
CMT	Charcot–Marie–Tooth (disease)
CMV	cytomegalovirus
CN	Crigler–Najjar (CN1, CN2)
CNC	Carney complex
CNS	central nervous system
CNV	copy number variant
COACH	cerebellar vermian hypoplasia–oligophrenia–ataxia–coloboma–hepatic fibrosis (syndrome)
Coarct	coarctation of the aorta
COD–MD	cerebro-ocular dysplasia–muscular dystrophy
COFS	cerebro-oculo-facial-skeletal (syndrome)
CORS	cerebello-oculo-renal syndrome
COX	cytochrome oxidase
CP	cerebral palsy
CP	cleft palate
CPAP	continuous positive airway pressure
CPEO	chronic progressive external ophthalmoplegia
CPHD	combined pituitary hormone deficiency
CPK	creatine phosphokinase
CPM	confined placental mosaicism
CPVT	catecholaminergic polymorphic ventricular tachycardia
CR	cumulative risk
CRC	colorectal cancer
CRF	chronic renal failure
CRL	crown–rump length
CRS	congenital rubella syndrome
CS	Cockayne syndrome
CSF	cerebrospinal fluid
CT	computerized tomography
CTA	computed tomographic angiography
CTC1	conserved telomere maintenance component 1
CTSK	cathepsin K (gene)
CTX	cerebrotendinous xanthomatosis
CVID	common variable immunodeficiency
CVS	chorionic villus sampling
D	diversity (region of an immunoglobulin chain)
D	dioptre
D & C	dilatation and curettage
DA	distal arthrogryposis
dB	decibel

DCIS	ductal carcinoma *in situ*		EAU	examination under anaesthesia
DCM	dilated cardiomyopathy		EBD	epidermylosis bullosa dystrophica
DDAVP	1-deamino-8-D-arginine vasopressin		EBP	emopamil binding protein
DDD	Deciphering Developmental Disorders (study)		EBV	Epstein–Barr virus
			ECC	ectrodactyly–ectodermal dysplasia–clefting (syndrome)
DDH	developmental dysplasia of the hip		ECG	electrocardiogram
DDS	Denys–Drash syndrome		echo	echocardiography
DEB	diepoxybutane		ECMO	extracorporeal membrane oxygenation
DGS	di George syndrome		ED	ectodermal dysplasia
DHA	dehydroepiandosterone		EDA-ID	anhidrotic ectodermal dysplasia with immunodeficiency
DHCR	7-dehydrocholesterol reductase× (gene)			
DHH	desert hedgehog (gene)		EDD	estimated date of delivery
dHPLC	denaturing high-performance liquid chromatography		EDS	Ehlers–Danlos syndrome
			EDTA	ethylenedinitrilotetraacetate
DHT	dihydrotestosterone		EEC	ectrodactyly–ectodermal dysplasia–clefting (syndrome)
DI	dentinogenesis imperfecta			
DIDMOAD	diabetes insipidus–diabetes mellitus–optic atrophy–deafness (syndrome)		EEG	electroencephalography
			EFE	endocardial fibroelastosis
dl	decilitre		*EFNB1*	ephrin-B1 (gene)
DM	myotonic dystrophy		eGFR	estimated glomerular filtration rate
DMD	Duchenne muscular dystrophy		EIEE	early infantile epileptic encephalopathy
DMPK	dystrophia myotonica protein kinase (gene)		eIF2B	eukaryotic translation initiation factor 2B
DMR	differentially methylated region			
DMSA	dimercaptosuccinic acid		EIMFS	epilepsy of infancy with migrating focal seizures
DNA	deoxyribonucleic acid			
DNM	*de novo* mutation		EM	electron microscopy
DOOR	deafness–onychodystrophy–onycholysis–retardation (syndrome)		EMEE	early myoclonic epileptic encephalopathy
			EMG	electromyography
DORV	double-outlet right ventricle		EMG	exomphalos–macroglossia–gigantism (syndrome)
DPNH	dinitrophenylhydrazine			
DR	MHC class 2		ENaC	epithelial sodium channel
DRD	dopa-responsive dystonia		*ENG*	endoglin
DRE	digital rectal examination		ENT	ear, nose, and throat
DRPLA	dentatorubropallidoluysian atrophy		EPL	early pregnancy loss
DSA	digital subtraction angiography		ERG	electroretinography
DSBR	double-strand break repair		ERT	enzymatic replacement therapy
DSM-5	*Diagnostic and statistical manual for mental disorders*, fifth edition		ESAC	extrastructurally abnormal chromosome
			ESR	erythrocyte sedimentation rate
DSD	disorder of sex development		ESRD	end-stage renal disease
DSP	desmoplakin		ESHRE	European Society of Human Reproduction and Embryology
DTPA	diethyltriaminepentaacetic acid			
DTR	deep tendon reflex		ESRF	end-stage renal failure
DVLA	Driver and Vehicle Licensing Agency (UK)		EST	expressed sequence tag
			EVC	Ellis–van Creveld (syndrome)
DWI	diffusion-weighted imaging		FA	Fanconi anaemia
DWM	Dandy–Walker malformation		FACS	fetal anticonvulsant syndrome
DW-MRI	diffusion-weighted magnetic resonance imaging		FADS	fetal akinesia deformation sequence
			FAO	fatty acid oxidation (disorders)
DWV	Dandy–Walker variant		FAP	familial adenomatous polyposis
DZ	dizygotic (twin)		FAS	fetal alcohol syndrome

FBC	full blood count	GI	gastrointestinal
FBS	fetal blood sampling	GMC	General Medical Council
FCMD	Fukayama congenital muscular dystrophy	GnRH	gonadotrophin-releasing hormone
FDB	familial defective apoB-100	GP	general practitioner
FE1	faecal elastase 1	GPC	glypican 3
FECD	Fuchs endothelial dystrophy of the cornea	GPI	glycosylphosphatidylinositol
		GRE	gradient-echo (image)
FEV₁	forced expiratory volume in 1 second	GS	Gillespie syndrome
FEVR	familial exudative vitreoretinopathy	GSD	Gerstmann–Straussler disease
ffDNA	free fetal DNA	GSD	glycogen storage disease
ffRNA	free fetal RNA	GT	glutamyl transpeptidase
FFU	femur–fibula–ulna (complex)	GTP	guanosine triphosphate
FGF	fibroblast growth factor	GTT	gestational trophoblastic tumour
FH	familial hypercholesterolaemia	GTT	glucose tolerance test
FHL	familial haemophagocytic lymphohistiocytosis	GUCH	grown-up congenital heart disease (clinic)
FHS	Floating Harbor syndrome	GWAS	genome-wide association study
FIHP	familial isolated hyperparathyroidism	HADHB	hydroxyacyl-CoA dehydrogenase/ 3-ketoacyl-CoA thiolase/enoyl-CoA hydratase, beta-subunit
FISH	fluorescence in situ hybridization		
FKRP	fukutin-related protein		
FLAIR	fluid-attenuated inversion recovery (sequence in MRI)	HAL	haploid autosomal length
		HARD ± E	hydrocephalus–agyria–retinal dystrophy ± encephalocele (alternative name for WWS)
FMF	familial Mediterranean fever		
FMTC	familial medullary thyroid cancer		
FOP	fibrodysplasia ossificans progressiva	HARP	hypoprebetalipoproteinaemia, acanthocytosis, retinitis pigmentosa, and pallidal degeneration (syndrome)
FRAX	fragile X (syndrome)		
FRDA	Friedreich's ataxia		
FSH	follicle-stimulating hormone	Hb	haemoglobin (HbA, HbH, etc.)
FSHD	facioscapulohumeral muscular dystrophy	HbF	fetal haemoglobin
FSS	Freeman–Sheldon syndrome	HC	head circumference
FVC	forced vital capacity	hCG	human chorionic gonadotrophin
FXTAS	fragile X tremor ataxia syndrome	HCO₃⁻	bicarbonate ion
g	gram	HCM	hypertrophic cardiomyopathy
G6PD	glucose-6-phosphate dehydrogenase (deficiency)	HCU	homocystinuria
		HD	Huntington disease
GA1	glutaric aciduria type 1	HDGC	hereditary diffuse gastric cancer
GABA	gamma aminobutyric acid	HDL	high-density lipoprotein
GAD	glutamic acid decarboxylase	HDL-1	Huntington disease-like 1
GAG	glycosaminoglycan	HDL-2	Huntington disease-like 2
GALT	galactose-1-phosphate uridyl-transferase	HDN	haemolytic disease of the newborn
GAP	GTPase-activating protein	HDR	hypoparathyroidism– sensorineural deafness–renal dysplasia (syndrome)
Gb	gigabase		
GBM	glomerular basement membrane		
GCDH	glutaryl CoA dehydrogenase	HED	hypohidrotic ectodermal dysplasia
GCK	glucokinase (gene)	HEM	hydrops–ectopic calcification–moth- eaten appearance
G-CSF	granulocyte colony-stimulating factor		
GDH	glutamate dehydrogenase (gene)	HFEA	Human Fertilisation and Embryology Authority (UK)
GEFS(+)	generalized epilepsy with febrile seizures		
GFAP	glial fibrillary acidic protein	HH	hereditary haemochromatosis
GH	growth hormone	HHS	Hoyeraal–Hreidarsson syndrome
		HHT	hereditary haemorrhagic telangiectasia
		Hib	Haemophilus influenzae type b

HIE	hypoxic–ischaemic encephalopathy		idic	isodicentric marker chromosome
HIF	hypoxia-inducible factor-1		IDM	infant of diabetic mother
HII	hypoxic–ischaemic injury		IFNγ	interferon γ
HIV	human immunodeficiency virus		IgA	immunoglobulin A
HLA	human leucocyte antigen		IGF	insulin-like growth factor
HLCS	holocarboxylase synthetase		IGFR	insulin-like growth factor receptor
HLH	hypoplastic left heart		IgG	immunoglobulin G
HLHS	hypoplastic left heart syndrome		IgG2	immunoglobulin G2
HLRCC	hereditary leiomyomatosis and renal cell cancer		IgM	immunoglobulin M
HME	hereditary multiple exostoses		IH	isolated hemihypertrophy
HMG-CoA	hydroxymethyl glutaryl coenzyme A		IHC	immunohistochemistry
HMPS	hereditary mixed polyposis syndrome		*IHH*	Indian hedgehog (gene)
HMSN	hereditary motor and sensory neuropathy		IHH	isolated hemihyperplasia
HNF-1β	hepatocyte nuclear factor-1β		IHH	isolated hemihypertrophy
HNPCC	hereditary non-polyposis colorectal cancer		IL	interleukin
			ILNR	intralobar nephrogenic rest
HNPGL	head and neck paraganglioma		IL-7R	interleukin 7 receptor
HNPP	hereditary neuropathy with liability to pressure palsies		ILS	isolated lissencephaly sequence
			IM	intramuscular
HOCM	hypertrophic obstructive cardiomyopathy		INAD	infantile neuroaxonal dystrophy
			INCL	infantile neuronal ceroid lipofuscinosis
HOS	Holt–Oram syndrome		InSiGHT	International Society for Gastrointestinal Hereditary Tumours
HOX	homeobox (gene)			
HPA	human platelet antigen		INSR	insulin receptor
HPE	holoprosencephaly		IOSCA	infantile-onset spinocerebellar ataxia
HPFH	hereditary persistence of fetal haemoglobin		IP	incontinentia pigmenti
			IP	interphalangeal (joints)
HPS	Hermansky–Pudlak syndrome		IPD	interpupillary distance
HPT-JT	hyperparathyroidism–jaw tumour (syndrome)		IPEX	immunodysregulation–polyendocrinopathy–enteropathy, X-linked
HRC	HNPCC-related cancer			
HRT	hormone replacement therapy		*IPF1*	insulin promoter factor-1 (gene)
HSP	hereditary spastic paraplegia		IPHD	isolated pituitary hormone deficiency
HSS	Hallervorden–Spatz syndrome		iPSC	inducible pluripotent stem cell
HTLV-1	human T-lymphocytic virus 1		IQ	intelligence quotient
Hz	hertz		IR	insulin receptor
IC	imprinting centre		IRT	immunoreactive trypsinogen
ICA	intracranial aneurysm		IS	infantile spasm
ICC	intracranial calcification		ISH	infantile systemic hyalinosis
ICD	implantable cardioverter–defibrillator		ITP	idiopathic thrombocytopenic purpura
ICD-10	International Classification of Diseases, tenth revision		iu	international unit
			IUD	intrauterine (fetal) death
ICEGTC	intractable childhood epilepsy with generalized tonic–clonic seizures		IUGR	intrauterine growth retardation
			IV	intravenous/ly
ICR	imprinting control region		IVA	isovaleric acidaemia
ICSI	intracytoplasmic sperm injection		IVC	inferior vena cava
ID	intellectual disability		IVD	isovaleryl CoA dehydrogenase
IDD	intellectual developmental disorder		IVF	*in vitro* fertilization
IDDM	insulin-dependent diabetes mellitus		IVH	intraventricular haemorrhage
			IVU	intravenous urography

J	joining (region of an immunoglobulin chain)		LEOPARD	(syndrome comprising) lentigines–ECG abnormalities–ocular hypertelorism–pulmonary stenosis–abnormal genitalia–retardation of growth–deafness
JAG1	*jagged1* (gene)			
Jak-3	Janus-associated kinase 3			
JBS	Johanson–Blizzard syndrome			
JHF	juvenile hyaline fibromatosis		LFS	Li–Fraumeni syndrome
JME	juvenile myoclonic epilepsy		LFT	liver function test
JMML	juvenile myelomonocytic leukaemia		LGA	large for gestational age
JNCL	juvenile neuronal ceroid lipofuscinosis		LGMD	limb–girdle muscular dystrophy
JPS	juvenile polyposis syndrome		LGS	Lennox–Gastaut syndrome
JS	Joubert syndrome		LH	luteinizing hormone
JVP	jugular venous pressure		LHON	Leber hereditary optic neuropathy
K	potassium		LINCL	late infantile neuronal ceroid lipofuscinosis
KATP	ATP-sensitive potassium (channel)		LKS	Landau–Kleffner syndrome
kb	kilobase		*LMNA*	lamin A (gene)
KCS	Kenny–Caffey syndrome		LMPS	lethal multiple pterygium syndrome
kg	kilogram		LMWH	low-molecular-weight heparin
KID	keratosis–icthyosis–deafness (syndrome)		lncRNA	long non-coding ribonucleic acid
km	kilometre		LOD	logarithm of the odds ratio (score)
KOH	potassium hydroxide		LOF	loss of function
KS	Kallmann syndrome		LOH	loss of heterozygosity
KSS	Kearns–Sayre syndrome		LOI	loss of imprinting
KTS	Klippel–Trenauny syndrome		LPS	levator palpebrae superioris (muscle)
KTW	Klippel–Trenauney–Weber (syndrome)		LRP	LDL receptor protein
kU	kilounit		LS	Leigh syndrome
l	litre		LS	LEOPARD syndrome
LAAHD	lethal arthrogryposis with anterior horn cell disease		LS	Lynch syndrome
			LSA	learning support assistant
LAD	left axis deviation		LSCS	lower segment Caesarean section
LADD	lacrimo-auriculo-dental-digital (syndrome)		LTC	long-term culture
			LTE	laryngo-tracheo-(o)esophageal (defects)
LAM	lymphangioleiomyomatosis		LV	left ventricle/ventricular
LBC	liquid-based cytology		LVD	left ventricle diameter
LCA	Leber congenital amaurosis		LVH	left ventricular hypertrophy
LCC	leukoencephalopathy with calcifications and cysts		LVNC	left ventricular non-compaction cardiomyopathy
LCH	lissencephaly with cerebellar hypoplasia		LWD	Leri–Weill dyschondrosteosis
LCHAD	long-chain hydroxyacyl-CoA dehydrogenase		m	metre
			M:F	male-to-female (ratio)
LCM	lymphocytic choriomeningitis		MADD	multiple acyl-CoA dehydrogenation deficiency
LCR	low-copy repeat (LCR22 = LCR on chromosome 22)		MAE	myoclonic–astatic epilepsy
			MAP	*MUTYH*-associated polyposis
LDD	Lhermitte–Duclos disease		MAPK	mitogen-activated protein kinase
LDDB	London Dysmorphology Database		MASA	mental retardation–aphasia–shuffling gait–adducted thumbs
LDH	lactate dehydrogenase			
LDL	low-density lipoprotein		MASS	mitral valve prolapse–aortic involvement–skeletal anomalies–skin anomalies
LDLR	low-density lipoprotein receptor			
LDS	Loeys–Dietz syndrome			
			MatUPD7	maternal uniparental disomy 7

Mb	megabase
MCA	multiple congenital anomaly
MCAD	medium-chain acyl-CoA dehydrogenase (deficiency)
MCAP	megalencephaly–capillary malformation–polymicrogyria
MCAS	McCune–Albright syndrome
MCD	multiple carboxylase deficiency
MCDK	multicystic dysplastic kidney
MCH	mean corpuscular haemoglobin
mCi	millicurie
M-CM	macrocephaly–capillary malformation (syndromes)
M-CMTC	macrocephaly–cutis marmorata–telangiectatica congenita
MCP	metacarpophalangeal (joint)
MC4R	melanocortin 4 receptor
MCUG	micturating cystourethrogram
MCUL	multiple cutaneous and uterine leiomyomatosis
MCV	mean corpuscular volume
MDC1C	congenital muscular dystrophy 1C
MDFM	mandibulofacial dysostosis with microcephaly
MDK	multicystic dysplastic kidneys
MDS	Miller–Dieker syndrome
MEB	muscle–eye–brain (disease)
MED	multiple epiphyseal dysplasia
MELAS	mitochondrial myopathy–encephalopathy–lactic acidosis–stroke-like episodes
MEN	multiple endocrine neoplasia (MEN1 and MEN2)
MEON	multiple endocrine and other organ neoplasia
MERRF	myoclonic epilepsy with ragged red fibres
MFDM	mandibulo-facial dysostosis with microcephaly
MFS	Marfan's syndrome
mg	milligram
MGIA	multiple gastrointestinal atresias
MGS	Meckel (Gruber) syndrome
mGy	milligray
MH	malignant hyperthermia
MHC	major histocompatibility complex
MHC	myosin heavy chain
MICPCH	mental retardation and microcephaly with pontine and cerebellar hypoplasia
MIM	Mendelian Inheritance in Man (database)
min	minute
MIP	major intrinsic protein

MIRAS	mitochondrial recessive ataxia syndrome
MKKS	McKusick–Kaufman syndrome
ml	millilitre
MLC	megalencephalic leukoencephalopathy with subcortical cysts
MLD	metachromatic leukodystrophy
MLPA	multiplex ligation-dependent probe amplification
MLS	microphthalmia with linear skin defects
mm	millimetre
mM	millimolar
MMC	mitomycin C
MMF	mycophenolate mofetil
MMIH	megacystis–microcolon–intestinal hypoperistalsis (syndrome)
mmol	millimole
MMR	mismatch repair (genes)
MMR	measles, mumps, rubella (vaccine)
MNV	multi-nucleotide variant
MODED	microcephaly–oculo–digito–(o)esophageal–duodenal (syndrome)
MODY	maturity-onset diabetes of the young
MoM	multiple of the median
MOPD	Majewski osteodysplastic primordial dwarfism
mol	mole
mOsm	milliosmole
MPH	mid-parental height
MPPH	megalencephaly–polymicrogyria–polydactyly–hydrocephalus
MPNST	malignant peripheral nerve sheath tumour
MPS	mucopolysaccharide (disorders)/mucopolysaccharidoses
MR	mental retardation
MR/MCA	mental retardation/multiple congenital anomalies (syndrome)
MRA	magnetic resonance angiography
MRC	mitochondrial respiratory chain
MRI	magnetic resonance imaging
mRNA	messenger ribonucleic acid
ms	millisecond
MS	multiple sclerosis
MSI	microsatellite instability
MSMD	Mendelian susceptibility to mycobacterial disease
MS-MLPA	methylation-specific multiplex ligation-dependent probe amplification
MSUD	maple syrup urine disease
mSv	millisievert
MTC	medullary thyroid cancer
mtDNA	mitochondrial DNA

MTHFR	5,10-methylenetetrahydrofolate reductase (gene)		NIPD	non-invasive prenatal diagnosis
			NIPT	non-invasive prenatal testing
mTOR	mammalian target of rapamycin		NK	natural killer (cells)
MTS	Muir–Torre syndrome		NKH	non-ketotic hyperglycinaemia
MUL	Mulibrey (muscle–liver–brain–eye) nanism		*NLGN*	neuroligin (*NLGN3*, *NLGN4*; gene)
			nm	nanometre
mUPD7	maternal uniparental disomy of chromosome 7		NMD	nonsense-mediated decay
			NOAEL	no observed adverse effect level
MURCS	Müllerian duct anomalies–renal aplasia–cervicothoracic somite dysplasia (Klippel–Feil anomaly)		NOMID	neonatal-onset multisystem inflammatory disease
			NOR	nucleolar organizing region
MVA	mosaic variegated aneuploidy		NPS	nail–patella syndrome
MVP	mitral valve prolapse		NPV	negative predictive value
MVR	mitral valve replacement		NR	nephrogenic rest
MZ	monozygotic (twin)		NS	Noonan syndrome
Na	sodium		NS	neonatal screening
NAA	N-acetylaspartic acid		NSAID	non-steroidal anti-inflammatory drug
NAD	nicotinamide–adenine dinucleotide		NT	nuchal translucency
NADH	reduced nicotinamide–adenine dinucleotide		NTD	neural tube defect
			NTRK1	neurotrophic tyrosine kinase receptor type I (gene)
NADP	nicotinamide–adenine dinucleotide phosphate		NTx	N-telopeptide of type I collagen
NADPH	reduced nicotinamide–adenine dinucleotide phosphate		O_2^-	superoxide
			OA	oesophageal atresia
NAI	non-accidental injury		OAG	open-angle glaucoma
NAIT	neonatal alloimmune thrombocytopenia		OAV	oculoauriculovertebral (syndrome)
NAP	*NTHL1*-associated polyposis		OAVS	oculoauriculovertebral spectrum
NARP	neuropathy–ataxia–retinitis pigmentosa		OCA	oculocutaneous albinism
NBS	Nijmegen breakage syndrome		OCP	oral contraceptive pill
NBS	National Blood Service		ODD	oculodentodigital (syndrome)
NBSLD	Nijmegen breakage syndrome-like disorder		ODP	otopalatodigital syndrome (ODP-1)
NBT	nitroblue tetrazolium		OEIS	(combination of) omphalocele–exstrophy of the cloaca–imperforate anus–spinal defects
NC	non-collagenous (domain)			
NCCN	National Comprehensive Cancer Network		OFC	occipital–frontal circumference
NCL	neuronal ceroid lipofuscinosis		OFD	oral–facial–digital syndrome (OFD-1, OFD-2, etc.)
NCV	nerve conduction velocity (test)			
NE	Northern epilepsy		OGD	oesophagogastroduodenoscopy
NER	nucleotide excision repair		OHP	OH-progesterone
NF	neurofibromatosis (NF1 and NF2)		OHSS	ovarian hyperstimulation syndrome
ng	nanogram		OI	osteogenesis imperfecta
NHEJ	non-homologous end-joining		OMA	ocular motor apraxia
NHL	non-Hodgkin's lymphoma		OMIM	Online Mendelian Inheritance in Man (database)
NHS	National Health Service			
NHSBSP	NHS breast screening programme		OMLH	oromandibular–limb–hypogenesis (syndrome)
NIBA	neuronal degeneration with brain iron accumulation			
			ONH	optic nerve hypoplasia
NICE	National Institute of Care and Health Excellence		OPD	otopalatodigital syndrome (OPD-1 and OPD-2)
NICU	neonatal intensive care unit		OPG	optic pathway glioma
NIDDM	non-insulin-dependent diabetes mellitus		OPG	orthopantogram

OPMD	oculopharyngeal muscular dystrophy
OR	odds ratio
ORF	open reading frame
OSMED	otospondylomegaepiphyseal dysplasia
OTC	ornithine transcarbamylase
OXPHOS	oxidative phosphorylation
PA	posteroanterior
PABP2	poly(A) binding protein 2 (gene)
PAIS	partial androgen insensitivity syndrome
PA–JEB	pyloric atresia associated with junctional epidermolysis bullosa
PAP	post-axial polydactyly
PAPP-A	pregnancy-associated plasma protein A
PAR	pseudoautosomal region
PARPi	poly ADP ribose polymerase inhibitor
PAVM	pulmonary arteriovenous malformation
PAX	paired box (gene)
PCD	primary ciliary dyskinesia
PCH	pontocerebellar hypoplasia
PCP	Pneumocystis carinii pneumonia
PCP	planar cell polarity
PCR	polymerase chain reaction
PCS	premature chromatid separation
PCSK1	prohormone convertase-1
PDA	patent ductus arteriosus
PDAC	pulmonary hypoplasia, diaphragmatic eventration/hernia, anophthalmia/microphthalmia, cardiac defect
PDH	pyruvate dehydrogenase
PECS	picture exchange communication system
PEHO	progressive encephalopathy–(o)edema–hypsarrhythmia–optic atrophy (syndrome)
PESA	percutaneous epididymal sperm aspiration
PET	positron emission tomography
PET	pre-eclampsia
PFIC	progressive familial intrahepatic cholestasis
PFO	persistent foramen ovale
PGC	primordial germ cell
PGD	pre-implantation genetic diagnosis
PGH	pre-implantation genetic haplotyping
PGS	pre-implantation genetic screening
PHHI	persistent hyperinsulinaemic hypoglycaemia of infancy
PHP	pseudohypoparathyroidism
PHPV	persistent hyperplastic primary vitreous
PHSP	pure hereditary spastic paraplegia
PHTS	PTEN hamartoma tumour syndrome (also known as Cowden syndrome)
PI3K	phosphoinositide 3-kinase

PID	primary immunodeficiency disorder
PIND	progressive intellectual and neurological deterioration
PIP	proximal interphalangeal (joints)
PJP	Pneumocystis jiroveci pneumonia
PJS	Peutz–Jeghers syndrome
PKAN	pantothenate kinase-associated degeneration
PKD	polycystic kidney disease
PKU	phenylketonuria
PLAN	phospholipase A2 group 6-associated neurodegeneration
PLIC	posterior limb of the internal capsule
PLNR	perilobar nephrogenic rest
PM	partial hydatidiform mole
PMD	Pelizaeus–Merzbacher disease
PME	progressive myoclonic epilepsy
PMG	polymicrogyria
PMM	phosphomannomutase
pmol	picomole
PND	prenatal diagnosis
PNDM	permanent neonatal diabetes mellitus
PNET	primitive neuroectodermal tumour
PNH	periventricular nodular heterotopia
PNP	purine nucleoside phosphorylase
PO	per os (by mouth)
POADS	post-axial acrofacial dysostosis syndrome
POAG	primary open-angle glaucoma
POC	product of conception
POF	premature ovarian failure
Poly-T	polythymidine
POMC	pro-opiomelanocortin
PoO	parent of origin
PPCD	posterior polymorphous dystrophy
PPD	preaxial polydactyly
PPH	post-partum haemorrhage
PPHP	pseudo-pseudohypoparathyroidism
PPM-X	X-linked psychosis–pyramidal signs–macroorchidism
PPNAD	primary pigmented nodular adrenocortical disease
PPROM	prelabour, premature, preterm rupture of membranes
PPT	palmitoyl-protein thioesterase
PPV	positive predictive value
PRC2	Polycomb repressive complex 2
PRINS	primed in situ labelling
PROMM	proximal myotonic myopathy
PSA	prostate-specific antigen
psudic	pseudo-dicentric (marker chromosome)
PSV	paralogous sequence variant

PT	prothrombin time
PTH	parathyroid hormone
PUBS	periumbilical blood sampling
PUJ	pelvi-ureteral junction
PUV	posterior urethral valve
PVNH	periventricular nodular heterotopia
PWACR	Prader–Willi/Angelman syndrome critical region
PWS	Prader–Willi syndrome
qPCR	quantitative polymerase chain reaction
QF-PCR	quantitative fluorescence-polymerase chain reaction
QTL	quantitative trait locus
RAG	recombinase-activating gene (*RAG1*, *RAG2*)
RAS	renin–angiotensin system
RB	retinoblastoma
RCAD	renal cysts and diabetes
RCC	renal cell carcinoma
RCDP	rhizomelic chondrodysplasia punctata
Rcp	reciprocal translocations
RCM	restrictive cardiomyopathy
RFLP	restriction fragment length polymorphism
RhD	rhesus D
RIDDLE	Radiosensitivity, ImmunoDeficiency, Dysmorphic features and Learning difficulty (syndrome)
RNA	ribonucleic acid
RNAi	RNA interference
ROP	retinopathy of prematurity
RP	retinitis pigmentosa
RR	relative risk (or risk ratio)
RRBSO	risk-reducing bilateral salpingo-oophorectomy
RTA	renal tubular acidosis
RT-PCR	reverse transcriptase polymerase chain reaction
RTD	renal tubular dysgenesis
RTS	Rubinstein–Taybi syndrome
RV	right ventricle/ventricular
RVOT	right ventricular outflow tract obstruction
RYR	ryanodine receptor
s	second
SA	sinoatrial (node)
SACS	Charlevoix–Saguenay syndrome
SAGE	serial analysis of gene expression
SAH	subarachnoid haemorrhage
SALT	speech and language therapy
SAM	systolic anterior motion
SANDO	sensory ataxic neuropathy dysarthria and ophthalmoplegia
SaO_2	arterial oxygen saturation
SAP	SLAM-associated protein
SB	serum bilirubin (concentration)
SB	stillbirth
SBBYSS	Say–Barber–Biesecker–Young–Simpson syndrome
SBE	subacute bacterial endocarditis
SBH	subcortical band heterotopia
SCA	spinocerebellar ataxia
SCAN	spinocerebellar ataxia with axonal neuropathy (SCAN-1)
SCD	sudden cardiac death
SCD	sickle-cell disease
SCE	sister chromatid exchange
SCID	severe combined immunodeficiency
SCS	Saethre–Chotzen syndrome
SCT	stem cell transplantation
SCT	sacrococcygeal teratoma
SCTAT	sex cord tumour with annular tubules
SD	standard deviation
SDH	subdural haemorrhage
SDH	succinate dehydrogenase
SED	spondyloepiphyseal dysplasia
SEDC	spondyloepiphyseal dysplasia congenita
SEGA	subependymal giant cell astrocytoma
SEN	subependymal nodule
SGB	Simpson–Golabi–Behmel (syndrome)
SH2	Src homology 2
SH2B1	Src homology 2B adapter protein 1
SHH	sonic hedgehog (gene)
SIDS	sudden infant death syndrome
siRNA	small interfering ribonucleic acid
SLE	systemic lupus erythematosus
SLO	Smith–Lemli–Opitz (syndrome)
SMA	spinal muscular atrophy
SMARD	spinal muscular atrophy with respiratory distress
SMC	supernumerary marker chromosome
SMEI	severe myoclonic epilepsy in infancy
SMS	Smith–Magenis syndrome
SNP	single nucleotide polymorphism
SNV	single nucleotide variant
SNRP	small nuclear ribonuclear protein
SNRPN	small nuclear ribonuclear protein-associated polypeptide N (gene)
SOD	septo-optic dysplasia
SPG2	spastic paraparesis type 2
SRS	Silver–Russell syndrome
SSCP	single-strand conformational polymorphisms

SSRI	selective serotonin reuptake inhibitor		TSC	tuberous sclerosis
STC	short-term culture		TSH	thyroid-stimulating hormone
STR	short tandem repeat		TSHR	thyroid-stimulating hormone receptor
STS	sequence-tagged-sites		TTCE	transthoracic contrast echocardiography
STS	steroid sulfatase		TTD	trichothiodystrophy
SUDEP	sudden unexplained death in epilepsy		TYRP1	tyrosinase-related protein 1
SUR1	sulfonylurea receptor 1		U	unit
SVAS	supravalvular aortic stenosis		U & Es	urea and electrolytes
SW	susceptibility-weighted (image)		UBOs	unidentified bright objects (in MRI scan)
SXR	skull X-ray		UDS	unscheduled DNA synthesis (assay)
T1D	type 1 diabetes		uE3	unconjugated (o)estriol
T2D	type 2 diabetes		UFH	unfractionated heparin
T3	triiodothyronine		UFS	urofacial syndrome
T4	thyroxine		UG	urogenital
TA	transabdominal		UK	United Kingdom
TAPVD	total anomalous pulmonary venous drainage		UKFOCSS	UK Familial Ovarian Cancer Screening Study
TAR	thrombocytopenia–absent radius (syndrome)		UKHCDO	UK Haemophilia Centre Doctor's Organisation
TBS	Townes–Brocks syndrome		UK NSC	UK National Screening Committee
Tc	technetium		UKTIS	UK Teratology Information Service
TC	transcervical		UMOD	uromodulin (gene)
TCC	transitional cell carcinoma		UP	urticaria pigmentosa
TCS	Treacher–Collins syndrome		UPD	uniparental disomy
TD	thanatophoric dysplasia		USA	United States
TDP1	tyrosyl-DNA phosphodiesterase1		USS	ultrasound scan
tds	ter die sumendus (three times a day)		UTI	urinary tract infection
TEV	talipes equinovarus		UV	ultraviolet
TFT	thyroid function test		UVSS	ultraviolet-sensitive syndrome
TGA	transposition of the great arteries		V	variable (region of an immunoglobulin chain)
TGF-β	transforming growth factor beta		VA	visual acuity
THD	tyrosine hydroxylase deficiency		VACTERL	(combination of) vertebral defects–anal atresia–cardiac anomalies–tracheo-oesophageal fistula–(o)esophageal atresia–renal anomalies–limb defects
TIA	transient ischaemic attack			
TNBC	triple-negative breast cancer			
TNDM	transient neonatal diabetes mellitus			
TNSALP	tissue-non-specific alkaline phosphatase		VATER	(combination of) vertebral defects–anal atresia–tracheo-oesophageal fistula–(o)esophageal atresia–renal anomalies
TOC	tylosis oesophageal cancer			
TOF	tracheo-oesophageal fistula			
TOP	termination of pregnancy		VCE	video capsule endoscopy
TORCH	(screen for) toxoplasmosis, other (including syphilis, varicella-zoster, parvovirus), rubella, cytomegalovirus, and herpes simplex virus		VCFS	velocardiofacial syndrome
			VDP	vertical, deepest pocket
			VLDLR	very low-density lipoprotein receptor
TPP	tripeptidyl-peptidase		VEGF	vascular endothelial growth factor
TRAP	twin reverse arterial perfusion sequence		VEP	visual evoked potential
TRH	thyrotropin-releasing hormone		VER	visual evoked response
TrKB	tropomycin-related kinase B		VF	ventricular fibrillation
TRPS	trichorhinophalangeal syndrome		VHL	von Hippel–Lindau (disease)
TRUS	transrectal ultrasound		VIP	vasoactive intestinal peptide
TS	Turner syndrome		VLCFA	very-long-chain fatty acid

VLNT	venterolateral nucleus of the thalamus		WWS	Walker–Warburg syndrome
VMA	vanillylmandelic acid		X-ALD	X-linked adrenoleukodystrophy
VNTR	variable number tandem repeat		X-HMSN	X-linked hereditary motor and sensory neuropathies
VP	ventriculoperitoneal (shunt)		XIAP	X-linked inhibitor of apoptosis
VPA	valproate		Xic	X-chromosome inactivation centre
VSD	ventricular septal defect		XL	X-linked
VTE	venous thromboembolism		XLA	X-linked agammaglobulinaemia
VUR	vesicoureteral reflux		XLAG	X-linked lissencephaly with abnormal genitalia
VUS	variant of unknown significance		XLAS	X-linked Alport syndrome
vWD	von Willebrand disease		XLCDP	X-linked chondrodysplasia punctata
vWF	von Willebrand factor		XLD	X-linked dominant
vWF:Ag	von Willebrand factor antigen		XLEDMD	X-linked Emery–Dreifuss muscular dystrophy
vWF:RiCof	ristocetin cofactor of von Willebrand factor		XLI	X-linked ichthyosis
VWM	leukoencephalopathy with vanishing white matter		XLID	X-linked intellectual disability
			XLIS	X-linked isolated lissencephaly sequence
VWS	van der Woude (syndrome)		XLMR	X-linked mental retardation
VZV	varicella-zoster virus		XLOA	X-linked ocular albinism
WAGR	Wilms tumour–aniridia–genitourinary anomalies–mental retardation		XLOS	X-linked Opitz syndrome
WBC	white blood cell		XLP	X-linked lymphoproliferative (syndrome)
WES	whole exome sequencing		XLR	X-linked recessive
WGS	whole genome sequencing		XLRP	X-linked retinitis pigmentosa
WHO	World Health Organization		XP	xeroderma pigmentosum
WRS	Wiedemann–Rautenstrauch syndrome		XP-V	xeroderma pigmentosum variant
WS	Waardenburg syndrome		YAC	yeast artificial chromosome
WS	West syndrome		ZIG	zoster immune globulin
WSS	Wiedemann–Steiner syndrome			

Chapter advisers

The authors would like to thank the following experts who reviewed and offered in-depth advice for the cancer chapter.

Ian Frayling Consultant in Genetic Pathology, Cardiff, UK.

Marc Tischkowitz Reader in `Medical Genetics, Cambridge, UK.

Advisory editor to the first edition

The authors would like to thank Judith Hall for her work on the first edition.

Judith G. Hall Emeritus Professor of Pediatrics and Medical Genetics, University of British Columbia, Vancouver, Canada.

Expert advisers

The authors would like to thank the following experts who reviewed and offered advice for the topics in this book.

Carlo Acerini University Senior Lecturer, Department of Paediatrics, University of Cambridge, Addenbrooke's Hospital, Cambridge, UK

Hayley Archer Department of Medical Genetics, Cardiff University, University Hospital of Wales, Cardiff, UK

Topun Austin Consultant Neonatologist, Rosie Hospital, Cambridge University Hospitals NHS Foundation Trust, Cambridge, UK

Trevor Baglin Formerly Consultant Haematologist, Department of Haematology, Cambridge University Hospitals, Cambridge, UK

Angela Barnicoat Consultant Clinical Geneticist, Department of Clinical Genetics, Great Ormond Street Hospital NHS Foundation Trust, London, UK

Phil Beales Professor of Medical and Molecular Genetics, Genetics and Genomic Medicine Programme, University College London, Institute of Child Health, London, UK

Elijah Behr Reader in Cardiovascular Medicine, Consultant Cardiologist, Cardiology Clinical Academic Group, St George's University of London, St George's University Hospitals NHS Foundation Trust, London, UK

Jonathan Berg Senior Lecturer and Honorary Consultant in Clinical Genetics, University of Dundee, Ninewells Hospital and Medical School, Dundee, UK

Di Bilton Honorary Consultant in Respiratory Medicine, Royal Brompton Hospital, London, UK

Nick Bishop Professor of Paediatric Bone Disease, Academic Unit of Child Health, Department of Oncology and Metabolism, University of Sheffield, Sheffield Children's Hospital, Sheffield, UK

Maria Bitner-Glindzic Professor of Clinical and Molecular Genetics, Genetics and Genomic Medicine Programme, University College London, Great Ormond Street Institute of Child Health, London, UK

Graeme Black Strategic Director, Manchester Centre for Genomic Medicine, Institute of Human Development, University of Manchester and Central Manchester University Hospitals NHS Foundation Trust, Manchester Academic Health Sciences Centre, St. Mary's Hospital, Manchester, UK

Edward Blair Consultant Clinical Geneticist, Oxford University Hospitals NHS Foundation Trust, Churchill Hospital, Oxford, UK

Paula Bolton-Maggs Consultant Haematologist, Serious Hazards of Transfusion UK National Haemovigilance Scheme, Manchester Blood Centre, Manchester, UK

Nigel P. Burrows Consultant Dermatologist, Addenbrooke's Hospital, Cambridge University Hospitals NHS Foundation Trust, Cambridge, UK

Katie Bushby Act. Res. Chair of Neuromuscular Genetics, Institute of Genetic Medicine, Newcastle University, Newcastle, UK

Lucinda Carr Consultant Paediatric Neurologist, Departments of Neurology and Neurodisability, Great Ormond Street Hospital for Children, London, UK

Angus J. Clarke Consultant in Clinical Genetics, Institute of Medical Genetics, University Hospital of Wales, Cardiff, UK

Jill Clayton-Smith Consultant Clinical Geneticist, Manchester Centre For Genomic Medicine, Central Manchester Hospitals NHS Trust, Manchester, UK

Trevor Cole Consultant in Clinical and Cancer Genetics, Reader in Medical Genetics, West Midlands Regional Genetics Service, Birmingham Women's Hospital, Birmingham, UK

Andrew Copp Professor of Developmental Neurobiology, University College London, Institute of Child Health, London, UK

Timothy M. Cox Director of Research and Professor of Medicine Emeritus, University of Cambridge, Addenbrooke's Hospital, Cambridge, UK

David Craufurd Senior Lecturer and Honorary Consultant in Neuropsychiatric Genetics, Manchester Centre for Genomic Medicine, University of Manchester and Central Manchester University Hospitals NHS Foundation Trust, St. Mary's Hospital, Manchester, UK

Yanick Crow Consultant Clinical Geneticist, Institut Imagine, Necker-Enfants Malades Hospital, Paris Descartes University, Paris, France

Bert de Bries Clinical Geneticist, Department of Human Genetics, University Hospital Nijmegen, Nijmegen, The Netherlands

Anna David Professor and Consultant in Obstetrics and Maternal Fetal Medicine, Head of Research Department of Maternal Fetal Medicine, Institute for Women's Health, University College London, London, UK

Charu Deshpande Consultant Clinical Geneticist, Guy's and St Thomas' NHS Foundation Trust, London, UK

Koen Devriendt Clinical Geneticist, Centre for Human Genetics, University Hospital Leuven, Leuven, Belgium

Hal Dietz Director, Institute of Genetic Medicine, John Hopkins Hospital, Baltimore, USA

Dian Donnai Professor of Medical Genetics, Manchester Centre for Genomic Medicine, University of Manchester and Central Manchester University Hospitals NHS Foundation Trust, Manchester Academic Health Science Centre, Manchester, UK

Susan Downes Consultant Ophthalmologist, Associate Professor University of Oxford, Oxford Eye Hospital, Oxford University Hospital NHS Trust, John Radcliffe Hospital, Oxford, UK

Diana Eccles Head of Cancer Sciences, Faculty of Medicine, University Hospital Southampton, Southampton, UK

Rosalind Eeles Professor and Honorary Consultant in Clinical Oncology and Oncogenetics, Division of Genetics & Epidemiology, The Institute of Cancer Research & Royal Marsden NHS Foundation Trust, London, UK

Sian Ellard Consultant Clinical Scientist, University of Exeter Medical School, Exeter, UK

Gareth Evans Consultant, Manchester Centre for Genomic Medicine, Division of Evolution and Genomic Sciences, St Mary's Hospital, University of Manchester, Manchester, UK

Sadaf Farooqi Professor of Metabolism and Medicine, Wellcome Trust–MRC Institute of Metabolic Science, Addenbrooke's Hospital, Cambridge, UK

Rebecca Fitzgerald Professor of Cancer Prevention and Programme Leader, MRC Cancer Unit, Hutchison/ MRC Research Centre University of Cambridge; Director of Studies in Medicine, and College Lecturer in Medical Sciences, Trinity College, Cambridge, UK

David FitzPatrick Paediatric Geneticist, Royal Hospital for Sick Children, Edinburgh, UK

Frances Flinter Consultant Clinical Geneticist, Department of Clinical Genetics, Guy's and St Thomas' NHS Foundation Trust, Guy's Hospital, London, UK

Ian M. Frayling Consultant Genetic Pathologist, Cardiff and Vale University Health Board, Cardiff University, Institute of Medical Genetics, University Hospital of Wales, Cardiff, UK

Anne-Frédérique Minsart Obstetrician, Department of Obstetrics and Gynaecology, Laboratory of Human Reproduction, Brussels University, Brussels, Belgium

Ali Gharavi Professor of Medicine and Chief, Division of Nephrology, Columbia University, New York, USA

Richard Gibbons Professor of Clinical Genetics, Weatherall Institute of Molecular Medicine, Oxford University Hospital NHS Trust, John Radcliffe Hospital, Oxford, UK

Ruth Gilbert Professor of Clinical Epidemiology, UCL GOS Institute of Child Health, London, UK

Paul Gissen Head of Genetics and Genomic Medicine Programme, University College London Institute of Child Health, Great Ormond Street Hospital for Children, London, UK

Judith Goodship Formerly Professor of Medical Genetics, University of Newcastle, Newcastle upon Tyne, UK

Andrew Grace Consultant Cardiologist, Papworth Hospital, Cambridge University Health Partners, Cambridge, UK

David Greenberg Principal Investigator, Research Institute at Nationwide Children's Hospital, Columbus, USA

Judith Hall Professor Emerita of Paediatrics and Medical Genetics, UBC & Children's and Women's Health Centre of British Columbia, Department of Medical Genetics, British Columbia's Children's Hospital, Vancouver, Canada

Andrew Hattersley Professor of Molecular Medicine, University of Exeter Medical School, Exeter, UK

Karl Heinimann Consultant Medical Geneticist, Division of Medical Genetics, University Hospital Basel, Basel, Switzerland

Tessa Homfray Consultant Medical Genetics, St George's University Hospital, Harris Birthright Unit, Kings College Hospital & Royal Brompton Hospital, London, UK

Richard S. Houlston Professor, Division of Molecular Pathology, The Institute of Cancer Research, Surrey, UK

Steve E. Humphries Emeritus Professor Cardiovascular Genetics, Institute Cardiovascular Science, University College London, London, UK

Matthew Hurles Head of Human Genetics, Wellcome Trust Sanger Institute, Wellcome Trust Genome Campus, Hinxton, UK

Khalid Hussain Professor, Genetics & Epigenetics in Health & Disease, UCL, Great Ormond Street Institute of Child Health, London, UK

Andrew Jackson Professor of Human Genetics, MRC Human Genetics Unit, Institute of Genetics and Molecular Medicine, University of Edinburgh, Edinburgh, UK

Alison Jones Consultant Paediatric Immunologist, Department of Immunology, Great Ormond Street Hospital, London, UK

Wendy Jones Locum Consultant, Clinical Genetics Department, Great Ormond Street Hospital for Children, London, UK

Mark Kilby Lead for Birmingham Centre for Women's & New Born's Health, University of Birmingham, Birmingham, UK

Veronica Kinsler Consultant Paediatric Dermatologist, Great Ormond St Hospital for Children, London, UK

Manju Kurian Principal Research Associate, UCL Great Ormond Street Institute of Child Health, London, UK

Katherine Lachlan Consultant Clinical Geneticist, Wessex Clinical Genetics Service, University Hospital Southampton, Princess Anne Hospital, Southampton, UK

Nayana Lahiri Consultant Clinical Geneticist, SW Thames Regional Genetics Service, St. George's University Hospitals NHS Foundation Trust, St. George's Hospital, London, UK

Alison Lashwood Consultant Genetic Counsellor, Guy's and St Thomas' NHS Foundation Trust, London, UK

Christoph Lees Clinical Reader in Obstetrics, Imperial College London, Honorary Consultant in Obstetrics and Head of Fetal Medicine, Imperial College Healthcare NHS Trust, London, UK

Eric Legius Clinical Geneticist, Centre for Human Genetics, University Hospital Leuven, Leuven, Belgium

Alan R. Lehmann Research Professor, Genome Damage and Stability Centre, School of Life Sciences, University of Sussex, Brighton, UK

John H. Livingston Consultant Paediatric Neurologist, Leeds Teaching Hospital NHS Trust, Leeds, UK

Y. M. Dennis Lo Li Ka Shing Professor of Medicine and Professor of Chemical Pathology, Department of

Chemical Pathology, The Chinese University of Hong Kong, Prince of Wales Hospital, Shatin, New Territories, Hong Kong SAR, China

David Lomas Vice Provost (Health), University College London, London, UK

Anneke Lucassen Consultant in Clinical Genetics, Faculty of Medicine, Wessex Clinical Genetic Service, University of Southampton, Southampton, UK

Stan Lyonnet Clinical Geneticist, Department of Medical Genetics, Hôpital Necker-Enfants Malades, Paris, France

Deborah Mackay Professor of Medical Epigenetics, Southampton University, Southampton, UK

Fiona L. Mackie Clinical Research Fellow in Obstetrics and Gynaecology, University of Birmingham, Birmingham Women's Hospital, Birmingham, UK

Eamonn R. Maher Professor and Honorary Consultant, Department of Medical Genetics, University of Cambridge, Cambridge University Hospitals, Cambridge, UK

Laurent Mandelbrot Professor, Department of Obstetrics and Gynaecology, Hôpital Louis Mourier, Assistance Publique-Hôpitaux de Paris, Colombes, France

Sahar Mansour Consultant and Honorary Professor in Clinical Genetics, St George's Healthcare NHS Trust, London, UK

Elizabeth Marder Consultant Paediatrician, Community Child Health, Nottingham Children's Hospital, Nottingham University Hospitals NHS Trust, Nottingham, UK

Robert Mcfarland Clinical Senior Lecturer in Paediatric Neurology, Wellcome Trust Centre for Mitochondrial Research, Institute of Neuroscience, Newcastle University, Newcastle upon Tyne, UK

Amy McTague Research Fellow, Developmental Neurosciences Programme, University College London, Great Ormond Street Institute of Child Health, London, UK

Anna Middleton Head of Social Science and Ethics and Registered Genetic Counsellor, Wellcome Genome Campus, Cambridge, UK

David Mowat Clinical Geneticist, Centre for Clinical Genetics, Sydney Children's Hospital, Sydney, Australia

Max Muenke Chief, Medical Genetics Branch, National Institutes of Health, Bethesda, Maryland, USA

Stefan Mundlos Group Leader of the Research Group Development & Disease, Max Planck Institute for Molecular Genetics, Berlin, Germany

Elaine Murphy Consultant in Inherited Metabolic Disease, Charles Dent Metabolic Unit, National Hospital for Neurology and Neurosurgery, London, UK

Elani Nastouli Lead Consultant in Virology, University College Hospital, London, UK

Ruth Newbury-Ecob Lead Clinician, Department of Clinical Genetics, University Hospitals Bristol NHS Foundation Trust, Bristol, UK

Soo-Mi Park Consultant in Clinical Genetics, Department of Clinical Genetics, Cambridge University Hospitals NHS Foundation Trust, Cambridge, UK

Michael Parker Professor of Bioethics and Director, Ethox Centre, Nuffield Department of Population Health, University of Oxford, Oxford, UK

Michael A. Patton Emeritus Consultant Clinical Geneticist and Head of the Human Genetics Research Centre, Department of Medical Genetics, St Georges University of London, London, UK

Joanna Poulton Professor of Mitochondrial Genetics, University of Oxford, Oxford, UK

Sue Price Consultant in Clinical Genetics, Oxford Regional Genetics Service, Churchill Hospital, Oxford, UK

Nicola Ragge Consultant Clinical Geneticist, Birmingham Women's Hospital, Birmingham, UK; Professor in Medical Genetics, Oxford Brookes University, Oxford, UK

Anita Rauch Professor of Medical Genetics, Institute of Medical Genetics, University of Zurich, Schlieren, Switzerland

Lucy Raymond Professor of Medical Genetics and Neurodevelopment, University of Cambridge, Cambridge, UK

Andrew Read Emeritus Professor of Human Genetics, University of Manchester, Manchester, UK

Willie Reardon Consultant Clinical Medical Geneticist, Department of Clinical Genetics, Our Lady's Children's Hospital, Dublin, Ireland

Evan Reid University Lecturer and Honorary Consultant in Clinical Genetics, Department of Medical Genetics, University of Cambridge, Cambridge, UK

Rhys C. Roberts Consultant Neurologist, Department of Neurology, Cambridge University Hospitals NHS Foundation Trust, Addenbrooke's Hospital, Cambridge, UK

Stephen Robertson Clinical Geneticist, Dunedin School of Medicine, University of Otago, Dunedin, New Zealand

Mark T. Rogers Consultant Clinical Geneticist and Honorary Senior Research Fellow, Institute of Medical Genetics, University Hospital of Wales, Cardiff, UK

Elizabeth Rosser Consultant in Clinical Genetics, Department of Clinical Genetics, Great Ormond St Hospital, London, UK

Julian Sampson Professor and Honorary Consultant in Medical Genetics, Institute of Medical Genetics, Cardiff University Heath Park, Cardiff, UK

Richard Sandford University Reader in Renal Genetics, Academic Department of Medical Genetics, University of Cambridge, Cambridge, UK

Ravi Savarirayan Consultant Clinical Geneticist, Victorian Clinical Genetics Services, Parkville, Australia

Richard Scott Consultant in Clinical Genetics, Great Ormond Street Hospital NHS Foundation Trust, London, UK

Charles Shaw-Smith Consultant Clinical Geneticist, Peninsula Clinical Genetics Service, Royal Devon and Exeter Hospital NHS Trust, Exeter, UK

Deborah Shears Consultant in Clinical Genetics, Department of Clinical Genetics, Churchill Hospital, Oxford, UK

Eamonn Sheridan Professor of Clinical Genetics, University of Leeds, Leeds, UK

Sanjay M. Sisodiya Professor of Neurology, Department of Clinical and Experimental Epilepsy, University College London, London, UK

David Skuse Professor of Behavioural and Brain Sciences, Population, Policy and Practice Programme, Institute of Child Health, University College London, London, UK

Sarah Smithson Consultant, Department of Clinical Genetics, University Hospitals Bristol NHS Foundation Trust, Bristol, UK

Martin P. Snead Consultant Vitreoretinal Surgeon, Vitreoretinal Service, Addenbrookes Hospital, Cambridge, UK

Miranda Splitt Consultant Clinical Geneticist, Northern Genetics Service, Newcastle upon Tyne Hospitals NHS Trust, Newcastle upon Tyne, UK

Mohnish Suri Consultant Clinical Geneticist, Nottingham Clinical Genetics Service, Nottinghamshire University Hospitals NHS Trust, Nottingham, UK

Nicole Tartaglia Developmental–Behavioural Paediatrician, Associate Professor of Paediatrics, University of Colorado, School of Medicine, Children's Hospital Colorado, USA

Kate Tatton-Brown Consultant Clinical Geneticist, South Thames Regional Genetics Service, St George's Universities NHS Foundation Trust, London, UK

Amy Taylor Principal Genetic Counsellor, Cambridge University Hospital, Cambridge, UK

Malcolm Taylor Professor of Cancer Genetics, Institute of Cancer and Genomic Sciences, University of Birmingham, Birmingham, UK

Karen Temple Professor of Medical Genetics and Honorary Consultant in Clinical Genetics, University of Southampton, University Hospital Southampton NHS Trust, Southampton, UK

Rajesh Thakker May Professor of Medicine, Radcliffe Department of Medicine, University of Oxford, Oxford Centre for Diabetes, Endocrinology & Metabolism, Churchill Hospital, Oxford, UK

Swee-Lay Thein Senior Investigator, Sickle Cell Branch, National Heart, Lung and Blood Institute, NIH, Bethedsa, MD, USA

Marc Tischkowitz Reader and Honorary Consultant Physician in Medical Genetics, Department of Medical Genetics, University of Cambridge and East Anglian Medical Genetics Service, Cambridge, UK

Pat Tookey Honorary Senior Lecturer, Population Policy and Practice Programme, University College London, Institute of Child Health, London, UK

Peter Turnpenny Consultant Clinical Geneticist and Honorary Clinical Professor, University of Exeter, Medical School, Royal Devon & Exeter Healthcare NHS Trust, Exeter, UK

Julie Vogt Consultant Geneticist, West Midlands Regional Genetics Service, Birmingham Women's NHS Foundation Trust, Birmingham, UK

Emma Wakeling Consultant in Clinical Genetics, North West Thames Regional Genetics Service, London North West Healthcare NHS Trust, Harrow, UK

Jonathan Waters Consultant Clinical Scientist, Regional Genetics Service, Great Ormond Street Hospital NHS Trust, London, UK

Diana Wellesley Consultant Clinical Geneticist, Wessex Clinical Genetics Service, Princess Anne Hospital, Southampton, UK

Andrew Wilkie Nuffield Professor of Pathology, Weatherall Institute of Molecular Medicine, University of Oxford, Oxford, UK

Paul Wordsworth Professor of Rheumatology, Nuffield Department of Orthopaedics, Rheumatology and Musculoskeletal Sciences, Oxford University, Oxford, UK

Caroline Wright Senior Lecturer in Genomic Medicine, University of Exeter, UK

Laura Yates Consultant in Clinical Genetics (NGS) and Head of Teratology (UKTIS), Institute of Genetic Medicine, Newcastle upon Tyne Hospitals NHS Foundation Trust and Newcastle University, Newcastle upon Tyne, UK

Expert advisers to the first edition

Judith Allanson Professor of Pediatrics, University of Ottawa, Ottawa, Ontario, Canada

Derek Applegarth Emeritus Professor of Pediatrics, University of British Columbia, Vancouver, British Columbia, Canada

Trevor Baglin Formerly Consultant Haematologist, Addenbrooke's Hospital, Cambridge, England

Michael Baraitser Emeritus Consultant Clinical Geneticist, Great Ormond Street Hospital, London, England

Angela Barnicoat Consultant in Clinical Genetics, Institute of Child Health, London, England

Philip Beales Wellcome Trust Senior Research Fellow and Honorary Consultant, Institute of Child Health, London, England

Di Bilton Consultant Respiratory Physician and Director of the Adult Cystic Fibrosis Unit, Papworth Hospital, Cambridge, England

Nick Bishop Professor of Paediatric Bone Disease, University of Sheffield, Sheffield, England

Maria Bitner-Glindzicz Senior Lecturer and Honorary Consultant Geneticist, Institute of Child Health, London, England

Martin Bobrow Professor of Medical Genetics, University of Cambridge, Cambridge, England

Patrick Bolton Professor of Child and Adolescent Psychiatry, The Institute of Psychiatry, London, England

Paula Bolton-Maggs Consultant Haematologist, Manchester Comprehensive Care Haemophilia Centre, Manchester Royal Infirmary, Manchester, England

Patricia Boyd Associate Specialist in Clinical Genetics for Prenatal Diagnosis, John Radcliffe Hospital, Oxford, England

Garry Brown University Lecturer, Genetics Unit, Department of Biochemistry, University of Oxford, Oxford, England

Han G. Brunner Professor, Department of Human Genetics, University of Nijmegen, Nijmegen, The Netherlands

Nigel Burrows Consultant Dermatologist, Addenbrooke's Hospital, Cambridge, England

Kate Bushby Action Research Professor in Neuromuscular Genetics, Institute of Human Genetics, University of Newcastle, Newcastle-upon-Tyne, England

Carlos Caldas Professor, Cancer Genomics Programme, Department of Oncology, University of Cambridge, Cambridge, England

Hilary Cass Wolfson Centre, Great Ormond Street Children's Hospital NHS Trust, London, England.

Edwin Chilvers Professor of Respiratory Medicine, University of Cambridge, Cambridge, England

Lyn Chitty Consultant in Genetics and Fetal Medicine, University College Hospital, London, England

Angus Clarke Professor in Clinical Genetics, University of Wales College of Medicine, Cardiff, Wales

Jill Clayton-Smith Consultant Clinical Geneticist, St Mary's Hospital, Manchester, England

Trevor Cole Consultant Clinical Geneticist, Birmingham, England

Amanda Collins Consultant Clinical Geneticist, Wessex Regional Genetics Service, Southampton, England

Helen Cox Specialist Registrar in Clinical Genetics, University of Southampton, Southampton, England

T.M. Cox Professor of Clinical Medicine, University of Cambridge, Cambridge, England

John Crolla Clinical Molecular Cytogeneticist, Wessex Regional Genetics Laboratories, Salisbury, England

Melanie Davies Consultant Obstetrician and Gynaecologist (Reproductive Medicine), University College Hospital, London, England

Sally J. Davies Consultant in Medical Genetics, University Hospital of Wales, Cardiff, Wales

Bert B.A. de Vries Clinical Geneticist, University Medical Centre, Nijmegen, The Netherlands

Dian Donnai Professor of Medical Genetics, University of Manchester, Manchester, England

David Dunger Professor of Paediatrics, University of Cambridge, Cambridge, England

Douglas Easton Director Cancer Research UK Genetic Epidemiology Unit, Cambridge, England

Diana Eccles Consultant/Professor of Cancer Genetics, University of Southampton, Southampton, England

John Edwards Emeritus Professor of Genetics, University of Oxford, Oxford, England

Charis Eng Professor and Director, Clinical Cancer Genetics Program, Ohio State University, Columbus, Ohio, USA

Gareth Evans Professor of Cancer Genetics, University of Manchester, Manchester, England

Peter Farndon Professor of Clinical Genetics, University of Birmingham, Birmingham, England

Sadaf Farooqi Wellcome Clinician Scientist Fellow, Department of Clinical Biochemistry, University of Cambridge, Cambridge, England

John Firth Consultant Physician and Nephrologist, Addenbrooke's Hospital, Cambridge, England

David FitzPatrick Senior Clinical Scientist and Hon. Consultant Clinical Geneticist, Western General Hospital, Edinburgh, Scotland

Frances Flinter Consultant Clinical Geneticist, Guy's Hospital, London, England

Charles ffrench-Constant Professor of Neurogenetics, University of Cambridge, Cambridge, England

Ian M. Frayling Consultant in Clinical Genetics and Director of Clinical Genetics Laboratory, University Hospital of Wales, Cardiff, Wales

R.M. Gardiner Professor, Department of Paediatrics and Child Health, Royal Free and University College Medical School, London, England

Paul Giangrande Consultant Haematologist, Oxford Haemophilia Centre and Thrombosis Unit, Churchill Hospital, Oxford, England

Richard Gibbons Lecturer in Clinical Biochemistry and Honorary Consultant in Clinical Genetics, Oxford, England

Karen Goldstone Radiation Protection Advisor, Addenbrooke's Hospital, Cambridge, England

Frances R. Goodman Former Honorary Clinical Lecturer, Molecular Medicine Unit, Institute of Child Health, London, England

Judith Goodship Formerly Professor of Medical Genetics, University of Newcastle, Newcastle-upon-Tyne, England

Robert J. Gorlin Professor (retired), Department of Oral Pathology and Genetics, University of Minnesota, Minneapolis, Minnesota, USA

Andrew Grace Consultant Cardiologist, Papworth Hospital, Cambridge, England

Christine Hall Professor of Paediatric Radiology, Institute of Child Health, London, England

Judith G. Hall Emeritus Professor of Pediatrics and Medical Genetics, University of British Columbia, Vancouver, British Columbia, Canada

Ann Harding-Bell Speech Therapist to the Eastern Region Cleft Network, Addenbrooke's Hospital, Cambridge, England

Peter S. Harper Professor of Genetics, University of Wales College of Medicine, Cardiff, Wales

David Hilton-Jones Consultant Neurologist, Oxford Kadcliffe Hospitals NHS Trust, Oxford, England.

Lewis B. Holmes Professor of Pediatrics, Harvard Medical School and Chief, Genetics and Teratology Unit, Massachusetts General Hospital for Children, Boston, Massachusetts, USA

Tony Hope Professor, Director of Ethox, Institute of Health Sciences, University of Oxford, Oxford, England

Ieuan Hughes Professor of Paediatrics, University of Cambridge, Cambridge, England

Steve E. Humphries Professor of Cardiovascular Genetics, British Heart Foundation Laboratories, Royal Free and Universty College Medical School, London, England

Susan M. Huson Hon Consultant in Clinical Genetics, Oxford Regional Genetics Service, Manchester, England

Alison Jones Consultant Paediatric Immunologist/Honorary Senior Lecturer, Great Ormond Street Hospital/Institute of Child Health, University College, London, England

Alison Kerr Consultant Paediatrician and Senior Lecturer, Department of Psychological Medicine, University of Glasgow, Glasgow, Scotland

Samantha J.L. Knight University Research Lecturer and Wellcome Trust Research Fellow, Wellcome Trust Centre for Human Genetics, Oxford, England

Ian D. Krantz The Children's Hospital of Philadelphia, The University of Pennsylvania School of Medicine, Philadelphia, Pennsylvania, USA

Alison Lashwood Consultant Nurse in Preimplantation Genetic Diagnosis, Guy's Hospital, London, England

Alan Lehmann Professor and Chairman, Genome Damage and Stability Centre, University of Sussex, Brighton, England

Mary Linden Genetic Counsellor, Kimball Genetics Inc., Denver, Colorado, USA

David Lomas Professor, Department of Radiology, University of Cambridge, Cambridge, England

David A. Lomas Professor of Respiratory Medicine, Department of Medicine, University of Cambridge, Cambridge, England

Peter Lunt Consultant Clinical Geneticist, St. Michael's Hospital, Bristol, England

Stanislas Lyonnet Professor of Genetics, Hôpital Necker–Enfants Malades, Paris, France

Eamonn Maher Professor of Medical Genetics, University of Birmingham, Birmingham, England

Kenny McCormick Consultant Neonatologist, John Radcliffe Hospital, Oxford, England

Patricia McElhatton Consultant Teratologist and Head of National Teratology Information Service, Newcastle-upon-Tyne, England

R.J. McKinlay Gardner Medical Geneticist, Genetic Health Services Victoria and Murdoch Children's Research Institute, Melbourne, Australia

Peter Mortimer Professor of Dermatological Medicine, St George's Hospital, London, England

Hugo Moser Professor of Neurology and Pediatrics, Johns Hopkins University, Baltimore, Maryland, USA

Jessica Mozersky Cancer Research UK and UCL Cancer Trials Centre, University College, London, England

Maximilian Muenke Chief, Medical Genetics Branch, National Institutes of Health, Bethesda, Maryland, USA

Andrea Németh Consultant and Lecturer in Clincal Genetics, University of Oxford, Oxford, England

Ruth Newbury-Ecob Consultant in Clinical Genetics, St Michael's Hospital, Bristol, England

John Old National Haemoglobinopathy Reference Laboratory, Churchill Hospital, Oxford, England

John Optiz Professor of Human Genetics, Pediatrics, Obstetrics and Gynaecology, and Pathology, University of Utah, Salt Lake City, Utah, USA

Ingegerd Östman-Smith Professor of Paediatric Cardiology, Gothenburg University, Gothenburg, Sweden

Willem H. Ouwehand Lecturer in Haematology, University of Cambridge, Cambridge, England

Ozkan Ozturk Senior Lecturer in Obstetrics and Gynaecology (Reproductive Medicine), University College Hospital, London, England

Gilbert Park Director of Intensive Care Research, Addenbrooke's Hospital, Cambridge, England

Donald Peebles Consultant in Fetal Medicine, University College Hospital, London, England

Paul Pharaoh Cancer Research UK Senior Clinical Research Fellow, Strangeways Research Laboratory, Cambridge, England

Robin Phillips Professor, St Mark's Hospital, London, England

Daniela Pilz Consultant Clinical Geneticist, Institute of Medical Genetics, University Hospital of Wales, Cardiff, Wales

Bruce Ponder Professor of Oncology, University of Cambridge, Cambridge, England

Mary Porteous Consultant Clinical Geneticist, Edinburgh, Scotland

Joanna Poulton Professor of Mitochondrial Genetics, University of Oxford, Oxford, England

Sue Price Consultant Geneticist, Oxford Regional Genetics Service, Oxford, England

Kathy Pritchard-Jones Senior Lecturer and Honorary Consultant in Paediatric Oncology, Institute of Cancer Research and Royal Marsden Hospital, London, England

Nicola Ragge Consultant Paediatric Opthalmologist, Moorfields Eye Hospital, London, England

Nazneen Rahman Senior Lecturer and Honorary Consultant in Clinical Genetics, Institute of Cancer Research, Sutton, Surrey, England

Uma Ramaswami Consultant Paediatrician (Metabolic Disorders), Addenbrooke's Hospital, Cambridge, England

Evan Reid University Lecturer and Honorary Consultant in Medical Genetics, University of Cambridge, Cambridge, England

Elisabeth Rosser Consultant Clinical Geneticist, Great Ormond Street Hospital, London, England

David Rubinsztein Wellcome Senior Clinical Fellow, Cambridge Institute for Medical Research, Cambridge, England

Judy Rubinsztein Clinical Lecturer in Old Age Psychiatry, University of Cambridge, Cambridge, England

Richard Sandford Wellcome Trust Senior Fellow in Clinical Research and Honorary Consultant in Medical Genetics, University of Cambridge, Cambridge, England

David Savage Wellcome Trust Training Fellow, Department of Clinical Biochemistry, University of Cambridge, Cambridge, England

Ravi Savirirayan Professor, Murdoch Children's Research Institute and Department of Paediatrics, University of Melbourne, Parkville, Victoria, Australia

A. Schinzel Professor, Institute of Medical Genetics, University of Zurich, Schwerzenbach, Switzerland

Robert Semple Wellcome Clinical Research Training Fellow, Department of Clinical Biochemistry, University of Cambridge, Cambridge, England

S.M. Sisodiya Department of Clinical and Experimental Epilepsy, University College London Institute of Neurology, London, England

Roger Smith Honorary Metabolic Bone Physician, Nuffield Orthopaedic Centre, Oxford, England

Martin Snead Consultant Ophthalmologist, Addenbrooke's Hospital, Cambridge, England

Miranda P. Splitt Consultant in Clinical Genetics, Northern Genetics Service, Newcastle upon Tyne, England

Robert Surtees Professor of Paediatric Neurology, Institute of Child Health, London, England

Malcolm Taylor Professor of Cancer Genetics, University of Birmingham, Birmingham, England

Karen Temple Consultant Clinical Geneticist, Wessex Regional Genetics Service, Southampton, England

Rajesh Thakker May Professor of Medicine, University of Oxford, Oxford, England

Susan Thomas Information Team, Breast Test Wales, Cardiff, Wales

Hugh Watkins Professor of Cardiovascular Medicine, University of Oxford, John Radcliffe Hospital, Oxford, England

A.O.M. Wilkie Nuffield Professor of Pathology and Honorary Consultant in Clinical Genetics, University of Oxford, England

David I. Wilson Professor of Medical Genetics, University of Southampton, Southampton, England

Louise Wilson Consultant Clinical Geneticist, Great Ormond Street Hospital, London, England

the late Robin Winter Former Professor of Clinical Genetics and Dysmorphology, Institute of Child Health, London, England

C. Geoff Woods Lecturer in Medical Genetics, University of Cambridge, Cambridge, England

Paul Wordsworth Professor of Rheumatology, University of Oxford, Oxford, England

Tim Wreghitt Consultant Virologist, Addenbrooke's Hospital, Cambridge, England

John R.W. Yates Professor of Clinical Genetics, University of Cambridge, Cambridge, England

Ian D. Young Consultant Clinical Geneticist, Leicester, England

Introduction

Chapter contents

Adoption

Adoption
Is the legal transfer of parental responsibility from the birth family to a new adoptive family. In the United Kingdom (UK), the Adoption Act 1976 states that to be eligible for adoption, the child must be under the age of 18 years and there must be no possibility of continuing in the care of his/her birth parents. Should the child be married or have been married, he cannot be adopted. In the UK, an Adoption Order severs all legal ties with the birth family and confers parental rights and responsibilities on the new adoptive family. The birth parents no longer have any legal rights over the child and they are not entitled to claim him/her back. The child becomes a full member of the adoptive family; he/she takes the surname and assumes the same rights and privileges as if he/she had been born to his/her adoptive parents, including the right of inheritance.

Adoption continues to provide an important service for children, offering a positive and beneficial outcome. Research shows that, generally, adopted children make very good progress through their childhood and into adulthood and do considerably better than children who have remained in the care system throughout most of their childhood.

The British Society of Human Genetics report (2010) made similar recommendations but suggested there may (very occasionally) be circumstances when it would be reasonable to test a child being considered for adoption who might not otherwise be tested at the same age. However, this comes with the strong recommendation that there should be a discussion between genetics professionals and the (prospective) adoptive parents and/or social workers before any such test is performed. Discussion at that point will often correct misunderstandings, so that the request for testing may disappear.

An additional note of caution about the genetic testing of children being considered for adoption is that the newer, genome-based tests used for investigation of neurodevelopmental disorders (array CGH, clinical exome analysis and other high-throughout sequencing investigations) are substantially more likely to generate results of uncertain significance than the karyotype, which would have been used in the past. This matters in the context of adoption as adopting parents face a great deal of uncertainty in any case; the explicit uncertainty of such a genomic test result may prove much more daunting than the implicit uncertainty of an apparently normal karyotype.

Fostering
Is an agreement to offer a temporary home to children whose parents are unable to care for them. It is usually organized by social workers working for local authorities. The authority pays for the children's accommodation and food.

Adoption agency
This is the organization that has arranged the adoption and has had contact with the birth and adoptive parents. The agency may be a state-run organization, a charity, or a profit-making company. The agencies have a statutory obligation to keep records of the adoption process.

Confidentiality
In the UK, when an adopted individual reaches the age of 18, he/she can request the original birth certificate that will contain the mother's name and address at the time of the birth. A birth parent is not able to obtain details of the child's new family and name, though some contact between the birth and adoptive parents is more common now.

Genetic issues relating to adoption
(1) Genetic information given to adoptive parents

Family history

The birth parents are asked to give information about medical problems in the family. Often there is no contact with the father and this limits the information that can be given.

In the United States (USA), the American Society of Human Genetics (1991) endorsed a statement concerning the importance of including a genetic history as part of the adoption process. Their recommendations are as follows and were written to encourage state and private agencies to collect helpful genetic histories.

- Every person should have the right to gain access to his or her medical record, including genetic data that may reside therein.
- A child entering foster care or the adoption process is at risk of losing access to relevant genetic facts about himself or herself.
- The compilation of an appropriate genetic history and the inclusion of genetic data in the adoptee's medical files should be a routine part of the adoption process.
- Genetic information should be obtained, organized, and stored in a manner that permits review, including periodic updating, by appropriate individuals.
- When medically appropriate, genetic data may be shared among the adoptive parents, biological parents, and adoptees. This should be done with the utmost respect for the right to privacy of the parties. The sharing of information should be bidirectional between the adoptive and biological parents, mediated as appropriate through the adoption agency, until the child reaches an age to receive such information himself or herself.
- The right to privacy includes the right of any party to refuse to enter into, or cease to participate in, the process of gathering genetic information.

Known genetic disease prior to adoption

When there is a known genetic condition in the family (e.g. single gene or chromosomal disorder), the question of whether to test a healthy child for the condition may arise prior to adoption. 'It should not be assumed that genetic (predictive or carrier) testing will be required before a suitable placement can be achieved. In each case, we would advise discussion between the medical adviser to the adoption agency and a clinical geneticist. The important factors other than the possible laboratory test results need to be identified for future attention in advance of any test being performed' (ASHG). See (4) below for a further discussion of issues relating to genetic testing and adoption.

(2) Genetic disorder diagnosed in a child after adoption
The geneticist may be involved in the diagnosis of a genetic condition in an adopted individual that may be of importance to his/her birth family.

Some adopted adults are in contact with their birth families, but in most the route to passing on this information is through the adoption agency. The geneticist may write a brief letter stating the name of the condition that has been diagnosed in the adopted child and that this is a condition that could have genetic implications for the biological family and recommending referral to their local genetic service. The medical advisor to the agency can assess the information and it may be feasible for them then to contact the birth family. Records made many years ago are less complete and for individuals >18 years these may not be adequate to enable contact to be made with the birth family.

(3) Genetic disorder diagnosed in birth family after a child has been adopted out
The geneticist may be involved in the diagnosis of a genetic condition or carrier status in the biological parent of a child who has been adopted out of the family. In most situations, the route to passing on this information is through the adoption agency. The geneticist may write a brief letter stating the name of the condition that has been diagnosed in the biological family and that it could have genetic implications for the adopted child and recommending referral to their local genetic service. The medical adviser to the agency can assess the information and, for those who are still <18 years of age, should have the information to contact the parents of the adopted child. Records made many years ago are less complete and it may be more difficult to trace an individual, adopted as a child, who is now an adult.

(4) Genetic testing
In most circumstances, when a child is being considered for adoption, the guidelines for genetic testing should be followed as for other children. The American Society of Human Genetics (ASHG) (Botkin 2015) recommends the following.
• The ASHG recommends that both children awaiting adoption and adopted children be given the same consideration in genetic testing as children living with their biological parents.

• All genetic testing of newborns and children in the adoption process should be consistent with the tests performed on all children of a similar age for the purposes of diagnosis or of identifying appropriate prevention strategies.
• Because the primary justification for genetic testing of any child is a timely medical benefit to the child, genetic testing of newborns and children in the adoption process should be limited to testing for conditions that manifest themselves during childhood or for which preventive measures or therapies may be undertaken during childhood.

Support group: Adoption UK, http://www.adoptionuk.org.

Expert adviser: Angus J. Clarke, Consultant in Clinical Genetics, Institute of Medical Genetics, University Hospital of Wales, Cardiff, UK.

References
American Society of Human Genetics. American Society of Human Genetics Social Issues Committee report on genetics and adoption: points to consider. *Am J Hum Genet* 1991; **48**: 1009–10.

American Society of Human Genetics/American College of Medical Geneticists. Points to consider: ethical, legal, and psychological implications of genetic testing in children and adolescents. *Am J Hum Genet* 1995; **57**: 1233–41.

British Society for Human Genetics. *Genetic Testing of Children.* Report of a working party of the British Society for Human Genetics, 2010.

Department of Health (UK). *Adoption and fostering.* https://www.gov.uk/topic/schools-colleges-childrens-services/adoption-fostering.

Jansen LA, Ross LF. The ethics of preadoption genetic testing. *Am J Med Genet* 2001; **104**: 214–20.

Plumridge D, Burns J, Fisher NL. Heredity and adoption: a survey of state adoption agencies. *Am J Hum Genet* 1990; **46**: 208–14.

The American Society of Human Genetics Social Issues Committee, The American College of Medical Genetics Social, Ethical, and Legal Issues Committee. Genetic testing in adoption. *Am J Hum Genet* 2000; **66**: 761–7.

Turnpenny P (ed.). *Secrets in the genes. Adoption, inheritance and genetic disease.* London, British Agencies for Adoption and Fostering, 1995.

Approach to the consultation with a child with dysmorphism, congenital malformation, or developmental delay

Terminology

Dysmorphology is the recognition and study of birth defects and syndromes. The term was first used by David Smith from the USA in the 1960s to describe the study of human congenital malformations and patterns of birth defects.

Malformation is a non-progressive morphological abnormality of a single organ or body part that arises because of an abnormal developmental programme (a primary error in morphogenesis, e.g. cleft lip).

Syndrome is a pattern of anomalies, at least one of which is morphologic, known or thought to be causally related (from the Greek 'running together'). For example, a patient with the combination of exomphalos, a large tongue, and overgrowth has a combination of the cardinal features of the 'syndrome' described by Beckwith and Wiedemann (known as Beckwith–Wiedemann syndrome (BWS)).

Sequence is one or more secondary morphologic anomalies known or presumed to cascade from a single malformation, disruption, dysplasia, or deformation, e.g. Robin sequence describes the combination of micrognathia, a wide U-shaped cleft palate, and upper airway obstruction, with the cleft palate and airway compromise consequent upon failure of normal mandibular growth in the 8th–11th weeks of embryonic development.

Association is a pattern of anomalies, at least two of which are morphologic, that occur together more often than would be expected by chance and where a causal relationship has not been identified, e.g. VACTERL (vertebral defects–anal atresia–cardiac anomalies–tracheo-oesophageal fistula–(o)esophageal atresia–renal anomalies–limb defects) association.

Dysplasia is a morphologic anomaly arising either prenatally or postnatally from dynamic or ongoing alteration of cellular constitution, tissue organization, or function within a specific organ or a specific tissue type, e.g. within cartilage and bone in skeletal dysplasias.

Disruption is a non-progressive, congenital morphologic anomaly due to the breakdown of a body structure that had a normal developmental potential, e.g. interruption of the blood supply to a developing limb leads to ischaemia, necrosis, and sloughing, resulting in structural damage.

Deformation is an altered shape or position of a body part due to aberrant mechanical force(s) that distorts an otherwise normal structure, e.g. the flat nasal bridge that occurs in a fetus developing with severe oligohydramnios.

Congenital anomalies

Approximately 2–3% of singleton neonates have an obvious major congenital anomaly. However, with follow-up, this rate doubles. Results of several studies suggest that there is a 2- to 3-fold increase of congenital anomalies in monozygotic (MZ) twins, i.e. ~10% of MZ twins are born with a congenital anomaly. Congenital anomalies (birth defects) may arise due to a number of mechanisms defined under Terminology above. Determining the mechanism has important implications for prognosis and recurrence risk. Before considering genetic causes, consider whether there is evidence of:

(1) abnormal physical forces *in utero* causing a deformation;

(2) vascular interruption causing disruptions;

(3) teratogenic exposure, e.g. fetal alcohol syndrome (FAS), fetal anticonvulsant syndrome (FACS), diabetic embryopathy are other causes of *disruptions and malformations*.

Germline genetic alterations affect morphogenesis, i.e. abnormal programming of development (Donnai and Read 2003), and can cause *malformations and dysplasias*. For example:

• failure of structural integrity—qualitative or quantitative defects of structural molecules, e.g. mutations in COL2A1 in Stickler syndrome;

• failure to regulate cell numbers appropriately, e.g. mutations in MCPH5 (ASPM) causing primary autosomal recessive (AR) microcephaly;

• failure of cell migration such that cells do not reach their correct location, e.g. mutations in MID1 in Opitz syndrome;

• failure of a developmental switch—many developmental defects result from deficiencies in transcription factors or cell–cell signalling systems.

Very many genes may be involved, e.g. chromosomal aneuploidy, or a number of genes, e.g. chromosomal microdeletion disorders such as Williams syndrome, or a single gene. Some single gene mutations have devastating consequences for development, e.g. Lys650Glu mutations in FGFR3 cause the perinatal lethal condition thanatophoric dysplasia (TD) type 2.

The term 'dysmorphic' is used to describe children whose physical features are not usually found in a child of the same age or ethnic background. Some features are abnormal in all circumstances, e.g. premature fusion of the cranial sutures, whereas other features may be a non-significant familial trait, e.g. 2/3 toe syndactyly. The recognition of which features are good diagnostic aids comes with experience, but most trainees will be able to come to a differential diagnosis, if not the exact diagnosis, by pursuing a plan such as we outline here.

Although 'dysmorphic' is generally used to refer to visible malformations or distinctive features, the term more correctly means the presence of an abnormality of structure. Internal organs may therefore be affected by the same mechanism as the visible malformations. Knowledge of normal fetal development is necessary to an understanding of dysmorphology.

Background

The clinical geneticist is asked to see children for the following reasons:

(1) to give a diagnostic opinion;

(2) to interpret an existing genetic test to help understand the aetiology;

(3) to discuss the genetic aspects of the condition;

(4) to advise if there are other investigations pertinent to the diagnosis;

(5) to advise about the prognosis and suggest various therapeutic options;

(6) to discuss the risk of recurrence in another pregnancy;

(7) to discuss if prenatal testing is available.

This chapter will deal primarily with the diagnostic aspects of the consultation and the gathering of clinical information necessary to answer the other questions.

Next-generation sequencing (panel/WES/WGS) in the diagnosis of the dysmorphic child

Increasingly, patients will be referred with the results of an existing genetic test that has been arranged by another health professional. Furthermore, the scope of the new genome sequencing technology means that there will inevitably be many variants discovered where it may be difficult to determine whether they are causal or not. It will be even more important that clinical geneticists are able to make an informed, expert evaluation of the likely relevance of the genomic findings to the clinical presentation.

The consultation

A consultation starts with a referral or a request for a ward visit. Use the information you have been given. Determine what questions are being asked by the referrer. Ask for the hospital notes and X-rays. A call to the paediatrician, or indeed the family, may help your pre-clinic work-up.

A child will usually attend with his parents, but ask, not assume this, during introductions to save embarrassment later. Parents can give you the child's history and family history and also you are able to observe, and later ask, if they have features in common with their child. Family photographs may be helpful.

Structure of the consultation

This is dependent on the circumstances, place, and age of the child. Even if you recognize the diagnosis at first sight, hold back. Build up a rapport with the family and check that the history and examination support your diagnosis. Below is a suggested approach.

(1) Introductions. Explain why you have been asked to see the child. Ask the parents about their main concerns and what they would like you to help with.

(2) Observation. Watch the child during the consultation. Try to involve him/her in the history and take note of spontaneous language and interaction between the child and adults, as well as looking at the face.

(3) History.

- Family history. Draw the family tree, usually extending over three generations, but extend further if there are known affected individuals in one branch of the family. Photographs of family members may be helpful.
- Pregnancy history. Conception, bleeding, fever, medication, investigations, alcohol/non-prescription drugs (ask with tact), fetal movements, liquor volume, gestation, mode of delivery.
- Neonatal history. Birthweight, length, head circumference. Resuscitation, feeding difficulties, ventilation, malformations, surgery, seizures, other medical problems?

- Developmental milestones and current schooling provision (e.g. mainstream school with 1:1 learning support assistant (LSA), special needs nursery). If developmentally delayed, ask about agencies involved, e.g. physical therapist.
- Photographs of the child at various ages may be helpful, especially if assessing an older child/adult.
- Behavioural phenotype.
- Vision, hearing, seizures.
- Other questions. Any other questions that may be of relevance.

(4) Physical examination, including clinical photographs (face, profile of face, hands, and any unusual features. A photograph of the child with his/her parents is helpful in assessing any familial contribution to facial dysmorphology) (see 'Dysmorphology examination checklist' in 'Appendix', p. 670).

(5) Further investigations.

(6) Conclusions. Assessment of genetic risk and counselling.

(7) Correspondence.

(8) Follow-up.

Normal variation

Without a thorough knowledge of normal pregnancy, delivery, developmental milestones, and usual infant/child behaviour, you may miss many important diagnostic clues in the history. It is of equal importance to the physical examination in establishing the diagnosis.

Examination

In the examination, the key to good practice is meticulous and accurate observation, measurement, and documentation of your findings (photography is extremely helpful in providing an accurate record of unusual features). Syndrome features alter with age and the geneticist tries to overcome this problem by noting serial measurements, e.g. of head circumference, and by asking the parents to bring photographs of the child at different ages. A natural history of the condition can then be seen. Trainees may find it helpful to use an examination checklist, such as the one on p. 670. The descriptive terms used may seem like a completely new language. The 'Glossary' on p. xvii describes these, but if in doubt, use everyday words or draw a simple sketch in the notes.

Diagnostic 'handles'

Some features are more likely to be of diagnostic help. These are sometimes called good 'handles' and these are not found as normal or familial traits or variations but are only present in a small number of conditions. A poor handle may occur as a normal variant or be found in a large number of syndromes. Diagnostic databases assist you most when a child has one or more of these distinctive features.

Making a diagnosis

It takes several years to develop the confidence to come to a diagnosis and several more to know when you won't! Many senior colleagues talk about 'gestalt' diagnoses. Such a diagnosis is made on the basis of recognition of previously having seen the condition. Many syndromes have characteristic facial features, e.g. Down's syndrome. The trainee should be assisted by a senior colleague for the diagnostic conclusions and counselling, having first presented the history and demonstrated the physical signs. Further investigations are often necessary to establish a diagnosis. You will find these listed in the chapters of the book that refer to specific features, e.g. 'Short limbs' in Chapter 6, 'Pregnancy and fertility', p. 784. Approximately 5% of children with a difficult-to-diagnose developmental disorder will have a composite phenotype caused by the co-occurrence of two distinct genetic disorders (Deciphering Developmental Disorders Study 2015).

Making an accurate diagnosis is central to the practice of clinical genetics. With a diagnosis, the genetic advice is usually accurate, the prognosis and natural history can be discussed, surveillance can be targeted appropriately, prenatal diagnosis (PND) may be possible, and the family can be given details of support groups and are empowered to access further information. Although it is satisfying to make a diagnosis, time spent ensuring that the diagnosis is correct and establishing a rapport with the parents and making an assessment of their state of readiness to receive a diagnosis will be valuable when you come to give this news to the family.

Expert adviser: Karen Temple, Professor of Medical Genetics and Honorary Consultant in Clinical Genetics, University of Southampton, University Hospital Southampton NHS Trust, Southampton, UK.

References

Aase JM. *Diagnostic dysmorphology.* New York, Plenum, 1990.

Allanson JF, Cunniff C, Hoyme HE, McGaughran J, Muenke M, Neri G. Elements of morphology: standard terminology for the head and face. *Am J Med Genet A* 2008; **149A**: 6–28.

Biesecker LG, Aase JM, Clericuzio C, Gurrieri F, Temple IK, Toriello H. Elements of morphology: standard terminology for the hands and feet. *Am J Med Genet A* 2009; **149A**: 93–127.

Carey JC, Cohen MM Jr, Curry CJ, Devriendt K, Holmes LB, Verloes A. Elements of morphology: standard terminology for the lips, mouth, and oral region. *Am J Med Genet A* 2009; **149A**: 77–92.

Deciphering Developmental Disorders Study. Large-scale discovery of novel genetic causes of developmental disorders. *Nature* 2015; **519**: 223–8.

Donnai D. Advances in dysmorphology: from diagnosis to treatment. *Clin Med* 2009; **9**: 154–5.

Donnai D, Read AP. How clinicians add to knowledge of development. *Lancet* 2003; **362**: 477–84.

Genetics Home Reference. *Beckwith–Wiedemann syndrome,* 2016. http://ghr.nlm.nih.gov/condition/beckwith-wiedemann-syndrome.

Hennekam RC, Biesecker LG. Next-generation sequencing demands next-generation phenotyping. *Hum Mutat* 2012; **33**: 884–6.

Hennekam RC, Biesecker LG, Allanson JE, et al.; Elements of Morphology Consortium. Elements of morphology: general terms for congenital anomalies. *Am J Med Genet A* 2013; **161A**: 2726–33.

Hennekam RC, Cormier-Daire V, Hall JG, Mehes K, Patton M, Stevenson RE. Elements of morphology: standard terminology for the nose and philtrum. *Am J Med Genet A* 2009; **149A**: 61–76.

Hennekam RCM, Krantz ID, Allanson JE. *Gorlin's syndromes of the head and neck,* 5th edn. Oxford University Press, New York, 2010.

Hunter A, Frias JL, Gillessen-Kaesbach G, Hughes H, Jones KL, Wilson L. Elements of morphology: standard terminology for the ear. *Am J Med Genet A* 2009; **149A**: 40–60.

Jones KL (ed.). *Smith's recognisable patterns of human malformation,* 6th edn. Elsevier Saunders, Philadelphia, 2006.

Joseph LN, Elkin C, Martin TG, Possinghami HP. Modeling abundance using N-mixture models: the importance of considering ecological mechanisms. *Ecol Appl* 2009; **19**: 631–42.

Reardon W. *The bedside dysmorphologist.* Oxford University Press, New York, 2007.

Robinson PN, Kohler S, Bauer S, Seelow D, Horn D, Mundlos S. The human phenotype ontology: a tool for annotating and analyzing human hereditary disease. *Am J Hum Genet* 2008; **83**: 610–15.

Shalev SA, Hall JG. Behavioural pattern profile: a tool for the description of behaviour to be used in the genetics clinic. *Am J Med Genet A* 2004; **128A**: 389–95.

Winter RM, Baraitser M. *London Dysmorphology Database.* London Medical Databases v1.0.17s, 2009. http://www.lmdatabases.com.

Autosomal dominant (AD) inheritance

AD disorders are encoded on the autosomes and the disorder manifests in heterozygotes, i.e. when a single copy of the mutant allele is present. AD disorders are characterized by inter- and intrafamilial variability. Factors influencing this variability may include haplotype (*cis* effects), modifier genes (*trans* effects), environmental exposure, and stochastic effects.

The major molecular mechanisms giving rise to AD inheritance are haploinsufficiency, gain of function, structural disruption, protein-toxic, and dominant negative (see Table 1.1). Some AD disorders, such as retinoblastoma and von Hippel–Lindau (VHL) disease, are recessive at the cellular level. The mutation confers increased susceptibility to tumours because of a heritable germline mutation in one allele, but cell behaviour appears normal in the heterozygous state. Tumorigenesis requires inactivation of the second allele ('second-hit').

Aspects of AD inheritance

Penetrance

The percentage of individuals expressing the disorder to any degree, from the most trivial to the most severe. Many dominant disorders show age-dependent penetrance, e.g. hereditary motor and sensory neuropathies (HMSN), hereditary spastic paraplegia (HSP), Huntington disease (HD). Features of the condition are not present at birth but become evident over time. Some conditions show incomplete penetrance, i.e. not all mutation carriers will manifest the disorder during a natural lifespan, e.g. Lynch syndrome (hereditary non-polyposis colorectal cancer (HNPCC)).

Expressivity

The variation in the severity of a disorder in individuals who have inherited the same disease alleles. Many AD conditions show quite striking variation in severity between families (interfamilial variation) and also within families carrying the same mutation (intrafamilial variation). A mildly affected parent can have a severely affected child, and vice versa. For example, in tuberous sclerosis (TSC), a parent with minimal cutaneous signs may have a child who develops infantile spasms and severe developmental delay.

Somatic mosaicism

A new mutation arising at an early stage in embryogenesis can give rise to a partial phenotype, often present in a dermatomal distribution, e.g. segmental neurofibromatosis type 1 (NF1). If the mutation is also present in the germline (germline mosaicism), it can be transmitted to future generations.

Germline mosaicism (gonadal mosaicism)

A new mutation arising during oogenesis or spermatogenesis may cause no phenotype in the parent, unless the somatic cells are involved as well, but can be transmitted to the offspring. If a population of germ cells harbours the mutation, there may be a significant recurrence risk, e.g. well documented in severe osteogenesis imperfecta (OI) due to type 1 collagen mutations. In general, recurrence risks for siblings after an apparently sporadic mutation depend on the particular gene and thus require knowledge of empiric data, which are often lacking; in this situation, a 1–2% figure is reasonable (Rahbari 2016).

Reproductive fitness

Many AD disorders, e.g. those causing severe brain malformation and/or intellectual disability (ID), have a reproductive fitness of zero, i.e. mutation carriers do not reproduce. Such a condition is maintained in the population entirely by new mutations and the majority of cases occur sporadically (although parental germline mosaicism may sometimes lead to recurrence in a sibling). Many other AD disorders have only modest effects on reproductive fitness.

New mutation rate

The de *novo* mutation (DNM) rate varies considerably between different AD conditions. It is high in NF1 with as many as 50% of cases representing new mutations; whereas for some other conditions, a new mutation is unusual.

Paternal age effect

For some AD disorders, the chance of a new mutation increases with advancing paternal age. In Apert syndrome, this observation is explained by germ cell selection for the pathogenic *FGFR2* mutation. Sibling recurrence risks are much lower than 1% in paternal age effect disorders because the mutations arise in adulthood rather than the embryonic stage (Goriely et al. 2003). See 'Paternal age' in Chapter 6, 'Pregnancy and fertility', p. 772.

Anticipation

The worsening of disease severity in successive generations. This is a feature of a few AD conditions and characteristically occurs in triplet repeat disorders where there is expansion of the triplet repeat in the maternal or paternal germline, e.g. myotonic dystrophy (DM; maternal), HD (paternal). In addition to variable expressivity, the mutation itself is unstably transmitted and varies in size between different generations (dynamic mutation).

Table 1.1 Major categories and mechanisms of genetic dominance, with the types of mutation commonly responsible. See text for further examples and references.

Category of mutation	Mechanism	Types of mutation	Examples
Loss of function			
Haploinsufficiency	Subunit imbalance	D, T, S, (M)	α and β globins
	Metabolic rate determining step	D, T, S, (M)	LDL receptor
	Developmental regulator	D, T, S, (M), (Tr)	PAX3, PAX6
Gain of function			
↑Gene dosage	Duplication	Dup	PMP-22
	Amplification	A	MDM2
↑/Ectopic mRNA expression	Altered temporal pattern	P, Tr,(D)	γ globin, MYC
	Altered tissue distribution	P, Tr	Ubx, Antp, MYC
	↑mRNA stability	D	lin-14

Table 1.1 Continued

Category of mutation	Mechanism	Types of mutation	Examples
↑/Constitutive protein activity	↑ Stability (PEST deletion)	T	CLN3, glp-1
	Constitutive activation	M	RAS, Gsz, SCN4A
Dominant negative	Disruption of dimer	M, (T)	KIT, p53
	Competition for substrate	M, (T)	RAS
Structural protein	Disruption of structure	M, S, (T)	Collagen, fibrillin
Toxic protein	Disruptive interaction	M	Rhodopsin, amyloidoses
New protein	Altered substrate specificity	M	α, antitrypsin
	Exon shuffling	Tr	BCR/ABL
Other mechanisms			
	Recessive antioncogene	–	Retinoblastoma
	Genomic imprinting	–	Beckwith-Wiedemann syndrome

D = large deletion, T = truncation (nonsense or frameshift mutation), M = missense mutation or small in frame deletion, S = splice site mutation, P = promoter mutation, Tr = translocation or other rearrangement, Dup = duplication, A = amplification, () = inconsistent association.
Reproduced from *Journal of Medical Genetics*, Wilkie, volume 31, page 92, 1994 with permission from BMJ Publishing Group Ltd.

Typical family tree

Some conditions show incomplete and age-dependent penetrance and these factors can make it difficult to give accurate genetic advice where the familial mutation is unknown (see Figure 1.1).

Genetic advice

- Males and females are affected equally.
- Males and females can both transmit the disorder.
- There is a 50% risk to offspring in any pregnancy that they will inherit the mutation. (NB. Depending on penetrance and expressivity, the risk of becoming symptomatic may be less than this.) See Figure 1.2.
- The severity of the disorder in the offspring may vary, being similar, more severe, or less severe than in the parent.

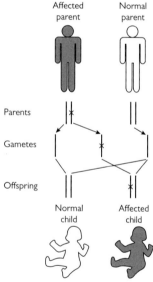

Figure 1.2 Diagram to show autosomal dominant inheritance.

- Examine parents very carefully before concluding that they are unaffected. For disorders with incomplete penetrance, apparently unaffected individuals will still be at some risk of transmitting the disorder (see Figure 1.1).

Expert adviser: Andrew Wilkie, Nuffield Professor of Pathology, Weatherall Institute of Molecular Medicine, University of Oxford, Oxford, UK.

References

Goriely A, McVean GA, Röjmyr M, Ingemarsson B, Wilkie AO. Evidence for selective advantage of pathogenic *FGFR2* mutations in the male germ line. *Science* 2003; **301**: 643–6.

Rahbari R, Wuster A et al. Timing, rates and spectra of human germline mutation. *Nat Genet* 2016; **48**: 126–33.

Strachan T, Read AP. *Human molecular genetics*, 4th edn. Garland Science, Philadelphia, 2010.

Young ID. *Introduction to risk calculation in genetic counselling*, 2nd edn. Oxford University Press, Oxford, 1999.

(a)

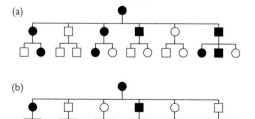

(b)

(c)

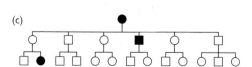

Figure 1.1 Family trees showing AD inheritance. (a) A typical family tree showing autosomal inheritance. An affected parent has a 50% risk of transmitting the condition to each child, whether they are male or female. (b) The same family tree showing AD inheritance with incomplete penetrance. In this example, the penetrance is reduced from 100% to 67%. (c) In this example, the family tree still shows AD inheritance, but with the penetrance reduced to 33%. The family tree then begins to look suggestive of a disorder following multifactorial inheritance (see 'Complex inheritance' in Chapter 1, 'Introduction', p. 14 for further discussion).

Autosomal recessive (AR) inheritance

See 'Carrier frequency and carrier testing for autosomal recessive disorders' in 'Appendix', p. 650.

AR disorders are encoded on the autosomes and the disorder manifests in homozygotes and compound heterozygotes, i.e. when both alleles at a given locus are mutated. Heterozygotes do not manifest a phenotype (e.g. cystic fibrosis (CF)), or if they do this is very mild in comparison with the disease state (e.g. sickle-cell trait versus sickle-cell disease). Affected siblings often follow a broadly similar clinical course which is more similar than for many AD disorders.

Aspects of AR inheritance

Consanguinity
AR disorders are associated with increased parental consanguinity, especially for rare AR disorders (see 'Consanguinity' in Chapter 3, 'Common consultations', p. 374).

Heterozygote advantage
For common recessive conditions, heterozygote advantage is usually much more important than recurrent mutation for maintaining the disease gene at high frequency, e.g. sickle-cell disease, where heterozygotes are less susceptible than normal individuals to malaria.

Founder effect
A high prevalence of a genetic disorder in an isolated or inbred population due to the fact that many members of the population are derived from a common ancestor who harboured a disease-causing mutation. The affected individuals in a given population are mostly homozygous for the same founder mutation. Examples include the recessive disorders Meckel syndrome, hydrolethalus syndrome, Cohen syndrome, and congenital Finnish nephropathy, which all occur with a disproportionately high incidence in Finland, compared with other European populations.

Carrier determination
For a relative of the proband, it is reasonably straightforward if the mutations in the proband are defined. Determining whether an unrelated partner is a carrier is usually more problematic. Unless the partner has a family history of the disorder, he/she will be at population risk for carrier status. Carrier testing usually involves DNA sequencing. Where certain specific mutations are common in a population, as in CF, these can readily be checked; otherwise it is necessary to examine the whole coding sequence. With advances in DNA sequencing, this is becoming increasingly feasible. In some cases, such as haemoglobinopathies, the gene product, rather than the gene itself, can be assayed, although for many inborn errors of metabolism, the levels of enzyme activity in heterozygotes and normals often overlap, making enzyme activity an unreliable test for carrier status. Tay–Sachs disease is a notable exception.

Deriving population risk for carrier status from disease frequency
See 'Carrier frequency and carrier testing for autosomal recessive disorders' in 'Appendix', p. 810— but note that, for conditions where most cases arise within consanguineous marriages, the simple Hardy–Weinberg calculation overestimates the population carrier risk.

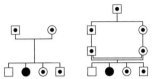

Figure 1.3 Family trees showing AR inheritance. If both parents are carriers, there is a 25% risk of an affected child in any pregnancy, independent of the sex of the child. The diagram on the right illustrates a consanguineous relationship between first cousins. A common ancestor is a carrier for a recessive mutation that may occur in homozygous form in a descendant as a consequence of consanguinity.

Family trees
See Figure 1.3.

Genetic advice
- Disease expressed only in homozygotes and compound heterozygotes.
- Parents are obligate carriers. Spinal muscular atrophy (SMA) is an exception to this rule as there is a significant new mutation rate of 1.7%. New array technology is also revealing deletion as a potential mechanism. If this occurs *de novo*, then the parent is not an obligate carrier, although there may be a small *gonadal mosaicism* risk.
- Risk to carrier parents for an affected child is 25% (1 in 4). See Figure 1.4.
- Healthy siblings of affected individuals have a two-third risk of carrier status.
- Risk of carrier status diminishes by one-half with every degree of relationship distanced from the parents of an affected individual, e.g. second-degree relatives (grandparents and aunts/uncles) and third-degree relatives (first cousins, great-grandparents, great-aunts, and great-uncles).

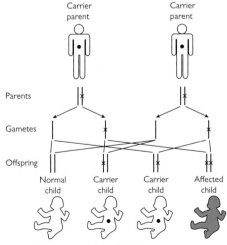

Figure 1.4 Diagram to show AR inheritance.

- All offspring of an affected individual whose partner is a non-carrier are unaffected but are obligate carriers.

Expert adviser: Andrew Read, Emeritus Professor of Human Genetics, University of Manchester, Manchester, UK.

References

Strachan T, Read AP. *Human molecular genetics*, 4th edn. Taylor & Francis, New York, 2010.

Young ID. *Introduction to risk calculation in genetic counselling*, 2nd edn. Oxford University Press, Oxford, 1999.

Communication skills

The genetics consultation

The success of any consultation depends on how well the patient and doctor communicate with each other. Time is limited, so it is important to ensure that it is used as effectively as possible. It may be helpful to think of the consultation as divided into three separate phases:

(1) establishing rapport and trust—building a relationship;

(2) collecting data;

(3) delivering information and agreeing a plan of action (management plan).

Key skills

(1) Setting an agenda for the consultation. Elicit the main issues at the outset of the consultation. Is the main issue finding a diagnosis, or determining whether an individual with a family history is themselves at risk of developing the condition, or reviewing the natural history if that is known? If the condition may have implications for future children, offer to discuss this. What do the family want to know?

(2) Determine the patients' perception. What is their interpretation of the child's problems, or family history?

(3) Explain the genetic basis of the condition if known or, if unknown, state whether you think it is likely to have a genetic basis or not. Check the family's understanding of the information you are giving as you go along. It is easier to change tack and alter the pitch of an explanation as you are going along.

(4) Assess the genetic risk to other family members. Discuss whether or not there is a significant risk to other family members not present at the consultation and, if an appreciable risk exists, agree a strategy for offering genetic advice and investigation.

(5) Use multiple communication tools. Good communication is an exchange *between* two people (not a monologue from one to the other). A patient needs to believe that you are really focussed on them and are clearly hearing their story. Listen, reflect, pause, rephrase, and focus on what the patient is saying, but also on their body language—are these congruent?

(6) Notice how your patient reacts. A consultation is pointless if the patient cannot see you properly, cannot hear you clearly, is translating what you are saying into a different language, or is crying too much to focus. Don't continue regardless; stop and change what you are doing.

Breaking bad news

Genetics health professionals are frequently called upon to give bad news to patients, whether it is a chorionic villus sampling (CVS) result indicating an affected fetus or an adverse result in a Huntington or *BRCA* predictive test, that the disorder just diagnosed has a progressive downhill course, or to tell parents that the disorder that has afflicted one of their children has a substantial recurrence risk.

When arranging prenatal or predictive tests, careful plans should be laid for the giving of results. Care should be taken to ensure the following.

- The individual is aware of the possibility of an adverse result and has thought through how they might handle this information and is prepared for this eventuality.
- The result is given by a member of staff well known to the individual, usually the person who has undertaken the pre-test counselling.
- The individual has a choice in how they receive the result and know when to expect the result, e.g. by telephone, in a clinic visit, or by letter.
- Ongoing support is offered following receipt of the test result.

Studies show that patients take in, and retain very little of, the information that is given after receiving a bad news result. Aim to keep the discussion simple and focussed on the patient's needs.

Communicating a diagnosis (after Unique—The Rare Chromosome Disorder Support Group)

Diagnosis and genetic counselling should be given:

- in private, in person, and with both partners present or with a supporter;
- with sensitivity, respect, compassion, understanding, and honesty;
- without being rushed and without jargon, using positive, sensitive language;
- with the contact details of relevant support groups;
- with the offer of a follow-up appointment to answer new questions and discuss new issues;
- with the offer of ongoing support to help the family cope and adjust.

Sometimes, it can be helpful to explain to the family that, although knowledge of the diagnosis is new, the genetic condition has in fact been present since conception and has always been a part of their child's life.

Arrange appropriate screening, if indicated. It may be necessary to explain and make referrals for multiple different screening strategies; it is important to not overload the patient with too much information but still present a clear plan of action. Standard leaflets and post-clinic letters are a useful way of ensuring practical information is delivered.

Expert adviser: Anna Middleton, Head of Social Science and Ethics and Registered Genetic Counsellor, Wellcome Genome Campus, Cambridge, UK.

References

Gask L, Usherwood T. ABC of psychological medicine: the consultation. *BMJ* 2002; **324**: 1567–9.

Maguire P, Pitceathly C. Key communication skills and how to acquire them. *BMJ* 2002; **325**: 697–700.

Unique—The Rare Chromosome Disorder Support Group. *Survey of 585 UK families*, 2003. http://www.rarechromo.org.

Wiggins J, Middleton A. *Getting the message across: communication with diverse populations in clinical genetics.* Oxford University Press, New York, 2013.

Complex inheritance

Many human characteristics show a tendency to run in families but do not show any of the simple Mendelian pedigree patterns. They depend on some combination of genetic susceptibility and environmental factors. The genetic susceptibility represents the cumulative effect of alleles at several or many different loci, each of which individually may have only a very small effect. From a clinical perspective, there is a continuous spectrum of disease from, at the one end, disorders that are strictly genetic and caused by fully penetrant mutations with minimal contribution from the environment to, at the other extreme, those caused predominantly by environmental factors (e.g. teratogens) with minimal contribution from genetic factors (see Figure 1.5). Between these two extremes lie the incompletely penetrant and the multifactorial disorders (Bomprezzi et al. 2003).

Complex characters come in two types. Traits such as height, weight, blood pressure (BP), and behavioural traits are *continuous characters*. We all have them, but to differing degrees. Their distribution in the general population approximates to a normal (Gaussian) distribution. Many genes are involved in determining these characteristics, together with environmental factors. For example, factors influencing height include parental height, nutrition, and chronic illness. Common birth defects, such as cleft lip/palate, congenital dislocation of the hip (CDH), congenital heart disease (CHD), and neural tube defect (NTD), are *discontinuous* or *dichotomous characters*. Some people have them, while most do not. Many such conditions tend to cluster in families, more than would be expected by chance (see Figure 1.6). The same is true for schizophrenia, ischaemic heart disease, and type 1 diabetes (T1D). The ratio λ (lambda) of the incidence of such a condition in the relatives of an affected person compared with its rate in the general population is a measure of relative risk and hence of disease heritability.

Polygenic threshold theory

A useful way of thinking about the genetics of discontinuous multifactorial characters is to postulate an underlying *genetic susceptibility* that is continuous (everybody has some degree of susceptibility) and normally distributed in the population. People whose susceptibility is above some threshold value manifest the condition. This formulation, from the geneticist DS Falconer, makes sense of much of the observed epidemiology of these conditions. Close relatives of an affected individual share genes with the affected person and therefore their distribution of liability is shifted towards higher liability. A greater proportion of them will exceed the critical threshold value and be affected (see Figure 1.7), hence the tendency to run in families. For first-degree relatives, the expected incidence approximates to the square root of the population incidence. Thus, for a condition affecting 1/1000 individuals (0.1%), the risk to sibs, parents, and children would be ~1/30 (3%), falling to 1/100 (1%) for second-degree relatives, and close to population risk for third-degree relatives. This is fairly close to the figures observed for NTDs and cleft palate.

Falconer's model makes sense of other features of the epidemiology. A couple with two affected children probably have more high susceptibility genes than a couple with only a single affected case, and so the risk of recurrence is higher. For most multifactorial disorders, the incidence differs between the sexes. This is accommodated by postulating different thresholds for the two sexes. Then, for a disorder with a male preponderance, the threshold for females is higher, and affected females will, on average, have a higher susceptibility than affected males. Accordingly, the risk to relatives (of either sex) of an affected female is greater than the risk to relatives of an affected male.

However, multifactorial conditions are unlikely to be homogeneous in terms of aetiology. Different causes will predominate in different affected individuals, and susceptibility is not necessarily the sum of large numbers of individually small effects, as in Falconer's model. A clinical label like 'schizophrenia' probably encompasses a heterogeneous collection of conditions with different causes including, in different individuals, major genes, chromosome structural abnormalities, and the accumulation of minor effects. Such conditions are described as complex. Counselling for multifactorial or complex conditions is therefore based on empirical (survey-based) risks, not on figures derived from any mathematical model. Refer to the individual topics in this resource for tables of data on specific conditions (e.g. cleft lip/palate). Several general principles affect the risk:

- relationship to the affected individual. The risk is greatest among close relatives and decreases rapidly with increasing distance of relationship (see above);
- severity of the disorder in the proband. The risks to relatives are greater if the proband is severely affected than if the proband is only mildly affected. The average liability in the siblings of affected individuals will be greater (further right-shifted) in such families (see Figure 1.7);

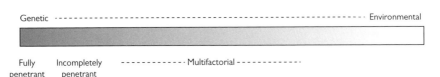

Figure 1.5 The spectrum of genetic causation.
Adapted by permission from BMJ Publishing Group Ltd., *Journal of Medical Genetics*, Bomprezzi R, Kovanen PE, Martin R., New approaches to investigating heterogeneity in complex traits, volume 40, issue 8, pp. 553–9, Copyright © BMJ Publishing Group Ltd 2003.

Multifactorial inheritance

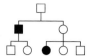

Figure 1.6 Family tree showing complex inheritance.

- the number of affected individuals in the family. If there are two or more close relatives affected, then the risks for other relatives are increased. If there are several affected close relatives, the possibility of an AD disorder with incomplete penetrance should be carefully considered.
- for disorders with an unequal sex ratio, e.g. Hirschsprung's disease, the sex of the proband will also affect the risk (see p. 453).

Identifying the susceptibility factors

A major thrust of twenty-first-century medical genetics research has been to try to identify individual susceptibility factors for complex diseases. The hope is

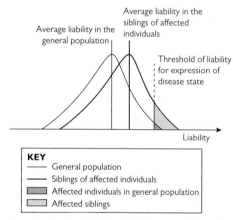

Figure showing the distribution of liability to a multifactorial trait/disease.

Figure 1.7 Falconer's model explains how multifactorial conditions tend to run in families.
Adapted with permission from D. S. Falconer et al., The inheritance of liability to certain diseases, estimated from the incidence among relatives, *Annals of Human Genetics*, Volume 29, Issue 1, pp.51–76, Copyright © 1965 John Wiley and Sons/University College London.

that this could lead to better prediction of risk and maybe suggest targets for new drugs. Primarily this has been through *genome-wide association studies* (GWAS)—case-control studies testing a large panel of common DNA polymorphisms spread across the genome for association with the disease. For diseases such as type 2 diabetes (T2D) and Crohn's disease, dozens of such factors have been identified—see http://www.genome.gov/gwastudies for summaries. However, virtually all the factors identified through GWAS confer only a very modest risk of the condition—typical relative risks are 1.05–1.3. Even in combination, all the known factors for a disease almost never allow clinically useful predictions of risk. Much of the heritability estimated from family studies remains unaccounted for. The cause and nature of this *missing heritability* are much debated (Manolio et al. 2009). Some characters, such as height, are probably truly polygenic, governed by very large numbers of individually very weak factors. In others, much of the susceptibility may be due to rare, but relatively strong, factors that cannot be detected by GWAS but might be found by sequencing. This is particularly the case for psychiatric conditions, including autism, schizophrenia, and ID, where a small percentage of cases are largely explained by individual mutations or chromosomal microdeletions/microduplications (Coe et al. 2012). For still others, strong interactions between factors, not readily detectable in case-control studies, may explain much of the missing heritability. Whatever the cause, the conclusion is that, for most complex conditions and most individuals, we are still a long way away from being able to identify specific causes or make clinically useful predictions of risk by genotyping susceptibility factors.

Expert adviser: Andrew Read, Emeritus Professor of Human Genetics, University of Manchester, Manchester, UK.

References

Bomprezzi R, Kovanen PE, Martin R. New approaches to investigating heterogeneity in complex traits. *J Med Genet* 2003; **40**: 553–9.

Coe BP, Girirajan S, Eichler EE. The genetic variability and commonality of neurodevelopmental disease. *Am J Med Genet C Semin Med Genet* 2012; **160C**: 118–29.

Manolio TA, Collins FS, Cox NJ, et al. Finding the missing heritability of complex diseases. *Nature* 2009; **461**: 747–53.

Strachan T, Read AP. *Human molecular genetics*, 4th edn. Garland Science, Philadelphia, 2010 (see Chapters 15 and 16).

Young ID. *Introduction to risk calculation in genetic counselling*, 2nd edn. Oxford, Oxford University Press, 1999.

Confidentiality

Confidentiality is a major issue for all doctors. Medical geneticists must particularly be on their guard against the potential for breaching confidentiality when their advice is sought by different members of the same family.

The general duty to maintain the confidential nature of personal genetic information is, however, not an absolute one. The Human Genetics Commission notes circumstances where it may be appropriate to disclose personal information. Wherever possible, this will be with the consent of the patient and will be in the interest of the patient, of relatives, or of the wider public.

Disclosure

The Human Genetics Commission recognizes that, exceptionally, 'disclosure of sensitive personal genetic information without consent may be justified in rare cases where a patient refuses to consent to such disclosure but the benefit to other family members or the wider public substantially outweighs the need to respect confidentiality'.

If you decide to disclose confidential information, you must be prepared to explain and justify your decision. In practice, such cases are usually discussed within a professional forum, such as a departmental meeting or with a group of consultant colleagues, so that the subjective decision about the balance of interests is shared and agreed.

However, a patient might refuse to consent to the disclosure of information that would benefit others, for example where family relationships have broken down, or if their natural children have been adopted. In these circumstances, disclosure might still be justified in the public interest (see paragraphs 36 to 56). If a patient refuses consent to disclosure, you will need to balance your duty to make the care of your patient your first concern against your duty to help protect the other person from serious harm. If practicable, you should not disclose the patient's identity in contacting and advising others of the risks they face (Point 69 GMC Confidentiality Guidance 2017).

Children

In 1985, Gillick challenged the right of a doctor to prescribe contraception to a girl under the age of 16 years without obtaining the consent of the girl's parents. This became an important case in English law and Lord Scarman gave the following ruling in the House of Lords, 'As a matter of law the parental right to determine whether or not their minor child below the age of 16 will have medical treatment terminates if and when the child achieves sufficient understanding and intelligence to enable him to understand fully what is proposed.' It is a doctor's responsibility to judge whether a child aged under 16 years is 'Gillick-competent', i.e. has sufficient maturity and understanding to make judgements about the particular aspect of their own medical care under considerations. This is not a global assessment of capacity, but an assessment in relation to a particular decision.

In the non-Gillick-competent child, authority must be given by whoever has parental responsibility under the provisions of the Children's Act 1989. In deciding whether to disclose information, the practitioner's overriding consideration must always be what is in the *best interests of the child.*

A child's biological parents both have parental responsibility if they were married at the time of the child's birth. In such circumstances, a practitioner will normally disclose all information concerning a young child to either parent without the other's consent. When such parents are separated or divorced, information may still be disclosed to either parent irrespective of who has custody, unless a court has removed parental responsibility from one or the other parent.

With parents who were unmarried at the time of the child's birth, only the mother automatically has legal parental responsibility. Her consent is therefore required before information may be disclosed to the father, unless he has been given parental responsibility either by agreement with the mother or by a court order. In England and Wales, an unmarried father can obtain parental responsibility for his child in one of three ways:

- jointly registering the birth of the child with the mother;
- obtaining a parental responsibility agreement with the mother;
- obtaining a parental responsibility order from a court.

Deceased patients

Seek consent from the next of kin. The Human Genetics Commission recognizes that 'There may be some clinical situations where genetic information about the dead is needed *in order to assess the risk to a living relative.* This information may be obtained by testing samples removed from an individual during life. The approach we favour is that a presumption should be made that the dead person would have consented in his or her lifetime to such testing and that this justifies post-mortem testing.'

Refusal of consent

While privacy and the right to refuse consent are an important proposition, it is not an absolute principle and it can be overridden if the harm to others outweighs the importance to the individual concerned, e.g. if the refusal of consent is capricious or vindictive.

Useful websites: General Medical Council (GMC), http://www.gmc-uk.org/guidance/ethical_guidance/confidentiality.asp; Joint Committee on Consent and Confidentiality in Medical Genetics, http://www.bsgm.org.uk/media/678746/consent_and_confidentiality_2011.pdf.

Expert adviser: Michael Parker, Professor of Bioethics and Director, Ethox Centre, Nuffield Department of Population Health, University of Oxford, Oxford, UK.

References

General Medical Council (GMC). *Confidentiality: good practice in handling patient information.* January 2017 www.gmc-uk.org/guidance

Gillick v. West Norfolk and Wisbech Area Health Authority [1985] 3 All ER 402 (HL).

Human Genetics Commission. *Inside information—balancing interests in the use of personal genetic data.* Human Genetics Commission, London, 2002.

Lucassen AM, Parker M, Wheeler R. Role of next of kin in accessing health records. *BMJ* 2004, **328**: 952–3.

Confirmation of diagnosis

See also 'Confirmation of diagnosis of cancer' in Chapter 4, 'Cancer', p. 562.

In order to provide precise genetic advice, it is essential to have an accurate diagnosis. If the diagnosis in your patient has been made by others, and the patient and his/her family are referred to you for genetic advice, you will need to seek confirmation of the diagnosis. If you are asked to give advice to a relative, without the opportunity to see and assess the proband, you will need to confirm the diagnosis in the proband before giving definitive genetic advice. The diagnosis is of such fundamental importance that there may be medico-legal implications if it turns out that the given diagnosis was wrong and appropriate steps were not taken to substantiate it. Some diagnoses such as 'cystic fibrosis' tend to be fairly reliable, whereas others such as 'achondroplasia' are notoriously unreliable. Depending on the circumstances, various options are available.

- Clinical assessment. Some genetic disorders have specific clinical features that enable a rapid confirmation of diagnosis. Take a history of the main features/symptoms and briefly examine the patient to confirm that you agree with the clinical diagnosis, e.g. NF1, TSC, etc., before giving genetic advice. Where possible, follow this up by seeking results of various key investigations that were instrumental in making the diagnosis, e.g. cranial magnetic resonance imaging (MRI) result, mutation result.
- Laboratory findings. Many genetic diagnoses depend on specific laboratory results. These may be the results of molecular genetic testing, e.g. HD, fragile X (FRAXA) syndrome, DM, or the results of biochemical investigations, e.g. Zellweger syndrome, phenylketonuria (PKU), etc., or histological assessment. Ensure that you have sight of the critical result(s) (or a copy of the result(s)) and that these are from a reliable source (e.g. an accredited laboratory) before giving definitive advice.
- Radiological investigations. Some genetic disorders, e.g. skeletal dysplasias, depend on radiological studies for diagnosis. Ensure that you see either the images or the radiologist's report confirming the radiological findings before giving definitive genetic advice.
- Death certificate. For deceased relatives, the death certificate may lend some support to diagnosis. This is generally less reliable than laboratory results but is helpful if, for example, hospital notes have been destroyed and it is otherwise difficult to obtain any confirmation of diagnosis.
- Family photographs. These are often helpful when determining familial involvement with a syndrome that has dysmorphic features and when other avenues fail.

Seeking confirmation of diagnosis in relatives

When advice is sought about a family history (and the proband is not seen in clinic), it is usual practice to obtain consent from the proband (their parents/guardians) to approach their doctor/genetics department for confirmation of the diagnosis. Many departments have a standard form for obtaining consent from relatives in these circumstances. Taking the family history and talking about affected family members may be a sensitive area—ensure that there is adequate time for this as it is often crucial to the provision of accurate genetic advice. Sometimes the genetic disorder is not openly discussed in the family, and not all families are on good speaking terms, so it often takes a lot of sensitivity to get accurate information and even so it can be difficult on occasion to establish the diagnosis truly accurately. Under such circumstances, you need to explain to the family the limits of the information that you have and document in the medical notes that you have done the best job possible under the circumstances. See also 'Confidentiality' in Chapter 1, 'Introduction', p. 16.

References

Douglas FS, O'Dair LC, Robinson M, Evans DG, Lynch SA. The accuracy of diagnoses as reported in families with cancer: a retrospective study. J Med Genet 1999; **36**: 309–12.

Consent for genetic testing

Consent is the agreement, free from coercion, to an action based on knowledge of what the action involves and its likely consequences.

Genetic information about a person (e.g. whether they are affected with a genetic disorder) should be considered confidential medical information and should generally not be obtained, held, or communicated without that person's consent.

The nature and extent of information provision that is required in seeking consent for a genetic test depends on the test in question. Those tests which are likely to reveal sensitive genetic information—information that has special significance for the patient or for the patient's relatives—will require greater attention to the consent process than, for example, tests that confirm information that is already known from clinical details.

Genetic testing of one person may reveal information about others, e.g. relatives who may have inherited the same condition, or unexpected information, e.g. about misattributed parentage. These wider implications of testing should therefore be considered and discussed before a genetic test is done.

Points to consider when obtaining consent for genetic testing

See also 'Testing for genetic status' in Chapter 1, 'Introduction', p. 38.

- What is the purpose of the test? Which test or tests are to be carried out?
- What are the nature and treatment of the condition and the way in which it is inherited (if appropriate)?
- What potential benefits might there be from having the test?
- What might be the potential disadvantages?
- Are there any alternatives to having the test that would achieve the same benefits? Does the test have to be done now or can it be delayed?
- What, if any, are the implications for the person's:
  - future health;
  - reproductive choices;
  - relatives;
  - family relationships (e.g. information about parentage);
  - present or future employment;
  - insurance prospects? (refer to the statement about the insurance moratorium, presumably elsewhere).
- How will the result be communicated to the patient and how long will it take from sampling to result?
- What are the arrangements for ensuring the confidentiality of the test result, e.g. arrangements for storing of the test result in the patient's individual medical record? What are the arrangements for sharing the test with the result with relatives to whom it might be relevant?
- Is any accompanying written information, particularly where this substitutes for face-to-face consultation, written in clear, simple, understandable language, objective, and without bias?
- Is there an awareness of the patient's level of understanding/cultural beliefs/language?
- Would the person like further information or access to other sources of advice (e.g. the opportunity to talk to other persons who have faced the same choice)?
- What provision is there for post-test support?

Consent to genomic testing

Because whole genome analysis is likely to provide much more information than targeted testing, there are several nuances to consent for whole genome analysis that require consideration:

(1) Consent may need to be broad because, unless the analysis is targeted, it will not be possible to predict all the possible outcomes;

(2) Consent will need to incorporate the possibility of uncertain result(s) and acknowledge that uncertainty may change as more evidence is acquired;

(3) That additional findings that are incidental to the clinical reason for doing the test may be acquired;

(4) That consent cannot be 'fully informed' and cannot do all the work in a decision about testing. Other elements, such as trust in the health service providing the test will also be necessary (see Nuffield Council on Bioethics report on biodata and Human Genetic Commission inside genetic information). Asking someone to decide what they would or would not want to know about beforehand may not constitute real consent.

Does consent need to be in writing?

General Medical Council (GMC) guidance (2008) states that it is good practice to document consent discussions in the patient's clinical notes. The GMC also states that 'you should get written consent from the patient if the investigation or treatment is complex or involves significant risks … '. The Joint Committee on Medical Genetics report (2011) gives examples of written consent forms that can sometimes be useful in genetic testing.

Competence to provide consent

Competence to make decisions depends on three broad capacities:

- the capacity for understanding and communication;
- the capacity for reasoning and deliberation;
- the capacity to develop and sustain a set of moral values.

In practice, 'capacity' means the ability to use and understand information to make a decision. This involves:

- being able to understand information about the test or procedure;
- remembering that information;
- using the information as part of the decision-making process;
- communicating the decision by talking, using sign language, or by any other means;
- being free from coercion about the decision by others.

Adults

Adults are presumed to have capacity to make decisions about their medical treatment, unless there is evidence to suggest otherwise.

The Mental Capacity Act (2005) is designed to protect people who cannot make decisions for themselves or lack the mental capacity to do so and to allow adults to make as many decisions as they can for themselves.

The Act also highlights that capacity is decision-specific and that some adults who lack capacity for complex decisions can still have the capacity to make other decisions.

If an adult lacks capacity to make a particular decision, then one must be made for them and it must be made in that person's *best interests* (the Mental Capacity Act sets out a checklist of issues to consider in a best interest assessment). Involvement of family and friends and any legally appointed representatives (e.g. a Lasting Power of Attorney) can inform health professionals what the patient would have wanted if they still had capacity.

Determining what is in a person's best interests in relation to consent for genetic testing

Where appropriate, seek advice from someone with experience and familiarity with local practices which, in some jurisdictions, may have a legal basis, e.g. a specialist nurse for vulnerable adults.

The decision-maker should:

(1) encourage the person to participate and support their ability to take part in making the decision;

(2) identify all relevant circumstances such as those of which the person is aware and those it would be reasonable to regard as relevant;

(3) find out the person's views as determined by their past and present wishes and feelings and past behaviour;

(4) avoid discrimination;

(5) assess whether they might regain capacity;

(6) consult others such as family carers, other close relatives, and any attorney appointed under a Lasting Power of Attorney;

(7) weigh up all of the above factors in order to determine their best interests.

Young people

The Family Law Reform Act 1969 states that children aged 16 and over are presumed to have capacity to consent to medical treatment. There is therefore no legal requirement to obtain consent from a parent or guardian.

As for adults over 18, if in fact there is evidence that the young person does not have capacity, then a best interest decision should be made.

Children

For young children and babies, parents can give or withhold consent on behalf of the child. (A parent who can give consent is one who holds parental responsibility.) Children under 16 years are presumed not to have capacity but can be found to have capacity for particular decisions on assessment. This is known as Gillick competence (see 'Confidentiality' in Chapter 1, 'Introduction', p. 16 for further discussion).

In practice, as children grow older and if they express an interest, competence, and desire to be involved in decision-making, they should participate in such decisions. Usually genetic tests that will have no impact on health care before adult life are deferred until the individual reaches an age when he/she is legally competent to make his/her own decisions regarding health care (British Society for Human Genetics 2010).

Children in care

When a child is the subject of a care order, the local authority acquires 'parental responsibility' under the Children Act 1989. The order does not, however, deprive parents of their parental responsibility and they are not deprived of their ability to authorize or refuse treatment.

Useful websites: General Medical Council (GMC), http://www.gmc-uk.org; Joint Committee on Consent and Confidentiality in Medical Genetics, http://www. bsgm.org.uk/media/678746/consent_and_confidentiality_2011.pdf.

Expert adviser: Anneke Lucassen, Consultant in Clinical Genetics, Faculty of Medicine, Wessex Clinical Genetic Service, University of Southampton, Southampton, UK.

References

British Society for Human Genetics. *Report on the genetic testing of children 2010*, 2010. http://www.bsgm.org.uk/media/678741/gtoc_booklet_final_new.pdf.

Department of Health. *Code of Practice Mental Health Act 1983*, 2008. http://www.mentalhealthlaw.co.uk/media/MHA_Code_of_Practice_2008.pdf.

General Medical Council. *Consent: patients and doctors making decisions together*, 2008. http://www.gmc-uk.org/guidance/ethical_guidance/consent_guidance_index.asp.

Royal College of Physicians, Royal College of Pathologists, British Society for Human Genetics. *Consent and confidentiality in clinical genetic practice: guidance on genetic testing and sharing genetic information*, 2nd edn. Report of the Joint Committee on Medical Genetics. Royal College of Physicians, Royal College of Pathologists, London, 2011. http://www.bsgm.org.uk/media/678746/consent_and_confidentiality_2011.pdf.

Genetic basis of cancer

Cancer is a common condition that affects ~1 in three of the population during their lifetime. All cancers arise as a result of changes that have occurred in the DNA sequence of the genomes of cancer cells (Stratton et al. 2009) (see Figure 1.8). The great majority of cancers are sporadic occurrences related to the gradual accumulation of somatic mutations with age and exposure to carcinogenic factors in the environment such as cigarette smoke, ultraviolet (UV) radiation, X-rays, etc. Genetic variation in (1) cellular repair mechanisms which affect the efficacy with which mutations in DNA are recognized and repaired together with (2) genetic variation affecting the likelihood of such cells surviving or undergoing apoptosis (programmed cell death) and (3) genetic variation in the metabolism of carcinogens will all affect an individual's likelihood of developing cancer.

Somatic mutations in human cancers show unevenness in genomic distribution that correlate with aspects of genome structure and function. These mutations are, however, generated by multiple mutational processes operating through the cellular lineage between the fertilized egg and the cancer cell, each composed of specific DNA damage and repair components and leaving its own characteristic mutational signature on the genome (Morganella et al. 2016).

Heritability of cancer

In 2016, Mucci et al. published a study of Nordic twins designed to estimate the familial risk and heritability of cancer types in a large cohort. For most cancer types, there were significant familial risks and the cumulative risks were higher in MZ than DZ twins. Heritability of cancer overall was 33% [95% confidence interval (CI) 30–37%].

Significant heritability was observed for skin melanoma (58%; 95% CI 43–73%), prostate (57%; 95% CI 51–63%), non-melanoma skin (43%; 95% CI 26–59%), ovary (39%; 95% CI 23–55%), kidney (38%; 95% CI

21–55%), breast (31%; 95% CI 11–51%), and corpus uteri (27%; 95% CI 11–43%) (Mucci et al. 2016).

Inherited cancer predisposition syndromes

A small, but important, minority of cancer cases arises in individuals predisposed to develop cancer by the inheritance of a mutation in a cancer susceptibility gene. Such cases are exemplified by:

- young age of onset;
- multiple affected members on the same side of the family;
- recognizable patterns of cancer occurring together in the same family, e.g. colorectal cancer (CRC) and endometrial cancer in Lynch syndrome or breast and ovarian cancer in BRCA1/BRCA2;
- multiple primaries in a single individual;
- rare and unusual tumour types, e.g. small bowel carcinoma in Lynch syndrome.

The majority of familial cancer susceptibility syndromes follow an AD pattern of inheritance. In a few instances, mutation in a single allele is sufficient to cause neoplasia, e.g. point mutation in RET in multiple endocrine neoplasia type 1 (MEN1) causes parathyroid hyperplasia through a dominant negative mechanism. However, in the great majority of tumours in inherited cancer predisposition syndromes, transformation to cancer usually requires a biallelic mutation at the cellular level. There are many different mechanisms by which the subsequent hits can be acquired (see Figure 1.9). These include:

(1) terminal deletion;

(2) mitotic recombination;

(3) loss of reduplication;

(4) loss of second allele, e.g. mitotic error resulting in monosomy;

(5) point mutation;

(6) interstitial deletion;

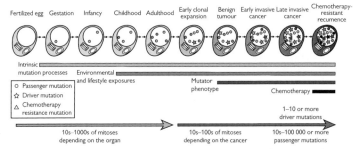

Figure 1.8 The lineage of mitotic cell divisions from the fertilized egg to a single cell within a cancer, showing the timing of the somatic mutations acquired by the cancer cell and the processes that contribute to them. Mutations may be acquired while the cell lineage is phenotypically normal, reflecting both the intrinsic mutations acquired during normal cell division and the effects of exogenous mutagens. During the development of the cancer, other processes, e.g. DNA repair defects, may contribute to the mutational burden. Passenger mutations do not have any effect on the cancer cell, but driver mutations will cause a clonal expansion. Relapse after chemotherapy can be associated with resistance mutations that often predate the initiation of treatment.

Reprinted by permission from Macmillan Publishers Ltd: Nature, Michael R. Stratton, Peter J. Campbell, and P. Andrew Futreal, The cancer genome, volume 458, issue 7239, pp. 719–24, copyright 2009.

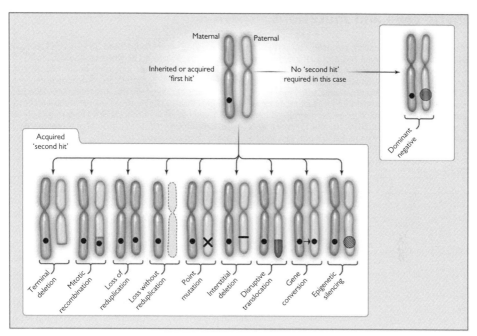

Figure 1.9 Mechanisms of loss of heterozygosity and inactivation of wild-type tumour suppressor genes.
From *New England Journal of Medicine*, Foulkes W, Inherited Susceptibility to Common Cancers, 359, pp. 2143–2153, Copyright © 2008 Massachusetts Medical Society. Reprinted with permission from Massachusetts Medical Society.

(7) translocation disrupting gene function;

(8) gene conversion;

(9) epigenetic silencing, e.g. methylation.

Predictive testing and effective surveillance are available for many of these conditions. Effective care relies on accurate diagnosis that, in turn, relies upon the clinical acumen of clinicians recognizing when their patient is a member of a family affected by a familial cancer syndrome and referring to clinical genetics for risk assessment and discussion of genetic testing and advice on surveillance and risk-reducing options (where applicable).

Obtaining a DNA sample from an affected member of such a family, along with appropriate consent for genetic testing, is crucial in order to define the genetic basis of the disease (e.g. *BRCA1* or *BRCA2*) and identify the causative mutation, thus enabling predictive testing for other members of the family.

If an affected member of a family likely to have a familial cancer syndrome is terminally ill, contact the local genetics service promptly to discuss obtaining a blood sample with consent for DNA storage and, where appropriate, genetic testing.

Expert adviser: Marc Tischkowitz, Reader and Honorary Consultant Physician in Medical Genetics, Department of Medical Genetics, University of Cambridge and East Anglian Medical Genetics Service, Cambridge, UK.

References

Foulkes W. Mechanisms of loss of heterozygosity and inactivation of wild-type tumour-suppressor genes. *N Engl J Med* 2008; **359**: 2143–53.

Morganella S, Alexandrov LB, Glodzik D, *et al.* The topography of mutational processes in breast cancer genomes. *Nat Commun* 2016; **7**: 11383.

Mucci LA, Hjelmborg JB, Harris JR, *et al.*; Nordic Twin Study of Cancer (NorTwinCan) Collaboration. Familial Risk and Heritability of Cancer Among Twins in Nordic Countries. *JAMA* 2016; **315**: 68–76.

Stratton MR, Campbell PJ, Futreal PA. The cancer genome. *Nature* 2009; **458**: 719–24.

Genetic code and mutations

DNA (deoxyribonucleic acid) contains four types of bases—two purines adenine (A) and guanine (G), and two pyrimidines cytosine (C) and thymine (T). RNA (ribonucleic acid) contains uracil (U) in place of thymine. The DNA double helix (Watson and Crick 1953) maintains a constant width and is faithfully replicated, because purines always face pyrimidines in the complementary A–T and G–C base pairs. Thus, it can: (1) serve as a template for replication that re-establishes the double helix and (2) open to be 'read' (transcribed to make an RNA copy, which can be a messenger RNA (mRNA) or an RNA with another function). In an mRNA, successive triplets of nucleotides carry the code for successive amino acids in a protein. Because there are more codons (61 plus three STOP codons) than there are amino acids (20), almost all amino acids are represented by more than one codon, i.e. the code is degenerate, particularly at the third base (see Table 1.2).

Table 1.2 Triplet codons and their corresponding amino acids and STOP sequences

	T	C	A	G
T	TTT = Phe	TCT = Ser	TAT = Tyr	TGT = Cys
	TTC = Phe	TCC = Ser	TAC = Tyr	TGC = Cys
	TTA = Leu	TCA = Ser	TAA = STOP	TGA = STOP
	TTG = Leu	TCG = Ser	TAG = STOP	TGG = Trp
C	CTT = Leu	CCT = Pro	CAT = His	CGT = Arg
	CTC = Leu	CCC = Pro	CAC = His	CGC = Arg
	CTA = Leu	CCA = Pro	CAA = Gln	CGA = Arg
	CTG = Leu	CCG = Pro	CAG = Gln	CGG = Arg
A	ATT = Ile	ACT = Thr	AAT = Asn	AGT = Ser
	ATC = Ile	ACC = Thr	AAC = Asn	AGC = Ser
	ATA = Ile	ACA = Thr	AAA = Lys	AGA = Arg
	ATG = Met	ACG = Thr	AAG = Lys	AGG = Arg
G	GTT = Val	GCT = Ala	GAT = Asp	GGT = Gly
	GTC = Val	GCC = Ala	GAC = Asp	GGC = Gly
	GTA = Val	GCA = Ala	GAA = Glu	GGA = Gly
	GTG = Val	GCG = Ala	GAG = Glu	GGG = Gly

Amino acid	Characteristic
Alanine (Ala, A)	Neutral
Arginine (Arg, R)	Basic
Asparagine (Asn, N)	Polar
Aspartic acid (Asp, D)	Acidic
Cysteine (Cys, C)	Polar, forms disulfide cross-links
Glutamine (Gln, Q)	Polar
Glutamic acid (Glu, E)	Acidic
Glycine (Gly, G)	Small, neutral
Histidine (His, H)	Basic (weak)
Isoleucine (Ile, I)	Hydrophobic
Leucine (Leu, L)	Hydrophobic
Lysine (Lys, K)	Basic
Methionine (Met, M)	Hydrophobic
Phenylalanine (Phe, F)	Hydrophobic, bulky
Proline (Pro, P)	Hydrophobic, helix breaker
Serine (Ser, S)	Polar
Threonine (Thr, T)	Polar
Tryptophan (Trp, W)	Hydrophobic, bulky
Tyrosine (Tyr, Y)	Polar, bulky
Valine (Val, V)	Hydrophobic
Nonsense (X)	(Stop)

Nomenclature of mutations

Descriptions of mutations are prefaced with p., c., or g., depending on whether they describe a change in protein, complementary DNA (cDNA), or genomic DNA sequence, respectively. For full nomenclature rules, including more complex sequence variants, see http://varnomen.hgvs.org/.

Nucleotide substitutions are described by a number representing the nucleotide in the DNA sequence (usually cDNA, rather than genomic), a letter representing the original nucleotide (A, C, G, T) followed by > and the new nucleotide, e.g. in the beta-globin gene (*HBB*) c.17A>T means that adenine at nucleotide 17 of the cDNA is replaced by thymine, while in the haemochromatosis gene (*HFE*) c.845G>A means that guanine at nucleotide 845 is changed to adenine. The number in a cDNA is the position of the nucleotide from the 5′ end, counting the A of the AUG initiating codon as 1. Numbering of a genomic sequence should cite the reference sequence being used.

If this results in an amino acid substitution, the mutation is termed a missense mutation. In protein annotation, the number of the changed amino acid is written between the one-letter codes for the old and new amino acids, e.g. in sickle-cell disease p.E6V (glutamic acid at amino acid 6 is replaced by valine); in *HFE*, p.C282Y (cysteine at amino acid 282 is changed to tyrosine) and p.H63D (histidine at amino acid 63 is changed to aspartic acid). A change that introduces a stop codon is shown with X or *, e.g. pG542X or p.G542*. If the nucleotide substitution does not alter the genetic code, it is termed a silent or synonymous substitution, but note this could still cause problems by affecting splicing, etc.

Most splice-site mutations occur in introns. In a cDNA, mutations in introns are referred to by the nearest nucleotide in an exon, e.g. in *CFTR* c.621+1G>T, the first nucleotide (G) in the intron which starts immediately after nucleotide 621 in the cDNA is replaced by T. In c.1717−1G>A, the last nucleotide (G) in the intron immediately preceding nucleotide 1717 in the cDNA is replaced by A.

Nucleotide deletions and insertions are described by the nucleotide number followed by del/ins and the letter for the relevant nucleotide, e.g. c.394delT. c.3905−3906insT means a T is inserted after nucleotide 3905 in the cDNA. Insertions/deletions involving single nucleotides or pairs of nucleotides cause a shift in the reading frame (*frameshift mutation*) which usually results in a complete lack of any protein product.

In protein annotation, an amino acid is specified followed by del or ins, e.g. the common CF mutation p.F508del where phenylalanine 508 is missing because of a three-nucleotide deletion in the DNA. A non-standard terminology using the term delta, or a small triangle, is still often used to denote a deletion, e.g. in CFTR, the p.F508del mutation is often described as ΔF508.

Types of mutation and assessment of their significance

Assessing the clinical significance of a DNA sequence change can be extremely difficult. Some mutations, e.g. p.F508del in CF, are well known and clearly pathogenic, and their interpretation is straightforward. In many cases, however, this is not so. A number of different computer programs are widely used to aid interpretation, but they are not infallible. Even with nonsense, frameshift, or splicing mutations that can be confidently predicted to abolish activity of a transcript, some caution is necessary before assuming they are necessarily pathogenic—are all transcript isoforms affected (see 'Truncating mutations' below) and would absence of that gene product matter? Thus, you are strongly advised to discuss the situation with a clinical molecular geneticist before using any novel result in clinical practice, especially in predictive or prenatal testing.

Missense mutations

A mutation that results in an altered amino acid in the encoded protein is termed a missense mutation. Many missense mutations are not pathogenic, as the nature of the amino acid change and its precise location in the three-dimensional protein structure will determine whether there is any effect on protein function. The following factors increase the likelihood that a missense mutation is pathogenic:

- it is a *de novo* change in the gene of interest (i.e. not present in either parent), or it segregates with the disease in the family;
- it changes an amino acid that is conserved in related genes in humans and other species into one that is not evolutionarily conserved;
- it causes a significant alteration in the predicted protein conformation, e.g. a hydrophobic amino acid is substituted for a polar one, or it occurs at a key site in the protein (e.g. a binding site);
- it has been reported previously on several occasions: see ClinVar database (www.ncbi.nlm.nih.gov/clinvar) and DECIPHER (see p. 44);
- it is not present at significant levels in the general population. Some 'missense mutations' are in reality polymorphisms. It is necessary to look at control data in the unaffected population (see ExAc and gnomAD databases on p. 44) to evaluate the significance.

Truncating mutations

These include single nucleotide substitutions that create STOP codons (nonsense mutations), frameshift mutations in which the reading frame is lost, and also large deletions/insertions. Despite the name, they do not usually result in production of a truncated protein—cells have a mechanism (nonsense-mediated RNA decay) for recognizing and degrading mRNA molecules containing premature termination codons. Truncating mutations will almost always completely inactivate any mRNA containing the mutation—but if a gene produces multiple alternatively spliced transcripts, as most genes do, only isoforms that include the exon in question will be affected. Thus, although truncating mutations in known disease genes are highly likely to be pathogenic, some degree of caution is still advised.

Splice-site mutations

Splicing is the process by which the introns are removed from the primary transcript and the exons are joined together (see Figure 1.10). A large multi-molecular machine, the spliceosome, recognizes the splice donor site at the start of an intron (the dinucleotide GT embedded in a consensus sequence) and the splice acceptor (AG in a consensus sequence) at the end. Splice sites are not all-or-nothing; they differ

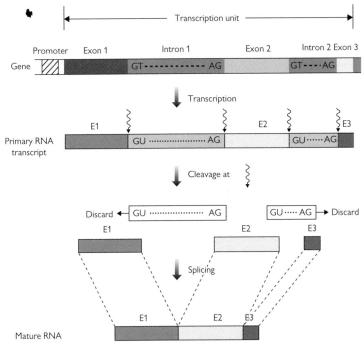

Figure 1.10 The process of RNA splicing.
Copyright 2011 from Human Molecular Genetics, 4th Ed. by Strachan et al. Reproduced by permission of Garland Science/
Taylor & Francis LLC.

in strength, so that a strong site is used in preference to a nearby weak site. The strength is modified by enhancers and suppressors of splicing—short DNA sequences nearby in the exon or intron. Most genes encode multiple splice isoforms that include or omit exons, often in a tissue-specific manner.

Splicing can be affected by mutations in different ways. Changes to the donor or acceptor sites (including changes to enhancers or suppressors of splicing) can weaken or abolish them. This may result in an exon being skipped, intronic material included, or a nearby alternative site being used, and it will often introduce a frameshift into the mRNA. Alternatively, a sequence in an exon or intron that is not normally used as a splice site may be changed, so that it is used in preference to the normal site (activation of a cryptic splice site). Again, the likely effect is to abolish gene function. Splicing effects, apart from changes to the standard GT … AG dinucleotides, are hard to predict without RNA studies.

Dynamic mutations (triplet repeat mutations)
Some genes contain runs of repeated nucleotides, e.g. CAGCAGCAGCAGCAG … In some cases, these repeats are meiotically unstable and tend to expand (or occasionally contract) on being passed from parent to child. For some genes, the repeat becomes pathogenic when it passes a certain threshold length. Triplet repeat diseases are highly heterogeneous in terms of

the nucleotide sequence, the location of the repeats (exon, intron, promoter, etc.), and the pathogenic mechanism.

Mechanisms by which mutations exert their effect on phenotype

Loss-of-function (LOF) mutation ('inactivating' mutation)
So-called truncating mutations almost always render the transcript non-functional, while many missense mutations cause LOF of the protein by disturbing the conformation or charge of a site critical in the interaction of the protein with other molecules. Most mutations in recessively inherited disease are LOF.

Gain-of-function mutation ('activating' mutation)
Specific missense mutations can cause a protein to function at the wrong time, in the wrong place or to ignore the normal controls on its activity. For example, in achondroplasia, two common mutations in the *FGFR3* gene c.1138G>A and c.1138G>C, both encoding p.G380R, account for 98% of mutations in affected individuals. The FGFR3 protein normally suppresses bone growth in response to bound fibroblast growth factor (FGF). The mutant protein is partially constitutively activated (i.e. activated even in the absence of its ligand), resulting in increased inhibition of growth of cartilage cells. Gain-of-function mutations usually cause dominant phenotypes.

Dominant negative mutation
Here a mutation in one copy of a gene results in a mutant protein that not only has lost its own function, but also prevents the heterozygously produced wild-type protein of the same gene from functioning normally. Usually an altered polypeptide (subunit) is produced that prevents or impairs the assembly of a multimeric protein, e.g. assembly of collagen triple helices in OI.

Haploinsufficiency
Arises when the normal phenotype requires the protein product of two alleles, and a reduction of 50% of the gene product as a result of LOF mutations results in an abnormal phenotype.

Expert adviser: Andrew Read, Emeritus Professor of Human Genetics, University of Manchester, Manchester, UK.

References

Dalgleish R, Flicek P, Cunningham F, *et al*. Locus reference genomic sequences: an improved basis for describing human DNA variants. *Genome Med* 2010; **2**: 24.

La Spada AR, Taylor JP. Repeat expansion disease: progress and puzzles in disease pathogenesis. *Nat Rev Genet* 2010; **11**: 247–58.

Strachan T, Read AP. Human genetic variability and its consequences. In: T Strachan, AP Read (eds.). *Human molecular genetics*, 4th edn. Garland Science, Philadelphia, 2010.

Wain HM, Bruford EA, Lovering RC, Lush MJ, Wright MW, Povey S. Guidelines for human gene nomenclature. *Genomics* 2002; **79**: 464–70. Also available at http://www.genenames.org.

Watson JD, Crick FHC. Molecular structure of nucleic acids: a structure for deoxyribose nucleic acid. *Nature* 1953; **171**: 737–8.

Genomes and genomic variation

Genomic variation is the major factor underlying the enormous diversity of the human race and, with the exception of MZ twins, the genetic uniqueness of every individual. Clinical geneticists diagnose and manage problems caused by mutations in the human genome. Their task is to identify the pathogenic genomic variant(s) and explain the implications of this to patients and their families. A working knowledge of the human genome, including an appreciation of the scale of genomic variation seen in healthy individuals, is therefore essential to the practice of genomic medicine.

Genome
A genome is the sum total of the haploid genetic material of an organism. The human genome includes both nuclear DNA and mitochondrial DNA and contains ~20 000 protein-encoding genes.

Genomic architecture
The structure, content, and organization of a genome, including the location and order of genes.

A question of scale
- 46 chromosomes—22 pairs of autosomes and two sex chromosomes (XY in males and XX in females).
- 3 000 000 000 base pairs (bp) of DNA, i.e. 3 gigabases (Gb) or 3 000 megabases (Mb) per haploid genome.
- 100 000 000 bp on the average chromosome, i.e. 100 Mb, with a 5-fold variation in size from the largest chromosome at 250 Mb to the smallest at 50 Mb.
- Only ~1–2% of the human genome is coding sequence (the 'exome'); the total length of coding and splicing regions is estimated to be ~35 Mb.
- Approximately 20 000 genes encoding proteins in the human genome (the 'exome').

The dimensions of DNA are measured in nanometres (thousands of millionths of a metre). To put this into perspective, each human cell has ~2 m of DNA, i.e. the equivalent of ~6 000 000 000 bp of DNA.

In genetic disease, pathology may involve anything from whole chromosome aneuploidy to a single base pair substitution or deletion, and the whole spectrum between these two extremes (see Table 1.3).

Table 1.3 Scales of genomic imbalance in the human genome

Type of imbalance	Approximate scale
Aneuploidy (e.g. trisomy 21)	Whole chromosome
Microscopically visible chromosomal imbalance (e.g. del 2q37)	Chromosome band (usually >5–10 Mb)
Submicroscopic imbalance (copy number variants, CNVs) detectable by genomic array analysis or fluorescence in situ hybridization (FISH)	Megabases of DNA (usually <5 Mb)
Whole gene deletion/duplication	Kilobases (kb) of DNA
Exon deletion/duplication	Often <1 kb
Base deletions or duplications	From one to several base pairs

Genomic variants in an individual human genome
Most people have around 4.1–5 million variants (sites where an individual's sequence differs from the reference genome) (1000 Genomes Project Consortium 2015), of which ~20 000 are in the exome, including around 400 rare variants that potentially impair the function of the encoded protein. Although 99.9% of variants consist of single nucleotide polymorphisms (SNPs) and short indels, structural variants affect more bases—the typical genome contains an estimated 2100–2500 structural variants (1000 large deletions, 160 copy number variants (CNVs), 915 Alu insertions, 128 L1 insertions, 51 SVA insertions, 4 NUMTs, and ten inversions), affecting 20 million bases of sequence (1000 Genomes Project Consortium 2015).

Variants in a human genome
- Approximately 3 400 000 SNVs (single nucleotide variants) ~1 every 1000 bases.
- Approximately 350 000 insertion/deletions (1000 Genomes Project Consortium 2012).
- Approximately 1000 larger scale deletions/duplications (CNVs).
- Approximately 100 genuine 'LOF' variants with ~20 genes completely inactivated (MacArthur et al. 2012).
- Approximately 50–100 variants that have previously been described as being disease-causing, although many are false assertions.
- Approximately 50 de novo mutations (DNMs) of which, on average, ~1.3 are located in the exome.

Rates of new mutation
Rate of SNV mutation
Recent publications (Campbell et al. 2012; Kong et al. 2012) have estimated a new mutation rate of ~1.2 × 10^{-8} substitutions per base per generation in the human genome. The paternal germline is ~4-fold more mutagenic than the maternal germline for base substitutions. Furthermore, Kong et al. delineate an approximately linear increase of ~2 mutations per year in the numbers of new base substitutions with advancing paternal, but not maternal, age. See also 'Paternal age' in Chapter 6, 'Pregnancy and fertility', p. 772.

Rate of CNV mutation
Using a 42 million-probe genomic array to characterize population variation of CNVs, it has been estimated at least one in 17 children will have a de novo CNV, in many cases with no obvious clinical consequences (Conrad et al. 2010).

Expert adviser: Matthew Hurles, Head of Human Genetics, Wellcome Trust Sanger Institute, Wellcome Trust Genome Campus, Hinxton, UK.

References
1000 Genomes Project Consortium. An integrated map of genetic variation from 1,092 human genomes. *Nature* 2012; **491**: 56–65.
1000 Genomes Project Consortium. A global reference for human genetic variation. *Nature* 2015; **526**: 68–74.

Campbell CD, Chong JX, Maliq M, *et al.* Estimating the human mutation rate using autozygosity in a founder population. *Nat Genet* 2012; **44**: 1277–81.

Conrad DF, Pinto D, Redon R, *et al.* Origins and functional impact of copy number variation in the human genome. *Nature* 2010; **464**: 704–12.

Kong A, Frigge ML, Masson G, *et al.* Rate of *de novo* mutations and the importance of father's age to disease risk. *Nature* 2012; **488**: 471–5.

MacArthur DG, Balasubramanian S, Frankish A, *et al.* A systematic survey of loss-of-function variants in human protein-coding genes. *Science* 2012; **335**: 823–8.

Xue Y, Chen Y, Ayub Q, *et al.* Deleterious- and disease-allele prevalence in healthy individuals: insights from current predictions, mutation databases, and population-scale resequencing. *Am J Hum Genet* 2012; **91**: 1022–32.

Genomic imprinting

Genomic imprinting is a genetic mechanism by which genes are *selectively silenced* from the *maternal or paternal homologue* of a chromosome, with the result that, for imprinted genes, there is expression of only one allele, depending on parental origin (Peters 2014). Imprinting invokes a variety of mechanisms, most notably methylation laid down on the DNA during the development of the male or female germ cells. This epigenetic 'mark' or imprint subsequently affects the chromatin structures that determine transcriptionally silent and active states of nearby genes in the embryo. The imprint is maintained throughout the life of the organism, in essentially all tissues; however germ cells erase and then reset imprints for transmission to offspring.

The majority of imprints are ubiquitous and permanent in humans; but transient imprinting or tissue-specific (e.g. placental) imprinting may also contribute to human development and disease (Prickett and Oakey 2012; Monk 2015). About 30 ICs (see below) are currently recognized, controlling parent of origin-specific expression of neighbouring genes: some ICs control single genes, some hundreds. These imprinted genes have diverse roles in growth, development, metabolism and behaviour, as well as in tumour suppression.

Imprinting disorders (IDs)

IDs result from changes in the expression of imprinted genes—either through genetic changes in the genes themselves, or epigenetic changes in their control. IDs are characterized by disordered growth which starts in fetal life, either overgrowth or restricted growth. This affects the life course of the individual and may be associated with poor feeding, altered timing of puberty and risk of the metabolic syndrome in adulthood. Some disorders are associated with intellectual disability. Structural congenital anomalies are relatively infrequent and the diagnosis may be missed if imprinting is not considered as a possible mechanism underlying a developmental disorder.

IDs can be caused by:
(a) mutation of the expressed genes;
(b) deletion or duplication of imprinted genes;
(c) uniparental disomy (UPD: see p. 31); or
(d) epigenetic errors at ICs causing mis-expression of imprinted genes, with or without an underlying genetic cause.

For example, Angelman syndrome is caused by loss of expression of UBE3A, normally expressed only from its maternal allele on chromosome 15. Mutation or deletion of maternal UBE3A leads to Angelman syndrome. Epigenetic errors or UPD15pat do not alter the gene sequence of UBE3A; but lead to loss of its expression.

In general, purely epigenetic errors are reset in subsequent generations and thus are not inherited; likewise, UPD is a reproductive error with a recurrence risk back to population levels. Coding mutations and copy number changes can be inherited, but may or may not result in an ID, depending on the sex of the parent transmitting them.

Eight IDs are well established (see Table 1.4), associated with altered expression of imprinted genes. However, new clinical entities and new genetic/epigenetic mutations continue to emerge (Eggermann 2015). For further information on imprinting disorders, see http://www.imprinting-disorders.eu/ Imprinting errors may be mosaic leading to body asymmetry and variable phenotypes.

Imprinting centre (IC)

An IC is a region of DNA that is epigenetically modified in development and controls the imprinted expression of neighbouring genes. The DNA methylation of ICs is reset during the development of germ cells. Gain or loss of genetic material, or of DNA methylation, can cause disordered expression of neighbouring genes.

Multi-locus imprinting disturbance (MLID)

MLID is present in a majority of patients with clinically defined imprinting disorders. Mutations of NLRP2 and

Table 1.4 Known human imprinted genes with disease associations (when normal imprinting mechanisms are disrupted)

Chromosome location		Gene	Maternally/paternally expressed gene	Disease association
6	6q24.2	ZAC/PLAGL1	Paternally expressed	Transient neonatal diabetes
7	7p21	GRB10	Maternally expressed	Russell–Silver syndrome
	7q21.3	SGCE	Paternally expressed	Myoclonic dystonia
	7q32.2	PEG1/MEST	Paternally expressed	Russell–Silver syndrome
11	11p15.5	H19	Maternally expressed	Russell–Silver syndrome and Beckwith–Wiedemann syndrome
	11p15.5	IGF2	Paternally expressed	
	11p15.5	p57kip2/CDkN1C	Maternally expressed	Beckwith–Wiedemann syndrome
14	14q32	DLK1	Paternally expressed	Pat UPD14 phenotypes (Wang Kagami syndrome) and Mat UPD 14 phenotypes (Temple syndrome)
	14q32	RTL1	Paternally expressed	
	14q32	GTL2/MEG3	Maternally expressed	
15	15q11-q13	SNRPN	Paternally expressed	Prader–Willi syndrome
	15q11-q13	UBE3A	Maternally expressed	Angelman syndrome
20	20q13.32	GNAS-AS	Maternally expressed	Pseudohypoparathyroidism type 1 B (PHP1B)

ZFP57 have been identified in rare causes of MLID, but in the majority the cause is unknown (Docherty 2015).

Uniparental disomy (UPD)

Describes the karyotype of a euploid cell or organism in which one of the chromosome pairs has been inherited exclusively from one parent. If two identical homologues are inherited, this is called *isodisomy*; if non-identical homologues are inherited, the term *heterodisomy* is used. This often results from non-disjunction during meiosis in one parent producing gametes with one or fewer chromosome than normal. Zygotes formed by such gametes are aneuploid and rescue of aneuploidy by loss or duplication of a chromosome from the other parent will cause UPD. If UPD occurs in an imprinted region, this may cause disease. For example, Angelman syndrome is due to mutations/deletions in the maternally expressed gene *UBE3A* or paternal UPD 15 where there is no functional *UBE3A* allele as the maternal allele is missing. Angelman syndrome can also be due to epigenetic modifications of the IC on chromosome 15q11 which results in loss of expression of *UBE3A*. These types of mechanisms explain most imprinting disorders reported to date.

Expert advisers: Karen Temple, Professor of Medical Genetics and Honorary Consultant in Clinical Genetics, University of Southampton, University Hospital Southampton NHS Trust, Southampton, UK and Deborah Mackay, Professor of Medical Epigenetics, Southampton University, Southampton, UK.

References

Demars J, Gicquel C. Epigenetic and genetic disturbance of the imprinted 11p15 region in Beckwith–Wiedemann and Silver–Russell syndromes. *Clin Genet* 2012; **81**: 350–61.

Docherty LE, Rezwan FI, et al. Mutations in NLRP5 are associated with reproductive wastage and multilocus imprinting disorders in humans. *Nat Commun* 2015; **6**: 8086.

Eggermann T, Perez de Nanclares G, Maher ER et al. Imprinting disorders: a group of congenital disorders with overlapping patterns of molecular changes affecting imprinted loci. *Clin Epigenetics* 2015; **7**: 123.

Eggermann T. Silver–Russell and Beckwith–Wiedemann syndromes: opposite (epi)mutations in 11p15 result in opposite clinical pictures. *Horm Res* 2009; **71**(Suppl 2): 30–5. geneimprint. http://www.geneimprint.com.

Krueger F, Kreck B, Franke A, Andrews SR. DNA methylome analysis using short bisulfite sequencing data. *Nat Methods* 2012; **9**: 145–51.

Mackay DJ, Callaway JL, Marks SM, et al. Hypomethylation of multiple imprinted loci in individuals with transient neonatal diabetes is associated with mutations in ZFP57. *Nat Genet* 2008; **40**: 949–51.

Monk D. Genomic imprinting in the human placenta. *Am J Obstet Gynecol* 2015; **213**(4 Suppl): S152–62.

Morison IM, Paton CJ, Cleverley SD. *The imprinted gene and parent-of-origin effect database*, 2001. http://igc.otago.ac.nz/home.html.

Murphy SK, Huang Z, Hoyo C. Differentially methylated regions of imprinted genes in prenatal, perinatal and postnatal human tissues. *PLoS One* 2012; **7**: e40924.

Peters J. The role of genomic imprinting in biology and disease: an expanding view. *Nature Rev Genet* 2014; **15**: 517–30.

Prickett AR, Oakey RJ. A survey of tissue-specific genomic imprinting in mammals. *Mol Genet Genomics* 2012; **287**: 621–30.

Genomic sequencing and interpretation of data from WES or WGS analyses

' ... whole-genome sequence data sets are in some ways more prone to misinterpretation than earlier analyses because of the sheer wealth of candidate causal mutations in any human genome, many of which may provide a compelling story about how the variant may influence the trait; a problem that has been referred to as the "narrative potential" of human genomes.'

(Reprinted by permission from Macmillan Publishers Ltd: Nature Publishing Group, MacArthur DG, Manolio TA et al. Guidelines for investigating causality of sequence variants in human disease. 508;7497:469–76 Copyright 2014.)

For many decades, Sanger sequencing was the mainstay of diagnosis for monogenic disorders. This approach required the clinician to select one (or a few) of ~20 000 genes to sequence. Where conditions have a very distinctive presentation, e.g. NF1, this is feasible and having selected the gene and sequenced it, there is a high chance of finding the causative mutation. However, many disorders are genetically heterogeneous, e.g. >50 genes can cause epilepsy, >70 genes can cause sensorineural deafness, and many hundreds (possibly thousands) of genes may cause ID. Choosing which gene to test in these disorders is problematic as each individual gene has a low probability of containing the causal variant(s). In these circumstances, testing genes sequentially one at a time becomes tedious, and there is a significant chance of finding a variant that is not causal but seems plausible among the small fraction of genes tested that could cause the phenotype.

By sequencing millions of fragments of DNA in parallel, 'next-generation' sequencing enables a much higher throughput approach to sequencing, making panel testing (a set of genes causing a particular phenotype/disease), whole exome analysis (all coding genes; whole exome sequencing (WES)), and whole genome analysis (whole genome sequencing (WGS)) feasible. This greatly improves the chance of making a genetic diagnosis but also hugely increases the number of variants observed. The opportunity of falsely assigning causality to a given variant (see above) is therefore much higher, as the prior chance of any given gene containing the causal variant is much lower when a large number of genes are sampled than when a single gene was selected for analysis based on the patient's phenotype.

Evaluation of sequence variants

Since every human genome contains 4–5 million variants, including rare functional variants with no known phenotypic consequences, interpretation of sequence variants can be challenging. A few well-known variants, e.g. c.1138G>A in FGFR3 in achondroplasia, are unequivocally pathogenic and can be interpreted in isolation, but the status of many variants is less certain and a holistic approach to evaluating a variant is appropriate, such as that outlined in Figure 1.11. This evaluation process is often undertaken as a multidisciplinary exercise involving scientists and clinical geneticists.

An analysis of 406 published severe disease mutations observed in 104 newly sequenced individuals reported that 122 (27%) of these were either common polymorphisms or lacked direct evidence for pathogenicity (Bell et al. 2011). Subsequently, guidelines for implicating sequence variants in human disease have been published, emphasizing the need for caution in assigning causality (see Box 1.1).

Expert adviser: Caroline Wright, Senior Lecturer in Genomic Medicine, University of Exeter, UK.

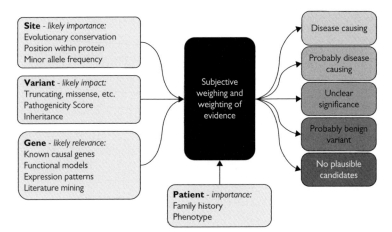

Figure 1.11 Factors to consider in evaluating a sequence variant as a cause of disease.

Box 1.1 Guidelines for implicating sequence variants in human disease

---

General guidelines
- Provide complete positive and negative evidence associated with the gene or variant implication, not just the results that are consistent with pathogenicity.
- In all cases in which it is possible, place genetic, informatic, and experimental results within a quantitative framework; determine the probability of observing this result by chance with a randomly selected variant or gene.
- Take advantage of public data sets of genomic variation, functional genomic data, and model organism phenotypes.
- Do not regard prior reports of gene or variant implication as definitive; to the degree that supporting data are available, reassess them as rigorously as your own data.
- Describe and assess clearly the available evidence supporting prior reports of gene or variant implication.

Assessment of evidence for candidate disease genes
- In presumed monogenic disease cases, evaluate genes previously implicated in similar phenotypes before exploring potential new genes.
- Report a new gene as confidently implicated only when variants in the same gene and similar clinical presentations have been confidently implicated in multiple unrelated individuals.
- In all cases in which it is possible, apply statistical methods to compare the distribution of variants in patients with large matched control cohorts or well-calibrated null models.

Assessment of evidence for candidate pathogenic variants
- Determine and report the formal statistical evidence for segregation or association of each variant, and its frequency in large control populations matched as closely as possible to patients in terms of ancestry.
- Recognize that strong evidence that a variant is deleterious (in an evolutionary sense) and/or damaging (to gene function) is not sufficient to implicate a variant as playing a causal role in disease.
- Predict variant deleteriousness with comparative genomic approaches, but avoid considering any single method as definitive or multiple methods as independent lines of evidence for implication.
- Validate experimentally the predicted damaging impact of candidate variants using assays of patient-derived tissue or well-established cell or animal models of gene function.
- Avoid assuming that implicated variants are fully penetrant, or completely explanatory in any specific disease case.

Publications and reporting
- Assess and report objectively the overall strength and cohesiveness of the evidence supporting pathogenicity for all variants listed in a publication.
- In all cases in which it is possible, ensure that the level of confidence of pathogenicity and supporting evidence are propagated in variant databases.
- Deposit genotype and phenotype data for both controls and disease patients, and for resultant analyses demonstrating associations, in publicly accessible databases, to the maximum degree permissible under study-specific participant consent and ethical approval.
- If returning results for clinical use, highlight strong, actionable findings, but also ensure that uncertain or ambiguous are clearly conveyed as such, along with appropriate supporting evidence.
- Provide clear cautions regarding decision-making based on variants with limited evidence when the potential for use in medical interventions is high.

Reprinted by permission from Macmillan Publishers Ltd: Nature Publishing Group, MacArthur DG, Manolio TA *et al.* Guidelines for investigating causality of sequence variants in human disease. 508;7497:469–76 Copyright 2014.

References

Bell CJ, Dinwiddie DL, Miller NA, *et al.* Carrier testing for severe childhood recessive diseases by next-generation sequencing. *Sci Transl Med* 2011; **3**: 65ra4.

MacArthur DG, Balasubramanian S, Frankish A, *et al.* A systematic survey of loss-of-function variants in human protein-coding genes. *Science* 2012; **335**: 823–8.

MacArthur DG, Manolio TA, Dimmock DP, *et al.* Guidelines for investigating causality of sequence variants in human disease. *Nature* 2014; **508**: 469–76.

Wright CF, Middleton A, Burton H, *et al.* Policy challenges of clinical genome sequencing. *BMJ* 2013; **347**: f6845.

Xue Y, Chen Y, Ayub Q, *et al.* Deleterious- and disease-allele prevalence in healthy individuals: insights from current predictions, mutation databases, and population-scale resequencing. *Am J Hum Genet* 2012; **91**: 1022–32.

Mitochondrial inheritance

Mitochondrial DNA (mtDNA) has unique genetic features that distinguish it from nuclear DNA, which follows a Mendelian pattern of inheritance. The mtDNA genome of humans is a double-stranded circular DNA, 16.6 kb in length and encoding 13 proteins (all subunits of respiratory chain complexes), two ribosomal RNAs, and 22 transfer RNAs. There are no introns and, except for the D loop region that is involved in the initiation of DNA replication and transcription, most of the mitochondrial genome is coding sequence. Mitochondria typically contain several copies of mtDNA and a typical human somatic cell can contain up to 1000 mitochondria (i.e. 5000–10 000 copies of mtDNA), representing >1% of the cell's total DNA. Mature oocytes contain a staggering ~100 000 copies of mtDNA, whereas sperm contain ~100.

The organs most often affected in mitochondrial disorders are highly energy-demanding tissues such as the central nervous system (CNS), skeletal and cardiac muscle, pancreatic islets, liver, and kidney (McFarland et al. 2010).

Aspects of mitochondrial inheritance

Maternal inheritance

mtDNA is exclusively maternally inherited, with very rare exceptions (Schwartz and Vissing 2002). Paternal mitochondria enter the egg on fertilization where they constitute a miniscule fraction (0.1%) of the total mitochondria. The paternal mitochondria and their mtDNA are rapidly eliminated early in embryogenesis. For the purposes of genetic counselling, the risk of paternal inheritance is essentially zero.

Homoplasmy

Is the existence of only one mtDNA type in the same cell, tissue, or individual, e.g. mitochondria containing only mtDNA carrying the m.1555A>G mutation associated with sensorineural deafness.

Heteroplasmy

Is the existence of more than one mtDNA type in the same cell, tissue, or individual, e.g. mitochondria containing a mixture of mtDNA carrying the m.3243A>G point mutation and mtDNA with the wild-type sequence. In mitochondrial disorders, because of the thousands of mitochondria in each cell, there are often variable percentages of mutant and wild-type mtDNAs between different cells and especially between different tissues. The different mtDNAs can vary between 0% and 100%.

Threshold effect

For some mtDNA mutations, there is a relatively narrow threshold below which mitochondrial function is normal, but above which mitochondrial function is greatly impaired. For some mtDNA mutations, e.g. the m.8993T>C/G mutation seen in neuropathy–ataxia–retinitis pigmentosa (NARP) syndrome and some patients with Leigh syndrome, the severity of clinical symptoms increases sharply above a relatively high threshold mutant load.

Mitochondrial bottleneck

The high variation in heteroplasmy levels of pathogenic mtDNA mutations present in oocytes (Brown et al. 2001), and therefore transmitted to offspring, can be explained by the presence of a genetic bottleneck. The bottleneck hypothesis states that the number of mtDNAs during oogenesis is either relatively small (Cree et al. 2008) or that only few mtDNAs are used as templates for amplification (Wai et al. 2008). Studies in mice suggest that the location of this genetic bottleneck is within the developing female germline (Freyer et al. 2012).

Tissue variation

In heteroplasmic disorders, the distribution of mutant load in tissues is often not uniform. In some tissues, the level of mutant mtDNA changes successively with time, for instance falling in blood and accumulating in non-dividing cells such as muscle.

Selection

Preferential accumulation of mutant mtDNA in affected tissues is a factor in their progressive nature (Poulton et al. 2003). However, in some cell lines, e.g. blood, cells with high mutant loads appear to be selected against and the mutant load may fall over time. In some instances, e.g. m.3243A>G, this appears to be at a predictable rate of ~1% per annum.

Mutation rate

Human mtDNA has a mutation rate 10–20 times that of nuclear DNA, probably due to replication repair systems that are less stringent than those in the nucleus. This has been exploited in a study of the migration of human populations (Sykes 2001).

Typical family tree

Figure 1.12 shows a typical family tree showing mitochondrial inheritance. Offspring of females in the maternal line are at risk; males do not transmit the condition.

Genetic advice

• Inheritance is matrilineal, i.e. the condition can only be transmitted by females in the maternal line.
• Males do not transmit mitochondrially inherited disorders, with extremely rare exceptions (Schwartz and Vissing 2002).
• Typically a mitochondrially inherited condition can affect both sexes.
• Point mutations are commonly maternally inherited, while deletions and duplications are most often sporadic, but see advice for specific mitochondrial

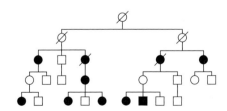

Figure 1.12 Family tree showing mitochondrial inheritance.

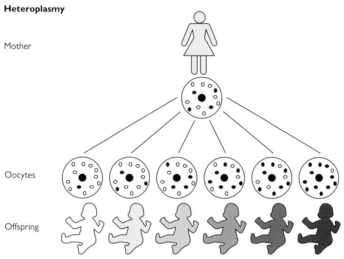

Figure 1.13 Schematic of homoplasmy and heteroplasmy in mitochondrial inheritance. NB. Correlation between phenotypic severity and level of mutant mtDNA (above threshold) is poor in many mitochondrial diseases, suggesting that nuclear genetic background and epigenetic factors are also important in disease expression.

disorders in 'Mitochondrial DNA diseases' in Chapter 3, 'Common consultations', p. 490.

- If the mother is heteroplasmic for a mutation, the proportion of mutant mtDNA in her offspring can vary considerably (see Figure 1.13).

Expert adviser: Robert Mcfarland, Clinical Senior Lecturer in Paediatric Neurology, Wellcome Trust Centre for Mitochondrial Research, Institute of Neuroscience, Newcastle University, Newcastle upon Tyne, UK.

References

Brown DT, Samuels DC, Michael EM, Turnbull DM, Chinnery PF. Random genetic drift determines the level of mutant mtDNA in human primary oocytes. *Am J Hum Genet* 2001; **68**: 533–6.

Cree LM, Samuels DC, de Sousa Lopes SC, *et al.* A reduction of mitochondrial DNA molecules during embryogenesis explains the rapid segregation of genotypes. *Nat Genet* 2008; **40**: 249–54.

Freyer C, Cree LM, Mourier A, *et al.* Variation in germline mtDNA heteroplasmy is determined prenatally but modified during subsequent transmission. *Nat Genet* 2012; **44**: 1282–5.

McFarland R, Taylor RW, Turnbull DM. A neurological perspective on mitochondrial disease. *Lancet Neurol* 2010; **9**: 829–40.

Poulton J, Macaulay V, Marchington DR. Transmission, genetic counselling and prenatal diagnosis of mitochondrial DNA disease. In: I Holt (ed.). *Genetics of mitochondrial disease. Oxford Monographs in Medical Genetics no. 47*, pp. 309–26. Oxford University Press, Oxford, 2003.

Schwartz M, Vissing J. Paternal inheritance of mitochondrial DNA. *N Engl J Med* 2002; **347**: 576–80.

Sykes B. *The seven daughters of Eve*. Corgi Books, London, 2001.

Thorburn DR, Dahl HH. Mitochondrial disorders: genetics, counselling, prenatal diagnosis and reproductive options. *Am J Med Genet* 2001; **106**: 102–14.

Wai T, Teoli D, Shoubridge EA. The mitochondrial DNA genetic bottleneck results from replication of a subpopulation of genomes. *Nat Genet* 2008; **40**: 1484–8.

Reproductive options

After a genetic disorder that has a significant sibling or offspring recurrence risk is diagnosed, many families are faced with a difficult choice about future pregnancies. It may be helpful for them to be introduced to the range of reproductive options available to them for future pregnancies. This is not always easy as such decisions are very personal. It may help to introduce the topic by explaining that some of the choices available may include options that they would not consider choosing.

Accepting the risk of another affected child
For some families, this will be their option of choice; for others an option they cannot bear to contemplate.

Electing against further pregnancies
The burden of caring for a child with a severe genetic disorder may be such that the family feel that they do not wish to extend their family because all of their energy is channelled into caring for their existing child(ren).

Adoption
Although this process can be frustrating and lengthy, some couples are successful in locating a baby or child to join their family. (Some couples may choose to adopt another affected child as sometimes happens in families who already have a child affected by achondroplasia or Down's syndrome.)

Donor gamete
Artificial insemination by donor (AID) is an option that can be used to minimize the risk of recurrence of an AR disorder for which both parents are carriers, or to evade the risk of a dominant disorder present in the father or the risk of unbalanced products of a balanced translocation present in the father. A donor ovum can also be used to minimize the risk of recurrence of an AR disorder and has the advantage that both parents play a biological role in bringing the baby into the world—technically this is much more demanding and the shortage of donor ova means that, in practice, AID is usually the more pragmatic option. A donor ovum is also an option to avoid the risk of a dominant disorder present in the mother, or a mitochondrial-encoded disorder carried by the mother, or the risk of unbalanced products of a balanced translocation present in the mother. If the gamete donor is related to either of the couple, it should have been demonstrated definitively that s/he is not a carrier of the condition. This is especially relevant for autosomal recessive disease or variable penetrance dominant disorders. For mitochondrial disorders, the woman's sister should generally not be used as an ovum donor.

Prenatal diagnosis
For many couples facing a high risk of recurrence for a serious disorder, this is the option of choice, but for others (particularly those with religious or moral objections to termination of pregnancy) it is ethically unacceptable. PND by CVS or amniocentesis is possible for cytogenetic disorders, monogenic disorders in which the pathogenic mutation is known, and the great majority of biochemical disorders. Prenatal diagnosis by ultrasound can be used in many conditions causing major structural malformations. PND by next-generation sequencing of free DNA in the maternal plasma, to infer the fetal genotype, is becoming available in some centres when the pathogenic mutation is known. Non-invasive prenatal diagnosis/testing (NIPD/T) is likely to become increasingly available (see 'Non-invasive prenatal testing' in Chapter 6, 'Pregnancy and fertility', p. 764).

Pre-implantation genetic diagnosis (PGD)
At first sight, this seems the most attractive option to many couples. In reality, PGD is only available in very few specialist centres and for a few severe genetic diseases (predominantly those in which single cell diagnosis is technically feasible, e.g. fluorescence in situ hybridization (FISH)-diagnosable conditions such as chromosome translocations or trisomies, or where there is a commonly occurring mutation such as the exon 7, 8 deletion in SMA). PGD entails ovarian hyperstimulation (and its attendant risks), egg retrieval, in vitro fertilization (IVF), embryo biopsy, and implantation of screened embryos. For single gene disorders, a pregnancy rate of 21% per egg retrieval and 25% per embryo transfer procedure has been reported. The costs are high (e.g. in the United Kingdom (UK), approximate current costs are £3500 for a first cycle plus the cost of the drugs (£800–1200)). There are limited data on safety and there may be unforeseen risks. See 'Assisted reproductive technology: *in vitro* fertilization (IVF), intracytoplasmic sperm injection (ICSI), and pre-implantation genetic diagnosis (PGD)' in Chapter 6, 'Pregnancy and fertility', p. 706. Approaches using a donor ovum and either pronuclear transfer or spindle transfer have been developed to enable couples to have a child with both their nuclear genetic contributions but the mitochondria of the donor ovum.

Adopt-out or foster-out an affected child In exceptional circumstances, this option may be considered.

Support group: coramBAAF Adoption & Fostering Academy, http://corambaaf.org.uk.

Expert adviser: Angus J. Clarke, Consultant in Clinical Genetics, Institute of Medical Genetics, University Hospital of Wales, Cardiff, UK.

Testing for genetic status

The great expansion in the number of disease genes or variants that have been identified, and for which mutation analysis is available, has led to a growth in the demand for genetic testing. On the one hand, a genetic test is much like any other investigation that might take place in response to symptoms or concern; on the other, there are some (albeit not unique) considerations:

- the results of a germline genetic test are permanent for the individual concerned;
- the results may have important implications for other family members, e.g. (future) offspring, siblings, or parents;
- occasionally, testing of other family members (e.g. linkage or testing of parents to confirm carrier status/array comparative genomic hybridization (aCGH) findings) may reveal that social relationships are not the same as biological ones, e.g. that paternity has been misattributed.

These issues need to be carefully thought through before embarking on genetic testing. Particular issues may arise with regard to genetic testing of children and MZ twins and these are discussed further below (see 'Predictive genetic testing of children' and 'Testing for genetic status in MZ twins' below).

Genetic testing for diagnostic indications

Genetic testing may be used as a diagnostic tool; for example, in a preterm neonate with meconium ileus in whom sweat testing is not feasible, molecular genetic testing for CF may enable a specific diagnosis of CF to be made and appropriate management to be instigated. Similarly, in a young boy presenting with delayed walking and a high creatine kinase (CK) level, genetic testing for Duchenne muscular dystrophy (DMD) may enable a specific diagnosis to be reached without the need to resort to an invasive test (muscle biopsy). Alternatively, in the young adult resuscitated from a ventricular fibrillation (VF) arrest or a young woman with triple-negative breast cancer, LQT or BRCA gene testing, respectively, may make a diagnosis.

Such testing is generally appropriate in adults or children, but those involved in the decision-making should consider the above bullet points at the outset.

Genetic testing to confirm or refine an existing clinical diagnosis

In this situation, there is a pre-existing clinical diagnosis and genetic testing serves to confirm and refine the diagnosis (but rarely to alter it). For example, an individual with tall stature, pectus carinatum, dilated aortic root, and dislocated lenses has a clinical diagnosis of Marfan's syndrome (MFS). If a fibrillin mutation (FBN1) is identified on genetic testing, this confirms the clinical diagnosis. For a child with sensorineural deafness diagnosed by audiometry, the finding of homozygosity for the del 35G mutation in connexin 26 serves to further refine the clinical diagnosis. In HMSN, the finding of a duplication of PMP22 serves to refine the diagnosis from HMSN type 1 to HMSN type 1A. There are very few situations in which this is inappropriate in adults or in children.

Predictive testing for disorders in which clinical management is affected by the test results

Examples of such disorders are familial adenomatous polyposis (FAP), HNPCC/Lynch syndrome, VHL, or retinoblastoma (RB).

These are disorders where effective screening and/or treatments are available and 'at-risk' individuals may choose to determine whether or not they have inherited the disease risk in order to avoid unnecessary screening.

Testing should be offered in the context of a clinic consultation at which the following are discussed:

(1) the natural history of the condition;

(2) the implications of a 'high risk' result;

(3) the screening programme/treatment available to individuals with a 'high risk' result and the evidence for benefit. Where individuals do not want to have genetic testing, such screening is also available to 'at-risk' individuals);

(4) the possible implications of the test result for other family members;

(5) the hypothetical future implications for financial arrangements (e.g. mortgages, pensions, and insurance)—discussion should include insurance industry moratorium on results of predictive genetic tests but the ability to use family history details.

If the individual wishes to proceed with predictive genetic testing, their consent (or parental consent) should usually be documented, the expected timescale for the results should be discussed, and arrangements made for the giving of the results (e.g. letter, phone call, clinic appointment). The 'Consent and confidentiality in clinical genetic practice' document (Royal College of Physicians (RCP), Royal College of Pathologists (RCPath), British Society for Human Genetics 2011) gives examples of suitable consent forms.

Predictive testing for disorders in which clinical management is not affected by the test result

Examples are HD and spinocerebellar ataxia (SCA).

Predictive testing for HD is usually only offered as part of a staged programme in which a series of three or more meetings between the individual at risk and a geneticist/genetic counsellor are held to explore the reasons why they wish to have the test and to discuss possible outcomes and future management. This is because of the considered decision of many who have requested testing and have decided not to proceed after considering the pros and cons (Royal College of Physicians (RCP), Royal College of Pathologists (RCPath), British Society for Human Genetics 2011).

- The predictive programme usually takes place over several months and includes a discussion of all points (1) to (5) raised above. This may be longer if awareness of the diagnosis in the family is very recent.
- A 'supporter' (often a partner or friend) is nominated by the patient who attends the clinic visits and makes a commitment to support the individual undergoing testing.

- If the individual wishes to proceed with genetic testing, *consent* for predictive testing may be obtained and documented and the expected timescale for results should be discussed. A clinic visit for the result is usually arranged, so that this can be given in person by a member of the team known to the patient. (Alternative arrangements for giving the result may be considered in some circumstances, e.g. letter, phone call.)
- Testing for dominant disorders in individuals at 25% risk (in which the result may reveal the status of an individual in a previous generation) is usually only undertaken if every effort has been made to provide genetic counselling to the individual at 50% risk, but they have declined or are unavailable.

Where the outcome of predictive genetic testing will not alter that person's medical management, care should be taken to ensure that patients understand this and that they are discouraged from making a rushed decision about testing. Encouraging patients to reflect on both the advantages and disadvantages of testing and the best timing of testing for them should be part of the process. Generally, this type of testing should be delayed until a person is old enough to make an informed decision themselves, rather than at the wish of parents who wish to know what their child might develop in the future.

Testing for carrier status

Examples are CF or chromosome translocations.

An individual's carrier status usually does not have health implications for them but may have potential implications for reproduction. These reproductive consequences should be carefully explained. Such testing is reasonable for any individual who has the competence (capacity) to consent to such testing.

Predictive genetic testing of children

Where children cannot themselves consent to testing, their best interests need to be considered. If the potential benefit of testing can reasonably be viewed as outweighing the disadvantages of testing (e.g. the removal of their future ability to choose whether or not to be tested, and the risk of stigmatization). It is usually undertaken when the child is at significant risk for a genetic disorder for which screening is burdensome and effective treatment is possible, e.g. RB, FAP, and VHL. Please refer to the websites listed at the end of this section for a thorough discussion of the ethical, legal, and psychological issues. In 2010, the British Society of Human Genetics issued new guidelines for the genetic testing of children. These summarize some of the issues to consider when making decisions about predictive testing in children:

(1) when a child is at risk of a genetic condition for which preventative or other therapeutic measures are available, genetic testing should be offered. Where the alternative screenings are burdensome, the direction to test may be stronger, e.g. in RB where genetic testing would remove the need for examinations under a general anaesthetic for 50% of at-risk children;

(2) when a child is at risk of a genetic condition with paediatric onset for which preventive therapeutic measures are not available, the best interests of the child are paramount in determining the appropriate course of action;

(3) when a child is at risk of a genetic condition with adult onset for which preventive or effective therapeutic measures in childhood are not available, genetic testing should generally be delayed until the child is old enough to decide for him/herself. Families should be informed of the existence of tests and given the opportunity to discuss the reasons why the tests are generally not offered for children;

(4) genetic testing for carrier status should generally be deferred until the child is old enough to decide for him/herself. In some cases, a baby may be found to be a carrier as an incidental result of a particular screening programme looking for affected individuals, but it does not follow that there are benefits to testing all young children for carrier status;

(5) testing for the benefit of a family member should generally be similarly delayed, unless such testing is necessary to prevent serious harm to the family member (GMC guidelines 2008).

Adoption

When a child is being considered for adoption, the same guidelines for genetic testing should generally be followed as for other children. Sometimes requests for testing are made to make children more 'adoptable' by removing uncertainty about their inheritance. Such testing is not recommended (ref court case; [2013] EWHC 953 (Fam)); see http://www.bailii.org/ew/cases/EWHC/Fam/2013/953.html).

The primary justification for genetic testing of any child should be a timely medical benefit and this is the same in children being considered for adoption.

Testing for genetic status in MZ twins

Genetic testing of MZ twins raises special ethical issues, particularly with respect to predictive testing. Where possible, try to ascertain that both twins wish to proceed with predictive testing and arrange for them to proceed through the predictive testing process simultaneously (perhaps with parallel consultations). When a diagnostic test is contemplated in one twin, this may be a predictive test for the other twin and this needs careful consideration. Where one twin wishes to proceed with genetic testing and the other does not, a discussion should be had about how the other's desire not to know can be respected in the light of testing of the other twin.

Paternity

Some genetic tests have the potential to reveal misattributed paternity. Unless this potential is recognized and discussed in advance of testing, such a test result can raise serious ethical issues (see Lucassen and Parker 2001, for a thorough discussion of this issue).

Where tests could potentially reveal misattributed paternity, a sensitive discussion of this possibility should be undertaken during pre-test counselling. Beware that certain results may suggest misattributed paternity, when this is not in fact the case, e.g. *de novo* deletion of a recessive gene.

Expert adviser: Anneke Lucassen, Consultant in Clinical Genetics, Faculty of Medicine, Wessex Clinical Genetic Service, University of Southampton, Southampton, UK.

References

American Medical Association. *Genetic testing of children*, Policy, E-2.138, June 1996.

American Society of Human Genetics Board of Directors, American College of Medical Genetics Board of Directors. Points to consider; ethical, legal, and psychological implications of genetic testing in children and adolescents. *Am J Hum Genet* 1995; **57**: 1233–41.

American Society of Human Genetics Social Issues Committee, American College of Medical Genetics Social, Ethical, and Legal Issues Committee. Genetic testing in adoption. *Am J Hum Genet* 2000; **66**: 761–7.

British Society for Human Genetics. *Report on the genetic testing of children 2010*, 2010. http://www.bsgm.org.uk/media/678741/gtoc_booklet_final_new.pdf.

Clarke A (ed.). *The genetic testing of children*. BIOS Scientific Publishers Ltd, Oxford, 1998.

Codori AM, Zawacki KL, Petersen GM, *et al.* Genetic testing for hereditary colorectal cancer in children: long-term psychological effects. *Am J Med Genet A* 2003; **116A**: 117–28.

General Medical Council. *Consent: patients and doctors making decisions together*, 2008. http://www.gmc-uk.org/Consent___English_1015.pdf_48903482.pdf.

Lucassen A, Parker M. Revealing false paternity: some ethical considerations. *Lancet* 2001; **357**: 1033–5.

Royal College of Physicians (RCP), Royal College of Pathologists (RCPath), British Society for Human Genetics. *Consent and confidentiality in clinical genetic practice: guidance on genetic testing and sharing genetic information*, 2nd edn. Report of the Joint Committee on Medical Genetics. RCP, RCPath, London, 2011. http://www.bsgm.org.uk/media/678746/consent_and_confidentiality_2011.pdf.

Timing and origin of new dominant mutations

De novo mutation (DNM) is the most prevalent cause of severe genetic developmental disorders in the offspring of non-consanguineous parents (McRae *et al.* 2016). In consanguineous families, where recessive disorders are the most common cause of developmental disorders, ~5% of children with a developmental disorder will have this as a consequence of a DNM.

Depending on the timing of mutations during embryonic development, different types of germline mosaicism can arise (see Figure 1.14); star signs

indicate different stages at which mutations can arise and the consequential types of mosaicism. Multiple arrows indicate separation of primordial germ cells (PGCs) from other tissues (suggesting that both blood and germ cell lineages are founded by multiple cells from the embryo). Germline mosaic variants, which are detectable in the parents' blood, were likely established before mesoderm tissue separation from PGCs in the parents (open stars). One possible explanation for mosaic mutations that are only shared by siblings is that the mutations occurred after

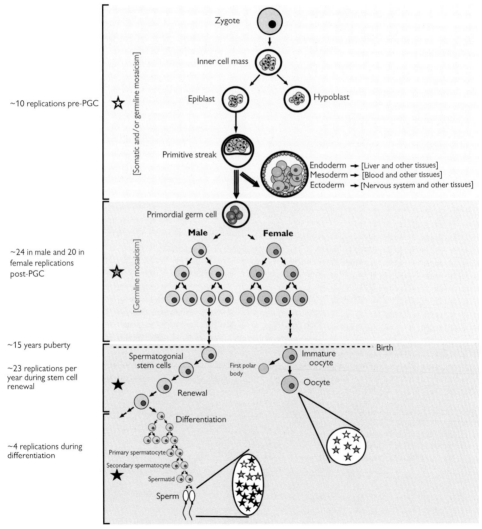

Figure 1.14 Schematic diagram depicting the different types of germline mosaicism that can occur depending upon the time in development at which a new mutation occurs.
Reprinted by permission from Macmillan Publishers Ltd: *Nature Genetics*, Raheleh Rahbari *et al.*, Timing, rates and spectra of human germline mutation, volume 48, issue 2, copyright 2015.

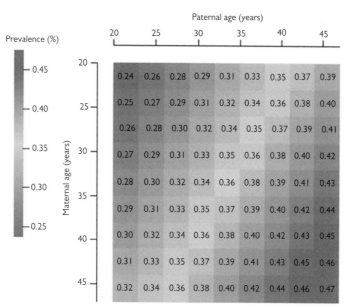

Figure 1.15 Prevalence of live births with developmental disorders caused by dominant *de novo* mutations (DNMs). The prevalence within the general population is provided as a percentage for combinations of parental ages, extrapolated from the maternal and paternal rates of DNMs. Distributions of parental ages within the DDD cohort and the UK population are shown at the matching parental axis.
Reprinted by permission from Macmillan Publishers Ltd: *Nature*, Deciphering Developmental Disorders Study, 'Prevalence and architecture of *de novo* mutations in developmental disorders', published online 25th January 2017, doi:10.1038/nature21062, copyright 2017.

separation of PGCs from the mesoderm in the mosaic parents (hatched stars).

Rahbari *et al.* (2016) estimated a sibling recurrence risk of 1.3% for across all DNMs; this figure is compatible with earlier empirical studies. If the mutation is not detectable on deep sequencing of the parents, the sibling recurrence risk is lower, perhaps ~0.5%, and the mutation is presumed to have arisen after separation of the PGCs.

Parental age

As a consequence of background mutational processes that occur in all cells, there is a slow acquisition of mutations over time. The marked differences in the number of mitotic divisions in paternal and maternal gametogenesis (see Figure 1.15) lead to an increased number of mutations present in male gametes in comparison with female gametes. (In addition, a very small fraction of mutations confer a selective advantage to spermatogonal progenitor cells; see 'Paternal age' in Chapter 6, 'Pregnancy and fertility', p. 772.) The prevalence of live births with developmental disorders arising as a consequence of new dominant mutations, increasing

with parental age, is shown in Figure 1.15. Note that the chance of a young couple in their early 20s having a child with a developmental disorder due to a DNM at 0.24% (~2.5/1000 live births) is approximately half of that of a couple in the mid 40s where the risk is 0.47% (~5/1000 live births). Note that the figure is asymmetric, showing a stronger influence of paternal age than maternal age on DNMs.

Expert adviser: Matthew Hurles, Head of Human Genetics, Wellcome Trust Sanger Institute, Wellcome Trust Genome Campus, Hinxton, UK.

References

Alexandrov LB, Jones PH, Wedge DC, et al. Clock-like mutational processes in human somatic cells. *Nat Genet* 2015; **47**: 1402–7.

McRae JF, Clayton S, Fitzgerald TW, et al. (2016, under review). Prevalence, phenotype and architecture of developmental disorders caused by *de novo* mutation. doi: http://dx.doi.org/10.1101/049056. http://biorxiv.org/content/early/2016/06/16/049056.

Rahbari R, Wuster A, Lindsay SJ, et al.; UK10K Consortium, Hurles ME. Timing, rates and spectra of human germline mutation. *Nat Genet* 2016; **48**: 126–33.

Useful resources

One of the frustrations in writing this Desk Reference has been the brevity with which each topic can be discussed. While this has been necessary in order to try to include the myriad of conditions that may be encountered in a general genetics clinic, we hope that we have included sufficient detail to enable the reader to make progress towards a diagnosis. Once a precise diagnosis is achieved, there is a wealth of sources from which further information can be obtained. Listed below is a selection of sources that we find particularly useful.

Databases/websites

ClinVar. A public archive of reports of the relationship among human variation and phenotypes, with supporting evidence. www.ncbi.nlm.nih.gov/clinvar

DECIPHER. Established in 2004 to serve the genetics community, it has grown to become a major global platform for the visualization of phenotypic and genomic relationships. DECIPHER is unique in displaying all scales of genomic variation, from a single base pair to megabases in size, in a single interface and has now developed an exciting visualization of phenotypic relationships based upon Human Phenotype Ontology (HPO) annotations. DECIPHER promotes flexible data sharing; it enables the extent of sharing to be tailored, so that it is proportionate to the clinical or scientific need to facilitate diagnosis or discovery. https://decipher.sanger.ac.uk.

Ensembl. Genome browser. http://www.ensembl.org.

Exome Aggregation Consortium (ExAC). A coalition of investigators seeking to aggregate and harmonize exome sequencing data from a variety of large-scale sequencing projects and to make summary data available for the wider scientific community. The data set provided on this website spans 60 706 unrelated individuals sequenced as part of various disease-specific and population genetic studies. ExAC has removed individuals affected by severe paediatric disease, so this data set should serve as a useful reference set of allele frequencies for severe disease studies. All of the raw data from these projects have been reprocessed through the same pipeline and jointly variant-called to increase consistency across projects. http://exac.broadinstitute.org.

Frequency of Inherited Disorders Database (FIDD). https://medicapps.cardiff.ac.uk/fidd.

Gene2Phenotype (G2P). A web-based interface of protein-coding genes annotated by allelic requirement, mutation consequence, and phenotype category designed for application in next-generation sequencing with provision to download system-based gene panels. http://www.ebi.ac.uk/gene2phenotype.

GeneReviews. An excellent source of accurate clinical genetics advice to guide practice for diagnosed patients. http://www.ncbi.nlm.nih.gov/books/NBK1116.

gnomAD (genome Aggregation Database). http://gnomad.broadinstitute.org. A resource developed by an international coalition of investigators with the goal of aggregating and harmonizing both the exome and genome sequencing data from a wide variety of large scale sequencing projects and making summary data available.

HUGO Gene Nomenclature Database. http://www.genenames.org.

Human Phenotype Ontology (HPO). Aims to provide a standardized vocabulary of phenotypic abnormalities encountered in human disease. Each term in HPO describes a phenotypic abnormality such as atrial septal defect. HPO is currently being developed using the medical literature, Orphanet, DECIPHER, and OMIM. HPO currently contains ~11 000 terms (still growing) and over 115 000 annotations to hereditary diseases. HPO also provides a large set of HPO annotations to ~4000 common diseases. http://human-phenotype-ontology.github.io.

Online Mendelian Inheritance in Man (OMIM). http://www.omim.org.

Orphanet. http://www.orpha.net.

POSSUMweb (Pictures Of Standard Syndromes and Undiagnosed Malformations). A dysmorphology database. http://www.possum.net.au.

PubMed. http://www.ncbi.nlm.nih.gov/pubmed.

University of California Santa Cruz (UCSC) Genome Browser. http://genome.ucsc.edu.

Support groups

Genetic Alliance UK. http://www.geneticalliance.org.uk.

National Organization for Rare Disorders (USA). http://www.rarediseases.org.

Syndromes Without A Name (SWAN UK). http://www.undiagnosed.org.uk.

Unique. http://www.rarechromo.org (excellent resource for patient leaflets about chromosomal conditions, e.g. XYY, 1p36 deletion, etc.).

References

Cassidy SB, Allanson JE. *Management of genetic syndromes*, 3rd edn. John Wiley & Sons, Hoboken, 2010.

Gardner RJM, Sutherland GR, Shaffer LG. *Chromosome abnormalities and genetic counseling*, Oxford monographs on medical genetics no. 31, 4th edn. Oxford University Press, New York, 2011.

Gorlin RJ, Cohen MM, Hennekam RCM (eds.). *Syndromes of the head and neck*, 5th edn. Oxford University Press, Oxford, 2010.

Hall JG, Froster-Iskenius I, Allanson J. *Handbook of physical measurement*. Oxford University Press, Oxford, 1989.

Harper PS. *Practical genetic counselling*, 7th edn. Arnold, London, 2010.

Hodgson SV, Foulkes WD, Eng C, Maher ER. *A practical guide to human cancer genetics*, 3rd edn. Cambridge University Press, Cambridge, 2013.

Jones KL (ed.). *Smith's recognizable patterns of human malformations*, 6th edn. WB Saunders, Philadelphia, 2006.

Read A, Donnai D. *New clinical genetics*, 3rd edn. Scion Publications, Banbury, 2015.

Reardon W. *The bedside dysmorphologist*. Oxford University Press, New York, 2007.

Rimoin DL, Pyeritz RE, Korf BR. *Emery and Rimoin's essential medical genetics*. Academic Press, Waltham, MA, 2013.

Sadler TW. *Langman's medical embryology*, 13th edn. Wolters Kluwer, Philadelphia, 2015.

Stevenson RE, Hall JG (eds.). *Human malformations and related anomalies*, 2nd edn. Oxford University Press, Oxford, 2006.

Strachan M, Read AP. *Human molecular genetics*, 4th edn. Taylor & Francis, New York, 2010.

Turnpenny P, Ellard S. *Emery's elements of medical genetics*, 14th edn. Elsevier Churchill Livingstone, Philadelphia, 2011.

Young ID. *Introduction to risk calculation in genetic counselling*, 3rd edn. Oxford University Press, Oxford, 2007.

X-linked dominant (XLD), semi-dominant, pseudoautosomal, and male-sparing inheritance

X-linked dominant (XLD) disorders are encoded on the X chromosome. An XLD disorder manifests very severely in males, often leading to spontaneous loss or neonatal death of affected male pregnancies. Typical examples include incontinentia pigmenti (IP) due to mutations in *NEMO*, Rett syndrome due to mutations in *MECP2*, oral–facial–digital syndrome type 1 (OFD-1) due to mutations in *CXORF5*, and otopalatodigital syndrome types 1 and 2 (OPD-1 and OPD-2) due to mutations in *FMNA* (filamin A).

An X-linked (XL) semi-dominant disorder manifests severely in males who are hemizygotes, and mildly or subclinically in females who have two X chromosomes (one normal and one mutated copy). Examples include Coffin–Lowry syndrome and X-linked hereditary motor and sensory neuropathy (X-HMSN) where a proportion of heterozygotes manifest features of the disorder. Where the disorder manifests only infrequently or not at all in heterozygotes, it is said to follow X-linked recessive (XLR) inheritance (see 'X-linked recessive (XLR) inheritance' in Chapter 1, 'Introduction', p. 50).

Male-sparing X-linked disorders

There are a few examples of male-sparing XL disorders—craniofrontonasal syndrome due to ephrin B1 mutation (*EFNB1*) and epilepsy and mental retardation (MR) limited to females (EFMR) due to *PCDH19*. Females are affected, whereas men carrying the mutation remain phenotypically normal. For *EFNB1*, Twigg *et al.* (2013) demonstrated a more severe outcome in mosaic than in constitutionally deficient males, providing further support for the cellular interference mechanism by which the differing expression of *EFNB1* generates abnormal tissue boundaries, a process that occurs in normal females (due to mosaicism related to X-inactivation) but which cannot occur in hemizygous males.

Recombination between the X and Y chromosomes is limited to the pseudoautosomal region (PAR) and is necessary for proper segregation of the sex chromosomes during spermatogenesis. Crossover between the sex chromosomes during male meiosis is restricted to the terminal pseudoautosomal pairing regions PAR1, a 2.6-Mb region on Xp/Yp, and PAR2, a 320-kb region on Xq/Yq. Genes in the PARs escape X-inactivation and exhibit pseudoautosomal inheritance. Genes encoded in PAR1 include *SHOX* which has an important role in growth. Under normal circumstances, the *SHOX* genes on both Xpters of a female are active, as are the *SHOX* genes on Xpter and Ypter in a male, and hence the severity of the phenotype is not sex-dependent. Mutations in *SHOX* therefore show pseudoautosomal inheritance, rather than XL semi-dominant inheritance. Deletions or mutations causing haploinsufficiency of *SHOX* are a common cause of idiopathic short stature (4/56 cases, i.e. ~7% in Morizio's series) and also cause Leri–Weill syndrome. Individuals homozygous for the deletion or homozygous or compound heterozygotes for inactivating mutations have the more severe Langer mesomelic dysplasia.

Aspects of XLD inheritance

Skewed X-inactivation

If there is complete skewing, the ratio is 100:0; often an intermediate value is found. Values <80:20 fall within values expected from normal variation in X-inactivation patterns in the general population; values >80:20 are suggestive of X-inactivation due to a selection bias due to a deleterious XLR mutation, but are seen in ~9% of normal females (see 'X-linked recessive (XLR) inheritance' in Chapter 1, 'Introduction', p. 50). This selection bias may not operate equally in all tissues and so variable degrees of skewing may be observed in different tissues.

Degree of manifestation in heterozygotes

Unfavourable skewing of X-inactivation in key tissues may be a major factor in determining the expression of an XLD disorder in heterozygotes. Skewing towards the X without the mutation may result in minimal features and it may not be clinically recognized that the individual is a heterozygote (and recurrence may be attributed erroneously to germline mosaicism).

Distribution of features in heterozygotes

The distribution of features in a female is a reflection of the X-inactivation pattern in specific tissues. Asymmetry is an important feature and this is well illustrated in XL chondrodysplasia punctata (XLCDP) where the limbs are shortened but not symmetrically. The skin lesions of IP are streaky and may follow the lines of Blaschko.

Germline mosaicism

As with XLR disorders, the risk of germline mosaicism needs to be considered. For example, in Rett syndrome, it is recommended that mothers and sisters of

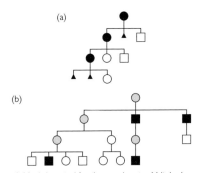

Figure 1.16 a) A typical family tree showing X-linked dominant inheritance. The condition is manifest in female heterozygotes and male hemizygotes. Many of these conditions cause spontaneous loss of affected male pregnancies. (b) A typical family tree showing X-linked semi-dominant inheritance. The condition is expressed severely in males and mildly in females. For a mildly affected female, on average, 50% of her sons will be severely affected and 50% of her daughters will be mildly affected. Daughters of an affected male are mildly affected and none of his sons inherit the condition.

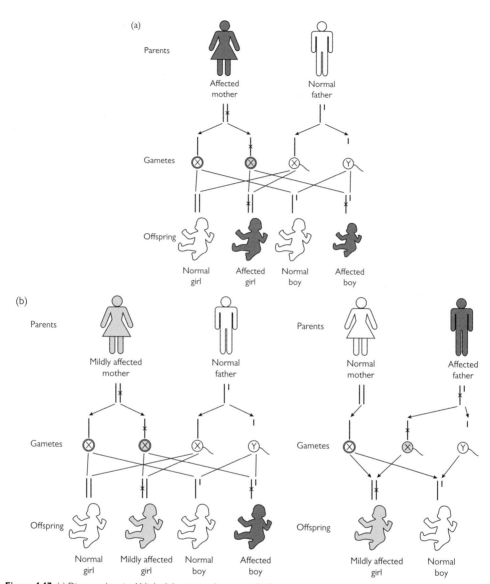

Figure 1.17 (a) Diagram showing X-linked dominant inheritance. (b) Diagram showing X-linked semi-dominant inheritance.

affected girls are tested for an *MECP2* mutation identified in the proband.

Typical family trees
See Figures 1.16 and 1.17.

Genetic advice
- Males carrying the mutation are severely affected, often leading to spontaneous loss or neonatal death of affected male pregnancies in XLD conditions.
- Female heterozygotes are affected but have less severe features than males.
- The degree to which females express the disorder is largely governed by X-inactivation patterns.

- When a heterozygous affected female has a pregnancy, there are four genetic possibilities at conception, each equally likely. These are: a normal daughter; an affected daughter; a normal son; and a severely affected son, e.g. XL hypophosphatasia (vitamin-D-resistant rickets) where affected males are viable. For many XLD disorders, e.g. IP, affected males are typically lost in early pregnancy, so at birth there are three possibilities: a normal daughter; an affected daughter; a normal son.
- When an affected male has a child, all of his daughters will inherit the mutation and none of his sons will be affected.
- The family tree shows no male-to-male transmission.

- If the mother of an affected female with a presumed DNM does not herself carry the mutation in her blood, female siblings of the proband should still be offered carrier testing by mutation detection because of the small possibility of germline mosaicism in the parent.
- Males who are born with features of a severe and normally lethal XLD condition should have a karyotype to exclude Klinefelter's syndrome.
- Females with unusually severe features of an XLD or an XL semi-dominant disorder may have this as a consequence of:
  - highly unfavourably skewed X-inactivation;
  - Turner syndrome where the girl is a hemizygote;
  - X-autosome translocation.

Hence a karyotype is indicated in these circumstances.

Expert adviser: Richard Gibbons, Professor of Clinical Genetics, Weatherall Institute of Molecular Medicine, Oxford University Hospital NHS Trust, John Radcliffe Hospital, Oxford, UK.

References

Dibbens LM, Tarpey PS, Hynes K, et al. X-linked protocadherin 19 mutations cause female-limited epilepsy and cognitive impairment. Nat Genet 2008; **40**: 776–81.

Morizio E, Stuppia L, Gatta V, et al. Deletion of the SHOX gene in patients with short stature of unknown cause. Am J Med Genet A 2003; **119A**: 293–96.

Shears DJ, Guillen-Navaro E, Sempere-Miralles M, et al. Pseudodominant inheritance of Langer mesomelic dysplasia caused by a SHOX homeobox missense mutation. Am J Med Genet 2002; **110**: 153–7.

Shi Q, Spriggs E, Field LL, et al. Absence of age effect on meiotic recombination between human X and Y chromosomes. Am J Hum Genet 2002; **71**: 254–61.

Strachan T, Read AP. Human molecular genetics, 4th edn. Taylor & Francis, New York, 2010.

Twigg SR, Babbs C, van den Elzen ME, et al. Cellular interference in craniofrontonasal syndrome: males mosaic for mutations in the X-linked EFNB1 gene are more severely affected than true hemizygotes. Hum Mol Gen 2013; **22**: 1654–62.

Twigg SR, Kan R, Babbs C, et al. Mutations of ephrin-B1 (EFNB1), a marker of tissue boundary foundation, cause craniofrontonasal syndrome. Proc Natl Acad Sci U S A 2004; **101**: 8652–7.

Young ID. Introduction to risk calculation in genetic counselling, 3rd edn. Oxford University Press, Oxford, 2007.

X-linked recessive (XLR) inheritance

X-linked recessive (XLR) disorders are encoded on the X chromosome. An XLR disorder manifests in males who are hemizygotes, but generally not in carrier females who have two X chromosomes (one normal and one mutated copy). Some XL disorders are almost never expressed in females, e.g. XL alpha-thalassaemia/mental retardation syndrome (ATRX). In some disorders, females have symptoms infrequently, e.g. DMD/Becker muscular dystrophy (BMD), whereas for others, e.g. X-HMSN and fragile X syndrome (FRAXA), manifestation in female carriers is fairly common but is usually less severe than in affected males. Disorders in which heterozygotes commonly manifest, e.g. X-HMSN and Coffin–Lowry syndrome, may be said to follow XL semi-dominant inheritance (see 'X-linked dominant (XLD), semi-dominant, pseudoautosomal, and male-sparing inheritance' in Chapter 1, 'Introduction', p. 46).

X-inactivation is the process by which dosage compensation of XL genes in females is achieved by the transcriptional silencing of one of the two X chromosomes during early development (from day 9 post-fertilization when the inner cell mass of the blastocyst contains 64 cells). As a result of X-inactivation, heterozygous females are mosaic for XL gene expression, with one population of cells expressing genes from the maternal X chromosome and the other population expressing genes from the paternal X chromosome (Nance 1964). The early events in X-inactivation are under the control of the X-chromosome inactivation centre (Xic). The *XIST* gene in the Xic at Xq13.2 is the only gene transcribed exclusively from the inactive X chromosome and is known to play an essential role in the initiation of X-inactivation. Initiation of X-inactivation involves a counting step in which the number of X chromosomes in the cell is counted relative to cell ploidy, so that only a single X chromosome is functional per diploid adult cell.

X-inactivation in the embryo is a random process, with ~50% of cells containing an inactivated maternal X chromosome and ~50% of cells containing an inactivated paternal X chromosome. Significant deviation from a 50:50 inactivation pattern is occasionally observed among normal females in the population, a phenomenon referred to as skewed X-inactivation (see Table 1.5). Skewing of X-inactivation is a feature of some XL disorders. In extra-embryonic tissues, e.g. placenta, there is imprinted inactivation of the paternal X chromosome.

X-inactivation patterns may be assessed by comparing the ratio of the two alleles at a highly polymorphic site, e.g. the CA repeat in the androgen receptor gene,

in a non-methylation-sensitive assay with the ratio of the same alleles in a methylation-sensitive assay. Usually the ratio approximates to 50%

Aspects of XLR inheritance

Skewed X-inactivation
If there is complete skewing, the ratio is 100:0; often an intermediate value is found. Values <80:20 fall within values expected from normal variation in X-inactivation patterns in the general population; values >80:20 are suggestive of X-inactivation due to a selection bias due to a deleterious XLR mutation, but are seen in ~9% of normal females (see Table 1.5). This selection bias may not operate equally in all tissues and so variable degrees of skewing may be observed in different tissues. Maternal X-inactivation skewing may be used to suggest that a sporadic affected male has an XL disorder.

Manifesting carriers
Unfavourable skewing of X-inactivation in key tissues may be a major factor in determining whether or not an XLR disorder is expressed in heterozygotes. As noted above, the penetrance in heterozygotes shows wide variation between different XLR disorders.

Germline mosaicism
A number of XLR disorders have substantial germline mosaicism risks—most notably DMD/BMD. For the mother of an affected boy with a known mutation that is not present in the mother's genomic DNA, there is a suggested 1 in 5 (20%) risk to a future son who inherits the same X chromosome as his affected brother (i.e. there is an overall 5% risk to future pregnancies). For androgen insensitivity syndrome (AIS), this risk is much smaller, but nevertheless germline mosaicism has been observed.

Typical family trees
See Figures 1.18 and 1.19.

Genetic advice

- Males carrying the mutation are severely affected; females carrying the mutation are generally either unaffected or more mildly affected than males.
- The degree to which females express the disorder is largely governed by X-inactivation patterns.
- When a carrier female has a pregnancy, there are four possible outcomes, each equally likely. These

Table 1.5 Frequency (%) of skewed X-inactivation in normal female controls

X-inactivation pattern	Frequency (%) of skewed X-inactivation in normal female controls
≥90:10	3
≥80:20	9
≥70:30	30

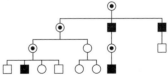

Figure 1.18 A typical family tree showing X-linked recessive inheritance. The condition is expressed in males, but not in females. For a carrier female, on average, 50% of her sons will be affected and 50% of her daughters will be carriers. All daughters of an affected male are obligate carriers and none of his sons inherit the condition.

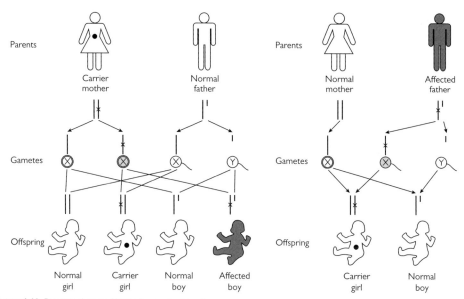

Figure 1.19 Diagram showing X-linked recessive inheritance.
Reprinted from *The American Journal of Human Genetics* Vol 64, Plenge *et al*, Evidence that mutations in the X-linked DDP gene cause incompletely penetrant and variable skewed X inactivation, Copyright 1999, with permission from Elsevier.

are: a normal daughter; a carrier daughter; a normal son; and an affected son. Another way of expressing this is that, in a female pregnancy, there is a 50% chance of a carrier daughter; in a male pregnancy, there is a 50% chance of an affected son.

- When an affected male fathers a pregnancy, all of his daughters will be carriers and none of his sons will be affected.
- The family tree shows no male-to-male transmission.
- Even if the proband is the only affected member, it is generally more likely that the mother is a carrier than that the proband has the condition as the result of a DNM. For XLR conditions where reproductive fitness is zero, there is a two-thirds chance that the mother is a mutation carrier and a one-third chance that the mutation is *de novo* for an apparently sporadic case.
- If the mother of a sporadic case with a presumed DNM does not herself carry the mutation in her blood, female siblings of the proband should still be offered carrier testing by mutation detection because of the small possibility of germline mosaicism in the mother.
- Females with unusually severe features of an XLR disorder may have this as a consequence of:

- highly unfavourably skewed X-inactivation;
- Turner syndrome where the girl is a hemizygote;
- X-autosome translocation.

Hence a karyotype is indicated in these circumstances.

Expert adviser: Richard Gibbons, Professor of Clinical Genetics, Weatherall Institute of Molecular Medicine, Oxford University Hospital NHS Trust, John Radcliffe Hospital, Oxford, UK.

References

Nance WE. Genetic tests with a sex-linked marker: glucose-6-phosphate dehydrogenase. *Cold Spring Harbor Symp Quant Biol* 1964; **29**: 415–52.

Plenge RM, Tranebjaerg L, Jensen PK, Schwartz C, Willard HF. Evidence that mutations in the X-linked *DDP* gene cause incompletely penetrant and variable skewed X inactivation. *Am J Hum Genet* 1999; **64**: 759–67.

Strachan T, Read AP. *Human molecular genetics*, 4th edn. Taylor & Francis, New York, 2010.

Young ID. *Introduction to risk calculation in genetic counselling*, 3rd edn. Oxford University Press, Oxford, 2007.

Clinical approach

Chapter contents

Ambiguous genitalia (including sex reversal)

Genetic sex is determined at fertilization. In sex chromosome aneuploidy, the presence of a Y chromosome promotes normal male sexual differentiation (e.g. 47,XXY and 47,XYY). Only a single X chromosome is required for female development, as in 45,X (although complete ovarian development requires XX). Up to 12 weeks' gestation, the external genitalia appear the same in both sexes; even up to 20 weeks' gestation, it can occasionally be difficult to reliably determine the fetal sex from the appearances of the external genitalia.

Under normal circumstances, genetic sex determines gonadal sex, which determines phenotypic sex (see Figure 2.1). Before 7 weeks' gestation, the gonadal precursor tissues are histologically identical. Both sexes possess paired Wolffian (precursors of the vas deferens and epididymis and seminal vesicles) and Müllerian ducts (precursors of the Fallopian tubes and uterus) (see Figure 2.2). The external genitalia are female in appearance. Towards the end of the first trimester, the indifferent gonad in males is stimulated to differentiate into a testis by the product of the *SRY* gene. If the *SRY* gene is absent (as in normal females), deleted, or mutated, the indifferent gonad fails to develop into a testis. The testis produces Müllerian inhibitory factor, which leads to Müllerian tract regression in males. The stabilization of Wolffian duct derivatives requires testosterone. Testosterone is important for the development of the internal genitalia, and dihydrotestosterone (DHT) has a key role in the development of the external genitalia. In the absence of testosterone (as in normal females), the Wolffian ducts regress.

Disorders of sex development (DSD) refer to congenital conditions in which the development of chromosomal, gonadal, or anatomic sex is atypical.

Clinical approach

Assessment and investigation of neonates with ambiguous genitalia are best done in close liaison with a paediatric endocrinologist.

History: key points
- Three-generation family tree (including consanguinity).
- Detailed enquiry about maternal health and drug exposure during pregnancy.
- Detailed documentation of pregnancy history.

Examination: key points
Document the findings carefully; clinical photographs may be helpful.
- The phallus—micropenis or clitoris; measure the length of the phallus.
- The labioscrotal folds—bifid scrotum or labial fusion.
- The gonads—palpable or impalpable (examine the labioscrotal folds and groins; if palpable, they are likely to be testes, or possibly ovotestes). Measure the length.
- The urethra—position, chordee (tethering of the penis).
- Other anomalies.
- Birthweight—strong association between low birthweight and hypospadias.

Special investigations
The *initial screen* should include:
- karyotype to determine the genetic sex (initial karyotype by interphase FISH or quantitative fluorescence-polymerase chain reaction (QF-PCR) if available), proceeding to full karyotype with mosaicism screen;

- genomic microarray (in the absence of a definitive endocrine diagnosis, e.g. congenital adrenal hyperplasia (CAH));
- pelvic ultrasound scan (USS) to determine whether a uterus is present and whether the gonads can be visualized;
- blood electrolytes sodium (Na)/potassium (K) and glucose;
- plasma 17OH-progesterone (*urgent* analysis);
- serum testosterone.

If 46,XX, the most likely diagnosis is CAH (see 'Congenital adrenal hyperplasia (CAH)' in Chapter 3, 'Common consultations', p. 370). There is an urgent need to determine if this is a salt-losing variety and further investigations should include:
- 11-deoxycortisol;
- androstenedione;
- testosterone;
- renin;
- aldosterone;
- 24-hour urine collection for urine steroid profile by specific chromatography in a specialist lab;
- blood for DNA studies.

If 45X/46XY, 95% of those diagnosed prenatally are phenotypically normal males, but potential exists for gonadal dysgenesis if both cell lines are present in the gonad. Testosterone level in the normal range within the first 8 weeks of life (when the neonatal gonads are very active) would be indicative of normal male gonadal development and be reassuring. If not detected antenatally and especially when ambiguous genitalia are present, the prognosis for normal masculinization is more guarded. Tests should include:
- testosterone level;
- consider follicle-stimulating hormone (FSH)/luteinizing hormone (LH) to see if gonad functional to suppress the pituitary.

If 46,XY, a specific diagnosis may be possible in only 25%. Testosterone implies the presence of testes. Measurement of testosterone, androstenedione, and DHT enables identification of the most common androgen biosynthetic defects, i.e. 17β-hydroxysteroid dehydrogenase and 5α-reductase. Proceed to a human chorionic gonadotrophin (hCG) stimulation test and measure:
- plasma 17OH-progesterone;
- testosterone;
- androstenedione;
- DHT;
- dehydroepiandosterone (DHA);
- 24-hour urine for urine steroid profile;
- blood for DNA studies.

In some laboratories, it may be possible to request anti-Müllerian hormone (AMH) and inhibin B.
For patients with a DSD that remains undiagnosed,
- consider panel/WES/WGS as available (Eggers *et al.* 2016).

Some diagnoses to consider

Congenital adrenal hyperplasia (CAH)
The most common cause of ambiguous genitalia in infants with a 46,XX karyotype. See 'Congenital adrenal hyperplasia (CAH)' in Chapter 3, 'Common consultations', p. 370.

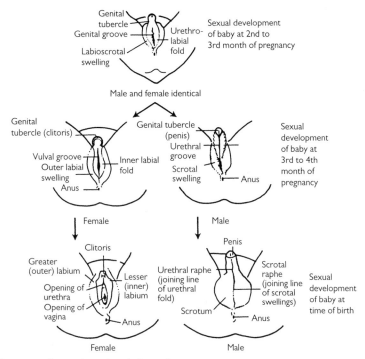

Figure 2.1 Differentiation of external genitalia in the human fetus.
Reproduced with permission from Judith G. Hall JG, Froster-Iskenius UG, and Allanson JE, *Handbook of Normal Physical Measurements*,
Figure 10.1, page 315, Copyright © 1989 Oxford University Press, New York, USA. www.oup.com.

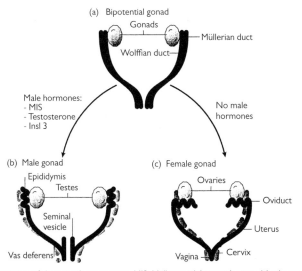

Figure 2.2 Sexual differentiation of the reproductive system. MIS, Müllerian inhibiting substance (also known as anti-Müllerian
hormone (AMH); Insl 3; insulin-like growth factor 3.
Reprinted by permission from Macmillan Publishers Ltd: *Nature Reviews Genetics*, Akio Kobayashi and Richard R. Behringer,
Developmental genetics of the female reproductive tract in mammals, volume 4, issue 12, p 969–80, copyright 2003.

Smith–Lemli–Opitz (SLO) disorder

An AR disorder caused by deficiency of 7-dehydro-cholesterol reductase (*DHCR7*). Males may have hypo-spadias, micropenis, and undescended testes, and also Y-shaped 2/3 syndactyly, microcephaly, cleft palate, congenital heart disease (CHD), developmental delay, etc. See 'Hypospadias' in Chapter 2, 'Clinical approach', p. 186.

Campomelic dysplasia (SOX9—an SRY-related gene on 17q23-ter)

Often *de novo* AD mutations. Bowing of the femur and tibia, narrow chest, short first metacarpals, and sex reversal in the majority of 46,XY infants. Cleft palate is common and one-third have CHD.

WAGR (Wilms tumour–aniridia–genitourinary anomalies–(mental) retardation)

A contiguous gene syndrome due to microscopic or submicroscopic interstitial deletion of 11p13. Specific FISH probes available. See 'Wilms tumour' in Chapter 4, 'Cancer', p. 620.

Drash syndrome or Wilms tumour and pseudohermaphroditism

Caused by mutations in the Wilms tumour receptor gene *WT1* that abolish DNA-binding capacity. Features are ambiguous genitalia, early-onset hypertension, and pro-teinuria with nephritic syndrome and mesangial sclerosis leading to progressive renal failure. See 'Wilms tumour' in Chapter 4, 'Cancer', p. 620.

Frasier syndrome

Ambiguous genitalia and nephropathy as for Drash syndrome, with low risk of Wilms tumour, but risk of gonadoblastoma. Due to dominant mutations causing defective alternative splicing of *WTI* (Klamt *et al.* 1998). See 'Wilms tumour' in Chapter 4, 'Cancer', p. 620.

5β-reductase deficiency

An AR defect in the testosterone biosynthetic pathway that converts testosterone to the more potent androgen DHT. Mutations in this gene can cause perineoscrotal hypospadias. In some instances, the genitalia may appear female, with a diagnosis made at puberty after presentation with primary amenorrhoea, lack of breast development, and deepening voice.

17β-hydroxysteroid dehydrogenase (17β-HSD) deficiency

An AR biosynthetic defect that impairs conversion of androstenedione to testosterone in the fetal testis. Defects in this conversion lead to a male form of DSD with gynaecomastia. The *HSD 17β3* gene maps to 9q22, and ambiguous genitalia are seen in 9q22 deletions.

Partial androgen insensitivity syndrome (PAIS)

Caused by mutations in the androgen receptor gene (*AR*) which impair androgen binding and signalling. See 'Androgen insensitivity syndrome (AIS)' in Chapter 3, 'Common consultations', p. 344.

Deletion of 9p24.3 or 10q26

Deletion of distal 9p has been reported in a number of cases to be associated with gonadal dysgenesis and XY sex reversal. This region contains the testis determining genes *DMR1* and *DMR2* (Raymond *et al.* 1999). Terminal 10q deletions appear to be associated with abnormal male genital development (Wilkie *et al.* 1993).

Genetic advice

Recurrence risk

Counsel for the specific diagnosis.

Carrier detection

Counsel for the specific diagnosis.

Prenatal diagnosis

Counsel for the specific diagnosis.

Natural history and further management (preventative measures)

If the genitalia are truly ambiguous, the issue of gender assignment needs to be discussed with a DSD team. Minto *et al.* (2003) have questioned whether surgical intervention in infancy is the best management or whether a more conservative approach should be followed initially, deferring surgery to allow the individual themselves to be actively involved in decisions that have such a profound effect on their own future (see also Reiner and Gearhart 2004). It is crucial to work with a specialist team at a tertiary referral centre.

Dysgenetic gonads should be removed because of the risk of gonadoblastoma.

Sex reversal

Complete discordance between the phenotypic and karyotypic sex. Usually comes to light when there is a discrepancy between the karyotypic sex reported from CVS/amniocentesis and the sex subsequently identified by prenatal USS or assessment of the newborn. Possibilities include:

• maternal contamination of CVS/amniocentesis (the most likely cause);
• sample mix-up;
• true discordance between phenotypic and genetic sex, as in XX males and XY females (rare);
• chimerism from twin or lost twin (rare).

Previous bone marrow transplantation (BMT) from a donor of the opposite sex may also give discrepant results between the phenotypic sex and the karyotypic sex, as determined by a blood sample (lymphocytes), and may sometimes come to light during the investigation of infertility.

XX males

Prevalence is 1/20 000. This is usually due to:

• cryptic translocations involving *SRY*-bearing Y material and the X chromosomes (FISH for *SRY*);
• mosaicism for XX and cell lines involving Y chromosome material;
• true XX hermaphroditism where both testicular and ovarian tissues persist (findings are variable but may have an ovary on one side and a testis on the other) may be due to mosaicism or chimerism or to mutations in genes in the pathway downstream of *SRY*.

XY females

• *SRY* mutations or deletions of *SRY* (explains only 15–20% of XY females).
• Complete AIS (see 'Androgen insensitivity syndrome (AIS)' in Chapter 3, 'Common consultations', p. 344).
• Camptomelic dysplasia (see above).
• 9p24 monosomy can cause abnormalities of testicular development.

- dup Xp21.2-p22.2 can cause female differentiation—dosage-sensitive sex reversal.
- Approximately 80% of XY females with gonadal dysgenesis are of unknown aetiology; often have uterus and streak gonads.

Support groups: Androgen Insensitivity Syndrome Support Group, http://www.aissg.org; Adrenal Hyperplasia Network, http://www.ahn.org.uk.

Expert adviser: Carlo Acerini, University Senior Lecturer, Department of Paediatrics, University of Cambridge, Addenbrooke's Hospital, Cambridge, UK.

References

Eggers S, Sadedin S et al. Disorders of sex development: insights from targeted gene sequencing of a large international patient cohort. *Genome Biol* 2016 Nov 29; **17**: 243.

Hall JG, Froster-Iskenius UG, Allanson JE. *Handbook of normal physical measurements.* Oxford University Press, Oxford, 1989.

Hughes IA. Female development—all by default? *N Engl J Med* 2004; **351**: 748–50.

Klamt B, Koziell A, Poulat F, et al. Frasier syndrome is caused by defective alternative splicing of *WT1* leading to an altered ratio of *WT1* +/− KTS splice isoforms. *Hum Mol Genet* 1998; **7**: 709–14.

Kobayashi A, Behringer RR. Developmental genetics of the female reproductive tract in mammals. *Nat Rev Genet* 2003; **4**: 969–80.

MacLaughlin DT, Donahoe PK. Mechanisms of disease: sex determination and differentiation. *N Engl J Med* 2004; **350**: 367–78.

Minto CL, Liao LM, Woodhouse CR, Ransley PG, Creighton SM. The effect of clitoral surgery on sexual outcome in individuals who have intersex conditions with ambiguous genitalia: a cross-sectional study. *Lancet* 2003; **361**: 1252–7.

Raymond CS, Parker ED, Kettlewell JR, et al. A region of human chromosome 9p required for testis development contains two genes related to known sexual regulators. *Hum Mol Gen* 1999; **8**: 989–96.

Reiner WG, Gearhart JP. Discordant sexual identity in some genetic males with cloacal exstrophy assigned to female sex at birth. *N Engl J Med* 2004; **350**: 333–41.

Simpson JL. Special issue: Sex determination and sex differentiation in humans. *Am J Med Genet C* 1999; **89C**: 175–248.

Wilkie AO, Campbell FM, Daubeney P, et al. Complete and partial XY sex reversal associated with terminal deletion of 10q: report of 2 cases and literature review. *Am J Med Genet* 1993; **46**: 567–600.

Anal anomalies (atresia, stenosis)

Anal anomalies affect 4/10 000 births (see Figure 2.3). Only one-third are isolated anomalies; two-thirds occur with other anomalies. Most anorectal anomalies result from abnormal development of the urorectal septum, resulting in incomplete separation of the cloaca into urogenital and anorectal portions. In the London Dysmorphology Database (LDDB) (Winter and Baraitser 2003), anal atresia/stenosis is a feature of 135 syndromes. Anal atresia also occurs in some chromosomal disorders (including trisomies). Of isolated anal anomalies, 75% are atresias, of which 10% are above and 90% below the level of the levator ani muscle ('high' and 'low' atresias). There is a predominance of males. The male-to-female (M:F) ratio for high lesions is 6.7, and for low lesions it is 2.3. Findings on examination are absence of the anus or abnormal placement of the anus. Other anal anomalies include congenital anal fistula (15%), ectopic anus (3%), and persistent cloaca (1%). Heij et al. (1996) undertook routine lumbosacral MRI in patients presenting with anorectal malformations and identified anomalies in 30% of those with low anorectal malformations and in 50% of those with high malformations. These included caudal regression syndrome, tethered cord, and other spinal anomalies.

Abnormalities of the external genitalia are often found in association with anal anomalies. In Heij et al.'s study, urogenital anomalies were found in 49% of patients presenting with anorectal malformation.

Clinical approach

History: key points

- Three-generation family tree, including specific enquiry regarding surgery in the neonatal period and history of colostomy.
- History of maternal diabetes and early bleeding.
- Feeding difficulties; any evidence of tracheo-oesophageal fistula (TOF) or laryngeal cleft.
- Floppy baby, delayed motor milestones, or developmental delay (syndromes and chromosomal abnormalities).
- Visual or hearing problems (cat-eye syndrome (CES), Townes–Brock syndrome (TBS)).

Examination: key points

- Carefully describe the anus and external genitalia and photograph prior to surgery.
- Bladder exstrophy (omphalocele–exstrophy of the cloaca–imperforate anus–spinal defects, OEIS; see 'Some diagnoses to consider' below).
- Look carefully for other dysmorphic features, but some, such as the anterior cowlicks of FG syndrome, are age-dependent.
- Carefully assess the external ear (TBS).
- Hypertelorism (Opitz G). Examine the heart (VACTERL (vertebral defects–anal atresia–cardiac anomalies–tracheo-oesophageal fistula–(o)esophageal atresia–renal anomalies–limb defects); see 'Some diagnoses to consider' below).
- Examine the limbs: thumb deficiency, occasionally duplication, and radial ray anomalies (VACTERL), triphalangeal or hypoplastic thumbs (TBS), polydactyly (Pallister–Hall syndrome).

Special investigations

- Genomic analysis in presence of features suggestive of a chromosomal or syndromic diagnosis, e.g. genomic array, gene panel, or WES/WGS as appropriate.
- X-rays of the spine, sacrum, pelvis, and chest (VACTERL).
- Consider lumbosacral MRI.
- Renal USS (genitourinary anomalies constitute 49% of associated anomalies).
- Additional radiology if a fistula is suspected.
- Echocardiogram (echo) (cardiovascular anomalies constitute 27% of associated anomalies).
- Endocrine referral (Pallister–Hall syndrome).
- DNA analysis/storage for panel/WES/WGS as available.

Some diagnoses to consider

VATER/VACTERL association

Incidence 1.6/10 000. Most children usually have 3–4 features present. Hall et al. (1989) suggest at least one anomaly from the limb, thorax, and pelvis/lower abdomen for a secure diagnosis and at least two anomalies in each of two of those regions for a probable diagnosis. Normal or near normal cognitive development expected. Usually sporadic with low recurrence risk. Chromosome 16q24.1 and 2q31.1 microdeletions may be associated with the VATER/VACTERL phenotype. The 16q24 deletion may rarely also have alveolar capillary malformation with misalignment of the pulmonary veins (Garci-Barcelo et al. 2008; Stankiewcz et al. 2009). VATER/VACTERL denotes combinations of the following anomalies:

- V, Vertebral defects—usually upper to mid-thoracic and lumbar regions. Usually hemivertebrae, but dyssegmented and fused vertebrae may occur—may be accompanying rib anomalies;
- A, Anal atresia (50–90%)—may be associated with genital defects (hypospadias, bifid scrotum) or fistulae;
- C, Cardiac anomalies—present in ~80%; any type, any severity;
- T, Tracheo-oesophageal fistula;
- E, (O)esophageal atresia—80% have an associated TOF;
- R, Renal anomalies—present in 80%, e.g. renal agenesis/dysplasia;
- L, Limb (radial defects)—preaxial with underdevelopment or agenesis of thumbs and radial bones; usually bilateral defects, but asymmetric. Reduced thenar muscle mass is the mildest end of the spectrum. The lower limbs are not affected.

X-linked VACTERL

Due to mutation of *ZIC3* on Xq26 (Wessels et al. 2010). Some have deletions identifiable on genomic array analysis.

OEIS (omphalocele–exstrophy of the cloaca–imperforate anus–spinal defects)

(Vlangos et al. 2011). Mostly sporadic.

Caudal regression

Most cases of caudal regression are sporadic or associated with maternal diabetes. The condition is thought to

Male

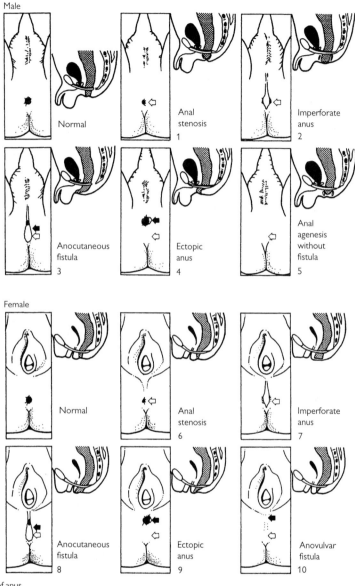

Figure 2.3 Anal anomalies.
Reprinted from *Journal of Pediatric Surgery*, volume 5, issue 3, Thomas V. Santulli, William B. Kiesewetter, Alexander H. Bili, Anorectal anomalies: A suggested international classification, pp. 281–287, Copyright 1970, with permission from Elsevier.

be part of a spectrum, including imperforate anus, sacral agenesis, and sirenomelia.

Currarino syndrome

AD sacral agenesis characterized by a partial agenesis of the sacrum, typically involving the sacral vertebrae S2–S5 only as a hemisacrum. Associated features include anorectal malformation (57%), a presacral mass (64%), and urogenital malformation. See 'Congenital cystic lung lesions, Currarino syndrome, and sacrococcygeal teratoma' in Chapter 6, 'Pregnancy and fertility', p. 712. Caused by dominant mutations in the *MNX1* gene (Merello *et al.* 2013).

Townes–Brock syndrome (TBS)

An AD condition with imperforate anus, hand anomalies (triphalangeal thumb, hypoplastic thumb), and ear malformations (dysplastic ears and ear tags) with sensorineural hearing loss. Within and between families, the phenotype displays striking variability. *SALL1*, a zinc finger transcription factor, is the disease-causing gene. There is a high incidence of new mutations. Cardiac anomalies have been reported.

Cat-eye syndrome (CES)

Anal anomalies (imperforate anus, anal atresia, or anteriorly placed anus), preauricular pits/tags, congenital heart defects, iris colobomata, renal anomalies, and variable learning disability. Results from a small marker chromosome containing a duplication of 22q11 resulting in tetrasomy 22q11. Can be an unbalanced product of the relatively common 11q23;22q11 reciprocal translocation. CES can occur in mosaic form and can also be inherited.

Pallister–Hall syndrome (anocerebrodigital syndrome)

Characterized by imperforate anus, mesoaxial (or post-axial) polydactyly, hypopituitarism, and hypothalamic hamartoblastoma. Some have a cleft larynx or a bifid epiglottis. An AD condition with very variable expression and caused by mutations in *GLI3* on 7p13 (allelic to Greig).

MED-12-related disorders (FG syndrome)

Difficult to diagnose without a strong family history. Hypotonia and constipation are common in infants. There may be a history of rectal biopsy to exclude short-segment Hirschsprung's disease. The anal defects reported are an imperforate, stenotic, and anteriorly placed anus; also perianal skin tags. Agenesis of the corpus callosum may be present. There is macrocephaly with a frontal upsweep of the hair (cowlick). A recurrent mutation R961W is responsible for the classical form of this condition (Risheg et al. 2007).

Opitz syndrome (also known as Opitz G or G/BBB)

Hypospadias is the major anomaly of urorectal development, but imperforate and ectopic anus are reported. There is striking hypertelorism and swallowing problems due to laryngeal clefts. There is an XL and an autosomal (22q) locus. The XL gene is *MID1* at Xp22.

STAR syndrome

Consider in girls with toe syndactyly with renal and anogenital malformation and sometimes telecanthus, due to mutation in the X-linked dominant gene *FAM58A*.

Mabry syndrome (hyperphosphatasia mental retardation syndrome)

An AR disease. Biallelic PIGV mutations are the main cause. Affected individuals may have anorectal anomalies e.g. anteriorly displaced anus or an anal fistula.

Genetic advice

Recurrence risk

After carefully excluding syndromic and chromosomal causes and those with a family history, isolated recto-anal malformations are rarely genetic. Both affected sibs and offspring have been reported, but overall the recurrence risk is about 1%.

Carrier detection

In syndromic cases, clinical examination combined with mutation analysis, if available.

Prenatal diagnosis

PND is possible for some of these conditions on the basis of:

• USS for structural abnormalities;

• chromosomal or mutation analysis if an abnormality has been identified in the proband.

Natural history and further management (preventative measures)

Surgical management

A colostomy is usually performed in the neonatal period with anastomosis at a later stage, depending on the anatomy and prognosis for continence.

Support groups: Many of the individual syndromes have their own support groups. See Contact a Family (UK), http://www.cafamily.org.uk and National Organization for Rare Disorders (USA), http://www.rarediseases.org.

Expert adviser: David Mowat, Clinical Geneticist, Centre for Clinical Genetics, Sydney Children's Hospital, Sydney, Australia.

References

Cho S, Moore SP, Fangman T. One hundred three consecutive patients with anorectal malformations and their associated anomalies. *Arch Pediatr Adolesc Med* 2001; **155**: 587–91.

Cuschieri A, EUROCAT Working Group. Descriptive epidemiology of isolated anal anomalies: a survey of 4.6 million births in Europe. *Am J Med Genet* 2001; **103**: 207–15.

Garci-Barcelo MM, Wong KK, Lui VC, et al. Identification of a *HOXD13* mutation in a VACTERL patient. *Am J Med Genet A* 2008; **146A**: 3181–5.

Hall JG, Froster-Iskenius UG, Allanson JE. *Handbook of normal physical measurements*. Oxford University Press, Oxford, 1989.

Heij HA, Nievelstein RA, de Zwart I, Verbeeten BW, Valk J, Vos A. Abnormal anatomy of the lumbosacral region imaged by magnetic resonance in children with anorectal malformations. *Arch Dis Child* 1996; **74**: 441–4.

Merello E, De Marco P, Raveegnani M, et al. Novel *MNX1* mutations and clinical analysis of familial and sporadic Currarino cases. *Eur J Med Genet* 2013; **56**: 648–54.

Risheg H, Graham JM Jr, Clark RD, et al. A recurrent mutation in *MED12* leading to R961W causes Opitz-Kaveggia syndrome. *Nat Genet* 2007; **39**: 451–3.

Santulli TV, Kiesewetter WB, Bill AH Jr. Anorectal anomalies: a suggested international classification. *J Pediatr Surg* 1970; **5**: 281–7.

Stankiewicz P, Sen P, Bhatt SS, et al. Genomic and genic deletions of the *FOX* gene cluster on 16q24.1 and inactivation mutations of *FOXF1* cause alveolar capillary dysplasia and other malformations. *Am J Med Genet* 2009; **84**: 780–91.

Vlangos CN, Siuniak A, Ackley T, et al. Comprehensive genetic analysis of OEIS complex reveals no evidence for a recurrent microdeletion or duplication. *Am J Med Genet A* 2011; **155A**: 38–49.

Wessels MW, Kuchinka B, Heydanus R, et al. Polyalanine expansion in the *ZIC3* gene leading to X-linked heterotaxy with VACTERL association: a new polyalanine disorder? *J Med Genet* 2010; **47**: 351–5.

Winter RM, Baraitser M. *London dysmorphology database*. London Medical Databases, London, 2003.

Anterior segment eye malformations

The cornea, iris, and trabecular meshwork together comprise the anterior segment of the eye (see Figure 2.4). Developmentally these structures are interdependent and, while gene expression may be spatially localized to one tissue, altered development of one structure can influence and disrupt the development of other components of the anterior segment.

There is a wide range of phenotypes associated with altered anterior segment development. While many of these are recognized clinically (e.g. Peters anomaly, Rieger anomaly), they do not necessarily represent different genetic or biological entities. In addition to such phenotypic heterogeneity, there is considerable allele heterogeneity among anterior segment phenotypes. For example, truncating mutations in *PAX6* have been found in aniridia, whereas missense mutations in the paired box domain are found in some cases of Peters anomaly. Lastly there is also genetic heterogeneity with similar phenotypes ascribed to mutations in different genes—for example, Peters anomaly may be caused by mutations in *PAX6, MAF, PITX2*, and *CYP1B1*. In approaching genetic counselling, precise phenotypic characterization and bilateral involvement may only be detected after careful examination of the apparently normal eye by an ophthalmologist.

A child may be referred to the geneticist for counselling after the identification of an anterior segment anomaly. The aim is to determine whether this is a purely ocular condition or if there are non-ocular features that suggest a syndrome diagnosis.

Clinical approach

History: key points

- Family history. At least three generations. Enquire about consanguinity. Ask about all visual difficulties. Affected individuals may be minimally affected.
- Exposure to teratogens and infections during pregnancy.
- Growth (most chromosomal conditions show poor growth; Rieger syndrome is associated with pituitary abnormalities).
- Developmental progress (allowing for visual difficulties).
- Dental history.
- Wilms tumour (WAGR: Wilms tumour–aniridia–genitourinary anomalies (hypospadias and cryptorchidism)–mental retardation).

Examination: key points

- Eye. Examination and photography of the eye and surrounding structures (usually performed by the ophthalmologist). Anomalies detected may include: aniridia, sclerocornea, megalocornea, microphthalmia, and/or lens abnormality. Ensure that patients are screened for glaucoma.
- Growth parameters (height, weight, and occipital–frontal circumference (OFC)):
  - short stature in Peters plus syndrome, SHORT syndrome, and Rieger syndrome.
- Face and mouth:
  - orofacial clefts (Peters plus syndrome, Kivlin syndrome);
  - abnormal dentition (Rieger syndrome).

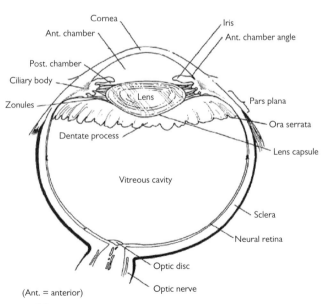

Figure 2.4 Anterior segment of the eye.
Reproduced with permission from Paul Dodson, *Diabetic Retinopathy: Screening to Treatment*, Figure 3.1, page 18, Copyright © 2008 Oxford University Press, New York, USA. www.oup.com.

- Skin:
  - lipoatrophy (SHORT syndrome);
  - patchy skin lesions with sclerocornea (Goltz syndrome, del Xp22);
  - redundant skin in the umbilicus (Rieger syndrome).
- Genitalia:
  - hypospadias and cryptorchidism in WAGR; hypospadias in Rieger syndrome.
- Neurological:
  - cerebellar ataxia (Gillespie syndrome);
  - olfaction abnormalities may be found with *PAX6* mutations.

Special investigations

- Genomic analysis in presence of features suggestive of a chromosomal or syndromic diagnosis, e.g. genomic array, gene panel, or WES/WGS as available.
- Store DNA for possible genetic testing.
- Renal USS in children with aniridia who have 11p–syndrome of loss of *WT1* suppressor gene on FISH, or mutations in *WT1*.
- Consider brain imaging (*PAX6* and Rieger syndrome).

Some diagnoses to consider

Peters anomaly

Defined as corneal opacification associated with lens–cornea or lens–iris adhesions.

Absence of the central corneal endothelium and Descemet's membrane leads to congenital central corneal opacities; 80% are bilateral but may be very asymmetrical. Lens abnormalities and microphthalmia are common. Associated glaucoma is extremely common.

- Ensure an array is performed if there are other congenital anomalies or developmental delay.
- If short stature and clefts, consider Peters plus/Kivlin syndrome (AR due to a disorder of glycosylation and caused by biallelic mutation in *B3GALTL*).
- Mutations of *PAX6* (aniridia gene), *PITX2* (Axenfeld–Rieger syndromes), and *CYP1B1* (congenital glaucoma) have been identified in some individuals. Hence recessive and dominant inheritance are both reported in isolated Peters anomaly.

Axenfeld–Rieger syndromes

A number of previously distinct eye phenotypes have now been grouped together under the heading of Axenfeld–Rieger malformation syndromes to eliminate arbitrary and confusing subclassification. They are associated with dominant mutation in the transcription factor genes *FOXC1* and *PITX2*. There are also loci on 13q14 and 16q24. Most Axenfeld–Rieger syndromes have AD inheritance. There is a ~50% risk of developing glaucoma.

Although now grouped together, the following may help in interpreting the literature:

- Axenfeld anomaly: defects limited to the peripheral anterior segment;
- Rieger anomaly: defects of the peripheral anterior segment and changes in the iris;
- Rieger syndrome: eye abnormalities and non-ocular defects (dental anomalies, midface hypoplasia, redundant periumbilical skin, hypospadias, and pituitary abnormalities):
  - type 1 Rieger syndrome: *RIEG1* mutations have been found in both *FOXC1* and *PITX2*;
  - type 2 Rieger syndrome: *RIEG2* is linked to 13q14. No gene identified;
  - posterior embryotoxon and Axenfeld anomaly can be found in apparently normal mutation carriers of Peters anomaly, and Alagille syndrome.

SHORT SYNDROME. Is the association of Rieger anomaly with short stature, deep-set eyes, and lipoatrophy. Previously thought to be AR, recent reports suggest AD inheritance is more likely.

Aniridia

One in 60–100 000 population frequency. Associated eye anomalies may include: corneal and lens opacities, cataract, foveal hypoplasia (100%), optic nerve hypoplasia, and glaucoma. Sixty-five per cent are familial (AD); extremely variable both within and between families.

- Arrange for examination of parents of sporadic cases. Such a genomic array or karyotype will screen for 11p13 deletions (WAGR locus) in *all* sporadic and familial cases. Using a panel of cosmids, encompassing the aniridia-associated *PAX6* gene, the Wilms tumour predisposition gene *WT1*, and flanking markers, in distal chromosome 11p13 to exclude a submicroscopic deletion (Crolla and van Heyningen 2002) found a high frequency (~40%) of chromosomal rearrangements in a cohort of 77 patients with sporadic and familial aniridia. Ensure follow-up and screening for Wilms tumour risk if a deletion is present.
- *PAX6* gene mutations at 11p13 causes aniridia. Where required, arrange mutation analysis. Prenatal diagnosis may be possible if the mutation is identified, but this is seldom requested. Counsel that this would not give guidance as to the clinical manifestations.

GILLESPIE SYNDROME. Aniridia plus cerebellar ataxia and intellectual disability caused by a restricted repertoire of dominant mutations in the ITPR1 gene.

Corneal malformations

MEGALOCORNEA. Defined as a cornea of ≥13 mm at birth, but which is still clear with normal other parameters. Exclude buphthalmos (congenital glaucoma) where the cornea is hazy. Developmental delay, cerebellar abnormalities, and short stature with megalocornea is sometimes known as Neuhauser syndrome and inherited as AR. Megalocornea can follow an XL, or occasionally a dominant, pattern of inheritance. XL megalocornea is caused by mutations in *CHRDL1* (Webb et al. 2012).

SCLEROCORNEA. A congenital non-progressive corneal opacification with vascularization and can be associated with glaucoma. It is commonly found in conjunction with other abnormalities of the anterior segment such as Peters anomaly, microphthalmia, coloboma, and cataract formation, and also in hypomelanosis of Ito and IP. It is a feature of del Xp22 in females who also have linear skin pigmentation on the face and neck. Sclerocornea in its mildest form is just peripheral corneal opacification but, if more extensive, is sometimes referred to as microcornea (see 'Microcornea' below).

MICROCORNEA. The cornea is <9–10 mm in diameter at birth. It may be associated with a normal-sized globe on ultrasound or microphthalmia. It may follow AD/AR inheritance. Microcornea may be a feature of Nance–Horan syndrome (XLR). See 'Cataract' in Chapter 2, 'Clinical approach', p. 88.

CORNEAL CLOUDING The cornea is opacified. It is important to exclude glaucoma (and rubella embryopathy in centres where this is common). Many of the causes are progressive metabolic conditions, rather than malformations. See 'Corneal clouding' in Chapter 2, 'Clinical approach', p. 120.

Genetic advice

Recurrence risk

- Arrange parental ophthalmological assessment of the anterior segment. Variability is well described for most of the anterior segment disorders and parents may have subtle features that are only detectable on careful assessment by a specialist.
- Check the literature for recent gene localizations. At present, known genes include *PAX6, PITX2, PITX3, FOXC1,* and *CHX10.* Most are transcription factor genes with AD inheritance. *CYP1B1* has been found to be a cause of AR congenital glaucoma and rarely Peters anomaly.

Carrier detection

- By ophthalmological examination.
- Is possible in families where a causative mutation has been identified.

Prenatal diagnosis

- By genetic testing where there is molecular or chromosomal confirmation of diagnosis.
- USS in mid trimester can visualize the eye and lens but is unlikely to be sensitive enough to detect recurrence.

Natural history and further management (preventative measures)

Long-term ophthalmological follow-up is indicated, particularly to screen for glaucoma.

Support groups: Many of the individual syndromes have their own support groups. See Contact a Family (UK), http://www.cafamily.org.uk and National Organization for Rare Disorders (USA), http://www.rarediseases.org.

Expert adviser: Graeme Black, Strategic Director, Manchester Centre for Genomic Medicine, Institute of Human Development, University of Manchester and Central Manchester University Hospitals NHS Foundation Trust, Manchester Academic Health Sciences Centre, St. Mary's Hospital, Manchester, UK.

References

Alward WL. Axenfeld–Rieger syndrome in the age of molecular genetics. *Am J Ophthalmol* 2000; **130**: 107–15.

Crolla JA, van Heyningen V. Frequent chromosome aberrations revealed by molecular cytogenetic studies in patients with aniridia. *Am J Hum Genet* 2002; **71**: 1138–49.

Traboulsi EI. Malformations of the anterior segment of the eye. In: EI Traboulsi (ed.). *Genetic diseases of the eye,* 2nd edn, pp. 81–98. New York, Oxford University Press, 1998.

Gregory-Evans K. Developmental disorders of the eye. In: A Moore (ed.). *Paediatric ophthalmology, fundamentals of clinical ophthalmology series,* pp. 53–61. BMJ Books, London, 2000.

Lesnik Oberstein, SA, Kriek M, White SJ, et al. Peters plus syndrome is caused by mutations in *B3GALTL*, a putative glycosyltransferase. *Am J Hum Genet* 2006; **79**: 562–6.

Lines MA, Kozlowski K, Walter MA. Molecular genetics of Axenfeld–Rieger malformations. *Hum Mol Genet* 2002; **11**: 1177–84.

McEntagart M, Williamson KA et al. A restricted repertoire of de novo mutations in ITPR1 cause Gillespie syndrome with evidence for dominant-negative effect. *Am J Hum Genet* 2016; **98**: 981–992.

Schimmenti LA, de la Cruz J, Lewis RA, et al. Novel mutations in sonic hedgehog in non-syndromic colobomatous microphthalmia. *Am J Med Genet A* 2003; **116A**: 215–21.

Van Heyningen V, Williamson KA. *PAX6* in sensory development. *Hum Mol Genet* 2002; **11**: 1161–7.

Webb TR, Matarin M, Gardner JC, et al. X-linked megalocornea caused by mutations in *CHDRL1* identifies an essential role for ventropin in anterior segment development. *Am J Hum Genet* 2012; **90**: 247–2011.

Arthrogryposis

See also 'Fetal akinesia' in Chapter 6, 'Pregnancy and fertility', p. 724.

Arthrogryposis is a term used to describe multiple congenital joint contractures (usually non-progressive) that are associated with lack of fetal movement *in utero*. Its incidence is 1/3000 live births (see Figure 2.5). In general, more than one type of joint is involved—bilateral talipes in the absence of other joint involvement does not constitute arthrogryposis. Any condition that causes decreased fetal movement may lead to congenital contractures. The genetic basis of many of the arthrogryposis syndromes is now known.

Some types of arthrogryposis result from unique spatiotemporal patterns of expression of sarcomeric proteins in embryonic and fetal life. Distal arthrogryposis (DA) syndromes are the most common of the heritable congenital contracture disorders, and ~50% of cases are known to be caused by mutations in genes that encode contractile proteins of skeletal myofibres. Amyoplasia (see Figure 2.6) is one of the most common forms of generalized arthrogryposis and usually occurs sporadically.

Children of myasthenic mothers can have arthrogryposis and features of the fetal akinesia sequence, due to maternal transmission of antibodies of the acetylcholine receptor (AChR) to the fetus. Studies of children with a similar phenotype, but no maternal antibodies, lead to the discovery of recessive mutations in the embryonal AChR g subunit (*CHRNG*). A continuum of conditions has been shown to be due to mutations in endplate-specific presynaptic, synaptic, and post-synaptic proteins. Complete or severe functional disruption of fetal AChR causes lethal multiple pterygium syndrome, whereas milder alterations result in fetal hypokinesia with contractures or a myasthenic syndrome later in life (Michalk *et al.* 2008). Non-lethal multiple pterygium syndrome is also known as Escobar syndrome.

Arthrogryposis is immensely heterogeneous, and achieving a specific diagnosis is often difficult (possible in 50% after careful assessment). During clinical assessment, try to classify your patient into one or more of the following aetiological groups:
- muscle (5–10%), e.g. congenital myopathy, congenital myasthenia;
- neurological (90%), e.g. CNS anomaly;
- abnormal connective tissue, e.g. diastrophic dysplasia;
- uterine constraint, e.g. bicornuate uterus, twins;
- maternal illness, e.g. myasthenia, myotonic dystrophy, fever >39°C;
- environmental, e.g. early amniocentesis (<14 gestational weeks); drugs, e.g. misoprostol.

Clinical approach
History: key points
- Three-generation family tree. Enquire specifically for club-feet, joint dislocation, congenital hip dislocation, contractures, hyperextensibility.
- Enquire about maternal illness (myotonic dystrophy, myasthenia gravis, diabetes mellitus, etc.) and uterine anomaly.
- Detailed pregnancy history. Enquire about infection and fever (>39°C), fetal movement, polyhydramnios (may be secondary to poor fetal swallowing), oligohydramnios, or amniotic fluid leak.
- Detailed history of the delivery, e.g. abnormal presentation or difficulty in delivery due to fixed joints; fracture may occur (5–10%).

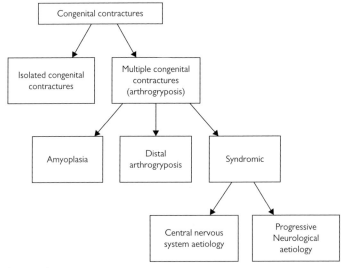

Figure 2.5 Types of congenital contractures.
Reproduced from M Bamshad *et al.*, Arthrogryposis: A Review and Update, *Journal of Bone and Joint Surgery*, 91, Supplement 4, pp. 40–46, Copyright 2009, with permission from The British Editorial Society of Bone & Joint Surgery.

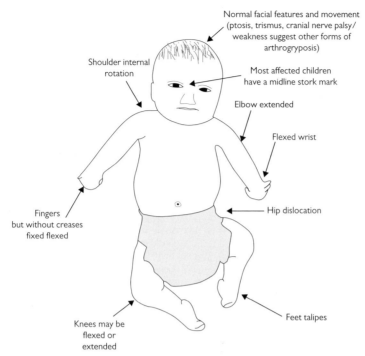

Figure 2.6 Child with amyoplasia. Sketch showing internal rotation of the shoulders, extended elbows, and flexed wrists. Fingers are flexed over the thumbs and are difficult to open. The hips may be dislocated; the knees may be flexed or extended, and the feet often show severe talipes equinovarus. Most children have symmetrical limb involvement.

- Detailed history of the limb position of the baby after delivery (obtain photos if available).

Examination: key points
- Photographs are extremely helpful in documenting the position of contractures at birth, as well as over time.
- Examine the rest position and the range of passive and active movements in each joint—take great care to avoid causing a fracture!
- Ulnar deviation of fingers is often present in distal arthrogryposis.
- Document carefully which joints are involved, including the jaw and spine (this may be helpful in achieving a specific diagnosis).
- Look for skin dimples overlying contractures and document flexion creases.
- Look for skin webs across joints with joint limitation.
- Examine for limitation of jaw opening (trismus). NB. Intubation.
- Detailed neurological assessment—level of alertness, tone, reflexes.
- Feel muscle texture (fibrous band, firm, soft).
- Examine carefully for other anomalies, e.g. cleft palate or jaundice (arthrogryposis multiplex congenita, renal dysfunction, and neonatal cholestasis (ARC) syndrome).
- Examine both parents carefully for joint contractures and lack of flexion creases.
- Examine the mother for features of myotonic dystrophy or myasthenia.

Special investigations
- Genomic analysis in presence of features suggestive of a chromosomal or syndromic diagnosis, e.g. genomic array, gene panel, or WES/WGS as available (if the child has developmental delay and deep furrows on the palms/soles, consider skin biopsy for trisomy 8).
- Store DNA (the list of arthrogryposis syndromes for which the causative gene has been defined is growing rapidly).
- Consider hip USS in the neonate if clinical suspicion of hip involvement.
- Consider TORCH (toxoplasmosis, other (including syphilis, varicella-zoster, parvovirus), rubella, cytomegalovirus, and herpes simplex virus) screen if neonate or <6 months old; include viral studies for enterovirus and Coxsackie.
- Consider CK if clinical assessment compatible with primary muscle aetiology.
- Consider electromyography (EMG) and nerve conduction velocity (NCV) tests to clarify whether lower motor neuron involvement or primary muscle pathology is likely.
- Consider muscle biopsy if primary muscle pathology seems likely (biopsy both involved and apparently uninvolved muscle and do electron microscopy (EM) and multiple stains).
- Consider radiographs if suspicion of chondrodysplasia or other skeletal dysplasia.

- Consider muscle USS/MRI of an affected limb if considering diagnosis of amyoplasia (muscle is replaced by fat/fibrous tissue).
- Consider cranial MRI scan if CNS involvement with normal chromosomes.
- Consider testing the mother for myotonic dystrophy (DNA for triplet repeat expansion).
- Consider testing the mother for myasthenia (anticholinesterase receptor antibodies). Rarely, the mother generates antibodies against the fetal receptor which affect the fetus in the absence of maternal disease. Inexpensive test, positive in 1–2% of mothers ascertained through a single affected infant (Polizzi et al. 2000).

For lethal forms of arthrogryposis, an autopsy with detailed neuropathology and muscle biopsy and storage of DNA will offer the best chance of making a specific diagnosis.

Some diagnoses to consider

Fetal akinesia deformation sequence (FADS)

A descriptive diagnosis of a usually lethal condition with multiple joint contractures, pulmonary hypoplasia, micrognathia, intrauterine growth retardation (IUGR), short umbilical cord, and polyhydramnios. A consequence (deformation) of severely reduced fetal movement. Includes the multiple pterygium syndromes and lethal congenital contractural syndromes. See 'Fetal akinesia' in Chapter 6, 'Pregnancy and fertility', p. 724).

Amyoplasia

'Classical arthrogryposis'. The most common condition with severe multiple congenital contractures (one-third of all cases). Characterized by very specific positioning with symmetrical limb involvement. Muscle tissue is replaced by fibrous bands/fatty tissue; firmly fixed joints with a fusiform shape to the limbs in the neonate. Flexion creases shallow/absent. Feet in equinovarus, wrists flexed, shoulders internally rotated, elbows in fixed extension at birth but may later develop some flexion with growth. Hips may be flexed or extended and are often dislocated. Knees fixed in extension/flexion. No sensory loss. Deep dimples often present over joints. Vascular birthmarks over midface are common. Mild syndactyly is often found. Normal intelligence quotient (IQ). There is an increase of bowel atresia and gastroschisis in amyoplasia. Fifteen per cent have some vascular compromise of the digits. Sporadic (possibly due to vascular disruption). Increased occurrence in one of MZ twins. Recurrence risk <1%.

Distal arthrogryposis type 1

AD with marked variability characterized largely by camptodactyly and club-foot. Characteristic positioning of the hands (+18 like with clenched fist and overlapping fingers) in the newborn period with primarily distal contractures of the limbs. Responds well to physiotherapy and generally improves with time. Feet may be in equinovarus or calcaneovalgus. Both hand and foot anomalies appear to be due to misplaced tendons. Causative genes include TNN12, TNT3, TPM2, and MYBPC1.

Distal arthrogryposis type 2A (Freeman–Sheldon syndrome, FSS) and 2B (Sheldon–Hall syndrome)

Can be caused by mutations in the gene MYH3 (Toydemir et al. 2006). FSS was the proof of concept to show that candidate genes for Mendelian disorders can be identified by exome sequencing of a small number of unrelated affected individuals (Ng et al. 2009).

Congenital contractural arachnodactyly (CCA, Beal's syndrome)

An AD disorder characterized by congenital contractures, long thin extremities, crumpled ear helix, and kyphoscoliosis. May have cardiac involvement, e.g. mitral valve prolapse (MVP), but generally less severe than in MFS. Due to mutations in fibrillin 2 (FBN2).

Multiple pterygium syndromes

Webbing (pterygia) of the neck, elbows, and/or knees and arthrogryposis. They are phenotypically and genetically heterogeneous but are traditionally divided into prenatally lethal and non-lethal (Escobar) types (Vogt et al. 2008).

Cerebro-oculo-facial-skeletal syndrome (COFS)

A lethal condition with contractures, microcephaly, structural brain anomalies, microphthalmia/cataracts. Some are due to mutations in DNA repair genes, as in Cockayne. See 'DNA repair disorders' in Chapter 3, 'Common consultations', p. 398.

Arthrogryposis multiplex congenita–spinal muscular atrophy association

Approximately 50% are homozygous for SMN deletions. Most SMN abnormalities are hypotonic at birth. Larger deletions of 5q are associated with contractures. See 'Spinal muscular atrophy (SMA)' in Chapter 3, 'Common consultations', p. 526.

XL spinal muscular atrophy

Leads to death in early infancy. Arthrogryposis, hypotonia, absent reflexes, loss of anterior horn cells. Mutations in the UBE1 gene of the ubiquitin–proteasome pathway. Consider testing when the features and investigations suggest SMA (see 'Spinal muscular atrophy (SMA)' in Chapter 3, 'Common consultations', p. 526), but SMN MLPA testing is normal and there is evidence for XL inheritance. There are several other types of XL arthrogryposis.

Arthrogryposis multiplex congenita, renal dysfunction, and neonatal cholestasis (ARC) syndrome

An AR condition characterized by arthrogryposis and cholestasis with bile duct hypoplasia (see 'Prolonged neonatal jaundice and jaundice in infants below 6 months' in Chapter 2, 'Clinical approach', p. 288).

Schaaf-yang syndrome

Truncating variants in the maternally imprinted, paternally expressed gene MAGEL2 located in the PWS critical region on 15q11–13. The phenotype overlaps with that of PWS, with developmental delay, hypotonia, feeding difficulties, autism spectrum and in most contractures ranging from fetal akinesia and arthrogryposis multiplex congenita to contractures of the small finger joints (Fountain 2017).

Genetic advice

Recurrence risk

- As for specific diagnosis. If a specific diagnosis is not possible, consider the following:
  - distal forms of arthrogryposis are often AD;
  - in arthrogryposis with CNS involvement, many cases are AR, so the recurrence risk for subsequent pregnancies after one affected child is 10–15%;

- amyoplasia is sporadic with no appreciable recurrence risk; however, care should be used when making this diagnosis and this recurrence risk is given only if there are classical features.

Prenatal diagnosis

PND is possible in many types of arthrogryposis by real-time USS to assess fetal movement. Studies at 16, 20, 24, and 32 weeks are recommended. Care must be taken to look at each major joint for range of movement. Need to discuss the limitations of USS and the small possibility of failure to detect significant joint contracture.

Natural history and further management (preventative measures)

This varies depending on the specific diagnosis. Physiotherapy with passive stretching is often useful (but avoid in diastrophic dysplasia). Surgery may be required as an adjunct to physiotherapy in most children with amyoplasia.

If there is a primary muscle pathology, you need to be cautious about anaesthesia. NB. Multiple pterygium with malignant hyperthermia (scoliosis, torticollis, myopathic facies, cleft palate).

Support groups: The Arthrogryposis Group, http://www.arthrogryposis.co.uk; Arthrogryposis Multiplex Congenita Support, Inc., http://amcsupport.org.

Expert adviser: Judith Hall, Professor Emerita of Paediatrics and Medical Genetics, UBC & Children's and Women's Health Centre of British Columbia, Department of Medical Genetics, British Columbia's Children's Hospital, Vancouver, Canada.

References

Bamshad M, Van Heest AE, Pleasure D. Arthrogryposis: a review and update. *J Bone Joint Surg Am* 2009; **91**(Suppl 4): 40–6.

Fountain MD, Atem E et al. The phenotypic spectrum of Shcaaf-Yang syndrome—18 new affected individuals from 14 families. *Genet Med* 2017; **19**: 45–52.

Hall JG. Arthrogryposes (multiple congenital contractures). In: DL Rimoin, RE Pyeritz, BR Korf (eds.). *Emery and Rimoin's principle and practice of medical genetics*, 6th edn, pp. 1–102. Elsevier, Oxford, 2013.

Hall JG, Aldinger KA, Tanaka KI. Amyoplasia revisited. *Am J Med Genet A* 2014; **164A**: 700–30.

Laugel V, Dalloz C, Tobias ES, et al. Cerebro-oculo-facio-skeletal syndrome: three additional cases with CSB mutations, new diagnostic criteria and an approach to investigation. *J Med Genet* 2008; **45**: 564–71.

Hall JG, Kiefer J. Arthrogryposis as a syndrome: gene ontology analysis. *Mol Syndromology* 2016; **7**: 101–9.

Michalk A, Stricker S, Becker J, et al. Acetylcholine receptor pathway mutations explain various fetal akinesia deformation sequence disorders. *Am J Hum Genet* 2008; **82**: 464–76.

Ng S, Turner EH, Robertson PD, et al. Targeted capture and massively parallel sequencing of 12 human exons. *Nature* 2009; **461**: 272–6.

Polizzi A, Huson SM, Vincent A. Teratogen update: maternal myasthenia gravis as a cause of congenital arthrogryposis. *Teratology* 2000; **62**: 332–41.

Ramser J, Ahearn ME, Lenski C, et al. Rare missense and synonymous variants in UBE1 are associated with X-linked infantile spinal muscular atrophy. *Am J Hum Genet* 2008; **82**: 188–93.

Toydemir RM, Rutherford A, Whitby FG, Jorde LB, Carey JC, Bamshad MJ. Mutations in embryonic myosin heavy chain (MYH3) cause Freeman–Sheldon syndrome and Sheldon–Hall syndrome. *Nat Genet* 2006; **38**: 561–5.

Vogt J, Harrison BJ, Spearman H, et al. Mutation analysis of CHRNA1, CHRNB1, CHRND, and RAPSN genes in multiple pterygium/fetal akinesia patients. *Am J Hum Genet* 2008; **82**: 222–7.

Vogt J, Morgan NV, Marton T, et al. Germline mutation in DOK7 associated with fetal akinesia deformation sequence. *J Med Genet* 2009; **46**: 338–40.

Ataxic adult

An individual with ataxia has poor coordination of his/her movements. This affects walking; the gait is wide-based and unsteady. Speech and eye movements may also be affected.

Ataxia may be caused by abnormalities that affect the function of the cerebellum ('cerebellar ataxia'), spinal cord, and the peripheral sensory system ('sensory ataxia').

The neurologist will investigate to determine the likely aetiology and particularly to differentiate acquired from genetic causes of ataxia. The geneticist may be involved in the diagnostic process when there is no definitive diagnosis or otherwise at a later stage to counsel an individual and the family.

Clinical approach

The approach here is primarily to distinguish between the hereditary ataxias.

History: key points

- Three-generation pedigree. Ask about signs of a similar problem in parents and sibs. Note if they have been investigated and if there is consent to ask for results.
- Consanguinity in parents may indicate an AR ataxia.
- Ethnic origin. Some ataxias are found in specific geographical areas, e.g. Charlevoix–Saguenay (autosomal recessive spastic ataxia of Charlevoix–Saguenay (ARSACS)) in Quebec, Canada.
- Onset and description of symptoms; document the disability stage.
- Visual loss.
- Cognitive disturbance (dementia).
- Non-neurological features.

Examination: key points

- There is an overlap in the clinical features of SCA genes (*SCA1–37*).
- Gait ataxia. Observe the patient walking. Ataxic patients typically have a wide-based gait.
- Tremor/parkinsonian features (SCA3). Titubation.
- Eye movement disorder. Slow saccadic eye movement (SCA2). Oculomotor apraxia.
- Examine with the finger–nose test and heel–shin test, and test the ability to perform rapid alternating movements.
- Reflexes. Increased in SCA1 and 3. Decreased in SCA2.
- Sensory signs. Sensory axonal neuropathy may occur in some dominant families.
- Eyes and fundus. Retinopathy in SCA7. Cataract in Marinesco–Sjögren syndrome.
- Cardiac. Cardiomyopathy in Friedreich's ataxia (FRDA).

Special investigations

Prioritizing investigations depends on the family history and clinical features. In individuals with a family history, proceed to genetic testing.

- Brain MRI scan, e.g. for cerebellar atrophy (SCA), other structural abnormalities, tumours (bilateral acoustic neuromas indicate a diagnosis of NF2), white matter abnormalities (found in metabolic disorders and fragile X tremor ataxia syndrome (FXTAS) as well as acquired conditions such as multiple sclerosis (MS)).
- Peripheral nerve conduction studies.
- Ophthalmic assessment, including electroretinography (ERG).
- Electrocardiogram (ECG)/cardiac echo (cardiomyopathy in FRDA).
- Consider further biochemical screening, such as vitamin E, alpha-fetoprotein (AFP), cholesterol, and albumin, and additional tests for metabolic disorders such as white cell enzymes (late-onset GM2 gangliosidosis).
- Antigliadin antibodies. A positive antibody test is found in 10–15% of patients with ataxia, but it is uncertain whether this is a consequence, rather than a cause, of cerebellar degeneration.
- DNA analysis: *SCA1, 2, 3, 6, 7, 12,* and *17, DRPLA, FRDA (frataxin)*, ataxia with vitamin E deficiency, Refsum's disease, GM2 gangliosidosis, FXTAS (*FMR1*), mitochondrial DNA analysis. Consider HD and Gerstmann–Straussler disease (GSD).
- Genomic analysis in presence of features suggestive of a genetic diagnosis, e.g. gene panel, genomic array, or WES/WGS as appropriate (note triplet repeat disorders and mitochondrial encoded disorders may not be detected by next-generation sequencing approaches).
- DNA storage for future testing.
- Consider cytogenetic analysis for breakage disorders such as ataxia telangiectasia (AT). These more typically have a childhood presentation.

Some diagnoses to consider

In individuals in whom acquired non-genetic conditions have been excluded as far as possible, a genetic aetiology needs to be considered, even in the absence of a family history. Abele *et al.* (2002) reported a 13% probability that an individual with a sporadically occurring ataxia has SCA1, SCA2, SCA3, SCA6, SCA7, SCA17, or FRDA. For young adults, see also 'Ataxic child' in Chapter 2, 'Clinical approach', p. 74.

Autosomal dominant cerebellar ataxias (ADCAs)

SPINOCEREBELLAR ATAXIA (SCA). The most likely diagnostic group for adult cerebellar ataxias. It is extremely genetically heterogeneous. All have gait ataxia and are slowly progressive. There is overlap in the clinical features, but some of the useful differentiating features are listed under 'Examination: key points'. GeneReviews® (http://www.ncbi.nlm.nih.gov/books/NBK1138) has useful reviews of many of the individual SCA types.

- Because of the clinical overlap, laboratories usually perform testing for several SCA genes, unless the familial type is known. Molecular testing is available for SCA1, 2, 3, 6, 7, 12, and 17. In the absence of a known type, testing is done in a stepwise fashion, excluding the most common first.
- The majority are $(CAG)_n$ trinucleotide expansion disorders. The remainder are caused by non-coding expansions or conventional mutations.
- Intermediate alleles may cause problems in genetic counselling and predictive testing of relatives.
- Anticipation. SCA7 has a particularly unstable $(CAG)_n$ repeat and children may have early-onset disease that presents prior to any signs in the parent. Expansion of the $(CAG)_n$ is more likely with paternal transmission.

EPISODIC ATAXIA. In episodic ataxias, patients experience more distinct attacks of incoordination lasting from minutes to hours. Recognition of these disorders is important, particularly as the patients may be responsive to therapy. There are several loci (EA1–8) and they are generally caused by mutations in ion channel genes. EA2 (*CACNA1A*) is allelic to SCA6 and to familial hemiplegic migraine.

HUNTINGTON DISEASE (HD). An AD neurodegenerative disorder characterized by a progressive involuntary movement disorder, psychiatric disturbance, and dementia. See 'Huntington disease (HD)' in Chapter 3, 'Common consultations', p. 454.

DENTATORUBROPALLIDOLUYSIAN ATROPHY (DRPLA). An AD neurodegenerative disorder that causes symptoms and signs very like those of HD.

GERSTMANN–STRAUSSLER DISEASE (GSD). A rare AD familial prion disorder characterized by cerebellar ataxia, progressive dementia, and absent reflexes in the legs and, pathologically, by amyloid plaques throughout the CNS. Onset is usually in the fifth decade, and in the early phase ataxia is predominant. Dementia develops later. The course ranges from 2 to 10 years. The disorder is caused by mutations in the prion protein gene (*PRNP*) on 20pter–p12.

Autosomal recessive

Particularly important is a history of parental consanguinity and/or affected sibs.

FRIEDREICH'S ATAXIA (FRDA). FRDA is caused by a GAA repeat in the *FRDA* gene coding for frataxin protein. The usual presentation is in childhood, but the disease may be mild with later presentation. Some patients present in adulthood. Prior to molecular genetic testing, there were strict diagnostic criteria for FRDA that included onset prior to age of 20 years. Since genetic testing became possible, many patients have been diagnosed with FRDA where the onset has occurred at ages of >20 years. There is no evidence for anticipation.

Typical clinical features are absent or reduced reflexes with upgoing plantars, loss of vibration sense and proprioception, and cardiomyopathy. Adult-onset patients may have retained reflexes and a much milder clinical course. See 'Ataxic child' in Chapter 2, 'Clinical approach', p. 74.

ATAXIA WITH VITAMIN E DEFICIENCY. It is important to recognize this, as the disorder can be treated with vitamin E supplements. It has clinical features similar to those of FRDA and is caused by biallelic mutation in the TTPA gene.

AUTOSOMAL RECESSIVE CEREBELLAR ATAXIA (ARCA). ARCA1 is a pure cerebellar ataxia with a relatively late onset (17–46 years) which shows slow progression. The disorder was identified in a French Canadian population and is caused by LOF mutations in *SYNE1*. ARCA3, caused by mutations in *ANO10*, is also a relatively pure recessive cerebellar ataxia and has its onset between 15 and 45 years.

AUTOSOMAL RECESSIVE SPASTIC ATAXIA OF CHARLEVOIX–SAGUENAY (ARSACS). Onset is usually <10, but later onset is possible. See 'Ataxic child' in Chapter 2, 'Clinical approach', p. 74.

METABOLIC DISORDERS. Refsum's disease; Tay–Sachs (GM2 gangliosidosis); Wilson's disease.

ATAXIA TELANGIECTASIA (AT). An AR condition usually presenting in childhood. See 'DNA repair disorders' in Chapter 3, 'Common consultations', p. 398.

ATAXIA WITH OCULOMOTOR APRAXIA (AOA). Ataxia and oculomotor apraxia. Patients may also display mild choreoathetosis or dystonia. See 'Ataxic child' in Chapter 2, 'Clinical approach', p. 74 and 'DNA repair disorders' in Chapter 3, 'Common consultations', p. 398.

CEREBROTENDINOUS XANTHOMATOSIS. Other features include pyramidal or extrapyramidal signs, seizures, dementia, juvenile cataract, and tendon xanthomas. Onset is usually <20 years, but late onset is possible. Increased levels of bile alcohols in the urine are suggestive. It is caused by mutations in *CYP27*.

SENSORY ATAXIC NEUROPATHY DYSARTHRIA AND OPHTHALMOPLEGIA/MITOCHONDRIAL RECESSIVE ATAXIA SYNDROME (SANDO/MIRAS) (POLG1). Ataxia with other neurological features, including ophthalmoplegia, neuropathy, myoclonus, dystonia, and encephalopathy. Onset is usually between the ages of 15 and 40 years.

X-linked (XL) disorders

FRAGILE X PREMUTATION TREMOR/ATAXIA SYNDROME (FXTAS). Individuals with a fragile X premutation are at risk of developing a multisystem progressive neurological disorder characterized by cerebellar ataxia and/or intention tremor, with a variety of other neurological features, e.g. cognitive decline, parkinsonism, etc. White matter lesions on MRI in the middle cerebellar peduncles and/or brainstem are features of the condition. Both males and females with a premutation are at increased risk for FXTAS; however, the penetrance is higher in males. The prevalence is estimated at ~45% overall for males with premutations who are older than 50 years of age and <20% in females. Onset before 50 years appears rare. See 'Fragile X syndrome' in Chapter 3, 'Common consultations', p. 424.

Mitochondrial disorders

Ataxia is found in association with other organ involvement. Note if deafness or diabetes mellitus are present.
• Myoclonic epilepsy with ragged red fibres (MERRF).
• Neuropathy, ataxia, and retinitis pigmentosa (NARP).
See 'Mitochondrial DNA diseases' in Chapter 3, 'Common consultations', p. 490.

Genetic advice
Recurrence risk

OFFSPRING AND SIBLING RISK, SPORADIC PROGRESSIVE CEREBELLAR ATAXIA. If testing to exclude syndromic and acquired causes is negative:
• the inheritance pattern may be found from close questioning of the family history, e.g. if there is parental consanguinity and no history in preceding generations, then an AR aetiology is likely;
• consider if non-paternity is a possibility.
Offspring risks in sporadic adult-onset ataxia are unknown, but it is likely that some are due to unknown genetic mutations. A 5% offspring risk is usually given, but there are no firm data to support this.

Pre-symptomatic predictive testing in AD ataxia families (mainly SCA)

Confirm the mutation in an affected family member before arranging predictive testing. It is not of use in predicting the age of onset or the severity and progression of the disease. Follow the guidelines for predictive testing of asymptomatic at-risk individuals. See 'Testing for genetic status' in Chapter 1, 'Introduction', p. 38.

Carrier detection in AR/XL ataxia
- By molecular testing in families in which a causative mutation has been identified.
- Analysis of the family history in XL ataxia.

Prenatal diagnosis and pre-implantation genetic diagnosis
May be available for families where the genetic basis is known.

Natural history and further management (preventative measures)

Management is essentially supportive; affected individuals should be under the care of a multidisciplinary neurological team with expertise in disability.

Support groups: National Ataxia Foundation, 2600 Fernbrook Lane, Suite 119, Minneapolis, MN 55447, USA, http://www.ataxia.org; Ataxia UK, http://www.ataxia.org.uk.

Expert adviser: Nayana Lahiri, Consultant Clinical Geneticist, SW Thames Regional Genetics Service, St. George's University Hospitals NHS Foundation Trust, St. George's Hospital, London, UK.

References

Abele M, Burk K, Schöls L, et al. The aetiology of sporadic adult-onset ataxia. *Brain* 2002; **125**: 961–8.

Bird TD. *Hereditary ataxia overview*, 2016. GeneReviews®. http://www.ncbi.nlm.nih.gov/books/NBK1138.

Durr A. Autosomal dominant cerebellar ataxias: polyglutamine expansions and beyond. *Lancet Neurol* 2010; **9**: 885–94.

Rodriguez-Revenga L, Madrigal I, Pagonabarraga J, et al. Penetrance of FMR1 premutation associated pathologies in fragile X syndrome families. *Eur J Hum Genet* 2009; **17**: 1359–62.

van de Warrenburg BP, van Gaalen J, Boesch S, et al. (2014) EFNS/ENS Consensus on the diagnosis and management of chronic ataxias in adulthood. *Eur J Neurol* 2014; **21**: 552–62.

Vermeer S, van de Warrenburg BP, Willemsen MA, et al. Autosomal recessive cerebellar ataxias: the current state of affairs. *J Med Genet* 2011; **48**: 651–9.

Ataxic child

Individuals with ataxia have poor coordination of their movements. This affects walking and the gait is wide-based and unsteady. In children, it is important to distinguish ataxia from an unsteady gait due to immaturity or muscle weakness. Speech and movement of the eyes may also be affected. Ataxia may be caused by abnormalities that affect the function of the cerebellum, spinal cord, and the peripheral sensory system such as structural lesions, metabolic disturbance, and inherited genetic disorders.

In congenital ataxia, clinical features of ataxia do not become apparent until between 1 and 2 years of age. Infants are hypotonic with poor sucking and delayed motor milestones; ataxia becomes apparent once the child is walking. To test for ataxia in an older child, assess heel–toe walking (gait ataxia), finger–nose and heel–shin tests (dysmetria), and rapid alternating movements (dysdiadochokinesis), and observe for a wide-based gait and unsteady walking (e.g. chair walking or walking with support). A significant proportion of children with congenital ataxia have a degree of learning disability.

The child requires assessment by a paediatric neurologist who will investigate to determine the likely aetiology. The geneticist may be involved in the diagnostic process when there is no definitive diagnosis or otherwise at a later stage to counsel the family. The approach here is to consider the differential diagnosis of the genetic causes of ataxia based on the age of presentation.

Clinical approach

History: key points

- Three-generation pedigree. Ask about signs of a similar problem in parents and sibs. Some of the autosomal AD ataxias caused by SCA can present in childhood, particularly SCA7. For more detail on the adult ataxias, see 'Ataxic adult' in Chapter 2, 'Clinical approach', p. 70.
- Consanguinity in parents may indicate an AR ataxia or a metabolic condition.
- Ethnic origin. Some ataxias are found in specific geographical areas.
- Pregnancy history with detailed account of delivery and perinatal period.
- Developmental milestones, in particular early motor milestones and the age at which the child walked, in order to try to distinguish between congenital and later-onset ataxias.
- Speech and swallowing difficulties. Dysarthria. Language is very delayed in Angelman syndrome (AS) and affected children usually have little language acquisition.
- Visual loss.
- Intermittent ataxia is suggestive of metabolic decompensation, particularly:
  - urea cycle defects (dietary protein intolerance is a feature of the manifesting female carriers of the XL urea cycle defect ornithine transcarbamylase (OTC) deficiency);
  - organic acidaemia;
  - maple syrup urine disease (MSUD);
  - pyruvate dehydrogenase (PDH) deficiency.

Examination: key points

- Head circumference; note any change in the rate of growth.
- Gait ataxia.
- Hand flapping, jerky limb movement, laughter (AS).
- Reflexes. Classically absent in FRDA and vitamin E deficiency with extensor plantars.
- Sensory signs. Vibration sense and joint position sense usually impaired in FRDA.
- Eyes and fundus. Conjunctival telangiectasia in AT. Retinopathy in SCA7, abetalipoproteinaemia, and the mitochondrial disorder NARP. Cataract in Marinesco–Sjögren syndrome. Optic atrophy in FRDA and infantile-onset SCA (IOSCA).
- Eye movement disorder in AT, Gaucher's disease, Leigh syndrome (LS) and Niemann–Pick disease type C. Oculomotor apraxia ('head thrusts') in ataxia with oculomotor apraxia (AOA).
- Cardiac. Cardiomyopathy in FRDA.
- Muscle weakness in NARP, Leigh encephalopathy, and late-onset GM2 gangliosidosis.
- Extrapyramidal signs seen in AOA, IOSCA, mitochondrial diseases, late-onset GM2 gangliosidosis, and infantile, late-infantile, and juvenile variants of neuronal ceroid lipofuscinosis (NCL).

Special investigations

Investigate in conjunction with a paediatric neurologist, who will have investigated the child for acquired, as well as genetic, causes for the ataxia (unless there is a strong family history of an inherited form of ataxia presenting at a similar age). Genomic analysis can be very helpful in establishing a diagnosis.

- Biochemical screening. Basic biochemical screening has usually already been performed but should include plasma electrolytes, liver function tests (LFTs), acid/base status, fasting glucose, pyruvate and lactate, ammonium, amino acids, and a urine screen for amino and organic acids.
- Further biochemical testing to consider: white cell enzymes (metachromatic leukodystrophy, Krabbes, gangliosidoses, galactosialodosis); very-long-chain fatty acids (VLCFAs) and phytanic acid (Refsum's disease); AFP (elevated in AT); vitamin E; cholesterol and albumin; abetalipoprotein B (abetalipoproteinaemia), transferrin isoelectrophoresis (congenital disorders of glycosylation).
- Lysosomal inclusions if there is a suspected metabolic aetiology, e.g. infantile NCL.
- Brain MRI scan. Cerebellar hypoplasia suggests a congenital cause. White matter abnormalities are found in metabolic disorders (see 'Developmental regression' in Chapter 2, 'Clinical approach', p. 128).
- Peripheral nerve conduction studies (FRDA, Charlevoix–Saguenay syndrome (SACS), Roussy–Levy syndrome, NARP).
- Ophthalmic assessment, including ERG.
- ECG and cardiac echo (cardiomyopathy in FRDA).
- Electroencephalography (EEG) in children with suspected AS, IOSCA, Unverricht–Lundborg progressive myoclonic epilepsy, and NCL.

- Endocrinology; exclude hypogonadotrophic hypogonadism.
- DNA analysis: frataxin (FRDA), mitochondrial DNA analysis (NARP, LS). Storage for future testing. In the older child, consider SCA and DRPLA (see 'Ataxic adult' in Chapter 2, 'Clinical approach', p. 70).
- Genomic analysis in presence of features suggestive of a chromosomal or syndromic diagnosis, e.g. genomic array, gene panel, or WES/WGS as appropriate.
- Cytogenetic analysis for breakage disorders if there are signs of AT or xeroderma pigmentosum (XP).
  - small nuclear ribonuclear protein-associated poly-peptide N (SNRPN) methylation studies for AS if there is severe developmental delay.

Some diagnoses to consider

Presumed congenital ataxia

STRUCTURAL ABNORMALITIES OF THE CEREBELLUM. See 'Cerebellar anomalies' in Chapter 2, 'Clinical approach', p. 92.

ATAXIC CEREBRAL PALSY. A descriptive term for a het-erogeneous group of disorders where the child presents with ataxia, but degrees of global developmental delay and hypotonia are often present. Be wary of this diag-nosis; it is a diagnosis of exclusion of other causes of a congenital ataxia. Take a careful birth history to assess if there is a history of hypoxia or injury to account for the problems. A high-resolution brain MRI scan is man-datory prior to definitive counselling. Congenital struc-tural lesions of the cerebellum, such as hypoplasia or a Dandy–Walker cyst, may be found and aid estimation of recurrence risks. See 'Cerebral palsy' in Chapter 2, 'Clinical approach', p. 96.

ANGELMAN SYNDROME (AS). See 'Angelman syndrome' in Chapter 3, 'Common consultations', p. 346.

INBORN ERRORS OF METABOLISM. 'Small molecule dis-orders', such as urea cycle disorders, MSUD, and PDH deficiency, have ataxia, along with other manifestations of metabolic decompensation including altered conscious-ness/encephalopathy/acidosis/hyperammonaemia.

Childhood-onset disorders

FRIEDREICH'S ATAXIA (FRDA). This is the most common inherited ataxia. The mean age at onset is 15.5 years ± 8 years, with a range of 2–51 years. It is AR and caused by mutations in frataxin (FRDA) on 9q. Frataxin is a nuclear-encoded mitochondrial protein. It is characterized by the longest and largest myelinated fibres (e.g. large fibres aris-ing in dorsal root ganglia) dying back from the periph-ery. The carrier frequency in the Caucasian population is ~1:85, with a disease prevalence of 1/29 000; FRDA is rare in Africans and Asians. Ninety-eight per cent of mutations are triplet repeat expansions of $(GAA)_n$ in intron 1 and 2% are point mutations or deletions. Normal triplet repeat allele size is 6–34; mutations have 67–1700 repeats. Repeat size is unstable, with a tendency to decrease in size when paternally transmitted and increase or decrease when maternally transmitted. The disease is slowly, but relentlessly, progressive with loss of walk-ing ~15 years after onset and the mean age of death is ~37.5 years (usual cause is cardiomyopathy). Late-onset FRDA (onset >25 years) has been recognized since the onset of molecular testing.

The clinical features of FRDA are:
- progressive gait and limb ataxia;
- dysarthria;
- absent lower limb reflexes;
- extensor plantar responses;

CEREBELLAR ATAXIA, MENTAL RETARDATION AND DYSEQUILIBRIUM. An AR disorder caused by biallelic vari-ants in CA8, VLDLR, ATP6A2, and WDR81.
- reduced vibration sense and proprioception (posterior columns);
- cardiomyopathy (hypertrophic cardiomyopathy (HCM) usually), diabetes, scoliosis, pes cavus, and optic atrophy are common features;
- -NCV studies show absent sensory nerve action potentials. Motor conduction velocities are reduced but >40 m/s.

Carrier testing is possible for relatives and their partners. If the partner of a carrier does not have a $(GAA)_n$ expan-sion, then since only 2% of mutations are point muta-tions, carrier risk falls to ~1/5000. PND is possible by CVS if mutations in parents are both defined.

ATAXIA WITH VITAMIN E DEFICIENCY. Clinical picture very similar to that for FRDA. It is AR, resulting from mutations in the alpha-tocopherol transfer protein gene (TTPA) on chromosome 8. It is treatable, and it is there-fore important to exclude this diagnosis by measure-ment of vitamin E levels if molecular testing for FRDA is negative.

CHARLEVOIX–SAGUENAY SYNDROME (SACS). This is AR with hypermyelinated retinal nerve fibres and mixed peripheral neuropathy. It presents with ataxia, dysar-thria, and nystagmus, with spasticity in the lower limbs. Consider in the differential diagnosis of FRDA if genetic tests for FRDA are negative. SACS is common in north-eastern Quebec where the carrier frequency reaches 1/22 in one region. SACS is caused by mutations in a gene encoding the protein sacsin on 13q11 (Engert et al. 2000).

ATAXIA WITH OCULOMOTOR APRAXIA (AOA). AOA type 1 is the most frequent cause of AR ataxia in Japan and is second only to FRDA in Portugal. It shares several neuro-logical features with AT, including early-onset ataxia, ocu-lomotor apraxia, and cerebellar atrophy, but does not share its extraneurological features (immune deficiency, chromosomal instability, and hypersensitivity to X-rays). AOA1 is also characterized by axonal motor neuropathy and decrease of serum albumin levels and elevation of total cholesterol. Caused by mutations in AOA1 on 9p encoding aprataxin. The gene has a DNA single-strand break repair domain. A second gene senataxin on 9q causes AOA2, characterized by onset between 11 and 22 years (Moreira et al. 2001). See also 'DNA repair dis-orders' in Chapter 3, 'Common consultations', p. 398.

INBORN ERRORS OF METABOLISM. Progressive ataxia is one of the features of a number of inborn errors. Consider hypobetalipoproteinaemia and abetalipopro-teinaemia, Refsum's disease, L-2 hydroxyglutaric aciduria, NCL, and GM2 (Tay–Sachs), and investigate further if necessary.

MITOCHONDRIAL DISORDERS. See 'Mitochondrial DNA diseases' in Chapter 3, 'Common consultations', p. 490.

Ataxia is found in association with involvement of other organs and other brain areas, e.g. basal ganglia (dystonia). There may be a family history of deafness and/or diabe-tes mellitus or early infantile death.
- MERFF, NARP, Kearns–Sayre syndrome (KSS), and LS.

DNA REPAIR DISORDERS. See 'DNA repair disorders' in Chapter 3, 'Common consultations', p. 398.

- AT (ataxia usually evident from 1 year of age; telangiectasia from 4 to 8 years).
- XP.

HEREDITARY SPASTIC PARAPLEGIA (HSP). See 'Hereditary spastic paraplegias (HSP)' in Chapter 3, 'Common consultations', p. 448.

ROUSSY–LEVY SYNDROME. AD form of HMSN1 with ataxia and tremor. See 'Charcot–Marie–Tooth disease (CMT)' in Chapter 3, 'Common consultations', p. 362.

SPINOCEREBELLAR ATAXIA (SCA). The triplet repeat in SCA7 is particularly unstable and large expansions in the triplet repeat can occur. SCA7 can present in childhood before signs appear in the parent. See 'Ataxic adult' in Chapter 2, 'Clinical approach', p. 70.

Genetic advice

Recurrence risk

If after investigation there is no known aetiology, the precise genetic risks are unknown.

- Assume AR inheritance is likely if there is an affected sibling or parental consanguinity.
- Progressive ataxia suggests a metabolic or genetic aetiology with a high recurrence risk.
- Ataxic cerebral palsy. There is a genetic subgroup within this disorder and the recurrence risk may be as high as 25%. An estimate of 10–15% may be used if there is no family history or parental consanguinity. See 'Cerebral palsy' in Chapter 2, 'Clinical approach', p. 96.

Carrier detection

This is possible where there is a known mutation with the usual restrictions on the genetic testing of children. See 'Testing for genetic status' in Chapter 1, 'Introduction', p. 38.

Prenatal diagnosis

PND by CVS can be offered to families at risk for some of the syndromic causes of ataxia if the causative familial mutations are known. Prenatal testing for mitochondrial disorders is rarely straightforward, but PND is available for some mutations; see 'Mitochondrial DNA diseases' in Chapter 3, 'Common consultations', p. 490. USS or fetal MRI may be of some value if there are structural abnormalities of the cerebellum. See 'Cerebellar anomalies' in Chapter 2, 'Clinical approach', p. 92.

Natural history and further management (preventative measures)

These are dependent on the diagnosis. Most are progressive conditions, so follow-up by a paediatric neurologist and a childhood disability team is appropriate.

Support groups: National Ataxia Foundation, 2600 Fernbrook Lane, Suite 119, Minneapolis, MN 55447, USA, http://www.ataxia.org; Ataxia UK, http://www.ataxia.org.uk.

Expert adviser: Robert Mcfarland, Clinical Senior Lecturer in Paediatric Neurology, Wellcome Trust Centre for Mitochondrial Research, Institute of Neuroscience, Newcastle University, Newcastle upon Tyne, UK.

References

Bird TD. *Hereditary ataxia overview*, 2016 GeneReviews®, http://www.ncbi.nlm.nih.gov/books/NBK1138.

Delataycki MB, Williamson R, Forrest SM. Friedreich's ataxia: an overview. *J Med Genet* 2000; **37**: 1–8.

Engert JC, Bérubé P, Mercier J, *et al*. ARSACS, a spastic ataxia common in northeastern Quebec, is caused by mutations in a new gene encoding an 11.5-kb ORF. *Nat Genet* 2000; **24**: 120–5.

Moreira MC, Barbot C, Tachi N, *et al*. The gene mutated in ataxia–ocular apraxia 1 encodes the new HIT/Zn-finger protein aprataxin. *Nat Genet* 2001; **29**: 189–93.

Moreira MC, Klur S, Watanabe M, *et al*. Senataxin, the ortholog of a yeast RNA helicase, is mutant in ataxia-ocular apraxia 2. *Nat Genet* 2004; **36**: 225–7.

Brachydactyly

Brachydactyly is shortening of the digits due to anomalous development of the phalanges or metacarpals.

Brachydactyly can be divided into the following categories:

- predominantly isolated brachydactyly;
- brachydactyly as part of a skeletal dysplasia;
- brachydactyly as part of a syndrome. In particular, we will discuss those syndromes where brachydactyly is a distinctive diagnostic feature, e.g. Albright, de Lange, Robinow.

Brachydactyly should be distinguished from small, but structurally normal, hands and feet (as seen in Prader–Willi syndrome (PWS), Smith–Magenis syndrome (SMS), and UPD14).

Brachydactyly was the first human trait to be interpreted as a Mendelian dominant by Farabee in 1903. The most commonly used classification is the clinical descriptive system devised by Julia Bell (1951). She classified the published pedigrees into seven groups on the basis of the anatomy (see Figure 2.7 and Box 2.1). Molecular analysis has shown that many are genetically heterogeneous. It has also been found that one gene produces several different phenotypes, depending on the action of the mutation, e.g. the ROR2 gene, where heterozygous truncating mutations thought to produce a specific gain of function, cause AD brachydactyly B (which predominantly affects the distal phalanges and nails) and homozygous LOF mutations lead to AR Robinow syndrome.

Clinical approach

History: key points

- At least three-generation family tree. The phenotype may vary in severity (variable expressivity) and gene carriers may be non-penetrant.
- Parental stature.
- Developmental delay.
- Other medical problems.

Examination: key points

- Measure the height, arm span, and upper and lower body lengths. Assess for short stature and disproportion. If limbs are short, is the shortening rhizomelic or mesomelic?
- Make measurements of the hands: total length (tip of the middle finger to the distal wrist crease), middle finger length (tip of the middle finger to the proximal

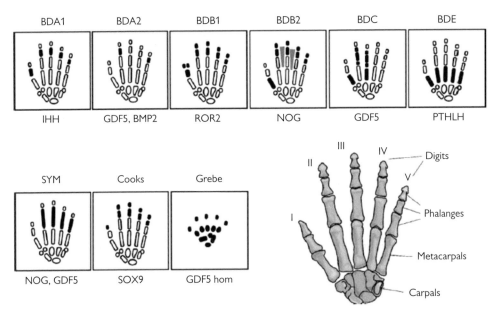

Figure 2.7 Schematic of human brachydactylies. The disease nomenclature is given on top, the mutated gene(s) below. All are inherited in dominant manner, with the exception of Grebe syndrome. BDA1, small/absent middle phalanges of digits I–V; BDA2, small/absent middle phalanges of digits II and V; BDB1, small/absent distal phalanges of digits II–V, joint fusions of distal interphalangeal joint, duplication of distal phalanx of digit I; BDB2, small/absent distal and middle phalanges, syndactyly (large variability in phenotype); BDC, short metacarpal I, short metacarpal and phalanges of digit III, short phalanges, hyperphalangy (additional phalanx) digit II and near normal digit IV; BDE, short metacarpals, most common in IV and V but may be present in all; SYM, symphalangism (fusion of joints) at various locations, most common in phalangeal joints of digits IV and V; Cooks syndrome, missing middle phalanges, relatively long proximal and distal phalanges, missing nails; Grebe syndrome, all elements affected, very short bones, missing phalanges. Right side shows schematic of human hand skeleton. Note the round shape of carpal bones which is in stark contrast to the other long bones. All digits show one metacarpal and three phalanges with the exception of the first digit (thumb) which has only two phalanges.

Reproduced from Stricker & Mundlos, *Developmental Dynamics, Mechanisms of digit formation: Human malformation syndromes tell the story*, pp. 990–1004, copyright 2011, with permission from John Wiley and Sons.

Box 2.1 Classification of isolated brachydactylies (most are AD)[*]

Type A. Shortening confined mainly to middle phalanges.
- A1 (MIM 112500 and 607004). Short/absent middle phalanges in all digits. May be short proximal phalanges in thumbs and halluces, plus short stature. Genetically heterogeneous. Can be caused by heterozygous missense mutations in the *IHH* gene. (Homozygous *IHH* mutations cause acrocepaitofemoral dysplasia.)
- A2 (MIM 112600). Short middle phalanges in the second fingers and toes only. Caused by heterozygous mutations in the *BMPR1B* gene.
- A3 (MIM 112700). Short middle phalanges in fifth fingers only.

Type B (MIM 113000). Hypoplastic/absent nails, short/absent distal phalanges and short middle phalanges in second to fifth digits. May be broad/bifid thumbs and halluces, central syndactyly, and characteristic face. Genetically heterogeneous. Can be caused by heterozygous truncating mutations in the *ROR2* gene.

Type C (MIM 113100). Short middle phalanges in second, third, and fifth fingers; hyperphalangism (extra phalanges) in second and third fingers; relative sparing of fourth fingers; short first metacarpals. May be short stature. Genetically homogeneous. Caused by heterozygous mutations in the *GDF5* gene—probably LOF mutations. (Homozygous *GDF5* mutations cause two very similar recessive chondrodysplasias—Grebe type and Hunter–Thompson type.)

Type D (MIM 113200). Short broad distal phalanges in thumbs and halluces.

Type E (MIM 113300). Shortening of one or more metacarpals/metatarsals. May be short stature. Genetically heterogeneous. Specific heterozygous missense mutations in the *HOXD13* gene can cause phenotypes overlapping with brachydactylies types D and E.

[*] MIM numbers are taken from the Online Mendelian Inheritance in Man® database.

---

crease at the base of the finger), and palm length (proximal crease at the base of the middle finger to the distal wrist crease).
- Observe and document palmar creases, finger contractures (camptodactyly), nail morphology/absence, and syndactyly (bony and skin).
- Carefully examine both feet.
- Dysmorphic features (syndromal causes of brachydactyly).
- Measure BP (brachydactyly/hypertension).

Special investigations
- Photography.
- X-rays of the hands and feet are required to investigate the structure of the bones. This is important in classification as there are recognizable patterns of malformation.
- Skeletal survey, if indicated from clinical assessment.
- DNA investigations may be possible to confirm the diagnosis.
- Genomic analysis in presence of features suggestive of a chromosomal or syndromic diagnosis, e.g. genomic array, gene panel, or WES/WGS as appropriate.

Some diagnoses to consider
Predominantly isolated brachydactyly
See p. 78 for classification and 'Genetic advice' below for genetic advice.
BRACHYDACTYLY, HYPERTENSION. This AD condition, characterized by brachydactyly, severe essential hypertension, and mild short stature, is caused by heterozygous mutations in PDE3A.
BRACHYDACTYLY TYPE 2 E2. Caused by heterozygous variants in the PTHLH gene on chromosome 12p.

Skeletal dysplasias
See Table 2.1 for some that should be considered.

Syndromic diagnoses (overlap with the skeletal dysplasias)
AARSKOG SYNDROME. Short stature (rhizomelic), ptosis in some, hypermetropia, shawl scrotum, brachydactyly with hyperextendable proximal interphalangeal (PIP) joints. Facial features tend to normalize with age. XL inheritance, caused by mutations in the *FGD1* gene.
ALBRIGHT HEREDITARY OSTEODYSTROPHY (AHO). This term describes a phenotype characterized by short adult stature with generalized obesity and relative microcephaly, brachydactyly particularly involving the distal phalanges (especially of the thumbs) and metacarpals/metatarsals, mild to moderate learning disability, and cutaneous ossifications (subcutaneous or intradermal lumps or flakes) in around 60%. The facial features are subtle, but usually these patients have a round face with a short neck, a short nose, and mild midface hypoplasia. The obesity is not usually associated with hyperphagia. The brachydactyly is associated with cone epiphyses and disharmonic bone age. Stature may be normal or above average in childhood, but there is reduced longitudinal growth and early epiphyseal closure. The condition tends to be overdiagnosed, largely because, with the exception of the cutaneous ossifications, the physical findings are non-specific. See 'Obesity with and without developmental delay' in Chapter 2, 'Clinical approach', p. 254. Caused by heterozygous mutation in GNAS.
NB. Some patients with an AHO-like phenotype, including brachydactyly type E and developmental delay, have a 2q37 deletion encompassing HDAC4 (see below).
HAND–FOOT–GENITAL SYNDROME. An AD condition caused by mutations in *HOXA13* on 7p15. Hands are small with hypoplastic proximally placed thumbs, and feet

Table 2.1 Skeletal dysplasia diagnoses to consider

Name	Gene	Helpful diagnostic features
AchondroplasiaAD	FGFR3	A 'starfish' or 'trident' configuration to the hands is found as the metacarpals are of an even size
Acrodysostosis	PRKAR1A, PDE4D	Short snub nose. Cone epiphyses in metacarpals
Acromesomelic dysplasia (AMD) AR	AMD Maroteaux type (AMDM), NPR2 gene AMD Grebe type (AMDG) and AMD Hunter–Thompson type (AMDH) are similar, both caused by GDF5 mutations	Mesomelic limb shortening. Broad hands with short stubby fingers
Geleophysic dysplasiaAR	ADAMTSL2	Heart valve thickening, tiptoe gait, developmental delay
HypochondroplasiaAD	FGFR3	Clinical features resemble those of achondroplasia but are milder with less involvement of the face, skull, and spine
PseudoachondroplasiaAD	COMP	Short stature not apparent until after 12 months. Early arthritic problems with joint pain
Robinow syndrome	ROR2	Hypertelorism, cardiac anomalies
Ter HaarAR	TKS4	Large fontanelle, glaucoma, hypertelorism, valvular heart lesions, prominent coccyx

are small with short halluces. Males have hypospadias and females have duplication of the uterus, and sometimes of the cervix, and may have a septate vagina. Urinary tract malformations are common in both sexes.

HDAC4 BRACHYDACTYLY MENTAL RETARDATION SYN-DROME (LOCUS 2Q37). Overlapping phenotype with AHO, but without endocrine dysfunction. Caused by mutation of the chromatin-modifying gene HDAC4.

PMRMT7 SYNDROME. Characterized by developmental delay with short metacarpals/metatarsals, obesity, and short stature and caused by heterozygous variants in PMRMT7 gene (Akawi 2015).

ROBINOW SYNDROME. Mesomelia (short limbs), characteristic facies (fetal face), vertebral abnormalities, small penis. The AR form is due to homozygous LOF mutations in the ROR2 gene.

SMALL HANDS AND FEET. Found in PWS and maternal UPD14.

Genetic advice

Recurrence risk
- Isolated brachydactyly is inherited as an AD trait, and in the majority of affected individuals, there is a family history. Mild short stature is frequently part of the phenotype. After classifying the form of brachydactyly, counsel appropriately.
- Syndromic brachydactyly. Counsel as appropriate for the specific syndrome diagnosed.

Carrier detection
Note that, in dominant kindreds, there is often marked variability in expression and sometimes incomplete penetrance.

Prenatal diagnosis
This is technically feasible if the familial mutation is known, but not usually requested or appropriate for isolated forms of brachydactyly.

Support group:
Many of the syndromes have their own support groups. See Contact a Family, http://www.cafamily.org.uk.

References
Akawi N, McRae J et al. Discovery of four recessive developmental disorders using probabilistic genotype and phenotype matching among 4,125 families. *Nat Genet* 2015; **47**: 1363–69.

Bell J. On brachydactyly and symphalangism. In: LS Penrose (ed.). *The treasury of human inheritance*, **Vol. 5**, part 1, pp. 1–31. Cambridge University Press, Cambridge, 1951.

Everman DB, Bartels CF, Yang Y, et al. The mutational spectrum of brachydactyly type C. *Am J Med Genet* 2002; **112**: 291–6.

Fitch N. Classification and identification of inherited brachydactylies. *J Med Genet* 1979; **16**: 36–44.

Gong M, Zhang H, Schulz H, et al. Genome-wide linkage reveals a locus for human essential (primary) hypertension on chromosome 12p. *Hum Mol Genet* 2003; **12**: 1273–7.

Mundlos S. The brachydactylies: a molecular disease family. *Clin Genet* 2009; **76**: 123–36.

Online Mendelian Inheritance in Man®. http://www.omim.org.

Patton MA, Afzal AR. Robinow syndrome. *J Med Genet* 2002; **39**: 305–10.

Poznanski AK. *The hand in radiologic diagnosis with gamuts and pattern profiles*. Saunders, Philadelphia, 1984.

Stricker S, Mundlos S. Mechanisms of digit formation: human malformation syndromes tell the story. *Dev Dyn* 2011; **240**: 990–1004.

Temtamy S, McKusick VA. The genetics of hand malformation. *Birth Defects Orig Art Series* 1978; **14**: 187–225.

Broad thumbs

There are some distinctive syndromes with broad thumbs as a key diagnostic feature. If there is difficulty in deciding whether the thumb is significantly broad, then it is unlikely to be a good diagnostic 'handle'. The degree of thumb involvement may be variable, especially in the AD syndromes.

A bifid thumb may be described as broad, and X-ray examination is necessary in most affected individuals unless they clearly have a syndromic cause such as Rubinstein–Taybi syndrome (RTS). There is considerable overlap between some of these syndromes and those described in 'Polydactyly' in Chapter 2, 'Clinical approach', p. 284.

Clinical approach

History: key points
- At least three-generation pedigree; explain to parents about the minimal signs that could indicate a gene carrier.
- Consanguinity.
- Neurological/developmental problems (RTS).

Examination: key points
- Thumb. Document structure and function:
  - number of phalanges (three phalanges known as 'triphalangeal');
  - if duplicated;
  - if broad;
  - opposition.
- Hallux (great or big toe). Document structure as above.
- Hands and feet. Examine for anomalies affecting the other digits such as syndactyly, brachydactyly, or pre-/post-axial polydactyly (refer to these sections on p. 254, p. 56, p. 218, and p. 214, respectively).
- Head and skull shape: macrocephaly and broad/high forehead (Greig syndrome); craniosynostosis (Pfeiffer syndrome).
- Features suggestive of any other skeletal abnormalities, talipes, or limb shortening (diastrophic dysplasia).
- Prominent nose (RTS).
- Cysts within the ear pinnae (diastrophic dysplasia).
- Atresia of the lacrimal punctae, causing overflow tears (lacrimo-auriculo-dental-digital (LADD) syndrome).
- Cardiac murmurs (RTS and TBS).
- Genital and renal anomalies (TBS).
- Remember to examine the parents!

Special investigations
- X-rays of the hands and feet are essential to assess the skeletal elements and to detect minor features not seen on clinical examination. The X-ray will assist in the process of definition.
- Skull X-rays and further skeletal films, if indicated from clinical assessment.
- Renal scan or cardiac echo, if indicated.
- Consider gene panel/WES/WGS as appropriate.

Some diagnoses to consider

Brachydactyly type B
The thumbs and halluces may be broad or bifid. There is central syndactyly and a characteristic face. Hypoplastic/ absent nails, short/absent distal phalanges, and short middle phalanges in the second to fifth digits are other digital anomalies. AD but genetically heterogeneous. Can be caused by heterozygous truncating mutations in the *ROR2* gene.

Brachydactyly types D and E
TYPE D (MIM 113200). Short broad distal phalanges in thumbs and halluces.

TYPE E (MIM 113300). Shortening of one or more metacarpals/metatarsals. May be short stature. Genetically heterogeneous. Specific heterozygous missense mutations in the *HOXD13* gene can cause phenotypes overlapping with brachydactyly types D and E.

Greig cephalopolysyndactyly
An AD condition, characterized by a high forehead with frontal bossing, macrocephaly, hypertelorism, and a broad base to the nose. In the hands, both post-axial polydactyly (type B) and, less commonly, preaxial polydactyly (PPD) (broad thumbs with bifid nails and distal phalanges) can occur; also often central syndactyly. In the feet, usually PPD (duplicated hallux), with syndactyly in toes 1–3. Caused by mutations/deletions of *GLI3* on 7p13. The facial features of Greig can be subtle, especially in infancy. It is generally considered that type IV PPD is part of the spectrum of Greig syndrome and caused by mutations in *GLI3*. Mutation analysis will help to determine if the cause is a new mutation in situations where there is clinical doubt. Children with a deletion have additional developmental delay and often do not have macrocephaly.

Lacrimo-auriculo-dental-digital syndrome
An AD condition, characterized by absence or atresia of the lacrimal punctae causing overflow of tears (epiphora) and recurrent eye infection, simple cup-shaped ears with sensorineural or conductive deafness, and hypoplastic teeth. The thumbs are usually bifid or triphalangeal with clinodactyly.

Otopalatodigital syndrome type 1 (Taybi syndrome)
Otopalatodigital syndrome type 1 (OPD-1) is a rare XL disease with diagnostic skeletal features, conductive deafness, cleft palate, and mild MR. Affected individuals have 'pugilistic facies'. The thumbs are broad. The feet have a particularly characteristic appearance with a large sandal gap, a short hallux, and lateral curvature of the toes. Caused by mutation in the *FLNA* gene on Xq 28 (Robertson *et al.* 2004).

Pfeiffer syndrome
An AD condition with coronal craniosynostosis, broad thumbs and halluces, and soft tissue syndactyly. The halluces are usually in the varus position, and a variety of anomalies are found including broad halluces, bifid halluces, and PPD. The face is similar to that in Crouzon syndrome, but clover leaf skull is a more frequent complication. Sometimes the thumbs and halluces are broad and there may be a degree of skin syndactyly. Mutations are found in either *FGFR1* or *FGFR2*. *FGFR2* mutations may lead to a more severe craniofacial phenotype.

Robinow syndrome
Both AD and AR types. Skeletal survey to assess mesomelia, costovertebral abnormalities, and distinctive

phalangeal changes. There is brachydactyly with abnormal orientation of the thumbs and occasional bifid thumbs. Large mouth and tongue, gingival hypertrophy, micropenis, and congenital heart defects. The AR type is due to homozygous abnormality in the *ROR2* gene. Different heterozygous mutations in *ROR2* cause brachydactyly type B.

Rubinstein–Taybi syndrome
Children with RTS usually have a normal birthweight, but subsequent growth is poor, with most children being of short stature with microcephaly. MR is usually moderate to severe, but some have mild learning difficulties. The most striking physical feature is broad, sometimes angulated, thumbs and first toes. The facial features vary with age and include a prominent beaked nose with the columella below the alae nasae and downslanting eyes. Cryptorchidism occurs in males. Other variable features include CHD (~30%) and kidney abnormalities, eye and hearing problems, feeding difficulties in infancy, and constipation. Seizures may occur. Most people with RTS are very sociable, even overfriendly, and enjoy adult attention. See Wiley *et al.* (2003) for medical guidelines for individuals with RTS. Two genes have been identified. The gene *CRBBP* at 16p13.3 is the major cause of RTS, either by truncating mutations or as part of a microdeletion. *EP300* causes a somewhat milder phenotype but probably accounts for <5% of mutations in individuals with the RTS phenotype.

Teunissen–Cremers (congenital ankylosis of the stapes with broad thumbs)
An AD condition with conductive deafness due to ankylosis of the auditory ossicles, together with mild skeletal anomalies, e.g. broad thumbs and halluces, short distal phalanges, fused cervical vertebrae, and syndactyly, but symphalangism is usually absent. Hypermetropia is a common feature. Caused by heterozygous mutation in the *NOG* gene (heterozygous mutation in this gene can cause other phenotypes, e.g. multiple synostoses or symphalangism).

Genetic advice

Recurrence risk
Counsel as appropriate for the underlying syndrome.

Prenatal diagnosis
- Genetic testing for some of these syndromes may be available.
- USS. Ultrasound markers, additional to the broad thumbs, should be used to confirm a diagnosis.

Support group:
Many of the syndromes have their own support groups. See Contact a Family, http://www.cafamily.org.uk.

References
Petrij F, Dauwerse HG, Blough RI, *et al.* Diagnostic analysis of the Rubinstein–Taybi syndrome: five cosmids should be used for microdeletion detection and low number of protein truncating mutations. *J Med Genet* 2000; **37**: 168–76.

Robertson SP, Twigg SR, Sutherland-Smith AJ, *et al.* Localised mutations in the gene encoding the cytoskeletal protein filamin A cause diverse malformations in humans. *Nat Genet* 2004; **33**: 487–91.

Temtamy SA, McKusick VA. *The genetics of hand malformations*. Alan R Liss, New York, 1978.

van Belzen M, Bartsch O, Lacombe D, Peters DJ, Hennekam RC. Rubinstein-Taybi syndrome (CREBBP, EP300). *Eur J Hum Genet* 2011;**19**: preceding 118–20.

Wiley S, Swayne S, Rubinstein JH, Lanphear NE, Stevens CA. Rubinstein–Taybi syndrome medical guidelines. *Am J Med Genet A* 2003; **119A**: 101–10.

Cardiomyopathy in children under 10 years

Cardiomyopathy (CM) is defined as a disease of the myocardium associated with cardiac dysfunction and/ or abnormal cardiac structure. CM is a major cause of cardiac mortality and is the leading cause of cardiac transplantation in children. The five main groups include dilated (DCM), hypertrophic (HCM), restrictive (RCM), arrhythmogenic right ventricular cardiomyopathy/dysplasia (ARVC/D), and unclassified cardiomyopathies, which include left ventricular non-compaction (LVNC) and endocardial fibroelastosis (EFE). Complications include worsening cardiac failure, arrhythmias, systemic or pulmonary emboli, or sudden death.

Severe peripartum asphyxia can cause an ischaemic CM—'transient myocardial ischaemia of the newborn'. These neonates usually do not have ischaemic encephalopathy or serious renal problems—the dilated heart with impaired function is the major manifestation. Usually these infants have some degree of IUGR and are small-for-dates, and usually there has been a hypoglycaemic episode as well as asphyxial stress.

Infants of diabetic mothers may have asymmetric septal hypertrophy (ASH) or left ventricular hypertrophy (LVH) in the neonatal period. ASH is present in 38.8% of large-for-gestational-age (LGA) infants of diabetic mothers, compared with 7.1% of LGA infants of non-diabetics. HCM in infants of diabetic mothers is generally transient and benign.

In utero ritodrine exposure may cause neonatal ventricular hypertrophy.

The annual incidence of CM in Australian children is 1.2 per 100 000 and it is over ten times higher in children aged <1 year, compared to 1–18 years (0.7 per 100 000 versus 8.3 per 100 000; Nugent et al. 2003). DCM is the most frequently found type and HCM the second most common. The differential diagnosis in infants is different from that in adults, mainly due to the contribution of metabolic disease and dysmorphic syndromes.

The geneticist is asked to see children in whom there is no evidence of an infective or other environmental cause, and to discuss recurrence risks with parents after a genetic aetiology has been identified.

Clinical approach

Carefully review the child's notes and the results of cardiac investigations, e.g. echo and ECG, MRI or cardiac biopsy.

History: key points
- Three-generation family tree, with a special note of CHD and neonatal or infant deaths. Any evidence for X-linkage or mitochondrial inheritance?
- Consanguinity (metabolic conditions, AR conditions).
- Pregnancy, diabetes, medication, infections, polyhydramnios.
- Birth asphyxia.
- Valvular heart defect (pulmonary stenosis in Noonan and LEOPARD (lentigines–ECG abnormalities–ocular hypertelorism–pulmonary stenosis–abnormal genitalia–retardation of growth–deafness) syndromes).
- Muscle weakness (skeletal muscle involvement, e.g. muscular dystrophies and mitochondrial myopathy).

- Developmental delay—differentiate between motor delay (muscular weakness) and global developmental delay.
- Fluctuation in level of consciousness, especially with intercurrent infections.
- Regression (multiple acyl-CoA dehydrogenase deficiency (MADD), mitochondrial disorders).
- Deafness (LEOPARD, Alstrom syndrome).
- Visual problems (mitochondrial disorders, though unlikely in infants).

Examination: key points
- Look carefully for facial features of Noonan, cardiofaciocutaneous (CFC), Costello, and LEOPARD syndromes.
- Hypotonia or weakness (skeletal muscle involvement).
- Skin, acanthosis nigricans (Alstrom syndrome), lentigines (LEOPARD syndrome), hyperkeratosis and woolly hair (Naxos disease).

Special investigations
- 24-hour tape to investigate heart rhythm disturbances.
- CK (skeletal muscle involvement, e.g. muscular dystrophies).
- Plasma carnitine.
- Dried blood spot on Guthrie card for acyl carnitine profile (fatty acid oxidation defects).
- Glucose (to exclude hypoglycaemia). Controlled and monitored fasting studies may be required.
- Blood lactate.
- Ammonia (raised in carnitine deficiency and disorders of fatty acid oxidation).
- Enzyme analysis (alpha-glucosidase deficiency, type II glycogen storage disease (GSD)).
- Full blood count (FBC) and differential count: neutropenia (Barth syndrome).
- Lactate dehydrogenase (LDH) is often markedly raised in fatty acid oxidation defects, and low cholesterol with high uric acid is typical for Barth syndrome (see 'Some diagnoses to consider' below).
- Urine organic acids (methylmalonic aciduria, malonyl-CoA decarboxylase, 3-methylglutaconic aciduria)—preferably early-morning urine before any diuretic dose.
- Urine dicarboxylic acids.
- Cardiolipin (in males to exclude Barth syndrome).
- Brain MRI scan if there are CNS features or regression (mitochondrial disorders, MADD).
- Genomic analysis if presentation suggestive of a syndromic diagnosis, e.g. genomic array, gene panel, or WES/WGS as appropriate.
- Ensure DNA is stored. Consider medium-chain acyl-CoA dehydrogenase (MCAD) deficiency.
- Consider skeletal muscle biopsy—may be informative in the absence of clinical skeletal muscle weakness. Do histochemistry and histology and assay mitochondrial enzyme function.
- Consider ophthalmology review (nystagmus/retinal dystrophy may suggest Alstrom syndrome).

Some diagnoses to consider

Dysmorphic syndromes

NOONAN SYNDROME (NS). HCM, pulmonary valve stenosis, and secundum atrial septal defect (ASD) are the most frequently found cardiac anomalies. Short stature and a characteristic facies with hypertelorism, and short webbed neck are characteristic. Fifty per cent have mutations in *PTPN11*, and in other genes from the Ras-MAPK pathway, e.g. *SOS1, SHOC2, KRAS, CBL*, and *RIT1*. Colquitt and Noonan (2013) found HCM in 14% which is often stable.

LEOPARD (LENTIGINES–ECG ABNORMALITIES–OCULAR HYPERTELORISM–PULMONARY STENOSIS–ABNORMAL GENITALIA–RETARDATION OF GROWTH–DEAFNESS) SYNDROME. Is caused by mutations in the *PTPN11* gene.

CARDIOFACIOCUTANEOUS SYNDROME. Hair is sparse; there is relative macrocephaly, and there can be cardiac defects, most commonly pulmonary stenosis and HCM. The skin is rough, dry, and hyperkeratotic. Polyhydramnios in pregnancy is common, perhaps a prenatal presentation of the severe feeding problems and failure to thrive that are common in the first year of life. Development is usually delayed. CFC is associated with mutations in *BRAF, KRAS*, and *MEK1/2* genes.

COSTELLO SYNDROME. Characterized by prenatally increased growth, postnatal growth retardation, coarse face, loose skin resembling cutis laxa, non-progressive CM (sometimes with arrhythmia), developmental delay, and an outgoing, friendly behaviour. There are very characteristic wrinkled palms and ulnar deviation of the hands. Patients can develop papillomas, especially around the mouth, and have a predisposition for malignancies (mainly abdominal and pelvic rhabdomyosarcoma in childhood). Consider USS surveillance. Costello syndrome is caused by mutations in the *HRAS* gene. Sixty-one per cent of patients have chronic or progressive HCM, emphasizing the need for lifelong screening in this group of patients.

RAS-MAPK (MITOGEN-ACTIVATED PROTEIN KINASE) SIGNALLING PATHWAY. Mutations are found in 6.4% of cases presenting with non-syndromic HCM.

BECKWITH–WIEDEMANN SYNDROME (BWS). HCM is a rare component of BWS. In Nugent *et al.*'s (2003) study, it accounted for only ~1% of HCM presenting before the age of 10 years. See 'Beckwith–Wiedemann syndrome (BWS)' in Chapter 3, 'Common consultations', p. 358.

Metabolic disorders

CARNITINE DEFICIENCY. Systemic carnitine deficiency is AR and due to mutation in *SLC22A5*. The cardiac features are CM, often with striking T-wave abnormalities on ECG, and EFE. Hypoglycaemia may be found and it is a cause of sudden infant death. It is important to recognize, as therapeutic treatment with L-carnitine is lifesaving. Many other conditions have moderately low carnitine and may benefit from carnitine, even though they do not have *SLC22A5* mutations.

FATTY ACID OXIDATION ABNORMALITIES

• HADHB (hydroxyacyl-CoA dehydrogenase/3-ketoacyl-CoA thiolase/enoyl-CoA hydratase, beta-subunit). Also known as LCHAD (long-chain hydroxyacyl-CoA dehydrogenase) deficiency;
• MADD. CM and leukodystrophy;

• MCAD. Sudden death due to hypoglycaemia, rather than CM, is the typical serious complication.

GLYCOGEN STORAGE DISEASE (GSD). Hepatomegaly is an important feature. Typically the ECG shows large voltages and prolonged activation time.

• Type II, alpha-glucosidase deficiency, was previously known as acid maltase deficiency (Pompe disease). Infants are breathless and floppy due to skeletal muscle involvement and cardiac failure. AR due to mutations in the gene *GAA* on 17q23.
• Type IIb. XL *LAMP2* gene at Xq24.

METHYLMALONIC ACIDURIA. AR methylmalonic aciduria (cobalamin deficiency). Type A is caused by mutations in *MMAA* on 4q31.1 and type B is caused by mutations in *MMAB* on 12q24. Toxic metabolites accumulating in methylmalonic acidurias can inhibit adenosine triphosphate (ATP) synthase, which is normally actively regulated in cardiac muscle in response to cellular energy demand (Das 2003).

MALONYL-COA DECARBOXYLASE DEFICIENCY. This AR disorder may present with sudden cardiac failure or death in the first year. Dietary manipulation is unlikely to prevent the development of CM. Mutation in *MLYCD*.

BARTH SYNDROME. Cardioskeletal myopathy with neutropenia occurring in males. An XL cause of a DCM due to mutation in 'taffazin', the *TAZ* gene, at Xq28. Affected boys have neutropenia.

ALSTROM SYNDROME. A rare AR syndrome caused by mutations in *ALMS1* on 2p13. Alstrom syndrome is characterized by childhood obesity with T2D (hyperinsulinism and chronic hyperglycaemia) and neurosensory deficits, e.g. cone–rod retinal dystrophy. A subset of individuals have DCM, hepatic dysfunction, hypothyroidism, male hypogonadism, short stature, and mild/moderate developmental delay.

Mitochondrial disorders (usually HCM)

A number of mitochondrial disorders, such as complex 1 (mitochondrial respiratory chain) deficiency (DCM), KSS, cytochrome C deficiency, and Leigh's disease, may have cardiac involvement. The mitochondrial mutation may be difficult to confirm and in some instances may only be detected in the myocardium. There is overlap between these conditions and the disorders of fatty acid oxidation. See 'Mitochondrial DNA diseases' in Chapter 3, 'Common consultations', p. 490.

Neuromuscular disorders

DMD and BMD, Emery–Dreifuss muscular dystrophy, and limb-girdle muscular dystrophy (LGMD) all have an associated CM. Typically the CM becomes apparent in adolescence or later. See 'Duchenne and Becker muscular dystrophy (DMD and BMD)', p. 402 and 'Limb–girdle muscular dystrophies', p. 476 in Chapter 3, 'Common consultations'.

FRIEDREICH'S ATAXIA (FRDA). Sometimes the characteristic HCM is diagnosed before the neurological symptoms present. FRDA is caused by a triplet expansion in the nuclear *FXN* gene. See 'Ataxic child' in Chapter 2, 'Clinical approach', p. 74.

Genetic advice

Recurrence risk

There will be a genetic aetiology in some children who have an isolated CM, in whom there is no clear aetiology.

The presentation, family history, and cardiac features may give guidance as to the likelihood of a genetic condition. Mitochondrial conditions may have matrilineal inheritance or AR inheritance, or may be sporadic.

Overall, approximately one-third of HCM cases detected in childhood have familial AD HCM, with mutations in the usual sarcomere protein gene. Genetic testing using multiplex gene panels is available (see UK Genetic Testing Network).

Carrier detection

Both parents of a child with CM should have an ECG and an echo. (There is a considerable risk of HCM, and even DCM, being familial with AD inheritance.)

Carrier detection is possible in families where a causative mutation has been defined and may be possible for some biochemical abnormalities.

Prenatal diagnosis

This is available to those families where there is molecular or biochemical confirmation of the diagnosis.

Natural history and further management (preventative measures)

Prevent hypoglycaemia in children with carnitine deficiency or MCAD with dietary advice and a management plan for adequate carbohydrate intake during intercurrent illnesses.

Support group:

Cardiomyopathy UK, http://www.cardiomyopathy.org.

Expert adviser: Ruth Newbury-Ecob, Lead Clinician, Department of Clinical Genetics, University Hospitals Bristol NHS Foundation Trust, Bristol, UK.

References

Colquitt JL, Noonan JA. Cardiac findings in Noonan syndrome on long-term follow-up. *Congenit Heart Dis* 2014; **9**: 144–50.

Das AM. Regulation of the mitochondrial ATP-synthase in health and disease. *Mol Genet Metab* 2003; **79**: 71–82.

Lin AE, Alexander ME, Colan SD, *et al.* Clinical, pathological, and molecular analyses of cardiovascular abnormalities in Costello syndrome: a Ras/MAPK pathway syndrome. *Am J Med Genet A* 2011; **155A**: 486–507.

Lipshultz SE, Sleeper LA, Towbin JA, *et al.* The incidence of pediatric cardiomyopathy in two regions of the United States. *N Engl J Med* 2003; **348**: 1647–55.

Nugent AW, Daubeney PE, Chondros P, *et al.*; National Australian Childhood Cardiomyopathy Study. The epidemiology of childhood cardiomyopathy in Australia. *N Engl J Med* 2003; **348**: 1639–46.

Ostman-Smith I, Brown G, Johnson A, Land JM. Dilated cardiomyopathy due to type II X-linked 3-methylglutaconic aciduria: successful treatment with pantothenic acid. *Br Heart J* 1994; **72**: 349–53.

UK Genetic Testing Network. http://ukgtn.nhs.uk.

van der Burgt I. Noonan syndrome. *Orphanet J Rare Dis* 2007; **2**: 4.

Vela-Huerta MM, Vargas-Origel A, Olvera-López A. Asymmetrical septal hypertrophy in newborn infants of diabetic mothers. *Am J Perinatol* 2000; **17**: 89–94.

Cataract

A cataract is an opacity of the lens of the eye. The birth incidence is 1–15 per 10 000 births; 22–27% of congenital cataracts are inherited, higher in bilateral cases (Rahi et al. 2001). Genetic causes of isolated cataracts are highly heterogeneous and show considerable intra- and interfamilial variation. Cataracts may be isolated or associated with other anterior segment malformations, e.g. aniridia or congenital glaucoma, or associated with syndromes. Lens opacities develop as part of the natural ageing process and cataracts are common in the elderly and conditions with premature ageing or DNA repair defects. Sixty per cent of children with trisomy 21 develop cataracts.

Ophthalmologists describe the type of cataract by its morphology and position in the lens and this will help with the differential diagnosis and classification. A totally opaque lens is the end point of all the pathological types and classification is not then possible. Screening for cataracts is part of the routine neonatal examination. Even after early detection, infants with bilateral cataracts may be significantly visually impaired; however, many of these may have their cataracts as a feature of a multisystem condition.

The geneticist is asked to see infants with cataract to assess if it is part of a metabolic or genetic condition. In adults, the indication is usually to estimate offspring risks.

Clinical approach

History: key points

- Three-generation family tree, with specific enquiry about cataract, visual impairment, retinal detachment, deafness, neurological, joint, renal, and gastrointestinal (GI) problems, and consanguinity.
- At what age were the cataracts first detected?
- Are there other eye anomalies?
- Are there other congenital anomalies or is there a known chromosomal condition?
- Non-genetic factors: infections during pregnancy, congenital and acquired infections, drugs, e.g. steroids, radiation, diabetes mellitus.
- Sun sensitivity (DNA repair defects, e.g. Cockayne syndrome).
- Deafness (Cockayne syndrome, NF2, Stickler syndrome).
- Neonatal jaundice (galactosaemia, cerebrotendinous xanthomatosis (CTX)).
- Developmental milestones. Is there any evidence of developmental delay?

Examination: key points

- Eyes. Detailed assessment for additional ophthalmological features or malformations, including photographs.
- Growth parameters, including head OFC. Investigate:
  - any evidence of deceleration (metabolic disease);
  - failure to thrive (metabolic disease, COFS syndrome, Cockayne syndrome);
  - short stature (skeletal conditions, e.g. Stickler syndrome, Kniest syndrome, chondrodysplasia punctata (CDP)).
- Head and face:
  - large fontanelle (Wiedemann–Rautenstrauch syndrome (WRS));

- hair (hypotrichosis in Hallermann–Streiff syndrome);
- deep-set eyes (Cockayne syndrome);
- 'beaked nose' (Hallermann–Streiff syndrome, WRS);
- coarse features, macroglossia (alpha-mannosidosis).
- Mouth:
  - cleft palate (Stickler and Kniest syndromes);
  - teeth ('screwdriver' incisors in Nance–Horan syndrome).
- Skin:
  - blisters (IP);
  - sun sensitivity (Cockayne);
  - poikiloderma (Rothmund Thomson);
  - ichthyosis (CDP);
  - premature ageing (progeria);
  - lipoatrophy (WRS);
  - xanthomas and xanthelasma (CTX).
- Limbs:
  - asymmetry of limb lengths in a female (Conradi–Hünermann–Happle type of CDP);
  - talipes, floppiness or myotonia (DM).

Special investigations

In an *otherwise normal child*, the basic screen is:
- TORCH (toxoplasmosis, other (including syphilis, varicella-zoster, parvovirus), rubella, cytomegalovirus, and herpes simplex virus) screen;
- urinary reducing substances (e.g. galactosaemia);
- urinary amino and organic acids;
- examination of parents and siblings. Many gene carriers are asymptomatic because of variable expression and mild involvement. Female carriers for Lowe syndrome have characteristic punctate lens opacities; carriers for Nance–Horan syndrome have posterior sutural lens opacities.

Other investigations, as dictated by systemic findings, include the following.
- Metabolic:
  - urinary reducing substances. If reducing substances are found, proceed to enzyme analysis (galactosaemia);
  - urinary protein. Proteinuria may indicate renal Fanconi syndrome which is found in Lowe syndrome. If present, investigate further with urine osmolality, phosphate, and urine and plasma amino acids;
  - urinary amino acids. May need repeating, as sometimes in Lowe syndrome a very early screen is negative;
  - serum calcium and phosphate;
  - peroxisomal analysis (plasma VLCFAs) if features suggest rhizomelic CDP or Zellweger syndrome;
  - sterol analysis (CTX) has elevated plasma cholestanol, Conradi–Hünermann–Happle or XLD CDP due to emopamil binding protein (EBP) mutation).
- Radiological investigations. Consider a skeletal survey to exclude:
  - rickets (Lowe syndrome);
  - epiphyseal stippling (CDP);
  - skeletal dysplasia (Kniest and Stickler syndromes).

- Genomic array analysis.
- DNA analysis:
  - targeted gene testing where a specific genetic condition is recognized, e.g. Lowe syndrome or Cockayne syndrome;
  - gene panel/WES/WGS as appropriate;
  - consider myotonic dystrophy (DM).
- TORCH screen in congenital or early-infancy cataracts.
- Audiology (Cockayne syndrome, NF2).
- Skin biopsy. Consider a skin biopsy to detect DNA repair defects if the clinical picture is suggestive.

Some diagnoses to consider

Congenital or early-infancy cataracts

GALACTOSAEMIA. Classic galactosaemia is an AR condition caused by a deficiency of galactose-1-phosphate uridyl-transferase (GALT). The infants are unwell and fail to thrive. See 'Prolonged neonatal jaundice and jaundice in infants below 6 months' in Chapter 2, 'Clinical approach', p. 288.

GALACTOKINASE DEFICIENCY. An AR condition caused by mutations in *GALK1* on 17q24. They may develop cataracts (as in galactosaemia due to accumulation of galactitol in the lenses, which may resolve with dietary management).

LOWE OCULO-CEREBRO-RENAL SYNDROME. There is renal dysfunction and generalized aminoaciduria. Failure to thrive, developmental delay, and rickets are features. Affected males have dense cataracts present from birth. Glaucoma may be a later feature that follows cataract surgery. Inheritance is XLR. Mutation testing of *OCRL* on Xq25–26.1 is available. Carrier females typically have characteristic punctate lens opacities. If the familial mutation is known, mutation analysis enables definitive assignment of carrier status.

PEROXISOMAL DISORDERS. Rhizomelic CDP and Zellweger syndrome are both AR disorders that present in infancy with a poor prognosis. See 'Floppy infant' in Chapter 2, 'Clinical approach', p. 154.

CEREBRO-OCULO-FACIAL-SKELETAL SYNDROME (COFS). An AR, rapidly progressive neurological disorder, leading to brain atrophy with calcifications, cataracts, microcornea, optic atrophy, progressive joint contractures, and growth failure. See 'DNA repair disorders' in Chapter 3, 'Common consultations', p. 398.

HALLERMANN–STREIFF SYNDROME. Microcornea is present. The nose is thin and the mandible small, and there is hypotrichosis.

WIEDEMANN–RAUTENSTRAUCH SYNDROME (WRS). This condition is also known as neonatal progeria. The facial features can be confused with those of Hallermann–Streiff syndrome, but WRS is a progressive condition leading to early death. Lipoatrophy, prominent veins, and wide fontanelles are features. The inheritance is AR.

NANCE–HORAN SYNDROME. A rare XL semi-dominant syndromic cause of cataract due to mutations in the *NHS* gene on Xp22.13 (Burdon et al. 2003). Males have severe cataracts from birth; other features include screwdriver incisors and dental anomalies of shape and number, and a long face with a prominent chin. Deletions comprise a significant proportion of mutations in *NHS*. Mild/moderate MR is seen in ~80% of males (Toutain

et al. 1997). Carrier females have characteristic sutural cataract; ~5% of carrier females have no ocular signs.

Infancy or childhood-onset cataracts

In a fit child with normal development and stature, the likelihood of finding a syndromic cause is much less than in a neonate. Screening of children with syndromes known to have a cataract as a component will lead to detection in this age group.

STICKLER SYNDROME. Short stature, joint pain (especially the hip), deafness (sensorineural and conductive), and myopia are features. See 'Stickler syndrome' in Chapter 3, 'Common consultations', p. 528.

CHONDRODYSPLASIA PUNCTATA (CDP). Milder types of CDP (AD, XLD, and XLR). See 'Chondrodysplasia punctata' in Chapter 2, 'Clinical approach', p. 98.

CEREBROTENDINOUS XANTHOMATOSIS (CTX). Biallellic mutation in *CYP27A1*. May present with congenital cataract, but more typically in infancy and childhood. It is a lipid storage disease with abnormality of the cholesterol pathway, and the high cholestanol level can be detected by most laboratories offering sterol analysis. Untreated, there is progressive neurological deterioration and atherosclerosis. Early detection important as treatment with bile acids and statins can arrest, though probably not reverse, symptoms.

PREMATURE AGEING AND/OR DNA REPAIR DEFECTS. Examples are progeria and Cockayne syndrome. A skin biopsy will be required to confirm DNA repair defects by UV irradiation of cultured fibroblasts. DNA mutation analysis may also be available. See 'DNA repair disorders' in Chapter 3, 'Common consultations', p. 398.

Juvenile-onset cataracts

NEUROFIBROMATOSIS TYPE 2 (NF2). Children with NF2 can present with embryonal, posterior subcapsular, and cortical lenticular opacities. This is sometimes in association with retinal hamartomas, nerve palsies, or other systemic features, e.g. schwannomas, café-au-lait (CAL) patches. See 'Neurofibromatosis type 2 (NF2)' in Chapter 4, 'Cancer', p. 596.

Adult-onset cataracts

Age-related cataract is a common finding in the elderly. In cross-sectional studies, the prevalence of cataracts is 50% in people aged 65–74 years, increasing to 70% in the over 75s. See 'Myotonic dystrophy' in Chapter 3, 'Common consultations', p. 496.

MYOTONIC DYSTROPHY (DM). Cataracts are found in otherwise asymptomatic individuals with DM, so test for this condition if any clinical suspicion or a positive family history.

Genetic advice

Recurrence risk

If, after careful exclusion of syndromic and environmental causes of cataract, the cataracts appear to be isolated, consider the following.

- Ophthalmological examination of first-degree relatives may detect cataracts and determine the mode of inheritance.

- There are many different forms of inherited cataract and the morphology is not always the same within a family.

- The most common mode of inheritance of familial isolated cataract is AD and these are generally caused by mutations in the structural proteins, such as crystallins. Mutations in the γ-, β-, and α-crystallin-encoding genes are the most frequent cause of isolated congenital cataract; also abnormalities in the erythropoietin-producing hepatocellular receptor tyrosine kinase class A2 (*EphA2*), the gap junction connexins (Cx43, Cx46, and Cx50), paired-like homeodomain transcription factor 3 (PITX3), avian musculoaponeurotic fibrosarcome (MAF), heat shock transcription factor 4 (HSF4), and major intrinsic protein (MIP), and abnormalities in the forkhead transcription factor FOXE3 can cause cataract if dominantly inherited or congenital aphakia in recessive families.
- Consanguinity suggests AR and metabolic abnormalities.
- XL inheritance has been reported.

If the cataracts are a component of a syndrome or chromosomal anomaly, counsel as appropriate for the specific diagnosis.

Carrier detection
- Identification of early cataracts by slit-lamp examination.
- Possible by DNA analysis in families where a causative mutation has been identified.
- May be possible for some biochemical abnormalities.

Prenatal diagnosis
This is technically feasible in those families where there is molecular or biochemical confirmation of diagnosis.

Natural history and further management (preventative measures)

Long-term ophthalmological follow-up and surgery where appropriate. Patients with isolated inherited congenital cataract have a better visual and surgical outcome than those with coexisting ocular and systemic abnormalities (Francis *et al.* 2001).

Support groups: Climb (Children Living with Inherited Metabolic Diseases), http://www.climb.org.uk; Lowe Syndrome Association, http://www.lowesyndrome.org.

Expert adviser: Nicola Ragge, Consultant Clinical Geneticist, Birmingham Women's Hospital, Birmingham, UK; Professor in Medical Genetics, Oxford Brookes University, Oxford, UK.

References

Bermejo E, Martinez-Frias ML. Congenital eye malformations: clinical–epidemiological analysis of 1,124,654 consecutive births in Spain. *Am J Med Genet* 1998; **75**: 497–504.

Burdon KP, McKay JD, Sale MM, et al. Mutations in a novel gene, NHS, cause the pleiotropic effects of Nance-Horan syndrome, including severe congenital cataract, dental anomalies, and mental retardation. *Am J Hum Genet* 2003; **73**: 1120–30.

Francis PJ, Ionides A, Berry V, Bhattacharya S, Moore AT. Visual outcome in patients with isolated autosomal dominant congenital cataract. *Ophthalmology* 2001; **108**: 1104–8.

Huang B, He W. Molecular characteristics of inherited congenital cataracts. *Eur J Med Genet* 2010; **53**: 347–57.

Khanna RC, Foster A, Krishnaiah S, Mehta MK, Gogate PM. Visual outcomes of bilateral congenital and developmental cataracts in young children in south India and causes of poor outcome. *Indian J Ophthalmol* 2013; **61**: 65–70.

Lim Z, Rubab S, Chan YH, Levin AV. Pediatric cataract: the Toronto experience. *Am J Ophthalmol* 2010; **149**: 887–92.

Rahi JS, Botting B; British Congenital Cataract Interest Group. Ascertainment of children with congenital cataract through the National Congenital Anomaly System in England and Wales. *Br J Ophthalmol* 2001; **85**: 1049–51.

Santana A, Waiswol M. The genetic and molecular basis of congenital cataract. *Arq Bras Oftalmol* 2011; **74**: 136–42.

Shiels A, Bennett TM, Hejtmancik JF. Cat-Map: putting cataract on the map. *Mol Vis* 2010; **16**: 2007–15.

Toutain A, Ayrault AD, Moraine C. Mental retardation in Nance-Horan syndrome: clinical and neuropsychological assessment in four families. *Am J Med Genet* 1997; **71**: 305–14.

Trumler AA. Evaluation of paediatric cataracts and systemic disorders. *Curr Opin Ophthalmol* 2011; **22**: 365–79.

Cerebellar anomalies

This section addresses the diagnostic approach to structural abnormality of the cerebellum and associated structures. It is difficult to differentiate between primary non-development (cerebellar hypoplasia) and an atrophic process (cerebellar atrophy) without serial MRI scans. This section is inclusive of both.

Where possible, always view the images and discuss the MRI report with a neuroradiologist to understand the terminology used in the report, so you have a clear anatomical picture of the abnormality. Determine whether the structural abnormality of the brain is restricted to the cerebellum or also involves the cerebral cortex or other neural tissues. Similarly, within the cerebellum, is the hypoplasia restricted to the vermis, or are the cerebellar hemispheres also involved?

For more details on Dandy–Walker malformation (DWM), see 'Posterior fossa malformations' in Chapter 6, 'Pregnancy and fertility', p. 776 and for Chiari malformation, see Box 2.2.

For SCA, see 'Ataxic adult' in Chapter 2, 'Clinical approach', p. 70.

The role of the geneticist is to try to establish a specific diagnosis and to offer genetic advice.

Clinical approach

History: key points

- Detailed three-generation family tree, with specific enquiry about consanguinity.
- Pregnancy: exposure to retinoic acid, cytomegalovirus (CMV), excess alcohol.
- History of episodic ventilation (hyperventilation alternating with hypoventilation).
- Developmental milestones, any loss of skills, hypotonia.
- Visual problems (chorioretinitis, retinal dystrophy, retinitis pigmentosa (RP)).

- Swallowing difficulties.
- Recurrent infections (Hoyeraal–Hreidarsson syndrome (HHS)).

Examination: key points

- OFC. Macrocephaly (rare; consider SNX14, PIGT) and microcephaly may be found, but each has different syndromic associations.
- Neurological examination: tone, posture, ataxia.
- Muscle weakness (muscular dystrophy in muscle–eye–brain (MEB) disease, mitochondrial/respiratory chain disorders).
- Nystagmus, ocular motor apraxia (ciliopathy).
- Tongue cysts and excessive oral frenulae (OFD syndromes, Joubert syndrome (JS)).
- Aniridia (Gillespie syndrome (GS)).
- Polydactyly (OFD, JS).

Special investigations

- Blood count (aplastic anaemia in HHS; also consider immunological investigations).
- LFTs (hepatic fibrosis in ciliopathies), CK (muscular dystrophy and myopathy).
- Renal function and USS (JS).
- Ophthalmology referral (retinal dystrophy or dysplasia in JS, retinal dysplasia in MEB, aniridia in GS).
- Genomic analysis in presence of features suggestive of a syndromic diagnosis, e.g. genomic array, gene panel, or WES/WGS as appropriate.
- 7-dehydrocholesterol (SLO syndrome).
- Isoelectric focussing of transferrins (carbohydrate-deficient glycoprotein syndrome).
- Assessment of plasma alkaline phosphatase (can be high or low in the glycosylphosphatidylinositol (GPI) anchor group of disorders, e.g. PIG).

Box 2.2 Glossary of terms

Cerebellar hypoplasia: a congenitally small cerebellum.

Cerebellar atrophy: progressive reduction in cerebellar size with increasing neurological sequelae.

Pontocerebellar hypoplasia: rare (mainly AR) genetic conditions with underdevelopment of the cerebellum and brainstem.

Dandy–Walker malformation (DWM): describes a triad of findings, including cystic dilatation of the fourth ventricle, complete or partial agenesis of the cerebellar vermis, and an enlarged posterior fossa with displacement of the tentorium.

Cerebellar vermis aplasia: neuroradiology demonstrates a midline defect between the cerebellar hemispheres, but the posterior fossa is not enlarged.

Molar tooth sign: seen on axial neuroimaging (magnetic resonance or computerized tomography (CT)) in Joubert syndrome but is not specific for this condition as it is also seen in other ciliopathies. It is characterized by a deep posterior interpeduncular fossa (best seen on transverse section), thick and elongated superior cerebellar peduncles (best seen on parasagittal section), and a hypoplastic or aplastic superior cerebellar vermis.

Chiari malformations:
- Chiari I. Downward displacement of the lower cerebellum, including the tonsils; rarely causes symptoms in childhood but may be associated with hydrocephalus and syringomyelia;
- Chiari II. Usually associated with myelomeningocele (see 'Neural tube defects' in Chapter 3, 'Common consultations', p. 500);
- Chiari III. Downward displacement of the cerebellum into a posterior encephalocele;
- Chiari IV. A form of cerebellar hypoplasia.

- Metabolic testing (lactate, pyruvate, etc.) if a respiratory chain disorder is suspected.
- EMG/nerve conduction: SMA-like disorder found with pontocerebellar hypoplasia (PCH).
- Mitochondrial studies, particularly where there is cerebellar atrophy, other neuromuscular features, and other organ involvement.

Some diagnoses to consider

With molar tooth sign

JOUBERT SYNDROME (JS). See 'Ciliopathies' in Chapter 3, 'Common consultations', p. 366.

Heterogeneous AR ciliopathy with diagnosis based on:
- hypotonia: present in all patients, moderately severe in infancy;
- ataxia: 75% learn to sit (average 19 months) and 50% to walk (average 4 years). Gait is unstable and tandem walking is poor;
- developmental delay: often severe, but very variable;
- neuroradiology shows cerebellar vermis hypoplasia and molar tooth sign.

Associated anomalies include: episodic hyperpnoea and/or apnoea in 50–75%, especially in infancy; distinctive facial features (high rounded eyebrows, broad nasal bridge and mild epicanthus, anteverted nostrils, triangular-shaped open mouth with an irregular tongue protrusion, low-set and coarse ears); eye anomalies (retinal dysplasia, colobomas, nystagmus, strabismus, and ptosis); oculomotor apraxia; microcystic renal disease; occasionally polydactyly; and a variety of other features. JS is genetically heterogeneous and caused by mutations in genes encoding components of the ciliary apparatus. Surveillance of renal function required. See 'Ciliopathies' in Chapter 3, 'Common consultations', p. 366.

Other ciliopathy syndromes with overlapping features and gene mutations with Joubert syndrome

CEREBELLO-OCULO-RENAL SYNDROMES (ARIMA, SENIOR–LOKEN, AND CEREBELLAR VERMIAN HYPOPLASIA–OLIGOPHRENIA–ATAXIA–COLOBOMA–HEPATIC FIBROSIS (COACH)). These forms of JS include retinal dysplasia and cystic dysplastic kidneys.

LEBER CONGENITAL AMAUROSIS (LCA). Presents with nystagmus and variable neurological involvement; the patient may have seizures. The fundus is normal in infancy, but the ERG is very subnormal or, more usually, non-recordable. Later there are signs of retinal degeneration. Genetic heterogeneity. Mostly AR. See 'Nystagmus' in Chapter 2, 'Clinical approach', p. 252.

ORAL–FACIAL–DIGITAL (OFD) SYNDROMES TYPE MOHR (2) AND VARADI (6). OFD types 2 and 6 are AR malformation syndromes. The features in the hands are syndactyly (usually skin syndactyly affecting variable digits), brachydactyly, and post-axial polydactyly (PAP). Craniofacial anomalies are midline cleft lip, tongue cysts, and excess oral frenulae; the nasal tip may be bifid in type 2. A central Y-shaped metacarpal is typically found in type 6.

Other neuroradiological features and neuronal migration defects

LISSENCEPHALY WITH CEREBELLAR HYPOPLASIA (LCH). This is genetically heterogeneous and tubulinopathies are a major cause.

MICROLISSENCEPHALY WITH SEVERE CEREBELLAR ABNORMALITY AND HIPPOCAMPAL INVOLVEMENT. Suggests an AR condition with mutation in *RELN* in some affected infants.

MUSCLE–EYE–BRAIN DISEASE (MEB) (INCLUDING WALKER–WARBURG SYNDROME (WWS)). AR disorders that share the combination of cerebral neuronal migration defects (cobblestone lissencephaly) and cerebellar abnormalities, ocular abnormalities, and a congenital muscular dystrophy. Mutations in *POMT1* (WWS) and *POMGnT1* (MEB) have been identified. See 'Floppy infant' in Chapter 2, 'Clinical approach', p. 154.

Pontocerebellar hypoplasia

NEURODEGENERATIVE PHENOTYPE WITH MICROCEPHALY AND SEVERE DEVELOPMENTAL DELAY. Feeding/swallowing problems are typical and there may be additional neurological features/weakness consistent with infantile SMA (Renbaum et al. 2009). The causative genes are involved in the development and survival of nerve cells and the processing of RNA molecules. At least eight known genes to date, type 1A probably most frequently diagnosed and due to mutation in *VRK1*. All PCH syndromes to date have AR inheritance, though consider *CASK* mutation in females and mitochondrial disorders in the differential diagnosis.

MENTAL RETARDATION AND MICROCEPHALY WITH PONTINE AND CEREBELLAR HYPOPLASIA (MICPCH). XL due to mutation in *CASK*. Congenital and marked postnatal microcephaly, severe ID, disproportionate pontine and cerebellar hypoplasia. Brain MRI: reduced number and complexity of gyri, thin brainstem, and severe cerebellar hypoplasia. Mostly females; males with this phenotype are more severe with poor survival (Najm et al. 2008).

CEREBELLAR ATAXIA, MENTAL RETARDATION, AND DYS-EQUILIBRIUM SYNDROME (CAMRQ1–4 NON-PROGRESSIVE ATAXIA). Cerebellar hypoplasia and sometimes some simplification of cerebral gyri. Consider in the differential of ataxic cerebral palsy. Biallelic mutation in the very low-density lipoprotein receptor gene (*VLDLR*) causes CAMRQ1. VLDLR is part of the reelin signalling pathway, which guides neuroblast migration in the cerebral cortex and cerebellum (Boycott et al. 2005). See 'Ataxic child' in Chapter 2, 'Clinical approach', p. 74.

Macrocephaly

The unusual combination of macrocephaly with progressive cerebellar hypoplasia may be caused by biallelic mutations in *SNX14* (Thomas et al. 2014) or the GPI anchor disorder PIGT.

Mitochondrial and respiratory chain disorders

These are conditions that reduce the amount of energy available to the developing brain and this may lead to congenital structural defects of the brain (complex 1 deficiency, PDH deficiency), PCH syndromes, and progressive neurological conditions (mitochondrial and autosomally encoded mitochondrial conditions).

Carbohydrate-deficient glycoprotein syndrome

Congenital disorders of glycosylation (CDG) are a group of AR metabolic disorders that are characterized biochemically by defective glycosylation of proteins (abnormal transferrin isoelectrophoresis). The most common type is CDG-Ia, which is a multisystem disorder affecting the nervous system (cerebellar atrophy and encephalopathy), liver, kidney, heart, adipose tissue (lipodystrophy and abnormal fat pads), bone, and genitalia. It is caused by phosphomannomutase (PMM) deficiency, and mutations have been identified in the gene *PMM2*.

GPI deficiency syndromes

Glycosylphosphatidylinositol (GPI) is a glycolipid that anchors >150 various proteins to the cell surface. At least 27 genes are involved in biosynthesis and transport of GPI-anchored proteins. These cause a wide range of multi-system disorders usually with a severe neurological component e.g. delay and seizures. Amongst others, PIGG and PIGT cause cerebellar hypoplasia. PIGT may have the unusual combination of macrocephaly with cerebellar hypoplasia.

Gillespie syndrome (GS)

GS is characterized by bilateral iris hypoplasia, congenital hypotonia, non-progressive ataxia, and progressive cerebellar atrophy, with mild/moderate developmental delay. It is caused by a restricted repertoire of DNMs in *ITPR1* with a dominant negative effect.

Genetic advice

Recurrence risk

After careful evaluation and exclusion of syndromic and single gene disorders, consider the following:

- many of the syndromic causes of cerebellar structural abnormalities have AR inheritance. For apparently isolated cerebellar hypoplasia or vermian agenesis, the recurrence risk may be as high as 25%. Empiric risk data are not available;
- CASK mutation-X-linked;
- AD inheritance of vermis aplasia is also reported; scan any parent with ataxia, nystagmus, or other neurological abnormalities. Phenotype overlaps with SCA. Tubulinopathy may be AD;
- DWM. When the evidence suggests that DWM has not occurred as part of a Mendelian or chromosomal disorder, then the recurrence risk is relatively low at 1–5% (Murray et al. 1985).

Carrier detection

This is possible in families with a known mutation.

Prenatal diagnosis

- This is possible by CVS in families with a known mutation.
- PND of cerebellar hypoplasia based on early USS is not reliable. Detailed USS is often offered in a subsequent

pregnancy, but these limitations must be carefully discussed with the parents.

- DWM. Refer to 'Posterior fossa malformations' in Chapter 6, 'Pregnancy and fertility', p. 776.

Support group:

Many of the syndromes have their own support groups. See Contact a Family, http://www.cafamily.org.uk.

References

Boycott KM, Flavelle S, Bureau A, et al. Homozygous deletion of the very low density lipoprotein receptor gene causes autosomal recessive cerebellar hypoplasia with cerebral gyral simplification. *Am J Hum Genet* 2005; **77**: 477–83.

Drouin-Garraud V, Belgrand M, Grünewald S, et al. Neurological presentation of a congenital disorder of glycosylation CDG-Ia: implications for diagnosis and genetic counseling. *Am J Med Genet* 2001; **101**: 46–9.

Ferland RJ, Eyaid W, Collura RV, et al. Abnormal cerebellar development and axonal decussation due to mutations in AHI1 in Joubert syndrome. *Nat Genet* 2004; **36**: 1008–13.

Makrythanasis P, Kato M, et al. Pathogenic variants in PIGG cause intellectual disability with seizures and hypotonia. *Am J Hum Genet* 2016 Apr 7; **98**(4): 615–26.

Maria BL, Boltshauser E, Plamer SC, Tran TX. Clinical features and revised diagnostic criteria in Joubert syndrome. *J Child Neurol* 1999; **14**: 583–90.

Murray JC, Johnson JA, Bird TD. Dandy–Walker malformation: etiologic heterogeneity and empiric recurrence risks. *Clin Genet* 1985; **28**: 272–83.

Najm J, Horn D, Wimplinger I, et al. Mutations of CASK cause an X-linked brain malformation phenotype with microcephaly and hypoplasia of the brainstem and cerebellum. *Nat Genet* 2008; **40**: 1065–7.

Parisi MA, Dobyns WB. Human malformations of the midbrain and hindbrain: review and proposed classification scheme. *Mol Genet Metab* 2003; **80**: 36–53.

Renbaum P, Kellerman E, Jaron R, et al. Spinal muscular atrophy with pontocerebellar hypoplasia is caused by a mutation in the VRK1 gene. *Am J Hum Genet* 2009; **85**: 281–9.

Ross ME, Swanson K, Dobyns WB. Lissencephaly with cerebellar hypoplasia (LCH): a heterogeneous group of cortical malformations. *Neuropediatrics* 2001; **32**: 256–63.

Satran D, Pierpont ME, Dobyns WB. Cerebello-oculo-renal syndromes including Arima, Senior–Loken and COACH syndromes: more than just variants of Joubert syndrome. *Am J Med Genet* 1999; **86**: 459–69.

Thomas AC, Williams H, Setó-Salvia N, et al. Mutations in SNX14 cause a distinctive autosomal-recessive cerebellar ataxia and intellectual disability syndrome. *Am J Hum Genet* 2014; **95**: 611–21.

Cerebral palsy

Cerebral palsy (CP) is a term used to describe a *non-progressive* physical disorder that affects movement. CP is not a progressive disorder because there is no ongoing pathological process. The features do alter with the age of the child and brain maturity, e.g. children who later develop spasticity may be very floppy as neonates.

Brain imaging, particularly MRI, is required before counselling to assess for features of hypoxic–ischaemic injury (HII) secondary to perinatal asphyxia and to exclude other CNS causes of the neurological deficit. The images need expert assessment as the findings in HII are highly variable and depend on a number of factors, including gestation/brain maturity, severity and duration of insult, and type and timing of imaging studies.

- Spastic CP. The muscle tone is increased and the reflexes are brisk. Muscle strength is reduced.
  - Hemiplegic CP: non-symmetrical. The contralateral limbs are affected.
  - Diplegic CP: symmetrical. The legs are affected more than the arms.
  - Quadriplegic CP: all four limbs are affected.
- Athetoid (extrapyramidal, dystonic, choreoathetoid, dyskinetic) CP. Involuntary movements and loss of control of posture.
- Ataxic CP. There is poor coordination of movements with balance difficulties. These patients have a wide-based gait and a tremor may be observed.

CP affects about one in 400 births. This figure is not reducing with better obstetric care because more premature infants are surviving. Prematurity, low birthweight, abnormal birth history, infections (pre- and postnatal), and vascular events are considered as aetiological factors when paediatricians assess children with CP. Birth trauma is not a frequent cause; perinatal asphyxia is a major factor in <5%. CP is more common in the first child and then from the fifth or subsequent child and in twins. The aetiology is unknown for most children with CP. There may be predisposing genetic factors, e.g. thrombophilia.

The challenge for the geneticist is to ensure that genetic conditions are detected, while recognizing that, in the majority of children with CP, there is a non-genetic aetiology. Some clinical features are more closely associated with a genetic aetiology and it is important to recognize these.

Clinical approach

History: key points

- Family history. Enquire about consanguinity and previously affected sibs. Birth order.
- Paternal age. A raised paternal age has been associated with athetoid CP in one study.
- Pregnancy: bleeding in the first trimester (vascular event, loss of twin), invasive testing, infections, drug exposure, twinning, fetal movements.
- Birth history risk factors:
  - prematurity—the lower the gestational age, the greater the risk of CP;
  - birthweight <1500 g;
  - twins;
  - birth history suggestive of anoxia, e.g. low Apgar scores, resuscitation and admission to a neonatal

intensive care unit (NICU), seizures, irritability, and poor feeding in the neonatal period (see 'Neonatal encephalopathy and intractable seizures' in Chapter 2, 'Clinical approach', p. 246).
- OFC measurement at birth and subsequent records.
- Seizures. Found in 25–30% of children and 10% of adults. Could indicate an underlying structural brain malformation or a metabolic condition with genetic implications.
- Developmental milestones. Global delay or, particularly, motor problems.
- Evidence of regression. CP by definition is a non-progressive disorder.

Examination: key points

- Head circumference. Plot and compare with previous readings.
- Neurological signs:
  - muscle power and tone;
  - reflexes are brisk in association with spasticity;
  - are the signs symmetrical?
  - movement disorder—athetosis, dystonia;
  - ataxia: assess for both fine and gross motor ataxia.
- Dysmorphic features, other congenital anomalies, skin pigmentary disturbances (investigate for genetic and chromosomal conditions), ichthyosis (Sjögren–Larsen syndrome).

Investigations

- Brain imaging, preferably MRI scan, to:
  - confirm that any lesions are compatible with asphyxia, prematurity, etc.;
  - exclude possibly genetically determined structural brain malformations such as migrational abnormalities;
  - assess for features of metabolic or mitochondrial disease (e.g. basal ganglia lesions, agenesis of the corpus callosum);
  - may be helpful in establishing the timing of the insult;
  - *COL4A1* mutation can cause porencephaly and MRI features that overlap with HII.
- Ophthalmology—dislocated lenses (molybdenum cofactor deficiency), retinal arterial tortuosity, and cataract (*COL4A1*).
- Basic screen of biochemistry to include creatine phosphokinase (CPK; MEB disease), plasma urate, free T3, T4 and TSH.
- Urine for amino acids, organic acids, sulfite (fresh and frozen urine required), purine metabolites. Organic acidaemias can present with a spastic diplegia. Microscopic haematuria (*COL4A1*).
- Genomic array on all children with any features, except uncomplicated CP with no intellectual impairment and typical cranial MRI findings.
- Consider gene panel/WES/WGS as appropriate. Conditions with specific diagnostic tests have been confused with CP, even though the features of these conditions are not classical for CP. These include COL4A1, molybdenum cofactor deficiency, Angelman syndrome, Rett syndrome, Batten disease, lissencephalies, and XL MR conditions.

- Thrombophilia screen and factor V Leiden in children with a perinatal stroke as the cause of the CP.
- Consider investigating the mother for lupus.

Some diagnoses to consider

Maternal factors
Mothers with medical problems are at higher risk in each pregnancy. Make sure that maternal PKU is not a possibility. Teratogens, placental dysfunction, and autoimmune factors may need to be considered, particularly systemic lupus erythematosus (SLE).

Genetic advice
For all types of CP, the following features have been described in familial cases:
- microcephaly;
- significant and symmetrical spasticity;
- progression of symptoms;
- seizures;
- MR;
- other congenital anomalies;
- a positive family history and consanguinity;
- a *lack* of significant perinatal asphyxia and other known environmental risk factors;
- dysmorphic features.

Recurrence risk
If there is consanguinity, a sibling recurrence risk of 25% may be advised. Where there are two affected children, a 25% recurrence risk to further siblings may be appropriate.

Spastic CP
Bundey and Griffiths (1977) confirmed earlier studies that established that the major determinants of genetic risk were symmetry of the spasticity and microcephaly. The 1977 study gave a recurrence risk of 9% to siblings of a child with symmetrical CP and a normal birth history. Some of these children may have had recognized genetically determined conditions if MRI scans had been available to screen for structural brain malformations and signs suggestive of metabolic disorders. This risk figure may overestimate the risk, but it does highlight the children with a potential (AR or XL) genetic risk.

Children without an abnormal pregnancy, birth, or perinatal history should be investigated thoroughly to exclude metabolic and genetic conditions. If there is significant microcephaly, see 'Microcephaly' in Chapter 2, 'Clinical approach', p. 228.

Athetoid CP
Within the CP syndromes, athetosis is most commonly causally associated with serious perinatal complications. It can follow hypoxic–ischaemic encephalopathy and, in these children, the brain MRI shows characteristic features with atrophy in the caudate and putamen. Genetic disorders to consider are:
- mitochondrial disorders;
- organic acidaemias;
- dopa-responsive dystonia (DRD; Segawa syndrome). The phenotype in childhood may resemble athetoid CP and all children with this condition should have a trial of L-dopa. See 'Dystonia' in Chapter 2, 'Clinical approach', p. 138;
- *MECP2* mutations, Rett syndrome;

- XL *ARX* mutations with dystonia.

Genetic factors are thought to play a lesser role, although the risk of recurrence in siblings has been suggested to be as high as 10%. Amor et al. (2001) state that the genetic contribution to athetoid CP is small, with an overall recurrence risk of 1%; **many geneticists consider this risk is too low to use for counselling purposes.** The actual risk figure given in any individual case will depend on how compelling the evidence is for serious perinatal complications and how thoroughly genetic factors have been considered and excluded.

Ataxic CP
Be wary of this diagnosis as many are genetic e.g. cerebellar ataxia, mental retardation, and disequilibrium, an AR disorder caused by biallelic variants in CA8, VLDLR, ATP6A2 and WDR81. If there is no evidence of birth asphyxia, this is a diagnosis made after exclusion of other causes of a congenital ataxia (see 'Ataxic child' in Chapter 2, 'Clinical approach', p. 74). A high-resolution brain MRI scan is mandatory prior to definitive counselling as congenital structural lesions of the cerebellum, such as hypoplasia or a Dandy–Walker cyst, may be found and aid estimation of recurrence risks.

Conflicting recurrence risk figures are found in the literature. There are undoubtedly a number of AR conditions with congenital ataxia and these require careful consideration. Most authors and geneticists advise an up to 10% recurrence risk.

CP with dysmorphic features and no diagnosis
Accurate empiric figures are not available for this heterogeneous group. Unless there are factors suggesting a high recurrence risk (e.g. consanguinity), a risk of ~5% for siblings of a female and ~5–10% for siblings of a male proband seems reasonable.

Carrier detection
Not possible unless a specific biochemical or genetic cause has been identified.

Prenatal diagnosis
Not possible unless a specific biochemical or genetic cause has been identified.

Natural history and further management (preventative measures)
Children should be under the care of a neurodevelopmental multidisciplinary team.

Support groups: Scope, PO Box 833, Milton Keynes, MK12 5NY, UK, http://www.scope.org.uk; Cerebral Palsy Foundation (USA), http://yourcpf.org.

References
Amor DJ, Craig JE, Delatycki MB, Reddihough D. Genetic factors in athetoid cerebral palsy. *J Child Neurol* 2001; **16**: 793–7.

Bundey S, Griffiths MI. Recurrence risks in families of children with symmetrical spasticity. *Dev Med Child Neurol* 1977; **19**: 179–91.

Colver A, Fairhurst C, Pharaoh PO. Cerebral palsy. *Lancet* 2014; **383**: 1240–9.

Hoon AH Jr, Reinhardt EM, Kelley RI, et al. Brain imaging in suspected extrapyramidal cerebral palsy: observations in distinguishing genetic–metabolic from acquired causes. *J Pediatr* 1997; **131**: 240–5.

Lynch JK, Nelson KB, Curry CJ, Grether JK. Cerebrovascular accidents in children with factor V Leiden mutation. *J Child Neurol* 2001; **16**: 735–44.

Chondrodysplasia punctata

In chondrodysplasia punctata (CDP), there is punctiform calcification (stippling) of bones, especially the epiphyses of the long tubular bones, patellae, and carpal and tarsal bones. Sites to look at specifically on a radiograph are the spine, knee joint, and shoulder. The larynx and tracheal rings may be affected. There may be paravertebral stippling. Stippling represents aberrant calcification of cartilage in the bones. Stippling is seen in fetuses, babies, and infants, but in older children >2 years, it is no longer present. It seems to be incorporated into the growing bone but may lead to disharmonic growth as in Conradi–Hünermann syndrome. It is important to request the early films when children and adults are referred for counselling.

CDP is a heterogeneous condition involving:
- genetic defects in:
  (1) peroxisomal metabolism;
  (2) cholesterol metabolism; or
  (3) vitamin K metabolism.
- acquired embryopathies caused by:
  (1) maternal malabsorption of vitamin K;
  (2) maternal use of warfarin;
  (3) maternal use of phenytoin; or
  (4) maternal SLE.
Table 2.2 gives a classification of the various CDPs.

Clinical approach

History: key points
- Three-generation family tree with specific enquiry for consanguinity (AR types of CDP).
- Pregnancy loss of males in the second trimester (XLD CDP).
- Male proband; consider XLR CDP.
- Detailed enquiry about maternal health, e.g. malabsorption, maternal SLE.
- Detailed enquiry about pregnancy history, e.g. fetal exposure to warfarin or phenytoin.
- Bleeding in the neonatal period (vitamin K deficiency).
- Growth delay (associated with failure to thrive in rhizomelic CDP (RCDP)).
- Developmental progress. Seizures?

Examination: key points
- Height or length, arm span, upper and lower body lengths.
- Limb shortening. Is it predominantly proximal (rhizomelic)?
- Asymmetry of limb shortening (XL CDP).
- Scoliosis.
- Congenital contractures.
- Flat nasal bridge/nasal hypoplasia (more severe in XLR CDP and acquired embryopathies).
- Cataracts.
- Hyperkeratosis and ichthyosis. Patchy or generalized?
- Alopecia (patchy in XLD CDP).
- Hands (hypoplasia of the distal phalanges in XLR CDP and warfarin embryopathy).
- Neurological signs of spinal stenosis.

Special investigations
- Full radiological survey, including lateral of the foot. Look for other characteristic features, e.g. vertebral coronal clefts in RCDP, hypoplasia of distal phalanges in XLR CDP, and warfarin embryopathy. These additional diagnostic features are important in children of age 3 years and over when stippling may no longer be seen. Patterns of stippling are characteristic for different disorders.
- Abnormalities of plasmalogen biosynthesis such as elevated phytanic acid.
- VLCFAs (Zellweger syndrome).
- Sterol analysis: elevation of 8-dehydrocholesterol and 8(9)-cholestenol in XLD CDP. Elevated 7-dehydrocholesterol in SLO syndrome.
- Arylsulfatase E analysis.
- DNA for diagnostic testing or storage.
- Genomic analysis in presence of features suggestive of a chromosomal or syndromic diagnosis, e.g. genomic array, gene panel, or WES/WGS as appropriate.
- Investigation of the mother for SLE (antinuclear factor (ANF) and antibodies to double-stranded DNA).

Some diagnoses to consider

Rhizomelic chondrodysplasia punctata (RCDP)

This is divided into three types. Classical RCDP is associated with mutation in *PEX7* that encodes peroxin 7. There is a correlation between low gene activity and a more severe clinical phenotype. Congenital contractures, typical facial features, symmetrical and predominantly proximal limb shortening, and cataracts. Failure to thrive, developmental delay, and seizures become apparent in the first year.

X-linked chondrodysplasia punctata (CDP)
- XLR (*ARSE* deficiency, brachytelephalangic). Males are affected. The nose is very flat and there is hypoplasia of the distal phalanges. The condition is caused by mutations in *ARSE* leading to arylsulfatase E deficiency. In children with additional features, consider a contiguous gene deletion syndrome of Xp22.
- XLD (Conradi–Hünermann or Conradi–Hünermann–Happle syndrome). Asymmetry of limb involvement is a useful diagnostic feature. Scoliosis can be a serious problem. Most affected females have hair and skin signs, which are patchy, in keeping with X-inactivation. The condition can be confirmed by sterol analysis; there is elevation of 8-dehydrocholesterol and 8(9)-cholestenol. The gene *EPB* is at Xp11.

Autosomal dominant (AD) CDP (tibia–metacarpal type)

In adults, the radiological features show improvement, compared to early films. Surveillance required for spinal stenosis.

Binder syndrome

The main feature is a hypoplastic nose with flattening of the tip and alae nasi and relative prognathism. There is debate as to whether this is a distinct entity or if it represents the adult phenotype of milder forms of CDP.

Table 2.2 Table to describe the different clinical phenotypes of CDP

CDP, X-linked dominant, Conradi–Hünermann type (CDPX2)	XLD	302960	Xp11	EBP	Emopamil-binding protein	
CDP, X-linked recessive, brachytelephalangic type (CDPX1)	XLR	302950	Xp22.3	ARSE	Arylsulfatase E	
Congenital hemidysplasia, ichthyosis, limb defects (CHILD)	XLD	308050	Xp11	NSDHL	NAD(P)H steroid dehydrogrenase-like protein	
Congenital hemidysplasia, ichthyosis, limb defects (CHILD)	XLD	308050	Xq28	EBP	Emopamil-binding protein	
Greenberg dysplasia	AR	215140	1q42.1	LBR	Lamin B receptor, 3-beta-hydroxysterol delta (14)-reductase	Includes hydrops–ectopic calcification–moth-eaten appearance dysplasia (HEM) and dappled diaphyseal dysplasia
Rhizomelic CDP type 1	AR	215100	6q22–24	PEX7	Peroxisomal PTS2 receptor	
Rhizomelic CDP type 2	AR	222765	1q42	DHPAT	Dihydroxyacetone phosphate acyltransferase (DHAPAT)	
Rhizomelic CDP type 3	AR	600121	2q31	AGPS	Alkylglycerone-phosphate synthase (AGPS)	
CDP tibial–metacarpal type	AD/AR	118651				Nosologic status uncertain
Astley–Kendall dysplasia	AR?					Relationship to OI and to Greenberg dysplasia unclear

Note that stippling can occur in several syndromes such as Zellweger, Smith–Lemli–Opitz, and others. See also desmosterolosis as well as SEMO short limb—abnormal calcification type in group 11.

Reproduced from Warman ML et al., International Nosology and Classification of Genetic Skeletal Disorders (2010 revision), *American Journal of Medical Genetics Part A*, copyright 2011, with permission from Wiley.

CHILD syndrome (congenital hemidysplasia–ichthiosiform erythroderma–limb defects)

An XLD disorder with clinical similarities to XLD CDP; indeed some patients originally thought to have CHILD had mutation in *EPB*. CHILD syndrome has been found to be due to mutation in *NSDHL*, another gene involved in cholesterol biosynthesis.

Zellweger syndrome

AR peroxisomal disorder often presenting in the neonatal period with central hypotonia ± seizures. The fontanelle is large and the forehead high. Punctate calcification is typically seen in the patellae. The stippled epiphyses are most commonly seen at the knees. See 'Floppy infant' in Chapter 2, 'Clinical approach', p. 154.

Smith–Lemli–Opitz (SLO) syndrome

Failure to thrive, microcephaly, hypospadias in males, and 2/3 toe syndactyly are important features. Stippled epiphyses are not a constant feature. See 'Hypospadias' in Chapter 2, 'Clinical approach', p. 186.

Stickler syndrome

There is no stippling in Stickler syndrome, but there may be some diagnostic difficulties as the facies of Stickler is similar to that of CDP. See 'Stickler syndrome' in Chapter 3, 'Common consultations', p. 528.

Acquired embryopathies

WARFARIN EMBRYOPATHY. Warfarin and other coumarin derivatives are vitamin K antagonists that cross the placenta and, after exposure at 6–12/40 weeks' gestation, can cause an embryopathy (CDP with nasal hypoplasia and/or stippled epiphyses). The nasal hypoplasia may be severe.

MATERNAL MALABSORPTION LEADING TO VITAMIN K DEFICIENCY. This can cause an embryopathy clinically indistinguishable from warfarin embryopathy.

PSEUDO-WARFARIN EMBRYOPATHY. This is due to an inborn deficiency of vitamin K epoxide reductase. Phenotype includes hypoplasia of the distal phalanges, which is a characteristic feature of XLR CDP due to arylsulfatase E deficiency, and helped establish that there is a common metabolic aetiology for XLR CDP, pseudo-warfarin embryopathy, and the acquired embryopathies.

MATERNAL SLE. This has been associated with a similar phenotype to that of warfarin embryopathy.

Genetic advice

Recurrence and offspring risk

If the cause of the stippling is unknown after careful investigation and expert analysis of the radiological features, consider:

- the possibility of mildly affected parents. X-rays of adults will not show stippling but may show irregular bone growth;
- the need to investigate the mother for evidence of malabsorption or SLE;
- the adult asking for offspring risks may be unaware of his/her own mother's pregnancy history.

Carrier detection

Possible where there is a causative mutation, biochemical test, or radiological features.

Prenatal diagnosis
- The two main techniques are USS and CVS/amniocentesis.
- Early prenatal testing may be possible using molecular or biochemical analysis.
- USS examination of the epiphyses combined with limb measurements may be used in pregnancies at risk due to maternal medication or SLE.

Natural history and further management (preventative measures)
- Arrange for ongoing medical supervision with particular attention to the spine (scoliosis and spinal stenosis).
- Rhizomelic CDP. In the study of White *et al.* (2003), 90% survived to 1.5–2 years and 50% to 6–6.5 years. They discuss surveillance based on the medical complications of the children studied.

Support group:
Many of the syndromes have their own support groups. See Contact a Family, http://www.cafamily.org.uk.

Expert adviser: Ravi Savarirayan, Consultant Clinical Geneticist, Victorian Clinical Genetics Services, Parkville, Australia.

References
Hall JG, Pauli RM, Wilson KM. Maternal and fetal sequelae of anticoagulation therapy during pregnancy. *Am J Med* 1980; **68**: 122–40.

Savarirayan R, Boyle RJ, Masel J, Rogers JG, Sheffield LJ. Longterm follow-up in chondrodysplasia punctata, tibia–metacarpal type, demonstrating natural history. *Am J Med Genet A* 2004; **124A**: 148–57.

Warman ML, Cormier-Daire V, Hall C, *et al.* Nosology and classification of genetic skeletal disorders: 2010 revision. *Am J Med Genet A* 2011; **155A**: 943–68.

White AL, Modaff P, Holland-Morris F, Pauli RM. Natural history of rhizomelic chondrodysplasia punctata. *Am J Med Genet A* 2003; **118A**: 332–42.

Cleft lip and palate

The development of the facial structures requires migration of cells and then fusion of adjacent areas (see Figure 2.8). Clefts of the lip and palate occur at the place where this fusion naturally occurs. At ~7 weeks' gestation, the maxillary prominences on each side of the face move into close proximity with the fused medial nasal prominences forming the labial grooves. Normally this groove is infilled by the mesenchyme. When this process is impaired, the labial groove persists and over time the thin residual tissue in the floor of the groove breaks down, forming a complete unilateral cleft. Cleft palate occurs when there is failure of the mesenchymal masses in the lateral palatine processes to meet and fuse with each other, with the nasal septum, and/or with the posterior margin of the median palatine process (see Figure 2.9). In the female, palatal processes fuse ~1 week later than in the male. Formation of the upper lip and palate is complete by 12 weeks' gestation.

Clefts of the lip and/or palate (CL/P) are common birth defects of complex aetiology (see Figure 2.10). CL/P can occur in isolation or as part of a broad range of chromosomal, Mendelian, or teratogenic syndromes. Although there has been marked progress in identifying genetic and environmental triggers for syndromic CL/P, the aetiology of the more common non-syndromic (isolated) forms remains poorly characterized (Dixon et al. 2011).

Cleft lip

With or without cleft palate, is found in 1/700 to 1/1000 births. It is unilateral in 80%, with the left side more commonly affected, and bilateral in 20%. Males are more likely to have severe disease with alveolar (gum) and palatal involvement. There is a spectrum of abnormality, ranging from a small notch in the upper lip lateral to the midline to a bilateral cleft extending up to the nostrils and into the gums and palate. Midline cleft lip is rare and may be a feature of OFD syndrome and Ellis–van Creveld (EVC) syndrome and holoprosencephaly.

Cleft palate

Occurs in 4 per 10 000 births. The spectrum goes from a bifid uvula to a submucous cleft palate (palatal mucosa intact but underlying muscle deficiency), with velopharyngeal insufficiency (regurgitation of milk through the nose in babies and nasal speech in older children), to a cleft soft palate, a narrow V-shaped cleft, and finally a wide U-shaped central cleft involving the hard palate.

Isolated midline cleft palate appears to represent a different malformation process to that of CL/P with different syndrome associations. We have attempted to show this by using the abbreviation CL/P for cleft lip and palate and CP for cleft palate.

In the majority of children, the cleft is an isolated malformation. In the newborn surveys of Stoll, 37% of children born with clefts had an associated malformation (47% CP; 37% CL/P; 13% CL) and Milerad's figures were 22% with CP, 28% with CL/P, and 8% in association with CL.

There are many syndromes that may have a cleft as a feature, and the aim of the clinic visit is to exclude these as far as possible prior to genetic counselling.

Pierre–Robin or Robin sequence

The Robin sequence is defined as a U-shaped palatal cleft in association with micrognathia and glossoptosis (retrodisplacement of the tongue in the pharynx) causing upper airway obstruction. It occurs with a frequency of 1/8500 births. In Robin sequence, micrognathia is present at the

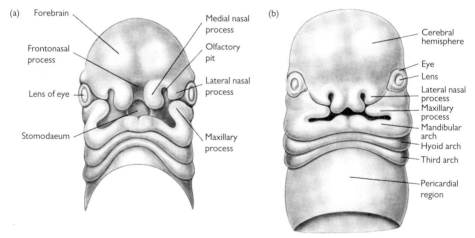

Figure 2.8 Schematic of facial features of embryos at stages 15 (33 days), 18 (45 days), 21 (52 days), and 23+ (60 days). The lip is a mosaic structure composed of the: (1) frontonasal, (2) left maxillary, (3) left mandibular, (4) right mandibular, and (5) right maxillary processes.

Reproduced with permission from G.J. Romanes, *Cunningham's Manual of Practical Anatomy*, Volume 3: Head, Neck and Brain, 15th Edition, 1986, Figure 300, Page 302, with permission from Oxford University Press.

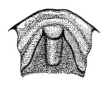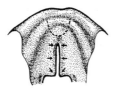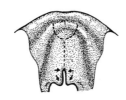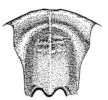

Figure 2.9 Schematic of closure of secondary palate.
This figure was published in *The Developing Human*, Fourth Edition, Moore KL, Copyright CV Mosby Co, St. Louis, 1988.

time that palate fusion is programmed to begin. Because of the mandibular anomaly, the tongue is not free to descend from between the vertical palatal shelves and prevents them from orientating horizontally and fusing in the midline. See 'Micrognathia and Robin sequence' in Chapter 2, 'Clinical approach', p. 232.

Clinical approach

History: key points

- Three-generation family tree, with specific enquiry about clefts and missing teeth.
- Pregnancy. Anticonvulsant medication, steroid treatment.
- Oligohydramnios (CP in Pierre–Robin or with micrognathia).

- Maternal diabetes.
- Vision (CP and myopia in Stickler syndrome).
- Delayed speech development and schooling difficulties (CP del 22q11).
- Hypocalcaemia, immune deficiency, cardiac abnormality (CP del 22q11).

Examination: key points

- Stature (short stature in 22q11, Stickler syndrome, bone dysplasia, e.g. Kniest).
- Skeletal abnormalities (skeletal dysplasias, OPD syndrome).
- Mouth:
  - lip pits (CL/P and CP/van der Woude (VWS) syndrome, popliteal pterygium syndrome);

(a) (b)

(c) (d)

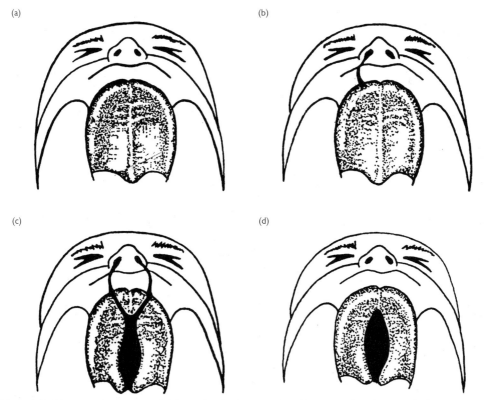

Figure 2.10 Schematics of various types of cleft lip with and without cleft palate. Orientation is from the tongue, looking upward. (a) Normal. (b) Unilateral cleft lip. (c) Bilateral cleft lip and palate. (d) Cleft palate.

- oral frenulae (OFD);
- ankyloglossia (XL CP and ankyloglossia).
- Face:
  - 'pugilistic' facies (OPD);
  - absent lacrimal punctae (ectrodactyly–ectodermal dysplasia–clefting (EEC) syndrome);
  - flat midface (Stickler syndrome).
- Chin. Robin sequence (CP, Stickler syndrome, del(22q); spondyloepiphyseal dysplasia congenital type (SEDC); abnormal fetal position pushing the tongue up on to the developing palate).
- Hands/feet:
  - polydactyly (OFD syndromes, SLO syndrome);
  - 'tree-frog' abnormality of the feet (OPD syndrome);
  - ectrodactyly (CL/P–ectrodactyly—EEC syndrome).
- Limbs. Contractures and webbing of knees, elbows (popliteal pterygium syndrome).
- Heart. Cardiac murmur/defects (22q11, other chromosomal conditions, SLO).
- Genital anomalies (SLO, popliteal pterygium syndrome).
- Examine parents for submucous cleft, bifid uvula, and lip pits.

Special investigations

- Genomic analysis in presence of features suggestive of a chromosomal or syndromic diagnosis (e.g. if cleft plus another abnormality), e.g. genomic array, gene panel, or WES/WGS as appropriate.
- Skull and/or skeletal survey if indicated from examination or pedigree.
- 7-dehydrocholesterol if any other features of SLO (e.g. growth deficiency, 2/3 toe syndactyly, cardiac defects, polydactyly, hypospadias).
- Cardiac echo if murmur present.
- Renal USS in OFD syndrome.
- Ophthalmology assessment in children with possible Stickler syndrome.
- DNA for *IRF6* analysis in VWS, *p63* in EEC, or for *TBX22* mutation analysis if XL CP with ankyloglossia.

Some diagnoses to consider

CL/P and CP are features of a large number of syndromes. Those listed below are selected because they are comparatively common and the presenting feature may be a cleft. In some individuals, the other features may be quite subtle.

van der Woude syndrome (VWS—CL/P and CP)
This is the most common syndromic form of CL/P and a condition where CL/P and CP can occur. It is a dominantly inherited condition caused in some families by mutations in the interferon regulatory factor 6 gene (*IRF6*). Mutation detection rate in *IRF6* is ~50%. Between 30% and 50% represent new mutations. It is characterized by bilateral indentations on the lower lips known as lip pits. Some gene carriers have missing teeth. Penetrance ranges between 89% and 99%, but expression can be *very* variable within a family and gene carriers may have lip pits as the only manifestation of the condition. Risks for clefts are less than the genetic risks and this is an example of a condition where prenatal genetic testing would not accurately predict the phenotype. Popliteal pterygium syndrome is allelic.

Stickler syndrome (CP)
An AD condition characterized by congenital and non-progressive myopia with abnormality of the vitreous gel,

flat midface and depressed nasal bridge, midline clefting ranging from a cleft of the soft palate to Pierre–Robin sequence, deafness, and hypermobility in youth with early degenerative arthritis in older individuals. See 'Stickler syndrome' in Chapter 3, 'Common consultations', p. 528.

22q del (CP)
Conotruncal heart defects, CP, or palatal insufficiency with nasal speech, speech delay, mild learning disability, immunodeficiency (usually mild), and hypocalcaemia in some. See '22q11 deletion syndrome' in Chapter 5, 'Chromosomes', p. 624.

SATB2 syndrome (CP)
All patients have significant neurodevelopmental impairment, most have absent/near absent speech with normal growth. Drooling and dental anomalies are common features. ~50% have cleft palate (Bengami 2017).

Treacher–Collins syndrome (CP)
AD due to mutations in *TCOF1* on 5q31. Severe micrognathia, ear anomalies including microtia, conductive deafness, malar hypoplasia, inferior lid colobomata. See 'Micrognathia and Robin sequence' in Chapter 2, 'Clinical approach', p. 232.

Opitz syndrome (CL/P)
XLR due to mutations in *MID1*. Associated features include hypertelorism and hypospadias. See 'Ocular hypertelorism' in Chapter 2, 'Clinical approach', p. 258.

Kabuki syndrome (CP)
Characterized by facial dysmorphism with long palpebral fissures and eversion of the lateral one-third of the lower lid, postnatal growth retardation. skeletal anomalies, MR, and persistent fetal finger pads. Joint laxity, highly arched palate or CP, dental anomalies, and recurrent otitis media are very common. Breast development in female infants is common. Congenital heart defects are seen in ~42% (Matsumoto and Niikawa 2003).

Smith–Lemli–Opitz (SLO) syndrome (CP)
The alveolar ridges are thickened. Prenatal-onset growth deficiency, failure to thrive, microcephaly, PAP, small proximally placed thumbs, and Y-shaped 2/3 toe syndactyly. See 'Hypospadias' in Chapter 2, 'Clinical approach', p. 186.

XL CP and ankyloglossia
An XL semi-dominant disorder caused by mutations in the T-box transcription factor gene *TBX22* on Xq21 (Braybrook et al. 2001).

Ectrodactyly, ectodermal dysplasia, and clefting syndrome (EEC; CL/P)
Due to mutations in *p63*. See 'Unusual hair, teeth, nails, and skin' in Chapter 2, 'Clinical approach', p. 330.

Non-syndromic CL/P due to MSX1
MSX1 mutations are found in 2% of cases of non-syndromic CL/P (Jezewski et al. 2003) and should be considered in those families in which AD inheritance patterns or dental anomalies appear to be co-segregating with the clefting phenotype.

Genetic advice

Recurrence risk

ISOLATED CL/P. The aetiology of isolated clefts, when syndromes and dominant families have been excluded, is a combination of genetic and environmental factors. A number of candidate genes have been identified, some

Table 2.3 Frequency of oral clefts in relatives based on the proband's phenotype

Relative	CL (%)	CL/P (%)	CP (%)
Sibling	2.5	3.9	3.3
Half sibling	1.0	0.5	1.0
Parent	2.5	2.5	2.1
Offspring	3.5	4.1	4.2
Niece/nephew	0.9	0.8	1.1
Aunt/uncle	0.6	1.1	0.6
First cousin	0.3	0.5	0.4

CL, cleft lip; CP, cleft palate; CL/P, cleft lip with or without cleft palate. Data from: Grosen,D, Chavrier, C, Skytthe, A, et al. A cohort study of recurrence patterns among more than 54,000 relatives of oral cleft cases in Denmark: support for the multifactorial threshold model of inheritance. J Med Genet 2009.

of which appear to play a major role in cleft development. Schliekelman et al. (2002) estimate that 3–6 major genetic loci may contribute to clefting. IRF6 plays a substantial role, with an attributable risk of 12% (Zucchero et al. 2004). See Table 2.3 for the recurrence risks.

ISOLATED CP. Infants with CP are more likely to have associated malformations and syndromes than those with CL/P. Examine and investigate carefully to exclude these prior to counselling. See Table 2.3 for the recurrence risk in *non-syndromic clefting*. The risks for syndromic forms and isolated clefting where a germline genetic diagnosis has been made are as for the given genetic diagnosis.

CP is difficult to detect on USS in pregnancy. The small jaw of Pierre–Robin sequence can be visualized on specialist scanning.

IDENTIFIED SYNDROMAL CAUSE. Counsel as indicated.

Carrier detection
Examine parents carefully for lip pits and a bifid uvula. If there is nasal speech, carefully examine for a submucous CP and ensure that del(22q11) has been excluded.

Prenatal diagnosis
Prenatal detection of cleft lip is possible on USS at 20 weeks' gestation. It may not be detected on routine obstetric scans and a small cleft may be missed, even with expert scanning. CP is difficult to detect on USS in pregnancy, even with three-dimensional (3D) imaging. The small jaw of Pierre–Robin sequence may be visualized with specialist scanning.

Natural history and further management
• Feeding is a priority in the neonatal period. Involvement of a specialist cleft team should ensure that appropriate support and advice is available with provision of specially adapted nipple shields and teats as required. Babies with Robin syndrome and significant upper airway obstruction

may require nasogastric feeding initially. The nasogastric tube may be sufficient to stent the tongue forward and the airway open, allowing the baby to breathe and gain weight by nasogastric feeding for several days/weeks.
• Surgery is usually undertaken at 3 months of age for a primary repair of cleft lip, alveolus, and anterior palate and at 6–8 months of age for a primary repair of the posterior palate. Further palate surgery may be required later to optimize speech production.
• Hearing. Children with CP have a high incidence of 'glue ear'.
• Orthodontics. Children with a cleft lip involving the alveolus often have missing teeth. Orthodontic treatment is not typically initiated until the early mixed dentition stage at 7–8 years of age.

Support groups: Cleft Lip and Palate Association (CLAPA), https://www.clapa.com; American Cleft Palate–Craniofacial Association (ACPA), http://www.acpa-cpf.org/.

Expert adviser: David FitzPatrick, Paediatric Geneticist, Royal Hospital for Sick Children, Edinburgh, UK.

References
Bengami H, Handley M et al. Clinical and molecular consequences of disease-associated de novo mutations in SATB2. Genet Med 2017 (in press).
Braybrook C, Dondney K, Marçano AC, et al. The T-box transcription factor gene TBX22 is mutated in X-linked cleft palate and ankyloglossia. Nat Genet 2001; 29: 179–83.
Dixon MJ, Marazita ML, Beaty TH, Murray JC. Cleft lip and palate: understanding genetic and environmental influences. Nat Rev Genet 2011; 12: 167–78.
Grosen D, Chavrier C, Skytthe A, et al. A cohort study of recurrence patterns among more than 54,000 relatives of oral cleft cases in Denmark: support for the multifactorial threshold model of inheritance. J Med Genet 2009; 47: 162–8.
Jezewski PA, Vieira AR, Nishimura C, et al. Complete sequencing shows a role for MSX1 in non-syndromic cleft lip and palate. J Med Genet 2003; 40: 399–407.
Matsumoto N, Niikawa N. Kabuki make-up syndrome: a review. Am J Med Genet C 2003; 117C: 57–65.
Saal HM. Robin sequence. In: SB Cassidy, JE Allanson (eds.). Management of genetic syndromes, 3rd edn. pp. 693–704. Wiley-Liss, New York, 2011.
Schliekelman P, Slatkin M. Multiplex relative risk and estimation of the number of loci underlying an inherited disease. Am J Hum Genet 2002; 71: 1369–85.
Schutte BC, Murray JC. The many faces and factors of orofacial clefts. Hum Mol Genet 1999; 8: 1853–9.
Tolarova MM, Cervenka J. Classification and birth prevalence of orofacial clefts. Am J Med Genet 1998; 75: 126–37.
van Rooij IA, Ocke MC, Straatman H, et al. Periconceptual folate intake by supplement and food intake reduces the risk of non-syndromic left lip with or without cleft palate. Prev Med 2004; 39: 689–94.
Zucchero TM, Cooper ME, Maher BS, et al. Interferon regulatory factor 6 (IRF6) gene variants and the risk of isolated cleft lip and palate. N Engl J Med 2004; 351: 769–80.

Coarse facial features

The facial features appear thickened and heavy. The fleshy parts of the nose, mouth, lips, and gums are enlarged. There may be periorbital oedema. In disorders such as the mucopolysaccharidoses (MPS), the progressive coarsening is due to deposition of material in the tissues, but there are syndromal causes for which, at present, there is no metabolic explanation.

The history and photographic evidence are particularly important when dealing with a progressive condition and to establish when the signs were first apparent.

One approach to this difficult diagnostic problem is to consider the following.

(1) Have the investigations for known metabolic disorders been performed?

(2) Do the features fit with any of the known presumed metabolic conditions that do not have a confirmatory test? Would additional investigations, such as skeletal survey, histochemistry of skin biopsy, be helpful?

(3) Does the child have one of the syndromal causes of a coarse face such as Noonan syndrome?

Clinical approach

History: key points

- Three-generation family tree, with specific enquiry for consanguinity (many of the conditions have recessive inheritance) and ethnic background (many of the conditions are more common in certain areas, e.g. Salla disease in Finland).
- When were the facial features first considered coarse? Explain the term to the parents. Establish who first noticed the feature and if there has been progression.
- Development. Any slow-down in progress or loss of skills?
- Visual difficulties.
- Hearing loss.
- Seizures. Are they becoming more difficult to control?
- Upper respiratory tract infections with enlargement of tonsils and adenoids and tracheal involvement.
- Medication. Antiepileptic medication can change facial features and lead to gum hypertrophy.

Examination: key points

- Growth parameters. Height, weight, and OFC. Children with storage disorders may develop macrocephaly.
- Hair. Coarse? Thick or sparse? Hypertrichosis and hirsuitism?
- Face:
  - describe the facial features carefully;
  - are there horizontal creases of the ear lobules (BWS)?
- Mouth. Is there gum hypertrophy?
- Skin. Does it feel as though there is deposition of an abnormal metabolite in the subcutaneous layers? Is it stiff or ichthyotic? Are there any papillomas (Costello syndrome)? Is there acanthosis nigricans (Donohue syndrome)? Is there pigment in Blaschko's lines (Pallister–Killian)?
- Hands:
  - contractures (storage disorders);
  - nail hypoplasia (Coffin–Siris syndrome).

- Heart. Is there a cardiac murmur?
- Abdomen:
  - enlargement of the liver and spleen;
  - umbilical hernia (storage diseases and Beckwith syndrome).
- Neurological examination.
- Eyes. Fundi, for lesions such as cherry red spots, corneal clouding.

Special investigations

If the diagnosis seems likely on the basis of your examination, e.g. Hurler's syndrome, then proceed directly to the confirmatory enzymatic and molecular analysis. If the diagnosis is uncertain, start with baseline tests and then more targeted testing can follow on when these results are through. These children should be under the care of a paediatrician with an interest in metabolic conditions and investigations should be done under his or her guidance. The investigations here have a bias towards rarer conditions, those of unknown aetiology, and syndromal causes, which are the usual reasons for the involvement of a geneticist in the diagnostic process.

- Baseline:
  - thyroid function;
  - urine metabolic screen (mucopolysaccharides, oligosaccharides, amino and organic acids);
  - plasma amino acids; basic biochemistry including CK and glucose; alkaline phosphatase and phosphate;
  - vacuolated lymphocytes.
- Photography to document features over time—this can be valuable in determining whether there is progression.
- Ophthalmology assessment. Consider conjunctival biopsy for storage deposits.
- Cranial MRI scan. In practice, brain imaging is performed on most children to clarify the diagnosis and prognosis.
- White cell enzymes. These need to arrive in the laboratory within a few hours. Please discuss your differential diagnosis with the lab, so that the correct analyses are performed. Relatively large volumes are required.
- Skeletal survey. This is a useful investigation to assess if there are features of a storage disease such as abnormal bone modelling. A feature such as rib thickening may suggest a rare syndrome such as Cantu syndrome. See 'Skeletal dysplasias' in Chapter 2, 'Clinical approach', p. 316 for a list of films to arrange.
- Skin biopsy. To assess if there is deposition of an abnormal compound. Storage of tissue for possible future analysis. Also to investigate for Pallister–Killian syndrome (mosaic 12p tetrasomy).
- Echo to assess for CMs and valvular abnormalities.
- Abdominal USS. Organomegaly, renal enlargement, or structural abnormality.
- Genomic analysis e.g. genomic array, gene panel, or WES/WGS as appropriate.
- Endocrine studies. Insulin level if Donohue syndrome suspected.
- VLCFAs.

Some diagnoses to consider

Confirmed metabolic conditions

- Mucopolysaccharide (MPS) disorders (typically present with glue ear, coarse facial features, and finger contractures).
- Gangliosidoses.
- Sialic acid storage diseases.

With short stature

NOONAN SYNDROME (NS). Typically, pulmonary valve stenosis, peripheral pulmonary artery stenosis, or HCM with short stature and characteristic facies (*PTPN11* mutations are found in ~40%). A stenotic, and often dysplastic, pulmonary valve is found in 20–50% of affected individuals. See 'Noonan syndrome and the Ras/MAPK pathway syndromes: neuro-cardio-facial-cutaneous syndromes' in Chapter 3, 'Common consultations', p. 512.

WILLIAMS SYNDROME. Microdeletion on 7q11.23, which encompasses the elastin gene (*ELN*). CHD occurs in 80%. Infants and young children have periorbital fullness, a bulbous nasal tip, a long philtrum, a wide mouth, full lips, full cheeks, and small widely spaced teeth. Older children and adults have a more gaunt appearance with coarser facial features. Very variable MR, over-friendly personality, short attention span, and anxiety. See 'Congenital heart disease' in Chapter 2, 'Clinical approach', p. 112.

SMITH–MAGENIS SYNDROME (SMS). Some patients have square and rather heavy facies and are short and obese with small hands and feet. They may have a history of hypotonia in infancy, developmental delay, behaviour disturbance (especially sleep), and sometimes food-searching behaviour. Some individuals with SMS have mutations in *RAI1*, a gene encompassed by the common 17p11.2 microdeletion.

PALLISTER–KILLIAN SYNDROME (TETRASOMY 12P). Individuals with Pallister–Killian syndrome are mosaic for an isochromosome of 12p that is present in skin fibroblasts, but not in blood lymphocytes; hence skin biopsy is necessary to make the diagnosis. They tend to have coarse features, with a broad forehead, normal OFC, apparent hypertelorism, sagging cheeks, and a prominent full philtrum. There may be additional folds of skin around the neck. Hair seems sparse, especially over the temporal areas. Birthweight is often normal or above average. MR is usually severe.

With failure to thrive

See 'Failure to thrive' in Chapter 2, 'Clinical approach', p. 150.

DONOHUE SYNDROME (LEPRECHAUNISM). An AR disorder due to mutations in the insulin receptor gene. Pre- and postnatal failure to thrive, hirsutism, aged face with thick lips and prominent ears, enlargement of the breast and genitalia; acanthosis nigricans may be present. The serum insulin level is grossly elevated.

COSTELLO SYNDROME. Macrosomia, coarse facial features, and cardiac defects usually presenting in the neonatal period or early infancy. With time, failure to thrive may supervene and papillomas develop around the nose and periorally. There are very characteristic wrinkled palms and ulnar deviation of the hands. Caused by activating mutations in the *HRAS* gene. See 'Failure to thrive' in Chapter 2, 'Clinical approach', p. 150.

With overgrowth

BECKWITH–WIEDEMANN SYNDROME (BWS). Macrosomia, anterior abdominal wall defects, macroglossia, anterior earlobe creases, and posterior helical pits. Complex genetics. See 'Beckwith–Wiedemann syndrome (BWS)' in Chapter 3, 'Common consultations', p. 358.

SIMPSON–GOLABI–BEHMEL (SGB) SYNDROME. An XLR disorder due to mutations in *glypican 3* (Xq26). Overgrowth is of prenatal onset and continues postnatally. Birthweight and birth OFC of affected males are usually both >97th centile. Other findings include hypertelorism, macroglossia, central groove of the lower lip, supernumerary nipples, advanced bone age, vertebral segmentation defects, and coarse facies in adults; most have a normal IQ. May have cardiac/GI malformations; refer for echo/ECG. Diagnostic overlap with BWS, but combination of minor facial anomalies, skeletal/hand anomalies, and supernumerary nipples only occurs in SGB. Small risk of Wilms tumour—consider periodic renal USS, as for BWS, i.e. USS of the kidneys, liver, and adrenals at 4-monthly intervals (triannually) until 8 years of age.

With severe developmental delay (without regression)

COFFIN–LOWRY SYNDROME (CLS). Mutation in the *RSK2* gene. The facial features become more pronounced with time and can also be recognized in some female carriers. Examine the hands, as these are large and 'soft' with tapering of the distal phalanges. Scoliosis and kyphosis develop. X-rays of the hands, chest, and spine may help confirm the diagnosis.

NICOLAIDES–BARAITSER SYNDROME. Seizures, sparse hair. X-ray and clinical abnormalities of the phalanges with brachydactyly and swelling of the interphalangeal (IP) joints. Caused by mutation in the *SMARCA2* gene (van Houdt *et al.* 2012).

GPI DEFICIENCY SYNDROMES. Glycosylphosphatidylinositol (GPI) is a glycolipid that anchors >150 various proteins to the cell surface. At least 27 genes are involved in biosynthesis and transport of GPI-anchored proteins. These cause a wide range of multi-system disorders usually with a severe neurological component e.g. delay and seizures. Mabry syndrome (hyperphosphatasia mental retardation syndrome) has coarse features, nail hypoplasia, and sometimes anorectal anomalies. Biallelic variants in PIGV cause Mabry syndrome.

With hypertrichosis

COFFIN–SIRIS SYNDROME. Caused by heterozygous mutation in components of the SWI/SNF chromatin remodelling complex (Santen *et al.* 2012; Tsurusaki *et al.* 2012). Characterized by developmental delay with sparse hair, coarse facial features, and nail hypoplasia, especially of the fifth finger. Carefully exclude chromosomal abnormalities.

CANTU SYNDROME. An AD condition with slightly coarse facial features caused by heterozygous mutation in the *ABCC9* gene (Harakalova *et al.* 2012). Facial hair is abundant and there is generalized hypertrichosis. Thick ribs may be a helpful diagnostic feature; other aspects of the accompanying osteochondrodysplasia may be subtle. Growth and development may be delayed in early infancy but subsequently normalize. DCM may be a feature.

Genetic advice

Recurrence risk
When a diagnosis remains unknown, counselling is difficult. If there is clear progression of the signs and symptoms, an AR risk should be considered. When the condition is non-progressive and there are other malformations, the cause may be a syndrome with a lower risk of recurrence.

Carrier detection
This can be performed for some of the metabolic conditions by DNA and enzymatic methods. General population testing, i.e. for the partners of siblings of the parents, may not be possible.

Prenatal diagnosis
This can be offered to those parents in whom a diagnosis has been confirmed. Consult closely with the laboratory to ascertain the type of sample (direct or cultured CVS, amniocytes, etc.) that is required.

Natural history and further management (preventative measures)
Therapy such as enzymatic replacement therapy (ERT) and bone marrow transplantation (BMT) may be possible and these children should be under the care of a paediatrician to ensure up-to-date advice. ERT is currently under trial for MPS I (Hurler's), MPS II (Hunter's), MPS VI, and infantile Pompe disease.

Support groups: Climb (Children Living with Inherited Metabolic Diseases), http://www.climb.org.uk, Tel. 0870 770 0326; Contact a Family, http://www.cafamily.org.uk; The Society for Mucopolysaccharide Diseases, http://www.mpssociety.org.uk, Tel. 01494 434 156.

Expert adviser: Dian Donnai, Professor of Medical Genetics, Manchester Centre for Genomic Medicine, University of Manchester and Central Manchester University Hospitals NHS Foundation Trust, Manchester Academic Health Science Centre, Manchester, UK.

References
Clarke JTR. *A clinical guide to inherited metabolic diseases*, 3rd edn. Cambridge University Press, Cambridge, 2005.

Harakalova M, van Harssel JJ, Terhal PA, et al. Dominant missense mutations in ABCC9 cause Cantu syndrome. *Nat Genet* 2012; **44**: 793–6.

Hennekam R, Allanson J Krantz I. *Gorlin's syndromes of the head and neck*, 5th edn. Oxford University Press, Oxford, 2010.

Horn D, Wieczorek D, et al. Delineation of PIGV mutation spectrum and associated phenotypes in hyperphosphatasia with mental retardation syndrome. *Eur J Hum Genet* 2014 Jun; **22**(6): 762–7.

Santen GW, Aten E, Sun Y, et al. Mutations in SWI/SNF chromatin remodeling complex gene *ARID1B* cause Coffin–Siris syndrome. *Nat Genet* 2012; **44**: 379–80.

Tsurusaki Y, Okamoto H, Ohashi H, et al. Mutations affecting components of the SWI/SNF complex cause Coffin–Siris syndrome. *Nat Genet* 2012; **44**: 376–8.

Van Houdt JK, Nowakowska BA, Sousa SB, et al. Heterozygous missense mutations in *SMARCA2* cause Nicolaides–Baraitser syndrome. *Nat Genet* 2012; **44**: 445–9, S1.

Coloboma

A coloboma is a segmental ocular defect, most commonly a 'keyhole' deficiency in the iris. A typical coloboma arises from a defective closure of the optic fissure during the sixth week post-conception. The line of closure of the primitive fissure is along the inferior and medial sides of the optic cup; iris colobomata are usually seen in the inferior 6 o'clock position of the iris, giving the pupil a 'keyhole' appearance. True colobomata only occur in this position. The gap or notch may be limited to the iris or may extend deeper and involve the ciliary body and retina. If the coloboma affects the retina, this may give rise to a visual field defect. Optic nerve involvement is associated with visual impairment.

Ocular (uveoretinal) colobomata occur in 71/10 000 individuals. Ocular colobomata may be unilateral or bilateral and are most commonly seen in otherwise normal children. A family history is uncommon. Colobomata are a common finding in some chromosomal disorders and a number of dysmorphic syndromes.

Coloboma of the eyelid

Defects in the eyelid are seen in Treacher–Collins syndrome (TCS), Nager syndrome, and oculoauriculovertebral (OAV) syndrome (Goldenhar). See 'Ear anomalies' in Chapter 2, 'Clinical approach', p. 142. They also occur in some rare facial clefting syndromes and occasionally in amnion disruption sequence.

Clinical approach

History: key points

- Three-generation family tree, with specific enquiry regarding coloboma and visual difficulties and renal failure.
- Developmental milestones.

Examination: key points

- Growth parameters, including OFC.
- Careful assessment for dysmorphic features.
- Look carefully for subtle microphthalmia.
- Detailed examination of both eyes by an ophthalmologist.
- Examine the ears carefully for pits/tags/abnormal morphology (CHARGE (coloboma–heart defects–atresia choanae–retardation of growth and/or development–genital defect–ear anomalies and/or deafness) association, CES, branchio-oculo-facial (BOF) syndrome).
- Examine for anal anomalies (CHARGE, CES).

Special investigations

- Arrange ophthalmological examination for parents (even in apparently sporadic cases). Subtle retinal colobomata may be easily missed by a non-specialist.
- Genomic analysis in presence of features suggestive of a chromosomal or syndromic diagnosis, e.g. genomic array, gene panel, or WES/WGS as appropriate.
- DNA for mutation analysis or storage.
- Consider renal function tests, e.g. plasma creatinine if optic nerve coloboma (renal-coloboma syndrome).

Some diagnoses to consider

CHARGE (coloboma–heart defects–atresia choanae–retardation of growth and/or development–genital defect–ear anomalies and/or deafness) syndrome

CHARGE has a prevalence of ~1/12 000. It is caused by mutation in the gene *CHD7* on 8q12 which acts in early embryonic development by affecting chromatin structure and gene expression (Vissers *et al.* 2004). Some children have a whole gene deletion (detection may require FISH or dosage sensitive analysis). Empiric data suggest that most are sporadic with a low recurrence risk (2–3%), but if a mutation is identified, this risk can be clarified. Note that chromosomal imbalance can mimic CHARGE syndrome—ensure high-quality chromosome analysis, including telomere screen/array–comparative genomic hybridization (CGH) in mutation-negative individuals.

Baraitser-Winter syndrome

AD disorder characterized by short stature, hypertelorism, bilateral ptosis, ocular coloboma, prominent metopic suture, and neuronal migration disorder. Caused by heterozygous mutation in ACTB or ACTG1. A recurrent *de novo* variant in ACTG1 has been detected in isolated coloboma and no features of Baraitser-Winter syndrome (Rainger 2017).

Cat-eye syndrome (CES)

Anal anomalies (imperforate anus, anal atresia, or anteriorly placed anus), preauricular pits/tags, congenital heart defects, iris colobomata, renal anomalies, and variable learning disability. Only 41% of CES patients have the combination of iris coloboma, anal anomalies, and preauricular anomalies (Berends *et al.* 2001). The remainder of CES patients are hard to recognize by their phenotype alone. Mild to moderate MR is found in 32%; MR occurs more frequently in male CES patients. There is no apparent phenotypic difference between mentally retarded and mentally normal CES patients. CES results from a small marker chromosome containing a duplication of 22q11, resulting in tetrasomy 22q11. It can be an unbalanced product of the relatively common 11q23;22q11 reciprocal translocation.

4p (Wolf–Hirschorn syndrome)

Characterized by low birthweight and postnatal failure to thrive, microcephaly, developmental delay, and hypotonia. There is a characteristic facial appearance with sagging everted lower eyelids, a 'Greek-helmet' profile, a short nose, and a very short philtrum. Patients may have iris colobomata. Seizures are common. Some have a visible deletion with varying breakpoints on 4p; others have a cryptic deletion requiring FISH to make the diagnosis.

Colobomatous microphthalmia

Mild degrees of microphthalmia are difficult to detect. This has been reported in families, so consider the possibility of AD inheritance with variable penetrance. It is genetically heterogeneous with heterozygous mutation in *SOX2*, *SHH*, etc. Biallelic mutation in *c12orf57* has been reported in a syndromic form associated with severe global delay (Zahrani *et al.* 2013).

Focal dermal hypoplasia (Goltz syndrome)

XLD (due to mutations in, or deletions encompassing, the *PORCN* gene at Xp11.23). Areas of focal dermal hypoplasia may be found on the trunk and limbs where there may be fat herniation through the skin deficiency. The eyes are frequently affected, mostly asymmetrically, with chorioretinal or iris colobomata, but unilateral anophthalmos has been reported.

Branchio-oculo-facial syndrome (BOF; haemangiomatous branchial clefts)

An AD condition with distinctive areas of thin, erythematous, wrinkled skin in the neck or infra-/supra-auricular regions, in addition to craniofacial, auricular, ophthalmologic (coloboma of the iris and/or retina), and oral anomalies. Some phenotypic overlap with branchio-oto-renal (BOR) syndrome since both can have nasolacrimal duct stenosis, deafness, prehelical pits, malformed pinnae, and renal anomalies, but the two conditions are not allelic.

Renal coloboma syndrome (papillorenal syndrome)
An AD condition caused by mutations in *PAX2*, characterized by colobomata of the optic nerve (and occasionally the retina), together with renal anomalies (vesicoureteral reflux (VUR) and renal hypoplasia with loss of corticomedullary differentiation). Ophthalmic and renal characteristics of the renal coloboma syndrome are highly variable. The need for dialysis or renal transplantation can occur early in life or several years later. A wide range of ocular abnormalities located in the posterior segment can be observed. Mild optic disc dysplasia or pit have no functional consequence and can be underdiagnosed. More severe colobomata or related abnormalities, such as morning glory anomaly, often lead to poor visual acuity.

Aicardi syndrome
Optic nerve colobomata, retinal lacunae, CNS abnormalities, and seizures. XLD.

Genetic advice
Recurrence risk
Isolated bilateral colobomata of the iris may follow an AD pattern of inheritance. The empiric recurrence risk is ~10% (~5% if the parents have a normal ocular examination) (Morrison *et al.* 2002).

Carrier detection
Careful ophthalmological examination of parents is essential.

Prenatal diagnosis
If the proband has a chromosomal disorder or a single gene mutation, PND by CVS or amniocentesis is possible.

Natural history and further management (preventative measures)
Chorioretinal colobomata are associated with a significant risk of rhegmatogenous retinal detachment.

Retinal tears can occur in the thinned retina overlying the colobomatous defect. Lens colobomata may also be associated with giant retinal tears. Children with large defects should be under the care of a paediatric ophthalmologist.

Support group:
MACS (Micro and Anophthalmic Children's Society), http://www.macs.org.uk, Tel. 0870 600 6227.

Expert adviser: David FitzPatrick, Paediatric Geneticist, Royal Hospital for Sick Children, Edinburgh, UK.

References
Berends MJ, Tan-Sindhunata G, Leegte B, van Essen AJ. Phenotypic variability of cat-eye syndrome. *Genet Couns* 2001; **12**: 23–34.

Dureau P, Attie-Bitach T, Salomon R, *et al.* Renal coloboma syndrome. *Ophthalmology* 2001; **108**: 1912–16.

Ford B, Rupps R, Lirenman D, *et al.* Renal-coloboma syndrome: prenatal detection and clinical spectrum in a large family. *Am J Med Genet* 2001; **99**: 137–41.

Liu C, Widen SA, *et al.* A secreted WNT-ligand-binding domain of FZD5 generated by a frameshift mutation causes autosomal dominant coloboma. *Hum Mol Genet* 2016 Apr 1; **25**(7): 1382–91.

Lin AE, Semina EV, Daack-Hirsch S, *et al.* Exclusion of the branchio-oto-renal syndrome locus (*EYA1*) from patients with branchio-oculo-facial syndrome. *Am J Med Genet* 2000; **91**: 387–90.

Ming JE, Russell KL, Bason L, McDonald-McGinn DM, Zackai EH. Coloboma and other ophthalmologic anomalies in Kabuki syndrome: distinction from charge association. *Am J Med Genet A* 2003; **123A**: 249–52.

Morrison D, FitzPatrick D, Hanson I, *et al.* A national study of microphthalmia, coloboma and anophthalmia in Scotland. *J Med Genet* 2002; **39**: 16–22.

Rainger J, Williamson KA, *et al.* A recurrent de novo mutation in ACTG1 causes isolated ocular coloboma. *Hum Mut* 2017; **38**: 942–6.

Stoll C, Viville B, Treisser A, Gasser B. A family with dominant oculoauriculovertebral spectrum. *Am J Med Genet* 1998; **78**: 345–9.

Vissers LE, van Ravenswaaij CM, Admiraal R, *et al.* Mutations in a new member of the chromodomain gene family cause CHARGE syndrome. *Nat Genet* 2004; **36**: 955–7.

Zahrani F, Aldahmesh MA, Alshammari MJ, Al-Hazzaa SA, Alkuraya FS. Mutations in c12orf57 cause a syndromic form of colobomatous microphthalmia. *Am J Hum Genet* 2013; **92**: 387–91.

Congenital heart disease

Structural heart malformations (see Table 2.4 for nomenclature) occur in 7/1000 live births (0.7%). An echo is the single most useful investigation to define the cardiac anatomy. Most commonly, congenital heart disease (CHD) occurs as an isolated finding in an otherwise normal individual. However, CHD can occur as part of an enormous number of chromosomal disorders or specific syndromes, or as a consequence of teratogenic exposure. Where a second anomaly is identified, this increases the chance of making a specific diagnosis.

The task of the geneticist is to determine whether the CHD is:

(1) isolated;

(2) isolated, but with a significant family history (other close relatives with similar CHD);

(3) syndromic;

(4) chromosomal;

(5) the result of a teratogenic exposure or maternal illness (see Tables 2.5 and 2.6).

Exome studies (Sifrim 2015) show an excess of *de novo* protein truncating variants in syndromic congenital heart disease.

Table 2.4 Nomenclature

Abbreviation	Definition
ASD	Atrial septal defect
AVSD	Atrioventricular septal defect (AV canal defect). A 'complete AVSD' involves underdevelopment of the lower part of the atrial septum and the upper part of the ventricular septum with a single common AV valve, resulting in unrestricted communication between the atria and ventricles. A 'partial AVSD' or 'ostium primum ASD' has a deficiency of the atrial septum. Defects of the inlet muscular ventricular septum and isolated cleft mitral valve are also part of the clinical spectrum
Coarct	Coarctation of the aorta
DORV	Double-outlet right ventricle (RV) (aorta lies predominantly over the RV)
Fallot's tetralogy	Aorta overriding a VSD with RVOT (e.g. pulmonary stenosis) and RV hypertrophy
HLH	Hypoplastic left heart
MVP	Mitral valve prolapse
PDA	Patent ductus arteriosus (common in preterm infants)
PFO	Persistent foramen ovale
RVOT	Right ventricular outflow tract obstruction
SVAS	Supravalvular aortic stenosis
TAPVD	Total anomalous pulmonary venous drainage
TGA	Transposition of the great arteries
VSD	Ventricular septal defect

Table 2.5 Teratogens and the risk of congenital heart disease

Alcohol (fetal alcohol syndrome (FAS))	Up to 25–30%	Mainly VSD and/or ASD; also Fallot's tetralogy
Anticonvulsants	1.8%	3-fold increased risk over baseline
Lithium	Equivocal (see 'Drugs in pregnancy' in Chapter 6, 'Pregnancy and fertility', p. 718	Ebstein anomaly, tricuspid atresia, ASD
Retinoic acid	10–20%	Conotruncal heart defects
Rubella	35%	PDA, peripheral pulmonary artery stenosis, septal defects

Clinical approach

History: key points

- Three-generation family tree, with a special note of CHD and neonatal or infant deaths.
- History of twinning. Monozygotic (MZ) twins have a ~3-fold excess risk for CHD, compared with singletons; dizygotic (DZ) twins have a slight excess risk of ~1.3-fold).
- History of alcohol or drug exposure in pregnancy (e.g. anticonvulsants).
- History of chronic maternal illness (e.g. maternal diabetes, maternal PKU; maternal SLE may cause congenital heart block).
- History of maternal infection (e.g. rubella).
- History of prematurity (patent ductus arteriosus (PDA)), birth, and subsequent development.

Examination: key points

- Growth parameters. Height, weight, and OFC. Abnormal growth parameters raise concerns that the cardiac defect is not isolated, provided the infant/child is not in heart failure or cyanosed which may both cause failure to thrive.
- Assess the index case carefully for any dysmorphic features or facies suggestive of Noonan, Williams, Turner, 22q, trisomies, etc.
- Assess the index case for nasal speech and submucous palate (22q deletion).
- Examine the index case for limb anomalies, e.g. hypoplastic thumb and thenar eminence (Holt–Oram

Table 2.6 Maternal illness and the risk of congenital heart disease*

Maternal diabetes	3–5%	VSD, coarct, TGA, truncus arteriosus, tricuspid atresia, and a variety of other defects including L-isomerism sequence
Maternal PKU	~15%	Fallot's tetralogy, coarct
Maternal SLE	20–40%	Complete heart block

*See 'Maternal diabetes mellitus and diabetic embryopathy', p. 756 and 'Maternal phenylketonuria (PKU)', p. 758 in Chapter 6, 'Pregnancy and fertility'.

(HOS)), radial ray defects (VACTERL and Fanconi), or polydactyly (EVC).
- Examine both parents. Detailed clinical examination of the cardiovascular systems of both parents.

Special investigations
- Genomic analysis in presence of features suggestive of a chromosomal or syndromic diagnosis, e.g. genomic array, gene panel, or WES/WGS as available, for all complex defects or if any accompanying learning disability or congenital anomaly.
- Urgent chromosome analysis with 22q11 FISH may be required in the sick neonate for prognosis and surgical management.
- Echo and ECG for the parent if any abnormality noted on cardiovascular history or examination; cardiology referral if abnormality detected.
- Storage of DNA prior to open heart surgery/extra-corporeal membrane oxygenation (ECMO).

Some diagnoses to consider
See Table 2.7.

Trisomies
Forty to 50% of individuals with Down's syndrome have a CHD, with perimembranous VSD the most common defect, followed by PDA and ASD. At least 90% of individuals with trisomy 18 have CHD, usually VSD with/without valve dysplasia. Eighty per cent of individuals with trisomy 13 have a cardiac malformation, e.g. ASD or VSD. See 'Down's syndrome (trisomy 21)', p. 666, 'Edwards' syndrome (trisomy 18)', p. 670, and 'Patau syndrome (trisomy 13)', p. 678 in Chapter 5, 'Chromosomes'.

Table 2.7 Congenital heart disease with dysmorphic features, developmental delay, or other congenital anomalies—syndromic diagnoses to consider

VSD	Perimembranous VSD is the most common cardiac defect seen in trisomy 21; VSD is also common in trisomy 18 and trisomy 13. Also seen in del 22q11, FAS, maternal diabetes
ASD	Trisomy 21, trisomy 13, FAS
AVSD	Sixty per cent have Down's syndrome; SLO, SMS, EVC, CHARGE syndrome, hydrolethalus, Kaufman–McKusick, HOS, OFD-2 (Mohr syndrome), and 3p syndrome and other ciliopathies
	AVSD may be caused by heterozygous mutation of *NR2F2*, possibly with an AD family history of septal defects or coarct or HLH syndrome (Al Turki *et al.* 2014)
Aortic stenosis	Williams syndrome (SVAS), TS
Coarctation of aorta	TS, Kabuki syndrome
Ebstein/tricuspid valve	del 1p36
Fallot's tetralogy	del 22q11, Alagille syndrome
Interrupted aortic arch	del 22q11
Pulmonary stenosis	NS, NF1-NS, Williams (supravalvular PS), del 22q11
Peripheral pulmonary artery stenosis	Williams, Alagille
Truncus arteriosus	del 22q11

22q11 deletion
CHD with short stature, cleft palate, or velopharyngeal insufficiency (nasal speech) and speech delay, may have low calcium, mild learning disability, and immunodeficiency (typically reduced T-cell subsets). Outflow tract anomalies are characteristic, including Fallot's tetralogy, truncus arteriosus, interrupted aortic arch, pulmonary atresia/stenosis, tricuspid atresia, TGA, vascular rings, aberrant major vessels, e.g. right-sided aorta. VSD is common in 22q11 deletion, but, since VSD is such a common anomaly, the pickup rate is tiny in apparently normal children with isolated VSD. ASD and PDA also occur in 22q, but, as above, a 22q screen is not usually indicated in otherwise normal children. A significant proportion of children with Fallot's tetralogy have 22q11 deletions. See '22q11 deletion syndrome' in Chapter 5, 'Chromosomes', p. 624.

Chromosomal deletions/microdeletion with recognizable phenotypes
Examples are 4p (Wolf–Hirschorn syndrome), 5p (cri-du-chat), and del(1p36). See 'Deletions and duplications (including microdeletions and microduplications)' in Chapter 5, 'Chromosomes', p. 660.

Noonan syndrome (NS)
Typically, pulmonary valve stenosis, peripheral pulmonary artery stenosis, or HCM with short stature and characteristic facies. (*PTPN11* mutations are found in ~40%.) A stenotic, and often dysplastic, pulmonary valve is found in 20–50% of affected individuals. Seven per cent of children with pulmonary stenosis have NS. See 'Noonan syndrome and the Ras/MAPK pathway syndromes: neuro-cardio-facial-cutaneous syndromes' in Chapter 3, 'Common consultations', p. 512.

Smith–Lemli–Opitz (SLO)
Cardiac defects are present in just <40%, especially AVSD and TAPVD. Prenatal and postnatal growth deficiency, developmental delay (almost all), cleft palate (37–52%), hypospadias and/or cryptorchidism (90–100%) in affected males, Y-shaped 2/3 toe syndactyly (>95%), and PAP post-axial polydactyly (~50%). Facial features include: narrow bifrontal diameter, ptosis (50%), downslanting palpebral fissures, and a short nose with a depressed nasal bridge and anteverted nares. See 'Hypospadias' in Chapter 2, 'Clinical approach', p. 186.

Turner syndrome (TS; 45,X)
CHD occurs in 17–45%. Coarctation of the aorta and bicuspid aortic valve or other aortic valve anomaly, e.g. stenosis. See 'Turner syndrome, 45,X and variants' in Chapter 5, 'Chromosomes', p. 696.

Williams syndrome
Microdeletion on 7q11.23 which encompasses the elastin gene (*ELN*). CHD occurs in 80%: Seventy-five per cent have supravalvular aortic stenosis (SVAS) and ~25% have a discrete supravalvular pulmonary stenosis. Peripheral pulmonic stenosis is found in 50–75% of infants but improves with time. The elastin anomaly is generalized and almost any artery can be narrowed, e.g. renal artery stenosis (40%). Aortic insufficiency (20%) and MVP (15%) may occur in some adults. As to characteristic facial features, infants and young children have periorbital fullness, a bulbous nasal tip, a long philtrum, a wide mouth, full lips, full cheeks, and small widely spaced teeth; older children and adults have a more gaunt appearance with coarser

facial features. Developmental delay with very variable MR from severe to low-average, with most having mild MR, strengths in language but poor visuospatial skills, overfriendly personality, short attention span, and anxiety. Approximately 15% of infants have hypercalcaemia.

Alagille syndrome

Caused by haploinsufficiency of *JAG1* on 20p11.2–20p12. Characterized by hypoplasia of the intrahepatic bile ducts (often presenting with prolonged neonatal jaundice). Approximately 90% have single or multiple areas of peripheral pulmonary artery stenosis, and one-third have other cardiac malformations, especially Fallot's tetralogy. Other features include butterfly vertebrae and posterior embryotoxon (slit-lamp examination). Facial features are subtle with a prominent forehead, deep-set eyes, and a long nose; adults have a prominent chin. See 'Prolonged neonatal jaundice and jaundice in infants below 6 months' in Chapter 2, 'Clinical approach', p. 288.

Holt–Oram syndrome

An AD heart–hand syndrome caused by mutations in *TBX5*. Penetrance is 100%. *Cardiac defects* include ASD (34%), VSD (25%), MVP (7%), with ECG changes only in 39% (long PR interval, bradycardia, and left or right axis deviation being the most frequent). Pectus deformity occurs in 40%. Cardiac defects (including minimal ECG changes) occur in 95%. *Skeletal defects* affect the upper limbs exclusively and are invariably bilateral and usually asymmetrical. They range from clinodactyly, limited supination, and narrow, sloping shoulders to absent, hypoplastic, or triphalangeal thumb and severe reduction deformities of the upper arm (4.5%). See 'Radial ray defects and thumb hypoplasia' in Chapter 2, 'Clinical approach', p. 296.

Kabuki syndrome

Characterized by facial dysmorphism with long palpebral fissures and eversion of the lateral one-third of the lower lid, postnatal growth retardation, skeletal anomalies, MR, and persistent fetal finger pads. Joint laxity, a highly arched palate or CP, dental anomalies, and recurrent otitis media are very common. Breast development in female infants is common. CHD are seen in ~42% (Matsumoto *et al.* 2003). Aortic coarctation, ASD, and VSD are the most common defects (Digilio *et al.* 2001). The majority of cases of Kabuki syndrome are caused by mutation of the *KMT2D* (*MLL2*) gene; a smaller number are caused by mutation of the *KMD6A* gene.

VACTERL (vertebral defects–anal atresia–cardiac anomalies–tracheo-oesophageal fistula–(o)esophageal atresia–renal anomalies–limb defects) association

Secure diagnosis requires at least one anomaly in each of the three anatomical domains (limb, thorax, and pelvis/lower abdomen) and at least two anomalies in each of two domains for a probable diagnosis. Sporadic with a low recurrence risk (2–3%).

CHARGE (coloboma–heart defects–atresia choanae–retardation of growth and/or development–genital defect–ear anomalies and/or deafness)

CHARGE syndrome (coloboma–heart defects, etc.) is caused by heterozygous mutations of the *CHD7* gene; 50% of affected individuals have CHD, e.g. ASD, AVSD. See 'Coloboma' in Chapter 2, 'Clinical approach', p. 110.

Table 2.8 Recurrence risk for isolated non-syndromic defects

Cardiac malformation	Risk in siblings (%)	Risk in offspring (%)[*]
Situs inversus (check for Kartagener)	3	
Isomerism sequence—non-syndromic	5–10	
Tricuspid atresia	1	
Mitral atresia	2	
Transposition of great arteries	2	
Truncus arteriosus	1	
Pulmonary atresia	1	
Secundum ASD	3	
AVSD	2	7.7 (M); 7.9 (F)
Ebstein anomaly (check for fetal exposure to lithium)	1	
VSD	3	
Pulmonary stenosis	2	
Tetralogy of Fallot	2	1.6 (M); 4.7 (F)
Aortic stenosis	3	
Coarctation of aorta	2	
Patent ductus arteriosus (PDA)	2.5	
Hypoplastic left heart	Low (1/77 in Birmingham study)	

[*] (F), risk to offspring of an affected father; (F), risk to offspring of an affected mother.

This table was published in *Emery and Rimoin's Principles and Practice of Medical Genetics*, Fourth Edition, D. Rimoin (ed.), Burn J and Goodship J, Congenital heart disease, pp. 1239–326, Copyright Churchill Livingstone, Edinburgh, 2001.

Isomerism sequence

See 'Laterality disorders including heterotaxy and isomerism' in Chapter 2, 'Clinical approach', p. 206.

Genetic advice

Isolated heart malformations are usually sporadic, but occasionally particular defects can be shown to be inherited as a simple Mendelian trait. The risks quoted in Table 2.8 are not appropriate in the latter case, when advice should be given according to the apparent inheritance in the family, with reference to Online Mendelian Inheritance in Man (OMIM).

Siblings

Oyen *et al.* (2009) undertook a cohort study of >18 000 individuals with CHD in Denmark, in which the sibling recurrence risks were summarized as 1.4% for the same heart defect and 1% for a different heart defect. Oyen *et al.* also found the approximated relative risks (RR) for MZ and DZ twins were 15.17 and 3.33, respectively.

Offspring

In general, the risks are greater in the offspring of affected mothers (overall risk 6.5%) than in the offspring of affected fathers (overall risk 2.2%) (Burn and Goodship 2001). However for AVSD, the risk in offspring were similar for mothers and fathers at ~8%. For tetralogy of Fallot the risks were 1.6% (father) and 4.5% (mother).

PRENATAL DIAGNOSIS. Fetal echo can be used for ante-natal diagnosis of the most complex CHD (not TGA), with scans at 14, 19, and 22 weeks' gestation.

Natural history and further management (preventative measures)

If an affected woman is contemplating pregnancy, check that she is under review at a GUCH (grown-up congeni-tal heart disease) clinic and that the effects of pregnancy on her health have been assessed. Also offer PND by fetal echo. Note increased miscarriage in mothers with CHD (20% with maternal proband, compared with 10% with paternal proband).

Support group:

Children's Heart Federation, http://www.chfed.org.uk.

Expert adviser: Judith Goodship, formerly Professor of Medical Genetics, University of Newcastle, Newcastle upon Tyne, UK.

References

Al Turki S, Manickaraj AK, Mercer CL, et al. Rare variants in NR2F2 cause congenital heart defects in humans. *Am J Hum Genet* 2014; **94**: 574–85.

Burn J, Brennan P, Little J, et al. Recurrence risks in offspring of adults with major heart defects. *Lancet* 1998; **351**: 311–15.

Burn J, Goodship J. Congenital heart disease. In: D Rimoin (ed.). *Emery and Rimoin's principles and practice of medical genetics*, 4th edn, pp. 1239–326. Churchill Livingstone, Edinburgh, 2001.

Digilio MC, Marino B, Toscano A, Giannotti A, Dallapiccola B. Congenital heart defects in Kabuki syndrome. *Am J Med Genet* 2001; **100**: 269–74.

Eldadal ZA, Hamosh A, Biery NJ, et al. Familial tetralogy of Fallot caused by mutation in the jagged 1 gene. *Hum Mol Genet* 2001; **10**: 163–9.

Goldmuntz E, Bamford R, Karkera JD, dela Cruz J, Roessler E, Muenke M. CFC1 mutations in patients with transposition of the great arteries and double-outlet right ventricle. *Am J Hum Genet* 2002; **70**: 776–80.

Lin AE, Pierpont ME. Heart development and the genetic aspects of cardiovascular malformations. *Am J Med Genet* 2000 Winter; **97**: 235–7.

Matsumoto N, Niikawa N. Kabuki make-up syndrome: a review. *Am J Med Genet C* 2003; **117C**: 57–65.

Oyen N, Poulsen G, Boyd HA, Wohlfahrt J, Jensen PK, Melbye M. Recurrence of congenital heart defects in families. *Circulation* 2009; **120**: 295–301.

Robinson SW, Morris CD, Goldmuntz E, et al. Missense muta-tions in CRELD1 are associated with cardiac atrioventricular septal defects. *Am J Hum Genet* 2003; **72**: 1047–52.

Sanlaville D, Romana SP, Lapierre JM, et al. A CGH study of 27 patients with CHARGE association. *Clin Genet* 2002; **61**: 135–8.

Sifrim A, Hitz MP, et al. Distinct genetic architectures for syn-dromic and nonsyndromic congenital heart defects identified by exome sequencing. *Nat Genet* 2016 Sep; **48**(9): 1060–5.

Wren C, Birrell G, Hawthorne G. Cardiovascular malformations in infants of diabetic mothers. *Heart* 2003; **89**: 1217–20.

Congenital hypothyroidism

Congenital hypothyroidism (CH) is detected at a rate of one in 3000–4000 live births, making it the most common congenital endocrine disorder. On a worldwide basis, hypothyroidism, including CH, results most commonly from iodine deficiency. In up to 10% of cases, CH is transient and self-limiting, lasting up to a few months. Some of these cases can be accounted for by the presence of anti-thyroid-stimulating hormone receptor (TSHR) antibodies in the mother, with transplacental passage to the fetus. Otherwise, CH results from developmental abnormalities at any level of the hypothalamic–pituitary–thyroid axis. CH is most commonly caused by defects in thyroid development leading to thyroid dysgenesis (85%), thyroid agenesis (40%), ectopy(40%), and hypoplasia (5%). The remaining cases are associated with either a goitre or a normal thyroid gland. Rarely, central (secondary) hypothyroidism may be caused by pituitary or hypothalamic disease leading to deficiency of thyrotropin (thyroid-stimulating hormone (TSH)) or thyrotropin-releasing hormone (TRH), respectively.

The essential role of thyroid hormones in CNS maturation has been clearly demonstrated, and CH is eminently treatable by thyroxine replacement. Screening for neonatal hypothyroidism was established in the UK in 1982, which revolutionized the development of infants with CH with the institution of early and adequate treatment. This is witnessed by the normal growth and neurological development in affected children, and by a dramatic increase in IQ, from an average of <80 to the mean of the general population.

Most cases of CH occur sporadically. However, cases with dyshormonogenesis are mostly recessively inherited, and recent cohort analyses estimate that ~2% of cases with thyroid dysgenesis are familial. It is also noteworthy that CH is associated with an increased incidence of birth defects, with surveys in the UK reporting a nonthyroidal congenital anomaly rate of 7% and an increased prevalence of chromosomal anomalies (1.5%).

The candidate genes associated with primary CH can be divided into two main groups: those causing thyroid gland dysgenesis and those associated with defects in the organification of iodide, leading to dyshormonogenesis.

Clinical approach

History: key points

- Family history: three-generation family tree, parental consanguinity, CH (permanent or transient), non-autoimmune hypothyroidism, goitre, or a history of any extrathyroidal congenital anomalies (e.g. cleft palate—FOXE1, renal anomalies—PAX8, neonatal respiratory distress and movement disorders—NKX2-1).
- Antenatal history of goitre detected on USS treated by intra-amniotic injections of thyroxine or tri-iodothyronine to shrink the gland (thyroid peroxidase defects).
- CH-associated features in the neonate including prolonged jaundice, coarse facial features, macroglossia, hoarse cry, goitre, airway obstruction, and umbilical hernia on examination.
- Age of diagnosis of hypothyroidism—as part of neonatal screening or afterwards. (NB. Central CH will not be detected on routine neonatal screening which measures elevated serum TSH.)

- Age when L-thyroxine replacement started.
- Developmental history including milestones.

Examination: key points

- Growth parameters, including OFC.
- In the neonate, look for respiratory distress, prolonged jaundice, macroglossia, and umbilical hernia.
- Presence or absence of goitre and any upper airway compromise if significantly enlarged.
- The presence of any other congenital malformations (e.g., cleft palate, spiky hair, and choanal atresia suggest FOXE1) and careful assessment for dysmorphic features.

Special investigations

BIOCHEMICAL INVESTIGATIONS

- Review thyroid function tests (TFTs) by obtaining the original diagnostic TFTs from the neonatal blood spot screening card and from the first venous serum measurements, before the onset of L-thyroxine treatment. CH is normally associated with elevated TSH and reduced FT4 and FT3 levels. Exceptions include MCT8 defects where FT3 is elevated with a normal or slightly raised TSH, and thyroid hormone receptor alpha gene mutations where FT4 levels are low-normal or subnormal, FT3 levels are high-normal or elevated, and TSH levels are normal.
- Check TFTs (circulating TSH, FT4, and FT3) in all first degree-relatives of a proband.
- Thyroid autoantibodies to rule out an autoimmune thyroid disease. Measure anti-TSHR antibodies in the mother if CH in the baby is transient (hyperthyroid mothers with Graves' disease can give birth to infants with transient CH).
- The measurement of serum thyroglobulin in all patients with suspected organification disorders or severe TSHR resistance, who have raised levels when their circulating TSH is increased. Exceptions are cases with thyroglobulin synthesis defects where the thyroglobulin level is usually low. If serum thyroglobulin is measurable where there is apparent athyreosis on thyroid imaging, this suggests the presence of radiologically undetectable hypoplastic thyroid tissue.

RADIOLOGICAL INVESTIGATIONS

- Thyroid scintigraphy, using either technetium (Tc) or radioactive iodine—provides information about the size and location of the gland.
- Perchlorate discharge test—if positive, CH is due to dyshormonogenesis.
- USS of the neck by an experienced radiologist to assess thyroid gland size (appropriateness for age and sex, and its location along the embryological line of development between the base of the tongue and thorax). If there is discordance between thyroid isotope scanning (no tracer uptake) and USS (normal or an enlarged thyroid gland), CH due to a sodium iodide symporter (SLC5A5) defect is likely.
- Consider renal USS to rule out renal anomalies (AD CH with renal dysgenesis suggest PAX-8) or temporal bone CT or MRI scanning (CH with goitre and sensorineural deafness suggests Pendred syndrome).

SPECIALIST INVESTIGATIONS

SPECIALIST INVESTIGATIONS

- Investigation of thyroid gland resistance to TSH involves the administration of TRH, with measurement of both the pituitary TSH response and the subsequent rise in circulating T3 following this increase in TSH.
- Defective iodide trapping by the thyroid gland caused by sodium iodide symporter defects can be confirmed by measuring the saliva-to-plasma (S/P) ratio of iodide 1 hour after oral administration of a small dose of radiolabelled iodide (25–50 mCi of either ^{125}I or ^{131}I-labelled sodium iodide; normal S/P ratio is 25–140). NB. Thyroxine treatment need not be stopped or reduced before this test, as it does not affect salivary gland iodide trapping.

GENETIC INVESTIGATIONS

- Genomic analysis in presence of features suggestive of a chromosomal or syndromic diagnosis, e.g. genomic array, gene panel for CH genes, or WES/WGS as available.

Some diagnoses to consider

Thyroid dysgenesis and non-syndromic CH

THYROID-STIMULATING HORMONE RECEPTOR DEFECTS (TSHR MUTATIONS LEADING TO TSH RESISTANCE). Homozygous or compound heterozygous mutations in the human *TSHR* gene leading to variable TSH resistance—compensated TSH resistance was associated with euthyroid hyperthyrotropinaemia, mild or borderline hypothyroidism, severe hypothyroidism associated with a hypoplastic thyroid gland, or even apparent athyreosis. Mildly raised TSH levels in individuals who are heterozygous for LOF germline mutations in the TSHR have also been reported.

BOREALIN ASSOCIATED THYROID DYSGENESIS. Biallelic mutation in the Borealin gene is a cause of thyroid dysgenesis (Carré et al. 2016).

Thyroid dysgenesis and syndromic CH

FOXE1 (FKHL15 OR TITF2) DEFECTS. AR inheritance leads to CH associated with thyroid agenesis (hypoplasia also reported), cleft palate, spiky hair, and in some cases bilateral choanal atresia and bifid epiglottis.

NKX2-1 (TITF-1) DEFECTS. *De novo* or dominantly inherited *NKX2-1* mutations (including interstitial deletions in chromosome 14q) have been reported with compensated CH (raised TSH, normal FT4 and FT3) and unexplained respiratory distress in term babies in the neonatal period who have normal bronchial morphology with hypotonia, persistent ataxia and dysarthria, microcephaly, choreoathetosis, global developmental delay, and major feeding difficulties, and in families with isolated benign hereditary chorea, an AD movement disorder. In addition to dysgenesis, decreased iodide trapping with a positive perchlorate discharge test suggestive of dyshormonogenesis suggest the basis for CH.

ALBRIGHT HEREDITARY OSTEODYSTROPHY. The degree of TSH resistance tends to be mild, and overt clinical hypothyroidism is not always present. The TSH response to TRH is exaggerated and the degree of TSH resistance may increase with age. Affected children develop rapidly progressive obesity in the first year of life. Caused by heterozygous mutation in GNAS, see 'Obesity with and without developmental delay' in Chapter 2, 'Clinical approach', p. 254.

PAX8 DEFECTS. AD or *de novo* CH of varying severity with hypoplastic, and sometimes ectopic, thyroid glands in non-syndromic form or with renal hemiagenesis associated with hypercalciuria. When present, renal agenesis is ipsilateral to thyroid hemiagenesis.

KAT6B-RELATED DISORDERS. Say–Barber–Biesecker–Young–Simpson syndrome (SBBYSS or Ohdo syndrome) is a multiple anomaly syndrome characterized by severe intellectual disability, blepharophimosis, and a mask-like facial appearance. A number of individuals with SBBYSS also have thyroid abnormalities and cleft palate (Clayton-Smith et al. 2011). Individuals with genito-patellar syndrome, an allelic KAT6B-related disorder, may also have hypothyroidism/thyroid agenesis.

Dyshormonogenesis and CH

Except in rare cases, these are all inherited in an AR manner and associated with varying degrees of congenital goitre with a positive perchlorate discharge test.

THYROID PEROXIDASE DEFECTS (TPO MUTATIONS LEADING TO THYROID DYSHORMONOGENESIS 2A). The most prevalent cause of dyshormonogenesis causing CH by a total iodide organification defect. Serum thyroglobulin is elevated.

THYROGLOBULIN DEFECTS (TG MUTATIONS LEADING TO THYROID DYSHORMONOGENESIS 3). Moderate to severe CH, usually with low serum thyroglobulin concentrations. Affected individuals often have abnormal iodoproteins in their serum, especially iodinated albumin, and they excrete iodopeptides of low molecular weight in the urine.

SODIUM IODIDE SYMPORTER DEFECTS (SLC5A5 MUTATIONS LEADING TO THYROID DYSHORMONOGENESIS 1). Hereditary iodide transport defect associated with goitrous hypothyroidism of varying severity and absent thyroidal radioiodine uptake. Not surprisingly, individuals with a higher dietary iodine intake (e.g. in Japan) are less likely to have severe hypothyroidism than those with iodine-deficient diets. This condition is therefore preferably treated with iodine supplementation, rather than thyroid hormone replacement.

PENDRED SYNDROME (SLC26A4 MUTATIONS LEADING TO THYROID DYSHORMONOGENESIS 2B). Characterized by sensorineural deafness and goitre. Classically associated with a Mondini cochlear defect together with an enlarged vestibular aqueduct. Thyroid disease usually presents as a multinodular or diffuse goitre in most affected individuals and is typically not evident until the second decade of life. Despite the goitre, individuals are likely to be euthyroid and only rarely present with CH. TSH levels, however, are often in the upper end of the normal range, and hypothyroidism of variable severity may eventually develop.

DUAL OXIDASE 2 DEFECTS (DUOX2 MUTATIONS LEADING TO THYROID DYSHORMONOGENESIS 6). Heterozygous truncation mutations are associated with transient CH and a partial iodide organification defect, whereas homozygosity for such defects are associated with severe CH and a complete iodide organification defect. Goitre is not described in these patients.

IODOTYROSINE DEIODINASE DEFECTS (IYD MUTATIONS LEADING TO THYROID DYSHORMONOGENESIS 4). Homozygous mutations lead to goitrous CH associated with ID where the hallmark diagnostic biochemical feature is that of elevated iodotyrosines in serum and urine. Heterozygosity can sometimes be associated with later-onset goitrous hypothryoidism.

Iodothyronine transporter defects and syndromic CH

Allan–Herdon–Dudley syndrome (SLC16A2 mutations). XL ID disorder associated with CH associated with an unusual biochemical signature consisting of low FT4 and raised levels of FT3 and TSH, which may not be found at the time of neonatal screening but detected within the first 2 years of life. Other reported features include central hypotonia, peripheral hypertonia, dystonia, rotary nystagmus, dysconjugate eye movements, feeding difficulties, vomiting, recurrent aspiration, irritability, and subsequent spastic quadriplegia resulting in severe developmental delay with absent speech. Brain MRI and EEG are normal. Female carriers can display milder thyroid phenotypes without the neurological features.

Central hypothyroidism

X-LINKED SYNDROME OF CENTRAL HYPOTHYROIDISM AND TESTICULAR ENLARGEMENT (IGFS1 MUTATIONS). Congenital central hypothyroidism, either in isolation or in conjunction with other pituitary hormone deficits including variably reduced prolactin and growth hormone levels, associated with testicular enlargement. Some female carriers also demonstrated central hypothyroidism.

ISOLATED AND COMBINED PITUITARY HORMONE DEFICIENCY (IPHD AND CPHD). Central hypothyroidism can occur as part of IPHD with TSHB or TSHR gene defects or as part of disorders of CPHD (e.g. caused by mutations in POU1F1, PROP1, HESX1, LHX3, LHX4, SOX3, LEPR).

THYROID HORMONE RECEPTOR ALPHA DEFECTS (THRA MUTATIONS). The few reported cases have not been detected by neonatal screening, as the TSH levels are not elevated. However, this condition (de novo or AD) presents in early childhood with disproportionate short stature, delayed tooth eruption, raised body mass index (BMI) associated with a reduced basal metabolic rate, severe chronic constipation, and impaired cognitive development. The biochemical profile is characterized by low-normal or subnormal FT4 levels, high-normal or elevated FT3 levels, and normal TSH levels. Skeletal survey shows delayed fusion of cranial sutures with a patent anterior fontanelle, multiple wormian bones, together with femoral epiphyseal dysgenesis and delayed bone age. The heart rate and BP are low for age. Serum sex hormone-binding globulin is markedly elevated. Some of these features improve with L-thyroxine treatment.

Genetic advice

Recurrence risk

Low recurrence risk if CH is isolated and sporadic. Twenty-five per cent risk if there is evidence of dyshormonogenesis or presence of parental consanguinity (the main exceptions are with DUOX2 mutations where if both parents carry a mutation, then the risk of transient CH is 2 in 3 and the risk of severe permanent CH is 1 in 4, and with TSHR mutations where inheritance is AR but carriers can present with frank or compensated hypothyroidism). As appropriate for individual syndromes or diagnoses.

Carrier detection

Where the familial mutations are known, this is possible by molecular testing.

Prenatal diagnosis

This is generally not a consideration, as the national neonatal screening programme detects the vast majority, enabling initiation of treatment early enough to prevent any significant developmental delay. Where there is a previous pregnancy affected with antenatal goitre, this can be screened with USS in subsequent pregnancies from the second trimester onwards.

Natural history and further management

Management is by a paediatric endocrinologist. L-thyroxine replacement is the norm. However, in sodium iodide symporter or dual oxidase 2 defects, iodine replacement is an alternative option that may be more effective.

Support groups: The British Thyroid Foundation, http://www.btf-thyroid.org; British Society for Paediatric Endocrinology and Diabetes, http://www.bsped.org.uk; Child Growth Foundation, http://www.childgrowth-foundation.org.

Expert adviser: Soo-Mi Park, Consultant in Clinical Genetics, Department of Clinical Genetics, Cambridge University Hospitals NHS Foundation Trust, Cambridge, UK.

References

Baris I, Arisoy AE, Smith A, et al. A novel missense mutation in human TTF-2 (FKHL15) gene is associated with congenital hypothyroidism but not athyreosis. J Clin Endocrinol Metab 2006; **91**: 4183–7.

Bochukova E, Schoenmakers N, Agostini M, et al. A mutation in the thyroid hormone receptor alpha gene. N Engl J Med 2012; **366**: 243–9.

Campeau PM, Lee BH. KAT6B-related disorders. In: RA Pagon, MP Adam, TD Bird, CR Dolan, CT Fong, K Stephens (eds.). GeneReviews™ [Internet]. University of Washington, Seattle, 2012.

Carré A, Stoupa A, et al. Mutations in BOREALIN cause thyroid dysgenesis. Hum Mol Genet 2016; epub Dec 26.

Castanet M, Park SM, Smith A, et al. A novel loss-of-function mutation in TTF-2 is associated with congenital hypothyroidism, thyroid agenesis, and cleft palate. Hum Mol Genet 2002; **11**: 2051–9.

Clayton-Smith J, O'Sullivan J, Daly S, et al. Whole-exome-sequencing identifies mutations in histone acetyltransferase gene KAT6B in individuals with the Say-Barber-Biesecker variant of Ohdo syndrome. Am J Hum Genet 2011; **89**: 675–81.

Dumitrescu AM, Liao XH, Best TB, Brockmann K, Refetoff S. A novel syndrome combining thyroid and neurological abnormalities is associated with mutations in a monocarboxylate transporter gene. Am J Hum Genet 2004; **74**: 168–75.

Park SM, Chatterjee VKK. Genetics of congenital hypothyroidism. J Med Genet 2005; **42**: 379–89.

Park SM, Clifton-Bligh RJ, Betts P, Chatterjee VK. Congenital hypothyroidism and apparent athyreosis with compound heterozygosity or compensated hypothyroidism with probable hemizygosity for inactivating mutations of the TSH receptor. Clin Endocrinol 2004; **60**: 220–7.

Park SM, Persani L, Beck-Peccoz P, Chatterjee VKK. Non-autoimmune thyroid disease. In: PE Harris, PMG Bouloux (eds.). Endocrinology in clinical practice, 1st edn. pp. 247–68. CRC Press, New York, 2001.

Sun Y, Bak B, Schoenmakers N, et al. Loss-of-function mutations in IGSF1 cause an X-linked syndrome of central hypothyroidism and testicular enlargement. Nat Genet 2012; **44**: 1375–81.

Corneal clouding

Corneal clouding is opacification of the cornea. It is a sign of several different systemic disorders, many of which are inherited metabolic conditions. Corneal clarity is maintained by the endothelium, which functions abnormally in the endothelial dystrophies, leading to corneal opacification. The corneal dystrophies are classified according to the corneal layer which is predominantly affected. The cornea has five layers: epithelium (outermost), Bowman's membrane, stroma, Descemet's membrane, and endothelium (innermost). The geneticist may be asked for advice during the diagnostic process, in particular to consider rare conditions of unknown aetiology and syndromic causes of corneal clouding.

Clinical approach

History: key points

- Family history. At least three generations; consider all forms of autosomal and mitochondrial inheritance and with specific enquiry for consanguinity.
- Exposure to teratogens, and infections during pregnancy.
- Growth (syndromic conditions).
- Developmental progress. Evidence of loss of skill/regression (metabolic/mitochondrial disorders)?
- Polyuria, polydipsia, renal disease (cystinosis).

Examination: key points

- Eyes. Ophthalmological confirmation, biomicroscopy and examination with fundoscopy for lesions such as cherry red spots (mucolipidoses), and USS to observe the intraocular structure. It is essential to exclude congenital glaucoma and other developmental ophthalmological disorders that might be associated with corneal opacification, e.g. Peters anomaly, or congenital aphakia (*FOXE3*).
- Head circumference. Macrocephaly in storage disorders.
- Height. Assess for disproportion.
- Hands. Contractures (storage disorders, Winchester syndrome).
- Hair. Coarse? Thick or sparse? Hypertrichosis and hirsuitism?
- Skin. Does it feel as though there is deposition of an abnormal metabolite in the subcutaneous layers? Is it stiff or ichthyotic?
- Cardiac murmur.
- Enlargement of the liver and spleen, umbilical hernia (storage diseases).
- Nail hypoplasia (Fryns syndrome).
- Neurological assessment.

Special investigations

If a diagnosis seems likely on the basis of your examination, e.g. Hurler's syndrome, then proceed directly to the confirmatory enzymatic and molecular analysis. If the diagnosis is uncertain, start with baseline tests and then more targeted testing can follow on when these results are through.

- Baseline: thyroid function; urine metabolic screen (MPS, oligosaccharides, amino and organic acids); plasma amino acids; basic biochemistry; vacuolated lymphocytes, ammonia, and lactate.

- Congenital infection screen.
- White cell enzymes. These need to arrive in the laboratory within a few hours. Please discuss your differential diagnosis with the laboratory, so that the correct analyses are performed.
- Skeletal survey. This is a useful investigation to assess if there are features of a storage disease such as abnormal bone modelling or if there are features of a skeletal dysplasia.
- VLCFAs.
- Abdominal USS (organomegaly, renal enlargement, or structural abnormality).
- Genomic analysis in presence of features suggestive of a chromosomal or syndromic diagnosis, e.g. genomic array, gene panel, or WES/WGS as appropriate.
- DNA testing/storage.
- Skin or muscle biopsy to assess if there is deposition of an abnormal compound or evidence of mitochondrial dysfunction. Storage of tissue for possible future analysis.

Some diagnoses to consider

Congenital

- Structural malformation of the eye. Many of the anterior segment dysgenesis or anophthalmia/microphthalmia conditions are associated with corneal opacification. For example, congenital corneal opacification or sclerocornea, in association with congenital aphakia, can be caused by mutations in *FOXE3*. For a full description of the genes that have now been identified, see particularly 'Microphthalmia and anophthalmia', p. 236 and 'Anterior segment eye malformations', p. 62 in Chapter 2, 'Clinical approach'.
- Fryns syndrome. A rare lethal AR condition with nail/digital hypoplasia and diaphragmatic hernia.
- Zellweger syndrome. An AR disorder of peroxisome metabolism.
- Rare congenital corneal dystrophies, e.g. congenital endothelial dystrophies (CHED) and congenital stromal dystrophy. CHED has AD and AR forms—CHED1 and CHED2, respectively. Some cases of CHED2 have been shown to be due to mutations in *SLC4A11*. CHED1 patients present in the first or second year of life with corneal clouding which progresses until age 5–10 years; CHED2 presents at birth or within the neonatal period. CHED1 maps to a locus on chromosome 20. Congenital hereditary stromal dystrophy can be caused by mutations in the decorin (*DCN*) gene on 12q22 (Bredrup et al. 2005). A family with XL corneal dystrophy has been described.
- Congenital infection and trauma.

Childhood

- Arrange for thorough metabolic investigations.
- MPS:
  - type I. Hurler's, Hurler's/Scheie, and Scheie syndromes;
  - type II. Hunter's syndrome;
  - type IV. Morquio syndrome;
  - type VI. Maroteaux–Lamy;
  - type VII. Sly;
  - but *not* type III. Sanfilippo.

- Mucoliposes (other eye findings include cherry red spot).
- Cystinosis. AR. Check for renal and thyroid involvement
- Fabry disease, XL semi-dominant with manifestation in females. Mutation in the alpha-galactosidase A gene (*GLA*). In addition to corneal dystrophy ('cornea verticillata'), there are tortuous retinal vessels. The cutaneous signs are angiokeratoderma (vascular skin lesions) in a truncal distribution. Neuropathic pain with acroparaesthesia and abdominal pain, fatigue, autonomic dysfunction, and renal failure are additional features. Treatment with ERT currently under clinical trial. See 'Hypertrophic cardiomyopathy (HCM)' in Chapter 3, 'Common consultations', p. 460.
- Skeletal dysplasia.
- Harboyan syndrome (congenital corneal endothelial dystrophy and progressive sensorineural deafness), follows AR inheritance and is caused by biallelic mutation in the borate transporter *SLC4A11* gene (this gene also causes CHED—see above).
- Winchester syndrome.

Adult corneal dystrophy
The corneal dystrophies are bilateral, genetic, and usually slowly progressive conditions. Many manifest in adulthood. They rarely present to the geneticist, but families may be seen in genetic eye clinics. Most are dominantly inherited and have a family history.

- Several clinical subtypes are caused by mutations in the *BIGH3* gene at 5q31. Fuchs endothelial dystrophy of the cornea (FCED) and posterior polymorphous dystrophy (PPCD) are AD disorders. Missense mutations in *COL8A2* (which may be '*de novo*') are found in some individuals (Biswas *et al.* 2001).
- Check the precise type of dystrophy and inheritance prior to counselling.
- The disease may recur after corneal grafting.
- Most are limited to the cornea.
- Exclude Fabry disease and adult cystinosis.

Genetic advice
Recurrence risk
Dependent on the aetiology. For adult corneal dystrophy, see above.

Carrier detection
- By ophthalmological examination (corneal dystrophy, Fabry disease).
- Is possible in families where a causative mutation has been identified; also within families with enzyme deficiencies.

Prenatal diagnosis
- By CVS or amniocentesis where there is molecular or biochemical confirmation of diagnosis.
- USS in mid trimester for syndromes with structural abnormalities, e.g. Fryns syndrome.

Natural history and further management (preventative measures)
- Long-term ophthalmological and/or medical follow-up.
- Corneal grafting may be possible.

Support group:
Climb (Children Living with Inherited Metabolic Diseases), http://www.climb.org.uk.

Expert adviser: Nicola Ragge, Consultant Clinical Geneticist, Birmingham Women's Hospital, Birmingham, UK; Professor in Medical Genetics, Oxford Brookes University, Oxford, UK.

References
Bredrup C, Knappskog PM, Majewski J, Rødahl E, Boman H. Congenital stromal dystrophy of the cornea caused by a mutation in the decorin gene. *Invest Ophthalmol Vis Sci* 2005; **46**: 420–6.
Biswas S, Munier FL, Yardley J, et al. Missense mutations in COL8A2, the gene encoding the alpha2 chain of type VIII collagen, cause two forms of corneal endothelial dystrophy. *Hum Mol Genet* 2001; **10**: 2415–23.
Iseri SU, Osborne RJ, Farrall M, et al. Seeing clearly: the dominant and recessive nature of FOXE3 in eye developmental anomalies. *Hum Mutat* 2009; **30**: 1378–86.
Mataftsi A, Islam L, Kelberman D, et al. Chromosome abnormalities and the genetics of congenital corneal opacification. *Mol Vis* 2011; **17**: 1624–40.
Reis LM, Semina EV. Genetics of anterior segment dysgenesis disorders. *Curr Opin Ophthalmol* 2011; **22**: 314–24.
Schmid E, Lisch W, Philipp W, et al. A new X-linked endothelial corneal dystrophy. *Am J Ophthalmol* 2006; **141**: 478–87.
Weiss JS, Meller HU, Lisch W, et al. The IC3D classification of the corneal dystrophies. *Cornea* 2008; **27**(Suppl 2): S1–83.

Deafness in early childhood

Severe or profound deafness affects ~1/1000 infants at birth or during early childhood (prelingual period). Acquisition of speech is a major difficulty for these children, and many with severe and profound deafness are considered for cochlear implantation. A further 2–3/1000 children have moderate/progressive deafness requiring aiding. In developed countries, deafness has an important genetic origin and at least 60% of cases are inherited. The pattern of inheritance can be AD, AR, XLR, or mitochondrial.

- In sensorineural deafness (nerve deafness, perceptive deafness), the abnormality lies between the hair cells of the cochlea and the auditory regions of the brain. Most sensorineural hearing loss is due to dysfunction of the hair cells themselves but rarely may be caused by pathology of the auditory nerve itself or its synapses with hair cells (auditory neuropathy). This is diagnosed by the presence of otoacoustic emissions (intact outer hair cells) in the presence of deafness, i.e. absent or abnormal auditory brainstem responses.
- In conductive deafness, the abnormality lies in the external or middle ear.

Causes of severe deafness are the following.

- Environmental (35%):
  - congenital infection (rubella, CMV); checking for congenital CMV infection is now part of routine diagnostic investigations of those with deafness confirmed by newborn hearing screening;
  - perinatal asphyxia;
  - hyperbilirubinaemia (serum bilirubin (SB) >250 μmol/l for prolonged period);
  - infection, e.g. meningitis;
  - drugs, e.g. aminoglycosides.
- Genetic—syndromic (about 35% of genetic causes).
- Genetic—non-syndromic (65% of genetic causes). There is huge genetic heterogeneity with >60 AD loci and >90 AR. The majority (~80–85%) follow AR inheritance.

Aim to identify syndromic causes of deafness in order to enable assessment for associated problems (e.g. visual impairment) and to permit accurate genetic counselling. Methods of assessing deafness include the following.

- Pure tone audiogram. Comprehensive test of the auditory pathway from the tympanic membrane to the auditory cortex.
- Otoacoustic emissions (newborn hearing test). Outer hair cell function (possible for this to be normal neonatally and yet the baby is unable to hear due to a problem with the VIIIth nerve). Mutations in OTOF (encoding otoferlin) and PJVK (pejvakin) can give a non-syndromic auditory neuropathy.
- BAER/BSER (brainstem auditory evoked response/brainstem evoked response). Testing nerve and brainstem pathways.
- MRI or CT scan. Some genetic conditions may give rise to characteristic malformations of the inner ear which may aid diagnosis (in Pendred syndrome there are often dilated vestibular aqueducts and enlarged endolymphatic sacs, and in BOR syndrome there may be a Mondini cochlea dysplasia with or without dilated vestibular aqueducts). XL deafness caused by POU3F4 mutations gives a pathognomonic appearance.

Connexin 26 (GJB2) and connexin 30 (GJB6) (DFNB1 locus)

Connexins are transmembrane proteins that form channels, allowing passage of ions or small molecules between cells. There are two types, named GJA or GJB followed by a number. Mutations in the gap junction protein connexin 26 Cx26 (GJB2) on 13q12 may account for up to 50% of all cases of prelingual AR non-syndromic hearing loss and 10–40% of sporadic cases. GJB2 which encodes Cx26 has a single coding exon. The carrier frequency in European, North American, and Mediterranean populations is ~1/50. A hotspot at c.35delG accounts for 70% of GJB2 mutations in these populations; c.167delT accounts for 3–4% in Ashkenazi Jews; the mild mutation p.V37I is very common in South East Asia and c.235delC is the most common mutation among Japanese; p.W77X, p.W24X, and p.Q124X are the most common in the Asian subcontinent.

There is no structural abnormality of the inner ear in Cx26 deafness and no vestibular pathology. The most common mutations generally cause severe to profound prelingual sensorineural deafness, but there is considerable variation, particularly with missense and non-truncating mutations. Twenty per cent of sib pairs may show significant variation in the degree of hearing loss, differing by two or more classes of severity (mild/moderate/severe/profound).

Connexin 30 (Cx30) (GJB6) is a gene lying adjacent to GJB2 at the DFNB1 locus on 13q12. Cx30 encodes a protein that is co-expressed with connexin 26 in the inner ear. A 342-kb deletion in Cx30 is the second most common mutation, causing prelingual deafness among Mediterranean populations. The deletion extends distally to GJB2, the coding region of which remains intact. Mutations in the complex locus containing the genes for Cx26 and Cx30 can result in deafness which is secondary to deletion of a distant regulatory element for GJB2 lying with GJB6. Sensorineural deafness is found in individuals who are homozygotes or compound heterozygotes for mutations in GJB2, homozygotes for the deletion in GJB6, and heterozygotes for both GJB2 and GJB6 deletions.

Auditory neuropathy (auditory neuropathy spectrum disorders).

This is characterized by normal otoacoustic emissions but abnormal auditory nerve function, as measured by auditory brainstem response. Patients with auditory neuropathy describe difficulty with hearing and understanding speech, out of proportion to the degree of pure tone hearing loss. Outcomes and prognosis are different from environmental hearing impairments. The commonest cause is factors surrounding prematurity especially hyperbilirubinaemia. For the term baby consider OTOF, including temperature sensitive mutation. Syndromic causes include neuropathies (e.g. CMT) and OPA1.

Deafness due to mutations in mtDNA

m.1555A>G is the most common mutation (Bitner-Glindzicz et al. 2009) but usually only causes hearing impairment in early life if there has been exposure to aminoglycosides (e.g. gentamicin); m.74445A>G is the second most common mitochondrial mutation (sometimes associated with palmoplantar keratoderma).

m.7472insC can cause isolated progressive deafness or deafness with ataxia/dysarthria/myoclonus. Overall, mitochondrial mutations have been found in up to 30% of families with affected members in two or more generations related through the maternal line, but only 1% of sporadic early-onset non-syndromic deafness. The age of onset of deafness can be very variable (Estivill *et al.* 1998). m.1555A>G is homoplasmic in nearly all pedigrees.

Clinical approach

Prior to the consultation, try to obtain the child's audiograms (if old enough) to determine whether the deafness is sensorineural or conductive, and the severity, i.e. mild (20–40 dB), moderate (40–60 dB), severe (60–80 dB), or profound >80 dB, and which frequencies are affected. Occasionally an audiometric pattern may be the key diagnostic clue (low-frequency hearing loss is unusual and may be caused by mutations in *WFS1* or *HDIA1*; 'U'-shaped or 'cookie-bite' hearing losses are usually dominant and may be caused by mutations in *COL11A2* or *TECTA*) and a ski-slope pattern by *TMPRSS3A*. If not available, you may need to repeat the audiogram; it is difficult to provide accurate advice without this information. The level of conversational speech is 45–60 dB.

If either parent is congenitally profoundly deaf, you may need to arrange for a communicator skilled in sign language to facilitate the consultation.

History: key points

- Family history. Three-generation (or more) family tree, with specific enquiry about:
  - hearing loss—age of onset, unilateral/bilateral, progressive/not;
  - sudden death or fainting (Jervell–Nielsen), goitre (Pendred), renal disease (Alport, BOR), poor vision (Usher, peroxisomal, mitochondrial), pigmentary anomalies (Waardenburg, piebaldism);
  - consanguinity (if present, counsel as for AR inheritance if rest of assessment is negative).
- Pre-, peri-, and postnatal history:
  - viral infections (CMV, rubella)—enquire about rash, arthralgia;
  - severe jaundice, meningitis, aminoglycosides. Aminoglycosides tend to cause a steep high-frequency hearing loss; hearing loss secondary to jaundice and perinatal factors would be expected to cause neurological problems and learning difficulties, in addition to deafness, i.e. the brain is more sensitive to hypoxia and jaundice than the inner ear).
- Developmental delay (delay in motor milestones is common in deaf children who are otherwise neurologically normal, probably due to involvement of the vestibular system). The vestibular system is involved in Usher type 1, Jervell and Lange–Nielsen syndrome, sometimes in Pendred syndrome, and sometimes in BOR or other non-syndromic genes. Thus, a history of profound congenital hearing loss, in association with vestibular problems/delayed motor milestones, should prompt specific investigations to exclude these syndromes (ECG, ERG, MRI/CT, etc.).
- Vestibular symptoms (Ménière-like symptoms are seen in families with *COCH* mutations; clues to this are an AD family history of adult-onset hearing loss, which is mainly high-frequency, in contrast to the hearing loss

in 'sporadic Ménière's which is predominantly low-frequency, and the association with Ménière-like symptoms). *MYO7A* mutations have also been reported in families with dominant deafness and mild vestibular symptoms.

Examination: key points

- Ear. Look for external ear malformations, e.g. tags, pits, atretic ear canal (BOR, TCS).
- Eyes. Look for dystopia canthorum and heterochromia or hypoplastic irides (Waardenberg), coloboma in the lower eyelid (TCS), and retinal pigmentation (Usher and peroxisomal disorders). Retinal pigmentation in Usher syndrome is unlikely to be visible before puberty. Check for optic atrophy if there is also diabetes (*WFS1*) or auditory neuropathy (*OPA1*).
- Neck. Look for branchial cysts (BOR); check for goitre (Pendred).
- Hair. Look for pigmentary disturbance (white forelock).
- Skin. Piebaldism and subtle pigmentary disturbances seen in Waardenburg.
- Abnormal neurological signs.

Special investigations

- Parental audiograms in all and sibling audiograms if any clinical suspicion of hearing loss.
- Mutation analysis in *GJB2/GJB6*.
- Consider mitochondrial mutation analysis if progressive sensorineural deafness in families consistent with maternal inheritance, i.e. without male–male transmission. Also if there has been a sudden deterioration or diagnosis of deafness following aminoglycoside exposure.
- Consider gene panel/WES/WGS as appropriate.
- Ophthalmology referral for refractive errors and fundoscopy in all cases (fundal assessment for RP, optic atrophy). ERG if delayed motor milestones have raised suspicion of Usher type I. Individuals with severe hearing impairment will rely heavily on visual function, so comprehensive ophthalmology assessment is important in all. If normal, suggest annual optician reviews with return to the ophthalmologist if any abnormality is detected.
- TORCH screen for congenital infections. CMV can be cultured from urine in the first few weeks of life or detected by polymerase chain reaction (PCR); rubella serology may be useful in children <6 months old.
- CT/MRI scan of the temporal bone in children (80% of those with Pendred have structural cochlear malformations, e.g. enlarged vestibular aqueducts and many, especially in childhood, do not have goitre and therefore appear non-syndromal.
- Renal USS if abnormalities of the pinnae, ear pits or tags, or branchial sinus (BOR), or multiple congenital anomalies, or low serum calcium (hypoparathyroidism–sensorineural deafness–renal dysplasia (HDR) syndrome).
- Urine dipstick for glucose (diabetes mellitus–optic atrophy–deafness (DIDMOAD) and mitochondrial myopathy–encephalopathy–lactic acidosis–stroke-like episodes (MELAS) 3243) and blood (Alport); send to lab if positive for confirmation.
- ECG for QT interval if severe/profound deafness (Jervell and Lange–Nielsen long QT syndromes). JLNS causes severe/profound deafness with delayed motor

milestones. If there is a suggestion of QT prolongation, assessment by a cardiologist is indicated. See 'Long QT and other inherited arrhythmia syndromes' in Chapter 3, 'Common consultations', p. 480.

- Thyroid function (thyroxine (T4)/TSH), if goitre present (Pendred syndrome—but diagnosis not excluded by normal results). Goitre is rare in children before puberty.

Some diagnoses to consider

Waardenburg syndrome (WS)
Accounts for >2% of childhood deafness and typically follows AD inheritance (see below for exceptions). Auditory–pigmentary syndromes are caused by physical absence of functional melanocytes from the skin, hair, eyes, and stria vascularis of the cochlea. All forms of Waardenburg show marked variability, from minor pigmentary changes to profound deafness, even within families, and at present it is not possible to predict the severity, even when a mutation is detected.

- WS1. In type 1, there is dystopia canthorum and 25% of patients have deafness. Type 1 patients tend to have the distinctive facial features of a high nasal bridge, synophrys, and hypoplasia of the alae nasi. Type 1 is caused by LOF mutations in PAX3 on 2q35.
- WS2. In type 2, there is no dystopia canthorum and over 50% of patients have deafness (Liu et al. 1995). It is a heterogeneous group; 20% are caused by mutations in the microphthalmia-associated transcription factor gene (MITF) (type 2A) and others by genes including homozygous mutations in SNAI2. Risk for clinically important deafness in MITF mutation carriers is around 1/3. The remainder have minor pigmentary anomalies, and some have mild hearing impairment which is not clinically significant. Deafness is thought to be non-progressive. There is little or no risk of Hirschsprung's in MITF mutation carriers.
- WS3 (Klein–Waardenburg (rare)) with upper limb anomalies, including flexion contractures of the fingers, is an extreme presentation of type 1; caused by mutations in PAX3. Some patients have been reported to be homozygotes, but not all; at least two parent–child transmissions are reported in the literature.
- WS4 (Shah–Waardenburg syndrome with Hirschsprung's disease) is genetically heterogeneous and can be caused by homozygous endothelin pathway mutations (genes for endothelin-3 or one of its receptors, EDNRB) and heterozygous SOX10 mutations. In the latter case, various neurological symptoms with demyelination might occur (Inoue et al. 2004). Some of these SOX10 patients have been reported to have dysplastic semicircular canals).

Pendred syndrome
Pendrin (SLC26A4). AR congenital severe/profound deafness, particularly affecting high frequencies with stepwise progressive fluctuating hearing loss. Speech/language is usually well developed for the degree of deafness identified on the audiogram. CT/MRI may show dilated vestibular aqueducts in ~80%. Goitre develops from puberty, so imaging is important in making the diagnosis in childhood. Approximately 5% of all severe/profound deafness in childhood.

Branchio-oto-renal syndrome (BOR)
An AD disorder with variable expressivity, but high penetrance caused by mutations in EYA1 and also rarely SIX1. Branchial, otic, and renal anomalies. Ear pits are a common feature. Hearing loss can be mixed or sensorineural and those with hearing impairment may have characteristic changes on their cochlear CT (Mondini dysplasia (fewer turns—normal is 2½)). BOR affects an estimated 2% of profoundly deaf children. Point mutations in EYA1 are present in ~50%. Complex rearrangements, such as inversions or large deletions, appear to be common and evade detection by direct sequencing methods (Vervoort et al. 2002). Renal anomalies vary from normal to mild dysplasia to agenesis. Branchial clefts or sinuses are less common than the otic or renal features.

Hypoparathyroidism–sensorineural deafness–renal dysplasia syndrome (HDR)
An AD disorder caused by mutations in a transcription factor GATA3 on 10p. Renal spectrum varies from normal through mild dysplasia to aplasia. HDR syndrome is primarily caused by GATA3 haploinsufficiency and is associated with a wide phenotypic spectrum (Muroya et al. 2001).

Treacher–Collins syndrome (TCS)
Caused by mutations in TCOF1 or more rarely by POLR1C and POLR1D. Deafness is mixed or sensorineural. Abnormal external ear, malar hypoplasia, inferior lid colobomata and downslanting palpebral fissures, cleft palate, Pierre–Robin sequence. AD; very variable expressivity, but fairly high penetrance. See 'Ear anomalies' in Chapter 2, 'Clinical approach', p. 142.

Usher syndrome
Characterized by sensorineural hearing loss and progressive RP. There are three clinical types (all AR), each with an underlying molecular heterogeneity.

- Type 1. Congenital severe/profound deafness with absent vestibular function. Delayed motor milestones, poor head control, late sitting, rarely walk before 18 months of age.
  - Type 1B is the most common type and is caused by mutation in MYO7A.
  - There are patients described with type 1D who have normal motor milestones.
- Type 2. Also congenital moderate/severe with sloping audiogram. Patients wear aids and develop speech.
- Type 3. Common in Finland, usually post-lingual and progressive. Vestibular function may be normal or absent. Also common among Ashkenazi Jews (specific mutations).

RP is usually not visible until the teenage years, by which time symptoms will be present (night blindness and loss of peripheral vision). The ERG is abnormal years before. In type 1, the ERG is likely to be abnormal within the first few years of life. For types 2 and 3, there are little data on when ERGs become abnormal and may be variable.

Keratosis–icthyosis–deafness (KID) syndrome
Dominant mutations in the Cx26 gene GJB2 have been shown to cause KID syndrome (skin thickening and fissuring with multiple hyperkeratotic plaques), palmo-plantar keratoderma associated with hearing loss, and Vohwinkel syndrome. Missense mutations in the closely related Cx30 gene GJB6 underlie Clouston syndrome (AD hidrotic ectodermal dysplasia).

Genetic advice
Many genes are involved in the different types of deafness (syndromic and non-syndromic). Non-syndromic

hereditary deafness in early childhood is mainly (80%) due to recessive genes.

Recurrence risk
- If sporadic case and all the above are normal, i.e. no environmental or syndromic diagnosis can be made, recurrence risk for future pregnancies is 10% (empiric figure; in reality, some families will have 25% recurrence risk, and others much lower risks, but it is not possible to discriminate).
- If two affected sibs or consanguinity, assume AR—25% risk in future pregnancies.
- If affected parent and child, assume AD—50% risk in future pregnancies.
- If parent has severe congenital hearing loss and environmental and syndromic forms have been excluded as far as possible, empiric risk to offspring is 5%.
- If both parents have severe congenital hearing loss (neither with environmental or syndromic form) and there is no consanguinity or likelihood of consanguinity, empiric risk to offspring is 10%. NB. If the first child is deaf, consider the possibility that both parents have allelic AR deafness (risk to offspring 100%), as well as the possibility of one or other or both parents having AD deafness.

Carrier detection
- Parental audiograms in all and sibling audiograms if any clinical suspicion of hearing loss.
- For connexin 26 deafness and other types where the mutations are defined, it is possible to offer accurate carrier detection to family members.

Prenatal diagnosis
PND for hearing loss is highly contentious but is technically feasible by CVS if the causative mutations are known.

Natural history and further management (preventative measures)
- Hearing aids. Skilled assessment by an audiologist is required to ensure good results. In young children, the ear moulds need to be changed periodically as the ear canal grows.
- Cochlear implants. These represent an established treatment in the management of very young children with profound hearing loss. They are best suited to children in the preschool years who, with optimal hearing aid correction, still have a loss >65 dB.
- Education. Provision needs to be carefully matched to the child's level of hearing loss.

Support groups: The National Deaf Children's Society (NDCS), http://www.ndcs.org.uk; Action on Hearing Loss, https://www.actiononhearingloss.org.uk/default.aspx; DeafPLUS, http://www.deafplus.org.

Expert adviser: Maria Bitner-Glindzic, Professor of Clinical and Molecular Genetics, Genetics and Genomic Medicine Programme, University College London, Great Ormond Street Institute of Child Health, London, UK.

References
Bitner-Glindzicz M. Hereditary deafness and phenotyping in humans. *Br Med Bull* 2002; **63**: 73–94.

Bitner-Glindzicz M, Pembrey M, Duncan A, et al. Prevalence of mitochondrial 1555A-->G mutation in European children. *N Engl J Med* 2009; **360**: 640–2.

Del Castillo I, Villamar M, Moreno-Pelayo MA, et al. A deletion involving the connexion 30 gene in nonsyndromic hearing impairment. *N Engl J Med* 2002; **346**: 243–9.

Dror AA, Avraham KB. Hearing impairment: a panoply of genes and functions. *Neuron* 2010; **68**: 293–308.

Duman D, Tekin M. Autosomal recessive nonsyndromic deafness genes: a review. *Front Biosci (Landmark Ed)* 2012; **17**: 2213–36.

Estivill X, Govea N, Barceló E, et al. Familial progressive sensorineural deafness is mainly due to the mtDNA A1555G mutation and is enhanced by treatment of amnoglycosides. *Am J Hum Genet* 1998; **62**: 27–35.

Fraser GR. *The causes of profound deafness in children*. John Hopkins University Press, Baltimore, 1976.

Hutchin TP, Thompson KR, Parker M, Newton V, Bitner-Glindzicz M, Mueller RF. Prevalence of mitochondrial DNA mutations in childhood/congenital onset non-syndromal sensorineural hearing impairment. *J Med Genet* 2001; **38**: 229–31.

Inoue K, Khajavi M, Ohyama T, et al. Molecular mechanism for distinct neurological phenotypes conveyed by allelic truncating mutations. *Nat Genet* 2004; **36**: 361–9.

Kimberling WJ. Special issue: Hereditary deafness. *Am J Med Genet C* 1999; **89C**: 121–74.

Liu XZ, Newton VE, Read AP. Waardenburg syndrome type II: phenotypic findings and diagnostic criteria. *Am J Med Genet* 1995; **55**: 95–100.

Milunsky JM. Waardenburg syndrome type I. In: RA Pagon, MP Adam, HH Ardinger, et al. (eds.). *GeneReviews®* [Internet]. University of Washington, Seattle, 2001 (updated 2011). http://www.ncbi.nlm.nih.gov/books/NBK1531.

Muroya K, Hasegawa T, Ito Y, et al. GATA3 abnormalities and the phenotypic spectrum of HDR syndrome. *J Med Genet* 2001; **38**: 374–80.

Parker MJ, Fortnum H, Young ID, Davis AC. Variations in genetic assessment and recurrence risks quoted for childhood deafness: a survey of clinical geneticists. *J Med Genet* 1999; **36**: 125–30.

Read AP, Newton VE. Waardenburg syndrome. *J Med Genet* 1997; **34**: 656–65.

Sanchez-Martin M, Rodriguez-Garcia A, Pérez-Losada J, Sagrera A, Read AP, Sánchez-García I. SLUG (SNAI2) deletions in patients with Waardenburg disease. *Hum Mol Genet* 2002; **11**: 3231–6.

Shearer AE, Smith RJ. Genetics: advances in genetic testing for deafness. *Curr Opin Pediatr* 2012; **24**: 679–86.

Steel K. Science, medicine, and the future: new interventions in hearing impairment. *BMJ* 2000; **320**: 622–5.

Vervoort VS, Smith RJ, O'Brien J, et al. Genomic rearrangements of EYA1 account for a large fraction of families with BOR syndrome. *Eur J Hum Genet* 2002; **10**: 757–66.

Willems PJ. Genetic causes of hearing loss. *N Engl J Med* 2000; **342**: 1101–9.

Developmental delay in the child with consanguineous parents

The incidence of AR disorders is increased in the offspring of consanguineous unions. However, it is important not to forget that non-genetic, chromosomal, AD, and XL conditions also occur in consanguineous populations. Approximately 5% of children with developmental delay who are the offspring of consanguineous parents will have a *de novo* dominant mutation responsible for their condition (McRae *et al.* 2016). There is strong evidence that developmental delay, chronic disease, and neonatal death are more common in children of related parents (Bittles and Black 2010). In communities which have long-standing traditions of consanguinity, the risks of congenital disorders may be higher than anticipated from a simple three-generation family tree. The genetic conditions are well described in the work of McKusick and colleagues (Khoury *et al.* 1987) in the American Amish community and of Bundey and Alam (1993) within the British Pakistani community. See 'Consanguinity' in Chapter 3, 'Common consultations', p. 374. AR intellectual delay is genetically very heterogeneous (Najmabadi *et al.* 2011).

Clinical approach

History: key points

As consanguinity is practised more commonly in migrant communities, it may be necessary to arrange for an interpreter to obtain a full history.

- Three-generation family tree. Ask specifically about consanguinity and define the relationships. Ask specifically if any child has/had schooling difficulties and about pregnancy, deaths in childhood, and early adult life as proxy markers for malformations and neurological disability.
- Developmental history. Trajectory of developmental delay, normal early development, followed by a fall-off in the trajectory is common in primary microcephaly. Ensure that screening for PKU and MCAD have occurred and are normal; these are the common causes of delay in consanguineous communities (Ropers 2010). Ask particularly about loss of skills; disorders associated with childhood dementia are much more common in the context of consanguinity (Verity *et al.* 2010).

Other key features are visual and hearing problems and the presence of seizures.

Examination: key points

Careful physical and neurological examination

- Growth parameters. Height, span, weight, and OFC; plot the centile. Note any disproportion.
- Neurological examination. Spasticity, hypotonia, ataxia, reflexes.
- Face. Coarse features (storage disorders, congenital thyroid disease).
- Abdomen. Organomegaly (storage disorders).
- Eyes. Fundal examination, particularly for pigmentary retinopathy.
- Skin. Pigmentation abnormalities, sun sensitivity, premature ageing (DNA repair defects).
- Skeletal and limbs (skeletal dysplasia, radial defects).
- Other features and malformations.

Special investigations

In this group of patients, with a higher prior risk of metabolic disease, more extensive metabolic screening is indicated. If the karyotype is normal, there is a better chance of diagnostic yield in this group of patients from investigating to exclude metabolic/AR single gene conditions than proceeding straight to specialized chromosome analysis, e.g. microarray studies; however, WES/WGS approaches may cover both. SNP arrays may be helpful to target/exclude candidate genes prior to single gene sequencing/dosage studies.

- Genomic analysis in presence of features suggestive of a chromosomal or syndromic diagnosis, e.g. genomic array, gene panel, or WES/WGS as available.
- Chromosomes. Consider if there are any signs of AR conditions that can be confirmed by cytogenetic testing, e.g. Fanconi anaemia, AT, Bloom syndrome, Roberts syndrome.
- Consider AR conditions with a high carrier frequency within the population and exclude, for example, Tay–Sachs disease.
- DNA for FRAXA and storage.
- Baseline biochemistry plus fasting lactate and pyruvate.
- Urine for amino acids and organic acids. Plasma amino acids. Some children will have been born in areas of no neonatal screening for PKU.
- Urine MPS screen; when there are coarse features, add oligosaccharides.
- Vacuolated lymphocytes.
- White cell enzymes, DNA testing for NCL (Battens): often not done as a first-line investigation, unless evidence for regression or other neurological features. Discuss with paediatric neurologists, if in doubt.
- Consider VLCFAs to exclude a peroxisomal disorder.
- Consider 7-dehydrocholesterol (SLO syndrome).
- CK. Muscular dystrophies in this group are heterogeneous and may be associated with significant developmental delay.
- If there are significant dysmorphic features, look in the appropriate section of this chapter.
- Brain MRI imaging to look for structural genetic brain abnormality, e.g. neuronal migration abnormalities.
- Additional radiological investigations if clinically indicated (cardiac, renal, skeletal).
- Ophthalmological referral for detailed assessment, including fundoscopy, in children with regression, syndromes with eye involvement, and in the presence of visual difficulties and squint.
- Children with undiagnosed neurological disorder: refer to a paediatric neurologist.

KNOWN AR CONDITIONS.

- Metabolic disorders: late-onset milder phenotypes more difficult. In children with progressive intellectual and neurological deterioration (PIND), the commonest diagnostic groups to consider are leukoencephalopathies, NCL, mitochondrial diseases, MPS, gangliosidoses, and peroxisomal disorders.
- Recognizable syndromes with known AR inheritance. Each ethnic group will have particular syndromes and conditions that are more common.

PROBABLE AR CONDITIONS.

- The same phenotype in two affected sibs of different sexes or two female sibs.
- Developmental regression. See 'Developmental regression' in Chapter 2, 'Clinical approach', p. 128.

POSSIBLE AR.
- Similar features to those of a known recessive condition.
- Severe MR with no environmental risk factors.

Genetic advice
Recurrence risk

When a diagnosis remains unknown, counselling is difficult. Consider if the diagnosis falls into the probable or possible AR group and advise accordingly.

When the condition is non-progressive and there are other malformations, remember that chromosome anomalies and dysmorphic syndromes which do not follow AR inheritance can also occur in consanguineous families.

Carrier detection
- This can be performed for some of the metabolic conditions by DNA and enzymatic methods. General population testing, i.e. for the partners of the parents' sibs, may not be possible.
- Mutational or linkage analysis may be possible.
- Pedigree analysis.

Prenatal diagnosis
- Biochemical or molecular testing by CVS or amniocentesis can be offered to those parents in whom a diagnosis has been confirmed. Consult closely with the laboratory to ascertain the type of sample (direct or cultured CVS, amniocytes, etc.) that is required.
- USS for structural anomalies.

Natural history and further management (preventative measures)
Information, education, and the offer of genetic advice to members of the extended family. Dual language information.

Support groups: Climb (Children Living with Inherited Metabolic Diseases), http://www.climb.org.uk; National Organization for Rare Disorders (USA), http://www.rare-disease.org; Syndromes Without A Name (SWAN UK) http://www.undiagnosed.org.uk, (SWAN USA) http://www.swanusa.org.

Expert adviser: Eamonn Sheridan, Professor of Clinical Genetics, University of Leeds, Leeds, UK.

References
Bittles AH, Black ML. Consanguinity, human evolution, and complex diseases. *Proc Natl Acad Sci U S A* 2010; **107**: 1779–86.

Bundey S, Alam H. A five-year prospective study of the health of children in different ethnic groups, with particular reference to the effect of inbreeding. *Eur J Hum Genet* 1993; **1**: 206–19.

Khoury MJ, Cohen BH, Diamond EL, Chase GA, McKusick VA. Inbreeding and prereproductive mortality in the Old Order Amish. I. Genealogic epidemiology of inbreeding. *Am J Epidemiol* 1987; **125**: 453–61.

McRae JF, Clayton S, Fitzgerald TW, et al. (2016, under review). Prevalence, phenotype and architecture of developmental disorders caused by de novo mutation. doi: http://dx.doi.org/10.1101/049056. http://biorxiv.org/content/early/2016/06/16/049056.

Najmabadi H, Hu H, Garshasbi M, et al. Deep sequencing reveals 50 novel genes for recessive cognitive disorders. *Nature* 2011; **478**: 57–63.

Ropers HH. Genetics of early onset cognitive impairment. *Annu Rev Genomics Hum Genet* 2010; **11**: 161–87.

Verity C, Winstone AM, Stellitano L, Will R, Nicoll A. The epidemiology of progressive intellectual and neurological deterioration in childhood. *Arch Dis Childhood* 2010; **95**: 361–4.

Developmental regression

This typically presents with a loss of previously acquired cognitive and/or motor skills. Other signs, such as behavioural changes or the onset of seizures, usually accompany it. In older children, the presentation may be schooling difficulties with emotional lability and immaturity.

These children should be under the care of a paediatric neurologist, who will work closely with a child development team for the assessment of developmental skills. It may take a period of observation to determine the pattern of developmental loss and to diagnose conditions such as autism. Geneticists become involved:

- as many of the neurodegenerative conditions have a genetic aetiology;
- during the period of investigation to help establish the diagnosis;
- with ethical discussions such as whether to offer pre-symptomatic testing to siblings and how much intensive support to give to the child;
- to give genetic advice after the diagnosis has been made.

Clinical approach

History: key points
- Three-generation family tree with specific enquiry about consanguinity and other similarly affected relatives.
- Family history of neurological disease. Consider that conditions usually found in adults can present in the neonatal period or in childhood due to anticipation (maternal DM and HD, respectively).
- Full developmental history. Obtain copies of assessments and school reports.
- Age of onset and mode of presentation.
- Sex of the child. Females: consider Rett syndrome; males: consider XL conditions such as XL adreno-leukodystrophy (X-ALD) and Pelizaeus–Merzbacher disease (PMD).
- Ethnic group, e.g. Tay–Sachs in the Ashkenazi Jewish population, Salla disease in Finns.
- Fluctuation with intercurrent illnesses may indicate an underlying metabolic disturbance such as mitochondrial disorders or MSUD.
- Seizures. Poorly controlled seizures can lead to apparent regression that is reversed on good control. This is a difficult assessment area because the development of seizures may be part of the progressive nature of a neurodegenerative process.
- Loss of vision and hearing, and timing of this in relation to the course of regression.

Examination: key points
- Head circumference and note any change in the rate of growth.
- Deceleration of head growth (Rett, Cockayne syndromes).
- Macrocephaly (Canavan, Alexander disease, other storage diseases, megalencephalic leukoencephalopathy with subcortical cysts (MLC)).
- Hypotonia or hypertonia (spasticity and/or dystonia).
- Ataxia, a useful diagnostic feature.
- Coarsening of facial features. See 'Coarse facial features' in Chapter 2, 'Clinical approach', p. 106.

- Eyes and eye movements: deep-set in Cockayne syndrome, conjunctival telangiectasia in AT. Kayser–Fleischer ring in Wilson's disease. Supranuclear gaze palsy in Niemann–Pick C. Nystagmus in PMD and where vision is lost.
- Optic fundi: optic atrophy, cherry red spots, pigmentary changes (Refsum's disease, GM2-gangliosidosis, mitochondrial disorders).
- Stereotypical hand movements such as wringing (Rett syndrome).
- Skin: increased pigment (Addison's disease in adrenoleukodystrophy (ALD)), chilblain lesions (Aicardi–Goutières syndrome).
- Hepatosplenomegaly (storage disorders).
- Scoliosis (Rett syndrome and FRDA).

Special investigations
The list of investigations will differ, depending on the differential diagnosis. This list is a guide but is not comprehensive.
- Baseline biochemistry: glucose, lactate, urate (Lesch–Nyhan syndrome), CK, copper and caeruloplasmin (Wilson's disease), and urine metabolic screen for MPS disorders and urinary oligosaccharides. Also amino and organic acid screens.
- Vacuolated lymphocytes (storage disorders such as Pompe's disease, juvenile neuronal ceroid lipofuscinosis (JNCL; NCL3)
- AFP and immunoglobulins (AT).
- Adrenal function.
- VLCFAs (peroxisomal disorders).
- White cell enzymes (lysosomal enzyme and storage diseases, infantile and late-infantile NCLs).
- EM studies of tissue (storage disorders; particularly used in the investigation of NCLs).
- MRI brain scan. An expert paediatric neuroradiologist will be needed to interpret, for example, the pattern of white matter disease, to establish a small list of differential diagnoses. Conditions like MLC have a characteristic appearance.
- EEG. Specific patterns may be associated with certain conditions such as NCLs and Rett disease.
- Ophthalmological assessment, including visual evoked responses (VERs).
- Brainstem evoked potentials and other electrophysiological studies.
- DNA analysis and storage. Consider any specific tests such as *MeCP2* for Rett syndrome, *CLNC3* in Batten disease, and mitochondrial DNA analysis. Also, in children with a proven enzyme defect, enquire if mutation analysis would make prenatal testing easier and offer the potential of carrier detection.
- Genomic analysis, e.g. genomic array, gene panel, or WES/WGS as appropriate.
- Consider the need for skin biopsy for conditions such as Cockayne syndrome.
- ECG and cardiac echo: mitochondrial diseases.
- Lumbar puncture (lactate level as a marker for disorders of the respiratory chain; Aicardi–Goutières syndrome has cerebrospinal fluid (CSF) lymphocytosis and high interferon levels).

- Skeletal survey for signs of dysostosis multiplex in many storage disorders or calcific stippling of the epiphyses in peroxisomal disorders.

Some diagnoses to consider

Non-genetic conditions
Non-genetic conditions where *the diagnosis should not be made by a geneticist* include environmental factors such as severe emotional deprivation, psychiatric conditions such as disintegrative psychosis, vascular disorders, tumours, and infections. There may be a genetic predisposition and recurrence risks to consider with many of these.

Autism
This complex condition usually presents with early regression (<3 years) but may develop later as a disintegrative disorder (<10 years) when it can be difficult to differentiate from developmental regression. A standardized multidisciplinary assessment is needed to confirm the diagnosis and some baseline investigations, such as EEG and MRI scan, will probably be needed in these late-presenting cases. There are genetic issues in this condition and these are discussed in 'Autism and autism spectrum disorders' in Chapter 3, 'Common consultations', p. 350.

Metabolic and storage disorders
The group of conditions known as the NCLs have particular diagnostic difficulties and are discussed in more detail.

NEURONAL CEROID LIPOFUSCINOSES (NCLS). Often collectively known as Batten disease, these are lysosomal storage disorders characterized by mental and motor deterioration, seizures, and visual loss. They may initially present to ophthalmologists where the classic retinal changes and abnormal neurophysiology should prompt referral for a diagnostic assessment. This will include EM study of vacuolated lymphocytes and lysosomal enzyme testing of palmitoyl-protein thioesterase (PPT)-1 and tripeptidyl-peptidase (TPP)-1. This screen can then be extended to check the *CLCN* genes.
- Infantile NCL (INCL). Gene *CLCN1*. Movement disorder, dementia, and retinal blindness by 2 years. Mainly seen in Finnish population. The enzyme PPT-1 is encoded by *CLCN1*.
- Late-infantile NCL. Gene *CLCN1* (8%) and *CLCN2* (80%). TPP-1 is encoded by *CLCN2*. Presents at age 2–4 years with epilepsy and regression.
- Juvenile NCL (JNCL; Batten disease). Gene *CLCN1* (21%), *CLCN2* (7%), and *CLCN3* (72%). Presents with visual loss between the ages of 4 and 10 years. Myoclonic seizures and regression. Vacuolated lymphocytes are seen. Common 1-kb deletion in *CLCN3* removes exons 7 and 8, which is offered as a diagnostic service to most clinicians.
- Adult NCL, Kufs disease (*CLN4*). Onset around 30 years.
- Although still classified as untreatable, there are ongoing clinical trials for enzyme replacement and gene therapy in *CLN2*.

SANFILIPPO SYNDROME (MPS III). Sanfilippo A and B syndromes are lysosomal storage disorders caused by the deficiency of heparin sulfaminidase and alpha-N-acetylglucosaminidase, respectively, which are enzymes involved in the degradation of heparan sulfate. Accumulation of the substrate in lysosomes leads to degeneration of the CNS, with progressive dementia often combined with hyperactivity and aggressive behaviour. Age of onset and rate of progression vary considerably, while diagnosis is often delayed due to the absence of pronounced skeletal changes observed in other MPS.

Progressive myoclonic epilepsy (PME)
PME is the triad of: stimulus-sensitive myoclonus; grand mal and absence epilepsy; and progressive neurological deterioration/regression.

Most causes of PME are rare AR conditions; exclude NCLs (e.g. Batten), Unverricht–Lunborg disease (cystatin B), Lafora disease (laforin gene), and sialodosis. Other genetic conditions to consider are MERFF and DRPLA.

Rett syndrome
This occurs almost exclusively in females. The clinical criteria for classical Rett syndrome are:
- normal development to 6 months;
- regression 6 months–2 years;
- deceleration of head growth;
- stereotypical hand movements develop;
- acquisition of severe developmental delay;
- gait ataxia and apraxia.

MECP2 mutations are detected in ~80% of girls with classical Rett syndrome. See 'Rett syndrome' in Chapter 3, 'Common consultations', p. 520.

Macrocephaly
ALEXANDER DISEASE. The most notable features of the infantile form of Alexander disease, which begins during the first 2 years of life, are macrocephaly and sometimes hydrocephaly (either of which may develop later in the course of the disease), psychomotor regression, seizures, and spasticity. See 'Macrocephaly' in Chapter 2, 'Clinical approach', p. 224.

CANAVAN DISEASE. Clinical features of the disease are macrocephaly, head lag, progressive severe MR, and hypotonia in early life, which later changes to spasticity. See 'Macrocephaly' in Chapter 2, 'Clinical approach', p. 224.

Rare AR disorders
Cockayne syndrome. An AR condition with progressive microcephaly, deep-set eyes, retinal pigmentary abnormalities and cataract, sun sensitivity, peripheral neuropathy, and deafness. Confirmed by abnormal DNA repair to UV irradiation of fibroblasts. See 'DNA repair disorders' in Chapter 3, 'Common consultations', p. 398.

NEURONAL DEGENERATION WITH BRAIN IRON ACCUMULATION (NIBA). The two major phenotypes presenting in childhood are (Kurian et al. 2011):
- pantothenate kinase-associated degeneration (PKAN), formally known as Hallervorden–Spatz syndrome. This is caused by mutations in the *PANK2* gene; mutations have been identified in all seven exons of the gene preventing phosphorylation of pantothenate, a rate-limiting step in the production of coenzyme A. Classical PKAN presents before 6 years of age with emerging dystonia, particularly involving oromandibular muscles. Children become non-ambulant in their teens. RP and late cognitive deterioration are common. Brain MRI characteristically show 'eye of the tiger' in the globus pallidus. Part of this spectrum includes hypobetalipoproteinaemia, acanthocytosis, RP, and pallidal degeneration (HARP syndrome) are part of this spectrum;

- phospholipase A2 group 6-associated neurodegeneration (PLAN) comprises a spectrum of disorders secondary to defects in the *PLA2G6* gene. Most commonly it presents in infancy as infantile neuroaxonal dystrophy (INAD), initially with axial hypotonia before peripheral spasticity develops. Visual signs with new-onset squint and evolving optic atrophy are common. Mean age of death is around 9 years. Diagnostic features are of progressive cerebellar hypoplasia on MRI scan with increasing iron accumulation in the globus pallidus. Neurophysiology shows fast activity on EEG and sensorimotor neuronopathy on EMG studies. Skin biopsy shows axonal swelling and spheroid body.

Mitochondrial disorders
These may follow a mitochondrial, sporadic, or AR pattern of inheritance. See 'Mitochondrial DNA diseases' in Chapter 3, 'Common consultations', p. 490.

XL disorders
ADRENOLEUKODYSTROPHY (ALD). XLR inheritance. Known to show variability within families of the age of onset, ranging from childhood to adult males. Although the diagnosis can be made on the basis of biochemical testing, this is not reliable for carrier testing. See 'X-linked adrenoleukodystrophy (X-ALD)' in Chapter 3, 'Common consultations', p. 538. BMT is offered to boys with early cerebral disease.

Genetic advice

Recurrence risk
- For those families in whom a definitive diagnosis has not been made after thorough investigation, there is a high recurrence risk and AR inheritance is the most likely mode of inheritance.
- XL conditions should be considered if there have been two or more affected boys and/or there is a family history compatible with X-linkage.
- Mitochondrial conditions pose difficult counselling problems. See 'Mitochondrial DNA diseases' in Chapter 3, 'Common consultations', p. 490.
- Store DNA and/or fibroblast cell line for future diagnostic use.

Carrier detection
This is possible in those families in whom a causative mutation has been identified. It may be possible for some biochemical abnormalities.

Prenatal diagnosis
This is available to those families in whom there is molecular or biochemical confirmation of diagnosis.

Pre-symptomatic testing of other siblings
Parents may wish to have apparently unaffected siblings tested for the condition that has been diagnosed in a child. Expert psychological help is needed to explain the pros and cons of such testing and the issue of consent. Please refer to guidelines on genetic testing of children. If there is a therapeutic intervention, then the issues are somewhat clearer.

Natural history and further management (preventative measures)
Unfortunately, there is usually progression of these conditions with early death. Symptomatic treatment of epilepsy and tone and maintenance of adequate nutrition are offered, often with the input of symptom care teams. Hospice care and family support are very important.

Support groups: Climb (Children Living with Inherited Metabolic Diseases), http://www.climb.org.uk, Tel. 0870 770 0326; National Organization for Rare Disorders (NORD), http://www.rarediseases.org.

Expert adviser: Lucinda Carr, Consultant Paediatric Neurologist, Departments of Neurology and Neurodisability, Great Ormond Street Hospital for Children, London, UK.

References
Aicardi J. *Diseases of the nervous system in childhood*, 3rd edn. Wiley, 2009.

Valle D, Beaudet AL, Vogelstein B, *et al.* (eds.). *The online metabolic and molecular bases of inherited diseases.* http://ommbid.mhmedical.com/book.aspx?bookID=971.

Kurian MA, McNeill A, Lin JP, Maher ER. Childhood disorders of neurodegeneration with brain iron accumulation (NBIA). *Dev Med Child Neurol* 2011; **53**: 394–404.

Mole SE, Williams RE. Neuronal ceroid-lipofuscinoses. In: RA Pagon, MP Adam, HH Ardinger, *et al.* (eds.). *GeneReviews®* [Internet]. University of Washington, Seattle, 2001 (updated 2013). http://www.ncbi.nlm.nih.gov/books/NBK1428.

Surtees R. Understanding neurodegenerative disorders. *Curr Paediatr* 2002; **12**: 191–8.

Duane retraction syndrome

This is also known as the Duane anomaly.

Strabismus is a misalignment of the visual axes. It is found in 4–5% of children and a much higher frequency is seen in children with neurodevelopmental delay. Duane anomaly accounts for 1% of strabismus. There is aberrant innervation of the horizontal external ocular muscles.

- Duane 1. Marked or complete limitation of abduction, with minimal or no limitation of adduction.
- Duane 2. Marked or complete limitation of adduction, with minimal or no limitation of abduction.
- Duane 3. Marked or complete limitation of adduction *and* abduction.

In addition, there is retraction of the globe and narrowing of the palpebral fissure on adduction on the affected side(s). The condition is bilateral in 20%.

Clinical approach

History: key points
- Family history, particularly for evidence of AD inheritance.
- Developmental delay (chromosome abnormalities).
- Other CNS features, e.g. seizures.
- Hearing loss (Wildervanck syndrome, Okihiro syndrome).
- May be associated with other miswiring symptoms, e.g. crocodile tears.

Examination: key points
- Exclude congenital cranial nerve palsies (Moebius syndrome).
- Ear tags and malformation of the external ear.
- Short neck (Klippel–Feil anomaly, Wildervanck syndrome).
- Thumb: structural abnormalities and hypoplasia; radial ray deficiencies (Okihiro syndrome).
- Heart: structural malformations are occasional features of Okihiro syndrome and some the overlap syndromes; some patients with an initial clinical diagnosis of HOS have been later identified as Okihiro-related.

Special investigations
- X-ray of the cervical spine for fusion abnormalities in children with a short neck (Klippel–Feil anomaly).
- Abdominal USS (renal abnormalities in del (8)(q13), invdup(22)(q11), Wildervanck syndrome, and Klippel–Feil anomaly).
- Echo.
- Hearing test.
- Consider imaging of the inner ear in the presence of a hearing loss.
- Genomic analysis in presence of features suggestive of a chromosomal or syndromic diagnosis, e.g. genomic array, gene panel, or WES/WGS as available.

Some diagnoses to consider

Klippel–Feil anomaly
Klippel–Feil anomaly of the cervical spine (fusion of one or more cervical vertebrae).

Wildervanck syndrome
Wildervanck syndrome is the triad of Duane retraction syndrome, Klippel–Feil anomaly, and sensorineural deafness. More females are affected than males. The inheritance pattern is unclear. Most cases are sporadic, but there are reports of other affected family members having one or more components of the condition.

Okihiro syndrome (Duane radial ray syndrome)
An AD condition with degrees of radial ray hypoplasia and Duane anomaly. It results from mutation in the *SALL4* gene.

Chromosomal anomalies
Duane has been associated with a number of cytogenetic anomalies. In particular, consider CES due to an inv dup (22)(q11) and a contiguous gene deletion syndrome at 8q13 that results in type 1 Duane anomaly and BOR syndrome.

Moebius syndrome
The congenital cranial nerve palsies of Moebius syndrome may be confused with Duane retraction syndrome.

Other
- Absence of external ocular muscles may occur in craniosynostosis syndromes.
- The squint caused by thalidomide embryopathy is similar to Duane anomaly.

Genetic advice

Recurrence risk
Most cases are sporadic. Approximately 10% of isolated Duane anomaly is familial with AD inheritance. Type 1 is linked to 8q13 and type 2 to 2q31.

Carrier detection
This may be available when Duane anomaly is part of a syndrome with a known mutation or cytogenetic abnormality.

Prenatal diagnosis
This may be available when Duane anomaly is part of a syndrome with a known mutation or cytogenetic abnormality.

Natural history and further management (preventative measures)

Amblyopia is a common complication.

Support group: Many of the individual syndromes have their own support groups. See Contact a Family, http://www.cafamily.org.uk.

Expert adviser: Willie Reardon, Consultant Clinical Medical Geneticist, Department of Clinical Genetics, Our Lady's Children's Hospital, Dublin, Ireland.

References

Al Baradie R, Yamada K, St Hilaire C, *et al.* Duane radial ray syndrome (Okihiro syndrome) maps to 20q13 and results from mutation in *SALL4* a new member of the *SAL* family. *Am J Hum Genet* 2002; **71**: 1195–9.

Chung M, Stout JT, Borchert MS. Clinical diversity of hereditary Duane's retraction syndrome. *Ophthalmology* 2000; **107**: 500–3.

Kohlhase J, Heinrich M, Schubert L, *et al.* Okihiro syndrome is caused by *SALL4* mutations. *Hum Mol Genet* 2002; **11**: 2979–87.

Dysmorphic child

This section describes the clinical approach to the infant/child/adult with dysmorphic features of unknown cause, so that the useful and significant diagnostic signs can be documented. Other sections in this chapter and diagnostic databases will be of help when the dysmorphic features have been carefully assessed.

The term 'dysmorphic' is used to describe children whose physical features, particularly facial, are not usually found in a child of the same age or ethnic background. Some features are abnormal in all circumstances, e.g. premature fusion of the cranial sutures. These are called good diagnostic 'handles', as they are not found as normal or familial traits or variations and are only present in a small number of conditions. In contrast, a feature such as 2/3 toe syndactyly may be a useful diagnostic tool or be a non-significant familial trait. The recognition of which features are good diagnostic aids comes with experience.

Clinical approach

The key points of the history are of equal importance to the physical examination in establishing the diagnosis.

History: key points

- Three-generation family tree. Enquire specifically for consanguinity and other members of the family with similar problems.
- Pregnancy history. Bleeding, fever, medication, investigations, alcohol/non-prescription drugs (ask with tact), fetal movements, liquor volume, gestation, mode of delivery.
- Neonatal history. Birthweight, length, head circumference. Resuscitation, feeding difficulties, ventilation, malformations, surgery, seizures, other medical problems.
- Developmental milestones and current schooling provision (e.g. mainstream school with 1:1 LSA, special needs nursery). If developmentally delayed, ask about agencies involved, e.g. physical therapist.
- Any specific difficulties with vision or hearing.
- Past medical and surgical history (previous hospital admissions) and current medication.
- Behavioural phenotype. Ask about unusual patterns of behaviour.

Examination: key points

- Observation. Look carefully at the child. Some conditions are immediately recognizable, e.g. Down's syndrome. Watch the child during the consultation. Try to involve him/her in the history and take note of spontaneous language and interaction between the child and adults, as well as looking at the face.
- Growth parameters. Height, weight, and OFC. In general, the further measurements deviate from the normal centile ranges, the greater the chance of making a genetic diagnosis. Plot measurements on a centile chart. For measurements outside the normal ranges, estimate by how many standard deviations (SDs). The statement 'the OFC is <0.4th centile at −5.5 SD' conveys far more information than simply noting that 'the OFC is <0.4th centile'.
- Use an examination checklist to ensure that all the systems have been adequately examined and the findings

documented. See 'Dysmorphology examination checklist' in 'Appendix', p. 829.
- Enquire specifically about 'birthmarks' and examine for skin pigmentary abnormalities (chromosomal mosaicism).
- Assess the need for more extensive investigation of systems, e.g. the skeletal system in an individual with short or tall stature.
- Review any photographs of the child that are in the notes or supplied by the family.

Special investigations

- Genomic analysis in presence of features suggestive of a chromosomal or syndromic diagnosis, e.g. genomic array, gene panel, or WES/WGS as appropriate.
- Molecular genetic analysis. FRAXA in children with developmental delay.
- Other specific testing, as indicated. Databases can be used to identify laboratories offering specific gene tests such as http://ukgtn.nhs.uk and http://www.orpha.net.
- Clinical photography. Document any significant features and use the photos to observe the evolution of the features with age (natural history). Photographs of the child with both parents can be useful in determining which of the distinctive features are potentially significant and which may just be family characteristics. Consider making a video record of movement. Many syndromes, particularly microdeletion disorders, have unusual expression of facial movement (trisomy 18 and trisomy 21 have been shown to have abnormal facial muscle attachments).
- Metabolic testing. Curry *et al.* (1997) found an extremely low pickup of abnormalities when metabolic screening was performed without specific signs of a metabolic disorder. However, many children with a dysmorphic appearance and developmental delay are offered testing for thyroid function and urine amino and organic acid abnormalities. If a child is microcephalic with no normal sibs, test the mother for PKU and organic acid abnormalities.
- Brain imaging. This is not routinely performed in children with a normal head circumference and no abnormal neurological signs, but the number having such scans is increasing since MRI is better than CT at detecting more subtle features that can be of diagnostic significance. Neuroimaging should be considered in patients without a known diagnosis, especially in the presence of neurological symptoms, cranial contour abnormalities, microcephaly, or macrocephaly (Curry *et al.* 1997). In most situations, MRI is the testing modality of choice.
- Further investigations to help establish a diagnosis and to evaluate the significance of a physical feature, e.g. echo if a heart murmur is noted.
- Skin biopsy. Consider a skin biopsy for karyotype if the following features are present:
  - streaky skin pigmentation, especially if following lines of Blaschko (hypomelanosis of Ito);
  - asymmetry;
  - 3/4 finger syndactyly with 2/3 finger syndactyly and bulbous fingertips (diploid/triploid mosaicism).

Making a diagnosis

It is useful in these situations to have a diagnostic framework.

(1) Ask some basic questions.
  - Are you dealing with a single malformation or multiple malformations?
  - Is the child likely to have a multiple anomaly syndrome?
  - Are there deformations that might tie in with the pregnancy history?
  - Does the family history help?

(2) Think about the various mechanisms by which birth defects come about.
  - Chromosomal anomalies.
  - Single gene defects (consider different types of genes, e.g. those encoding structural proteins, transcription factors, etc.). Also consider disturbances in gene expression, e.g. imprinted genes.
  - Effects of multiple gene mutations/polymorphisms, e.g. Hirschsprung's disease.
  - Multifactorial disorder (a combination of genetic predisposition and environmental factors, e.g. NTDs).
  - Mainly environmental, e.g. mechanical compression and teratogens (although, in the latter, genetic predisposition may play a part, e.g. in drug metabolism).
  - Mosaicism: chromosomal, single gene mutation, or in gene expression.

(3) Think whether you have seen this before.
  - Personal experience is helpful and people get better and more experienced at dysmorphology over time. You may be able to recognize a 'gestalt' that is familiar to you from a previous consultation or from the literature.

(4) Seek help from the literature.
  - See 'Useful resources' in Chapter 1, 'Introduction', p. 44.

(5) Search online resources. See 'Useful resources' in Chapter 1, 'Introduction', p. 44.
  - Databases are most useful if you search on distinctive features ('hard' diagnostic handles), e.g. midline cleft lip, rather than common or subjective features such as 'low-set ears'. With experience, it becomes easier to 'sift out' syndromes that are least likely matches with your patient.

(6) Seek help from colleagues.
  - Share information and photographs/images with other colleagues in your department and with specialists in the field.

Approximately 5% of children with a difficult-to-diagnose developmental disorder will have a composite phenotype caused by the co-occurrence of two distinct genetic disorders (Deciphering Developmental Disorders Study 2015).

Genetic advice for a known diagnosis

If you are able to make a specific diagnosis, take steps to confirm it, where possible, by suitable laboratory tests. Genetic advice about recurrence risk or offspring risk is usually relatively straightforward in this situation.

Genetic advice for an unknown diagnosis

The clinical geneticist may need to give advice in the absence of a specific diagnosis. Studies have shown that follow-up of children may lead to a diagnosis, as genetic and biochemical testing improves and syndrome delineation is clearer. The practice of sharing knowledge within a genetics department by the use of clinical photography sessions ensures that expertise and experience of rare syndromes are shared for the benefit of the patients and the training of junior staff.

When a diagnosis remains unknown, it is important to spend time in the counselling session explaining the reasons for this and the fact that genetic advice is derived from the probability that the child's problems have a genetic cause.

Recurrence risk

Certain features, or patterns of features, suggest a high recurrence risk of up to 25%. These include (but this is *not* a complete list):
- previous affected child;
- previous stillbirth/late miscarriages due to fetal abnormalities;
- family history of a similarly affected individual (XL, chromosomal, variable dominant condition);
- consanguinity;
- neurodevelopmental regression;
- coarsening of facial features;
- symmetrical structural defects previously noted in AR conditions;
- maternal influences, such as immunological conditions like myasthenia where the antibodies cross the placenta, have a very high risk in a subsequent pregnancies.

In the absence of features suggesting a high risk (see above), an *empiric risk* of ~5% may be advised. Explain that this is a composite risk—for the majority of families the risks are very low, but for some they will be high (25%). Also emphasize that this risk figure could change substantially if a specific diagnosis is subsequently made.

Carrier detection

Individuals at high risk may be determined from the pedigree, e.g. where there is evidence of XL inheritance.

Prenatal diagnosis

In the absence of a specific diagnosis it is not usually possible to offer PND, unless there are congenital malformations, e.g. CHD, polydactyly. If malformations are present (and these are thought to be part of the child's condition, rather than coincidental), it may be possible to look for structural abnormalities in the fetus by USS in the second trimester. Consult a fetal medicine specialist if there is any doubt over the timing of scanning or the ease with which the specific structural anomalies in question can be visualized. Explain the limitations of this approach.

Natural history and further management

Observation of the natural history is an extremely important part of the management of a child with an undiagnosed dysmorphic syndrome. Follow up the first consultation with another to establish that the investigations are complete and that all of this information has been exchanged.

Subsequent follow-up at 1 year is suggested and thereafter by discussion with the family, depending on such issues as their plans to have more children.

Surveillance and follow-up

Review appointments can help in the following ways:
- to offer newly available diagnostic tests;

- to establish that there are no additional medical problems and that there is forward developmental progress;
- to increase the chance of syndrome recognition. Some dysmorphic syndromes are not easy to diagnose until a few years of age;
- to discuss recurrence risks.

Support group: Contact a Family, http://www.cafamily.org.uk (puts families in touch with others with similar features).

References

Aase JM. *Diagnostic dysmorphology*. Plenum, New York, 1990.

Bi W, Borgan C, Pursley AN, *et al.* Comparison of chromosome analysis and chromosomal microarray analysis: what is the value of chromosome analysis in today's genomic array era? *Genet Med* 2013; **15**: 450–7.

Biesecker LG. The end of the beginning of chromosome ends. *Am J Med Genet* 2002; **107**: 263–6.

Bundey S, Carter C. Recurrence risks in severe undiagnosed mental deficiency. *J Ment Defic Res* 1974; **18**: 115–34.

Curry CJ, Stevenson RE, Aughton D, *et al.* Evaluation of mental retardation: recommendations of a Consensus Conference: American College of Medical Genetics. *Am J Med Genet* 1997; **72**: 468–77.

Deciphering Developmental Disorders Study. Large-scale discovery of novel genetic causes of developmental disorders. *Nature* 2015; **519**: 223–8.

Jones KL, Jones MC, Del Campo M (eds.). *Smith's recognizable patterns of human malformation*, 7th edn. WB Saunders, Philadelphia, 2013.

Knight SJ, Flint J. Screening chromosome ends for learning disability. *BMJ* 2000; **321**: 1240.

Knight SJ, Regan R, Nicod A, *et al.* Subtle chromosomal rearrangements in children with unexplained mental retardation. *Lancet* 1999; **354**: 1676–81.

Kotzot D. Review and meta-analysis of systematic searches for uniparental disomy (UPD). *Am J Med Genet* 2002; **111**: 366–75.

Ness GO, Lybaek H, Houge G. Usefulness of high-resolution comparative genomic hybridization (CGH) for detecting and characterizing constitutional chromosome abnormalities. *Am J Med Genet* 2002; **113**: 125–36.

POSSUMweb (Pictures Of Standard Syndromes and Undiagnosed Malformations). http://www.possum.net.au/

Rosenthal ET, Biesecker LG, Biesecker BB. Parental attitudes toward a diagnosis in children with unidentified multiple congenital anomaly syndromes. *Am J Med Genet* 2001; **103**: 106–14.

Turner G, Partington M. Recurrence risks in undiagnosed mental retardation. *J Med Genet* 2000; **37**: E45.

Winter RM, Baraitser M. *London dysmorphology database*. London Medical Databases v1.0.17s, 2009. http://www.lmdatabases.com.

Dystonia

Dystonia is defined as a movement disorder characterized by sustained or intermittent muscle contractions causing abnormal, often repetitive, movements, postures, or both. Dystonic movements are typically patterned and twisting and may be tremulous. Dystonia is often initiated or worsened by voluntary action and is associated with overflow muscle activation (Albanese *et al.* 2013).

Prevalence figures have varied between 127 and 329 per million, but it is probably more common than this. Focal dystonia that affects a single body part is the most common type, but dystonia may also be a component of some complex multisystem neurodevelopmental disorders.

Clinically, the dystonias are usually classified by:

(1) age of onset (early onset versus adult onset);
(2) distribution of affected body parts (focal, multifocal, segmental, or generalized);
(3) the underlying cause (primary, secondary, or heredodegenerative);
(4) special clinical features (paroxysmal, exercise-induced, task-specific, or dopa-responsive).

In the paediatric genetics clinic, dystonia is most frequently seen in the context of a complex neurodevelopmental disorder. It may present as unusual posturing, difficulties with swallowing, or variable tone/rigidity on a background of profound delay, hypotonia, and seizures. See Box 2.3 for features suggestive of a non-primary dystonia.

Clinical approach

The investigation of the child/adult with dystonia is primarily by a paediatric neurologist/neurologist and the clinical approach of this section is primarily to detect genetic forms of dystonia.

History: key points

- Three-generation family tree; consider AD, AR, XL, and mitochondrial forms of inheritance.
- Ethnic origin. AD, early-onset torsion dystonia is 5–10 times more common in Ashkenazi Jews. XL dystonia–parkinsonism in Filipinos.
- Age of onset.
- Site of onset and progression, both in severity and to other parts of the body. Presentation with dystonia involving the legs is more likely to progress.

- Reaction to alcohol (alcohol can improve the symptoms and signs in myoclonic dystonia).
- Constant or paroxysmal?
- Other neurological features (epilepsy, MR, regression or loss of acquired skills).
- Exposure to neuroleptic medication.

Examination: key points

- Abnormal posturing; distribution of dystonia—is it predominantly focal or generalized?
- Myoclonus.
- Parkinsonism (tremor, rigidity).
- Choreoathetosis (some heredodegenerative dystonias).
- Brisk or reduced reflexes, extensor plantars?
- Eyes. Eye movement disorder and nystagmus. Kayser–Fleischer rings (Wilson's disease).
- Fundal examination. Pigmentary retinopathy (Hallervorden–Spatz syndrome (HSS), mitochondrial disorders), optic atrophy (HSS, XL deafness–dystonia–optic atrophy syndrome, mitochondrial disorders).
- Muscle or cardiac involvement?
- Dementia.
- Hearing.
- Ataxia (patients with FRDA may have dystonia).

Special investigations

- Brain imaging, preferably MRI scan. Basal ganglia calcification (Fahr disease, Aicardi–Goutières disease, mitochondrial disorders), 'eye of the tiger' sign in HSS.
- EEG.
- ERG (retinal dysfunction).
- Electrophysiology (myoclonus).
- Genomic array in children (*FOXG1* deletion).
- Consider panel/WES/WGS as appropriate. In patients with an age of onset <26 years with any site of involvement, test for *DYT1* mutation and sequencing of *KMT2B*. DRD *GCH1* and *TH* (see below). Store with consent for future testing when there is no genetic testing available.
- Response to L-dopa—if positive, consider specialist neurometabolic tests, e.g. CSF metabolites of dopamine degradation pathway (tyrosine hydroxylase deficiency (THD)).

Box 2.3 Features suggestive of non-primary dystonia

- Abnormal birth or perinatal history
- Dysmorphic features
- Delayed developmental milestones
- Seizures. Dystonia is a component of several of the severe early-onset epilepsy syndromes
- Hemidystonia
- Sudden onset or rapidly progressive dystonia
- Prominent oro-bulbar dystonia
- The presence of another movement disorder (except tremor)
- Neurological signs suggesting involvement of other neurological systems (pyramidal signs, cerebellar signs, neuropathy, cognitive decline)
- Signs suggesting disease outside of the nervous system (hepatomegaly, splenomegaly)

Second-line testing/consider:

- metabolic investigations (amino acids in plasma and urine, urine organic acids (L-2-hydroxyglutaric aciduria, glutaric aciduria)), white cell enzymes (GM2, Niemann–Pick type C, Krabbe's), lipoproteins (hypobetalipoproteinaemia and abetalipoproteinaemia), NCL, CSF pyruvate/lactate, and investigate further with CSF neurotransmitters if necessary. See 'Developmental regression' in Chapter 2, 'Clinical approach', p. 128 for further details on the investigation of metabolic disorders.
- TSH, T4, and freeT3 (Allan–Herndon–Dudley syndrome).
- Acanthocytes (neuroacanthocytosis).
- Copper studies to exclude Wilson's disease.
- Manganese, CK.
- Consider AT. See 'DNA repair disorders' in Chapter 3, 'Common consultations', p. 398.
- Consider HD, SCA, DRPLA, and GSD, especially if there is a dominant family history or if other neurological features develop.

Some diagnoses to consider

The primary dystonias

AUTOSOMAL DOMINANT EARLY-ONSET TORSION DYSTONIA (IDIOPATHIC TORSION DYSTONIA, DYSTONIA 1). A predominantly generalized dystonia, it typically presents in children and young adults. The arms or legs are often the primary focus of dystonia and it then spreads to affect other areas. It is an extremely variable condition and some obligate carriers have minimal symptoms. Individuals with *DYT1* mutation obtain symptom relief with deep brain stimulation.

The gene locus is *DYT1*. The GAG deletion mutation, which leads to a loss of glutamic acid, accounts for all known mutations and is usually referred to as the '*DYT1* mutation'. Penetrance is 30–40%.

Empirical recurrence risks were calculated prior to the availability of *DYT1* testing. The sib recurrence risk given in familial cases was 21% and for an isolated case 14%. Observed risks are slightly lower. There is no figure for the risk of a severely affected child.

ADULT-ONSET IDIOPATHIC TORSION DYSTONIA. A predominantly focal or segmental dystonia. The main differentiating features from early-onset idiopathic torsion dystonia are:

- later presentation, typically mid-adult life;
- symptoms do not usually spread to become generalized.

The genetic contribution to this condition is uncertain, but there has been an estimate that 25% of affected individuals have a significant family history.

Genetic testing is not possible, unless there is a family history of early onset, in which case arrange for *DYT1* analysis.

'Dystonia-plus'

MYOCLONIC DYSTONIA. This group includes patients with variable degrees of dystonia and myoclonus. An important feature in the history is that there may be a dramatic improvement in symptoms with alcohol.

Inheritance is AD with reduced penetrance. There is >1 locus and one gene has been characterized (epsilon-sarcoglycan).

Childhood genetic dystonia syndromes

Investigate for metabolic and mitochondrial disorders. In addition, the following have recognizable phenotypes and should be considered.

DOPA-RESPONSIVE DYSTONIA (DRD, DYT5) (SEGAWA SYNDROME). This is a rare condition (prevalence of 0.5–1.0 per million), but important to recognize as it is treatable. Onset is usually in childhood/adolescence and dystonia is the presenting feature. Parkinsonism may also occur. Reflexes may become brisk with extensor plantars. There is a 4F:1M ratio. Diurnal fluctuation is a prominent feature.

The phenotype in childhood may resemble athetoid cerebral palsy and all children with this condition should have a trial of L-dopa.

Inheritance is usually AD with reduced penetrance. The gene *GCH1* codes for an enzyme in the tetrahydrobiopterin pathway.

KMT2B-ASSOCIATED COMPLEX EARLY ONSET DYSTONIA. Heterozygous variants in and deletions encompassing KMT2B cause a complex progressive childhood onset dystonia often with distinctive cranial MRI findings. This condition is predicted to be a common cause of childhood dystonia. Cervical, cranial, and laryngeal dystonia are typical. Deep brain stimulation (DBS) may be beneficial (Meyer 2016).

OTHER DOPA-RESPONSIVE DYSTONIAS. An AR form of DRD with or without hyperphenylalaninaemia is caused by mutation in the same gene *GCH1*.

Another AR type (THD) is due to mutation in the tyrosine hydroxylase gene. The severe type of THD is associated with early encephalopathy. Diagnosis is by CSF metabolites of the dopamine degradation pathway and *TH* mutation analysis.

Metabolic/storage disorders presenting with dystonia as a prominent feature

KRABBE'S DISEASE. Or globoid cell leukodystrophy, is an AR disorder involving the white matter of the peripheral and central nervous systems. Mutations in the gene for the lysosomal enzyme galactocerebrosidase (*GALC*) result in low enzymatic activity and decreased ability to degrade galactolipids found almost exclusively in myelin. While most patients present with symptoms within the first 6 months of life, others present later in life, including adulthood. Infantile Krabbe's disease can present with dystonia (lead-pipe rigidity of the limbs and abnormal posturing), together with irritability, poor feeding, motor regression, and seizures. MRI may show white matter changes and calcification, particularly affecting the basal ganglia.

NEURONAL BRAIN IRON ACCUMULATION SYNDROMES. E.g. pantothenate kinase-associated neurodegeneration syndrome (HSS): *PANK2* AR. Characteristic MRI features. Refer to specialist centre for deep brain stimulation.

XL DEAFNESS–OPTIC ATROPHY SYNDROME. (Mohr–Tranebjaerg syndrome.) *DDP* gene.

NEUROACANTHOCYTOSIS. Distinguish between McLeod syndrome (XLR) and choreoacanthocytosis (AR).

Dystonia with epilepsy/dyskinesia
See Table 2.9.

Paroxysmal dystonia/dyskinesia
Intermittent episodes of dystonia or dyskinesia, usually with no neurological features in between attacks. As for episodic ataxia and some forms of epilepsy, mutations in ion channel genes may be the underlying cause.

Table 2.9 Genetic epilepsy/dystonia syndromes

Condition	Gene	Key features	Age of onset
GLUT1	*SLC2A*—heterozygous mutation (rarely compound heterozygous and homozygous)	Variable presentation with intermittent movement disorder and epilepsy often with nystagmus. Symptoms may be aggravated by fatigue and fasting	Infancy and early childhood
		Low CSF glucose and low CSF lactate are essentially diagnostic for this disorder. Paired CSF and plasma glucose are also helpful in diagnosis	
		Transport defect of glucose across the blood–brain barrier	
		Responds to ketogenic diet	
ARX	*ARX*	Variable phenotypes:	Infancy
		(1) Infantile spasms, hypsarrythymia, normal brain MRI, expansion of poly-A tract in ARX	Childhood
		(2) Partington syndrome ID with focal dystonia and dysarthria, smaller poly-A expansion in ARX	
Allan–Herndon–Dudley	*SLC16A2*	XLR disorder presenting in male infants with profound hypotonia and progresses with severe feeding problems, evolving to dystonic posturing. Measure free T3; also T4 and TSH	Infancy
Congenital Rett syndrome	*FOXG1*	Severe developmental delay, hypotonia with or without seizures (onset after 3 months). Dystonic/choreiform movements from second year. Hypoplasia of corpus callosum. NB. Autosomal locus, affects males and females. *De novo* due to deletion/sequence variant in *FOXG1*	Infancy

Genetic advice

If the exact diagnosis is unknown, aim to place into one of the above groups.

- Most of the primary dystonias and 'dystonia-plus' syndromes show AD inheritance, often with reduced penetrance and clinical variability.
- Heredodegenerative conditions may have AD, AR, XL, or mitochondrial inheritance.
- Referral to specialist centre to consider deep brain stimulation therapy in individuals with DYT1, KMT2B, GNAO1 and secondary conditions such as PANK2.

Recurrence risk

As for the underlying diagnosis.

Carrier detection

Pedigree analysis or using a specific biochemical or genetic test.

Prenatal diagnosis

Not possible unless a specific biochemical or genetic cause has been identified.

Natural history and further management (preventative measures)

- Specific treatment for DRD and Wilson's disease.
- Medication may help the symptoms.
- Injection of the affected muscles with botulinum toxin.
- Peripheral or central stereotatic surgery.

Support group: The Dystonia Society, http://www.dystonia.org.uk/.

Expert adviser: Manju Kurian, Principal Research Associate, UCL Great Ormond Street Institute of Child Health, London, UK.

References

Albanese A, Bhatia K, Bressman SB, *et al*. Phenomenology and classification of dystonia: a consensus update. *Mov Disord* 2013; **28**: 863–73.

Bressman SB, Sabatti C, Raymond D, *et al*. The DYT1 phenotype and guidelines for diagnostic testing. *Neurology* 2000; **54**: 1746–52.

Fahn S, Marsd CD, Calne DB. Classification and investigation of dystonia. In: CD Marsden, S Fahn (eds.). *Movement disorders*, 2nd edn, pp. 332–58. Butterworths, London, 1987.

Fletcher NA. The genetics of idiopathic torsion dystonia. *J Med Genet* 1990; **27**: 409–12.

Kurian MA, Dale RC. Movement disorders presenting in childhood. *CONTINUUM: Lifelong Learning in Neurology* 2016; **22**: 1159–85.

Meyer E, Carss KJ, *et al*. Mutations in the histone methyltransferase gene KMT2B cause complex early-onset dystonia. *Nat Genet* 2016 Dec 19. doi: 10.1038/ng.3740. [Epub ahead of print].

Meyer E, Carss KJ, Rankin J, et al. Mutations in the histone methyltransferase gene KMT2B cause complex early-onset dystonia. *Nature Genet* 2017; **49**: 223–37.

Németh AH. The genetics of primary dystonia and related disorders. *Brain* 2002; **125**: 695–721.

Wenger DA, Rafi MA, Luzi P, Datto J, Costantino-Ceccarini E. Krabbe disease: genetic aspects and progress toward therapy. *Mol Genet Metab* 2000; **70**: 1–9.

Willemsen MA, Verbeek MM, Kamsteeg EJ, *et al*. Tyrosine hydroxylase deficiency: a treatable disorder of brain catecholamine biosynthesis. *Brain* 2010; **133**(Pt 6): 1810–22.

Ear anomalies

The external auricle (pinna) develops from the six auricular hillocks that arise as mesenchymal derivatives of the first and second branchial arches. The external ears begin to develop around the first branchial groove and ascend up to the level of the eyes during embryonic and early fetal life.

Accurate description of ear anomalies (see Table 2.10 for terminology used) is not always straightforward—photography provides the best documentation (see Figure 2.11). The ear of newborns, especially in premature babies, is sometimes rather 'crumpled' and the helix may appear deficient. If there is a major anomaly, this is usually obvious, but otherwise it may be best to review when the infant is a few weeks older.

This section describes the approach to the diagnosis in children where the ear anomalies are a major diagnostic feature. There are many syndromes where the abnormality of the ear is a component of the condition, e.g. low-set and posteriorly rotated ears in NS and ear creases in Beckwith syndrome, but is not the presenting or main diagnostic feature, nor is it always present.

Clinical approach

History: key points

- Three-generation family tree, including specific enquiry regarding ear anomalies, deafness, renal problems, and unusual facial appearance.
- History of maternal diabetes, early bleeding, teratogenic agents, e.g. retinoic acid, alcohol.
- Delayed motor milestones or developmental delay.
- Visual or hearing problems.

Examination: key points

- Carefully describe the ear morphology, and photograph if appropriate.
- Look carefully for ear pits. Take the hearing aids out as the tubes are perfectly positioned to obscure preauricular ear pits, if present.
- Carefully assess the external auditory meatus. Is it normal in diameter or atretic?
- Examine the eyes for lower lid colobomata (TCS) or epibulbar dermoid (OAV syndrome), upper lid colobomata (OAV), iris and retinal colobomata (CHARGE association).
- Assess the face for malar hypoplasia (TCS, Nager, and Miller syndromes).
- Examine the neck for branchial sinuses/cysts or pigmented branchial patches or spots (BOR syndrome).
- Measure the OFC (mandibulofacial dysostosis with microcephaly (MFDM)).
- Examine the heart (CHARGE).
- Examine the limbs: thumb duplications and deficiency (OAV syndrome), triphalangeal or hypoplastic thumbs (TBS), radial ray anomalies (Nager syndrome), ulnar ray anomalies (Miller syndrome).

Special investigations

- Genomic analysis in presence of features suggestive of a chromosomal or syndromic diagnosis, e.g. genomic array, gene panel, or WES/WGS as appropriate/available.
- Store blood for DNA if a diagnosis of TCS, TBS, CHARGE, or BOR is possible.

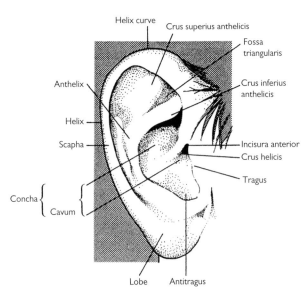

Figure 2.11 Landmarks of the external ear.
Reproduced with permission from Judith G. Hall JG, Froster-Iskenius UG, and Allanson JE, *Handbook of Normal Physical Measurements*, Figure 7.52, page 161, Copyright © 1989 Oxford University Press, New York, USA. www.oup.com.

Table 2.10 Terminology

Anomaly	Description
Simple ear	Lack of interior detail such as anthelix and crus inferius anthelicus, rather than showing the sculpting and moulding usually seen. The pinna is largely flat and the helix may be partly deficient
Dysplastic ear	Loosely used to describe any form of ear malformation
Microtia	Vestiges of the external ear are present, but it is very small. Complete absence of the external ear (anotia) is very rare
Ear tags	These result from the development of accessory auricular hillocks. Usually fleshy but may contain cartilage and may be sessile or pedunculated. In OAV, they occur in the line between the tragus and angle of the mouth (line of junction of the mandibular and maxillary processes)
'Cupped ear'	Caused by deficiency of the posterior auricular muscle
'Lop ear'	Caused by deficiency of the superior auricular muscle
'Ear pits'	Blind-ending pits typically found in the preauricular region
'Ear creases'	Usually found on the earlobe and on the back of the ear, particularly along the rim
'Low-set ear'	The upper attachment of the ear is below a line connecting the outer canthus of the eye and the occiput
'Posteriorly rotated ear'	The longitudinal axis of the ear is rotated towards the occiput

- Audiogram. Is hearing loss purely conductive or is there a sensorineural component? NB. Malformations of the tympanic membrane almost always result in a conductive hearing loss.
- Ophthalmology opinion, epibulbar dermoid (OAV syndrome), coloboma of choroids and/or retina (CHARGE).
- Renal USS, unless clear diagnosis of TCS in which renal anomalies are not found; renal anomalies are rare in OAV.
- Chest X-ray, ECG, cardiac echo in suspected CHARGE or if signs of a cardiac abnormality.
- Consider cervical spine films if a diagnosis of OAV is possible (cervical vertebral fusion in 20–35%).

Some diagnoses to consider

Treacher–Collins syndrome (TCS; mandibulofacial dysostosis)
An AD disorder with extremely variable expressivity caused by mutations in the *TCOF1* gene at 5q32–33.1, or more rarely *POLR1D* (dominant) or *POLR1C* (recessive). The ear anomalies are bilateral. They are malformed and displaced towards the angle of the mandible. One-third have atresia of the external auditory meatus or abnormality of the ossicles. The facial features tend to be symmetrical. Conductive hearing loss is common, but also screen for sensorineural deafness. Malar hypoplasia, coloboma (V-shaped notch) of the inferior eyelid at the junction of the medial two-thirds and lateral one-third. Choanal atresia may be a feature of severe

TCS. Intelligence is normal. Consider mutation analysis of *TCS1*. Approximately 17% have a 5-nucleotide deletion towards the 3′ end of the gene. Sixty to 70% are the result of DNMs.

If there is mandibulofacial dysostosis with microcephaly, developmental delay, and TOF/oesophageal atresia (OA), consider *EFTUD2* mutation.

Oculoauriculovertebral spectrum (OAVS)
Also known as Goldenhar syndrome, hemifacial microsomia, first and second arch syndrome, and craniofacial microsomia.

In the majority of children, the disorder is unilateral. When bilateral, there is a difference in severity between the right and left sides. The right is more often involved than the left. OAV syndrome is extremely variable, ranging from isolated, unilateral ear anomalies as the mildest form to an expanded form with malformations in the CNS, vertebrae, heart, and kidneys. Ear abnormalities are present in 65%. Microtia with preauricular skin tags and additional skin tags in the line between the tragus and the angle of the mouth. The ear abnormalities may be bilateral but are asymmetric. See 'Facial asymmetry' in Chapter 2, 'Clinical approach', p. 146.

CHARGE (coloboma–heart defects–atresia choanae–retardation of growth and/or development–genital defect–ear anomalies and/or deafness) syndrome
Distinctive ear anomalies and/or deafness occur in 85–100%. Usually bilateral but asymmetrical, with low-set, prominent, posteriorly rotated ears with deficient cartilage and hypoplastic lobes. The ears may be 'cup-shaped' or lop, but the variation in morphology is very wide and often quite marked between the two ears of an individual patient. Deafness is variable, most usually a moderate to severe progressive mixed loss, with defects of the ossicles and 'glue ear' causing the conductive component. Absent or hypoplastic semicircular canals appear to be a common and important feature.

CHARGE has a prevalence of ~1/12 000. It is caused by a mutation in the gene *CHD7* which acts in early embryonic development by affecting chromatin structure and gene expression (Vissers *et al.* 2001). See 'Coloboma' in Chapter 2, 'Clinical approach', p. 110 for further details.

Branchio-oto-renal (BOR) syndrome
An AD disorder caused by mutations in *EYA1* on 8q13. Ear anomalies include ear pits (highly penetrant), dysplastic pinnae, and conductive, sensorineural, or mixed hearing loss. Branchial fistulae or cysts (60%) usually found on the medial border of the sternomastoid muscle. Renal anomalies include a duplex collecting system, hydronephrosis, cystic kidneys, and unilateral or bilateral renal agenesis. The nasolacrimal duct may be blocked. Rarely also caused by mutations in the *SIX1* and possibly *SIX5* genes.

Townes–Brock syndrome (TBS)
An AD disorder caused by mutations in the *SALL1* transcription factor gene, which is expressed in the developing ear, limb buds, and excretory organs. Phenotypic expression is extremely variable but includes two or more of: bilateral ear malformation, e.g. dysplastic ears; ear tags; sensorineural hearing loss (71%); hand malformations, e.g. triphalangeal or hypoplastic thumbs (56%); imperforate anus or rectovaginal/rectourethral fistula (47%); and renal anomalies. High incidence of new mutations. Cardiac anomalies have been reported.

Mandibulofacial dysostosis with microcephaly (MFDM)

MFDM is a multiple malformation syndrome with microcephaly, first and second arch malformations, craniofacial malformations (including a wide spectrum of ear malformations such as microtia, multiple ear tags, and hearing loss in some). Oesophageal atresia is present in 27% (Huang et al. 2016). It is caused by heterozygous variants in the EFTUD2. Microcephaly is virtually universal in childhood but some show 'catch-up' growth and may have a normal OFC as adults.

Nager acrofacial dysostosis

TCS-like facial features with marked micrognathia. Radial ray anomalies (hypoplastic or absent thumbs and radii) are the main distinguishing features. Ninety-five per cent have hearing impairment. Haploinsufficient dominantly acting *SF3B4* mutations are responsible for about 60% of cases (either *de novo* or inherited from an affected parent).

Miller syndrome

An AR condition with TCS-like facial features with lower lid colobomata, malar hypoplasia, and micrognathia. Ulnar ray hypoplasia (ulnar hypoplasia or fifth finger hypoplasia/aplasia) is the key distinguishing feature. Twenty per cent have hearing impairment. Biallelic *DHODH* mutations are responsible. Miller syndrome was the first example where exome sequencing identified the gene for a rare Mendelian disorder of unknown cause (Ng et al. 2010).

Cat-eye syndrome (CES)

Variable pattern of multiple anomalies, including iris colobomata, anal atresia, and preauricular anomalies (triad only present in 40%). Mild to moderate mental retardation in 32%. Bisatellite marker chromosome derived from inverted dicentric duplication of 22q. Occasionally inherited. See 'Supernumerary marker chromosomes (SMCs)—postnatal', p. 690 and 'Supernumerary marker chromosomes (SMCs)—prenatal', p. 692 in Chapter 5, 'Chromosomes'.

18q−

Patients with subtelomeric deletions of 18q typically have narrow slit-like ear canals, together with MR, midface hypoplasia, and a carp-shaped mouth.

Genetic advice

Recurrence risk

As for specific condition.

Carrier detection

Clinical examination combined with mutation analysis, if available.

Prenatal diagnosis

Is possible for some of these conditions, e.g.:

• USS for structural abnormalities;

• chromosomal or mutation analysis if an abnormality has been identified in the proband.

Support group: Many of the conditions have their own support group. See Contact a Family, http://www.cafamily.org.uk.

Expert adviser: Maria Bitner-Glindzic, Professor of Clinical and Molecular Genetics, Genetics and Genomic Medicine Programme, University College London, Great Ormond Street Institute of Child Health, London, UK.

References

Devriendt K, de Smet L, Casteels I. Oculo-auriculo-vertebral spectrum. In: SB Cassidy, JE Allanson (eds.). Management of genetic syndromes, 3rd edn, pp. 587–96. John Wiley & Sons, Inc., Hoboken, 2010.

Gripp KW, Slavotinek AM, Hall, JG, Allanson JE. *Handbook of physical measurements*, 3rd edn. Oxford University Press, Oxford, 2013.

Huang L, Vanstone MR et al. Mandibulofacial dysostosis with microcephaly: mutation and database update. *Hum Mutat* 2016; **37**(2): 148–54.

Ng SB, Buckingham KJ, Lee C, et al. Exome sequencing identifies the cause of a mendelian disorder. *Nat Genet* 2010; **42**: 30–5.

Oley CA. CHARGE syndrome. In: SB Cassidy, JE Allanson (eds.). *Management of genetic syndromes*, 3rd edn, pp. 157–68. John Wiley & Sons, Inc., Hoboken, 2010.

Powell CM, Michaelis RC. Townes–Brock syndrome. *J Med Genet* 1999; **36**: 89–93.

Rainger J, Bengani H, Campbell L, et al. Miller (Genee–Wiedemann) syndrome represents a clinically and biochemically distinct subgroup of postaxial acrofacial dysostosis associated with partial deficiency of DHODH. *Hum Mol Genet* 2012; **21**: 3969–83.

Vissers LE, Ravenswaaij CM, Admiraal R, et al. Mutations in a new member of the chromodomain gene family cause CHARGE syndrome. *Nat Genet* 2004; **36**: 955–7.

Wang RY, Earl DL, Ruder RO, Graham JM Jr. Syndromic ear anomalies and renal ultrasounds. *Pediatrics* 2001; **108**: E32.

Facial asymmetry

Although all faces show some asymmetry, significant facial asymmetry is a well-recognized feature of a number of distinctive conditions, including the oculoauriculovertebral spectrum (OAVS), which is one of the most common malformations seen in babies.

If there is a size difference without malformation, a common difficulty is distinguishing which side is 'normal'.

Also see 'Ear anomalies', p. 108 and 'Plagiocephaly and abnormalities of skull shape', p. 280 in Chapter 2, 'Clinical approach'.

Clinical approach

History: key points

- Family history, particularly to exclude AD conditions with variable expression.
- Pregnancy. Diabetes, early bleeding, teratogenic agents, e.g. retinoic acid, alcohol (OAVS), bleeding, placental abnormality (disruption), decreased liquor, abnormal fetal presentation, persistent discomfort and sensation of 'head being stuck', twin pregnancy (deformation).
- Uterine abnormalities such as bicornuate uterus, precipitate delivery, sleeping position (deformation).
- Obstructed labour (pre-existing craniosynostosis, syndromes with macrocephaly).
- Was asymmetry noted at birth? If not, at what age?
- Progression of deformity.
- Delayed motor milestones or developmental delay.
- Visual or hearing problems.
- Seizures (structural brain malformations, hemimegalencephaly, raised intracranial pressure from craniosynostosis).

Examination: key points

Careful measurements and clinical photography should be used to document the visual impression.

- Overall shape of the face and supraorbital area. Is any abnormality unilateral or is it bilateral with asymmetry?
- Is it possible to differentiate the normal from the affected side of the face?
- Are all the structures normally formed or are malformations present?
- Ears. Shape, size, symmetry.
- Ear malformations: accessory auricles, skin tags between the tragus and the angle of the mouth (OAVS), preauricular ear pits (BOR syndrome).
- Mid-facial (malar) flattening?
- Mandibular asymmetry.
- Eye spacing (measure) and/or exorbitism.
- Eye malformations: epibulbar dermoid (OAVS), microphthalmia (OAVS), coloboma or notch in the outer third of the lower eyelid (TCS).
- Mouth. Macrostomia in OAVS, facial clefting.
- Facial weakness/palsy gives an asymmetric appearance (CHARGE syndrome).
- Fontanelle. Position, size, and tension.
- Palpable sutures, compensatory bulging/bossing (craniosynostosis).
- Describe the skull shape. Examine the head from both sides, from above, and from the front (differentiating postural plagiocephaly and craniosynostosis). Ear position, used in conjunction with the skull shape, to assess if deformation is likely.
- Facial clefts (developmental disruptions, malformation syndromes) and cleft palate (deformations, OAVS).
- Neck: torticollis, branchial cyst (BOR).
- Skin pigmentary abnormalities and haemangiomas.
- Cardiac murmur.
- Hands and feet:
- Thumb duplications and deficiency (OAVS), triphalangeal or hypoplastic thumbs (TBS).
- Minor degrees of syndactyly in Saethre–Chotzen syndrome (SCS).
- Movement asymmetric?

Special investigations

- Clinical photographs are valuable, especially for documenting changes over time.
- Audiology in children with ear anomalies.
- Ophthalmology review: delineate structural lesions, epibulbar dermoid (OAVS), coloboma of the choroid and/or retina (CHARGE).
- Cervical X-rays in children with OAVS (cervical vertebral fusion in 20–35%). Consider imaging the entire spine, as vertebral anomalies may exist below the cervical level.
- Skull X-ray. Posteroanterior (PA); lateral if there is cranial asymmetry:
  - orbital asymmetry (OAVS);
  - sphenoid wing dysplasia (NF1);
  - the signs of synostosis are partial or total absence of the suture, indistinct zones along the suture, and perisutural sclerosis. Assess for evidence of a harlequin sign (elevation of the lesser wing of the sphenoid) in coronal synostosis. Interpretation is difficult in infants and requires good-quality films and expert reporting.
- Consider cranial USS in infants.
- Chest X-ray, ECG, cardiac echo in syndromes with a high incidence of cardiac abnormality.
- Consider the need for a renal USS.
- Referral to a specialist surgical centre, if appropriate, for detailed assessment and further imaging.
- Assessment of parents.
- Genomic analysis in presence of features suggestive of a chromosomal or syndromic diagnosis, e.g. genomic array, gene panel or, WES/WGS as appropriate. Routine cytogenetic analysis in the normally developing infant with no features other than facial asymmetry is not usually indicated.
- Molecular analysis in infants with TBS, BOR, and SCS and *FGFR3* for Muenke syndrome.
- Consider video to demonstrate asymmetric facial movement.

Some diagnoses to consider

With features that usually lead to presentation at birth or during infancy

OCULOAURICULOVERTEBRAL SPECTRUM (OAVS). Also known as Goldenhar syndrome, hemifacial microsomia, first and second arch syndrome, and craniofacial microsomia. Gorlin (2001) recommends the use of the term oculoauricularvertebral spectrum for this heterogeneous condition that affects primarily the development of the ear, oral structures, and mandible. In the majority of children, the disorder is unilateral. When bilateral, there is a difference in severity between the right and left sides. The right is more often involved than the left. OAVS is extremely variable, ranging from isolated, unilateral ear anomalies as the mildest form to an expanded form with malformations in the CNS, vertebrae, heart, and kidneys.

Facial asymmetry is severe in 20% but evident to some extent in 65%. This is due to a combination of hypoplasia of the bony structures of the face and abnormalities of the ear. The ear abnormalities are more fully described in 'Ear anomalies' in Chapter 2, 'Clinical approach', p. 142.

Gorlin (2001) estimates the frequency to be about one in 5600 births. OAVS is usually a sporadic disorder, and a vascular event in early pregnancy is a possible mechanism. There are some dominant families, so it is important to examine parents.

SYNDROMES WITH OVERLAPPING FEATURES OF OAVS. Asymmetry may be present, but the bilateral features help differentiate these from OAVS.

- TCS. An AD condition characterized by a distinctive facial appearance with ear anomalies, malar hypoplasia, and micrognathia and caused by mutations in the *TCS1* gene, or more rarely in the *POLR1D* or *POLR1C* genes. The symmetry of TCS is not found in OAVS. For more detail, see 'Ear anomalies' in Chapter 2, 'Clinical approach', p. 142.
- TBS. Caused by mutation in the *SALL1* transcription factor gene, which is expressed in the developing ear, limb buds, and excretory organs. Phenotypic expression is extremely variable but includes two or more of: bilateral ear malformation, e.g. dysplastic ears; ear tags; sensorineural hearing loss (71%); hand malformations, e.g. triphalangeal or hypoplastic thumbs (56%); imperforate anus or rectovaginal/rectourethral fistula (47%); and renal anomalies. High incidence of new mutations. Cardiac anomalies have been reported. Consider screening patients with overlapping features of OAVS for mutations in *SALL1*.
- BOR syndrome. AD disorder caused by mutations in *EYA1* on 8q13. More rarely, mutations are found in *SIX5* or *SIX1*. Preauricular pits and branchial fistulae are useful diagnostic craniofacial features. See 'Ear anomalies' in Chapter 2, 'Clinical approach', p. 142.
- CHARGE syndrome (coloboma–heart defects–atresia choanae–retardation of growth and/or development–genital defect–ear anomalies and/or deafness). Asymmetry of the ears is commonly seen in CHARGE syndrome. Facial asymmetry and unilateral facial palsy are also common in this condition which is caused by mutations in the gene *CHD7*. See 'Coloboma' in Chapter 2, 'Clinical approach', p. 110 for further details.
- Oculocerebrocutaneous (Delleman) syndrome. A rare syndrome with orbital cysts, focal dermal malformations, periorbital skin tags, and agenesis of the corpus callosum.
- Auriculo-condylar syndrome is characterized by variable micrognathia, temporomandibular joint ankylosis, cleft palate, and a characteristic 'question-mark' ear malformation. It is inherited by dominant mutations in the *PLCB4* or *GNAI3* genes.

- Mutations in the *EFTUD2* gene cause a wide spectrum of anomalies, with features observed in OAVS including microtia, mandibular hypoplasia, and sometimes epibulbar dermoids. This represents a recently described disorder, previously recognized as otofacial syndrome, acrofacial dysostosis type Guion–Almeida, and syndromic OA and is now called mandibulofacial dysostosis with microcephaly (MFDM).

MOEBIUS SYNDROME. The face is asymmetric if there is unilateral weakness of the VIIth (facial) nerve. Moebius sequence/syndrome is a rare disorder characterized by congenital palsy of the VIth and VIIth cranial nerves. Other cranial nerves may be affected, together with skeletal and orofacial anomalies. In Stromland et al.'s survey (2002) of 25 patients with Moebius syndrome, associated anomalies included: limb malformations (10); Poland anomaly (2); hypodontia (7); microglossia (6); cleft palate (4); hearing impairment (5); and external ear malformation (1). Pronounced functional abnormalities were observed involving: facial expression (16); speech (13); eating and swallowing (12); and difficulty in sucking in infancy (11). Six patients had an autistic syndrome, one an autistic-like condition, and intellectual disability was found in all these patients. Bouwes-Bavinck and Weaver (1986) propose that Moebius syndrome results from vascular disruption of the primitive trigeminal arteries before the establishment of sufficient blood supply for the brainstem by the vertebral arteries. Moebius is usually sporadic (especially when there are accompanying limb defects), but there are some reports of dominant transmission in the literature.

DEFORMATION. See 'Plagiocephaly and abnormalities of skull shape' in Chapter 2, 'Clinical approach', p. 280.

DISRUPTIONS. Unusual facial clefts, possibly associated with amniotic bands.

CRANIOSYNOSTOSIS. See 'Craniosynostosis' in Chapter 3, 'Common consultations', p. 378.

- Unilateral coronal craniosynostosis.
- SCS: facial asymmetry is a major feature of SCS, unlike the other syndromal craniosynostosis syndromes.
- *FGFR3*-associated coronal synostosis (Muenke syndrome). The mutation Pro250Arg in *FGFR3* causes AD inheritance of unilateral or bilateral craniosynostosis (Reardon et al. 1997).

CHROMOSOMAL ABNORMALITIES

- Abnormalities of chromosome 22, including trisomy 22, del 22q, ring and duplication (CES), are particularly associated with ear tags and facial asymmetry.
- Mosaic chromosome abnormalities.

VASCULAR ANOMALIES. Arteriovenous malformations (AVMs) and haemangiomas.

With features that usually lead to presentation in childhood

HEMIHYPERPLASIA OR OVERGROWTH (AND TUMOURS).

- Encephalocraniocutaneous lipomatosis and Proteus syndrome. There is disagreement as whether to classify these as separate disorders. Features are multiple lipomas of the head and neck, hyperostosis of the skull, macrocephaly, and streaks of yellow-brown pigmentation.
- NF1 sphenoid wing dysplasia, plexiform neurofibromata.
- Isolated hemihypertrophy. Examine for features of BWS and Silver–Russell syndromes (SRS).

HEMIATROPHY. Less common than hyperplasia.
- Consider mosaicism for single gene and chromosomal disorders.
- Progressive hemiatrophy/Parry–Romberg syndrome in older children.
- Post-radiation damage.

Genetic advice

Recurrence risk
As for specific condition.

Carrier detection
Clinical examination combined with mutation analysis, if available.

Prenatal diagnosis
This is possible for some of the conditions.
- USS for structural abnormalities.
- Chromosomal or mutation analysis.

Natural history and further management (preventative measures)
- Deformational disorders improve with time once the deformational force has been lost.
- Specialist surgical assessment by a craniofacial centre.

Support group: Many of the syndromes have their own support groups. See Contact a Family, http://www.cafamily.org.uk.

Expert adviser: Koen Devriendt, Clinical Geneticist, Centre for Human Genetics, University Hospital Leuven, Leuven, Belgium.

References
Bouwes-Bavinck J, Weaver D. Subclavian artery disruption sequence—hypothesis of vascular etiology for Poland, Klippel–Feil and Moebius anomalies. *Am J Med Genet* 1986; **23**: 903–18.

Devriendt K, de Smet L, Casteels I. Oculo-auriculo-vertebral spectrum. In: SB Cassidy, JE Allanson (eds.). *Management of genetic syndromes*, 3rd edn, pp. 587–96. John Wiley & Sons, Inc., Hoboken, 2010.

Keegan CE, Mulliken JB, Wu BL, Korf BR. Townes–Brocks syndrome versus expanded spectrum hemifacial microsomia: review of eight patients and further evidence of a 'hot spot' for mutation in the *SALL1* gene. *Genet Med* 2001; **3**: 310–13.

Kelberman D, Tyson J, Chandler DC, et al. Hemifacial microsomia: progress in understanding the genetic basis of a complex malformation syndrome. *Hum Genet* 2001; **109**: 638–45.

Reardon W, Wilkes D, Rutland P, et al. Craniosynostosis associated with *FGFR3* pro250arg mutation results in a range of clinical presentations including unisutural sporadic craniosynostosis. *J Med Genet* 1997; **34**: 632–6.

Sanlaville D, Romana SP, Lapierre JM, et al. A CGH study of 27 patients with CHARGE association. *Clin Genet* 2002; **61**: 135–8.

Strömland K, Sjögreen L, Miller M, et al. Mobius sequence—a Swedish multidiscipline study. *Eur J Paediatr Neurol* 2002; **6**: 35–45.

Voigt C, Mégarbané A, Neveling K, et al. Oto-facial syndrome and esophageal atresia, intellectual disability and zygomatic anomalies – expanding the phenotypes associated with *EFTUD2* mutations. *Orphanet J Rare Dis* 2013; **8**: 110.

Failure to thrive

This section describes the genetic investigation of babies who are small at birth and infants who fail to gain weight normally and are relatively proportionate, but small and thin, with a weight below the 0.4th centile. They are usually short, though their height/length centile may be slightly better than the weight centile. Their head size may be normal for age or in proportion to their body size. If the child's weight is on a similar or higher centile to the height/length centile, see 'Short stature' in Chapter 2, 'Clinical approach', p. 312 and Wit et al. 2016.

One of the most useful features is the differentiation between pre- and postnatal onset of growth retardation. Early embryonic growth is largely driven by insulin-like growth factors 1 and 2 (IGF-1 and IGF-2), fetal and early neonatal growth by IGF-1, and growth in later childhood by growth hormone (GH) and IGF-1.

It is assumed that a paediatrician has excluded the most common medical causes of failure to thrive (coeliac disease, cows' milk protein intolerance, etc.). Often the referral letter will query whether the child has Silver–Russell (Russell–Silver) syndrome (SRS).

Clinical approach

History: key points
- Three-generation family tree, with specific enquiry for consanguinity, parental heights, and birthweights and current size (in relation to their peers) of other children in the family.
- Pregnancy.
  - Did USS indicate growth problems and at what gestation were they noted?
  - Liquor volume. Oligohydramnios (placental insufficiency), polyhydramnios (CFC syndrome, Costello and Bartter syndromes).
- Birthweight, length, and head circumference. Copy the growth record chart into the genetic files.
- Feeding history (SRS babies with little interest in feeding).
- Developmental milestones. Children with SRS may have mild delay in motor milestones because of the relatively large head size, compared to body size and strength. Also allow for prematurity.
- Medical history. Recurrent infections?

Examination: key points
- Accurate measurement of weight, length, and head circumference. Note any disproportion.
- Limb or body asymmetry (SRS). Compare the length and circumference of the limbs (align thumbs and feet for comparison).
- Skin pigmentation abnormalities. CAL patches (SRS and Fanconi), telangiectasias (Bloom), acanthosis nigricans (lipoatrophic conditions and Donohue syndrome).
- Dry or lax skin (CFC and Costello syndromes).
- Polyps and papillomas around mucous membranes (Costello syndrome).
- Coarse facial features (Costello syndrome, CFC syndrome, Donohue syndrome, and other metabolic disorders).
- Blue sclerae (SRS).
- Sparse, curly hair (CFC syndrome).
- Fifth finger clinodactyly (SRS).
- Cardiac murmurs (pulmonary stenosis is the most common lesion in CFC and Costello syndromes).

Special investigations
- Basic investigations (usually performed by the paediatrician): serum urea and electrolytes (U & Es), thyroid function, antigliadin antibodies, FBC, and erythrocyte sedimentation rate (ESR).
- Bone age (wrist X-ray) and other skeletal films if a skeletal dysplasia is a possibility.
- Genomic analysis in presence of features suggestive of a chromosomal or syndromic diagnosis, e.g. genomic array, gene panel, or WES/WGS as appropriate.
- DNA for UPD-7 (see below). Consider PWS methylation assay if hypotonic. Consider CF screen.
- Cardiac echo for valvular and heart muscle abnormalities.
- Metabolic investigations. Ensure a basic screen has been performed. Further specific testing, e.g. insulin levels (Donohue syndrome), if clinically indicated.
- Consider tests of exocrine pancreatic function if clinically indicated, e.g. faecal elastase 1 (FE1; Shwachman–Diamond and Johanson–Blizzard syndromes). FE1 is a simple, non-invasive, highly specific, and sensitive test for determining pancreatic function. FE1 levels in meconium are low and reach normal levels by day 3 in term newborns and by 2 weeks in infants born before 28 weeks' gestation (Kori et al. 2003).
- Consider plasma aldosterone level if history of polyhydramnios (Bartter syndrome).
- Consider lymphocyte subsets and immunoglobulins to exclude a primary immunodeficiency.

Some diagnoses to consider

With prenatal onset of growth retardation

NON-SYNDROMIC OR IDIOPATHIC INTRAUTERINE GROWTH RETARDATION (IUGR). These children may remain below the 2nd or 0.4th centile throughout childhood, though some catchup is usual after birth. This group includes infants whose mothers had significant medical problems, as well as babies who are undernourished for a variety of non-genetic causes such as deprivation and drug and/or alcohol abuse.

SILVER–RUSSELL SYNDROME (SRS). The head is proportionately large, but usually between the 3rd and 25th centiles. The face is triangular and the mouth downturned. Asymmetry is a key diagnostic feature. The children are notoriously fussy eaters. Parents may comment on excessive sweating. There have been a few dominant families described with a milder phenotype, but the condition is generally sporadic. Discordant identical twins have been described. The development is usually within normal limits, but about one-third have late cognitive impairment. Approximately 10% of children have maternal UPD-7. DNA samples from the parents and child are required. Up to 60% of cases have hypomethylation of the imprinting control region (ICR) 1 on chromosome 11p15.

FETAL ALCOHOL SYNDROME (FAS). Growth retardation is a cardinal feature of FAS. Affected children have a low birthweight for gestational age (<2.5 centile), with decelerating weight over time not due to nutrition and disproportionately low weight to height. See 'Fetal alcohol syndrome (FAS)' in Chapter 6, 'Pregnancy and fertility', p. 728.

DUBOWITZ SYNDROME An AR condition characterized by pre- and postnatal growth retardation, eczema, telecanthus, epicanthal folds, blepharophimosis, ptosis, and broadening of the bridge and tip of the nose. Dubowitz syndrome is a complex of multiple, genetically distinct, and phenotypically overlapping disorders including dyskeratosis congenita and LIG4 (Stewart et al. 2014).

BARTTER SYNDROME. A condition characterized by hypokalaemic alkalosis with hypercalciuria. Genetically heterogeneous with mutations in SLC12A1, KCNJ1, and SLC12A3. History of polyhydramnios and often of preterm delivery with low birthweight and severe failure to thrive. Large head with prominent forehead, triangular face, large pinnae, and large eyes. Plasma K may be normal.

DONOHUE SYNDROME (LEPRECHAUNISM). An AR disorder due to mutations in the insulin receptor gene. Pre- and postnatal failure to thrive, hirsutism, aged face with thick lips and prominent ears, enlargement of the breasts and genitalia; acanthosis nigricans may be present. Serum insulin is grossly elevated. The prognosis is poor.

DNA REPAIR DEFECTS. Rare syndromes with chromosome breaks, etc., e.g. Bloom syndrome and Cockayne syndrome. Patients have short stature and microcephaly and developmental delay. See 'DNA repair disorders' in Chapter 3, 'Common consultations', p. 398.

With predominantly postnatal failure to thrive and developmental delay/learning disability

WILLIAMS SYNDROME. These children may have terrible feeding difficulties and it is worth considering the diagnosis. See 'Congenital heart disease' in Chapter 2, 'Clinical approach', p. 112.

PRADER–WILLI SYNDROME (PWS). Central hypotonia and feeding difficulties with failure to thrive in infancy. See 'Obesity with and without developmental delay' in Chapter 2, 'Clinical approach', p. 254.

METABOLIC AND MITOCHONDRIAL DISORDERS. Assess for other features of these conditions and investigate accordingly, in close collaboration with paediatric colleagues.

CARDIOFACIOCUTANEOUS (CFC) SYNDROME. The hair is sparse; there is relative macrocephaly, and there can be cardiac defects, most commonly pulmonary stenosis and CM. The skin is rough, dry, and hyperkeratotic. Noonan-like facies. Polyhydramnios in pregnancy is common; perhaps a prenatal presentation of the severe feeding problems and failure to thrive that are common in the first year of life. Development is delayed. PTPN11 mutations are not found, but many other mutations in the Ras/MAPK pathway defined.

COSTELLO SYNDROME. Characterized by prenatally increased growth, postnatal growth retardation, coarse face, loose skin resembling cutis laxa, non-progressive CM (sometimes with arrhythmia), developmental delay, and an outgoing, friendly behaviour. There are very characteristic wrinkled palms and ulnar deviation of the hands. Patients can develop papillomata, especially around the mouth, and have a predisposition for malignancies (mainly abdominal and pelvic rhabdomyosarcoma in childhood). Consider USS surveillance. Costello syndrome is often caused by heterozygous mutations in HRAS.

JOHANSON–BLIZZARD SYNDROME. An AR condition with IUGR, scalp defects, and exocrine pancreatic insufficiency (FE1 is a useful screen), combined with dysmorphic features, notably a 'pinched' nose and notching of the alae nasi. CHD and deafness may occur. The hair is often spiky. Usually associated with some learning disability, but not in all cases. Caused by biallelic mutations in the gene UBR1.

DNA REPAIR DEFECTS. See above.

With predominantly postnatal failure to thrive and normal cognitive development

METABOLIC AND MITOCHONDRIAL DISORDERS. Assess for other features of these conditions and investigate accordingly, in close collaboration with paediatric colleagues.

LIPODYSTROPHIES. There is loss of subcutaneous fat. Insulin resistance is common. Syndromic diagnoses include Beradinelli and SHORT syndromes. See 'Diabetes mellitus' in Chapter 3, 'Common consultations', p. 390.

SHWACHMAN–DIAMOND SYNDROME. An AR condition characterized by pancreatic exocrine insufficiency, haematological dysfunction, and skeletal anomalies (metaphyseal dysplasia). Caused by mutations in SBDS on 7q11 (Boocock et al. 2003).

Genetic advice

Recurrence risk

When the diagnosis is unknown, consult carefully with the paediatricians to establish the likelihood of non-genetic factors. If there has been severe IUGR, this may recur in the absence of a known cause. The presence of significant developmental delay and other dysmorphic features would suggest a syndromal cause. Beware that some of the conditions listed above have recessive inheritance and try to exclude these.

Prenatal diagnosis

Growth USS, but growth retardation is rarely detectable before 28 weeks' gestation.

Natural history and further management (preventative measures)

Children should remain under the care of a paediatrician or a paediatric endocrinologist to ensure optimal nutrition and growth.

Support groups: Child Growth Foundation, http://www.childgrowthfoundation.org, Tel. 0208 994 7625; CostelloKids, http://www.costellokids.org.uk.

Expert adviser: Sue Price, Consultant in Clinical Genetics, Oxford Regional Genetics Service, Churchill Hospital, Oxford, UK.

References

Boocock GR, Morrison JA, Popovic M, et al. Mutations in SBDS are associated with Shwachman–Diamond syndrome. *Nat Genet* 2003; **33**: 97–101.

Eggermann T, Begemann M, Binder G, Spengler S. Silver–Russell testing:genetic basis and molecular genetic testing. *Orphanet J Rare Dis* 2010; **5**: 19.

Hennekam RC. Costello syndrome: an overview. *Am J Med Genet C* 2003; **117C**: 42–8.

Kofoed EM, Hwa V, Little B, et al. Growth hormone insensitivity associated with a STAT5b mutation. N Engl J Med 2003; **349**: 1139–47.

Kori M, Maayan-Metzger A, Shamir R, Sirota L, Dinari G. Faecal elastase 1 levels in premature and full term infants. Arch Dis Child Fetal Neonatal Ed 2003; **88**: F106–8.

Lepri FR, Scavelli R, Digillo MC, et al. Diagnosis of Noonan syndrome and related disorders using target next generation sequencing. BMC Med Genet 2014; **15**: 14.

Stewart DR, Pemov A, et al. Dubowitz syndrome is a complex comprised of multiple, genetically distinct and phenotypically overlapping disorders. PLoS One 2014 Jun 3; **9**(6): e98686. doi: 10.1371/journal.pone.0098686.eCollection 2014.

Tartaglia M, Gelb BD, Zenker M. Noonan syndrome and clinically related disorders. Best Pract Res Clin Endocrinol Metab 2011; **25**: 161–79.

Price SM, Stanhope R, Garrett C, Preece MA, Trembath RC. The spectrum of Silver–Russell syndrome: a clinical and molecular genetic study. J Med Genet 1999; **36**: 837–42.

Wakeling E. Silver-Russell syndrome. Arch Dis Child 2011; **96**: 1156–61.

Wit JM, Oosterdilk W, van Duvvenvoorde HA, et al. Mechanisms in Endocrinology: Novel genetic causes of short stature. Eur J Endocrinol 2016; **174**: R145–73.

Floppy infant

You may be asked to see a baby on a NICU or on the postnatal wards who appears floppy. The paediatricians will usually have already excluded sepsis and hypoglycaemia as possible causes and are asking your opinion because they are considering a metabolic or neuromuscular cause. Central hypotonia is much more common than peripheral neuromuscular disease as a cause for presentation as a floppy infant. The most common neuromuscular cause of floppiness in the neonatal period is congenital DM. Other causes include neonatal myasthenia, congenital muscular dystrophy (CMD), and congenital myopathies (nemaline or myotubular). Rarely severe cases of SMA type 1 may present neonatally. Other types of SMA may also present in the neonatal period.

General points

- Distribution of weakness. In truncal hypotonia of central origin, there is relative sparing of the face and limbs. Although the baby may appear very floppy when picked up, with exaggerated head lag, when laid supine it will be able to kick quite powerfully.
- Facial muscle involvement. This is common in some of the congenital myopathies and congenital DM, but not SMA.
- Sucking and swallowing difficulty. This presents with poor feeding. If swallowing is impaired, there is a risk of aspiration. Sucking and swallowing difficulty are common features of severe SMA (with bulbar involvement), congenital DM, myotubular myopathy, nemaline myopathy, and neonatal myasthenia, as well as PWS and hypoxic–ischaemic encephalopathy (HIE).
- Respiratory difficulty. Respiratory problems soon after birth are rare in SMA type 1, but common in congenital DM, severe nemaline myopathy, and myotubular myopathy. Diaphragmatic weakness may be an early feature of SMA with respiratory distress (SMARD).

Clinical approach

History: key points

- Three-generation family history, with specific enquiry for consanguinity and for any neuromuscular problems, e.g. muscle weakness, and for features suggestive of DM, e.g. cataracts, diabetes, sudden cardiac death, unexplained infant deaths in offspring of other relatives (AD pattern for DM, XL for myotubular myopathy).
- Normal fetal movements in pregnancy?
- Was there polyhydramnios (poor fetal swallowing)?
- Normal labour and delivery or is there evidence of asphyxia and poor Apgar scores?
- Term or preterm delivery?
- When was the baby first noted to be floppy; did the baby handle normally immediately after delivery? Did it cry and kick?
- Is the floppiness getting worse or remaining static?
- Is the baby able to feed?

Examination: key points

If the labour was prolonged and/or the delivery traumatic and if there is an impression that the situation is improving, it may be appropriate to observe closely before launching into extensive investigations. If there is any hint that the situation is deteriorating, it is important to initiate investigations and to work in conjunction with your paediatric colleagues who will need to decide if the baby needs transfer to the NICU.

- Peripheral neuromuscular cause more likely if the baby is alert and responsive and the floppiness appears static over a period of hours/days. In SMA type 1, there is preservation of facial movement, compared to limb movement. The presence of reflexes does not exclude SMA.
- A strikingly myopathic face is characteristic of DM or myotubular myopathy. The face is generally less myopathic in babies with CMD.
- Central or metabolic cause more likely if the baby is not alert, but lethargic and sleepy. Progression of floppiness over a period of hours/days is suggestive of a metabolic cause.
- Describe the posture of the baby. Is it frog-legged?
- Look carefully for fasciculation: tongue and limbs (SMA type 1 can present in the neonatal period but more usually evolves over a period of weeks).
- Examine for contractures and talipes, suggestive of reduced fetal movement *in utero*.
- Observe spontaneous movements. Does the baby make any? Does the baby grimace or cry?
- Check for head lag, usually present in the newborn but can be very marked truncal hypotonia in some conditions of central origin.
- Check deep tendon reflexes (DTRs). Are they present? If absent, suggests a peripheral neuromuscular cause (but may be reduced in PWS and can be present in SMA).
- OFC, cry, drooling, swallowing, facial and eye movement, level of alertness.
- Document the muscle strength and changes over time.
- *Examine the mother* for features of DM or myasthenia gravis.

Special investigations

The paediatric team will probably have completed glucose, ammonia, and blood gas (to check for metabolic or respiratory acidosis) before you are asked to assess the baby. A paediatric neurologist should also be involved in the diagnosis and ongoing care of the infant.

(1) Clinical picture suggestive of central cause for hypotonia.
   - Genomic array.
   - Urine for amino and organic acids.
   - Consider lactate.
   - VLCFAs, transferrin isoelectric focussing, alkaline phosphatase and phosphate.
   - DNA for SNRPN (small nuclear ribonuclear protein-associated polypeptide N) methylation status (PWS) if central hypotonia, poor suck, and no other cause likely. Typical facies include delicate features and thin upper lip.
   - DNA for DM expansion (usually >1000 (CTG) repeats), especially if the face is myopathic and examination of the mother is suggestive. Rarely a baby can have congenital DM when examination of the mother is apparently normal.
   - CK. Should be normal in all central causes of hypotonia. Re-evaluate if raised and consider congenital muscular dystrophies, e.g. WWS and MEB syndrome, where the hypotonia is of mixed origin.

- Consider gene panel/WES/WGS where appropriate.
(2) Clinical picture suggestive of a peripheral cause for hypotonia.
  - CK (will be elevated in most forms of CMD, but normal or only slightly elevated in SMA or congenital myopathies).
  - EMG and NCVs. Fibrillation in SMA; if myopathic, proceed to muscle biopsy.
  - DNA for *SMN1* exons 7 and 8 deletion for SMA type 1 if a peripheral cause evident.

When most of these results are available, you should be in a position to decide whether this is likely to be a peripheral neuromuscular, central, or metabolic problem and proceed with further investigations accordingly.

For a central cause for hypotonia, consider:
- brain MRI scan;
- DNA storage.
- For a peripheral cause for hypotonia, consider:
- muscle biopsy with histology and immunohistochemistry (IHC);
- echo to exclude CM if suggestive of a primary muscle disorder;
- DNA storage.

Some diagnoses to consider

Prader–Willi syndrome (PWS)
The neonatal period is dominated by hypotonia, lethargy, and weak suck leading to feeding difficulties. Central hypotonia may manifest as reduced fetal movement, abnormal fetal position, e.g. breech, and difficulty at the time of delivery, often necessitating delivery by lower segment Caesarean section (LSCS). Reflexes may be reduced. The baby has to be awakened for feeds and sucks poorly, and frequently nasogastric feeding or other special feeding techniques may be needed in the early weeks of life. Breastfeeding is rarely possible. The facial features are delicate with a thin upper lip. The baby is quiet and sleeps for long periods and has a weak cry. Birthweight and length are usually within normal limits. See 'Obesity with and without developmental delay' in Chapter 2, 'Clinical approach', p. 254 for further details.

Congenital myotonic dystrophy
Pregnancy often complicated by polyhydramnios. At delivery, severely affected infants are floppy and often have respiratory problems with diaphragmatic hypoplasia and may require ventilatory support. There is a confusing combination of central and peripheral hypotonia. The diagnosis is usually apparent following a careful history and examination of the mother for signs of DM (typical facies, weak sternomastoids, grip myotonia, etc.). See 'Myotonic dystrophy (DM1)' in Chapter 3, 'Common consultations', p. 496 for further details.

Spinal muscular atrophy (SMA)
See 'Spinal muscular atrophy (SMA)' in Chapter 3, 'Common consultations', p. 526.

SMARD—see 'Spinal muscular atrophy (SMA)' in Chapter 3, 'Common consultations', p. 526.

Zellweger syndrome
An AR peroxisomal disorder, often presenting in the neonatal period with central hypotonia ± seizures. The fontanelle is large and the forehead high. There may be stippled epiphyses (especially the knees). VLCFAs are elevated. Prognosis is poor and most die in the first year of life. Zellweger syndrome is genetically heterogeneous and is caused by mutations in any of several genes involved in peroxisome biogenesis, e.g. peroxin-1, 2, 3, 5, 6, and 12 (*PEX1, 2, 3, 5, 6,* and *12*).

GPI DEFICIENCY SYNDROMES. Glycosylphosphatidylinositol (GPI) is a glycolipid that anchors >150 various proteins to the cell surface. At least 27 genes are involved in biosynthesis and transport of GPI-anchored proteins. These cause a wide range of multi-system disorders usually with a severe neurological component that may present with/without seizures and with/without congenital anomalies.

Pompe disease
AR acid maltase deficiency—CM. See 'Cardiomyopathy in children under 10 years' in Chapter 2, 'Clinical approach', p. 84.

Congenital myopathy
Types of congenital myopathy typically presenting at birth include severe nemaline myopathy and myotubular myopathy (which may clinically resemble congenital DM). CK levels are normal or marginally raised. Diagnosis requires muscle biopsy, which shows no necrosis or degenerative changes but may have characteristic structural features. Specialized examination of the muscle biopsy is indicated if a congenital myopathy is suspected.

X-linked myotubular myopathy
A rare congenital muscle disorder that usually presents at birth with hypotonia, severe generalized muscle weakness, and respiratory distress in affected males. Caused by hemizygous mutation in the *MTM1* gene. It is usually fatal in the neonatal period, although some families have a milder phenotype.

SCHAAF-YANG SYNDROME. Truncating variants in the maternally imprinted, paternally expressed gene *MAGEL2* located in the PWS critical region on 15q11-13. The phenotype overlaps with that of PWS, with developmental delay, hypotonia, feeding difficulties, autism spectrum, and in most contractures ranging from fetal akinesia and arthrogryposis multiplex congenita to contractures of the small finger joints (Fountain 2017). See 'Arthrogryposis' in Chapter 2, 'Clinical approach', p. 66.

Congenital muscular dystrophy (CMD)
These are a heterogeneous group of severely disabling AR disorders that affect the skeletal muscle and have an overall frequency of 71/10 000 live births. Affected children present with muscle weakness and hypotonia at birth, or within the first 6 months of life, and progressive joint contractures. Motor development is delayed. Progression of the disease is variable and dependent on the disease subtype, and some children never achieve the ability to walk without support and remain wheelchair-dependent for life. Brain involvement in the form of mental retardation and abnormal formation of different parts of the brain is a feature of several forms of CMD. The prognosis varies and some die early of respiratory failure. CK is variable in these disorders and diagnosis requires muscle biopsy, and often also cranial MRI.

CMD WITHOUT BRAIN INVOLVEMENT. Of cases without intellectual impairment or major structural brain abnormalities, half of the cases show deficiency of laminin alpha-2 (merosin) due to mutations of the laminin alpha-2 chain gene. These children typically have a very high CK and white matter changes visible on brain MRI from the age of 6 months. Mutations in the fukutin-related protein (*FKRP*) gene can cause a secondary deficiency of laminin alpha-2 and a severe form of congenital muscular dystrophy 1C (MDC1C), also associated with a very high CK. Other causes of secondary laminin alpha-2 deficiency are yet to be elucidated. Of the types of CMD with normal laminin alpha-2, the best defined is Ullrich CMD, due to AR mutations in the collagen VIA genes. These children typically have distal joint laxity and proximal contractures. Most have absence of collagen VI in their muscle biopsies.

WITH BRAIN INVOLVEMENT—LISSENCEPHALY. Fukuyama CMD, MEB, and WWS are associated with eye abnormalities and neuronal migration defects, and result from mutations in *FKTN*, *POMGnT1*, and *POMT1*, respectively. See 'Lissencephaly, polymicrogyria, and neuronal migration disorders' in Chapter 2, 'Clinical approach', p. 216. Abnormalities of alpha-dystroglycan are a common feature, reflecting the role of these proteins in glycosylation.

• White matter changes. Another glycosyltransferase, encoded by the gene *LARGE*, causes CMD and profound MR, with white matter changes and subtle structural abnormalities on brain MRI (MDC1D). In several cases, the gene localization remains unknown.

Genetic advice

Recurrence risk
This is dependent on the diagnosis—see relevant section.

Carrier detection
This may be possible if the causative mutation is defined in the proband.

Prenatal diagnosis
This may be possible if the causative mutation is defined in the proband.

Natural history and further management (preventative measures)
Babies should be under the care of a paediatric neurologist for ongoing care.

Support group: Many of the individual conditions have their own support groups. See Contact a Family, http://www.cafamily.org.uk.

References

Dubowitz V. The floppy infant syndrome. In: V Dubowitz. *Muscle disorders in childhood*, 2nd edn, pp. 457–72. WB Saunders, Philadelphia, 1995.

Gunay-Aygun M, Schwartz S, Heeger S, O'Riordan MA, Cassidy SB. The changing purpose of Prader–Willi syndrome clinical diagnostic criteria and proposed revised criteria. *Pediatrics* 2001; **108**: E92.

Longman C, Brockington M, Torelli S, *et al.* Mutations in the human *LARGE* gene cause MDC1D, a novel form of congenital muscular dystrophy with severe mental retardation and abnormal glycosylation of alpha-dystroglycan. *Hum Mol Genet* 2003; **12**: 2853–61.

Miller SP, Riley P, Shevell MI. The neonatal presentation of Prader–Willi syndrome revisited. *Pediatrics* 1999; **134**: 226–8.

Prasad AN, Prasad C. Genetic evaluation of the floppy infant. *Semin Fetal Neonatal Med* 2011; **16**: 99–108.

Tubridy N, Fontaine B, Eymard B. Congenital myopathies and congenital muscular dystrophies. *Curr Opin Neurol* 2001; **14**: 575–82.

Fractures

One-third to one-half of children have one fracture during childhood; 20% have two or more. A geneticist may be asked to see the child, usually to determine if the cause is osteogenesis imperfecta (OI; brittle bone disease). The severe forms of OI have marked clinical and radiological changes that present either prenatally on USS or in the neonatal period. Most (85–90%) patients harbour heterozygote germline mutations in the *COL1A1* or *COL1A2* genes that encode the chains of type I procollagen, the major protein in bone.

The clinical approach described here is to assist in the diagnosis of milder forms of OI. Sometimes the possibility of a non-accidental injury (NAI) has been raised, so sensitive questioning is appropriate.

Clinical approach

History: key points
- Three-generation family tree with specific enquiry about fractures, blue sclerae, dental problems, hearing loss, short stature, and osteoporosis (fractures and getting shorter with age, kyphosis); age at walking.
- Child's age at each fracture. Were fractures present at birth? (Babies with arthrogryposis often sustain fractures during delivery.)
- Number of fractures and which bones were fractured. Fractures occurring with apparently trivial trauma are highly relevant.
- Did anyone observe the events? Is the story consistent? (NAI has to be considered.)
- Did the fracture heal normally? (Occasionally children with OI have a large mass of callus at the site of a healing fracture that is mistaken for a malignant lesion; this is now recognized as a specific form of OI—type V.)
- Is there any limb deformity?
- Joint dislocations (ligamentous laxity is a feature of OI) or joint contractures.
- Hearing loss (stapedial fixation occurs in OI, as does sensorineural deafness).
- Teeth that chip or crack (dentinogenesis imperfecta (DI)).

Examination: key points
Mainly for features of OI.
- Height (reduced in OI).
- Limb deformity (may be none with mild OI).
- Blue sclerae (often said to be more striking when the fractures occur; note infants up to age of 6 months often have blue sclerae).
- Scoliosis (due to lax ligaments and osteoporosis/vertebral crush fractures in older children and adults).
- Ligamentous laxity; estimate the 'Beighton score'. Ten per cent of population score >5. See 'Hypermobile joints' in Chapter 2, 'Clinical approach', p. 176.
- Skin. Is it smooth, soft, easily bruised? Does it show poor wound healing or scarring (consider Ehlers–Danlos syndrome (EDS))?
- Teeth for DI (discoloration, poor growth, defective dentin).
- Heart (in adults, MVP more common).
- Neurological if spinal abnormality (unusual) or basilar invagination.

Special investigations
Osteogenesis imperfecta (OI). The presence of Wormian bones is the main diagnostic feature in type I OI, as the rest of the skeletal survey may be normal. Bone density may be reduced but is often normal in type I. In more severe forms, bony deformity and low bone mass are common. Basilar invagination is the key skull base abnormality resulting in morbidity.
- Radiology:
  - a full radiological survey is used to document old fractures and is important in distinguishing between genetic conditions and child abuse;
  - skull X-ray (SXR) is useful to look for Wormian bones if mild OI is suspected in a child with a known family history (teeth with poor roots may also be visible on the SXR);
  - lateral spine X-ray has a role in the assessment of a baby <12 months old with OI—looking for biconcavity of vertebral bodies and wedge fractures, prior to consideration of bisphosphonate therapy.
- Hearing test.
- Bone biochemistry, including alkaline phosphatase (reduced/absent in hypophosphatasia, normal or increased in OI).
- Urine, for amino acids (homocystinuria) and/or markers of collagen breakdown (N-telopeptide of type I collagen (NTx) is the most useful).
- Blood for DNA storage. Molecular confirmation, especially useful in prenatal situations. Next-generation sequencing for all known OI genes is now available; consider panel/WES/WGS as appropriate.
- Skin biopsy for collagen studies may occasionally be useful to confirm a suspected diagnosis or to help with PND, but there is limited availability of collagen protein analysis.
- Bone density scans may help to determine if osteoporotic complications are likely. This should be done in conjunction with a physician with a special interest in bone metabolic disorders.

Some diagnoses to consider

Osteogenesis imperfecta (OI)
See below for more details.

Non-accidental injury (NAI)
See 'Suspected non-accidental injury' in Chapter 2, 'Clinical approach', p. 326.

Juvenile osteoporosis
Reduced bone density; can resolve spontaneously and may rarely be familial. Can be caused by heterozygous *LRP5* and *wnt-1* mutations.

Premature osteoporosis
Search for endocrine causes. The increased use of bone density scanning in young women has resulted in the identification of some individuals who have such reduced density that they may have a mild form of OI.

Hypophosphatasia
An inherited disorder characterized by defective bone mineralization and a deficiency of tissue non-specific alkaline phosphatase (*TNSALP*) activity. The disease is highly variable in its clinical expression, depending on

the specific mutation in *TNSALP*. Levels of alkaline phosphatase in blood are very low. The disease usually follows an AR inheritance, but Lia-Baldini *et al.* (2001) provide evidence that some mutations may have a dominant negative effect and so be transmitted in an AD, rather than an AR, pattern. Expression of the disease may be highly variable, with parents of even severely affected children showing no or extremely mild symptoms of the disease. Parental molecular genetic analysis and parental alkaline phosphatase levels may be helpful. Early referral for recombinant enzyme therapy is needed in severe cases.

Skeletal dysplasias with Wormian bones
Distinguished on the basis of their other features.

Osteoporosis–pseudoglioma syndrome
Rare AR disorder characterized by severe juvenile-onset osteoporosis and congenital or early-onset blindness. Other manifestations include muscular hypotonia, ligamentous laxity, mild mental retardation, and seizures. The gene responsible is *LRP5* on chromosome 11q11–12. (Abnormalities in the canonical wnt signalling pathway through LRP5 are becoming apparent as causes of dominant osteoporosis.)

Short stature, optic atrophy, and Pelger–Huet anomaly
An AR disorder caused by biallelic mutation in the *NBAS* gene on chromosome 2p24. This can present with bone fractures accompanied by recurrent infections, neutropenia, and elevated alanine aminotransferase (ALT) (Segarra 2015).

Bruck syndrome (BS)
An AR syndrome presenting with OI (blue sclerae and Wormian bones are found) and congenital contractures of the large joints, often with bilateral talipes equinovarus. Webbing (pterygia) is seen at the elbows and knees. Bank *et al.* (1999) reported that the molecular defect underlying BS is a deficiency of bone-specific telopeptide lysyl hydroxylase that results in aberrant cross-linking of bone collagen. BS is caused by mutations in the *FKBP10* gene on 17p12 (BS1) or by mutations in the *PLOD2* gene on 3q23-q24 (BS2).

Arthrogryposis
Multiple congenital contractures, often with gracile long bones that are poorly ossified and so frequently fracture during delivery (8–10%) or iatrogenically when trying to move limbs with contractures. See 'Arthrogryposis' in Chapter 2, 'Clinical approach', p. 66.

Genetic advice
Osteogenesis imperfecta (OI)
In types I–IV OI, excessive bone fragility is caused by mutations in the A1 and A2 chains of type I collagen (Ward *et al.* 2001). Type I OI is the most common and has a frequency of 2–5 per 100 000. In *type I*, there may be mutations that cause non-functional alleles (null alleles), giving a 50% reduction in collagen (reduced amount of normal collagen), whereas in *type II and other severe forms*, there are often glycine substitutions that disturb the helical structure and stability of collagen (dominant negative) and thus lead to a more severe phenotype.

The clinical classification of Sillence is used to describe types I–IV OI; there are now 15 forms of OI described, associated with specific genetic defects that encompass defects in the type I collagen genes themselves, factors

Table 2.11 Expanded Sillence classification of osteogenesis imperfecta[*]

Type	Severity	Clinical description	Genetic basis
I	Mild, non-deforming	Normal height or mild short stature; blue sclerae; no dentinogenesis imperfecta	AD; premature stop codon in *COL1A1*
II	Perinatal lethal	Multiple rib and long bone fractures are present at birth. Deformities. Dark sclerae. Radiographs show low density of skull bones and broad long bones. Lethal in perinatal period, usually due to respiratory failure from multiple rib fractures	Glycine substitutions in *COL1A1* or *COL1A2*
IIA	Lethal	Broad, crumpled long bones; broad ribs with continuous beading	
IIB	Lethal	Broad, crumpled long bones, but ribs have discontinuous or no beading	
IIC	Lethal	Thin, fractured long bones and thin, beaded ribs	
III	Severely deforming	Very short stature; limb and spine deformity due to multiple fractures. Severe scoliosis can lead to respiratory difficulty which is a leading cause of death in type III OI; greyish sclerae; dentinogenesis imperfecta; triangular facies	Mostly *de novo* AD due to glycine substitutions in *COL1A1* or *COL1A2*
IV	Moderately deforming	Moderate short stature; mild/moderate scoliosis; greyish/white sclerae; dentinogenesis imperfecta	AD; glycine substitutions in *COL1A1* or *COL1A2*
V	Moderately deforming	Mild/moderate short stature; interosseous membrane of forearm calcifies early in life, limiting hand movement and sometimes causing dislocation of the radial head; hyperplastic callus; white sclerae; no dentinogenesis imperfecta	AD; *IFITM5*
VI	Moderately/severely deforming	Moderately short; scoliosis; accumulation of osteoid in bone tissue, 'fish-scale' pattern of bone lamellation; white sclerae; no dentinogenesis imperfecta	AR; *SERPINF1*
VII	Moderately deforming	Mild short stature; proximal shortening of limbs; coxa vara; white sclerae. No dentinogenesis imperfecta. Rare.	AR; *CRTAP*
VIII	Severe to lethal	Overlaps with type II/severe type III	AR; *LEPRE1*

[*] The range of clinical severity in OI is a continuum; however, categorization of patients is helpful in determining prognosis and assessing treatment.

Reprinted from *The Lancet*, Vol 363, Rauch and Glorieux, Osteogenesis Imperfecta, pp. 1377–1385, copyright 2004, with permission from Elsevier.

involved in collagen protein processing, folding, or stability, and factors in osteoblast differentiation or activity-regulating pathways (see Table 2.11).

Recurrence risks

Types I and IV: AD inheritance.

- Most type II is caused by *de novo* dominant mutations and recurrences are due to germline mosaicism. Recurrence risk was traditionally given as 7% (Cole and Dalgleish 1995), suggesting a high rate of gonadal mosaicism. Some of these cases may have been due to AR forms with phenotypic overlap, but gonadal mosaicism remains an important consideration in AD forms of OI and justifies the offer of molecular PND in subsequent pregnancies (where possible).
- Type III: mostly AD, except for southern African where there is an AR form that is also reported in an Irish kindred and in several other consanguineous families. Germline mosaicism risk is likely to be similar to that of type II.
- Types V–VII are not caused by mutations in collagen I. Type V follows AD inheritance, types VI, VII, and VIII are AR.

Prenatal diagnosis

This is mostly requested by couples who have a child with type II or type III OI.

- USS will detect recurrence of type II and most of type III in the second trimester. Safe and effective, but relatively late diagnosis.
- CVS is possible when the diagnosis has been confirmed by molecular methods or collagen studies.
- Amniocentesis is not suitable for collagen studies.

Management of delivery

Cubert *et al.* (2001) reviewed the records of 167 babies affected by OI. There was an unusually high incidence of breech presentation at term (37%). In infants with non-lethal forms of OI, 40% delivered by LSCS and 32% delivered vaginally had new fractures. LSCS did not decrease the fracture rate at birth in infants with non-lethal OI nor did it prolong survival for those with lethal forms. If a baby is diagnosed to have OI antenatally, normal delivery is generally advised in the absence of obstetric indications for a Caesarean section. Unless progress through the second stage is normal, it may be best to avoid an instrumental delivery and proceed with LSCS if delivery needs to be expedited because of fetal distress.

Natural history and further management (preventative measures)

Bisphosphonates are a safe and effective therapy, as part of multidisciplinary management including occupational therapy and physiotherapy and orthopaedic and other surgical interventions. Bisphosphonates can be given by mouth or intravenously (IV); recent evidence using risedronate shows a clear and rapid reduction in fracture risk (Bishop *et al.* 2013).

Support groups: Brittle Bone Society (UK), http://www.brittlebone.org; Osteogenesis Imperfecta Foundation (USA), http://www.oif.org.

Expert adviser: Nick Bishop, Professor of Paediatric Bone Disease, Academic Unit of Child Health, Department of Oncology and Metabolism, University of Sheffield, Sheffield Children's Hospital, Sheffield, UK.

References

Bank RA, Robins SP, Wijmenga C, et al. Defective collagen crosslinking in bone, but not in ligament or cartilage, in Bruck syndrome: indications for a bone-specific telopeptide lysyl hydroxylase on chromosome 17. *Proc Natl Acad Sci, U S A* 1999; **96**: 1054–8.

Bishop N, Adami S, Ahmed SF, et al. Risedronate in children with osteogenesis imperfecta: a randomised, double-blind, placebo-controlled trial. *Lancet* 2013; **382**: 1424–32.

Bonadio J, Ramirez F, Barr M. An intron mutation in the human alpha 1(I) collagen gene alters the efficiency of pre-mRNA splicing and is associated with osteogenesis imperfecta type II. *J Biol Chem* 1990; **265**: 2262–8.

Byers PH, Cole WG. Osteogenesis imperfecta. In: PM Royce, B Steinmann (eds.). *Connective tissue and its heritable disorders*, 2nd edn, pp. 385–430. Wiley-Liss, New York, 2002.

Cole WG, Dalgleish R. Perinatal lethal osteogenesis imperfecta. *J Med Genet* 1995; **32**: 284–9.

Cubert R, Cheng EY, Mack S, Pepin MG, Byers PH. Osteogenesis imperfecta: mode of delivery and neonatal outcome. *Obstet Gynecol* 2001; **97**: 66–9.

Glorieux FH. Bisphosphonate therapy in severe osteogenesis imperfecta. *J Pediatr Endocrinol Metab* 2000; **13** (Suppl 2): 989–92.

Ha-Vinh R, Alanay Y, Bank RA, et al. Phenotypic and molecular characterization of Bruck syndrome (osteogenesis imperfecta with contractures of the large joints) caused by a recessive mutation in PLOD2. *Am J Med Genet A* 2004; **131A**: 115–20.

Lia-Baldini AS, Muller F, Taillandier A, et al. A molecular approach to dominance in hypophosphatasia. *Hum Genet* 2001; **109**: 99–108.

Plotkin H, Rauch F, Bishop NJ, et al. Pamidronate treatment of severe osteogenesis imperfecta in children under 3 years of age. *J Clin Endocrinol Metab* 2000; **85**: 1846–50.

Rauch F, Glorieux FH. Osteogenesis imperfecta. *Lancet* 2004; **363**: 1377–85.

Rauch F, Plotkin H, Zeitlin L, Glorieux F. Bone mass, size, and density in children and adolescents with osteogenesis imperfecta: effect of intravenous pamidronate therapy. *Bone Miner Res* 2003; **18**: 610–14.

Roughley PJ, Rauch F, Glorieux FH. Osteogenesis imperfecta—clinical and molecular diversity. *Eur Cell Mater* 2003; **5**: 41–7; discussion, 47.

Segarra NG, Ballhausen D, et al. NBAS mutations cause a multisystem disorder involving bone, connective tissue, liver, immune system, and retina. *Am J Med Genet A* 2015; **167A**(12): 2902–12.

Sillence DO, Senn A, Danks DM. Genetic heterogeneity in osteogenesis imperfecta. *J Med Genet* 1979; **16**: 101–16.

Tsipouras P. Osteogenesis imperfecta. In: P Beighton (ed.). *McKusick's heritable disorders of collagen*, 5th edn, pp. 281–314. Mosby, St Louis, 1993.

Ward LM, Lalic L, Roughley PJ, Glorieux FH. Thirty-three novel COL1A1 and COL1A2 mutations in patients with osteogenesis imperfecta types I–IV. *Hum Mutat* 2001; **17**: 434.

Zeitlin L, Fassier F, Glorieux FH. Modern approach to children with osteogenesis imperfecta. *J Pediatr Orthop B* 2003; **12**: 77–87.

Generalized disorders of skin pigmentation (including albinism)

The skin pigments (eumelanin and phaeomelanin) are produced in melanosomes by melanocytes, which are large cells found among the basal cells of the epidermis. The melanosomes are then transferred to keratinocytes. Melanocytes are of neural crest origin.

The first part of an assessment of skin pigmentation is to classify it as *generalized* or *only affecting a portion of the body* and then to decide whether the abnormality is of *hypo-* or *hyperpigmentation*. The non-generalized disorders are discussed elsewhere in 'Patchy pigmented skin lesions (including café-au-lait spots)', p. 278 and 'Patchy hypo- or depigmented skin lesions', p. 276 in Chapter 2, 'Clinical approach'. In many instances, the differentiation between hypo- and hyperpigmentation is not easy, and it may not be possible to establish which is the 'normal' skin colour.

Generalized hyperpigmentation

This is defined as an increased degree of skin pigmentation affecting the whole body.

Clinical approach

HISTORY: KEY POINTS
- Three-generation family tree. Enquire specifically for ethnicity and consanguinity.
- Always consider familial and racial background, as well as sun exposure and normal variation in skin tones (e.g. Futcher's line).

EXAMINATION: KEY POINTS
- Hair and eye colour.
- Skin on the palms and soles for pigmentation in the creases (endocrine abnormalities, e.g. Addison's).
- If appropriate, genital skin and areola of the nipple.
- Assess if there are any non-cutaneous features.

SPECIAL INVESTIGATIONS. Investigation is tailored to the likely underlying diagnosis (see below).

Some diagnoses to consider

- Endocrine causes such as Addison's disease, ALD, CAH.
- Metabolic disorders, including Wilson's disease, alkaptonuria, haemachromatosis.
- Syndromic conditions: Fanconi syndrome, insulin resistance syndromes, NF1.

Generalized hypopigmentation

Decreased pigmentation of the whole body.
- Albinism. Skin, hair, and eye pigment is absent or much reduced. The terms tyrosinase-positive (a milder phenotype) and tyrosinase-negative are older terms that have been replaced by OCA1A and OCA1B, respectively, since the genetic causes of oculocutaneous albinism (OCA) have been established.
- Albinoidism. The eye problems are not present. There may be features of other syndromes (see below).
- Generalized vitiligo. Common generalized vitiligo is an acquired depigmenting disorder characterized by a chronic and progressive loss of melanocytes from the epidermis and follicular reservoir. It sometimes clusters in families together with autoimmune thyroid disease, pernicious anaemia, lupus, Addison's disease, and adult-onset autoimmune diabetes.

Clinical approach

HISTORY: KEY POINTS
- Three-generation family tree with specific enquiry regarding consanguinity (OCA) and other affected family members.
- Visual problems.
- Easy bruising from toddlerhood (Hermansky–Pudlak syndrome (HPS)).
- Serious or recurrent infections (Chediak–Higashi syndrome (CHS)).
- Global developmental delay is not a feature of OCA.

EXAMINATION: KEY POINTS
- Skin, hair, and eye colour.
- Iris transillumination.
- Nystagmus and other indicators of poor visual acuity.
- Features of syndromes associated with reduced pigmentation.

SPECIAL INVESTIGATIONS
- Molecular testing for OCA syndromes is available but is rarely required for diagnostic reasons in those with a family history. Genomic analysis (e.g. panel/WES/WGS) may be helpful in the diagnosis of babies and young children with no family history.
- Ophthalmology referral for visual assessment, looking for albinism of the retina, and follow-up.
- Platelet testing if there are features to suggest HPS.
- Vacuolations in white cells in CHS.
- Additional diagnostic tests in presence of albinoid features rather than OCA.

Some diagnoses to consider

OCULOCUTANEOUS ALBINISM (OCA). OCA affects about one in 20 000. All types have generalized hypopigmentation (affecting skin, hair, and eyes). There are abnormalities in the decussation of the optic nerves. The visual problems are reduced acuity, nystagmus, and alternating strabismus (squint). The skin is more at risk from damage due to exposure to UV light.

- OCA1A and OCA1B. AR and caused by mutations in the *TYR* gene encoding tyrosinase on 11q14–21. Mutation detection rate is ~70–80%. OCA1 is divided into two types: type 1A, characterized by complete lack of tyrosinase activity due to production of an inactive enzyme; and type 1B (OCA1B), characterized by reduced activity of tyrosinase. Temperature-sensitive albinism is a subtype of OCA1B. Compound heterozygosity is common. OCA1 is the most common type of OCA in Caucasians but is uncommon in African-Americans and Africans. Together, OCA1A and OCA1B account for 40% of OCA. Most babies with tyrosine-deficient OCA have completely white hair at birth, even though in type 1B a certain amount of pigment may develop later.
- OCA2. This causes AR tyrosine-positive OCA and is caused by mutations in the *P* gene at 15q11–2. It accounts for about 50% of OCA worldwide. In OCA2, some pigment is present at birth and is lost later. Pigmented naevi may be another clue that the OCA is tyrosine-positive. OCA2 is common throughout sub-Saharan Africa where it is responsible for a high morbidity, with skin cancer and visual impairment

being important sequelae. OCA2 is uncommon in Caucasians. In blacks with this form of albinism, the hair is yellow and many pigmented spots develop in the skin. The occurrence of both brown oculocutaneous albinism (BOCA) and OCA2 within the same family suggest that these disorders are allelic. The 2.7-kb deletion on one allele in the *P* gene is the most frequent cause of OCA2 among southern African blacks.

- OCA3. This is often called rufous or red albinism due to reddish hair and skin colour. Some retinal pigment may be present on fundoscopy and sun sensitivity is less marked. In dark-skinned races, the diagnosis may not be obvious and signs such as nystagmus and red reflex on transillumination of the iris are important clues. AR and caused by mutations in *TYRP1* (tyrosinase-related protein 1) on 9p23.
- OCA4 (rare). Mutations have been reported in the *MATP* gene on 5p. AR.

It is thought that other OCA loci may be identified.

ALBINOID SYNDROMES.

- Phenylketonuria (PKU). PKU is a treatable AR inborn error of metabolism, resulting from a deficiency of phenylalanine hydroxylase and characterized by MR. It is caused by mutations in the *PAH* gene on 12q24.1. In the UK, neonates are screened for PKU using the Guthrie test ('heel-prick') on day 6 of life.
- Homocystinuria is an AR metabolic disorder due to deficiency of cystathionine beta-synthase, producing increased urinary homocystine and methionine. Major clinical manifestations involve the eyes (lens dislocation), the CNS (MR in untreated individuals), and the skeletal (Marfanoid habitus with long limbs and pectus excavatum, osteoporosis) and vascular systems (thrombotic lesions of arteries and veins, premature strokes).
- Prader–Willi syndrome (PWS) and Angelman syndrome (AS). Albinism occurs in association with PWS and AS where a del 15q11–12 has deleted one copy of the *P* gene and the child has an inherited *P* mutation on the other chromosome 15.
- Menkes syndrome. XLR disorder of copper metabolism. Main features are sparse, steely hair (with pili torti on microscopy) and progressive neurological impairment, often with seizures and spasticity.
- Chediak–Higashi syndrome (CHS). Rare AR disorder characterized by OCA, bleeding tendency, recurrent bacterial infections, and various neurological symptoms. This is a life-limiting condition, with children dying from infection or lymphoma, usually by 10 years. Intracellular vesicle formation is deficient, resulting in giant granules in many cells, e.g. giant melanosomes in the melanocytes. Diagnosis is by staining for giant lysosomal granules in the peripheral granulocytes or by mutation analysis of the *LYST* gene.
- Hermansky–Pudlack syndrome (HPS). Very rare AR disorder characterized by variable OCA, excessive bruising, nose bleeding and bleeding after dental extraction, progressive pulmonary fibrosis leading to death in the 4th or 5th decade, and granulomatous colitis. It is caused by mutations in *HPS* on 10q23. There is a founder effect in Puerto Ricans where the carrier rate is 1/18. Diagnosis is by EM of platelets which show absent platelet dense bodies.
- Griscelli syndrome. Rare AR disorder caused by mutations in the gene *myosin-Va* on 15q21. The disorder is similar to CHS. Infants have silver-grey hair and generalized hypo- or hyperpigmentation of the skin, immunodeficiency with recurrent infections, and lymphadenopathy, neutropenia, and low immunoglobulins.
- Cystinosis. Cystinosis presents in the first year of life with severe failure to thrive and photophobia with corneal crystals. There is renal tubular dysfunction with proteinuria, glycosuria, and a generalized aminoaciduria progressing to end-stage renal failure (ESRF). Affected individuals have lighter skin and hair pigmentation than their unaffected siblings. Incidence 1/100 000–1/200 000 live births. AR condition caused by mutations in the cystinosin gene (*CTNS*) on 17p13. A 65-kb deletion is present in either the homozygous or heterozygous state in 76% of cystinotic patients of European origin. Three types of cystinosis are recognized: (1) infantile nephropathic; (2) juvenile or adolescent nephropathic; and (3) adult non-nephropathic.

Genetic advice

RECURRENCE RISK. All the above-mentioned forms of OCA plus CHS and HPS follow AR inheritance.

CARRIER DETECTION. Some carriers of OCA type 1 are fairer than the population norm. Strabismus may be more prevalent, but generally carriers do not have problems.

PRENATAL DIAGNOSIS. Potentially possible by CVS if familial mutations are known.

Natural history and further management (preventative measures)

- Use of sun block is critical for individuals with OCA—risk of cutaneous malignancy with UV exposure.
- Protect the skin from UV damage by using broad-spectrum sunscreens with a sun protection factor of 45 or greater.
- Protect the eyes with sunglasses and hats with broad brims or peaks.

Support group: Albinism Fellowship, http://www.albinism.org.uk.

References

Dotta L, Parolini S, Prandini A, *et al*. Clinical, laboratory and molecular signs of immunodeficiency in patients with partial oculo-cutaneous albinism. *Orphanet J Rare Dis* 2013; **8**: 168.

Sybert VP. *Genetic skin disorders, Oxford monographs in medical genetics*. Oxford University Press, New York, 1997.

Hemihypertrophy and limb asymmetry

Hemihyperplasia, hemiatrophy, hemihypoplasia.

This may affect the face, or a single limb, or half the body. If facial asymmetry is the only feature, see 'Facial asymmetry' in Chapter 2, 'Clinical approach', p. 146. Some degree of asymmetry is not unusual in the general population. A small percentage of normal children have a minor discrepancy of foot size when measured for shoes, but a difference sufficient to require differently sized shoes for each foot is unusual. Similarly leg length discrepancy is not an uncommon referral to a paediatric orthopaedic clinic. A discrepancy of >1 cm in limb length, together with a measurable difference in limb circumference, should be regarded as abnormal.

It is often not that easy to decide which side is normal and whether the fundamental abnormality is hyperplasia or hypoplasia. Hemihypertrophy is more common in a developmentally normal or large child; hemihypoplasia is more likely in a child with a mosaic chromosome problem who may have developmental delay, growth retardation, and dysmorphic features.

Making limb measurements

See Figure 2.12.

To measure total upper limb length

With arms hanging loosely down, measure between the acromion (most prominent posterior lateral bony prominence of the shoulder joint) and the tip of the middle finger.

To measure total lower limb length

If the child can stand, measure between the greater trochanter and the floor (with measure perpendicular to the floor); for a baby, measure between the greater trochanter and the lateral malleolus of the ankle.

To measure limb circumference

Circumference measurements are taken at the widest diameter of the limb or from a fixed bony point, e.g. 10 cm distal to the lower edge of the patella. In the upper arm, the widest point is at the middle of the biceps, just below the insertion of the deltoid. In the upper leg (thigh), the widest point is usually just below the gluteal crease. In the lower leg (calf), the widest point is in the mid-upper calf muscle.

Clinical approach

History: key points

- Three-generation family tree with specific enquiry about birthweights, height, and cancer.
- Pregnancy, neonatal, and developmental history.

Examination: key points

- Growth parameters. Height, weight, and OFC.
- Observe the upper limbs with both arms hanging loosely by the child's side and compare sides. Photograph and measure as above.
- Observe the lower limbs with the child sitting with the legs outstretched on the bed and compare sides. Photograph and measure as above.
- Look carefully for CAL patches, abnormal skin pigmentation, vascular birthmarks, connective tissue, and epidermal naevi (Proteus syndrome), lymphatic malformations, and lipomas.
- Assess tongue size and symmetry.

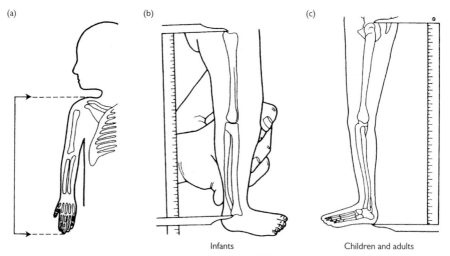

(a)   (b)   (c)

Infants   Children and adults

Figure 2.12 Measurement of limb length. (a) Total upper limb length. Measure between the acromion (the most prominent posterior lateral bony prominence of the shoulder joint) and the tip of the middle finger. (b) Total lower limb length. In infants, measure between the greater trochanter of the femur to the lateral malleolus of the ankle. (c) In older children and adults, measure from the greater trochanter to the plane of the sole of the foot (floor).
Reproduced with permission from Judith G. Hall JG, Froster-Iskenius UG, and Allanson JE, *Handbook of Normal Physical Measurements*, Figure 8.4, page 227 and Figure 8.34, page 253, Copyright © 1989 Oxford University Press, New York, USA. www.oup.com.

- Look for features of BWS (see below).
- Look for syndactyly and macrodactyly.

Special investigations
- Genomic analysis in presence of features suggestive of a chromosomal or syndromic diagnosis, e.g. genomic array, gene panel or WES/WGS as available.
  (1) Hemihypertrophy.
- Chromosome analysis by highest resolution available (looking especially for 11p15dup), including genomic array.
- DNA for 11p15 methylation and dosage studies, e.g. by methylation-specific multiplex ligation-dependent probe amplification (MS-MLPA), to look for UPD 11p15, isolated 11p15 methylation defects, and 11p15 copy number abnormalities.
- Renal USS at diagnosis. See later for advice on Wilms tumour.
  (2) Hemihypotrophy.
- Chromosome analysis with mosaicism screen by highest resolution available (including genomic array).
- Skin biopsy for chromosome analysis if developmental delay (especially with syndactyly or hypomelanosis of Ito) if blood karyotype is normal.

Some diagnoses to consider

Beckwith–Wiedemann syndrome (BWS)
Macrosomia (prenatal and/or postnatal), hemihypertrophy, macroglossia, abdominal wall defect (omphalocele, umbilical hernia, diastasis recti), ear anomalies. See 'Beckwith–Wiedemann syndrome (BWS)' in Chapter 3, 'Common consultations', p. 358.

Neurofibromatosis type 1 (NF1)
See 'Neurofibromatosis type 1 (NF1)' in Chapter 3, 'Common consultations', p. 506.

McCune–Albright syndrome
A syndromic association between polyostotic fibrous dysplasia, cutaneous pigmentation (coast of Maine areas of CAL-coloured pigmentation), and precocious puberty (50% of affected girls and some affected boys). Caused by mosaicism for somatic activating mutation in the *GNAS* gene. Recurrence risks are very low.

Proteus syndrome
A complex and variable disorder characterized by limb asymmetry, disproportionate overgrowth of hands and/or feet and especially digits, vascular and lymphatic malformations, and cranial hyperostosis (see Box 2.4). Proteus is sporadic and caused by somatic mosaicism for an *AKT* mutation. Most babies show comparatively little asymmetry at birth, although they may have vascular or lymphatic malformations. The condition is very progressive in early childhood but tends to change little after adolescence. IQ is usually normal.

Macrocephaly–capillary malformation syndrome and related disorders
An overlapping group of disorders are now recognized that cause regional overgrowth, including in some cases macrodactyly, together with other features including megalencephaly, neuronal migration defects/polymicrogyria. Capillary malformations (often philtral) and other vascular malformations are often present, as is lipoma. The course of the overgrowth may be progressive but is less aggressive than in Proteus syndrome and may be present prenatally. Syndactyly of toes 2–3 and polydactyly are recurrent features. The conditions are sporadic and somatic mosaic mutations in *PIK3CA*, *AKT3*, and *PIK3R2* have been identified.

Klippel–Trenaunay syndrome (KTS)
Combined capillary, lymphatic, and venous malformation, varicosities, and limb enlargement. Lower limb involved in 95%; upper limb in 5%. Fifteen per cent have combined upper and lower limb involvement. Trunk involvement is not common. Capillary malformations of the skin are purplish in colour. Lymphoedema is common. Lower limb enlargement is present in nearly all cases—the limb being thicker and longer. Macrodactyly may involve the toes on the affected foot. There is overlap with macrocephaly–capillary malformation syndrome.

Parkes Weber syndrome
Characterized by a cutaneous vascular flush due to capillary malformation often with arteriovenous malformations (CM-AVM) in association with soft tissue and skeletal hypertrophy of the affected limb. May be caused by heterozygous variants in *RASA1* gene (Revencu 2013).

Box 2.4 Diagnostic criteria for Proteus syndrome

Proteus syndrome = mosaic distribution of lesions + progressive course + sporadic + one from A, or two from B or three from C

A Connective tissue naevus (fibrous connective tissue with gyral pattern occurring most frequently on the soles, but also found on the palms and abdomen)

B i Epidermal naevus (linear, whorled, or verrucous and usually found on the neck, trunk, or extremities). Appear like areas of leathery discoloured skin and are present from infancy

ii Disproportionate overgrowth of the limbs (arms/legs/hands/feet/digits), skull, external auditory meatus, vertebrae, or viscera (spleen/thymus)

iii Specific tumours <20 years (bilateral ovarian cystadenomas, parotid monomorphic adenoma)

C i Dysregulated adipose tissue (lipomas, or regional absence of fat)

ii Vascular malformations (capillary malformation, venous malformation, lymphatic malformation)

iii Facial phenotype (dolicocephaly, long face, minor downslanting palpebral fissures and/or minor ptosis, wide or anteverted nares, open mouth appearance)

Silver–Russell syndrome (SRS)
Failure to thrive, proportionately large head, but usually between 3rd and 25th centiles, triangular face, and down-turned mouth. Asymmetry is a key diagnostic feature. See 'Failure to thrive' in Chapter 2, 'Clinical approach', p. 150.

Isolated hemihypertrophy
Isolated finding in an otherwise normal individual who after careful assessment has none of the features of the above conditions. Approximately 20% have an 11p15 abnormality as seen in BWS, i.e. it is a 'forme fruste' of these disorders. In Hoyme *et al.*'s (1998) multicentre study, tumours developed in 9/168 patients (5.9%). Tumours are of embryonal origin (similar to those seen in BWS), including Wilms tumour (3% in Hoyme *et al.*'s study). The risk of Wilms tumour is likely to be >5% in those with high-risk 11p15 defects and Wilms surveillance is recommended in these patients.

Genetic advice

Recurrence risk
As for the underlying diagnosis. If isolated hemihypertrophy, recurrence risk is likely to be low.

Prenatal diagnosis
As for the underlying diagnosis.

Natural history and further management (preventative measures)

- 3- to 4-monthly renal USS surveillance for Wilms tumour during first 7 years of life for BWS or isolated hemihypertrophy with molecular evidence of BWS (unless due to isolated KvDMR hypomethylation). See 'Wilms tumour' in Chapter 4, 'Cancer', p. 620.
- Regular clinical surveillance and imaging if Proteus syndrome.
- Otherwise manage as for specific diagnosis.

Support group: Many of the individual syndromes have their own support groups. See Contact a Family, http://www.cafamily.org.uk.

Expert adviser: Richard Scott, Consultant in Clinical Genetics, Great Ormond Street Hospital NHS Foundation Trust, London, UK.

References

Cohen MM Jr, Neri G, Weksberg R. *Overgrowth syndromes, Oxford monographs on medical genetics no. 43*. Oxford University Press, Oxford, 2002.

Hoyme HE, Seaver LH, Jones KL, *et al.* Isolated hemihyperplasia (hemihypertrophy): report of a prospective multicenter study of the incidence of neoplasia and review. *Am J Med Genet* 1998; **79**: 274–8.

Revencu N, Boon LM, Mendola A, *et al.* RASA1 mutations and associated phenotypes in 68 families with capillary malformation-arteriovenous malformation. *Hum Mutat* 2013; **34**: 1632–41.

Scott RH, Walker L, Olsen OE, *et al.* Surveillance for Wilms tumour in at-risk children: pragmatic recommendations for best practice. *Arch Dis Child* 2006; **91**: 995–9.

Weksberg R, Shuman C, Smith AC. Beckwith–Wiedemann syndrome. *Am J Med Genet C Semin Med Genet* 2005; **137C**: 12–23.

Holoprosencephaly (HPE)

During embryonic life, the forebrain vesicle divides along the dorsal midline to form the cerebral hemispheres. Failure, or partial failure, of this cleavage results in, respectively, *alobar holoprosencephaly* where the two lateral ventricles are replaced by a single midline ventricle (which is often greatly enlarged), and part fusion of the frontal lobes (*lobar holoprosencephaly*). Other midline forebrain structures, including the olfactory bulbs and tracts, optic bulbs and tracts, corpus callosum, thalamus, hypothalamus, and pituitary, are frequently also affected.

The development of the midface is related to that of the forebrain and there is a range of anomalies, particularly affecting the mid-facial structures (eyes, nose, midline cleft lip) associated with HPE. Cyclopia, where there is a single midline orbit with abnormal eye tissue, is the most severe malformation. The nose in cyclopic babies is usually represented by a proboscis that is sited above the orbit.

HPE occurs in ~1/10 000 live births, but in 1/250 during early embryogenesis, since most affected fetuses are miscarried. It is genetically heterogeneous—chromosomal in up to 50% (especially +13, and many other small deletions (including 7q36) and duplications), recognizable syndrome in 15%, familial AD in some, and *de novo* AD mutation in some of the remainder. To date, heterozygous mutations in 15 genes have been identified in HPE patients (see Box 2.5).

Associated facial features

HPE may be identified on USS in pregnancy, or a neonate is born with *hypotelorism* and *median (midline) cleft lip* in whom cranial USS or MRI reveals HPE. The most extreme form of craniofacial malformation is cyclopia (a single central eye) with a nose-like structure (proboscis) above it. More commonly, there is severe hypotelorism, a flat nose with a single nostril, ocular coloboma/microphthalmia, and median clefting of the upper lip. Milder cases can have bilateral or unilateral CL/P, slight hypotelorism, and a single central upper incisor. Up to 20% of children with major brain malformations have only minor dysmorphic features.

Alobar holoprosencephaly

In alobar HPE, the cerebrum is a single U-shaped mass, without division into right and left hemispheres. Most affected children die before, during, or soon after birth. Fifty per cent of live births with alobar HPE will have died by 4 months of age, but survival for several years is possible (such children have profound learning disability, seizures, and feeding difficulties often requiring gastrostomy). Pituitary and hypothalamic dysfunction is common.

Semilobar and lobar holoprosencephaly

In semilobar and lobar HPE, there is more complete development of the right and left cerebral hemispheres (see Figure 2.13). Many affected children live into adulthood, although early death is also common. Seizures are common. Some degree of learning disability is usual. There is a spectrum of severity, from children with severe semilobar HPE having problems similar to those seen in alobar HPE through to minimal disability and a normal lifespan in the mildest forms of lobar HPE.

Clinical approach

History: key points

- Three-generation family history.
- History of HPE, microcephaly, anosmia, or single central incisor tooth in other family members may indicate that this is a family with AD HPE.
- Maternal diabetes mellitus (infants of diabetic mothers have an overall ~1% risk for HPE—a 200-fold risk, compared with the general population).
- Raised maternal age (increased risk for trisomy 13).

Examination: key points

- Birthweight (reduced in most chromosomal imbalance).
- OFC. Shape of cranium, microcephaly, trigonocephaly.
- Eyes. Spectrum from hypotelorism through to cyclopia.
- Nose. Spectrum from midline proboscis through absence of the anterior nasal spine and nasal septum and a single nostril.
- Mouth. Spectrum ranging from poorly defined cupid's bow and an absent labial frenulum through to midline clefting of the upper lip with associated cleft palate (sometimes referred to as premaxillary agenesis).
- Agnathia (agnathia–HPE).
- Other midline anomalies, e.g. CHD, anal anomalies.
- Limbs. Polydactyly (Pallister–Hall syndrome, pseudotrisomy 13), 2/3 toe syndactyly (SLO syndrome).
- Examine the parents, including testing for anosmia.

Special investigations

- Chromosomes. Use QF PCR in pregnancy to exclude trisomy 13.
- MRI scan for better delineation of cranial anatomy if diagnosis based on cranial USS.
- Genomic array, gene panel, WES, WGS as appropriate. Due to genetic heterogeneity a gene panel approach with dosage enhances diagnostic detection rates.
- 7-dehydrocholesterol to exclude SLO syndrome.

Some diagnoses to consider

Chromosomal imbalance

Up to 50% of HPE has a chromosomal aetiology. Trisomy 13 is the most common abnormality, but many other anomalies have been described. Particularly exclude loci known to have been associated with HPE. Triploidy may be found in fetuses with HPE.

Box 2.5 Top 10 genes implicated in the pathogenesis of holoprosencephaly with their frequency (%), in a cohort of 257 HPE patients (Dubourg 2016)

SHH (5.8%)	AD
ZIC2 (4.7%)	AD
GLI2 (3.1%)	AD
SIX3 (2.7%)	AD
FGFR8 (2.3%)	AD
DISP1 (1.2%)	AD
DLL1 (1.2%)	AD
SUFU (0.4%)	AD

(a) 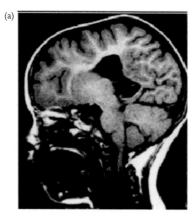 (b)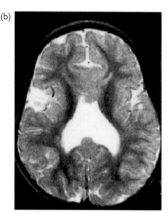

Figure 2.13 (a) Semilobar holoprosencephaly in a girl aged 2 years imaged with T1-weighted sagittal MRI. This midline view shows absence of the corpus callosum and fusion of the frontal lobes. (b) Semilobar holoprosencephaly in the same patient using T2-weighted axial MRI. There is fusion of the frontal lobes of both central hemispheres and a common central ventricle. Reproduced with permission from Verity CM, Firth H and Ffrench-Constant C, Developmental abnormalities of the central nervous system. In David A. Warrell, Timothy M. Cox, and John D. Firth, *Oxford Textbook of Medicine*, Fourth edition, 2003, Figure 2, page 1205, with permission from Oxford University Press.

AD HPE

AD HPE is characterized by incomplete penetrance and extreme intrafamilial variability. Variability may be due to a digenic/multigenic mode of inheritance. The transmitting parent may have a single central incisor as their only manifestation, or even be clinically normal. When a mutation is identified in an affected child, it is not uncommon to find that it is inherited from an unaffected parent.

The most common single gene associated with HPE is sonic hedgehog *SHH* detectable in 37% of AD families.

Environmental causes
Maternal diabetes: 200-fold increased risk for HPE.

Pallister–Hall syndrome
AD with mutation in *GLI3* at 7p13 which is a major downstream effector of *SHH* signalling. Hypothalamic hamartoblastoma, PAP, imperforate anus, hypospadias. Highly variable. Examine the parents for features.

Smith–Lemli–Opitz (SLO) syndrome
A rare, but testable, cause of HPE. The diagnostic test is measurement of 7-dehydrocholesterol in the blood. PAP, cleft palate, hypospadias, and 2/3 syndactyly are features that may suggest the diagnosis in a neonate. The frequency is ~1 in 20 000–30 000. HPE occurs in 75% of patients with SLO. See 'Hypospadias' in Chapter 2, 'Clinical approach', p. 186.

Pseudotrisomy 13 or HPE polydactyly syndrome
AR. PAP and heart defects. Similarities to hydrolethalus syndrome.

Agnathia–HPE
Carefully exclude a chromosomal imbalance. One report of possible dominant inheritance.

Fetal akinesia sequence
Features are microcephaly, poor fetal movement, and contractures. There are reports of families with XL inheritance.

Genetic advice

Recurrence risk
If after careful assessment the diagnosis is isolated HPE, consider if either parent could be minimally affected.

Enquire about family history. Enquire about missing teeth or anosmia. Careful clinical examination of both parents looking for hypotelorism, a poorly defined Cupid's bow, an absent labial frenulum, and a single central incisor. Arrange an MRI scan of both parents for any evidence of a midline lesion.

- For sporadic cases with no family history, normal genetic analysis and normal parents, recurrence risk counselling is difficult if the underlying cause has not been identified. Recurrence risk can range from as low as 0% to as high as 50% (but see comment below regarding risk for a severely affected child with AD inheritance).
- For AD families, the risk of an obligate carrier having a severely affected child is 16–21%; the risk of milder effects is 13–14%. Males may be at greater risk than females for major malformations outside the CNS.
- For chromosomal and syndromic cases, counsel as for the specific diagnosis.

Prenatal diagnosis
If a specific chromosomal defect or gene mutation has been identified, PND by CVS or amniocentesis would be possible.

If not, PND by detailed USS should enable detection of a severely affected fetus. Scanning could begin at 16 weeks when it should be possible to visualize the lateral ventricles, although repeat later scans will be required to exclude recurrence.

Prognosis
HPE is a serious developmental disorder, but the prognosis depends on the severity of the abnormality and the presence of other malformations. See Barr and Cohen (1999).

Support groups: Many of the individual syndromes have their own support groups. See Contact a Family, http://www.cafamily.org.uk.

Expert adviser: Max Muenke, Chief, Medical Genetics Branch, National Institutes of Health, Bethesda, Maryland, USA.

References

Barr M Jr, Cohen MM Jr. Holoprosencephaly survival and performance. *Am J Med Genet* 1999; **89**: 116–20.

Dubourg C, Carré W, Hamdi-Rozé H, *et al.* Mutational spectrum in holoprosencephaly shows that FGF is a new major signaling pathway. *Hum Mutat* 2016; **37**(12): 1329–39.

Goodman FR. Congenital abnormalities of body patterning: embryology revisited. *Lancet* 2003; **362**: 651–62.

Gropman AS, Muenke M. Holoprosencephaly. In: SB Cassidy, JE Allanson (eds.). *Management of genetic syndromes*, 3rd edn, pp. 441–59. John Wiley & Sons, Inc., Hoboken, 2010.

Kauvar EF, Muenke M. Holoprosencephaly: recommendations for diagnosis and management. *Curr Opin Pediatr* 2010; **22**: 687–95.

Muenke M, Solomon BD, Odent S. Introduction to the *American Journal of Medical Genetics Part C* on holoprosencephaly. *Am J Med Genet C Semin Med Genet* 2010; **154C**: 1–2.

Roessler E, Belloni E, Gaudenz K, *et al.* Mutations in the human sonic hedgehog gene cause holoprosencephaly. *Nat Genet* 1996; **14**: 357–60.

Roessler E, Muenke M. The molecular genetics of holoprosencephaly. *Am J Med Genet C Semin Med Genet* 2010; **154C**: 52–61.

Solomon BD, Gropman AS, Muenke M. Holoprosencephaly overview. In: RA Pagon, TD Bird, CR Dolan, K Stephens, MP Adam (eds.). *GeneReviews®* [Internet]. University of Washington, Seattle, 2000 (last updated 2013).

Solomon BD., Pineda-Alvarez DE, Mercier S, Raam MS, Odent S, Muenke M. Holoprosencephaly flashcards: a summary for the clinician. *Am J Med Genet C Semin Med Genet* 2010; **154C**: 3–7.

Whiteford M, Tolmie JL. Holoprosencephaly in the West of Scotland 1975–1994. *J Med Genet* 1996; **33**: 578–84.

Hydrocephalus

Congenital hydrocephalus comprises a diverse group of conditions in which there are impaired circulation and absorption of CSF. The incidence is 4–8/10 000 live births and stillbirths. Congenital malformations of the CNS, e.g. spina bifida, infections, e.g. congenital infection or meningitis, and haemorrhage can all give rise to hydrocephalus. Infants commonly present with progressive macrocephaly whereas children older than 2 years generally present with signs and symptoms of intracranial hypertension (Kahle 2016).

The CSF flows from the lateral ventricles into the third ventricle through the foramina of Monro, and then into the fourth ventricle via the aqueduct of Sylvius. The CSF leaves the ventricular system through the foramen of Magendie (into the cisterna magna) and the foramina of Luschka (into the pontine cistern). See Figure 2.14.

Hydrocephalus usually refers to *obstructive* or *non-communicating* hydrocephalus where all or part of the ventricular system is enlarged. In *aqueduct stenosis*, the lateral and third ventricles are enlarged, but not the fourth ventricle (see Figure 2.15). Bleeding into the ventricles may block the foramina, causing obstructive hydrocephalus, whereas bleeding into the subarachnoid space may impair resorption of CSF by the arachnoid villi, causing *non-obstructive* or *communicating* hydrocephalus.

Hydrocephalus causing increased intracranial pressure and progressive hydrocephalus are treated by insertion of a ventriculoperitoneal (VP) shunt.

Clinical approach

History: key points
- Detailed three-generation family tree. Extend further on the maternal side, if possible. Enquire specifically for other relatives with hydrocephalus, unexplained stillbirths, spasticity, mental handicap, or NTDs. (NTDs and hydrocephalus can occur in the same family.)

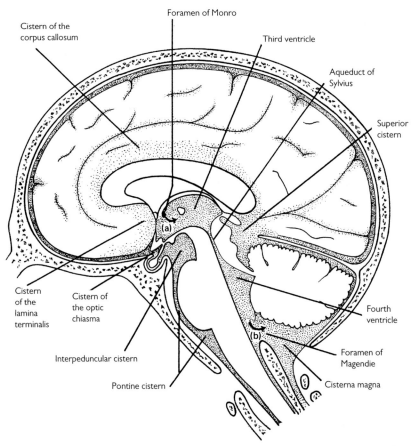

Figure 2.14 Subarachnoid cisterns. (a) Cerebrospinal fluid entering the third ventricle from the lateral ventricle through the foramen of Monro. (b) Cerebrospinal fluid entering the cisterna magna from the fourth ventricle through the foramen of Magendie.
Reproduced with permission from John Kiernan and Raj Rajakumar, *Barr's The Human Nervous System: An Anatomical Viewpoint*, p. 369, Lippincott Williams and Wilkins, 2013.

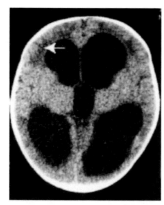

Figure 2.15 Aqueduct stenosis in a boy aged 1 month with a bulging anterior fontanelle and an increasing head circumference. Axial CT shows gross dilatation of the third and lateral ventricles (the fourth ventricle is not shown but was normal in size). Note the periventricular low density due to transependymal exudation of cerebrospinal fluid under pressure (arrow).
Reproduced with permission from Verity CM, Firth H and Ffrench-Constant C, Developmental abnormalities of the central nervous system. In David A. Warrell, Timothy M. Cox, and John D. Firth, *Oxford Textbook of Medicine*, Fourth edition, 2003, Figure 8, page 1213, with permission from Oxford University Press.

- Consanguinity. MEB and proliferative vasculopathy and hydranencephaly–hydrocephaly malformation.
- Enquire about infections in pregnancy.
- Was ventriculomegaly noted on antenatal scans? What was the OFC at birth?
- Detailed perinatal history enquiring for secondary causes of hydrocephalus. Was there intracranial haemorrhage, e.g. intraventricular haemorrhage (IVH), following premature delivery? Was there neonatal meningitis?
- Developmental milestones.
- Seizures.
- Exclude clinical features of raised intracranial pressure.

Examination: key points
- Height, OFC, and fontanelle size and tension. (Has the OFC crossed centiles?)
- Head shape.
- Palpate the VP shunt, if present.
- Eyes. 'Setting sun' sign, microphthalmia (MEB).
- Spina bifida?
- Other congenital malformations and dysmorphic features (syndromic and chromosomal conditions).
- In a male infant, look carefully for congenitally adducted thumbs, thumb/radial hypoplasia in XL VACTERL with hydrocephalus.
- In a male infant, detailed neurological exam looking for spasticity (increased tone, exaggerated DTRs, and extensor plantar response).
- CAL skin lesions (NF1).

Special investigations
- Review MRI scan for:
  - complications associated with prematurity, e.g. periventricular leucomalacia;

- tumours and cysts;
- structural malformations like aqueduct stenosis, Chiari malformation, DWM;
- cortical abnormality such as cobblestone (type II) lissencephaly;
- intracranial calcification (congenital infections;
- differentiation from hydranencephaly;
- to look for evidence of cerebral atrophy.
- Skull X-ray if there are features suggestive of premature cranial suture closure.
- CK (elevated CK ~3000 iu/l; MEB disease (WWS)).
- Ophthalmology opinion (papilloedema, optic atrophy, oculomotor palsy, retinal dysplasia (MEB), features of congenital infection).
- Genomic array, gene panel, WES, WGS as appropriate.
- TORCH screen for congenital infection in babies <6 months of age.
- Consider *L1CAM* mutation analysis if male infant with aqueduct stenosis and positive family history or suggestive clinical features (e.g. adducted thumbs, spasticity, agenesis or hypoplasia of the corpus callosum). Mutation detection rate is 75% in families with three affected male members, and 15% with a negative family history.
- Review brain histology of any affected individuals.

Some diagnoses to consider

Arnold–Chiari malformation
- Type I. Downward displacement of the lower cerebellum, including the tonsils; rarely causes symptoms in childhood but may be associated with hydrocephalus and syringomyelia.
- Type II. Downward displacement of the cerebellar vermis, tonsils, and medulla through the foramen magnum and associated with myelomeningocele (see 'Neural tube defects' in Chapter 3, 'Common consultations', p. 500). Counsel as for NTD.

Hydranencephaly

Scans show a small rim of cerebral cortex, but the cerebellum and brainstem may be normal. Disruption to the carotid artery supply is one cause. Enquire about early pregnancy and also consider the possibility of *COL4A1/2* mutation which classically presents with porencephaly. Biallelic mutations in *FLVCR2* are associated with proliferative vasculopathy and hydranencephaly–hydrocephaly malformation. Hydranencephaly may be confused with holoprosencephaly (HPE).

Arachnoid cyst

A cystic cavity within the arachnoid membrane. Hydrocephalus can occur by obstruction and reduced CSF resorption. The majority of arachnoid cysts are sporadic. See 'Structural intracranial anomalies (agenesis of the corpus callosum, septo-optic dysplasia, and arachnoid cysts)' in Chapter 2, 'Clinical approach', p. 320.

X-linked hydrocephalus
- The neural cell adhesion molecule *L1CAM* plays a key role during neurodevelopment. The gene encoding *L1CAM* maps to Xq28, and males with mutation in this gene have a phenotype characterized by a combination of corpus callosum hypoplasia, MR, adducted thumbs, spastic paraplegia, and hydrocephalus. There is a high degree of intra- and interfamilial variability.

- XL hydrocephalus with features of VACTERL. Two known genes: *FANCB* and *ZIC3*. *ZIC3* may have associated heterotaxy.

Muscle–eye–brain disease (MEB)
These are AR disorders that share the combination of cerebral neuronal migration defects (cobblestone lissencephaly), ocular abnormalities, and CMD. The features of MEB are hydrocephalus, agyria, retinal dystrophy, and sometimes an encephalocele—thus its alternate name of HARD ± E. Both are due to genes in the *O*-mannosylation pathway (*POMT1* gene in WWS and *POMGNT1* in MEB). See 'Lissencephaly, polymicrogyria, and neuronal migration disorders' in Chapter 2, 'Clinical approach', p. 216.

Neurofibromatosis type 1 (NF1)
Aqueduct stenosis is a rare, but well-recognized, complication in infancy. See 'Neurofibromatosis type 1 (NF1)' in Chapter 3, 'Common consultations', p. 506.

Achondroplasia
Most infants with achondroplasia are macrocephalic. OFC should be plotted on achondroplasia-specific charts and monitored serially (every 1–2 months) during the first years of life. Hydrocephalus is usually communicating but can also be due to cervicomedullary compression (small foramen magnum, displacement of the brainstem). See 'Achondroplasia' in Chapter 3, 'Common consultations', p. 334.

Craniosynostosis syndromes
Affected infants may have raised intracranial pressure from the synostosis, but ventricular dilatation is an additional reason. See 'Craniosynostosis' in Chapter 3, 'Common consultations', p. 378.

Genetic advice

The extent to which some degree of neurological impairment or abnormal neurological signs are attributed to sequelae of sustained hydrocephalus *in utero* may determine how exhaustive a search is made for an underlying cause. Discussion with a paediatric neurologist may be very helpful in making this judgement.

Recurrence risk
Review babies and young infants when older to exclude other signs of a genetic disorder, e.g. NF1.

After careful evaluation and exclusion of syndromic conditions:

- the empiric risk for sibs of an isolated case is up to 5%, all studies showing a higher risk for male sibs of an affected male;

- the risk for male sibs of an isolated male case with aqueduct stenosis is higher (5–10%), unless *L1CAM* has been excluded;
- children of consanguineous parents may have hydrocephalus as part of an AR condition.

Carrier detection
This is possible in families with a known mutation or by linked markers in XL families.

Prenatal diagnosis
PND based on early USS is often not reliable as ventriculomegaly usually starts after 20 weeks of gestation and may not appear until near term or after delivery. Serial USS is often offered in a subsequent pregnancy, but these limitations must be carefully discussed with the parents. See 'Ventriculomegaly' in Chapter 6, 'Pregnancy and fertility', p. 802.

Support group: Support and advice about hydrocephalus are available from Shine (charity for spina bifida and hydrocephalus), https://www.shinecharity.org.uk.

References

Kiernan JA, Rajakumar N. *Barr's the human nervous system. An anatomical viewpoint*, 10th edn. Lippincott Williams & Wilkins, Baltimore, 2014.

Burton BK. Recurrence risks for congenital hydrocephalus. *Clin Genet* 1979; **16**: 47–53.

Fransen E, Van Camp G, D'Hooge R, *et al*. Genotype–phenotype correlation in L1 associated diseases. *J Med Genet* 1998; **35**: 399–404.

Howard FM, Till K, Carter CO. A family study of hydrocephalus. *J Med Genet* 1981; **18**: 252–5.

Kahle KT, Kulkarni AV, *et al*. Hydrocephalus in children. *Lancet* 2016; **387**(10020): 788–99.

Kenwrick S, Jouet M, Donnai D. X-linked hydrocephalus and MASA syndrome. *J Med Genet* 1996; **33**: 59–65.

Meyer E, Ricketts C, Morgan NV, *et al*. Mutations in *FLVCR2* are associated with proliferative vasculopathy and hydranencephaly-hydrocephaly syndrome (Fowler syndrome). *Am J Hum Genet* 2010; **86**: 471–8.

Schrander-Stumpel C, Fryns JP. Congenital hydrocephalus: nosology and guidelines for clinical approach and genetic counselling. *Eur J Pediatr* 1998; **157**: 355–62.

Varadi V, Toth A, Torok O. Heterogeneity and recurrence risk for congenital hydrocephalus (ventriculomegaly): a prospective study, *Am J Med Genet* 1988; **29**: 305–10.

Warrell D (ed.). *Oxford textbook of medicine*, 4th edn. Oxford University Press, Oxford, 2003.

Hypermobile joints

Joint hypermobility syndrome, ligamentous laxity, joint laxity, loose-jointed, double-jointed.

Hypermobile joints have an excessive range of movement usually due to alterations in the soft tissues that surround the joint. The ligaments consist principally of collagen, but elastic tissue containing fibrillin and elastin is also important. Hypermobility is typically evaluated using the Beighton scoring system described below. Approximately 5–10% of school-age children are hypermobile, but the percentage decreases with age. It is more common in females at all ages. There is considerable normal variation in the range of joint movement between different ethnic groups.

Hypermobility is a diagnostic feature of Ehlers–Danlos syndrome (EDS) but also occurs in about 25% of patients with Marfan's syndrome (MFS). The benign joint hypermobility syndrome (EDS hypermobility type) is heterogeneous and generally differs from the other forms of EDS in that the skin involvement is less pronounced. Hypermobility needs to be differentiated from hypotonia of central or peripheral origin.

The 'Beighton scoring system' (see Table 2.12) assesses the degree to which specific joints can be hyperextended or hyperflexed. A point is given if an individual is able to perform the manoeuvre; the left and right are scored independently, giving a maximum score of 9. Generalized joint hypermobility is diagnosed when the Beighton score is:

≥ 6 pre-pubertal children and adolescents;
≥ 5 pubertal men and women to age 50;
≥ 4 men and women over the age of 50.

Clinical approach

History: key points

A child may be referred by a paediatrician or a bone and joint specialist who has noted the excessive hypermobility and asks if there are other conditions or associated features.

- Three-generation family tree. Ask about congenital dislocation of the hip (CDH), joint pain, and joint replacement surgery. Is there a history of premature cardiac death?
- Joint pain, dislocation, effusions.

Table 2.12 Beighton scoring system

Type of hypermobility	Score
Passive extension of the little finger metacarpophalangeal (MCP) joint to ≥90° (1 point for each hand)	2
Passive apposition of the thumb to the flexor aspect of the forearm (1 point for each hand)	2
Hyperextension of the elbow by >10° (1 point for each elbow)	2
Hyperextension of the knee by >10° (1 point for each knee)	2
Bend forward and flex the spine. Palms of the hands touch the floor with the knees extended	1
Total score	9

Reprinted with permission from Beighton P and MuKusick VA, *MuKusick's heritable disorders of connective tissue*, Fifth Edition, copyright 1993, with permission from Elsevier.

- Abnormal skin scarring after trauma. Easy bruising.
- Fractures after minor trauma (OI).
- Motor milestones may be delayed, but global developmental delay indicates the possibility of a central neurological problem.

Examination: key points

- Assessment of joint mobility. Beighton score.
- Skin: excessive stretching and abnormal scars that are often described as like cigarette paper; excessive bruising (EDS). Cutis laxa can sometimes be confused with EDS. Redundant skinfolds and pseudotumours.
- Skeletal signs associated with joint hypermobility: flat feet (pes planus), knock knees (genu valgum), scoliosis.
- Heart murmurs. Floppy mitral valves are particularly common. Aortic root dilatation is typically absent or non-progressive in EDS but may rupture in MFS. Rupture of blood vessels and internal viscera in EDS vascular type.
- Hernias. More likely to recur after repair.
- Eyes. Retinal detachment (EDS), dislocated lenses (MFS), myopia (MFS and Stickler syndrome), blue sclerae (OI).
- Palate. High with dental crowding (MFS), cleft (Stickler syndrome, Larsen syndrome).
- Many skeletal dysplasias are caused by collagen mutations, but only a few (particularly pseudoachondroplasia) also have joint laxity. Milder dysplasias, such as Stickler syndrome, may be missed, unless specifically considered.
- Muscle strength to exclude myopathies and other causes of peripheral hypotonia.

Special investigations

Individuals with benign hypermobility rarely require special investigations.

- Molecular testing is available for some specific forms of EDS which are usually evident clinically. See 'Ehlers–Danlos syndrome (EDS)' in Chapter 3, 'Common consultations', p. 406.
- Radiology if CDH or other orthopaedic complications are present.
- Skeletal survey or limited skeletal survey for diagnostic reasons, e.g. in the presence of features of pseudoachondroplasia, Stickler syndrome, or OI.
- Cardiac echo if there is a murmur or clinical suspicion of MFS.

Some diagnoses to consider

The differential diagnosis will depend on the age of presentation and the presence of other features.

Ehlers–Danlos syndrome (EDS)—hypermobility type (benign joint hypermobility syndrome)

In this condition, there is isolated joint hypermobility and the diagnosis is made after excluding other syndromic causes of hypermobility. The child may sometimes present with delayed motor milestones. Labels, such as poor muscle tone, may have been used to describe the signs as the condition may be severe enough to cause floppiness in infancy. Fine, as well as gross, motor milestones may be delayed and the older child may be described as clumsy. There is no intellectual impairment. There may be a dominant family history. It is not a major cause of degenerative joint disease, although joint injuries are more common due to instability. This may lead to secondary osteoarthritis. Examine parents and assess their joint mobility. The condition is variable, but girls are usually more affected than boys. Carefully exclude CDH in subsequent children. Chronic joint pain is a possible troublesome complication for some individuals in the absence of obvious structural joint damage. There is considerable debate about whether this is actually more common than in the general population. The risk of widespread pain, autonomic dysfunction, and chronic fatigue has almost certainly been exaggerated but has not been subjected to systematic population studies. A diagnostic checklist for hEDS can be downloaded from www.ehlers-danlos. com/heds-diagnostic-checklist

Ehlers–Danlos syndrome (EDS), except EDS hypermobility type

There are several other types of EDS: joint hypermobility, hyperextensible skin, and tissue fragility with abnormal scarring and easy bruising are the major features. See 'Ehlers–Danlos syndrome (EDS)' in Chapter 3, 'Common consultations', p. 406.

Marfan's syndrome (MFS)

An AD systemic disorder of connective tissue with a high degree of clinical variability. Cardinal manifestations involve the ocular (myopia, lens dislocation), skeletal (pectus excavatum, pectus carinatum, scoliosis, long limbs, arachnodactyly, high palate), and cardiovascular systems (aortic root dilatation and dissection, mitral and aortic regurgitation). Caused by mutations in *FBN1*, the gene encoding fibrillin, a component of the extracellular matrix. Use the Ghent criteria to establish the diagnosis. See 'Marfan's syndrome' in Chapter 3, 'Common consultations', p. 484.

Floppy infant

Floppiness in infancy can be caused by many disorders of the CNS that are associated with hypotonia; also myopathies, dystrophies, and peripheral nerve problems such as SMA. See 'Floppy infant' in Chapter 2, 'Clinical approach', p. 154.

Skeletal dysplasias

- In Larsen syndrome, there are multiple joint dislocations. There are both AD and AR types. A skeletal survey is required to establish the diagnosis. One of the characteristic features is that the tarsal bones show a bifid calcaneus in childhood.
- In Stickler syndrome, cleft palate, myopia, retinal detachment, and epiphyseal dysplasia are much more

definitive diagnostic handles than joint hypermobility. See 'Stickler syndrome' in Chapter 3, 'Common consultations', p. 528.
- OI. The cardinal features are fractures, reduced bone density, and blue sclerae. See 'Fractures' in Chapter 2, 'Clinical approach', p. 158.

Genetic advice

Recurrence risk

Counsel for the specific condition diagnosed. Specific diagnosis is usually impossible for the milder phenotypes. Some of the milder connective tissue disorders follow AD inheritance, with a 50% risk to offspring, and typically show quite wide inter- and intrafamilial variation. One recessive form of joint hypermobility (<5% of joint hypermobility type of EDS) may be caused by tenascin X deficiency. This should be particularly suspected if there is also 21-hydroxylase deficiency since contiguous deletions of chromosome 6 may be implicated.

Prenatal diagnosis

Possible only if the pathogenic mutation has been defined in a given family.

Natural history and further management (preventative measures)

The condition can be aggravated by repetitive activities and obesity. A physiotherapist can advise about posture and the benefit of orthoses, such as insoles to support the arches of the feet, and suggest a beneficial exercise regime (swimming, cycling, walking).

High-impact activities, e.g. trampolining, that place a severe stress on the joints are probably best avoided. The risk of joint injury in contact sports is increased.

Support group: Hypermobility Syndromes Association, http://hypermobility.org.

Expert adviser: Paul Wordsworth, Professor of Rheumatology, Nuffield Department of Orthopaedics, Rheumatology and Musculoskeletal Sciences, Oxford University, Oxford, UK.

References

Beighton P, McKusick VA. *McKusick's heritable disorders of connective tissue*, 5th edn. Mosby, St Louis, 1993.

Grahame R. Joint hypermobility and genetic collagen disorders: are they related? *Arch Dis Child* 1999; **80**: 188–91.

Raff ML, Byers PH. Joint hypermobility syndromes. *Curr Opin Rheumatol* 1996; **8**: 459–66.

Schalkwijk J, Zweers MC, Steijlen PM, *et al.* A recessive form of the Ehlers–Danlos syndrome caused by tenascin-X deficiency. *N Engl J Med* 2001; **345**: 1167–75.

Hypertrichosis

Hypertrichosis is excessive growth of hair (terminal, vellus, or lanugo) over and above what is normal for the age, sex, and ethnicity of the individual. Hypertrichosis may be generalized, in which case it occurs over the majority of the body, or localized. There is substantial ethnic diversity in the amount and distribution of hair among healthy newborns and infants. It is helpful to be familiar with this in assessing a child who is noted to have excessive hair.

It is important to distinguish hypertrichosis from hirsuitism. Hirsutism is a subclass of hypertrichosis caused by excess androgen-sensitive hair growth, resulting in excess body or facial hair in an adult male pattern. Although hirsuitism can occur in post-pubertal males, it is more difficult to detect, as there is a wide range of normal hair growth in men. Hirsutism affects ~10% of women in Western societies and is more common in women of Mediterranean and Middle Eastern descent.

Hypertrichosis may occur as an isolated feature or as part of a syndromic ID disorder when it can be a useful diagnostic handle. It is characteristic of some of the syndromes caused by mutation of chromatin-remodelling genes; it can be a feature of conditions associated with lipoatrophy and is seen in individuals with MPS.

Clinical approach

History: key points

- Three-generation family tree with specific enquiry for consanguinity and ethnic background. Did the parents or other family members have similar hair growth?
- When was excess hair first noted? Was it present from birth?
- Development milestones (delayed milestones in syndromic hypertrichosis), any slowdown in progress or loss of skills (MPS)?
- Visual difficulties.
- Hearing loss.
- Upper respiratory infections (enlargement of tonsils and adenoids, tracheal involvement).
- Ask about systemic symptoms (hypertrichosis can be a manifestation of a more generalized medical problem).
- Visual difficulties.
- Hearing loss.
- Drug history (some drugs, e.g. minoxidil or phenytoin, can cause hypertrichosis).

Examination: key points

- Growth parameters. Height, weight, and OFC. (Babies with Cornelia de Lange syndrome (CdLS) are typically very small for dates.)
- Skin. Distribution and pattern of hair growth. Thick or sparse? Vellus or terminal hair? Axillar, groin, and flexural surfaces for acanthosis nigricans (insulin resistance), lipodystrophy, muscular hypertrophy, and vasculomegaly (Berardinelli–Seip).
- Hands:
  - contractures (storage disorders);
  - nail hypoplasia (Coffin–Siris syndrome);
  - broad thumbs (RTS).

- Eyes. Narrow palpebral fissures (Wiedemann–Steiner syndrome (WSS)). Corneal clouding (MPS).
- Facial appearance. Coarse features (Coffin–Siris and Cantu syndromes)?
- Mouth. Is there gum hypertrophy?
- Heart. Is there a cardiac murmur?
- Spine. If hypertrichosis is over the spine, examine carefully for evidence of an underlying spinal abnormality.
- Abdomen:
  - enlargement of the liver and spleen (MPS disorders);
  - umbilical hernia (MPS disorders, Berardinelli–Seip syndrome).
- Neurological examination.
- Genitalia. Genital abnormalities (Schinzel–Giedion syndrome).

Investigations

- Genomic analysis in presence of features suggestive of a chromosomal or syndromic diagnosis, e.g. genomic array, gene panel, or WES/WGS as appropriate.
- Echo to assess for CM and valvular abnormalities.
- Abdominal USS (organomegaly, renal enlargement, or structural abnormality).
- Endocrine studies. Insulin level if Donohue syndrome suspected.
- Skeletal survey. To assess for features of a storage disease such as abnormal bone modelling. A feature such as rib thickening may suggest Cantu syndrome.
- Spinal MRI. If hypertrichosis is over the spine and an underlying spinal abnormality is suspected.

Some diagnoses to consider

Primary generalized hypertrichosis

HYPERTRICHOSIS UNIVERSALIS CONGENITA, AMBRAS TYPE. A rare syndrome characterized by excessive growth of long hair (thought to be vellus type) across the entire body, sparing only the palms, soles, and mucous membranes. Hypertrichosis is characteristically accentuated on the face, ears, and shoulders. Reported families suggest AD inheritance and rearrangements of 8q have been identified in some individuals.

CONGENITAL HYPERTRICHOSIS LANUGOSA (CHL). This is a very rare syndrome, characterized by an excess of fine blond lanugo hair that remains over most of the body after birth, sparing only the palms, soles, and mucous membranes. Hair shedding is reported to occur during childhood.

CONGENITAL GENERALIZED HYPERTRICHOSIS TERMINALIS (CGHT) WITH OR WITHOUT GINGIVAL HYPERPLASIA. This is a rare condition that is often accompanied by progressive gingival hyperplasia and is characterized by universal excessive growth of pigmented terminal hairs. There is evidence that inheritance is AD and that a copy number variant at 17q24.2-q24.3 is responsible for the condition (Sun et al. 2009).

X-LINKED CONGENITAL GENERALIZED HYPERTRICHOSIS. This is an extremely rare condition associated with deafness and dental and palatal anomalies linked to Xq24-27, which may be caused by a chromosomal insertion causing a position effect on *FGF13* (DeStefano *et al*. 2013).

Syndromic hypertrichosis

COFFIN–SIRIS SYNDROME. Caused by heterozygous mutation in components of the SWI/SNF chromatin-remodelling complex, e.g. *ARID1B* (Santen *et al*. 2012; Tsurusaki *et al*. 2012). Characterized by developmental delay, with sparse hair, coarse facial features, and nail hypoplasia, especially of the fifth finger. Carefully exclude chromosomal abnormalities.

CANTU SYNDROME. An AD condition with slightly coarse facial features caused by heterozygous mutation in the *ABCC9* gene (Harakalova *et al*. 2012). Facial hair is abundant and there is generalized hypertrichosis. Thick ribs may be a helpful diagnostic feature; other aspects of the accompanying osteochondrodysplasia may be subtle. Growth and development may be delayed in early infancy but subsequently normalize. DCM may be a feature.

CORNELIA DE LANGE SYNDROME (CDLS). A clinically and genetically heterogeneous developmental disorder characterized by growth retardation, ID, limb defects, hypertrichosis, typical facial dysmorphism including synophrys. Mutations in five genes (*NIPBL*, *SMC1A*, *SMC3*, *RAD21*, and *HDAC8*), all regulators or structural components of cohesin, have been identified. Approximately 60% of CdLS cases are due to *NIPBL* mutations.

WIEDEMANN–STEINER SYNDROME (WSS). An AD condition caused by heterozygous mutation of the *KMT2A* (*MLL*) gene (Jones *et al*. 2012). WSS is characterized by excessive growth of terminal hair around the elbows (hypertrichosis cubiti), back, and lower limbs, in association with ID, and a distinctive facial appearance.

RUBINSTEIN–TAYBI SYNDROME (RTS). Normal birthweight, postnatal short stature and microcephaly, moderate to severe learning difficulties in most, and broad thumbs and halluces. Approximately 10% of RTS caused by heterozygous microdeletions of *CREBBP*, 30–50% of *CREBBP* mutations, and 3% mutations in *EP300*.

SCHINZEL–GIEDION SYNDROME. Characterized by severe MR, wide open fontanelle, midface hypoplasia, choanal stenosis, hydronephrosis, genital abnormalities. AR resulting from mutations in *SETBP1* (Hoischen *et al*. 2010).

BARBER–SAY SYNDROME. A rare disorder characterized by a coarse face with bilateral ectropion, absent eyebrows and lashes, hypertelorism, atrophic skin with changes of premature ageing, and severe hypertrichosis of the forehead and back. The genetic basis is not defined.

MUCOPOLYSACCHARIDE (MPS) DISORDERS. Several of the MPS disorders are associated with hypertrichosis (typically present with glue ear, coarse facial features, and finger contractures).

BERARDINELLI–SEIP CONGENITAL LIPODYSTROPHY. Characterized by severe insulin resistance, near absence of adipose tissue from birth or early infancy, muscular hypertrophy, and hepatomegaly. An AR disorder caused by mutations in the gene encoding seipin (*BSCL2*).

DONOHUE SYNDROME (LEPRECHAUNISM). An AR disorder due to mutations in the insulin receptor gene. Pre- and postnatal failure to thrive, hirsutism, aged face with thick lips and prominent ears, enlargement of the breasts and genitalia; acanthosis nigricans may be present. The serum insulin level is grossly elevated.

Primary circumscribed hypertrichosis/localized hypertrichosis

SPINAL HYPERTRICHOSIS. If hypertrichosis is limited to the spinal region, consider the presence of underlying diastematomyelia such as a myelomeningocele, a dermal cyst or sinus, vertebral abnormalities, or a subdural or extradural lipoma. Consider spinal MRI to enable early treatment and prevent neurological sequelae.

HYPERTRICHOSIS CUBITI. Hairy elbows can be seen as an isolated finding or in association with a variety of other features, most commonly short stature; the underlying cause is likely heterogeneous. Consider WSS.

ANTERIOR CERVICAL HYPERTRICHOSIS. This can be an isolated finding but may be associated with a peripheral sensory and motor neuropathy as what is thought to be an AR trait.

POSTERIOR CERVICAL HYPERTRICHOSIS. Reported in association with underlying kyphoscoliosis as an AD disorder in one family.

Acquired disorders associated with hypertrichosis

Hair overgrowth may also be a manifestation of a more generalized medical problem and can be seen in association with hepatic porphyria, anorexia, juvenile hypothyroidism, juvenile dermatomyositis, and human immunodeficiency virus (HIV) infection. Acquired hypertrichosis lanuginosa can also occur as a paraneoplastic phenomenon.

Genetic advice

Recurrence risk
As for the specific genetic diagnosis.

Prenatal diagnosis
This can be offered to those parents in whom a syndromic genetic diagnosis has been confirmed by molecular tests.

Natural history and further management and therapy
As per the specific condition.

DONOHUE SYNDROME AND BERARDINELLI–SEIP CONGENITAL LIPODYSTROPHY. Individuals suspected of having Donohue syndrome or Berardinelli–Seip congenital lipodystrophy should be investigated and managed under the care of a metabolic physician.

MUCOPOLYSACCHARIDE (MPS) DISORDERS. ERT and BMT may be possible and these children should be under the care of a paediatrician to ensure up-to-date advice.

HAIR REMOVAL. Some individuals may opt for removal of excess body hair. As hair overgrowth may be a manifestation of a more generalized medical problem, accurate characterization of the hair growth must precede hair removal treatment. Multiple methods are available. Referral to dermatology may be helpful.

Support group: Many of the individual syndromes have their own support groups. See Contact a Family, http://www.cafamily.org.uk.

Expert adviser: Wendy Jones, Locum Consultant, Clinical Genetics Department, Great Ormond Street Hospital for Children, London, UK.

References

DeStefano GM, Fantauzzo KA, Petukhova L, *et al.* Position effect on *FGF13* associated with X-linked congenital generalised hypertrichosis. *Proc Natl Acad Sci U S A* 2013; **110**: 7790–5.

Jones WD, Dafour D, McEntagart M, *et al.* Dominant mutations in MLL cause Weidemann–Steiner syndrome. *Am J Hum Genet* 2012; **91**: 358–61.

Harakalova M, van Harssel JJ, Terhal PA, *et al.* Dominant missense mutations in *ABCC9* cause Cantu syndrome. *Nat Genet* 2012; **44**: 793–6.

Hoischen A, van Bon BW, Gilissen C, *et al. De novo* mutations of *SETBP1* cause Schinzel–Giedion syndrome. *Nat Genet* 2010; **42**: 483–5.

Miyake N, Tsurusaki Y, Koshimizu E, *et al.* Delineation of clinical features in Wiedemann–Steiner syndrome caused by *KMT2A* mutations. *Clin Genet* 2016; **89**: 115–19.

Santen GW, Aten E, Sun Y, *et al.* Mutations in SWI/SNF chromatin remodeling complex gene *ARID1B* cause Coffin–Siris syndrome. *Nat Genet* 2012; **44**: 379–80.

Sun et al.

Tsurusaki Y, Okamoto H, Ohashi H, *et al.* Mutations affecting components of the SWI/SNF complex cause Coffin–Siris syndrome. *Nat Genet* 2012; **44**: 376–8.

Hypoglycaemia in the neonate and infant

The definition of hypoglycaemia is one of the most contentious issues in paediatric clinical practice. Several groups have tried to define hypoglycaemia, but difficulties still exist, particularly in the neonatal period (Hawdon 2013). After 72 hours in term babies and after the first week in preterm babies, hypoglycaemia may be defined as plasma or whole blood glucose of <2.6 mmol/l, although a stricter definition is used by some (<2.5 mmol/l; Saudubray et al. 2000).

After feeding, the liver builds up stores of glycogen and triglyceride. During fasting, glucose and ketones are released to provide energy.

To maintain a normal blood glucose level, there must be:

- intact hepatic glycogenolytic and gluconeogenic enzyme systems to produce glucose from stored glycogen (impaired in glycogen storage disorders);
- adequate supply of amino acids, glycerol, and lactate;
- adequate energy from beta-oxidation of fatty acids to produce glucose and ketones (impaired in fatty acid oxidation disorders);
- a normal endocrine system (impaired in hyperinsulinism, GH, adrenocorticotrophic hormone (ACTH), and cortisol deficiency, and Laron syndrome).

In normal neonates, hypoglycaemia immediately after birth is associated with developmental immaturity of hepatic gluconeogenesis and ketogenesis. In the majority of babies with hypoglycaemia, there is a non-genetic aetiology (secondary) (prematurity, low birthweight, sepsis, infant of diabetic mother, etc.). This section is an approach to some of the genetic causes of hypoglycaemia.

Clinical approach

History: key points

- Three-generation family history with specific enquiry for consanguinity and unexplained infant/neonatal death or Reye's syndrome.
- Gestational diabetes.
- Birthweight is increased in congenital hyperinsulinism of infancy (CHI) and syndromes such as BWS.
- Apgar scores at delivery and was resuscitation required?
- Was the baby handling normally and feeding well before the onset of symptoms? Babies who appear normal at birth and handle and feed well and subsequently deteriorate are more likely to have an inborn error of metabolism.
- How old was the infant when hypoglycaemia was noted? Was it after a period of fasting? Was there any additional metabolic stress?
- Seizures.

Examination: key points

- Weight, length, and OFC.
- Assess the posture and tone of the infant and note any abnormal movements.
- Dysmorphic features and macrosomia (BWS).
- Hepatomegaly (moderate in CHI and fatty acid oxidation (FAO) disorders; severe in GSD I and III). You might not find hepatomegaly in the newborn period due to GSD I/III; this develops over time with increased glycogen storage (mostly in infants).

- CM and arrhythmia: FAO defects (see also 'Cardiomyopathy in children under 10 years' in Chapter 2, 'Clinical approach', p. 84).
- Micropenis (pituitary dysfunction). Midline lesions (cleft palate) indicating GH, ACTH, and cortisol deficiency.

Special investigations

Ensure that non-genetic causes of hypoglycaemia are being concurrently investigated. Usually, by the time the geneticist is called, a basic screen for glucose, calcium, sodium, metabolic acidosis (pH, base excess, and HCO_3^-), liver function, ammonia, uric acid, blood count, and urine dipstick for pH, ketones, and reducing substances will have been completed.

NB. The list below covers many of the likely causes but is not an exhaustive list of diagnostic investigations.

- Urine:
  - urine ketones. If there is significant ketonuria with no acidosis in a sick neonate, exclude MSUD. Ketosis is not an important fuel source in the normal neonate, due to liver immaturity. In the infant or older child, ketonuria is typically absent in hyperinsulinaemia and FAO disorders, moderate in association with fasting hypoglycaemia in GSD types I and III, and raised in idiopathic ketotic hypoglycaemia (but this does not present until 1–2 years). If ketonuria occurs in conjunction with metabolic acidosis, consider GSD type III;
  - urine organic acids and amino acids to pick up abnormal metabolites suggestive of an inborn error of metabolism.
- Blood:
  - DNA for storage and analysis. For further investigation of BWS, e.g. UPD;
  - genomic analysis in presence of features suggestive of a chromosomal or syndromic diagnosis, e.g. genomic array, gene panel, or WES/WGS as available;
  - acyl carnitines (dried blood spot on Guthrie card), total and free carnitine (FAO and carnitine transporter defects);
  - insulin level (record blood glucose level at time sample is taken);
  - GH/cortisol;
  - lactate: lactic acidosis in GSD type III (and see below);
  - ammonia: raised ammonia and lactate in hyperinsulinism/hyperammonaemic (lactate is not raised in this condition) syndrome, FAO, organic acidaemias, and mitochondrial cytopathies;
  - free fatty acids in blood and ketone bodies (disorders of beta-oxidation and hyperinsulinism);
  - neutropenia is a feature of GSD Ib.
- Imaging:
  - cardiac echo to exclude CM and ECG for arrhythmia—FAO (see also 'Cardiomyopathy in children under 10 years' in Chapter 2, 'Clinical approach', p. 84);
  - imaging of the liver and pancreas;
  - cranial USS/MRI of the brain for panhypopituitarism, agenesis of the corpus callosum.

Under the supervision of a paediatrician with expertise in metabolic/endocrine disease:

- glucose requirements (high in CHI; low in other causes); >8 mg/kg/min virtually diagnostic of CHI;
- response to glucagon (dramatic in CHI, absent in GSD, variable in FAO and endocrine disorders);
- response to diazoxide and hydrochlorothiazide (CHI);
- consider liver biopsy for specific enzyme abnormality (may not be necessary to perform liver biopsy to confirm diagnosis).

Some diagnoses to consider

Neonate

CONGENITAL HYPERINSULINISM. (See Table 2.13.) This is the most common cause of recurrent hypoglycaemia in early infancy. This term is now preferred to nesidioblastosis. It is characterized by dysregulation of insulin secretion. It occurs in ~1/40 000 to 1/50 000 live births, but much higher in some consanguineous regions (1/10 000). Approximately 95% of cases are sporadic; some cases are AR (Cohen 2003) and dominant forms. Birthweights are >90th centile in at least 45%. Most present in the first 72 hours with hypoglycaemia. A small number present later and these have adenomas. In the neonate, the diagnosis is made on the high glucose requirement. Response to glucagon is dramatic. There may be focal or diffuse abnormalities of the β-cells of the pancreas.

There is molecular heterogeneity in the sporadic forms of CHI; all patients with the focal type have somatic loss of maternal alleles at the imprinted domain on 11p15.

Integrity of the pancreatic β-cell ATP-sensitive potassium (KATP) channel depends on the interactions between the pore-forming inward rectifier potassium channel subunit (KIR6.2) and the regulatory subunit sulfonylurea receptor 1 (SUR1). The *ABCC8* and *KCJN11* genes (both localized to chromosome 11p15.1) encode the two components of the KATP channel and most of the severe forms of CHI are due to recessively inactivating mutations of these genes (Thomas *et al.* 1995).

This channel is involved in glucose-mediated insulin secretion, promoting insulin release when intracellular glucose levels are high, and preventing it when intracellular insulin levels fall. When this channel is faulty, insulin release is unregulated, leading to profound hypoglycaemia.

Early recognition of hypoglycaemia, correct differentiation between histological types (focal or diffuse), and

Table 2.13 Genes involved in congenital hyperinsulism of infancy (CHI)

Autosomal dominant (AD)	Autosomal recessive (AR)
GLUD1	ABCC8/KCNJ11
GCK	HADH
SLC16A1	
HNF4A	
HNF1A	
UCP2	
ABCC8/KCNJ11	

maintenance of adequate glucose levels are of critical importance for the outcome of these patients. If medical therapy is not effective, surgical removal of the pancreas (either partial or complete) is performed. Discuss management with a centre with expertise in CHI.

BECKWITH–WIEDEMANN SYNDROME (BWS). A somatic overgrowth and cancer predisposition syndrome estimated to affect 71/13 700 individuals. Eighty-five per cent of cases are sporadic and 15% are the result of vertical transmission. The genetic basis of BWS is complex but involves genes at 11p15. See 'Beckwith–Wiedemann syndrome (BWS)' in Chapter 3, 'Common consultations', p. 358.

KABUKI SYNDROME. A multiple congenital anomaly syndrome characterized by typical facial features, skeletal anomalies, mild to moderate ID, and postnatal growth deficiency. It is caused by heterozygous mutation in the *KMT2D* (*MLL2*) gene in the majority (usually *de novo*), but a minority has a mutation in the *KDM6A* gene and patients with the latter gene are more likely to present with hypoglycaemia (Banka 2015).

SOTOS SYNDROME. An overgrowth syndrome characterized by macrocephaly, hypotonia, developmental delay, and often neonatal jaundice. It is caused by heterozygous mutation of the *NSD1* gene.

FATTY ACID OXIDATION (FAO) AND KETOGENESIS DISORDERS. Hypoketotic hypoglycaemia and cardiac abnormalities. In infants, the presentation may resemble Reye's syndrome. It is important to recognize primary carnitine deficiencies, as therapeutic treatment with L-carnitine is lifesaving. (Secondary causes of carnitine deficiency include malnutrition and renal failure.)

ENDOCRINE ABNORMALITIES. Exclude GH deficiency in neonates, panhypopituitarism, disorders of cortisol metabolism, etc.

Infant and older child

AUTOSOMAL DOMINANT (AD) HYPERINSULINISM. Median age of onset is 1 year. Normal birthweight. May present with a seizure or a seizure-like disorder. Caused by mutation in the glucokinase gene (*GCK*) or mutations in the glutamate dehydrogenase gene (*GDH*). Hyperammonaemia is also found in the latter. In some families, the molecular cause is unknown.

ENDOCRINE ABNORMALITIES. Laron syndrome (mutation in growth hormone-releasing hormone receptor) can present with hypoglycaemia in infants. Short stature, micropenis, and obesity are additional features.

ABNORMALITIES OF GLYCOGEN SYNTHESIS AND DEGRADATION. Glycogen synthase deficiency and GSD IV prevent synthesis of glycogen, but these do not present in neonates. GSD IV typically causes hypoglycaemia and hyperketonuria in the mornings after night feeds are discontinued. Deficiencies of the enzymes involved in the degradation of glycogen cause hypoglycaemia 2–3 hours after a meal and present in infancy rather than in neonates.

Genetic advice

Recurrence risk

As for the given diagnosis. Thorough testing usually gives a clue to the aetiological group, even if a precise diagnosis is not possible.

For infants with sudden death in whom hypoglycaemia was suspected, the possibility of a genetic condition needs to be considered with a risk of up to 25% for recurrence.

Carrier detection
This is possible in families where a causative mutation has been identified. May be possible for some biochemical abnormalities.

Prenatal diagnosis
This is available to those families where there is molecular or biochemical confirmation of the diagnosis.

Natural history and further management (preventative measures)
Children with these problems require close medical and dietetic supervision to prevent death and neurological disability as a consequence of hypoglycaemia.

Support group: Climb (Children Living with Inherited Metabolic Diseases), http://www.climb.org.uk.

Expert adviser: Khalid Hussain, Professor, Genetics & Epigenetics in Health & Disease, UCL, Great Ormond Street Institute of Child Health, London, UK.

References
Banka S, Lederer D, Benoit V, *et al*. Novel KDM6A (UTX) mutations and a clinical and molecular review of the X-linked Kabuki syndrome (KS2). *Clin Genet* 2015; **87**(3): 252–8.

Cohen MM Jr. Persistent hyperinsulinemic hypoglycaemia of infancy. *Am J Med Genet A* 2003; **122A**: 351–3.

Cornblath M, Hawdon JM, Williams AF, *et al*. Controversies regarding definition of neonatal hypoglycemia: suggested operational thresholds. *Pediatrics* 2000; **105**: 1141–5.

Hawdon JM. Definition of neonatal hypoglycaemia: time for a rethink? *Arch Dis Child Fetal Neonatal Ed* 2013; **98**: F382–3.

Meissner T, Mayatepek E. Clinical and genetic heterogeneity in congenital hyperinsulinism. *Eur J Pediatr* 2002; **161**: 6–20.

Saudubray JM, de Lonlay P, Touati G, *et al*. Genetic hypoglycaemia in infancy and childhood: pathophysiology and diagnosis. *J Inherit Metab Dis* 2000; **23**: 197–214.

Saudubray JM, Nassogne MC, de Lonlay P, Touati G. Clinical approach to inherited metabolic disorders in neonates: an overview. *Semin Neonatol* 2002; **7**: 3–15.

Senniappan S, Arya VB, Hussain K. The molecular mechanisms, diagnosis and management of congenital hyperinsulinism. *Indian J Endocrinol Metab* 2013; **17**: 19–30.

Society for the Study of Inborn Errors of Metabolism. http://www.ssiem.org.

Thomas PM, Cote GJ, Wohllk N, *et al*. Mutations in the sulfonylurea receptor gene in familial persistent hyperinsulinemic hypoglycemia of infancy. *Science* 1995; **268**: 426–9.

Hypospadias

In hypospadias, the urethral meatus is abnormally located and is displaced proximally on to the ventral surface of the penis—in mild cases on the glans itself, and in more severe cases at some point along the ventral surface of the penile shaft. The foreskin is also almost always affected, being imperfectly formed beneath, and this deformity may be more obvious than the hypospadias itself. In a proportion of cases, there is also a downward bend on the shaft of the penis (chordee) which becomes exaggerated during penile erections and, as a general rule, the more severe the hypospadias, the greater the chance of significant chordee. It is classified as shown in Table 2.14 and Figure 2.16.

The male external genitalia develops from 8 weeks in the presence of dihydrotestosterone which is produced by the action of the enzyme 5-alpha-reductase on testosterone. Hypospadias is found in 6.4/1000 live male births. Stoll *et al.* (1990) established that 80% are of the mild phenotype and over 90% of these do not have any other malformations. The incidence of associated malformations is higher in the severe group and studies have established the aetiology in about one-third of these. In severely affected infants, the gender may be in doubt and careful counselling is required. A stepwise diagnostic approach is recommended to avoid unnecessary invasive and expensive testing.

EPISPADIAS. This occurs in ~1/117 000 live births and is much more common in boys (5M:1F). The urethral meatus is abnormally located and is displaced on to the dorsal surface of the penis. The penis is short and broad.

Clinical approach

History: key points
- Three-generation family tree.
- Birthweight (hypospadias is more common in low-birthweight babies).
- Medication during pregnancy, e.g. antiepileptic drugs.
- Developmental delay (syndromes and chromosomal conditions).

Examination: key points
- Position of the urethral meatus to classify severity.
- Presence of chordee, bifid scrotum, position of the testes.
- BP and renal masses (Wilms tumour).
- Growth parameters and head circumference.
- Hypertelorism, swallowing and laryngeal problems (Opitz G/BBB syndrome).
- Cleft palate (SLO syndrome and chromosomal anomalies).

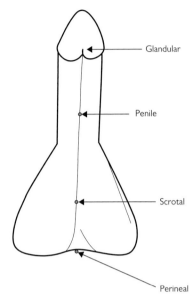

Figure 2.16 Types of hypospadias.

- Post-axial polydactyly and syndactyly between the second and third toes (SLO).

Special investigations
Stepwise diagnostic studies, usually coordinated by a paediatric endocrinologist working with a paediatric urologist.
- USS of the renal and urogenital (UG) systems in all affected boys.
- Karyotype (additional X chromosomes, XX males, triploidy, trisomy 13 and 18, many other visible cytogenetic abnormalities) including mosaicism screen. This is an essential investigation in infants with additional malformations and ambiguous genitalia, but not routine for the boy with isolated mild hypospadias. FISH investigation for del 11p in the presence of aniridia or Wilms tumour.
- Genomic analysis in presence of other malformations suggestive of a chromosomal or syndromic diagnosis, e.g. genomic array, gene panel, or WES/WGS as available.
- hCG stimulation to measure testosterone and dihydrotestosterone (5-alpha-reductase deficiency) in boys with moderate or severe hypospadias.
- Genital skin sample for androgen-binding studies at time of surgical repair.
- Consider molecular genetic analysis of the androgen receptor gene or 5-alpha-reductase gene if endocrine studies indicate an abnormality.
- 7-dehydrocholesterol if there are other features of SLO syndrome.

Some diagnoses to consider

In Albers *et al.*'s (1997) study, 33 patients with severe hypospadias were investigated and in 12 the cause was

Table 2.14 Classification of hypospadias

Severity	Position of urethral meatus
Mild	Glandular or coronal
Moderate	Penile (along the length of the shaft)
Severe	Perineal/scrotal

NB. The presence of chordee (ventral curvature of the penis due to fibrous tethering) may make it difficult to estimate the severity and extent of the hypospadias until the chordee is released at the first repair.

found. The diagnoses were Drash syndrome (three patients), androgen receptor mutations leading to partial androgen insensitivity (two patients), true hermaphrodite (two patients), chromosome abnormality (one patient), deficiency of AMH (one patient), gonadal dysgenesis (one patient), partial 5-alpha-reductase deficiency (one patient), and XX male (one patient). Boehmer *et al.* (2001) investigated 63 children with severe hypospadias and were able to find the underlying aetiology in about one-third. Of these, 17% had a complex genetic syndrome and 10% chromosomal anomalies.

Smith–Lemli–Opitz syndrome (SLO)
Hypospadias and/or cryptorchidism are found in 90–100% of males with SLO. The genitalia may be ambiguous with a hypoplastic scrotum. Other features are prenatal and postnatal growth deficiency (almost all), microcephaly, cleft palate (37–52%), thickened alveolar ridges, cardiac defects (36–38%; especially AVSD and TAPVD), Y-shaped 2/3 toe syndactyly (>95%), and PAP (~50%). Facial features include narrow bifrontal diameter, ptosis (50%), downslanting palpebral fissures, and a short nose with a depressed nasal bridge and anteverted nares. It is an AR condition. Plasma 7-dehydrocholesterol levels are elevated because mutations in the *DHCR7* gene on 11q13 lead to deficient activity of 7-dehydrocholesterol reductase (*DHCR7*), the final enzyme in the cholesterol biosynthetic pathway (Jira *et al.* 2003). The frequency is 71 in 20 000–30 000.

WAGR (Wilms tumour–aniridia–genitourinary anomalies–mental retardation)
A contiguous gene syndrome due to microscopic or submicroscopic deletion of 11p13. Specific FISH probes available. See 'Wilms tumour' in Chapter 4, 'Cancer', p. 620.

Drash syndrome or Wilms tumour and pseudohermaphroditism and Frasier syndrome
Usually have ambiguous genitalia. Caused by mutations in *WT1*. See 'Ambiguous genitalia (including sex reversal)' in Chapter 2, 'Clinical approach', p. 54.

Opitz syndrome
The key features of hypertelorism, hypospadias, swallowing difficulties, and developmental delay are found in both the AD and XL conditions. Anteverted nares and laryngeal clefts appear to be features found in the XL type. The AD locus is on 22q11.2 and the XL locus is on Xp22.3 (*MID1* gene).

Mowat–Wilson syndrome
Characteristic facial appearance (hypertelorism, pointed chin, prominent columella, open-mouthed expression, broad, medial flared eyebrows, and uplifted earlobes), together with severe MR. Microcephaly, seizures, congenital heart defects, aplasia/hypoplasia of the corpus callosum, and urogenital anomalies (especially hypospadias in boys) are frequent findings. Caused by 'de novo' truncating mutations in *ZEB2* on 2q22.

Hand–foot–genital syndrome
An AD condition caused by mutations in *HOXA13* on 7p15. Males have hypospadias and females have

duplication of the uterus and sometimes of the cervix and may have a septate vagina. Hands are small with hypoplastic proximally placed thumbs, and feet are small with short halluces. Urinary tract malformations are common in both sexes.

Genetic advice
Recurrence risk
- Syndromic hypospadias. Counsel as appropriate for the specific diagnosis.
- Isolated hypospadias. Stoll *et al.*'s (1990) study of births in north-eastern France found a 17% or 1 in 6 recurrence risk for brothers. There have been reports of dominant transmission and a couple of reports of recessive inheritance in consanguineous kindreds. Androgen receptor gene mutations are a rare cause of isolated hypospadias.

Prenatal diagnosis
Severe hypospadias may be detected if there is severe chordee or ambiguous genitalia by combining USS information with cytogenetic analysis showing a male karyotype.

Natural history and further management
Surgical treatment for the hypospadias as necessary. Moderate or severe hypospadias is usually repaired as a staged procedure. As a rule, the repair is undertaken some time between 12 months and 2 years of age or after toilet training between 3 and 4 years of age. Although repair is usually successful, there is an appreciable (15–30%) rate of complications requiring further surgery. Because the foreskin may be needed for the repair, the child should not be circumcised. In severe cases, gender assignment is a difficult problem. Patients at risk of malignancy or hormonal imbalance require long-term surveillance.

Support group: Hypospadias UK, http://www.hypospadiasuk.co.uk, Tel. 01925 496 510.

Expert adviser: Carlo Acerini, University Senior Lecturer, Department of Paediatrics, University of Cambridge, Addenbrooke's Hospital, Cambridge, UK.

References
Albers N, Ulrichs C, Gluer S, *et al.* Etiological classification of severe hypospadias: implications for prognosis and management. *J Pediatr* 1997; **131**: 386–92.

Boehmer AL, Nijman RJ, Lammers BA, *et al.* Etiological studies of severe or familial hypospadias. *J Urol* 2001; **165**: 1246–54.

Jira PE, Waterham HR, Wanders RJ, *et al.* Smith–Lemli–Opitz syndrome and the DHCR7 gene. *Am J Hum Genet* 2003; **67**(Pt 3): 269–80.

Klamt B, Koziell A, Poulat F, *et al.* Frasier syndrome is caused by defective alternative splicing of *WT1* leading to an altered ratio of *WT1* 9 KJS splice isoforms. *Hum Mol Genet* 1998; **7**: 709–14.

Stoll C, Alembik Y, Roth MP, Dott B. Genetic and environmental factors in hypospadias. *J Med Genet* 1990; **27**: 559–63.

Intellectual disability

Mental retardation, mental handicap, intellectual developmental disorder, intellectual handicap, learning difficulty, learning disability, developmental delay.

In the United States (USA), the formerly preferred term mental retardation (MR) was recently abandoned and changed to 'intellectual disability (ID)' by a federal statute (see Harris 2013 for discussion on terminology), but the Department of Health in the UK uses 'learning disability' and the Department of Education term is 'learning difficulties'.

The reported frequency of ID varies substantially across studies. Most studies report overall rates of 1–2.5% for intelligence quotient (IQ) <70, and 0.3–0.5% for IQ <50. Population studies show a preponderance of males (M:F = 1.3:1), mainly attributable to X-linked ID (XLID).

Definitions

ID was traditionally defined by an IQ <70 determined by standardized IQ testing with childhood onset and functional deficits. Based on IQ levels, the older literature describes four degrees of retardation, whereas more recently this has been simplified into 'mild' with an IQ range of 50–70 and 'severe' with IQ <50, reflecting the difficulties in IQ testing, especially in the lower range. The fifth edition of the *Diagnostic and statistical manual for mental disorders* (DSM-5) of the American Psychiatric Association (APA; 2013) dismisses the categorization by IQ levels and instead emphasizes the importance of clinically assessed levels of adaptive functioning, because it is the latter that determines the level of supports required. The DSM-5 categorizes ID as a 'neurodevelopmental disorder', in contrast to the group of late-onset 'neurocognitive disorders' (dementia), and defines it as 'a disorder with onset during the developmental period that includes both intellectual and adaptive functioning deficits in conceptual, social, and practical domains' (http://www.dsm5.org/documents/intellectual%20disability%20fact%20sheet.pdf).

The American Association on Mental Retardation has been a leader in the adoption of the term intellectual disability and changed its name into American Association on Intellectual and Developmental Disabilities (AAIDD). Their definition of ID is very similar to the DSM-5 definition: 'Intellectual disability is a disability characterized by *significant limitations in both intellectual functioning and in adaptive behaviour*, which covers many everyday social and practical skills. This disability originates *before the age of 18*.' (Schalock *et al.* 2010).

The *ICD-10 classification of mental and behavioural disorders* defines it as follows: 'Mental retardation is a condition of arrested or incomplete development of the mind, which is especially characterised by impairment of skills manifested during the developmental period, contributing to the overall level of intelligence—i.e. cognitive, language, motor and social abilities' (World Health Organization 1992). The ICD-11 is expected in 2018 and the working group proposed to replace MR by intellectual developmental disorders (IDDs) and defines it as 'a group of developmental conditions characterized by significant impairment of cognitive functions, which are associated with limitations of learning, adaptive behaviour and skills (Salvador-Carulla *et al.* 2011).

Idiopathic ID is ID of no known cause. Within this group is the subgroup of non-specific ID that refers to the normally grown, non-dysmorphic child with no problems other than ID. In this subgroup, there is an excess of males.

ID usually presents with delay in the developmental milestones, but those with complex medical problems will present accordingly. ID has significant comorbidity with other neurodevelopmental disorders and the most prevalent are epilepsy (22%), cerebral palsy (20%), anxiety disorder (17%), oppositional defiant disorder (12%), and autistic disorder (10%) (Oeseburg *et al.* 2011).

Mild intellectual disability

The prevalence figures for mild MR do vary from study to study, with an average of about 3% of the population. There is a higher rate in socially disadvantaged groups. Those with an IQ in the top of the range for this group live a relatively independent life. Some of this group represent individuals at the lower end of the normal distribution for IQ. On clinical and traditional cytogenetic grounds, the aetiology is unknown in about 70–80% (see Table 2.15). However, the recent widespread use of chromosomal microarray testing reveals an increasing number of relatively common recurrent CNVs being associated with mild or borderline ID with reduced penetrance and thus being commonly transmitted by a parent functioning in the normal range. See Table 2.16 for penetrance estimates for the most common of these CNVs.

Severe intellectual disability

In the moderate, severe, and profound groups, there is a more equal social class distribution. This group has special educational needs and will require long-term care as adults. Many have serious long-term health problems. The life expectancy is reduced by a combination of these health problems and the delay in getting appropriate and prompt treatment of acute problems due to communication difficulties. An explanation of the ID can be established in about 50%, with Down's syndrome as the most common condition (see Table 2.17). However, causes like 'brain malformation' or 'epilepsy' are usually heterogeneous conditions and are of limited help for genetic counselling.

ID has a complex genomic architecture (see Figure 2.17). When considering only diagnoses of distinct

Table 2.15 Cytogenetic and clinical diagnoses in mild mental retardation*

Diagnoses	Number (%)
Down's syndrome	25 (5.7)
Fragile X	20 (4.6)
Other chromosome abnormalities	2 (0.6)
Cerebral palsy, neonatal illness, intrauterine infection	12 (2.7)
Postnatal trauma and illness	14 (3.2)
Malformation or genetic syndrome	15 (3.4)
Unknown	88 (80)

*N = 439. In 88 (20%), a cause for the ID was identified.

Reproduced from *Journal of Medical Genetics*, Bundey *et al.*, vol 26, issue 4, copyright 1989 with permission from BMJ Publishing Group Ltd.

Table 2.16 Penetrance estimates with case and control frequencies for recurrent CNVs significantly associated with mild/borderline ID

Region (gene in region)	CNV	hg18 (Mb)	Cases (%)	Controls (%)	De novo in cases (%)	Pene-trance (%)
Proximal 1q21.1 (*RBM8A*)	Dup	Chr 1: 144.0–144.5	0.17	0.04	0	17
Distal 1q21.1 (*GJA5*)	Del	Chr 1: 145.0–146.4	0.29	0.03	18	37
Distal 1q21.1 (*GJA5*)	Dup	Chr 1: 145.0–146.4	0.20	0.03	17	29
15q11.2 (*NIPA1*)	Del	Chr 15: 20.3–20.8	0.81	0.38	0	10
16p13.11 (*MYH11*)	Del	Chr 16: 14.9–16.4	0.15	0.05	22	13
16p12.1 (*CDR2*)	Del	Chr 16: 21.85–22.4	0.19	0.07	4	12
Distal 16p11.2 (*SH2B1*)	Del	Chr 16: 28.65–29.0	0.14	0.005	33	62
Distal 16p11.2 (*SH2B1*)	Dup	Chr 16: 28.65–29.0	0.11	0.04	13	11
Proximal 16p11.2 (*TBX6*)	Del	Chr 16: 29.5–30.15	0.44	0.03	70	47
Proximal 16p11.2 (*TBX6*)	Dup	Chr 16: 29.5–30.15	0.28	0.04	23	27
17q12 (*HNF1B*)	Del	Chr 17: 31.8–33.3	0.09	0.01	56	34
17q12 (*HNF1B*)	Dup	Chr 17: 31.8–33.3	0.11	0.02	22	21
22q11.21 (*TBX1*)	Dup	Chr 22: 17.2–19.9	0.28	0.05	26	22

Adapted by permission from Macmilliam Publishers Ltd: *Genetics in Medicine*, Rosenfield *et al.*, Estimates of penetrance for recurrent pathogenic copy-number variations, vol 15, pp. 478–481, copyright 2012.

entities as diagnostic yield in ID, a clinically recognizable diagnosis is established in about 25% of cases (Rauch *et al.* 2006). In clinically non-specific cases, microscopic karyotyping reveals a diagnosis in about 4%, and high-resolution chromosomal microarray analysis (CMA) in another 14% of cases (Hochstenbach *et al.* 2011). WES is currently capable of revealing a disease causing single gene mutation in up to 50% of patients with sporadic severe ID.

Many of these disorders, while having a severe ID phenotype, do not have an otherwise distinctive phenotype, so that targeting a single gene to test has a low diagnostic yield. Early studies of WES in ID cohorts established that a limited number of recurrently mutated genes were common causes of ID (Rauch *et al.* 2012). More recent reports from large-scale studies of children with ID, such as the Deciphering Developmental Disorders (DDD) study in the UK, have confirmed the high prevalence of *de novo* dominant mutations as a common cause of previously undiagnosed predominantly syndromic ID. The DDD study (McRae *et al.* 2016) reported 94 genes enriched for damaging *de novo* mutation (DNM) at genome-wide significance ($P < 7 \times$

10^{-7}). In the DDD cohort, the factors that increased the chance of finding a new dominant mutation were female sex, increased paternal age (and to a lesser extent maternal age), and lack of consanguinity.

This high yield of WES is likely to increase, even more with ongoing improvement of sequencing techniques and data interpretation. Currently, >950 ID genes have been identified and the underlying pathways often affect either brain development or neural signalling (http://sysid.cmbi.umcn.nl/).

Clinical approach

The aim is to try and establish the aetiology so that precise, rather than empiric, recurrence risks can be discussed, as well as giving information about the natural history and respective management advice. Spend time making certain that the child is continuing to make forward progress and find out if there are areas of development where the child has particular difficulties. When dysmorphic features accompany ID, these should be used to help establish the diagnosis. Recognition of a specific

Table 2.17 Cytogenetic and clinical causes of severe mental retardation

Diagnosis	Percentage of cases
Chromosomal, including Down's syndrome	4–28
Fragile X	2–6
CNS anomalies	7–17
Environmental causes, prematurity	5–13
Malformation or genetic syndrome	10–20
Unknown	30–50

Adapted from Curry CJ, *et al.*, Evaluation of mental retardation: recommendations of a consensus conference, *American Journal of Medical Genetics Part A*, 72, pp. 468–72, copyright 1997, with permission from Wiley.

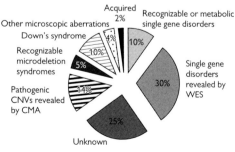

Figure 2.17 Causes of ID by means of distinct aetiological diagnoses. Adapted with permission from Otte and Rauch [Intellectual disability – a frequent reason for referral to medical gene cs], *Praxis* 2013, 102(24):1467–73, Hans Huber © 2013. Based on Rauch *et al.* 2006 and 2012, and Hochstenbach *et al.* 2011.

syndrome may prevent further extensive and invasive testing and allows optimization of care. Not only other neurodevelopmental, but also mental, medical, and physical, conditions are frequent in ID. The prognosis and outcome of co-occurring diagnoses may be influenced by the presence of ID since reduced perception and communication skills may hamper the diagnosis of an unexpected comorbidity. This section is primarily addressing the counselling problem of the child with no, or minor, dysmorphic features.

History: key points

- Three-generation family tree with enquiry about consanguinity. Try to establish if either parent had special educational needs. In other words, is the child's educational attainment similar to, or very different from, that of the rest of the family? Ask about the developmental and educational progress of siblings, uncles, and aunts. Look carefully at the family tree for evidence of XL inheritance. Premature ovarian failure (POF) or late-onset ataxia–tremor syndrome may indicate fragile X permutation carriers.
- Pregnancy, labour, delivery. Note any adverse events. Ask about alcohol, prescription medications, and recreational drugs. Note if there have been any previous pregnancy losses that might indicate a subtle chromosomal rearrangement.
- Developmental progress. Education/schooling. Evaluate for loss of skills (regression), autistic signs, seizure disorder, sleeping anomalies, reduced pain sensitivity.
- Does he/she have a recognizable behavioural phenotype?
- Other medical and neurological problems.

Examination: key points

- Measure the OFC to establish if microcephalic or macrocephalic. Refer also to 'Macrocephaly', p. 224 and 'Microcephaly', p. 228 in Chapter 2, 'Clinical approach'.
- Focal neurological signs such as hemiplegia.
- Neurocutaneous signs, particularly pigmentary changes (to exclude TSC and NF1 and chromosomal/genetic mosaicism).
- Presence of dysmorphic features. When there are minor dysmorphic features, are these familial? However, consider the possibility of mildly affected carrier parents. Always consider the three most frequent diagnoses after Down's syndrome: deletion 22q11.2 (2.4%), Williams–Beuren syndrome (1.3%), and FRAX (1.2%) (Rauch et al. 2006).

Investigations

Debate continues as to the usefulness of baseline general investigations, including electrolytes, uric acid, LFTs, FBC with indices and blood film, CPK, and urine metabolic screen (reducing substances, amino and organic acids, and mucopolysaccharides).

GENETIC TESTING.

- Genomic analysis in presence of features suggestive of a chromosomal or syndromic diagnosis, e.g. genomic array, gene panel, or WES/WGS as appropriate. According to a meta-analysis by Hochstenbach et al. (2011), high-resolution array testing results in an average diagnostic yield of 18% if used as a first-tier test.
- WES, if available, should currently be performed after exclusion of clinically recognizable single gene disorders

and CMA testing (Shashi et al. 2013). Current costs, as well as limitations in exon capturing, identification of certain mutations, and CNVs, hamper its actual use as a first-tier test. Due to the plethora of variants of unknown significance commonly detected by WES, data interpretation is greatly facilitated by analysis of patient–parent trios in sporadic patients and tight interaction between clinical and laboratory geneticists (de Ligt et al. 2012; Rauch et al. 2012).

- DNM is the most prevalent cause of severe genetic developmental disorders in the offspring of non-consanguineous parents (McRae et al. 2016). In consanguineous families, where recessive disorders are the most common cause of developmental disorders, ~5% of children with a developmental disorder will have this as a consequence of a DNM.

METABOLIC INVESTIGATIONS. As suggested by Garcia-Cazorla et al. 2009.

- In non-specific ID without dysmorphic features:
  - basic laboratory tests (blood glucose, lactate, ammonia, acid–base status, blood counts, LFTs, CK levels, phosphate, uric acid);
  - thyroid function, including free T3;
  - consider maternal phenylalanine;
  - creatine metabolites (urine—creatine transporter deficiency);
  - glycosaminoglycans in urine (by electrophoresis—Sanfilippo disease);
  - consider purines and pyrimidines (urine).
- Additional tests in ID with neurological abnormalities:
  - urine: simple tests, organic acids, oligosaccharides, sialic acid;
  - plasma/serum: quantitative amino acids, including homocysteine;
  - biotinidase activity, if not included in neonatal screening (dried blood spots);
  - consider purines and pyrimidines (urine), glycosylation disorders (CDG);
  - consider thiamine deficiency.
- Additional tests in ID with dysmorphic features:
  - maternal phenylalanine;
  - sterols, peroxisomal studies (VLCFAs, phytanic acids, plasmalogens);
  - transferrin isoelectric focusing for glycosylation studies (CDG).

MOLECULAR X-INACTIVATION STUDIES. May be considered in healthy mothers of affected boys as a screening tool for XL inheritance and guidance of interpretation of WES data. However, significant skewing in carrier mothers is only present in ~50% of XLID disorders and even highly significant skewing may be a chance finding (Plenge et al. 2002).

FRAXA. FMR1 molecular testing is considered in all individuals due to its non-specific presentation in early childhood and high recurrence risk. Moreover, recent studies and ongoing clinical trials are nourishing the hope for the possibility of improvement of intellectual and behavioural function by targeted drug treatment in the near future (Hagerman et al. 2012). In children over 6 and adults, a clinical checklist for the signs of FRAXA can reduce the number of tests. Commercially available multiplex ligation-dependent probe amplification (MLPA) kits for FRAXA methylation testing also detect FRAXE methylation. Note that WES is currently not capable of detecting higher-magnitude repeat mutations.

UPD SCREENING. There are a few recognizable phenotypes associated with UPD. CMA testing by SNP arrays are also capable of detecting long runs of homozygosity, which may indicate isodisomy if limited to a single chromosome or parental consanguinity if involving several chromosomes. The frequency of true UPDs detected by SNP array testing was <0.5% in various studies.

BRAIN IMAGING. Indicated in individuals with micro- or macrocephaly and/or neurological signs. There is currently no consensus on whether to arrange imaging in patients without neurological signs. MRI is preferred, except in cases of suspected craniosynostosis or congenital infection when CT is preferable.

EEG

• If any suspicion of seizures.
• If neurodevelopmental regression. See 'Developmental regression' in Chapter 2, 'Clinical approach', p. 128.

CONSIDER CK. In young males with developmental delay. Approximately one-third of boys with DMD will present with developmental delay in the first instance.

HAEMOGLOBIN H (HBH) INCLUSIONS. In males with abnormal genitalia (XL alpha-thalassaemia/mental retardation (ATRX) syndrome) if the required special staining is locally available.

Some diagnoses to consider

CHROMOSOMAL ABNORMALITIES. See 'Deletions and duplications (including microdeletions and microduplications)' in Chapter 5, 'Chromosomes', p. 660.

X-LINKED INTELLECTUAL DISABILITY. Including FRAXA. See 'Intellectual disability with apparent X-linked inheritance' in Chapter 2, 'Clinical approach', p. 194.

STRUCTURAL BRAIN LESION. See 'Structural intracranial anomalies (agenesis of the corpus callosum, septo-optic dysplasia, and arachnoid cysts)' in Chapter 2, 'Clinical approach', p. 320.

ENVIRONMENTAL FACTORS. For example, FAS. See 'Fetal alcohol syndrome (FAS)' in Chapter 6, 'Pregnancy and fertility', p. 728.

Genetic advice: non-specific mental retardation

Inheritance and recurrence risk

All studies have shown a risk of recurrence, but with widely different rates. Older studies did not include routine cytogenetic analysis or molecular testing for FRAXA. When the condition has recurred, all modes of Mendelian inheritance have been documented, but special mention needs to be made of the possibility of an XL condition. There is an excess of males with ID, but conflicting data about the contribution of XLID conditions. Turner and Partington (2000) have reviewed the data from a cohort of 429 subjects with ID. In about two-thirds, the IQ was

<50, 8% had no IQ assessment, and in the remainder the IQ was >50. Twenty-eight per cent were undiagnosed and recurrence risks in these families were ascertained (see Table 2.18). The M:F ratio was 1.76.

Turner and Partington's (2000) figures support the hypothesis that genes on the X chromosome contribute to ID. Ropers (2010) estimates that 10–12% of boys with ID are due to XL conditions.

Recent WES studies in sporadic severe non-specific ID patients from non-consanguineous parents detected autosomal or XL DNMs in up to 60% of cases, while XL inherited mutations were detected in up to 3% of boys (de Ligt *et al.* 2012; Rauch *et al.* 2012; Willemsen and Kleefstra 2013). Clear evidence of AR mutations was lacking in these studies, but this is likely to be changing with increasing knowledge about such disease genes. However, if parents are consanguineous, a 25% recurrence risk has to be assumed, unless otherwise disproven.

Be aware that not only obviously unbalanced translocations but also seemingly *de novo* interstitial CNVs may be caused by balanced insertional translocations in the parents in ~2% of cases (Nowakowska *et al.* 2012). The latter is only detectable by targeted FISH or breakpoint PCR testing in the parents, since dosage-based techniques, such as MLPA, quantitative PCR (qPCR), and CMA, will give normal results in carriers of a balanced cryptic translocation.

Variability and penetrance

There may be variability in the severity of problems, especially in the context of XL inheritance and in recurrent low-penetrant CNVs (see Tables 2.18 and 2.19). Turner and Partington (2000) believe that, if the mother or maternal aunt of an affected male has learning and educational difficulties, this is strongly suggestive of XLID.

Offspring risk to the siblings of ID individuals

The data of Bundey *et al.* (1989) probably overestimated the proportion of ID caused by FRAXA. For various counselling situations and further explanation, see Turner and Partington (2000) and Tables 2.18 and 2.19. Their calculations estimate the likelihood of XLID, as against other mechanisms of inheritance, and then add the risk that the ID is caused by a familial occult chromosomal abnormality, using the data of Knight *et al.* (1999).

Prenatal diagnosis

Unless a specific laboratory-based diagnosis has been made in the proband, no specific diagnostic tests are available. Parents may ask about sex selection or termination of males. Inform them of the risks of an affected female child and that such testing cannot distinguish between normal and affected boys.

Surveillance and follow-up

Review appointments can help:

Table 2.18 Observed recurrence risks for mental retardation in the sibs of index cases

Index case				
Gender	Number	Affected brothers	Affected sisters	All affected sibs
Male	69	11/83 (1 in 7.5) (13%)	3/60 (1 in 20) (5%)	14/43 (1 in 10) (10%)
Female	32	3/36 (1 in 12) (8%)	2/30 (1 in 15) (6.5%)	5/66 (1 in 13) (7.5%)

Reproduced from *Journal of Medical Genetics*, Turner and Partington, vol 37, copyright 2000, with permission from BMJ Publishing Group Ltd.

Table 2.19 Estimated risks for severe MR to the offspring of sibs of index cases (assuming normal intelligence and no learning difficulties in the consultant or the consultand's mother)

Index	Offspring risk (%)			
	Brother (cryptic translocation risk)	Brother (genomic array negative)*	Sister (XLMR and cryptic translocation risk)	Sister (genomic array negative)*
One affected male sib	1–2	~1	2–5	1.5–3
One affected female sib				
mild MR	~1[†]	~1	1.5–3[†]	1.5–3
severe MR	1–2	~1	1–2	~1
Two affected male sibs	1–2	~1	11–12[‡]	10
Two affected female sibs	Not known	Not known[§]	Not known	Not known[§]

NB. Use this table with caution; it is based on extrapolations from data from a small sample (101 families) and is not suitable for use in consanguineous families.

* Genomic array must be done in the proband, rather than the healthy sibling. (Dosage-based techniques, e.g. MLPA or array-CGH will give normal results in carriers of a balanced cryptic translocation.)

[†] Assuming that telomeric deletions are only very rarely a cause of mild MR.

[‡] Sister has 40% risk of carrier status for XLMR (since her mother has an 80% risk of being a carrier with two affected sons).

[§] Likely to be low if no consanguinity, once translocation risk excluded.

Table derived from data given in Turner and Partington 2000 to incorporate estimated risks after negative telomere screening.

- to offer newly available diagnostic tests;
- to establish that there are no additional medical problems and that there is forward developmental progress;
- to increase the chance of syndrome recognition;
- to discuss recurrence risks.

There are no absolute guidelines for review, but a reasonable approach would be a review 1 year after the initial completed consultation (which may involve more than one appointment) and another 2 years after this.

Genetic advice: mild mental retardation

The study of Bundey et al. (1989) investigated a group of 439 schoolchildren with mild ID. Although there were 274 boys and 165 girls in the group, the recurrence risks were not higher for male sibs. There were considerable contributions from familial, environmental, and cultural factors that make individual risks vary. The overall recurrence risk was high at between 1 in 4 and 1 in 5 (i.e. 20–25%).

Support groups: Mencap, http://www.mencap.org.uk, Tel. 0808 808 1111 (England and Wales); American Association on Mental Retardation (AAMR); Association of Retarded Citizens of the US (ARC).

Expert adviser: Anita Rauch, Professor of Medical Genetics, Institute of Medical Genetics, University of Zurich, Schlieren, Switzerland.

References

American Psychiatric Association (APA). *Diagnostic and statistical manual of mental disorders*, 5th edn. APA, Washington DC, 2013.

Bundey S, Thake A, Todd J. The recurrence risks for mild idiopathic mental retardation. *J Med Genet* 1989; **26**: 260–6.

Crow YJ, Tolmie JL. Recurrence risks in mental retardation. *J Med Genet* 1998; **35**: 177–82.

Curry CJ, Stevenson RE, Aughton D, et al. Evaluation of mental retardation: recommendations of a consensus conference. *Am J Med Genet* 1997; **72**: 468–72.

de Ligt J, Willemsen MH, van Bon BW, et al. Diagnostic exome sequencing in persons with severe intellectual disability. *N Engl J Med* 2012; **367**: 1921–9.

Garcia-Cazorla et al. Mental retardation and inborn errors of metabolism. *J Inherit Metab Dis* 2009; **32**(5): 597–608.

Gillberg C, Soderstrom H. Learning disability. *Lancet* 2003; **362**: 811–21.

Hagerman R, Lauterborn J, Au J, Berry-Kravis E. Fragile X syndrome and targeted treatment trials. *Results Probl Cell Differ* 2012; **54**: 297–335.

Harris JC. New terminology for mental retardation in DSM-5 and ICD-11. *Curr Opin Psychiatry* 2013; **26**: 260–2.

Hochstenbach R, Buizer-Voskamp JE, Vorstman JA, Ophoff RA. Genome arrays for the detection of copy number variations in idiopathic mental retardation, idiopathic generalized epilepsy and neuropsychiatric disorders: lessons for diagnostic workflow and research. *Cytogenet Genome Res* 2011; **135**: 174–202.

McRae JF, Clayton S, Fitzgerald TW, et al. (2016, under review). Prevalence, phenotype and architecture of developmental disorders caused by de novo mutation. doi: http://dx.doi.org/10.1101/049056. http://biorxiv.org/content/early/2016/06/16/049056.

Knight SJL, Regan R, Nicod A, et al. Subtle chromosomal rearrangements in children with unexplained mental retardation. *Lancet* 1999; **354**: 1676–81.

Miller DT, Adam MP, Aradhya S, et al. Consensus statement: chromosomal microarray is a first-tier clinical diagnostic test for individuals with developmental disabilities or congenital anomalies. *Am J Hum Genet* 2010; **86**: 749–64.

Nowakowska BA, de Leeuw N, Ruivenkamp CA, et al. Parental insertional balanced translocations are an important cause of apparently de novo CNVs in patients with developmental anomalies. *Eur J Hum Genet* 2012; **20**: 166–70.

Oeseburg B, Dijkstra GJ, Groothoff JW, et al. Prevalence of chronic health conditions in children with intellectual disability: a systematic literature review. *Intellect Dev Disabil* 2011; **49**: 59–85.

Otte C, Rauch A. [Intellectual disability—a frequent reason for referral to medical genetics]. *Praxis (Bern 1994)* 2013; **102**: 1467–73.

Plenge RM, Stevenson RA, Lubs HA, Schwartz CE, Willard HF. Skewed X-chromosome inactivation is a common feature of X-linked mental retardation disorders. *Am J Hum Genet* 2002; **71**: 168–73.

Rauch A, Hoyer J, Guth S, et al. Diagnostic yield of various genetic approaches in patients with unexplained developmental delay or mental retardation. *Am J Med Genet A* 2006; **140A**: 2063–74.

Rauch A, Wieczorek D, Graf E, et al. Range of genetic mutations associated with severe non-syndromic sporadic intellectual disability: an exome sequencing study. *Lancet* 2012; **380**: 1674–82.

Roelveld N, Zeilhuis GA, Gabreels F. The prevalence of mental retardation: a recent critical review of the literature. *Dev Med Child Neurol* 1997; **39**: 125–32.

Ropers HH. Genetics of early onset cognitive impairment. *Annu Rev Genomics Hum Genet* 2010; **11**: 161–87.

Rosenfeld JA, Coe BP, Eichler EE, Cuckle H, Shaffer LG. Estimates of penetrance for recurrent pathogenic copy-number variations. *Genet Med* 2013; **15**: 478–81.

Salvador-Carulla L, Reed GM, Vaez-Azizi LM, *et al*. Intellectual developmental disorders: towards a new name, definition and framework for 'mental retardation/intellectual disability' in ICD-11. *World Psychiatry* 2011; **10**: 175–80.

Schalock RL, Borthwick-Duffy SA, Bradley VJ, *et al*. *Intellectual disability: definition, classification, and systems of supports*, 11th edn. American Association on Intellectual and Developmental Disabilities (AAIDD), Washington DC, 2010.

Shashi V, McConkie-Rosell A, Rosell B, *et al*. The utility of the traditional medical genetics diagnostic evaluation in the context of next-generation sequencing for undiagnosed genetic disorders. *Genet Med* 2014; **16**:176–82.

Turner G, Partington M. Recurrence risks in undiagnosed mental retardation. *J Med Genet* 2000; **37**: E45.

van Bokhoven H. Genetic and epigenetic networks in intellectual disabilities. *Annu Rev Genet* 2011; **45**: 81–104.

Vissers LE, Gilissen C, Veltman JA. Genetic studies in intellectual disability and related disorders. *Nat Rev Genet* 2016; **17**: 9–18.

Willemsen MH, Kleefstra T. Making headway with genetic diagnostics of intellectual disabilities. *Clin Genet* 2014; **85**: 101–10.

World Health Organization (WHO). *The ICD-10 classification of mental and behavioural disorders. Clinical descriptions and diagnostic guidelines*. WHO, Geneva, 1992.

Intellectual disability with apparent X-linked inheritance

Intellectual disability (ID) and learning difficulties are more prevalent in males. There is a subtly different genomic burden and architecture in males and females presenting with ID (McRae 2017). Studies show a 20–40% excess of males with ID. Assuming this excess was caused by genes on the X chromosomes, XLID would account for about 10% of ID. This has not been proven in clinical surveys of individuals with ID, which may be due to the paucity of distinctive features in many of the conditions, the lack of confirmatory tests, and the presence of new mutations.

Fragile X syndrome (FRAXA) is the most common form of XLID.

This section addresses the approach to the investigation of the family where only males are affected by ID (or males are much more severely affected than females) and there is no evidence of male-to-male transmission, i.e. a family history consistent with an XL mode of inheritance.

The number of genes that have been identified as causing XLID syndromes is rapidly growing. Most of the genetic defects that underlie syndromic XL mental retardation (XLMR) (which is associated with additional phenotypes) are either known or have been mapped to small regions of the X chromosome. It has become apparent that different mutations in one gene may give a spectrum of phenotypes; thus, some XLID syndromes that were considered to be distinct are now known to be allelic. The distinction between syndromic XLID and non-syndromic XLID is becoming increasingly blurred.

This is a very fast moving field. The review by Piton et al. (2013) provides an excellent overview. Readers may need to supplement this by reference to the current literature.

The approach is to:
- assess the affected individuals in the family;
- confirm that the inheritance is compatible with X-linkage;
- divide into syndromic or non-syndromic XLID;
- in syndromic XLID, compare the features with known XLID syndromes;
- not to forget that other mechanisms of inheritance, such as the segregation of an unbalanced chromosome rearrangement, could mimic apparent XL inheritance in small families.

Clinical approach

History: key points
- Family history. Look carefully at the family tree for evidence of XL inheritance. Aim to expand further than a three-generation pedigree, especially concentrating on the maternal line and the children of maternal aunts and the maternal grandmother.
- Establish if either parent had special educational needs. Is there evidence of girls with milder degrees of learning difficulties than boys? Ask about the developmental and educational progress of siblings, uncles, and aunts.
- Pregnancy, labour, delivery. Note if there have been any previous pregnancy losses that might indicate a subtle chromosomal rearrangement, rather than an XL genetic aetiology for the problems.
- Developmental progress. Education/schooling.

- Assess if there is loss of skills (regression).
- Seizure disorder in males and females (*ARX* mutations, bilateral periventricular nodular heterotopia (BPNH) in carrier females of the filamin A gene, subcortical band heterotopia (SBH) in carrier females with *XLIS/DCX*).
- Is there a recognizable behavioural phenotype (FRAXA, autism)?
- Severe constipation (Opitz FG syndrome)
- Associated spastic quadriplegia (SLC16A2).
- Other medical and neurological problems, including enquiry about vision and hearing.

Examination: key points

HEAD.
- Macrocephaly/relatively large OFC (CUL4B, OFC; FRAXA, Opitz FG, SGB, MPS IIA, Aitkin–Flaitz syndrome).
- Hydrocephalus (XL hydrocephalus).
- Microcephaly (Börjeson–Forssman–Lehmann syndrome, Renpenning syndrome, ATRX).
- Hair: cowlicks (Opitz FG syndrome).

EYES.
- Hypertelorism (CLS, ATRX, Opitz G).
- Structural abnormalities in Lenz microphthalmia, Norrie disease.

FACE.
- Coarse facial features with full/thick lips (CLS, Aitkin–Flaitz syndrome, SGB, Hunter's syndrome).
- Flat nasal bridge with a small triangular nose (ATRX).
- Mouth: tented/arched upper lip (ATRX, Chudley–Lowry syndrome). Wide mouth with a midline groove of the lower lip and tongue (SGB).
- Long, narrow face with prognathism (Renpenning).
- Relative macrocephaly, epilepsy, and pes cavus (CUL4B).

HANDS.
- Tapering fingers (CLS).
- Fetal fingertip pads (Opitz FG syndrome).
- Adducted thumbs (mental retardation–aphasia–shuffling gait–adducted thumbs (MASA) and XL hydrocephalus due to *L1CAM* mutations).
- PAP (SGB).
- Abnormal hand posturing (SLC9A6, MAOA and B deficiency).

CHEST.
- Accessory nipples (SGB).

ABNORMALITIES OF THE MALE GENITALIA.
- Macro-orchidism (FRAXA, XL psychosis–pyramidal signs–macro-orchidism (PPM-X) syndrome).
- Spectrum from undescended testes to apparently female external genitalia in males in ATRX and XL lissencephaly with abnormal genitalia (XLAG).
- Hypospadias (Opitz G).
- Small genitalia with hypogonadism (Börjeson–Forssman–Lehmann syndrome, CUL4B syndrome).
- Neurological signs (*L1CAM* mutations, Pelizaeus–Merzbacher disease (PMD), XL spastic paraplegia 2, Alan–Herndon–Dudley syndrome (SLC16A2 or MCT8)):

- hypotonia (FG);
- dystonia (*ARX* gene abnormalities);
- if there are minor dysmorphic features, are these familial?

Special investigations

- Baseline general investigations, including electrolytes, uric acid, LFTs, FBC with indices and blood film, CPK, and urine metabolic screen (reducing substances, amino and organic acids, and mucopolysaccharides). Consider measurement of free T3 (elevated free T3 levels are found in XLID due to mutations in *SLC16A2*) and urinary creatine (increased urinary creatine-to-creatinine ratio is found in XLID due to mutations in *SLC6A8*).
- Further biochemical screening is necessary if there is neurodevelopmental regression. See 'Developmental regression' in Chapter 2, 'Clinical approach', p. 128:
  - VLCFA abnormalities in ALD;
  - exclude MPS IIA.
- Molecular testing. Genomic analysis in presence of features suggestive of a chromosomal or syndromic diagnosis, e.g. genomic array, gene panel, or WES/WGS as appropriate. Routine testing is indicated, even in non-dysmorphic boys.
  - FRAXA. *FMR1* molecular testing in all individuals;
  - specific mutation testing may be available for other conditions, e.g. *RPS6KA3* in CLS, ATRX; CUL4B, SLC16A2;
  - store DNA for future analysis (obtain consent).
- Brain imaging (preferably MRI). Should be performed on individuals with:
  - microcephaly or macrocephaly, except those with an established diagnosis such as FRAXA;
  - neurological signs;
  - seizures.
- EEG. If any suspicion of seizures.
- HbH inclusions in erythrocytes (males with abnormal genitalia to exclude ATRX).
- Consider X-inactivation studies in female carriers from large kindreds, but note that, unless there is consistent almost complete skewing (>95%) in all obligate carriers in a large kindred, then using this information for carrier testing is risky. See 'X-linked recessive (XLR) inheritance' in Chapter 1, 'Introduction', p. 50.

Diagnoses to consider

Syndromic XLMR

See Table 2.20.

COFFIN–LOWRY SYNDROME (CLS). Males with CLS show ID (usually severe) with characteristic dysmorphism, most notably affecting the face and hands. The typical facial features consist of a prominent forehead, hypertelorism, a flat nasal bridge, downward sloping palpebral fissures, and a wide mouth with full lips. Mild progression in facial coarsening occurs during childhood and adult life. The hands are broad with soft, stubby, tapering fingers. Other clinical findings include short stature (95%), pectus deformity (80%), kyphosis and/or scoliosis (80%), mitral valve dysfunction, and sensorineural hearing loss. The facial features become more pronounced with time and can also be recognized in some female carriers. X-rays of the hands, chest, and spine may help confirm the diagnosis. CLS is caused by mutations in the *RPS6KA3* gene. See

Table 2.20 Some additional clinical features found in syndromic XLMR

Absent speech	*ATRX, SLC16A2, SLC6A8, SLC9A6*
Abnormal genitalia	*ATRX*
Autistic behaviour	*NLGN3, NLGN4, AGTR2, SLC6A8*
Cerebellar hypoplasia	*OPHN1*
Cleft lip and palate	*PQBP1, PHF8*
Congenital heart disease	*PQBP1*
Dystonia	*ARX, SLC16A2*
Free T3 elevated	*SLC16A2*
Hypertelorism	*RSK2*
Infantile spasms	*ARX*
Microcephaly	*ATRX, MECP2, PQBP1, SMCX*
Macrocephaly	*CUL4B, SGB*
Scoliosis	*RSK2, ATRX, SLC9A6*
Seizures	*AGTR2, SYN1, ATRX, SLC6A8, ARX, PQBP1*
Short stature	*PQBP1, SMCX*
Spastic paraplegia	*SLC16A2, ATRX, SMCX, MECP2*
Tapering fingers	*RSK2*
Nystagmus	*CASK*

Hunter (2002) for information on long-term outcome in CLS.

SIMPSON–GOLABI–BEHMEL (SGB) SYNDROME. There is prenatal and postnatal overgrowth. The facial features appear coarse with wide thick lips. Macrocephaly is present. The development can vary from normal to mildly delayed. Other physical features are described above. Surveillance for malignancy (Wilms tumour, neuroblastoma, and others have been described) should be considered. Mutations in glypican 3 (*GPC3*). See 'Overgrowth' in Chapter 2, 'Clinical approach', p. 272.

X-LINKED ALPHA-THALASSAEMIA INTELLECTUAL DISABILITY (ATRX). Mutations in the *ATRX* gene. The key facial features are the characteristic tenting of the upper lip associated with a small triangular-shaped nose and a flat nasal bridge. Abnormalities of the genitalia in males, ranging from hypoplasia of the external genitalia to ambiguous genitalia, are found (these are not seen in CLS). Search carefully for HbH inclusions in erythrocytes stained with brilliant cresyl blue, although not always present in mutation-positive individuals. The facial features have been confused with those of CLS, but in ATRX carrier females do *not* have physical or intellectual manifestations of the condition. The phenotype in mild mutation males may be less syndromic. Carrier women may have some HbH inclusions, but it is not a reliable method of carrier detection (Gibbons and Higgs 2000).

OPITZ FG SYNDROME. Hypotonia and constipation are common in infants. Agenesis of the corpus callosum may be present. There is macrocephaly with a frontal upsweep of the hair (cowlick). Most cases are associated with a *de novo* mutation (DNM) in *MED12* and this now defines the classical FG syndrome. Some XL mutation-negative families are described where the gene has yet to be identified. Rare mutations in *ZDHHC9* (Lujan–Fryns syndrome) and *UPF3B* are also described as FG syndrome, but these are no longer regarded as classical FG.

OPITZ SYNDROME (ALSO KNOWN AS OPITZ G OR G/BBB). These families are usually referred for a dysmorphology opinion, rather than because of a family history of ID. There is striking hypertelorism, swallowing problems due to laryngeal clefts, and hypospadias. There is an XL and an autosomal (22q) locus. The XL gene is *MID1* at Xp22.

BÖRJESON–FORSSMAN–LEHMANN SYNDROME. Mutations in the *PHF6* gene. Affected males are short with microcephaly, deep-set eyes, obesity, and hypogonadism. Carrier females have milder physical features with some impairment of cognitive function.

RENPENNING SYNDROME. This term was previously used to describe all types of *XLID*. Stevenson et al. (2000) consider that Renpenning syndrome should be reserved for the condition caused by mutations in *PQBP1* on Xp11.2-11.4 (Lenski et al. 2004). Renpenning syndrome is characterized by severe mental impairment, microcephaly, and a tendency to short stature and small testes. Patients have a striking facial appearance with a long narrow face, malar hypoplasia, prognathism, and nasal speech.

CUL4B. Absent speech, relative macrocephaly, some seizures, and Parkinsonian features.

ALLAN–HERNDON–DUDLEY Hypotonic in the neonatal period, later evolving to dystonic posturing associated with severe developmental delay. Low free T3 (not detected by routine neonatal screening). Due to mutation in the *SLC16A2* gene encoding a thyroid hormone-specific transporter.

ARX (ARISTALESS-RELATED HOMEOBOX) GENE ABNORMALITIES. A spectrum of clinical phenotypes have been described with mutation in *ARX*.
• XLAG and agenesis of the corpus callosum in females.
• XL infantile spasms (West syndrome).
• XLID.
• Partington syndrome (XLMR with dystonia).

PELIZAEUS–MERZBACHER DISEASE (PMD) AND X-LINKED SPASTIC PARAPLEGIA 2. These two conditions are caused by mutations in the proteolipid protein gene *PLD*. There is striking hypomyelination in PMD. A duplication within the gene can sometimes be detected with a specific FISH probe.

X-LINKED ISOLATED LISSENCEPHALY SEQUENCE (XLIS OR DCX). Mutations leading to SBH in heterozygous females and predominantly anterior lissencephaly in hemizygous males.

BILATERAL PERIVENTRICULAR NODULAR HETEROTOPIA (BPNH). Lethal in the perinatal period in males; focal epilepsy in carrier females who have BPNH on MRI scan. Filamin A (*FLNA*) gene at Xq28.

MECP2. A number of phenotypes have now been associated with this gene.
• MECP2 duplication: the cardinal features include early infantile hypotonia, severe ID with absent speech, seizures, spasticity, and recurrent respiratory infections with GI motility problems (pseudo-obstruction). Most are inherited; carrier females are asymptomatic due to extreme X-skewing. This condition is estimated to affect ~2% of males with severe ID.
• Triplication of MECP2 is also reported resulting in an even more severe phenotype.
• Rett syndrome. See 'Rett syndrome' in Chapter 3, 'Common consultations', p. 520.
• Neonatal encephalopathy in males. See 'Neonatal encephalopathy and intractable seizures' in Chapter 2, 'Clinical approach', p. 246.
• PPM-X. Parkinsonian features are also found.
• An A140V mutation in *MECP2* has been identified. A140V can also result in severe non-syndromic XLID in males.

OLIGOPHRENIN-1. Moderate/severe MR with neonatal hypotonia and variable cerebellar hypoplasia. Cranial MRI shows some degree of vermic hypoplasia and cystic dilatation of the cisterna magna (Philip et al. 2003).

Non-syndromic XLMR

Fragile X syndrome (FRAXA). See 'Fragile X syndrome (FRAX)' in Chapter 3, 'Common consultations', p. 424.

FRAXE. See 'Fragile X syndrome (FRAX)' in Chapter 3, 'Common consultations', p. 424.

X-LINKED AUTISM. Mutations have been found in neuroligins 3 and 4 (*NLGN3* and *NLGN4*) in some families with both autism and Asperger's syndrome affecting males and where the family tree is consistent with XLR inheritance (Jamain et al. 2003).

XLID. A number of genes are reported with mutations where there are few syndromic features: *DLG3*, *ACSL4*, *HUWE1* (most commonly associated with whole gene duplications), *BRWD3*, *GDI1*, *GRIA3*, *IQSE2*, *PAK3*, *PTCHD1*, *RAB39B*, *SYN1*, *SYP*, *UBE2A*, *UPF3B*, and *ZNF711*.

Genetic advice

Recurrence risk

• Carefully exclude other causes for the apparent XLID.
• For families with established XL inheritance (affected males in more than one generation linked through the maternal line) but no diagnosis, calculate the carrier risk and counsel as appropriate. Assess the likelihood of females manifesting signs and symptoms, particularly ID, by careful family history questioning (but note the vagaries of X-inactivation and the wide variation seen, e.g. in women with FRAXA who carry a full mutation). Discuss the fact that prenatal sexing will not differentiate between an affected and unaffected male. Ensure that DNA is stored from affected members of the family.
• The offspring risk to sisters of two affected boys, but no other affected male relatives, is 5–10% (see 'Intellectual disability' in Chapter 2, 'Clinical approach', p. 188) but can be reduced if extensive sequence analysis of the X chromosome is performed to identify the causative mutation in the affected male. (This family structure is consistent with both XLR and AR inheritance.)

Carrier detection

• Possible where the causative mutation has been established.
• The carrier risk may be calculated from the pedigree.
• Carriers may be detectable on the basis of similarities in phenotype to the affected males.

Prenatal diagnosis

- If the causative mutation in the family has been defined, PND by CVS is possible.
- Where there is no defined mutation, sex determination by maternal free fetal DNA (ffDNA), CVS, or amniocentesis can be offered. This approach necessitates stringent evidence that the disorder is XL, e.g. affected males in more than one generation linked through the maternal line, and cannot distinguish between affected and unaffected male pregnancies.
- If there is a definite diagnosis of an XLMR syndrome and the familial mutation is unknown, PND by linkage may be an option, although risky due to the heterogeneity of the condition.
- USS for associated anomalies and biochemical markers may give additional information.

Support groups: Mencap (England and Wales), http://www.mencap.org.uk, Tel. 0207 454 0454; ENABLE (Scotland), http://www.enable.org.uk, Tel. 0141 226 4541.

Expert adviser: Lucy Raymond, Professor of Medical Genetics and Neurodevelopment, University of Cambridge, Cambridge, UK.

References

Frints SGM, Froyen G, Marynen P, Fryns J-P. X-linked mental retardation: vanishing boundaries between non-specific (MRX) and syndromic (MRXS) forms. *Clin Genet* 2002; **62**: 423–32.

Froyen G, Belet S, Martinez F, et al. Copy-number gains of HUWE1 due to replication- and recombination-based rearrangements. *Am J Hum Genet* 2012; **91**: 252–64.

Gibbons RJ, Higgs DR. Molecular-clinical spectrum of the ATR-X syndrome. *Am J Med Genet* 2000; **97**: 204–12.

Hanauer A, Young ID. Coffin–Lowry syndrome: clinical and molecular features. *J Med Genet* 2002; **39**: 705–13.

Hu H, Haas SA, Chelly J, et al. X-exome sequencing of 405 unresolved families identifies seven novel intellectual disability genes. *Mol Psychiatry* 2016; **21**: 133–48.

Hunter AGW. Coffin–Lowry syndrome: a 20-year follow-up of long-term outcomes. *Am J Med Genet* 2002; **111**: 345–55.

Jamain S, Quach H, Betancur C, et al. Mutations of the X-linked genes encoding neuroligins NLGN3 and NLGN4 are associated with autism. *Nat Genet* 2003; **34**: 27–8.

Klank SM, Lindsay S, Beyer KS, Splitt M, Burn J, Poustka A. A mutation hot spot for non-specific X-linked mental retardation in the MECP2 gene causes PPM-X syndrome. *Am J Hum Genet* 2002; **70**: 1034–7.

Lenski C, Abidid F, Meindl A, et al. Novel truncating mutations in the polyglutamine tract binding protein 1 gene (PQBP1) cause Renpenning syndrome and X-linked mental retardation in another family with microcephaly. *Am J Hum Genet* 2004; **74**: 777–80.

Lower KM, Turner G, Kerr BA, et al. Mutations in PHF6 are associated with Börjeson–Forssman–Lehmann syndrome. *Nat Genet* 2002; **32**: 661–5.

McRae JF, Clayton S, et al. Prevalence, phenotype and architecture of developmental disorders caused by de novo mutation. *Nature* 2017; in press.

Philip N, Chabrol B, Lossi AM, et al. Mutations, in the oligophrenin-1 gene (OPHNI) cause X-linked congenitial cerebellar hypoplasia. *J Med Genet* 2003; **40**: 441–6.

Piton A, Redin C, Mandel JL. XLID-causing mutations and associated genes challenged in light of data from large-scale human exome sequencing. *Am J Hum Genet* 2013; **93**: 368–83.

Raymond FL. X-linked mental retardation: a clinical guide. *J Med Genet* 2006; **43**: 193–200.

Stevenson RE, Schwartz CE, Schroer RJ. *X-linked mental retardation, Oxford monographs on medical genetics no. 39*. Oxford University Press, Oxford, 2000.

Tarpey PS, Smith R, Pleasance E, et al. A systematic, large-scale resequencing screen of X-chromosome coding exons in mental retardation. *Nat Genet* 2009; **41**: 535–43.

Tarpey PS, Raymond FL, O'Meara S, et al. Mutations in CUL4B, which encodes a ubiquitin E3 ligase subunit, cause an X-linked mental retardation syndrome associated with aggressive outbursts, seizures, relative macrocephaly, central obesity, hypogonadism, pes cavus, and tremor. *Am J Hum Genet* 2007; **80**: 345–52.

Turner G. Intelligence and the X chromosome. *Lancet* 1996; **347**: 1814–15.

van Esch H. MeCP2 duplication syndrome. *Mol Syndromology* 2012; **2**: 128–36.

Veltman JA, Yntema HG, Lugtenberg D, et al. High resolution profiling of X chromosomal aberrations by array comparative genomic hybridisation. *J Med Genet* 2004; **41**: 425–32.

Vissers LE, Gilissen C, Veltman JA. Genetic studies in intellectual disability and related disorders. *Nat Rev Genet* 2016; **17**: 9–18.

Whibley AC, Plagnol V, Tarpey PS, et al. Fine-scale survey of X chromosome copy number variants and indels underlying intellectual disability. *Am J Hum Genet* 2010; **87**: 173–88.

Increased bone density

Skeletal X-rays may reveal increased bone density and generalized skeletal changes consistent with a skeletal dysplasia. These disorders are known as sclerosing skeletal dysplasias. The International Nomenclature of Constitutional Disorders of Bone divides these conditions into four groups:

(1) increased bone density without modification of bone shape;

(2) increased bone density with diaphyseal involvement;

(3) increased bone density with metaphyseal involvement;

(4) neonatal severe osteosclerotic disorders.

There is an underlying disturbance of bone metabolism and many of these conditions have a progressive natural history. They are rare, and expert radiological advice is extremely important. As this is such a diverse group of conditions, the radiological findings need to be interpreted along with the clinical and biochemical data.

Sclerosis refers to a generalized disturbance with increased bone density. Hyperostosis refers to an overgrowth process localized to a part of the bone. In osteopetrosis, the bone cortex and the cancellous bone cannot be differentiated radiologically.

Clinical approach

History: key points

- Three-generation family history with enquiry about consanguinity and affected relatives.
- Age of onset of symptoms and signs.
- Progression of symptoms and signs.
- Ethnic group (van Buchem disease in Holland, sclerosteosis in Afrikaaners).
- Muscle weakness/pain (Cammurati–Engelmann syndrome).
- Visual and hearing problems, headaches (cranial nerve compression).
- Osteomyelitis of the mandible (osteopetrosis).
- Developmental delay.
- Easy fracturing (or no fractures after significant trauma).

Examination: key points

- Height (reduced in pycnodysostosis, increased in sclerosteosis).
- Head circumference (increased in many of these conditions).
- Bony overgrowth of the nasal bridge, forehead, and upper face (craniometaphyseal dysplasia, craniodiaphyseal dysplasia, and frontometaphyseal dysplasia).
- Overgrowth of the mandible (infantile cortical hyperostosis; in adults van Buchem disease, sclerosteosis, and Worth type dominant endosteal hyperostosis).
- Prominent eyes and large fontanelle (Melnick–Needles syndrome and pycnodysostosis).
- Teeth. Eruption or retention of primary dentition.
- Choanal stenosis.
- Cranial nerves for evidence of compression.
- Fundal examination for papilloedema.
- Digits for contractures and expansion.
- Limb and joint abnormalities due to bone expansion and modelling anomalies.
- Secondary sexual development (pituitary compression).

- Hepatosplenomegaly (AR osteopetrosis due to extramedullary haematopoiesis).
- Non-skeletal anomalies in rare syndromes, e.g. Raine, Schinzel–Giedion, Lenz–Makewski, oculodentodigital (ODD) syndrome.
- Torus palatinus. High bone mass phenotype families with activating mutations of *LRP5*.

Special investigations

- Bone biochemistry will often be normal, but the following may help with classification:
  - alkaline phosphatase, increased in Van Buchem disease but not in Worth endosteal hyperostosis;
  - acid phosphatase increased in AD osteopetrosis.
- Blood count (anaemia and bone marrow failure due to loss of bone marrow).
- Urinalysis, renal function (AR type of osteopetrosis due to carbonic anhydrase deficiency).
- Visual assessment (optic atrophy, papilloedema, squints).
- Hearing tests.
- Consider endocrine investigations.
- Exclude raised intracranial pressure due to medullary compression.
- Genomic analysis e.g. genomic array, gene panel or WES/WGS as appropriate.

Some diagnoses to consider

The age of onset, severity of the condition, and the presence of non-skeletal features should all be considered.

From the neonatal period to 2 years

Severe precocious AR osteopetrosis. Rapidly progressive with bone marrow failure with distinctive clinical and skeletal features. Infants may present with macrocephaly, hepatosplenomegaly, and visual inattention. It is a heterogeneous disorder and homozygous/compound heterozygous mutations have been described at six loci leading to severe infantile forms, with two further loci leading to intermediate AR phenotypes. Genes mutated include *CLCN7* and *CA2* (encoding carbonic anhydrase).

GHOSAL SYNDROME. AR. Hyperostosis of tubular bones and pancytopenia. Mutations in *TBXAS1* encoding thromboxane synthetase.

PYCNODYSOSTOSIS. AR, gene *CTSK*, cathepsin K. Large fontanelles, facial dysmorphic features, bone fragility, and short limbs.

SEVERE CRANIOMETAPHYSEAL DYSPLASIA. AR. There is progressive bony overgrowth of the nasal bridge and forehead. Some have mutations in *GJA1*.

CRANIODIAPHYSEAL DYSPLASIA. AR or AD (mutations in *SOST*). Non-skeletal features include raised intracranial pressure. Some have developmental delay.

RARE OSTEOSCLEROTIC CONDITIONS. Conditions in which the other non-skeletal features will aid the diagnosis.

- Blomstrand dysplasia. AR. Perinatal lethal. Advanced skeletal maturation. Inactivating mutations in the *PTHR1* gene.
- Raine syndrome. AR intracranial calcification. Choanal stenosis, proptosis, cleft palate, usually lethal. Mutations in *FAM20C*.

- Schinzel–Giedion syndrome. AD (DNMs in *SETBP1*). Wide fontanelle, midface hypoplasia, choanal stenosis, hydronephrosis, genital anomalies.
- Lenz–Majewski syndrome. AD (DNMs in *PTDSS1*). Wide cranial sutures, loose skin, choanal stenosis, developmental delay.
- Melnick–Needles syndrome. XL. Skull base sclerosis; features overlap with OPD syndrome. Caused by gain-of-function mutations in the gene encoding filamin A (*FLNA*) (Robertson *et al.* 2003). Most cases occur in females; lethal in males.
- Otopalatodigital (OPD) syndrome. XL. Skull base sclerosis is seen. Allelic conditions due to gain-of-function mutation in *FLNA*.

2–12 years

CRANIOMETAPHYSEAL DYSPLASIA. AR (GJA1 mutations) and AD (ANKH mutations) forms. Cranial nerve compression occurs as the child grows older, with optic atrophy and facial nerve palsy.

FRONTOMETAPHYSEAL DYSPLASIA. XL and AD forms. Prominent brow, cervical vertebral abnormalities, digital contractures. Features overlap with OPD-1. XL cases have mutations in *FLNA*; AD cases have mutations in MAP3K7 or TAB2.

CAMURATI–ENGELMANN SYNDROME. AD, *TGFB1* gene. Diaphyseal dysplasia, muscular weakness and pain, anaemia.

PYLE DYSPLASIA. AR and caused by biallelic variants in the SFRP4 gene (Simsek Kiper *et al.* 2016). Metaphyseal dysplasia distinguished from craniometaphyseal dysplasia by mild skull involvement.

SCLEROSTEOSIS. AR, *SOST* gene mutations. Endosteal hyperostosis, tall stature, syndactyly.

JUVENILE PAGET'S DISEASE AND IDIOPATHIC HYPERPHOSPHATASIA. AR, mutations in *TNFRSF11B*. Rapidly remodelling woven bone, osteopenia, fractures, progressive long bone deformities with bowing, vertebral collapse, skull enlargement, and deafness.

OSTEOPATHIA STRIATA WITH CRANIAL SCLEROSIS. XL. Usually female. Cranial stenosis, metaphyseal, pelvic striations in females. Lethal hyperostotic multiple congenital anomalies syndrome in males. Mutations in *WTX*.

DYSOSTEOSCLEROSIS. AR (mutations in *SLC29A3*). Short stature, skin atrophy; may fracture.

OSTEOPETROSIS. Mild AD type; see '12 years to adult' below.

KENNY–CAFFEY SYNDROME. AD (mutations in *FAM111A*; allelic to osteocranioscleroisis) short stature, hypoparathyroidism, microphthalmia, gracile bones.

MELNICK–NEEDLES SYNDROME. XL. Skull base sclerosis; features overlap with those of OPD. Caused by gain-of-function mutations in the gene encoding filamin A (*FLNA*) (Robertson *et al.* 2003). Most cases occur in females; usually lethal in males.

12 years to adult

CAMURATI–ENGELMANN SYNDROME. See '2–12 years' above.

PYLE DYSPLASIA. See '2–12 years' above.

VAN BUCHEM DISEASE. AR. Elevated alkaline phosphatase; slowly progressive enlargement of the mandible and other cranial bones. Allelic to sclerosteosis.

ENDOSTEAL HYPEROSTOSIS. Worth type. AD. Usually no cranial nerve compression. Gain-of-function mutations in *LRP5*.

OSTEOPETROSIS. Mild AD type; two loci: *LRP5* and *CLCN7*.

OTOPALATODIGITAL SYNDROME (OPD). XL. Skull base sclerosis is seen. Allelic conditions due to gain-of-function mutations in *FLNA* on Xq28. OPD is allelic in frontometaphyseal dysplasia and Melnick–Needles syndrome.

Genetic advice

These conditions are rare and genetic mutation analysis may only be available on a research basis.

A number of different conditions and phenotypes with increased bone density have been associated with mutation in the low-density lipoprotein (LDL) receptor protein 5 (*LRP5*). See Van Westenbeeck *et al.* (2003) for additional information.

Recurrence or offspring risk

As appropriate for each diagnosis.

Carrier detection

- Possible in families in whom causative mutations have been identified in the proband.
- Clinical and radiological examination may be informative in the XL and AD conditions.

Prenatal diagnosis

- By mutation analysis if a causative mutation has been identified in the proband.
- USS may detect increased bone density and other skeletal features, but usually not until the second or third trimester. Please check the literature carefully relating to the specific condition prior to counselling.

Support group: Many of the syndromes have their own support groups. See Contact a Family, http://www.cafamily.org.uk.

Expert adviser: Stephen Robertson, Clinical Geneticist, Dunedin School of Medicine, University of Otago, Dunedin, New Zealand.

References

de Vernejoul MC, Kornak U Heritable sclerosing bone disorders: presentation and new molecular mechanisms. *Ann N Y Acad Sci* 2010; **1192**: 269–77.

Holman SK, Daniel P, Jenkins ZA, *et al.* The male phenotype in osteopathia striata congenita with cranial sclerosis. *Am J Med Genet A* 2011; **155A**: 2397–408.

International Skeletal Dysplasia Society (for nomenclature and genetic information). http://www.isds.ch.

Robertson SP, Twigg SR, Sutherland-Smith AJ, *et al.* Localized mutations in the gene encoding cytoskeletal protein filamin A can cause diverse malformations in humans. *Nat Genet* 2003; **33**: 487–91.

Simsek Kiper PO, Saito H, Gori F, *et al.* Cortical-bone fragility insights from sFRP4 deficiency in Pyle's disease. *New Eng J Med* 2016; **374**: 2553–62.

Stark Z, Savarirayan R. Osteopetrosis. *Orphanet J Rare Dis* 2009; **4**: 5.

Van Westenbeeck L, Cleiren E, Gram J, *et al.* Six novel missense mutations in the LDL receptor related protein 5 (*LRP5*) gene in different conditions with increased bone density. *Am J Hum Genet* 2003; **72**: 763–71.

Waterval JJ, Borra VM, Van Hul W, Stokroos RJ, Manni JJ. Sclerosing bone dysplasias with involvement of the craniofacial skeleton. *Bone* 2013; **60C**: 48–67.

Intracranial calcification

Intracranial calcification (ICC) refers to calcification within the cranial cavity and generally is taken to mean calcification within the parenchyma of the brain and/or its vasculature. There is probably no pathological process that cannot, in some circumstances, result in ICC, so that there is a potentially endless list of causes of ICC. However, for poorly understood reasons, certain disorders exist in which ICC is prominent/characteristic, and thus of diagnostic value.

Focal calcification is common in CNS tumours and following acquired brain insults such as HII, CNS infection, or cerebrovascular compromise. Usually, there is no diagnostic difficulty in these situations—although it is important to bear in mind that cerebrovascular disease may have a genetic basis, e.g. with mutations in *COL4A1* or *SAMHD1*.

One of the first diagnostic considerations when ICC is identified in a neurologically abnormal child is congenital infection, especially CMV infection. However, the geneticist needs to be aware of the large number of genetic disorders that may result in ICC, some of which closely resemble congenital infection.

ICC is identified radiologically and may be demonstrated by X-ray, USS, CT, or MRI. Each of these modalities has different sensitivities and specificities for the identification of ICC. CT has the highest sensitivity and remains the gold standard investigation. However, for most children, MRI is the first imaging modality performed. MRI has a lower sensitivity than CT, so that (even quite extensive) calcification may be missed. For this reason, performing a CT should be considered in any child with an undiagnosed neurological condition, especially an undiagnosed white matter disorder.

It may not be possible to unequivocally distinguish haemorrhage from calcification on imaging. Follow-up scanning may be necessary to demonstrate the resolution of haemorrhage. Gradient-echo (GRE) and susceptibility-weighted (SW) images are much more sensitive than conventional T1 and T2 MRI sequences for detecting haemorrhage and mineralization, including calcification.

Once ICC is identified, its pattern and distribution should be considered since certain disorders have characteristic calcification phenotypes. The presence of other radiological features, such as cortical malformations, leukoencephalopathy, or the presence of cysts, can provide useful diagnostic information, and sometimes these other features allow a diagnosis to be made.

Clinical approach

History: key points giving clues to the diagnosis
- Family history of a previous affected child, stroke, cataract.
- Parental consanguinity.
- Pregnancy and labour (congenital infections, perinatal/prenatal asphyxia).
- Birthweight and OFC.
- Neonatal history (e.g. seizures, fever, coagulopathy, hepatosplenomegaly).
- Vision and hearing loss.
- Motor abnormalities (weakness, ataxia, spasticity, dystonia).

Examination: key points giving clues to the diagnosis
- Eye involvement (e.g. chorioretinopathy in congenital infection, Coats disease with *CTC1* mutations, cataract or microphthalmia in *COL4A*-related disease).
- Deafness in congenital infection.
- Skin signs (e.g. photosensitivity in Cockayne syndrome (CS), chilblains in Aicardi–Goutières syndrome (AGS), dyskeratosis congenita in telomere disorders).
- Short stature.
- Bone involvement (e.g. osteoporosis with *CTC1* mutations, osteopetrosis in carbonic anhydrase deficiency type 2).

Initial investigations
Neuroimaging is central to diagnosis. If the calcification pattern is not clear on MRI, a CT scan should be performed. Before proceeding to further investigations, an expert paediatric neuroradiology opinion should be sought. Many characteristic phenotypes can be recognized which may immediately suggest the diagnosis and avoid unnecessary or expensive tests.
- U & Es.
- Calcium, phosphate, and parathyroid hormone (PTH) levels.
- Serology for congenital infection.
- CMV PCR on neonatal blood spot (Guthrie).
- Urine organic acids, amino acids.
- Plasma lactate, amino acids.
- CSF examination (cells, protein, lactate, interferon alpha, pterins).
- Genomic analysis, e.g. genomic array, gene panel, or WES/WGS as available, unless a specific single gene disorder is suspected.
- Specific mutation testing guided by clinical and radiological features.
- Store DNA.

Some diagnoses to consider

Endocrine disorders
Parathyroid disorders and nephrogenic diabetes insipidus should be readily diagnosable by corresponding electrolyte or mineral abnormalities detectable on routine testing.

Congenital infections
Distinguishing congenital infection from genetic disorders associated with intracranial calcification may be difficult. ICC is common, but not invariable, in congenital infection and has been described following congenital CMV, rubella, Zika, toxoplasma, parvovirus, varicella, herpes, lymphocytic choriomeningitis (LCM) virus, and HIV. The diagnosis may be straightforward when there is active neonatal infection with identification of the virus by serology or PCR. After the neonatal period, diagnosis becomes more difficult, and in this situation careful consideration of the radiological phenotype may enable specific genetic disorders to be recognized. The MRI appearances of congenital CMV have been well characterized, although atypical cases do occur.

Cystic leukoencephalopathy without megalencephaly due to *RNASET2* mutations
May mimic congenital CMV infection. This is an AR disorder characterized by early-onset severe developmental

problems, often microcephaly and seizures and sometimes hearing impairment. It is important to be aware of this condition as it may be clinically and radiologically indistinguishable from congenital CMV.

Aicardi–Goutières syndrome (AGS)
Caused by mutations in any one of the genes *TREX1, RNASEH2A, RNASEH2B, RNASEH2C, SAMHD1, ADAR1* and *IFIH1*. The typical presentation is either as a neonatal encephalopathy resembling a congenital infection or with an infantile onset of an initially progressive disorder. The neonatal presentation is frequently characterized by fever, seizures, hepatosplenomegaly, thrombocytopenia, and anaemia, with or without microcephaly. The infantile form sometimes occurs after a period of apparently normal development, followed by the onset of a severe encephalopathy with irritability, fevers, loss of skills, and acquired microcephaly. Characteristic ICC and white matter disease (the early onset form can demonstrate marked temporal lobe cysts and a frontal gradient of abnormal white matter) are seen in many patients.

Coats plus disease due to CTC1 mutations
Mutations in the gene encoding conserved telomere maintenance component 1 (CTC1) were recently identified as the cause of Coats plus disease. This is a multisystem disorder characterized by: retinal telangiectasia and exudates (Coats disease), ICC with an associated leukoencephalopathy and brain cysts, osteopenia with a tendency to fractures and poor bone healing, and a high risk of life-limiting GI bleeding and portal hypertension caused by the development of vascular ectasias in the stomach, small intestine, and liver. The radiological appearances are striking with a diffuse leukoencephalopathy, dense rock-like calcification involving the basal ganglia, thalami, cerebellum, and deep cortex, and intraparenchymal space-occupying cysts.

Leukoencephalopathy with calcifications and cysts (LCC)
The neuroradiological features of LCC are identical to those of Coats plus, but this condition is a purely neurological disorder characterized by motor dysfunction, epilepsy, and cognitive difficulties. The disease is due to biallelic mutations in SNOR118, a small nucleolar RNA gene (Jenkinson 2016).

Band-like calcification with simplified gyration and polymicrogyria
Previously known as pseudo-TORCH syndrome, this is a rare AR disorder caused by mutations in the *OCLN* gene encoding the tight junction protein occludin. It is a severe condition presenting at birth or shortly after with epileptic seizures, feeding difficulties, microcephaly, quadriplegia, and bulbar palsy. The imaging features are highly characteristic and are best appreciated by considering both CT and MRI. There is generalized malformation of the cerebrum with very primitive sulcation and abnormal gyration. On CT, the calcification is seen as a symmetrical continuous or semi-continuous ribbon of cortical calcification, and also symmetrical thalamic calcification and sometimes central pontine calcification. The brain malformation and the pattern of calcification are distinct from those seen in congenital CMV, which is the most common cause of the association of ICC with polymicrogyria.

COL4A1 and COL4A2 mutation-related disease
Mutations in the gene encoding the alpha 1 chain of type IV collagen (*COL4A1* and *COL4A2*), a major component of vascular basement membranes, are a recognized cause of a genetic small-vessel disease affecting the brain, eyes, and kidneys. *COL4A1* mutations lead to intracerebral haemorrhage and ischaemic damage that may have an ante-, peri-, or postnatal onset. Most characteristically, but not exclusively, the disorder is associated with the presence of porencephaly. Recently, *COL4A1* mutations have also been demonstrated in patients with schizencephaly and focal cortical dysplasia. Children with *COL4A1*-related disease often present with early-onset seizures, developmental delay, and cerebral palsy, with or without extraneurological features such as cataract or other eye abnormalities. On MRI, there is often evidence of periventricular leukomalacia. Subtle spot-like calcification in the white matter or basal ganglia may occur.

Idiopathic basal ganglia calcification (syn. Fahr disease)
There is much confusion surrounding the use of Fahr disease as a diagnostic term. Fahr disease is not a single entity but describes a common and non-specific, albeit very striking, pattern of calcification which is usually symmetrical and is predominantly in the grey matter involving the caudate, putamen, globus pallidus, thalamus, deep cortex, dentate, and sometimes cerebellar folia. White matter calcification is not prominent but may occur. Familial and apparently non-familial forms occur; some patients are asymptomatic, but in others a wide spectrum of clinical manifestations have been described, most commonly movement disorders, cognitive impairment, or psychiatric disease. The molecular causes of some forms of Fahr disease have recently been identified due to mutations in *SLC20A2, PDGFRB, PDGFB* and *XRN1*.

Cockayne syndrome (CS)
An AR nucleotide excision repair disorder caused by mutations in either the *CSA* or *CSB* genes. CS comprises a spectrum of overlapping phenotypes which may present antenatally through to adult life. It is a multisystem disorder most typically recognized by the combination of facial features ('sunken eyes'), retinopathy, deafness, cutaneous photosensitivity, short stature, and (sometimes only slowly) progressive neurological features. ICC develops in the majority of patients. The MRI frequently demonstrates hypomyelination and cerebellar atrophy.

Other genetic causes of ICC
There are many other genetic disorders in which ICC may occur. These include: Nasu–Hakola disease, hereditary diffuse leukoencephalopathy with spheroids, Fried syndrome/AP1S2, dihydropteridine reductase deficiency, cerebrotendinous xanthomatosis, oculodentodigital dysplasia, Papillon–Lefèvre syndrome, Adams–Oliver syndrome, Gorlin syndrome, and Raine syndrome.

Expert advisers: Yanick Crow, Consultant Clinical Geneticist, Institut Imagine, Necker-Enfants Malades Hospital, Paris Descartes University, Paris, France and John H. Livingston, Consultant Paediatric Neurologist, Leeds Teaching Hospital NHS Trust, Leeds, UK.

References

Anderson BH, Kasher PR, Mayer J, et al. Mutations in CTC1, encoding conserved telomere maintenance component 1, cause Coats plus. *Nat Genet* 2012; **44**: 338–42.

Briggs TA, Abdel-Salam GMH, Balicki M, et al. Cerebroretinal microangiopathy with calcifications and cysts (CRMCC). *Am J Med Genet A* 2008; **146A**: 182–90.

Crow YJ, Livingston JH. Aicardi–Goutières syndrome: an important Mendelian mimic of congenital infection. *Dev Med Child Neurol* 2008; **50**: 410–16.

Henneke M, Diekmann S, Ohlenbusch A, *et al*. RNASET2-deficient cystic leukoencephalopathy resembles congenital cytomegalovirus brain infection. *Nat Genet* 2009; **41**: 773–5.

Jenkinson EM, Rodero MP, *et al*. Mutations in SNORD118 cause the cerebral microangiopathy leukoencephalopathy with calcifications and cysts. *Nature Genet* 2016; **48**: 1185–92.

Keller A, Westenberger A, Sobrido MJ, *et al*. Mutations in the gene encoding PDGF-B cause brain calcifications in humans and mice. *Nat Genet* 2013; **45**: 1077–82.

Koob M, Laugel V, Durand M, *et al*. Neuroimaging in Cockayne syndrome. *AJNR Am J Neuroradiol* 2010; **31**: 1623–30.

Livingston JH, Doherty D, Orcesi S, *et al*. COL4A1 mutations associated with a characteristic pattern of intracranial calcification. *Neuropediatrics* 2011; **42**: 227–33.

Livingston JH, Stavros S, van der Knaap MS, Crow YJ. Recognizable phenotypes associated with intracranial calcification. *Dev Med Child Neurol* 2013; **55**: 46–57.

Nicolas G, Pottier C, Maltête D, *et al*. Mutations of the *PDGFRB* gene as a cause of idiopathic basal ganglia calcification. *Neurology* 2013; **80**: 181–7.

O'Driscoll MC. Daly SB. Urquhart JE, *et al*. Recessive mutations in the gene encoding the tight junction protein occludin cause band-like calcification with simplified gyration and polymicrogyria. *Am J Hum Genet* 2010; **87**: 354–64.

van der Knaap MS, Vermeulen G, Barkhof F, Hart AAM, Loeber JG, Weel JFL. Pattern of white matter abnormalities at MR imaging: use of polymerase chain reaction testing of Guthrie cards to link pattern with congenital cytomegalovirus infection. *Radiology* 2004; **230**: 529–36.

Wang C, Li Y, Shi L, *et al*. Mutations in SLC20A2 link familial idiopathic basal ganglia calcification with phosphate homeostasis. *Nat Genet* 2012; **44**: 254–6.

Yoneda Y, Haginoya K, Kato M, *et al*. Phenotypic spectrum of *COL4A1* mutations: porencephaly to schizencephaly. *Ann Neurol* 2013; **73**: 48–57.

Large fontanelle

The fontanelles are the spaces in the immature and incompletely ossified skulls of babies and infants that permit brain growth. They lie in the sutures between the bones of the skull. The bones of the skull base and vault are known as the neurocranium. There are intricate processes that control the pre- and postnatal growth of the neurocranium and coordinate it to brain growth. If the OFC is significantly increased please see 'Macrocephaly' in Chapter 2, 'Clinical approach', p. 224.

At birth, the anterior fontanelle should always be patent and is known as a constant fontanelle. Those not always present are known as accessory fontanelles. Charts are available showing age-related sizes for the anterior and posterior fontanelles (see Figure 2.18). The anterior fontanelle normally closes at 12 ± 4 months. The posterior fontanelle normally closes at birth ± 2 months.

Very delayed and/or deficient ossification of the skull leads to cranium bifidum and parietal foramina. Parietal foramina have also been called Caitlin marks after the name of an affected family. They are defects in the parietal bone found on each side of the sagittal suture.

The first diagnostic step is to exclude raised intracranial pressure and hydrocephalus. Paediatric conditions to exclude are hypothyroidism and congenital infections. The geneticist is usually called once structural brain lesions have been excluded and this chapter concentrates on:
- syndromic causes of fontanelle enlargement due to abnormalities of the neurocranium;
- genetic and chromosomal disorders that characteristically have enlarged fontanelles.

A mildly enlarged fontanelle with no other craniofacial features is not a good diagnostic handle, but the cause of gross enlargement is usually found.

Clinical approach

History: key points
- Three-generation family tree with specific enquiry about consanguinity (pycnodysostosis, AR Robinow) and other affected family members (cleidocranial dysplasia, parietal foramina).
- Pregnancy. Congenital infection, aminopterin or angiotensin-converting enzyme (ACE) inhibitor exposure.

- OFC at birth (hydrocephalus), macrocephaly ERF craniosynostosis, other craniosynostoses. See 'Craniosynostosis' in Chapter 3, 'Common consultations', p. 378.
- Neonatal screening to exclude hypothyroidism.
- Developmental delay (chromosomal abnormalities, hypothyroidism, congenital infections).

Examination: key points
- Measurement of the OFC and fontanelles.
- Palpation of the cranial sutures; assess if open or closed. Remember to feel over the metopic region and on either side of the midline back to the occiput for parietal foramina.
- Scalp defects.
- Asymmetry of the cranium and face.
- Exorbitism (Crouzon and ERF craniosynostosis).
- Orofacial clefts can delay midline suture closure.
- Spina bifida (hydrocephalus).
- In floppy neonates, look for dysmorphic features of Down's and Zellweger syndromes and monosomy 1p36.
- Height, span, and limbs (skeletal dysplasias).
- Clavicles (cleidocranial dysplasia).
- Hands and feet (in Apert and Pfeiffer syndromes, the metopic and sagittal sutures remain patent to allow the brain to grow).
- Bony exostoses (proximal 11p deletion syndrome).
- Features of a chronic medical or metabolic condition (organomegaly, failure to thrive, developmental delay).

Special investigations
- Radiology:
  - SXRs;
  - consider full skeletal survey;
  - a delayed bone age may be an indicator of a generalized condition delaying skull maturation.
- In conjunction with a craniofacial team, the following are often performed:
  - brain imaging;
  - CT reconstruction of the skull bones;
  - exclusion of raised intracranial pressure.
- Metabolic bone profile including calcium, phosphate, PTH.
- Genomic analysis in presence of features suggestive of a chromosomal or syndromic diagnosis, e.g. genomic array, targeted gene test, gene panel, or WES/WGS as appropriate.
- VLCFAs (Zellweger syndrome).
- Transferrin isoelectric focussing if features of cutis laxa or neurological impairment.

Check that medical conditions such as hypothyroidism, rickets, and congenital infections have been excluded.

Some diagnoses to consider

Craniosynostosis syndromes
Especially Saethre–Chotzen syndrome where it may be associated with parietal foramina. Do not confuse with multiple craniolacunae related to a dysplastic skull vault.

Cleidocranial dysostosis
AD, caused by mutations in *RUNX2*. In some families, there is severely delayed skull ossification with a cranium bifidum. Careful examination of relatives is required. In addition to the widely patent anterior fontanelle, the

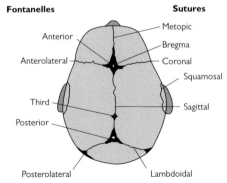

Fontanelles   **Sutures**

Anterior — Metopic
Bregma
Anterolateral — Coronal
Squamosal
Third — Sagittal
Posterior —
Posterolateral — Lambdoidal

Figure 2.18 View of the infant skull to show sutures and fontanelles.
Reproduced with permission from Pamela MacKinnon and John Morris, *Oxford Textbook of Functional Anatomy, Volume 3,* Second Edition, 2005, Figure 6.1.9, page 46, with permission from Oxford University Press.

clavicles are either absent or severely hypoplastic and there is delayed eruption of the dentition with dental enamel abnormalities. SXR may show Wormian bones, and chest X-ray displays hypoplastic or absent clavicles.

Osteogenesis imperfecta (OI)
Consider if mild/moderate enlargement of the fontanelle and fractures or Wormian bones present. See 'Fractures' in Chapter 2, 'Clinical approach', p. 158.

Pycnodysostosis
An AR condition caused by mutations in the gene cathepsin K (CTSK). Large fontanelles, increased bone density, facial dysmorphic features, and short limbs.

AR Robinow syndrome
Caused by mutations in ROR2 and characterized by a prominent forehead, large fontanelle, hypertelorism, a wide mouth, and a small nose with anteverted nostrils. There may be a cleft lip/palate and significant gum hypertrophy. Some affected individuals have CHD. There is mesomelic shortening of the limbs. Milder AD forms are caused by mutation in WNT5A, DVL1 or DVL3.

Hypophosphatasia
There are two forms, one presenting in utero or in infancy that is usually lethal, and the other presenting in childhood or adulthood. Both have reduced chondro-osseous mineralization with undermineralization of the skull and low levels of alkaline phosphatase in blood. Mutations in TNSALP on 1p36.1 are found in both severe and mild cases. The severe form is AR whereas milder forms can be either AR or AD.

Zellweger syndrome
An AR peroxisomal disorder often presenting in the neonatal period with central hypotonia ± seizures. The fontanelle is large and the forehead high. There may be stippled epiphyses (especially knees). VLCFAs are elevated. See 'Floppy infant' in Chapter 2, 'Clinical approach', p. 154.

Parietal foramina
AD with variable penetrance due to haploinsufficiency of MSX2 or ASLX4. Parental SXRs are helpful in evaluating possible mutation carriers. Rarely require active clinical management.

Proximal 11p deletion (Potocki-Shaffer) syndrome
Parietal foramina associated with exostoses, developmental delay, and mildly dysmorphic facial features may occur as part of a microdeletion syndrome at 11p11.2 that incorporates combined haploinsufficiency of EXT2 and ALX4. Parental karyotypes necessary.

Neonatal progeroid syndromes (WRS)
IUGR with relative macrocephaly, progeroid features, and an enlarged anterior fontanelle. Some overlap with AR cutis laxa with CDG and EDS—progeria type.

Renal tubular dysgenesis
AR renal tubular dysgenesis is a severe disorder of renal tubular development characterized by persistent fetal anuria and perinatal death, probably due to pulmonary hypoplasia from early-onset oligohydramnios. Absence or paucity of differentiated proximal tubules is the histopathologic hallmark of the disorder and may be associated with skull ossification defects. It is caused by biallelic mutation of genes in the renin–angiotensin pathway (Gribouval et al. 2005), REN, ACT, AGTR1 and ACE.

Kenny–Caffey syndrome (KCS)
In addition to delayed closure of the fontanelle, these children have short stature with cortical thickening and medullary stenosis of the long bones and transient hypocalcaemia in infancy. Intelligence is normal. It is caused by heterozygous mutation in FAM111A (allelic with gracile bone dysplasia, a perinatally lethal condition with very thin, brittle bones). A more severe AR form of KCS presents in the neonatal period with severe IUGR and congenital hypoparathyroidism is caused by biallelic mutation of TBCE.

Yunis-Varon syndrome
A very rare syndrome with some skeletal overlap with cleidocranial dysostosis. Although absent thumbs were thought to be a hallmark of the syndrome, they may be present. CMT-like peripheral neuropathy. Bi-allelic mutation in FIG4.

Vascular malformations
Vascular malformations of the brain have been associated with scalp defects and parietal foramina, as well as brain malformation.

Other rare syndromes
Skull ossification defects are a good handle for some rare syndromes, including Schinzel phocomelia, aminopterin syndrome sine amniopterin (ASSA) or 'pseudoaminopterin' syndrome and CYP26B1 deficiency.

Genetic advice
This is dependent on the diagnosis, but the following points may be useful for counselling.

Recurrence risk and carrier detection
It is important to consider the possibility that other family members may be affected in all the AD conditions described above. Examine parents and siblings and ask whether they were known to have any soft areas in the skull as a child. Radiology may help to detect parietal foramina or other skeletal features.

Prenatal diagnosis
May be requested by families at risk of the conditions with MR where molecular, cytogenetic, or molecular genetic testing is available.

Natural history and further management (preventative measures)
The large fontanelles usually close during childhood. Parents are understandably concerned about the risk of trauma and management advice from a craniofacial surgeon may be reassuring. Surgical intervention is usually contraindicated.

Expert adviser: Andrew Wilkie, Nuffield Professor of Pathology, Weatherall Institute of Molecular Medicine, University of Oxford, Oxford, UK.

References
Campeau PM, Lenk GM, et al. Yunis-Varón syndrome is caused by mutations in FIG4, encoding a phosphoinositide phosphatase. Am J Hum Genet 2013; **92**: 781–91.

Gribouval O, Gonzales M, Neuhaus T, et al. Mutations in genes in the renin–angiotensin system are associated with autosomal recessive renal tubular dysgenesis. Nat Genet 2005; **37**: 964–8.

Hall JG, Froster-Iskenius I, Allanson J. Handbook of normal physical measurements. Oxford University Press, Oxford, 1989.

Mavrogiannis LA, Antonopoulou I, Baxová A, et al. Haploinsufficiency of the human homeobox gene ALX4 causes skull ossification defects. Nat Genet 2001; **27**: 17–18.

Wilkie AO, Tang Z, Elanko N, et al. Functional haploinsufficiency of the human homeobox gene MSX2 causes defects in skull ossification. Nat Genet 2000; **24**: 387–90.

Laterality disorders including heterotaxy and isomerism

The left–right (L–R) axis of the embryo is defined as soon as the rostrocaudal and dorsoventral axes are established. Curvature of the heart loop to the right is the first morphological sign of asymmetry in embryogenesis.

- Terminology:
  - situs solitus. The usual L–R body plan with the heart, spleen, and stomach on the left and the liver and gall bladder on the right;
  - situs inversus. Approximately 1/10 000 individuals have a mirror image arrangement of the L–R body plan, with the heart, spleen, and stomach on the right and the liver and gall bladder on the left. There is an increased incidence of CHD (3–9%), compared with 0.7% in situs solitus;
  - situs ambiguus/visceral heterotaxy. Discordance between situs of asymmetric organs often accompanied by complex cardiovascular malformation;
  - R isomerism sequence. Asplenia syndrome, Ivemark syndrome, right atrial isomerism. Right isomerism sequence is the consequence of bilateral right-sided signalling pathways in early development which invariably leads to complex CHD. There are two morphologically right atria, often with a single ventricle, AVSD, and TGA and anomalous pulmonary venous drainage. The spleen is absent and there may be abnormal folding of the intestines that may present as intestinal obstruction.
  - L isomerism sequence (polysplenia syndrome) is the consequence of bilateral left-sided signalling pathways in early development. Absence of the sinoatrial (SA) node may cause complete heart block. There are two morphologically left atria. There may be an ASD or AVSD, but usually the heart defects are not as severe as in R isomerism sequence. Multiple small spleens may be found and there may be abnormal folding of the intestines, which may present as intestinal obstruction.

Isomerism sequence (see Table 2.21) accounts for ~1% of CHD and occurs with an incidence of ~1/24 000.

In humans, relatively few genes have been associated with a small percentage of human situs defects. These include: *ZIC3*, *LEFTB*, *ACVR2B* (activin-binding receptor 2), and *CFC1* encoding the cryptic protein. The structural anomalies typical of left and right isomerism are shown in Table 2.22.

Clinical approach

History: key points

- Detailed three-generation family tree with specific enquiry for consanguinity and CHD.
- Enquire for maternal diabetes. (In Splitt *et al.*'s (1999) study, 50% of cases of L isomerism occurred in infants of diabetic mothers.)

Examination: key points

Careful cardiovascular assessment.

Special investigations

- Echo to define the cardiac anatomy.
- USS to define the position of the liver and the presence/absence of the spleen.
- DNA to store or, if the family tree is suggestive of XL inheritance, for *ZIC3* mutation analysis.
- Genomic analysis (e.g. genomic array, panel, WES, WGS as available).

Some diagnoses to consider

Primary ciliary dyskinesia (immotile cilia syndrome, Kartagener's syndrome)

Primary ciliary dyskinesia (PCD) with situs inversus, nasal polyps, and bronchiectasis. A genetically heterogeneous

Table 2.21 Heart defects in patients with isomerism sequence[*]

Heart defect (%)	Left isomerism (%)	Right isomerism (%)
Interruption of IVC with azygos continuation	75	7
TAPVD	35	
Common atrium	47	67
Single ventricle	30	70
AVSD	68	93
DORV	7	47
Pulmonary stenosis/atresia	48	78

[*] See also Table 2.22.

AVSD, atrioventricular septal defect; DORV, double-outlet right ventricle; IVC, inferior vena cava; TAPVD, total anomalous pulmonary venous drainage.

This article was published in *Emery and Rimoin's Principles and Practice of Medical Genetics*, Congenital Heart Disease, Burn and Goodship, pp. 1239–1326, copyright Elsevier 2001.

Table 2.22 Structural anomalies typical of right and left isomerism

	Left isomerism	Right isomerism
Cardiovascular features		
Great vessels		Right aortic arch
		Transposition
Pulmonary circulation	Partial anomalous pulmonary venous drainage	Total anomalous pulmonary venous drainage
Atria	Bilateral left atrial appendages	Bilateral right atrial appendages
		Common atrium
Valves		Pulmonary stenosis
Ventricles	AVSD	AVSD
		Double-outlet right ventricle
Conduction	AV block	
	Sick sinus syndrome	
Abdomen		
	Polysplenia	Asplenia
	Bilateral bilobed lungs	Bilateral trilobed
	Biliary atresia	Malrotation
Other		
		Ciliary dysfunction

AR disorder; there are currently 17 genes identified. All affected individuals have ciliary dyskinesia and half of affected individuals have situs inversus (see 'Ciliopathies' in Chapter 3, 'Common consultations', p. 366).

MMP21-related heterotaxy

Biallelic mutations in the *MMP21* gene cause visceral heterotaxy with complex heart malformations. MMP21 may modulate cell proliferation and migration through regulating extracellular matrix remodelling (Akawi 2015).

X-linked laterality sequence. A rare XL condition in which laterality disturbance may be combined with sacral agenesis or NTDs caused by mutations in ZIC3 on Xq28.

Genetic advice

Recurrence risk

Overall, an empiric 5% sibling recurrence risk is given where no specific diagnosis is possible (if there is no family history and no consanguinity). If there is consanguinity, a sibling recurrence risk of 25% may be appropriate.

Prenatal diagnosis

Fetal echo can be used for antenatal diagnosis of most laterality disorders with scans at 14, 19, and 22 weeks' gestation.

Natural history and further management (preventative measures)

If the spleen is absent, prophylactic penicillin should be prescribed.

Support group: Children's Heart Federation, http://www.chfed.org.uk.

Expert adviser: Miranda Splitt, Consultant Clinical Geneticist, Northern Genetics Service, Newcastle upon Tyne Hospitals NHS Trust, Newcastle upon Tyne, UK.

References

Akawi N, McRae J, Ansari M, *et al*.; DDD study. Discovery of four recessive developmental disorders using probabilistic genotype and phenotype matching among 4,125 families. *Nat Genet* 2015; **47**: 1363–9.

Bamford RN, Roessler E, Burdine RD, *et al*. Loss-of-function mutations in the EGF-CFC gene *CFC1* are associated with human left–right laterality defects. *Nat Genet* 2000; **26**: 365–9.

Burn J. Disturbance of morphological laterality in humans. In: GR Bock, J Marsh (eds.). *Biological asymmetry and handedness*, pp. 282–99. Wiley, Chichester, 1991.

Burn J, Goodship J. Congenital heart disease. In: D Rimoin (ed.). *Emery and Rimoin's principles and practice of medical genetics*, 4th edn, pp. 1239–326. Churchill Livingstone, Edinburgh, 2001.

Gebbia M, Ferrero GB, Pilia G, *et al*. X-linked situs abnormalities result from mutations in *ZIC3*. *Nat Genet* 1997; **17**: 305–8.

Guimier A, Gabriel GC, Bajolle F, *et al*. MMP21 is mutated in human heterotaxy and is required for normal left–right asymmetry in vertebrates. *Nat Genet* 2015; **47**: 1260–3.

Splitt M, Wright C, Sen D, Goodship J. Left-isomerism sequence and maternal type-1 diabetes. *Lancet* 1999; **354**: 305–6.

Leukodystrophy/leukoencephalopathy

Leukodystrophy is a genetic condition primarily affecting the white matter of the brain. The term leukoencephalopathy is used to denote the broader number of pathologies that may cause abnormal white matter on neuroimaging. These may be non-genetic, i.e. they may have an environmental basis such as hypoxic–ischaemic damage or a congenital infection (most particularly with CMV). It should be noted that genetic disorders can mimic such environmental causes (e.g. consider the 'destructive' brain injury and leukoencephalopathy associated with COL4A1 mutations). Differentiating genetic and non-genetic causes of white matter disease is important, and not infrequently difficult, so that we emphasize here the value of an expert radiological opinion. Currently a molecular diagnosis can be made in up to 80% of patients with a leukodystrophy.

Leukodystrophy is usually suspected following MRI in a neurologically abnormal child. Some leukodystrophies demonstrate characteristic MRI patterns that suggest the diagnosis (e.g. the predominantly posterior cerebral involvement frequently observed in ALD versus the predominantly anterior involvement more typical of infantile Alexander disease). Furthermore, clues to the diagnosis may be obtained from other data seen in the context of white matter disease (e.g. a large head size in MLC1-related leukodystrophy, and basal ganglia calcification in AGS). Many conditions have different forms presenting at different ages, with clinical features that are specific to the age of presentation (e.g. metachromatic leukodystrophy, Alexander disease, Krabbe disease).

In about 50% of children with leukodystrophy, a precise aetiology is not identified.

Approach to the MRI

Many different MRI sequences can be performed and specialist advice is important when choosing the most appropriate sequences for a given child. Generally, T1-weighted, T2-weighted, and fluid-attenuated inversion recovery (FLAIR) images, with some images in each plane—axial, sagittal, and coronal—should be available. IV contrast enhancement and spinal cord imaging sometimes provide useful further information. Diffusion-weighted images and MRI spectroscopy may be of value in some cases. GRE and SW images are useful for detecting haemorrhage and mineralization, including calcification.

The first 2 years of life is the period when the majority of myelination occurs. During this time, the MRI appearances of the white matter alter considerably.

On normal T1-weighted imaging, unmyelinated white matter is dark (or low signal), whereas myelinated white matter is white (or high signal). The CSF is black (low signal).

On normal T2-weighted imaging, unmyelinated white matter is grey or white (relatively high signal), whereas myelinated white matter is black (or low signal). The CSF is white (high signal).

It is abnormal for cerebral white matter to have a high signal on T2-weighted images in a child over 1.5 years of age.

It is important to distinguish dysmyelinating disorders, where there is damage or abnormality of myelin, from hypomyelinating disorders where there is a defect in myelin production. Radiologically, hypomyelination is defined as an unchanged pattern of deficient myelination on two MRI scans at least 6 months apart.

Clinical approach

History: key points giving clues to the diagnosis

- Family history of a previous affected child.
- Parental consanguinity.
- Ethnicity (e.g. Canavan disease in a child of Ashkenazi Jewish ancestry).
- Pregnancy and labour (congenital infections, perinatal/prenatal asphyxia).
- Birthweight and OFC.
- Neonatal history (e.g. seizures, fever, coagulopathy, hepatosplenomegaly).
- Early developmental milestones (was there ever a period of normal development? If so, how long did it last?).
- Regression/loss of skills (e.g. deteriorating school performance, worsening gait, increasing feeding difficulties).
- Behavioural or psychiatric disturbances (e.g. irritability, aggression, hallucinations).
- Vision and hearing loss.
- Motor abnormalities (weakness, ataxia, spasticity, dystonia).

Examination: key points giving clues to the diagnosis

- Macrocephaly (e.g. Canavan disease, Alexander disease, megalencephalic leukoencephalopathy with cysts (MLC), gangliosidoses).
- Peripheral nerve involvement (e.g. metachromatic leukodystrophy (MLD), infantile Krabbe disease, mitochondrial disease, connexin 32 mutations, hyccin deficiency).
- Eye involvement (e.g. rotatory eye nystagmus in PMD, cherry red spots in GM1 and GM2 disease, retinal dystrophy in various disorders, cataract in hyccin deficiency, visual loss in many). A formal ophthalmology opinion is important.
- Gait abnormalities (e.g. progressive diplegia in late-infantile MLD).
- Movement disorder (e.g. dystonia and signs of cerebellar dysfunction, e.g. dysarthria and ataxia).
- Skin signs (e.g. photosensitivity in Cockayne syndrome (CS), increased skin pigmentation due to adrenal insufficiency in X-ALD, chilblains in AGS).
- Cognitive/developmental assessment (e.g. school decline with X-ALD).

Initial investigations

MRI is central to diagnosis. Before proceeding to further investigations, an expert paediatric neuroradiology opinion should be sought. Many characteristic phenotypes can be recognized which may immediately suggest the diagnosis and avoid unnecessary or expensive tests. Investigation should be targeted by the MRI findings. A blind trawl is often unhelpful.

- Urine organic acids, amino acids.
- Mucopolysaccharide and oligosaccharide screen.
- Plasma lactate, ammonia, amino acids.

- Biotinidase, VLCFAs, white cell enzymes.
- CSF examination (cells, protein, lactate, serine, glycine, interferon alpha, pterins).
- Electrophysiology (ERG, visual evoked potentials (VEPs), auditory evoked potentials, nerve conduction studies and EMG).
- Genomic analysis, e.g. genomic array, gene panel, or WES/WGS as available.
- Specific mutation testing guided by MRI features.
- DNA storage.

Some diagnoses to consider

Dysmyelinating disorders

AICARDI–GOUTIÈRES SYNDROME (AGS). Caused by mutations in any one of the genes *TREX1*, *RNASEH2A*, *RNASEH2B*, *RNASEH2C*, *SAMHD1*, *ADAR1* and *IFHI1*. The typical presentation is either as a neonatal encephalopathy resembling a congenital infection, or with an infantile onset of an initially progressive disorder. The neonatal presentation is frequently characterized by fever, seizures, hepatosplenomegaly, thrombocytopenia, and anaemia, with or without microcephaly. The infantile form sometimes occurs after a period of apparently normal development, followed by the onset of a severe encephalopathy with irritability, fevers, loss of skills, and acquired microcephaly. Characteristic ICC and white matter disease (the early-onset form can demonstrate marked temporal lobe cysts and a frontal gradient of abnormal white matter) are seen in many patients.

ALEXANDER DISEASE. Caused by mutations in the *GFAP* gene. It is AD and is usually sporadic, caused by DNMs. Infantile, juvenile, and adult forms occur. In infants, developmental delay, progressive motor difficulties, feeding problems, megalencephaly, seizures, and sometimes hydrocephalus occur. The MRI features are characteristic, and diagnostic criteria have been defined that allow the diagnosis to be strongly suspected on radiological grounds. However, atypical juvenile and adult forms can occur.

CANAVAN DISEASE. An AR condition that presents in the first year of life with hypotonia (which changes to spasticity), macrocephaly, head lag, and progressive cognitive delay. The disease is caused by mutations in the aspartoacetylase gene (*ASPA*) and there is an excess of *N*-acetylaspartate in the CSF, blood, and urine. Canavan disease occurs worldwide but is most prevalent in the Ashkenazi Jewish population where the E285A mutation accounts for 80–85% of mutant alleles.

KRABBE DISEASE, OR GLOBOID CELL LEUKODYSTROPHY. An AR disorder involving the white matter of the peripheral and central nervous systems. Mutations in the *GALC* gene encoding the lysosomal enzyme galactocerebrosidase result in low enzymatic activity and decreased ability to degrade galactolipids found almost exclusively in myelin. The infantile form is the most common, presenting within the first 6 months of life with rapid onset of irritability, loss of skills, and feeding problems. Death occurs by the age of 3 years. Later-onset forms, even in adulthood, occur. The characteristic imaging features of early-infantile Krabbe disease include high signal in the cerebellar white matter, brainstem, and internal capsule, with streaky high signal in the periventricular and deep cerebral white matter.

LEUKOENCEPHALOPATHY WITH VANISHING WHITE MATTER (VWM). An AR disorder caused by mutations in any of the five genes encoding the eukaryotic translation initiation factor 2B (eIF2B). The most common form presents between 2 and 6 years of age with progressive ataxia and later spasticity. Acute deterioration may be triggered by stresses such as fever, minor head injury, or fright. More severe early-onset forms occur, and an adult onset has also been described. In adult females, ovarian failure may occur. The diagnosis is suggested by striking MRI appearances where white matter rarefaction and cystic degeneration occur in a diffuse, melting-away fashion, leaving behind a cobweb of better preserved tissue strands (without any well-delineated isolated cysts).

MEGALENCEPHALIC LEUKOENCEPHALOPATHY WITH SUBCORTICAL CYSTS (MLC). This disease is caused by mutations in either the *MLC1* gene or the *HEPACAM* gene. Megalencephaly is usually present at birth, and patients may first be referred because of their large head size. Motor difficulties develop in infancy and progress slowly. Epilepsy is common and cognitive decline is slow and mild. MLC is characterized by a very abnormal-looking brain scan, in the presence of relatively mild physical signs. Cystic lesions, particularly in the temporal or frontal lobes, are characteristic, but not diagnostic. Some patients die in their teens, but others live into adult life. It has recently been demonstrated that patients with two *HEPACAM* mutations develop classical MLC, whereas remarkably, in those with a single mutation, the radiological appearances improve with age and patients have a non-progressive disorder (which may or may not be accompanied by MR and autistic features).

METACHROMATIC LEUKODYSTROPHY (MLD). An AR disorder due to arylsulfatase A deficiency with accumulation of the myelin lipid sulfatide in the brain and peripheral nerves. Late-infantile, juvenile, and adult-onset forms occur. In MLD, leukodystrophy primarily affects the periventricular and deep cerebral white matter, whereas the U-fibres are relatively spared. The late-infantile form is the most common form, presenting typically in the third year of life with spasticity, signs of peripheral neuropathy, high protein in the CSF, and eventual loss of intellectual function.

MITOCHONDRIAL DISEASES. Abnormal white matter on MRI is a common feature of mitochondrial disorders. In some conditions, this is subtle and minor; in others, the white matter changes are prominent. In mitochondrial defects, the abnormal white matter may be partially cystic, but here the cysts are usually isolated and well delineated. Mutations in genes encoding components of complex 1 may produce a striking cystic leukoencephalopathy. Leukoencephalopathy with brainstem and spinal cord involvement and elevated white matter lactate (LSBL) is caused by mutations in the mitochondrial aspartyl-tRNA synthetase (*DARS2*).

X-LINKED ADRENOLEUKODYSTROPHY (X-ALD). Due to mutations in the *ALDP* gene. Late-onset disease is called adrenomyeloneuropathy (AMN). Carrier females may develop AMN in middle age. Even within the same family, there may be extreme variation in the clinical presentation—though biochemical testing will detect all those at risk. Typically there is a posterior predominance in white matter involvement, but sometimes this pattern is reversed.

Hypomyelinating disorders

Hypomyelinating phenotypes currently represent the largest group of 'undiagnosed' leukodystrophies. The

MRI diagnosis of a hypomyelinating disorder can be challenging. Characteristically, the white matter signal on T2-weighted MRI is increased, but not as bright as in a dysmyelinating disorder, with a relatively normal appearance of the white matter on T1-weighted images.

COCKAYNE SYNDROME (CS). An AR nucleotide excision repair disorder caused by mutations in either the *CSA* or *CSB* genes. CS comprises a spectrum of overlapping phenotypes which may present antenatally through to adult life. It is a multisystem disorder, most typically recognized by the combination of facial features ('shrunken eyes'), retinopathy, deafness, cutaneous photosensitivity, short stature, and (sometimes only slowly) progressive neurological features. ICC develops in the majority of patients. The MRI frequently demonstrates hypomyelination and cerebellar atrophy.

PELIZAEUS–MERZBACHER DISEASE (PMD). An XLR condition due to duplication of, or mutation in, the *PLP1* gene that codes for proteolipid protein. The condition may present at birth with hypotonia, rotatory nystagmus, and stridor and follow a severe clinical course resulting in early death. More commonly, presentation is in infancy and the clinical course is slowly progressive with survival into adult life followed by a static motor disorder and later deterioration. Female carriers may have neurological abnormalities. Mutations in the *PLP1* gene may also cause XL spastic paraparesis type 2 (SPG2).

OTHER HYPOMYELINATING DISORDERS. Include: hypomyelination with congenital cataract (HYCCIN deficiency), hypomyelination, hypodontia and hypogonadotrophic hypogonadism (4H syndrome due to *POLR3A, POLR3B* and *POLR1C* mutations), Salla disease, fucosidosis, serine synthesis defects, MCT8 deficiency, and hypomyelination with atrophy of the basal ganglia (HABC) caused by a recurrent p.Asp249Asn DNM in the *TUBB4A* gene.

Genetic advice: known diagnosis

Recurrence risk
Counsel as appropriate.

Carrier detection
Within a family, carrier testing by genetic testing is possible when there is a known mutation. Screening of the partners of known carriers may present problems, except in populations where there are common mutations.

Enzyme testing within families can often detect carriers but is rarely discriminatory enough to use for partners of carriers.

Prenatal diagnosis
CVS and amniocentesis measuring enzyme levels or mutation analysis. Please check with your laboratory to ensure that the correct samples are taken.

Genetic advice: undiagnosed leukodystrophy
A recent and expert opinion on the MRI is important. There is an important role for panel/WES/WGS

approaches (with a clinical diagnostic rate of 42%) where these can be accessed (Vanderver *et al.* 2016). If, despite this, there is no known cause, counselling is given on the basis of the probability that the condition is genetic.

Recurrence risk
(1) If there is parental consanguinity, an AR aetiology is probable and recurrence risks are likely to be 25%.
(2) If there is a history of a previous affected sibling, then recurrence risks are likely to be 25%. AR inheritance is more likely than XL or germline mosaicism.
(3) If neither of the above apply, then consider the possibility of environmental factors or non-recurring genetic conditions such as DNMs, but counsel that the risk may be as high as 25%.

Carrier detection
Not available, other than a pedigree-based risk.

Prenatal diagnosis
Not possible.

Natural history and further management
These conditions are frequently progressive and in the undiagnosed group a review may bring about a diagnosis based on the features or after repeat testing, e.g. MRI, or by recent delineation of a phenotype.

Support groups: Climb (Children Living with Inherited Metabolic Diseases), http://www.climb.org.uk, Tel. 0870 770 0326; Contact a Family, http://www.cafamily.org.uk.

Expert advisers:
John H. Livingston, Consultant Paediatric Neurologist, Leeds Teaching Hospital NHS Trust, Leeds, UK and Yanick Crow, Consultant Clinical Geneticist, Institut Imagine, Necker-Enfants Malades Hospital, Paris Descartes University, Paris, France.

References
Schiffmann R, van der Knaap MS. Invited article: an MRI-based approach to the diagnosis of white matter disorders. *Neurology* 2009; **72**: 750–9.

Steenweg ME, Vanderver A, Blaser S, et al. Magnetic resonance image pattern recognition in hypomyelinating disorders. *Brain* 2010; **133**: 2971–82.

van der Knaap MS, Breiter SN, Naidu S, Hart AAM, Valk J. Defining and categorizing leukoencephalopathies of unknown origin: MR imaging approach. *Radiology* 1999; **213**: 121–33.

van der Knaap MS, Scheper GC. Vanishing white matter disease. *Lancet Neurol* 2006; **5**: 413–23.

van der Knaap MS, Valk J. Magnetic resonance of myelination and myelin disorders, 3rd edn. Springer, Berlin, 2005.

Vanderver A, Simons C, Helman G, et al. Whole exome sequencing in patients with white matter abnormalities. *Ann Neurol* 2016; **79**: 1031–7.

Limb reduction defects

See also 'Radial ray defects and thumb hypoplasia' in Chapter 2, 'Clinical approach', p. 296.

Congenital limb reduction defects are more common at the extremes of maternal age, but the age association is not a strong one. Matsunaga and Shiota (1979) found that the prevalence of limb reduction defects was 15 times greater where there was a history of first-trimester bleeding. Most major malformations are more common in multiple births than singletons. One small study reported a prevalence of limb anomalies as 1/252 twins (40/10 000) and 2/287 triplets (60/10 000). Possible mechanisms include amniotic bands, inequalities of blood supply in MZ twins, vascular disruption from a deceased co-twin. Malformations such as sirenomelia (fusion of the lower extremities) are increased in MZ twins (risk 100–150 times greater than for singletons). Table 2.23 outlines the stages in human limb development.

The fact that different aetiologies can cause a similar result makes the analysis of limb defects particularly challenging, e.g. *TBX5*, mutations in Holt-Oram syndrome (HOS), and thalidomide exposure can cause limb and cardiac defects that are clinically indistinguishable.

Overall, the minimum prevalence of limb reduction defects is ~5.6/10 000 live births (higher rates in miscarriages, intrauterine deaths (IUDs), and stillbirths (SBs)). About half of the defects are transverse. There are many ways of classifying limb defects (see Box 2.6) (Gold et al. 2011).

Table 2.23 Outline of stages in human limb development

Days from fertilization	Gestation	Upper limb	Lower limb
27 days	5 weeks, 6 days	Arm buds begin to appear	
28–30 days	6 weeks–6 weeks, 2 days	Well-developed arm buds	Lower limb bud appears
34–36 days	6 weeks, 6 days–7 weeks, 1 day	Elongated arm buds	
34–38 days	6 weeks, 6 days–7 weeks 3 days	Hand paddle formed	
38–40 days	7 weeks, 3 days–7 weeks, 5 days	Fingers begin to separate	
41–43 days	7 weeks, 6 days–8 weeks, 1 day	Fingers distinct	
44–46 days	8 weeks, 2 days–8 weeks, 4 days	Fingers separated	Toes distinguishable
52–53 days	9 weeks, 3 days–9 weeks, 4 days	Fingers fully separated	
54–55 days	9 weeks, 5 days–9 weeks, 6 days		Toes fully separated

Brown N, Lumley J, et al. Congenital limb reduction defects—clues from developmental biology, teratology and epidemiology. The Stationery Office, London, 1996.

TERATOGENS. Limb abnormalities are one of the most common and visible phenotypic effects of several human teratogens. The specific effects are different for most teratogens and include effects on limb morphogenesis (thalidomide, warfarin, phenytoin, valproic acid) and the effect of vascular disruption on a limb that had formed normally (misoprostol, CVS, and phenytoin). Procedures during pregnancy, including CVS and dilatation and curettage (D & C), produce defects of vascular disruption (Holmes 2003).

Clinical approach

History: key points

- Three-generation family tree with detailed enquiry regarding limb defects, CHD, deafness, or eye problems, e.g. squint/Duane (Okihiro), thalassaemia.
- Is there a history of maternal diabetes?
- Detailed history of pregnancy from 5 to 11 weeks' gestation:
  - vaginal bleeding;
  - drug exposure, e.g. misoprostol, vitamin A or other retinoids, cocaine; valproate;
  - twinning;
  - invasive procedures, e.g. CVS, attempted termination of pregnancy.
- Were fibrous bands attached to the affected limb(s) noted at delivery; did the placenta and membranes show amniotic bands?

Examination: key points

- Examine all four limbs. If the defect appears to be limited to a single limb, make certain that the other three limbs are truly normal (is there nail hypoplasia?). Defects are best documented with photos, supplemented with a sketch and written description.
- Examine the limbs for constriction bands.
- Examine the scalp for scalp defects (Adams–Oliver syndrome).
- Examine the tongue and mandible (oromandibular–limb–hypogenesis (OMLH) syndrome).
- Examine the eyes and face for VIth or VIIth cranial nerve palsy (very easily missed in a young baby).
- If there is an upper limb defect, examine the pectoral muscle and chest (Poland anomaly).
- Examine the heart.
- If there is a major limb reduction defect affecting the lower limb(s), examine the anus (anorectal malformation) and male genitalia (e.g. splenogonadal fusion–limb defect).
- Examine the hands and feet of the parents. If there is any suspicion of HOS, examine the parents' heart as well.

Special investigations

- Radiograph of both upper or both lower limbs, including the affected limb (also any other limbs where there is clinical suspicion of abnormality).
- Echo and ECG. Always indicated in babies and young children. Also indicated in adults if you suspect HOS or another hand–heart syndrome. Note that 15% of children with limb reduction defects have CHD.
- Genomic analysis in presence of other features suggestive of a chromosomal or syndromic diagnosis, e.g. genomic array, gene panel, or WES/WGS as available.

Box 2.6 Eurocat classification of congenital limb defects

Terminal transverse defects.* Absence of distal structures of the limb, with proximal structures more or less normal, e.g. absent hand. May vary from absence of a nail or distal phalange or finger through to absence of a whole limb.

Proximal intercalary defect. Absence or severe hypoplasia of proximal intercalary parts of the limb when the distal structures (i.e. the digits), whether normal or malformed, are present, e.g. radial aplasia with intact thumb, femoral hypoplasia.

Longitudinal absence or severe hypoplasia of lateral part of the limb, e.g. Radial aplasia with absent thumb or ulnar aplasia with absent fifth finger.

Split hand/foot. Absence of central digits, with or without absence of central metacarpal/metatarsal bones, usually associated with syndactyly of other digits (e.g. ectrodactyly–ectodermal dysplasia–clefting (EEC) syndrome).

Multiple types of reduction defect. Infants with more than one type of reduction, according to the classification given above.

* Not infrequently some soft tissue nubbins (rudimentary digits) are seen at the end of a proximal transverse limb defect. Only if there are significant skeletal elements present should this lead to classification as an intercalary defect.

Stoll C, Mastroiacovo P, et al. Eurocat guide 3: for the description and classification of congenital limb defects. Department of Epidemiology University of Louvain, Brussels, 1988. http://www.eurocat-network.eu/aboutus/publications/publications.

• In SHFM assure an array to investigate for 10q24 duplication and other rearrangements.
• DNA for single gene testing if a syndromic diagnosis with a known gene seems likely (e.g. HOS).
• Chromosome breakage only if other features of Fanconi or DNA repair disorder.
• Karyotype for chromosome 'puffing' if features of Roberts syndrome.

Some diagnoses to consider

NB. For many of these syndromes, the limb defect may fit into one of several types.

Terminal transverse defects

AMNIOTIC BANDS. Early rupture of the amnion may lead to the production of fibrous mesodermal cords that constrict or cleave parts of the fetus, causing disruption of an otherwise normal development. Another possible causal mechanism is the modification of fetal blood flow—the bands being a secondary phenomenon. Sometimes amniotic bands can be visualized by USS. There may be a clear history that at delivery fibrous cords were wrapped tightly round the affected digit(s). The defects are typically asymmetric (if defects are symmetric and/or involvement of multiple limbs, consider carefully the possibility of an underlying genetic disorder). Recurrence risk is very small (<2%). Investigations listed above may not be required if confident of this diagnosis.

ADAMS–OLIVER SYNDROME. Characterized by terminal transverse limb defects and scalp defect (cutis aplasia). Small defects underlying the scalp defect are sometimes seen. Most affected individuals have relatively minor limb defects (usually affecting fingers and toes), but considerable variability is seen and occasionally severe limb defects can be present. Serious bleeding from the scalp defects can occur in neonates. Cardiac malformations also form part of the syndrome. AOS is genetically heterogenous with 4 AD genes (ARHGAP31, RBPJ, NOTCH1, and DLL4) and two AR genes (EOGT and DOCK6). In non-consanguineous populations, ARHGAP31 is the most common gene.

MOEBIUS SYNDROME. Congenital cranial nerve palsies affecting VIth (abduction of the eye) and VIIth (facial movement) cranial nerves, in conjunction with terminal transverse defects and/or Poland anomaly. See 'Facial asymmetry' in Chapter 2, 'Clinical approach', p. 146.

POLAND ANOMALY. There is congenital absence of the sternal head of pectoralis major, often in association with hypoplasia of the breast on the ipsilateral side and sometimes with shortening of phalanges and other elements of the digits in association with cutaneous syndactyly. Poland anomaly is usually sporadic and is thought to have a multifactorial basis involving vascular disruption in early development. Occasional parent–child occurrences are reported (Shalev and Hall 2003).

OROMANDIBULAR–LIMB–HYPOGENESIS (OMLH) SYNDROME. This group of disorders includes hypoglossia–hypodactyly, splenogonadal fusion–limb defects, and Hanhart syndrome. The clinical expression is variable and the limb abnormalities can vary from absence of digits to absence of the distal part of a whole limb. The jaw is small (micrognathia) and the tongue may also be small. Those who survive usually have normal intelligence. There is a definite association with Moebius syndrome, in which there are bilateral facial and abducens nerve palsies. Most cases are sporadic and attributed to vascular disruption. OMLH has been reported after exposure to misoprostol in the first trimester of pregnancy and after very early CVS (prior to the tenth week).

Proximal intercalary defects

THROMBOCYTOPENIA–ABSENT RADIUS (TAR) SYNDROME. Characterized by bilateral absence of the radii and thrombocytopenia; the thumbs are present. The lower limbs, GI, cardiovascular, and other systems may also be involved. In a survey of 34 cases, Greenhalgh et al. (2002) found that all cases had a documented thrombocytopenia and bilateral radial aplasia, 47% lower limb anomalies, 47% cows' milk intolerance, 23% renal anomalies, and 15% cardiac anomalies. TAR syndrome is caused by either a microdeletion at 1q21.1 or a null RBM8A gene mutation in combination with one of two minor SNP alleles in the RBM8A gene at 5′ UTR or in intron 1.

Longitudinal absence or severe hypoplasia of lateral part of the limb

See 'Radial ray defects and thumb hypoplasia' in Chapter 2, 'Clinical approach', p. 296.

HOLT–ORAM SYNDROME (HOS). AD heart–hand syndrome caused by mutations in *TBX5*. Penetrance is 100%. *Skeletal defects* affect the upper limbs exclusively and are invariably bilateral and usually asymmetrical. They range from clinodactyly, limited supination, and narrow, sloping shoulders to absent, hypoplastic, or triphalangeal thumb and severe reduction deformities of the upper arm (4.5%). Hypoplasia of the thenar eminence accompanies thumb hypoplasia. The radial ray is predominantly affected and the left side is usually more severely affected than the right. *Cardiac defects* (including minimal ECG changes) occur in 95%. See 'Radial ray defects and thumb hypoplasia' in Chapter 2, 'Clinical approach', p. 296.

VACTERL (VERTEBRAL DEFECTS–ANAL ATRESIA–CARDIAC ANOMALIES–TRACHEO-OESOPHAGEAL FISTULA–(O) ESOPHAGEAL ATRESIA–RENAL ANOMALIES–LIMB DEFECTS) ASSOCIATION. Preaxial limb defects with underdevelopment or agenesis of thumbs and radial bones; usually bilateral defects, but may be asymmetric. Reduced thenar muscle mass is the mildest end of the spectrum. The lower limbs are not affected. Sporadic with low recurrence risk (2–3%). See 'Anal anomalies (atresia, stenosis)' in Chapter 2, 'Clinical approach', p. 58 for further details.

OKIHIRO SYNDROME (DUANE RADIAL RAY SYNDROME). An AD condition with degrees of radial ray hypoplasia and Duane anomaly. It results from mutation in the *SALL4* gene.

ACROFACIAL DYSOSTOSIS WITH LIMB DEFECTS (MILLER SYNDROME, POST-AXIAL ACROFACIAL DYSOSTOSIS SYNDROME (POADS)). An AR condition characterized by hypoplasia of the fifth ray of all limbs, together with malar hypoplasia and micrognathia ± cleft palate caused by biallelic mutation in *DHODH* gene.

ULNAR–MAMMARY SYNDROME. AD with variable penetrance. Ulnar ray defects varying from hypoplasia of the 5th digit to absence of the ulna and ulnar ray (occasionally may have PAP). In addition, females have small/absent breasts with hypoplastic nipples and males have a small penis, delayed puberty, and reduced fertility. Cardiac conduction defects may occur. Due to mutations in *TBX3*.

Split hand/foot malformation (SHFM)

A rare condition affecting 1 in 8000–25 000 newborns and accounting for ~15% of all limb reduction defects. SHFM can be isolated or syndromic and is genetically heterogeneous. AD, often with incomplete penetrance, is the most typical mode of inheritance.

AD ECTRODACTYLY. AD with high penetrance, but variable expressivity. One locus is on 7q21 due to mutation in *DLX5*.

ECTRODACTYLY–ECTODERMAL DYSPLASIA–CLEFTING (EEC) SYNDROME. An AD condition caused by mutations in *TP63*. Cleft lip and/or palate is common. Dry skin with variable hypohidrosis. Sparse fair, dry hair, often with absent eyebrows and eyelashes. Tear duct anomalies are common. Often have hypodontia. Nails are thin, brittle, and ridged. Mental development is usually normal. Limbs are affected to a markedly variable degree, ranging from no obvious defect to absence of the middle three rays (Rinne *et al*. 2006).

10Q DUPLICATION. A recurrent 0.5Mb duplication on 10q24q25 has been found in some affected families usually causing 4-limb involvement and sometimes associated with micrognathia, hearing problems, and renal hypoplasia (Dimitrov 2010).

MESOAXIAL SYNOSTOTIC SYNDACTYLY (MSSD). A rare AR disorder in which the middle and ring finger are replaced by a single digit. It is caused by biallelic variants in BHLHA9 gene (Malik *et al*. 2014).

Multiple types of reduction defect

CORNELIA DE LANGE SYNDROME (CDLS). Birth incidence ~1/50 000. The syndrome is characterized by MR, short stature (often with IUGR), limb anomalies, and distinctive craniofacial features (microbrachycephaly with a low anterior and posterior hairline, neat arched eyebrows often with synophyrys, a depressed nasal bridge with anteverted nares, a long, smooth philtrum, and thin lips often with downturned corners to the mouth, micrognathia). Cardiac septal defects, hirsutism, and feeding problems are common. The limb anomalies range from short forearms with small hands and tapering fingers to severe limb reduction defects with missing fingers, hands, and forearms. More minor hand anomalies include proximally placed thumbs, single palmar creases, and clinodactyly of the fifth finger. Occasionally fusion of two fingers or polydactyly may be seen. Upper limb defects are very much more common than lower limb defects. Most cases are sporadic and a recurrence risk of 1% is usually given. (NB. A milder form of the condition is recognized, which may follow a dominant pattern of inheritance.) The major gene for CdLS is *NIPBL* on 5p13.1 (Krantz *et al*. 2004) and other genes include *SMCl1*, *SMCA*, and *SMC3* (Mannini *et al*. 2013).

FEMUR–FIBULA–ULNA COMPLEX. A poorly defined condition with a spectrum of abnormalities affecting the ulnar ray, femur, and fibular ray. Upper limb anomalies are more common than lower limb anomalies. Overall, sibling recurrence risks seem to be low, but beware of the limitation of diagnostic uncertainty.

ROBERTS SYNDROME. An AR disorder characterized by growth failure, craniofacial anomalies, limb reduction defects, and loss of cohesion at heterochromatic regions of centromeres (chromosome 'puffing'). Limb defects vary from tetraphocomelia to radial ray defects. Caused by mutations in *ESCO2* (Vega *et al*. 2005). See 'Radial ray defects and thumb hypoplasia' in Chapter 2, 'Clinical approach', p. 296.

Genetic advice

Work systematically to try to establish an accurate diagnosis. Ask yourself the following questions.

• How many limbs are affected?
• What is the pattern of the limb defect (according to Stoll *et al*.'s (1988) classification)?
• Are there any other malformations or associated developmental delay?

You should then be in a position to reach a diagnosis and assess the recurrence risk.

Recurrence risk

Isolated transverse defects affecting only one limb are most likely to be sporadic, with a low recurrence risk for both siblings and offspring. *Think very carefully about a genetic aetiology for defects affecting more than one limb, especially if they are symmetrical.* (Defects affecting the middle ray of more than one limb are highly likely to be genetic.)

Carrier detection
Examine the hands and feet of the parents for subtle anomalies. Consider the possibility of incomplete penetrance and variable expressivity for an AD condition.

Prenatal diagnosis
Detailed fetal anomaly USS is the mainstay of PND. The limbs can be visualized on scanning by 13–14 weeks' gestation. It is usually not possible to visualize the digits clearly before ~20 weeks' gestation.

Support groups: Reach (for upper limb defects), http://www.reach.org.uk, Tel. 08451 306 225; STEPS (for lower limb defects), http://www.steps-charity.org.uk, Tel. 0871 717 0045.

Expert adviser: Ruth Newbury-Ecob, Lead Clinician, University Hospitals Bristol NHS Foundation Trust, Bristol, UK.

References
Albers CA, Newbury-Ecob R, Ouwehand WH, Ghevaert C. New insights into the genetic basis of TAR (thrombocytopenia-absent radii) syndrome. *Curr Opin Genet Dev* 2013; **23**: 316–23.

Brown N, Lumley J, Tickle C, Keene J. *Congenital limb reduction defects—clues from developmental biology, teratology and epidemiology.* The Stationery Office, London, 1996.

Dimitrov BI, de Ravel T, *et al.* Distal limb deficiencies, micrognatia syndrome and syndromic forms of split hand foot malformation (SHFM) are caused by chromosome 10q genomic rearrangements. *J Med Genet* 2010; **47**: 103–11.

Duijf PH, Van Bokhoven H, Brunner HG. Pathogenesis of split-hand/split-foot malformation. *Hum Mol Genet* 2003; **12**(Suppl. 1): R51–60.

Gold NB, Westgate MN, Holmes LB. Anatomic and etiological classification of congenital limb deficiencies *Am J Med Genet A* 2011; **155A**: 1225–35.

Gonzalez C, Vargas F, Perez AB, *et al.* Limb deficiency with or without Mobius sequence in seven Brazilian children associated with misoprostol use in the first trimester of pregnancy. *Am J Med Genet* 1993; **47**: 59–64.

Greenhalgh KL, Howell RT, Bottani A, *et al.* Thrombocytopenia–absent radius syndrome: a clinical genetic study. *J Med Genet* 2002; **39**: 876–81.

Holmes LB. Teratogen-induced limb defects. *Am J Med Genet* 2003; **112**: 297–303.

Fitzpatrick DR, Kline AD. Cornelia de Lange syndrome. In: SB Cassidy, JE Allanson (eds.). *Management of genetic syndromes,* 3rd edn, pp. 195–210. John Wiley & Sons, Inc., Hoboken, 2010.

Krantz ID, McCallum J, DeScipio C, *et al.* Cornelia de Lange syndrome is caused by mutations in NIPBL, the human homolog of Drosophila melanogaster Nipped-B. *Nat Genet* 2004; **36**: 631–5.

Malik S, Percin FE, Bornholdt D, *et al.* Mutations affecting the BHLHA9 DNA-binding domain cause MSSD, mesoaxial synostotic syndactyly with phalangeal reduction, Malik-Percin type. *Am J Hum Genet* 2014; **95**: 649–59.

Mannini L, Cucco F, Quarantotti V, Krantz ID, Musio A. Mutation spectrum and genotype-phenotype correlation in Cornelia de Lange syndrome. *Hum Mutat* 2013; **34**: 1589–96.

Matsunaga E, Shiota K. Threatened abortion, hormone therapy and malformed embryos. *Teratology* 1979; **20**: 469–80.

Newbury-Ecob RA, Leanage R, Raeburn JA, Young ID. Holt–Oram syndrome: a clinical genetic study. *J Med Genet* 1996; **33**: 300–7.

Rinne T, Hamel B, van Bokhoven H, Brunner HG. Pattern of p63 mutations and their phenotypes—update. *Am J Med Genet A* 2006; **140A**: 1396–406.

Shalev SA, Hall JG. Poland anomaly—report of an unusual family. *Am J Med Genet A* 2003; **118A**: 180–3.

Stoll C, Mastroiacovo P, Weatherall J, Lechat M. *EUROCAT Guide 3: for the description and classification of congenital limb defects.* Department of Epidemiology, University of Louvain, Brussels, 1988.

Vega H, Waisfisz Q, Gordillo M, *et al.* Roberts syndrome is caused by mutations in ESCO2, a human homolog of yeast ECO1 that is essential for the establishment of sister chromatid cohesion. *Nat Genet* 2005; **37**: 468–70.

Lissencephaly, polymicrogyria, and neuronal migration disorders

Lissencephaly may be identified on a cranial USS of a neonate with poor feeding and hypotonia or seizures. An MRI scan is the investigation of choice to confirm the diagnosis. Most children with lissencephaly have severe developmental delay and epilepsy. They often present with infantile spasms early in life.

Lissencephaly (Greek for 'smooth brain') is a genetically heterogeneous group of disorders characterized by a lack of normal gyri and sulci of the cerebral cortex (see Table 2.24). The abnormalities of gyration are a consequence of abnormal neuronal migration. In a normally developing brain, cells in the developing cortex migrate from the inner ventricular zone to the outer cortical plate. The contour of the normal fetal brain as seen on USS appears smooth until about 24 weeks of gestation; thereafter the first sulcal and gyral folds become visible and increase in number throughout the remainder of pregnancy. Various descriptive terms are used to describe the macroscopic appearance of the cortex. Agyria is an absence of gyral folds. Pachygyria describes a reduced number of very thick gyral folds. The disturbance of neuronal migration can create partially overlapping phenotypes, ranging from pachygyria to agyria. If the abnormal neuronal migration only affects a subset of neurons, this may be evident as subcortical band heterotopia (SBH).

The types of lissencephaly can be summarized as follows.

- 'Classical' lissencephaly (type I lissencephaly) (see Figure 2.19) is characterized by agyria and pachygyria and a thickened cortex. SBH is seen at the milder end of the spectrum. The genes involved are *PAFAH1B1* (17p13.3), *DCX* (Xq22.3), and *TUBA1A* (12q12-14). The proteins are associated with the cytoskeleton;

however, their exact mechanism in neuronal migration remains to be defined.

- 'Cobblestone' lissencephaly (type II lissencephaly) is characterized by a disorganized cortex, with migration of cortical cells through defects in the pia. It can be further subdivided according to the presence of other features such as NTD (see Table 2.24).
- Tubulinopathies are an important and recently delineated cause of lissencephaly/pachygyria/polymicrogyria (PMG) with other brain malformation (see below).
- Lissencephaly variants. Lissencephaly with cerebellar hypoplasia (LCH) is genetically heterogeneous, so far most commonly caused by mutations in *TUBA1A*, where it is also associated with dysmorphic basal ganglia and callosal abnormalities. A subset is caused by mutations in 'reelin' (*RELN*), which encodes an extracellular protein that regulates neuronal migration. XL lissencephaly with abnormal genitalia (XLAG) is associated with absence of the corpus callosum, ambiguous genitalia, and neonatal seizures. Mutations in the *ARX* gene have been identified.

Clinical approach

History: key points

- Three-generation family tree with specific enquiry regarding consanguinity, seizures, and developmental delay.
- History of pregnancy and delivery and neonatal period (polyhydramnios, feeding difficulties, level of alertness).
- Developmental milestones.
- Seizure activity: onset and type of seizures.

Examination: key points

- Measure the OFC (microcephaly is common), length, and weight.
- Examine for dysmorphic facial features (Miller–Dieker syndrome (MDS)) and other associated anomalies.

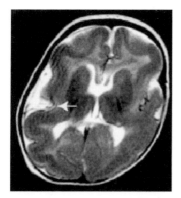

Figure 2.19 Lissencephaly type I in a girl aged 5 months who is visually and socially unresponsive and displays poor feeding and increased tone. The T2-weighted axial MRI shows a smooth cerebral cortex with absence of normal gyri and sulci. A vertically orientated shallow Sylvian fissure is seen (arrow). Reproduced with permission from Verity CM, Firth H and Ffrench-Constant C, Developmental abnormalities of the central nervous system. In David A. Warrell, Timothy M. Cox, and John D. Firth, *Oxford Textbook of Medicine*, Fourth edition, 2003, Figure 3a, page 1206, with permission from Oxford University Press.

Table 2.24 Types of lissencephaly

MRI appearances	Gene(s) to consider
Classical lissencephaly with posteriorly more severe gyral abnormality	*PAFAH1B1, TUBA1A*
Classical lissencephaly with anterior predominant gyral abnormality in males	*DCX*
Subcortical band heterotopia (SBH) in females	*DCX*
SBH in males (likely somatic mosaicism)	*DCX/PAFAH1B1*
Lissencephaly with cerebellar hypoplasia	*TUBA1A, TUBB2B* and other tubulinopathies, *RELN*, *CASK, CAMRQ 1–4*
Bilateral periventricular nodular heterotopia in females	*FLNA*
Lissencephaly with agenesis of corpus callosum and abnormal genitalia (XLAG)	*ARX*
Cobblestone lissencephaly	(See Figure 2.20)

(a)

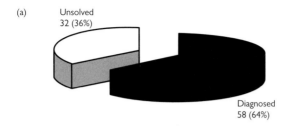

(b)

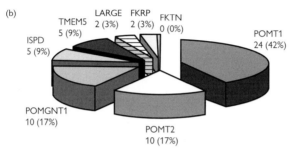

Figure 2.20 Results of molecular diagnosis of cobblestone lissencephaly fetuses.
Reprinted from *American Journal of Human Genetics*, 91, 6, S Vuillaumier-Barrot et al., Identification of Mutations in TMEM5 and ISPD as a Cause of Severe Cobblestone Lissencephaly, pp. 1135–1143, Copyright 2012, with permission from Elsevier.

- Examine for gaze palsy (tubulins).
- Examine for retinal dysplasia (MEB/WWS) and retinal dystrophy (JS).
- Assess for hypotonia or hypertonia.
- Examine the genitalia of males (XLAG).

Special investigations
- MRI scan if assessment based on cranial USS or CT scan.
- Ophthalmic examination for retinal dysplasia, cataracts, myopia (WWS, MEB disease, Fukayama congenital muscular dystrophy (FCMD)).
- Plasma CK (WWS, MEB, FCMD).
- VLCFAs (affected individuals may have lissencephaly and/or PMG).
- Genomic array or targeted deletion analysis with FISH of 17p13.3 and 22q11 or MLPA of *PAFAH1B1* or *DCX* in classical lissencephaly.
- Mutation analysis (in absence of deletion); *DCX* analysis in males, particularly if gyral abnormality is more severe anteriorly. If isolated affected male with apparent isolated lissencephaly sequence (ILS) and normal *DCX/PAFAH1B1* mutation analysis, consider MRI scan in the mother to look for SBH. Band heterotopia in female gene carriers usually causes seizures and learning difficulties but may be clinically unapparent. Note, however, that female *DCX* mutation carriers can have normal MRI scans; therefore, always consider *DCX* analysis first.
- Consider tubulin genes—heterozygous pathogenic variants in one of six genes (*TUBA1A, TUBB2A, TUBB2B, TUBB3, TUBB (TUBB5),* or *TUBG1*) or biallelic pathogenic variants in *TUBA8.*
- Consider *ARX* mutation analysis in males with lissencephaly and abnormal genitalia.

- If perisylvian PMG, consider GPR56, AKT3, PIK3CA, PIK3R2, WDR62, or 22q11DS.
- Consider gene panel/WES/WGS as appropriate. Due to phenotypic overlap and genetic heterogeneity a gene panel approach to investigations enhances diagnostic detection rates.
- Consider nerve conduction studies if hyporeflexia or foot deformities (DYNC1H1).

Some diagnoses to consider

Lissencephalies
See Figure 2.21.

ISOLATED LISSENCEPHALY SEQUENCE (ILS). If lissencephaly is the only abnormality after careful clinical assessment and the MRI is typical of classical (type I) lissencephaly, a diagnosis of ILS is made. About 80% of patients with ILS have a deletion or mutation of *PAFAH1B1* and a few in *TUBA1A*, and 12% (males) of *DCX*.

MILLER–DIEKER SYNDROME (MDS). Lissencephaly with dysmorphic features (see list below) due to a deletion at 17p13.3 that includes the *PAFAH1B1* gene. In about 12%, the deletion is due to a familial chromosome rearrangement.
- Tall prominent forehead with vertical furrowing, bitemporal narrowing.
- Hypertelorism; upslanting palpebral fissures.
- Short nose with anteverted nares.
- Inverted vermilion border of the upper lip with a long, broad, and thick upper lip.
- Associated anomalies such as CHD, omphalocele, joint contractures.

DOUBLECORTIN (DCX/XLIS). XL, semi-dominant ILS (XLIS) and SBH are allelic disorders caused by mutations in the doublecortin (*DCX*) gene. Most patients with SBH or XLIS are sporadic, representing *de novo* doublecortin

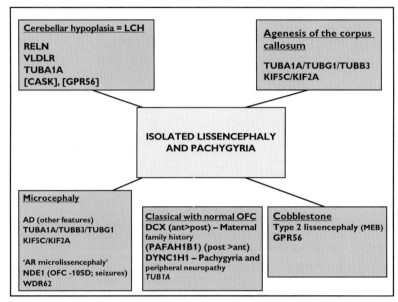

Figure 2.21 A simplified guide to clinical investigation of lissencephaly.

mutations. Females are functionally mosaic for the *DCX* mutation due to X-inactivation. A proportion of cortical neurons arrest early in migration, forming a subcortical band, whereas the remainder migrate normally to the cortical surface (hence 'double cortex').

Males with sporadic SBH may be somatic mosaics for *DCX*. There is a high rate of somatic mosaicism in male and female patients with variable penetrance of bilateral SBH. Incomplete penetrance (normal MRI scan) has been reported in a woman with a germline mutation in *DCX* who had three affected sons (Demelas *et al.* 2001).

X-LINKED LISSENCEPHALY WITH ABNORMAL GENITALIA (XLAG). Caused by loss of function mutations in the homeobox gene *ARX*. All affected individuals are genotypic males, with severe congenital or postnatal microcephaly, lissencephaly, agenesis of the corpus callosum, neonatal-onset intractable epilepsy, poor temperature regulation, chronic diarrhoea, and ambiguous or underdeveloped genitalia (Kitamura *et al.* 2002). In XLAG, the cortical thickness is only 6–7 mm, rather than the 15–20 mm cortical thickness seen in classical lissencephaly associated with mutations in *LIS1* or *DCX*. (In addition, mutations in *ARX* are associated with a wide range of phenotypes, including XL infantile spasms (polyA tract expansions), XL myoclonic epilepsy with spasticity and ID, and mild/moderate MR with or without dystonia, ataxia, or autism.)

TUBULINOPATHIES. Heterozygous variants in *TUBA1A, TUBB2A, TUBB2B, TUBB3, TUBB*, or *TUBG1* or biallelic variants in *TUBA8* cause a range of brain malformations. A disordered gyral pattern, in combination with abnormalities of the cerebellum/brainstem and/or corpus callosum and/or basal ganglia anomalies, together with lissencephaly/pachygyria/PMG, is characteristic of tubulin disorders. Clinical features include developmental delay and ID, seizures, and a variety of ocular findings.

LISSENCEPHALY WITH CEREBELLAR HYPOPLASIA (LCH). Features include a small head circumference (OFC) and cortical malformation ranging from agyria to simplification of the gyral pattern and from near-normal cortical thickness to marked thickening of the cortical grey matter. Cerebellar manifestations range from midline hypoplasia to diffuse volume reduction and disturbed foliation. DNMs in *TUBA1A* are so far the most common cause, and cerebral anomalies include dysmorphic basal ganglia and callosal abnormalities. LCH caused by mutations in 'reelin' (*RLN*) is distinguished by the severity of cerebellar and hippocampal involvement. When due to mutations in *RELN*, inheritance is AR.

WALKER–WARBURG SYNDROME (WWS), MUSCLE–EYE–BRAIN DISEASE (MEB), AND FUKAYAMA CONGENITAL MUSCULAR DYSTROPHY (FCMD). WWS, MEB, and FCMD are all associated with cobblestone lissencephaly and MR. They are all AR. Interference in O-mannosyl glycosylation appears to be the common pathological mechanism underlying both the muscular dystrophy and the neuronal migration disorder. These disorders are considered under the heading 'Dystroglycanopathies'.

- WWS is the most severe form of these conditions and is associated with ocular anomalies, like retinal dysplasia, and a markedly elevated CK. The prognosis is usually poor.
- MEB is comparatively common in Finland and is characterized by ocular anomalies and muscular dystrophy with an elevated CK.
- FCMD is characterized by CMD and myopia. It is comparatively common in Japan and is due to mutations in the fukutin gene at 9q31–33. There is a founder effect with a common 3-kb insertion.

MICROLISSENCEPHALY. Encompasses a wide range of cerebrocortical malformations, including simplified gyration, lissencephaly, and PMG. It is associated with severe congenital microcephaly (−3 SD and more below the mean). AR inheritance has been commonly reported. Genetic causes to consider include NDE1 and WDR62.

Other cortical dysplasias

PMG is characterized by the formation of multiple small gyri and can have genetic and non-genetic aetiologies The exact pathogenesis is yet unknown. A cleft from the cortex to the ventricle is known as schizencephaly (see below). The cleft in schizencephaly is usually lined with PMG.

POLYMICROGYRIA (PMG). (See Figure 2.22.) This is aetiologically heterogeneous. PMG has been associated with intrauterine infection, especially CMV, intrauterine hypoperfusion, and other teratogenic exposures in pregnancy (e.g. alcohol). A substantial proportion is genetic, with genetic heterogeneity including AR, XL, and AD PMG. PMG has been reported in several children with 22q11 deletions and a number of other chromosomal anomalies such as 1p36 deletions. A karyotype and 22q11 deletions analysis should be considered when assessing individuals with PMG. The molecular cause in a number of syndromes with PMG as a feature is known (JS; Goldberg–Shprintzen syndrome). Mutations in *PIK3CA* cause megalencephaly–capillary malformation–polymicrogyria (MCAP) syndrome; *GPR56* (AR) mutations are associated with cobblestone-like PMG.

PRIMARY MICROCEPHALY 2, WITH OR WITHOUT CORTICAL MALFORMATIONS (MCPH2). An AR neurodevelopmental disorder showing phenotypic variability. Patients with biallelic variants of this gene may have an OFC ranging from normal to severe microcephaly (e.g. -1SD to -10SD) and cranial MRI scans may show various types of cortical malformation including bilateral PMG.

SCHIZENCEPHALY. Has a wide anatomoclinical spectrum, including focal epilepsy in most patients. Association with an intrauterine CMV infection has been reported.

Heterozygous mutations in *EMX2* have been seen in a very small subset of patients.

MPPH SYNDROME. This disorder is characterized by megalencephaly (brain overgrowth) with the cortical malformation bilateral perisylvian PMG. Birth OFC ranges from normal to +6 SD. Most have ventriculomegaly and ~50% have hydrocephalus. All have ID that may be mild to severe and oromotor dysfunction. ~Five-% have seizures and ~50% have polydactyly. Heterozygous variants are found in AKT3, CCND, PIK3R2 in germline or mosaic state (see also 'Macrocephaly' in Chapter 2 'Clinical approach', p. 224).

Periventricular nodular heterotopia

In periventricular nodular heterotopia (PNH), a subset of neurons destined for the cerebral cortex fail to negotiate this complex developmental process. Failure of migration may occur due to LOF mutations in the gene *FLNA* on Xq28. Severe mutations in males lead to fetal death and usually cause epilepsy in females (sometimes with learning disability) (XL dominant inheritance). Approximately 10% of males with periventricular heterotopia also have mutations in *FLNA*, but these are mild mutations causing only partial LOF (Sheen *et al.* 2001). PNH with microcephaly is associated with mutations in *ARFGEF2* (AR).

Biallelic mutations in genes encoding the receptor–ligand cadherin pair *DCHS1* and *FAT4* may lead to a recessive syndrome in humans that includes periventricular neuronal heterotopia.

Genetic advice
Recurrence risk

ILS.

• If no genetic diagnosis, recurrence risks vary depending on the extent of the testing performed. In the pre-genomic era these were approximately 10%, but this

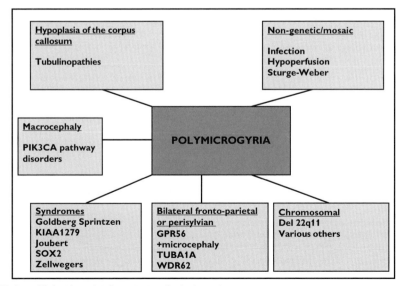

Figure 2.22 A simplified guide to clinical investigation of polymicrogyria.

figure should be used with caution as risk, particularly when associated with microcephaly, could be as high as 25%.

- If the ILS is caused by a *DCX* mutation (XLIS), the mother may be a carrier, in which case 50% of daughters will have SBH and 50% of sons will have XLIS. However, in an apparent *de novo* case, maternal germline mosaicism needs to be taken into account, with a possible recurrence risk of 10%, and PND should be offered (see 'Prenatal diagnosis' below).

MDS. If parental chromosomes are normal, recurrence risk is very low (<1%).

SBH. If an affected female carries a *DCX* mutation, 50% of daughters will have SBH and 50% of sons will have XLIS. Somatic and gonadal mosaicism is not uncommon. For a woman whose child has an apparently *de novo* *DCX* mutation, there is a significant (up to 10%) risk of recurrence on the basis of gonadal mosaicism and PND should be offered. Mosaic PAFAH1B1 mutations can cause SBH.

WWS, MEB, AND FCMD. All follow AR inheritance with 25% sibling recurrence risk.

LCH. When caused by mutations in *TUBA1A*, counsel as above; when caused by mutations in *RELN*, and WDR62, inheritance is AR with a 25% sibling recurrence risk.

PMG. Familial recurrence has been reported with PMG due to AR syndromic causes (see Figure 2.22). An intrauterine infection and an abnormal karyotype, e.g. del 22q11, should be excluded. In the absence of a family history or a causative mutation, the recurrence risk is uncertain. There appears to be a higher risk with perisylvian PMG, particularly in males, which has been quoted as up to 30%. Many cases are sporadic.

SCHIZENCEPHALY. Familial occurrence is rare; heterozygous *EMX2* mutations have been reported in some patients.

PERIVENTRICULAR NODULAR HETEROTOPIA. XL inheritance—women with an *FLNA* mutation will transmit the mutation to 50% of their daughters. At conception, 50% of male pregnancies will carry the *FLNA* mutation, but these will usually be lost prenatally or early in the postnatal period. PNH due to *ARFGEF2* mutations has a 1:4 recurrence risk for siblings and there are other recessive causes. Not infrequently a genetic diagnosis is not identified using current sequencing tests.

Carrier detection

OTHER GENETIC CAUSES. Counsel as appropriate. *DCX* mutation analysis in mothers of patients (XLIS, SBH) with *DCX* mutations. In the absence of a mutation, MRI scanning should be considered in mothers who have children with these conditions.

Prenatal diagnosis

If a specific diagnosis has been possible and the familial mutation(s) is known, PND by CVS at 11 weeks' gestation may be possible.

PND of lissencephaly by USS is *not reliable* and does not become possible before about 28 weeks' gestation; fetal MRI scanning in these cases is more accurate. However, there may be associated features, such as congenital microcephaly, hydrocephalus, or cerebellar hypoplasia, that may be a useful guide earlier in pregnancy.

Natural history and further management (preventative measures)

The child should be under the care of a paediatric neurologist.

References

Aigner L, Uyanik G, Couillard-Despres S, *et al.* Somatic mosaicism and variable penetrance in doublecortin-associated migration disorders. *Neurology* 2003; **60**: 329–32.

Allanson JE, Ledbetter DH, Dobyns WB. Classical lissencephaly syndromes: does the face reflect the brain? *J Med Genet* 1998; **35**: 920–3.

Allen KM, Walsh CA. Genes that regulate neuronal migration in the cerebral cortex. *Epilepsy Res* 1999; **36**: 143–54.

Barkovich AJ. Neuroimaging manifestations and classification of congenital muscular dystrophies. *Am J Neuroradiol* 1998; **19**: 1386–96.

Cappello S, Gray MJ, Badouel C, *et al.* Mutations in genes encoding the cadherin receptor-ligand pair DCHS1 and FAT4 disrupt cerebral cortical development. *Nat Genet* 2013; **45**: 1300–8.

Cardoso C, Leventre RJ, Dowling JJ, *et al.* Clinical and molecular basis of classical lissencephaly: mutations in the LIS1 gene (PAFAH1B1). *Hum Mutat* 2002; **19**: 4–15.

Demelas L, Serra G, Conti M, *et al.* Incomplete penetrance with normal MRI in a woman with germline mutation of the DCX gene. *Neurology* 2001; **57**: 327–30

Ehara H, Maegaki Y, Takeshita K. Pachygyria and polymicrogyria in 22q11 deletion syndrome. *Am J Med Genet A* 2003; **117A**: 80–2.

Gleeson JG, Minnerath S, Kuzniecky RI, *et al.* Somatic and germline mosaic mutations in the doublecortin gene are associated with variable phenotypes. *Am J Hum Genet* 2000; **67**: 574–81.

Guerrini R, Carrozzo R. Epileptogenic brain malformations: clinical presentation, malformative patterns and indications for genetic testing. *Seizure* 2002; **11**(Suppl. A): 532–43.

Kato M, Dobyns WB. Lissencephaly and the molecular basis of neuronal migration. *Hum Mol Gen* 2003; **12**(Suppl.): R89–96.

Kitamura K, Yanazawa M, Sugiyama N, *et al.* Mutation of ARX causes abnormal development of forebrain and testes in mice and X-linked lissencephaly with abnormal genitalia in humans. *Nat Genet* 2002; **32**: 359–69.

Olson EC, Walsh CA. Smooth, rough and upside-down neocortical development. *Curr Opin Genet Dev* 2002; **12**: 320–7.

Parrini E, Mei D, Wright M, Dorn T, Guerrini R. Mosaic mutations of the FLN1 gene cause a mild phenotype in patients with periventricular heterotopia. *Neurogenetics* 2004; **5**: 191–6.

Ross ME, Swanson K, Dobyns WB. Lissencephaly with cerebellar hypoplasia (LCH): a heterogeneous group of cortical malformations. *Neuropaediatrics* 2001; **32**: 256–63.

Sheen VL, Dixon PH, Fox JW, *et al.* Mutations in the X-linked filamin 1 gene cause periventricular nodular heterotopia in males as well as in females. *Hum Mol Genet.* 2001; **10**: 1775-83.

Vuillaumier-Barrot S, Bouchet-Séraphin C, Chelbi M, *et al.* Identification of mutations in TMEM5 and ISPD as a cause of severe cobblestone lissencephaly. *Am J Hum Genet* 2012; **91**: 1135–43.

Walsh CA. Genetic malformations of the human cerebral cortex. *Neuron* 1999; **23**: 19–29.

Warrell D (ed.). *Oxford textbook of medicine*, 4th edn. Oxford University Press, Oxford, 2003.

Lumps and bumps

Children and adults may be referred to a geneticist to determine if a 'lump or bump' is a marker for an inherited condition. There is often a dominant family history of similar lesions.

The history may be the first clue as to the underlying diagnosis, but the new mutation rate is significant and there is variability and incomplete penetrance for many of the dominantly inherited conditions.

Clinical approach

History: key points

- Three-generation family tree. Enquire whether any other family members have similar lesions.
- Family history of malignancy.
- At what age did the lesions first appear?
- Take a full medical history to identify any other problems.

Examination: key points

- Document the approximate number and location of the lesions (photographs if possible).
- Examine a typical lesion carefully and describe in detail.
- Is the lump in the soft tissues or is it hard and bony?
- If there is more than one type of lesion, record the various types.
- Examine carefully for other clues, e.g. CAL spots.

Special investigations

If the diagnosis is not evident, consider referring to a dermatologist or surgeon for consideration of biopsy of one of the lesions to obtain a histological diagnosis.

Some diagnoses to consider

Predominantly cutaneous syndromes

AUTOSOMAL DOMINANT LIPOMAS. These usually appear in adults, predominantly in a central distribution. They rarely affect the face. Usually the lipomas are benign, though progression to mixoid liposarcoma may rarely occur. Advise patients to report enlarging lesions.

NEUROFIBROMATOSIS TYPE 1 (NF1). Dermal neurofibromas are a characteristic feature of NF1 and occur in the majority of NF1 patients from early adolescence. They increase in number with time, especially during puberty and pregnancy. See 'Neurofibromatosis type 1 (NF1)' in Chapter 3, 'Common consultations', p. 506.

HEREDITARY LEIOMYOMATOSIS AND RENAL CELL CANCER (HLRCC). An AD condition that causes multiple small skin lumps (cutaneous leiomyomata), associated with uterine fibroids and renal cancer. Heterozygous mutations of the fumarate hydratase (*FH*) gene can be readily found in about 75% of HLRCC cases (Alam *et al.* 2003). Renal cancer with papillary type II morphology is sometimes part of the multiple cutaneous and uterine leiomyomatosis spectrum. Homozygosity or compound heterozygosity for mutations of the fumarate hydratase (*FH*) gene cause fumarase deficiency, a rare AR disorder of the citric acid cycle causing severe neurological impairment.

STEATOCYSTOMA MULTIPLEX. An AD condition characterized by multiple sebaceous cysts. Due to mutations in *KRT17*.

BROOKE-SPIEGLER SYNDROME. AD disorder characterized by multiple trichoepitheliomas (benign tumours of the hair follicle) and caused by heterozygous variants in CYLD.

MULTIPLE CYLINDROMATOSIS. AD disorder characterized by multiple cylindromas mainly affecting the face, trunk, and extremities. On the scalp they may coalesce into large turban tumours. Caused by heterozygous variants in CYLD (Rajan 2015).

AUTOSOMAL DOMINANT GLOMUS TUMOURS. These present as small, soft blue swellings, particularly on the limbs. They can be tender and ache and may increase in size. Mutations may be detected in glomulin (*GLML*) on 1p21-22. (They should not be confused with paragangliomas, which are sometimes called 'glomus tumours'.)

FAMILIAL ANGIOLIPOMATOSIS. Familial angiolipomatosis is a rare syndrome that may be confused clinically with NF1. Usually AD, but AR inheritance has been described. It is characterized by subcutaneous tumours at the wrists, knees, and ankles. There may be bone deformity near affected joints. Onset is usually in early adult life.

PROTEUS SYNDROME (DUE TO SOMATIC ACTIVATING MUTATIONS IN AKT1). Can be confused with NF1. Lipomas, pigmentary skin changes. Localized overgrowth of limbs and digits. Deep creases on the soles of the feet. See 'Overgrowth' in Chapter 2, 'Clinical approach', p. 272.

JUVENILE HYALINE FIBROMATOSIS (JHF) AND INFANTILE SYSTEMIC HYALINOSIS (ISH). AR conditions characterized by multiple subcutaneous skin nodules, gingival hypertrophy, joint contractures, and hyaline deposition. Allelic conditions caused by mutations in capillary morphogenesis protein 2 (*CMG2*) on 4q21.

Cancer syndromes

NEUROFIBROMATOSIS TYPE 2 (NF2). Cutaneous neurofibromas are found in nearly 30% of NF2 patients. See 'Neurofibromatosis type 2 (NF2)' in Chapter 4, 'Cancer', p. 596.

FAMILIAL ADENOMATOUS POLYPOSIS (FAP). Multiple sebaceous cysts, especially over the scalp and occurring in young individuals, may be a feature of FAP. It is caused by mutations in the *APC* gene. Mutations 3′ of codon 1400 are especially associated with desmoid tumours. See 'Familial adenomatous polyposis (FAP) and adenomatous polyposis due to *MUTYH, NTHL1, POLE,* and *POLD1*' in Chapter 4, 'Cancer', p. 568.

MUIR–TORRE SYNDROME (MTS). Co-occurrence of skin sebaceous tumours, adenomas, epitheliomas, or carcinomas with internal malignancy. Most of MTS is due to mutations in *MSH2* (Lynch syndrome), but it can occasionally be associated with mutations in *MLH1*. Other skin tumours, such as keratoacanthomas, can be seen in MTS, but there can often be a fine histological distinction between keratoacanthomas and squamous carcinomas, which may account for the latter also being associated with MTS.

BANNAYAN–RILEY–RUVALCABA/COWDEN SYNDROME. An AD disorder consisting of macrocephaly, vascular malformations, lipomas, and pigmented macules on the shaft of the penis, associated with malignancies (breast, thyroid, endometrial, and gut hamartomas). Birthweight usually >4000 g, OFC often >4.5 SD. Hypotonia, gross motor delay (60% have a mild proximal myopathy), learning disability, and speech delay occur in 70%; 25% have seizures. They may have mild hypertelorism. Sixty per cent have mutations in *PTEN*. See 'Cowden syndrome (PTEN hamartoma tumour syndrome (PHTS))' in Chapter 4, 'Cancer', p. 564.

CARNEY COMPLEX. An AD condition due to mutations in *CNC1*, characterized by skin pigmentary anomalies, cardiac and cutaneous myxomas, endocrine tumours, and schwannomas. Cutaneous myxomas are pale, smooth papules or subcutaneous nodules that appear between birth and the middle age on any part of the body, e.g. eyelid, except the hands and feet. See 'Multiple endocrine neoplasia' in Chapter 4, 'Cancer', p. 592.

Bony lumps

HEREDITARY MULTIPLE EXOSTOSES (HME). An AD disorder characterized by multiple exostoses that may be painful, most commonly arising from the juxtaepiphyseal region of the long bones. These start as cartilaginous lesions and then ossify. Other bones that can be involved include the pectoral and pelvic girdles and ribs. The skull is not usually involved. Abnormal bone modelling, particularly of the long bones, causes bowing, shortness, cortical irregularities, and metaphyseal widening of the involved bones, leading to deformities of the forearms and a disproportionate short stature in severe cases. Malignant transformation to sarcoma is uncommon (0.5–2% of cases) and usually occurs between the ages of 10 and 50 years; families should be told to report any enlarging or painful lesions. HME is genetically heterogeneous; most families have mutations in EXT1 (8q24) or EXT2 (11p12–p11) and around 10% of cases are caused by DNMs. Penetrance is >95% and around 5% are affected at birth. Males have more severe and frequent complications.

NB. Langer–Giedion syndrome is due to a microdeletion at 8q24 involving the genes for multiple exostoses 1 and trichorhinophalangeal syndrome.

ENCHONDROMATOSIS (MULTIPLE ENCHONDROMATOSIS, OLLIER DISEASE, MAFFUCCI SYNDROME). Enchondromas are common benign cartilage tumours of bone. They can occur as solitary lesions or as multiple lesions in enchondromatosis (Ollier and Maffucci diseases). Clinical problems caused by enchondromas include skeletal deformity and the potential for malignant change to chondrosarcoma. The extent of skeletal involvement is variable in enchondromatosis and may include dysplasia that is not directly attributable to enchondromas. When haemangiomata are associated, the condition is known as Maffucci syndrome. Neither condition seems to be genetically determined in a simple Mendelian manner. There are a few instances of familial occurrence of Ollier disease, however.

ALBRIGHT HEREDITARY OSTEODYSTROPHY (AHO; PSEU-DOHYPOPARATHYROIDISM, PSEUDOPSEUDOHYPOPAR-ATHYROIDISM). Subcutaneous gritty deposits of calcification, predominantly affecting the scalp, hands, and feet. Shortness of the 4th and 5th metacarpals, short distal phalanges of the thumb, cone-shaped epiphyses. AD, but with imprinting effect. Gs alpha (*GNAS*) gene. See 'Obesity with and without developmental delay' in Chapter 2, 'Clinical approach', p. 254.

FIBRODYSPLASIA OSSIFICANS PROGRESSIVA (FOP). An extremely rare and disabling genetic disorder characterized by ectopic ossification of the soft tissues. The hallux is short. Avoid surgery and dental work as these lead to significant acceleration of the ossification. The inheritance of FOP is new dominant and all cases of classic FOP are caused by a single recurrent mutation (*R206H*) in ACVR1, a bone morphogenetic protein (BMP) type I receptor. Other missense mutations have been seen in the ACVR1 glycine and serine residue activation domain in atypical FOP cases (Kaplan *et al.* 2009).

Other syndromes

MYOTONIC DYSTROPHY (DM). Rarely patients with DM may develop pilomatrixomas, benign tumours of the hair matrix. See 'Myotonic dystrophy (DM1)' in Chapter 3, 'Common consultations', p. 496.

Genetic advice

Recurrence risk

As for the specific disorder.

Carrier detection

Clinical examination combined with mutation analysis, if available.

Prenatal diagnosis

This is possible for some of these conditions.

Natural history and further management (preventative measures)

Many of the conditions require long-term medical surveillance.

Support group: Many of the individual syndromes have their own support groups. See Contact a Family, http://www.cafamily.org.uk.

Expert adviser: Marc Tischkowitz, Reader and Honorary Consultant Physician in Medical Genetics, Department of Medical Genetics, University of Cambridge and East Anglian Medical Genetics Service, Cambridge, UK.

References

Alam NA, Rowan AJ, Wortham NC, *et al*. Genetic and functional analyses of FH mutations in multiple cutaneous and uterine leiomyomatosis, hereditary leiomyomatosis and renal cancer, and fumarate hydratase deficiency. *Hum Mol Genet* 2003; **12**: 1241–52.

Hall CR, Cole WG, Haynes R, Hecht JT. Reevaluation of a genetic model for the development of exostosis in hereditary multiple exostosis. *Am J Med Genet* 2002; **112**: 1–5.

Hanks S, Adams S, Douglas J, *et al*. Mutations in the gene encoding capillary morphogenesis protein 2 cause juvenile hyaline fibromatosis and infantile systemic hyalinosis. *Am J Hum Genet* 2003; **73**: 791–800.

Hopyan S, Gokgoz N, Poon R, *et al*. A mutant PTH/PTHrP type I receptor in enchondromatosis. *Nat Genet* 2002; **30**: 306–10.

Kaplan FS, Xu M, Seemann P, *et al*. Classic and atypical fibrodysplasia ossificans progressiva (FOP) phenotypes are caused by mutations in the bone morphogenetic protein (BMP) type I receptor ACVR1. *Hum Mutat* 2009; **30**: 379–90.

Rajan N, Ashworth A. Inherited cylindromas: lessons from a rare tumour. *Lancet Oncol* 2015; **16**(9): e460–9.

Sybert VP. *Genetic skin disorders, Oxford monographs in medical genetics*. Oxford University Press, New York, 1997.

Macrocephaly

Megalencephaly, megacephaly.

Macrocephaly is the term used to describe a head circumference >3 SD above the mean for chronological age. It is compared with the length/height to determine if it is proportionate. Macrocephaly associated with large stature is found in the overgrowth syndromes (see 'Overgrowth' in Chapter 2, 'Clinical approach', p. 272). Here we address the problem of a head circumference disproportionately large in relation to stature. Neuroimaging has an especially important role in patients with developmental delay and macrocephaly. Large ventricles are frequently reported in children with macrocephaly; the ventricular volume needs to be assessed in relation to the degree of megalencephaly. If the predominant abnormality is hydrocephalus, see 'Hydrocephalus' in Chapter 2, 'Clinical approach', p. 172.

Bailey et al. in 1998 noted autism was associated with increased brain size at post-mortem. Bolton et al. (2001) found that idiopathic infantile macrocephaly was associated with an increased risk of developing autism spectrum disorders (odds ratio (OR) 5.44). This is well reviewed by Lainhart et al. in 2006. In Nevo et al.'s (2002) community-based study of >4000 children with neurodevelopmental disability in Israel, 1.4% of children had macrocephaly (OFC >98th centile). Children with developmental disability and macrocephaly had an increased risk of seizures (OR 7.7).

Clinical approach

History: key points

- Three-generation family history with specific enquiry about family history of large head circumference and family history of malignancy (especially breast cancer, colonic polyps, endometrial and thyroid disorders in Bannayan–Riley–Ruvalcaba/Cowden syndrome (BRR-PHTS)), and skin disorders (especially early or multiple basal cell carcinoma (BCC) and medulloblastoma) in Gorlin syndrome. Enquire specifically about consanguinity.
- Head circumference at birth.
- Developmental milestones.
- Regression.
- Seizures.

Examination: key points

- Measurement of head circumference, height/length, and weight. Exclude causes of a spuriously large head size such as hair arrangements, craniosynostosis, or other abnormalities of head shape.
- Coarse facial features (storage disorders).
- Prominent forehead, long face, and large jaw (Sotos syndrome and Van Bucham syndrome).
- Neurocutaneous lesions: CALs, capillary haemangiomata, depigmented lesions.
- Other skin lesions: lipomata, vascular lesions, and tricholemmomas (Bannayan–Riley–Ruvalcaba (BRR) syndrome), megalencephaly, capillary malformation, polymicrogyria syndrome (MCAP), BCC (Gorlin syndrome), papillomata around the nose and mouth and behind the ears (Cowden syndrome, Costello syndrome).

- Limb asymmetry and syndactyly, philtral haemangioma. Macrocephaly–capillary malformation syndromes (M-CM).
- Organomegaly.
- Penile or vulval freckling (BRR syndrome).
- Parental head circumferences which should be plotted against height (Bushby et al. 1992). See 'Centile charts for occipital–frontal circumference (OFC)' in 'Appendix', p. 823.

Special investigations

- Brain imaging. MRI preferable to identify white matter changes.
- Neurodevelopmental assessment.
- Metabolic screen. Urine organic acids and mucopolysaccharide screen.
- Fragile X.
- Genomic analysis in presence of other malformations suggestive of a chromosomal or syndromic diagnosis, e.g. genomic array, gene panel, or WES/WGS as appropriate. A number of different CNVs are associated with macrocephaly.
- Consider very high depth sequencing (>1000) in germline DNA or DNA affected tissue for mosaic disorders if there is a high clinical suspicion for a disorder of the PIK3CA/AKT pathway.
- Consider PTEN mutation analysis if consistent with BRR-PHTS.

Some diagnoses to consider

Structurally normal brain

Large ventricles are frequently reported in children with macrocephaly. Virchow–Robin spaces are perivascular extensions of the subarachnoid space. They are found normally and frequently seen on modern MRI scans. There are some individuals, especially those with macrocephaly, in whom these spaces are prominent and widespread.

FAMILIAL MACROCEPHALY. Diagnosis based on parental OFC and absence of any associated features or developmental delay; may follow AD inheritance. Beware that PTEN and PTCH gene mutations can present with few syndromic features.

NEUROFIBROMATOSIS TYPE 1 (NF1). An AD condition characterized by CALs, axillary freckling, dermal neurofibroma, and short stature. See 'Neurofibromatosis type 1 (NF1)' in Chapter 3, 'Common consultations', p. 506.

FRAGILE X SYNDROME. An XLR condition characterized by developmental delay. The head circumference, though relatively large, is usually nearer to 75th centile size. See 'Fragile X syndrome (FRAX)' in Chapter 3, 'Common consultations', p. 424.

SOTOS SYNDROME. Overgrowth from the prenatal stage through childhood, with advanced bone age, an unusual face with a large skull and a pointed chin, occasional seizures, and mild learning problems. Mutations in NSD1. See 'Overgrowth' in Chapter 2, 'Clinical approach', p. 272.

NFIX. Heterozygous mutation causes a Sotos-like overgrowth syndrome with advanced bone age, macrocephaly, developmental delay, scoliosis, and unusual facies (Malan *et al*. 2010).

WEAVER SYNDROME. Prenatal and postnatal overgrowth, advanced bone age, round face with a small, discrete chin, large ears, and frequent contractures. Often misdiagnosed with Sotos, but different gene (*EZH2*). Most, but *not all*, cases significant macrocephaly.

SIMPSON—GOLABI—BEHMEL SYNDROME. An XLR disorder with high birthweight, heavy facies, cleft lip and palate, digital anomalies, supernumerary nipples, bilateral undescended testes, and mild/moderate learning disability. Mutations in glypican 3. See 'Overgrowth' in Chapter 2, 'Clinical approach', p. 272.

SKELETAL DYSPLASIAS. A number of skeletal dysplasias may be associated with relative macrocephaly (due to sparing of the head circumference, e.g. multiple epiphyseal dysplasia (MED)) or absolute macrocephaly made more distinctive due to short stature (achondroplasia, WTX). Look for evidence of short stature, disproportionate stature, or limb length and digital anomalies. Consider a skeletal survey.

Also consider disorders of skull enlargement or thickening such as craniodiaphyseal or craniometaphyseal dysplasia and Van Buchem disease which may require a skeletal survey to confirm the diagnosis.

STORAGE DISORDERS. In association with developmental delay and regression. MPS, most typically type III (Sanfilippo), but may be associated with relative macrocephaly in other MPS disorders. Dysmorphic features may be less pronounced than in MPS III and other MPS. See 'Developmental regression' in Chapter 2, 'Clinical approach', p. 128.

GLUTARIC ACIDURIA TYPE 1. Detectable on urine organic acid screen.

BANNAYAN—RILEY—RUVALCABA/COWDEN SYNDROME (BRR-CS). An AD disorder consisting of macrocephaly, vascular malformations, lipomas, and pigmented macules on the vulva or glans of the penis. It is associated with malignancies (breast, thyroid, endometrial, and gut with hamartomas). Birthweight usually >4000 g; OFC often >4.5 SD. Hypotonia, gross motor delay (60% have a mild proximal myopathy), learning disability, and speech delay occur in 70%; 25% have seizures. May have mild hypertelorism. Sixty per cent have mutations in *PTEN*. See 'Cowden syndrome (PTEN hamartoma tumour syndrome (PHTS))' in Chapter 4, 'Cancer', p. 564.

GORLIN SYNDROME (BASAL CELL NAEVUS SYNDROME). An AD condition characterized in older individuals by BCCs and jaw cysts; mutations in *PATCH*. See 'Gorlin syndrome' in Chapter 4, 'Cancer', p. 576.

CARDIOFACIOCUTANEOUS (CFC) AND COSTELLO SYNDROMES. Feeding difficulties in infancy, coarse facies, loose skin over the hands, characteristic perinasal papillomata, and Noonan-like features. See 'Noonan syndrome and the Ras/MAPK pathway syndromes: neuro-cardio-facial-cutaneous syndromes' in Chapter 3, 'Common consultations', p. 512.

DISORDERS OF THE PIK3CA/AKT PATHWAY. (See Figure 2.30 in 'Overgrowth', Chapter 2, 'Clinical approach', p. 272.) Megalencephaly—capillary malformation polymicrogyria (MCAP), previously known as macrocephaly—cutis maramorata—telangiectatica congenita (M-CMTC) or macrocephaly—capillary malformation (M-CM). Macrocephaly (often with hydrocephalus that may require shunting), macrosomia, philtral haemangioma, cutis marmorata (vascular mottling of the skin), syndactyly of toes 2/3 and/or fingers 3/4; may have PAP and asymmetry. Perisylvian PMG is the classical brain phenotype in this condition. Variable developmental delay and expressivity of the physical phenotype. A further subgroup is megalencephaly—polymicrogyria—polydactyly—hydrocephalus (MPPH) which lacks vascular malformation and syndactyly. Mutations in both disorders have been identified in *AKT3*, *PIK3R2*, and *PIK3CA*, most commonly post-zygotic mutations in *PIK3CA*. All cases reported to date are sporadic. The timing and tissue distribution of post-zygotic mutations may influence the final phenotype. Riviere *et al*. (2013) provide a very useful review.

PROTEUS SYNDROME. May overlap with some of the clinical features seen in the PIK3CA/AKT pathway disorders and includes macrocephaly, but the skin, fat, and lipomatous overgrowth and skeletal manifestations are characteristic and due to somatic mutations in *AKT1*.

Structurally abnormal brain

The structural abnormality may guide further investigation, e.g. lissencephaly, pachygyria, or other migration anomaly.

If a diagnosis is suggested on the basis of brain imaging, ensure that any other investigations that may support the diagnosis are performed. Genetic counselling is as appropriate for the diagnosis.

NEUROFIBROMATOSIS TYPE 1 (NF1). Unidentified bright objects (UBOs) may be seen on a T2-weighted MRI scan in children with NF1, as may optic tract gliomas (seen in up to 15%, but only symptomatic in 71.5%). See 'Neurofibromatosis type 1 (NF1)' in Chapter 3, 'Common consultations', p. 506.

Metabolic with associated leukodystrophy

CANAVAN DISEASE (CD). An inherited AR leukodystrophy, with an increased prevalence in Ashkenazim (carrier frequency >1/40). The clinical features of the disease are macrocephaly, head lag, progressive severe MR, and hypotonia in early life, which later changes to spasticity. It is caused by aspartoacylase (ASPA) deficiency and accumulation of N-acetylaspartic acid (NAA) in the brain that result in disruption of myelin and spongiform degeneration of the white matter of the brain. The gene for ASPA has been cloned and there are two founder mutations in the Ashkenazi Jewish population.

ALEXANDER DISEASE. Regression and megalencephaly with leukodystrophy. The most notable features of the infantile form of Alexander disease, which begins during the first 2 years of life, are macrocephaly (and sometimes hydrocephaly), psychomotor regression, seizures, and spasticity. MRI shows signal changes in the white matter with frontal predominance. The patient dies within the first decade. Caused by heterozygous DNMs in the glial fibrillary acidic protein gene (*GFAP*).

Genetic advice

Recurrence risk

As appropriate for each identified condition.

For an isolated female with learning difficulties in whom all the above investigations do not reveal a diagnosis, a recurrence risk for sibs of ~3–5% may be appropriate but beware variable dominant disorders. For an isolated male, a recurrence risk of 5–10% may be used to cover the possibility of an XL condition.

Carrier detection
Not possible unless a familial mutation is identified.

Prenatal diagnosis
Not possible unless a familial mutation is identified.

Natural history and further management (preventative measures)

If there are seizures or abnormal features on MRI, the child should be assessed by a paediatric neurologist. If there are associated developmental problems, the child should be under the care of a child development team.

Support groups: M-CM Network, http://www.m-cm.net, Tel. 0808 808 3555. Many of the individual syndromes have their own support groups. See Contact a Family, http://www.cafamily.org.uk.

Expert adviser: Trevor Cole, Consultant in Clinical and Cancer Genetics, Reader in Medical Genetics, West Midlands Regional Genetics Service, Birmingham Women's Hospital, Birmingham, UK.

References

Bailey A, Luther P, Dean A, et al. A clinicopathological study autism. *Brain* 1998 **121**; 889–905.

Bolton PF, Roobol M, Allsopp L, Pickles A. Association between idiopathic infantile macrocephaly and autism spectrum disorders. *Lancet* 2001; **358**: 726–7.

Brenner M, Johnson AB, Boespflug-Tanguy O, et al. Mutations in GFAP, encoding glial fibrillary acidic protein, are associated with Alexander disease. *Nat Genet* 2001; **27**: 117–20.

Bushby KM, Cole T, Matthews JN, Goodship JA. Centiles for adult head circumference. *Arch Dis Child* 1992; **67**: 1286–7.

Franceschini P, Licata D, Di Cara G, et al. Macrocephaly–cutis marmorata telangiectatica congenital without cutis marmorata? *Am J Med Genet* 2000; **90**: 265–9.

Lainhart JE, Bigler ED, Boican M, et al. Head circumference and height in autism: a study by the Collaborative Program of Excellence in Autism. *Am J Med Genet A* 2006; **140A**: 2257–74.

Malan V, Rajan D, Thomas S, et al. Distinct effects of allelic NFIX mutations on nonsense-mediated mRNA decay engender either a Sotos-like or a Marshall-Smith syndrome. *Am J Hum Genet* 2010; **87**: 189–98.

Nevo Y, Kramer U, Shinnar S, et al. Macrocephaly in children with developmental disabilities. *Pediatr Neurol* 2002; **27**: 363–8.

Riviere JB, Mirzaa GM, O'Roak BJ, et al. De novo germline and postzygotic mutations in AKT3, PIK3R2 and PIK3CA cause a spectrum of related megalencephaly syndrome. *Nat Genet* 2013; **44**: 934–40.

Stevenson RE, Schroer RJ, Skinner C, Fender D, Simensen RJ. Autism and macrocephaly. *Lancet* 1997; **349**: 1744–5.

Microcephaly

The clinical finding of an abnormally small head. In practice, the term is applied if the OFC is −3 SD or <0.4th centile for age and sex.

Microcephaly is caused by a very heterogeneous group of conditions. The role of the geneticist is to exclude chromosomal and environmental causes and to attempt to identify syndromic associations. Microcephaly is a feature in >450 syndromes listed in the London Dysmorphology Database, so the number of possible diagnoses is frighteningly large; fortunately most will have other features that are obvious on careful clinical assessment.

Clinical approach

History: key points

- Three-generation family tree.
- History of infection, drug exposure, radiation, foreign travel, birth asphyxia, or excess alcohol during pregnancy.
- Enquire carefully for possible consanguinity.
- If antenatal USS was performed, was the estimated date of delivery (EDD) revised because the biparietal diameter (BPD) was smaller than expected?
- Birthweight.
- Ascertain the OFC at birth or the earliest record in infancy and plot longitudinally. Is the microcephaly static or progressive? (Primary microcephaly is evident at birth; secondary microcephaly occurs postnatally.)
- Developmental progress.
- Does the child have seizures?

Examination: key points

- Plot the OFC, height (or length), and weight accurately, and estimate how small the head is, e.g. −5 SD; exclude craniosynostosis. Particularly if the microcephaly is borderline −2 to 3 SD), establish if this is a dominant family trait by measuring parental OFCs.
- Assess carefully for dysmorphic features. Assessment of the facies can be difficult as these are distorted by severe microcephaly.
- Examine carefully for other congenital anomalies, e.g. CHD.
- Detailed neurological exam? Spasticity?

Special investigations

- Genomic analysis, e.g. genomic array and gene panel or WES/WGS as available.
- DNA for relevant molecular investigation if gene panel or WES/WGS not available (e.g. *MCPH5* mutation analysis in primary AR microcephaly).
- Karyotype for spontaneous rearrangements indicative of a DNA breakage disorder.
- MRI scan (look carefully for neuronal migration abnormalities).
- Urine for organic and amino acids.
- Ophthalmology referral (chorioretinopathy may not be symptomatic).
- TORCH screen. Consider congenital infection, including Zika virus.
- Maternal urine biochemistry to exclude maternal PKU.
- Consider testing for Angelman syndrome (may present with mild microcephaly in the first year of life,

before seizures or characteristic facies and movement become apparent).
- Consider lactate, VLCFAs if hypotonic.
- Consider plasma 7-dehydrocholesterol to exclude SLO syndrome if one additional suggestive feature, e.g. syndactyly, cleft palate.

Some diagnoses to consider

AR conditions

PRIMARY AR MICROCEPHALY. Marked microcephaly in the absence of other malformations or significant neurological deficits. Characterized by relatively normal development with respect to the severity of the microcephaly, resulting in typically mild to moderate MR. Head size is reduced at birth (≤−2 SD) and almost always <−4 SD postnatally (>6 months). The remainder of the examination and investigations are normal. Neuroimaging shows a small, but structurally normal, cerebral cortex with simplified gyral folding. Ten genes have been identified (*MCPH1, ASPM, CDK5RAP2, CENPJ, STIL, WDR62, CEP63, CEP135, CEP152, CASC5*). *ASPM* is the most common, with mutations in ~40% of patients across ethic groups. *WDR62* mutations are also common and may have additional cortical anomalies. Increased numbers of prophase-like cells on karyotyping are seen with *MCPH1* mutation (Trimborn et al. 2004).

MICROCEPHALIC PRIMORDIAL DWARFISM (SECKEL SYNDROME, MOPD I AND II). This group of disorders are recognized by IUGR and marked microcephaly in association with significant short stature (both OFC and height <−4 SD) (Klingseisen et al. 2011). The OFC may be in proportion to the height or more severely affected. Within this group, there are several recognizable entities. MOPD II caused by mutations in *PCNT* is the most common. Birthweight −4 SD, and later on the OFC and height typically reach −8 SD to −10 SD, alongside relatively normal developmental progression. Skeletal features may be mild, with brachydactyly and coxa vara. Often small, loose secondary dentition. High risk of moya moya/cerebral aneurysms and insulin resistance in childhood. Taybi–Linder (MOPD I) exhibit the most extreme growth failure accompanied by severe neurological impairment, cerebral cortical dysplasia, joint contractures/dislocations, bowed long bones, and absent/sparse hair with dry skin, often with death before 2 years. Mutations have been identified in *RNU4ATAC*. Mutations in the pre-replication complex genes (*ORC1, 4,* and *6, CDT1, CDC6*) are found in Meier Gorlin syndrome, recognized by the triad of short stature, microtia, and patella hypoplasia/aplasia. Seckel syndrome is a heterogeneous entity which, in its broadest sense, according to the original definition of 'nanocephalic dwarfism', encompassed all MOPD. However, now usually used to describe disproportionate microcephaly, accompanied by moderate/severe ID and characteristic facies of a slopping forehead and a beaked nose, associated with mutations in several genes (e.g. *ATR, ATRIP, CEP152*).

SMITH–LEMLI–OPITZ (SLO) SYNDROME. Prenatal and postnatal growth deficiency, developmental delay (almost all), cleft palate (37–52%), cardiac defects (36–38%), especially AVSD and TAPVD, hypospadias and/or cryptorchidism (90–100%) in affected males, Y-shaped 2/3 toe syndactyly (>95%), and PAP (~50%). See 'Hypospadias' in Chapter 2, 'Clinical approach', p. 186.

AICARDI–GOUTIÈRES SYNDROME (AGS). Characterized by progressive microcephaly and ICC. See 'Intracranial calcification' in Chapter 2, 'Clinical approach', p. 200.

PSEUDO-TORCH SYNDROME. An AR condition characterized by congenital microcephaly, congenital cerebral calcification, spasticity, and seizures. Also known as band-like calcification with simplified gyration and polymicrogyria and caused by biallelic variants in the OCLN gene. See 'Intracranial calcification' in Chapter 2, 'Clinical Approach', p. 200.

DNA REPAIR DEFECTS (FANCONI, COCKAYNE SYNDROME, NIJMEGEN BREAKAGE SYNDROME, LIGASE IV, ETC.). Growth retardation is also a feature of most of these conditions with proportionate microcephaly or minor microcephaly. Nijmegen breakage syndrome is an extremely rare AR condition, but affected children have moderate microcephaly with IUGR, short stature, a prominent midface, growth retardation, mild learning difficulties, and susceptibility to infections with panhypogammaglobulinaemia, and susceptibility to lymphoma and other tumours. See 'DNA repair disorders' in Chapter 3, 'Common consultations', p. 398.

AD conditions

Mild, non-progressive microcephaly associated with normal intelligence may be inherited as an AD trait that is likely genetically heterogeneous. Measurement of the parental head circumference is important in the assessment of individuals with mild microcephaly.

AD MICROCEPHALY WITH CONGENITAL LYMPHOEDEMA AND CHORIORETINOPATHY. Mild AD microcephaly variably associated with congenital lymphoedema and chorioretinopathy is caused by mutations in the KIF11 gene.

Chromosomal deletions/microdeletion with recognizable phenotypes

Examples are 5p– (cri-du-chat) and del (1p36).

WOLF–HIRSCHHORN SYNDROME (4P–). Prevalence is 1/ 50 000. Fifty-eight per cent are detectable with routine G-banded karyotype; the remainder require FISH or CGH. Microcephaly, growth retardation, and MR with dysmorphic features. Prominent nasal bridge with 'Greek helmet' profile in children and adults. They may have iris colobomata. Seizures are common, as is CHD. Frequent infections are common in infancy.

MOWAT–WILSON SYNDROME. Pre- or postnatal microcephaly with severe ID and seizures, associated with hypospadias, Hirschsprung's (67%), CHD, genitourinary anomalies, agenesis of the corpus callosum (35%), and short stature (Zweier et al. 2003). Affected individuals have a typical facies with upturned ear lobules. Eighty-two per cent have seizures. Results from large-scale deletions or truncating mutations in ZFHX1B (SMAD1P1) on 2q22.

Other syndromes

ANGELMAN SYNDROME. Severe MR, with little expressive language, seizures, ataxia, and wide-based gait. Characteristic jerky movement disorder with hand flapping and episodic laughter. Facial features include a wide mouth and a prominent chin. Severe microcephaly is not a feature, but most have an OFC <25th centile by 3 years of age. See 'Angelman syndrome' in Chapter 3, 'Common consultations', p. 346.

RUBINSTEIN–TAYBI SYNDROME (RTS). Normal birthweight, postnatal short stature and microcephaly, moderate to severe learning difficulties in most, broad thumbs and halluces. Caused by heterozygous mutation in CREBBP or EP300. See 'Broad thumbs' in Chapter 2, 'Clinical approach', p. 82.

Metabolic conditions

The OFC may be normal at birth. Regression of skills may be a feature. See other sections of this chapter, especially 'Developmental regression' in Chapter 2, 'Clinical approach', p. 128.

Environmental aetiology

Infections, trauma, teratogens (both pre- and postnatal). See other sections of this chapter, especially 'Cerebral palsy' in Chapter 2, 'Clinical approach', p. 96.

ZIKA VIRUS. The Zika virus has spread rapidly in the Americas since its first identification in Brazil in early 2015. Rasmussen et al. (2016) conclude that a causal relationship exists between prenatal Zika virus infection and microcephaly and other serious brain anomalies. See Centers for Disease Control and Prevention (2016), *Zika virus*, http://www.cdc.gov/zika. Intracranial calcification and brain malformation should prompt consideration of this diagnosis. Note Zika virus can be sexually transmitted.

Genetic advice

Recurrence risk

• After careful exclusion of syndromic and environmental causes, and if the MRI brain scan is structurally normal, there is a high proportion of primary AR microcephaly among the remainder and so, for primary microcephaly, a recurrence risk of 15–20% is appropriate for future pregnancies.

• If there is consanguinity, assume AR inheritance and advise a recurrence risk of 25%.

• Beware of genetic conditions mimicking environmental ones, e.g. pseudo-TORCH.

• If structural brain abnormality seen on MRI, investigate and counsel appropriately.

Carrier detection

Possible in families in whom causative mutations have been identified in the proband.

Prenatal diagnosis

With recurrence of primary microcephaly, head size often falls off only late in pregnancy, sometimes as late as 32–36 weeks' gestation. PND by USS is therefore unreliable, although in practice most subsequent pregnancies are scanned.

Support groups: Microcephaly Support Group, info@ cafamily.org.uk, Tel. 0808 808 3555; Walking With Giants Foundation (WWGF) for primordial dwarfism, http:// www.walkingwithgiants.org, Tel. 0151 526 0134.

Expert adviser: Andrew Jackson, Professor of Human Genetics, MRC Human Genetics Unit, Institute of Genetics and Molecular Medicine, University of Edinburgh, Edinburgh, UK.

References

Bond J, Roberts E, Mochida GH, et al. ASPM is a major determinant of cerebral cortical size. Nat Genet 2002; **32**: 316–20.

de Munnik SA, Bicknell LS, Aftimos S, *et al*. Meier–Gorlin syndrome genotype-phenotype studies: 35 individuals with pre-replication complex gene mutations and 10 without molecular diagnosis. *Eur J Hum Genet* 2012; **20**: 598–606.

Kaindl AM, Passemard S, Kumar P, *et al*. Many roads lead to primary autosomal recessive microcephaly. *Prog Neurobiol* 2010; **90**: 363–83.

Klingseisen A, Jackson AP. Mechanisms and pathways of growth failure in primordial dwarfism. *Genes Dev* 2011; **25**: 2011–24.

Majewski F, Goecke T. Studies of microcephalic primordial dwarfism I: approach to a delineation of the Seckel syndrome. *Am J Med Genet* 1982; **12**: 7–21.

Majewski F, Ranke M, Schinzel A. Studies of microcephalic primordial dwarfism II: the osteodysplastic type II of primordial dwarfism. *Am J Med Genet* 1982; **12**: 23–35.

Majewski F, Stoeckenius M, Kemperdick H. Studies of microcephalic primordial dwarfism III: an intrauterine dwarf with platyspondyly and anomalies of pelvis and clavicles--osteodysplastic primordial dwarfism type III. *Am J Med Genet* 1982; **12**: 37–42.

Mowat DR, Wilson MJ, Goossens M. Mowat–Wilson syndrome. *J Med Genet* 2003; **40**: 305–10.

Nagy R, Wang H, Albrecht B, W, *et al*. Microcephalic osteodysplastic primordial dwarfism type I with biallelic mutations in the *RNU4ATAC* gene. *Clin Genet* 2012; **82**: 140–6.

Nicholas AK, Swanson EA, Cox JJ, *et al*. The molecular landscape of *ASPM* mutations in primary microcephaly. *J Med Genet* 2009; **46**: 249–53.

Rasmussen SA, Jamieson DJ, Honein MA, Petersen LR. Zika virus and birth defects—reviewing the evidence for causality. *N Engl J Med* 2016; **374**: 1981–7.

Rauch A, Thiel CT, Schindler D, *et al*. Mutations in the pericentrin (*PCNT*) gene cause primordial dwarfism. *Science*. 2008; **319**: 816–19.

Rouse B, Matalon R, Koch R, *et al*. Maternal phenylketonuria syndrome: congenital heart defects, microcephaly, and developmental outcomes. *J Pediatr* 2000; **136**: 57–61.

Tolmie J. Prenatal diagnosis of microcephaly. *Prenat Diag* 1991; **11: 347**.

Trimborn M, Bell SM, Felix C, *et al*. Mutations in microcephalin cause aberrant regulation of chromosome condensation. *Am J Hum Genet* 2004; **75**: 261–6.

Verloes A, Drunat S, Gressens P, Passemard S. Primary autosomal recessive microcephalies and Seckel syndrome spectrum disorders. In: RA Pagon, MP Adam, TD Bird, CR Dolan, CT Fong, K Stephens (eds.). *GeneReviews®* [Internet]. University of Washington, Seattle, 2013.

Vivarelli R, Grosso S, Cioni M, *et al*. Pseudo-TORCH syndrome or Baraitser–Reardon syndrome: diagnostic criteria. *Brain Dev* 2001; **23**: 18–23.

Willems M, Geneviève D, Borck G, *et al*. Molecular analysis of pericentrin gene (PCNT) in a series of 24 Seckel/microcephalic osteodysplastic primordial dwarfism type II (MOPD II) families. *J Med Genet* 2010; **47**: 797–802.

Woods CG, Bond J, Enard W. Autosomal recessive primary microcephaly (MCPH): a review of clinical, molecular, and evolutionary findings. *Am J Hum Genet* 2005; **76**: 717–28.

Zweier C, Templet IK, Beemer F, *et al*. Characterisation of deletions of the *ZFHX1B* region and genotype–phenotype analysis in Mowat–Wilson syndrome. *J Med Genet* 2003; **40**: 601–5.

Micrognathia and Robin sequence

Micrognathia

Is the term used to describe a small mandible or a small chin. Mild micrognathia is seen in a large number of conditions and is rarely useful as a diagnostic handle. In some conditions, marked micrognathia is a major feature and can be a useful aid to diagnosis.

Micrognathia may occur as a deformation, as in oligohydramnios (e.g. Potter sequence: renal agenesis, micrognathia, pulmonary hypoplasia, talipes, crumpled ears), or as part of a genetically determined restriction of mandibular growth as in Treacher–Collins syndrome (TCS), or 22q11 deletion syndrome, or certain skeletal dysplasias.

Robin sequence

(Also termed Pierre–Robin sequence, Robin anomaly) describes a triad of micrognathia, cleft palate, and upper airway obstruction. In practice, many clinicians use the term when only two of these three features are present. In Robin sequence, micrognathia is present at the time that palate fusion is programmed to begin. Because of the mandibular anomaly, the tongue is not free to descend between the vertical palatal shelves and prevents them from orientating horizontally and fusing in the midline.

Typically, the cleft in Robin sequence is U-shaped, but the term is still often used when a V-shaped cleft is present (see Figure 2.23). Infants with Robin sequence may have airway and feeding problems in infancy and need specialist care as neonates. A deep pectus excavatum is commonly seen with each inspiration and may be accompanied by suprasternal and intercostal retraction. Careful monitoring by pulse oximetry is important. Management should be in conjunction with a neonatologist and a paediatric ear, nose, and throat (ENT) specialist.

In a retrospective survey of 74 patients with Robin sequence, van den Elzen *et al.* (2001) found that Robin sequence was the only anomaly in two-thirds but was part of a more complex phenotype in the remaining one-third. Stickler syndrome and 22q11 deletions were the most common diagnoses in the complex group. However, in Shprintzen's (2001) large case series, <20% were isolated. A 'diagnosis' of Robin sequence should therefore prompt a very careful search for an underlying aetiology.

• Stickler syndrome was the most common associated diagnosis (34%).
• Del (22q11) accounted for 11%.
• Deformation caused by restriction of fetal movement and growth due to oligohydramnios.
• Neurological problems such as CNS malformations and hypotonia where poor fetal movement and fetal akinesia are features, e.g. DM.

Normal mandibular growth is not typical for Robin sequence, unless it is secondary to mechanical constraint (deformation sequence), in which case the mandible has usually achieved normal size by 2 years of age. In syndromes that have intrinsic mandibular anomalies, mandibular growth remains deficient. In some syndromes, such as Stickler where there is also maxillary hypoplasia, the mandible and maxilla may become proportionate with time.

Clinical approach

History: key points
• Three-generation family tree with specific enquiry about small chin, cleft palate, osteoarthritis.

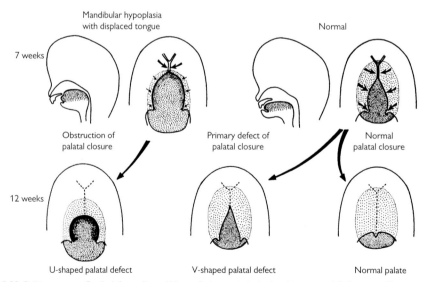

Figure 2.23 Robin sequence. On the left, small mandible results in a posteriorly placed tongue partially interposed between palatal shelves. This prevents closure and posterior growth of the soft palate, producing a U-shaped cleft palate. A V-shaped defect on the right is frequently seen in primary defects of palatal closure not secondary to mandibular involvement.
Reprinted from *The Journal of Pediatrics*, volume 87, issue 1, James W. Hanson, David W. Smith, U-shaped palatal defect in the Robin anomalad: Developmental and clinical relevance, p.30–33, Copyright 1975, with permission from Elsevier.

- Pregnancy history. Was there normal liquor volume on USS and at delivery?
- Neonatal history. Were there feeding problems?
- Developmental milestones.
- Specific enquiry regarding vision and hearing.

Examination: key points

If the baby has respiratory compromise, be careful not to disturb the position of the head and neck during your examination.

- Growth parameters. Height, weight, and OFC.
- Observe carefully for a cleft palate and consider the possibility of a submucous cleft.
- Heart. Listen for a murmur (22q).
- Limbs. Examine the digits and nails carefully for transverse limb deficiency.
- Ophthalmological assessment for features of Stickler syndrome (vitreoretinal and high myopia).
- Mandibulofacial dysostosis can be highly variable in expression, so careful assessment of parents is important.

Special investigations

- Genomic analysis in presence of features suggestive of a chromosomal or syndromic diagnosis, e.g. genomic array, gene panel, or WES/WGS as appropriate.
- DNA if mutation analysis is possible for specific syndromes, e.g. TCS.
- Consider chest X-ray or skeletal survey to look for rib gaps or signs of skeletal dysplasia.

Some diagnoses to consider

Stickler syndrome

A dominantly inherited disorder of collagen, resulting in a congenital vitreous gel anomaly, myopia, variable oro-facial features, deafness, and arthropathy. Stickler syndrome is caused by mutations in either COL2A1 or COL11A1. See 'Stickler syndrome' in Chapter 3, 'Common consultations', p. 528.

22q11 deletion

CHD with short stature, cleft palate or velopharyngeal insufficiency (nasal speech), and speech delay. Patients may have low calcium, mild learning disability, and immunodeficiency (typically reduced T-cell subsets). The single most common cardiac anomaly among children with 22q is VSD. Aortic arch anomalies, such as interrupted aortic arch or truncus arteriosus, are characteristic. A significant proportion of children with Fallot's tetralogy have 22q11 deletions. See '22q11 deletion syndrome' in Chapter 5, 'Chromosomes', p. 624.

SATB2 syndrome

All patients have significant neurodevelopmental impairment, most have absent/near absent speech with normal growth. Drooling and dental anomalies are common features. ~50% have cleft palate (Bengami 2017).

Treacher–Collins syndrome (TCS; mandibulofacial dysostosis)

This is most common and well-known mandibulofacial dysostosis and is caused by heterozygous mutation in one of at least three genes involved in pre-rRNA transcription *TCOF1*, *POLR1D*, and *POLR1C*. *TCOF1* is the most commonly mutated gene and is characterized by extremely variable expressivity. Ear anomalies are bilateral. They are malformed and displaced towards the angle of the mandible. One-third have atresia of the external auditory meatus and abnormality of the ossicles. Conductive hearing loss is common, but also screen for sensorineural deafness. Malar hypoplasia, coloboma (V-shaped notch) of the inferior eyelid at the junction of the medial two-thirds and the lateral one-third. Intelligence is normal. Sixty to 70% are the result of DNMs.

Mandibulofacial dysostosis with microcephaly (MFDM)

Recently described association with OA/TOF (Gordon *et al.* 2012) due to heterozygous mutations in the spliceosomal GTPase *EFTUD2*. Severe microcephaly, malar and mandibular hypoplasia, dysplastic ears/microtia, and cleft palate are typical findings.

Nager syndrome (acrofacial dysostosis)

An AD condition with TCS-like facies combined with radial ray limb defects, e.g. absent/hypoplastic thumbs and radial hypoplasia. Caused by heterozygous mutation of the *SF3B4* gene, a component of the pre-mRNA spliceosomal complex (Bernier *et al.* 2012).

Potter sequence

Deformation sequence arising from severe oligo- or anhydramnios—typically resulting from bilateral renal agenesis. In addition to severe micrognathia, the baby has talipes and severe pulmonary hypoplasia, usually resulting in neonatal death.

Oromandibular–limb–hypogenesis (OMLH) syndrome

Combination of micrognathia and/or hypoglossia (small tongue) with transverse limb reduction defects. Sometimes a U-shaped cleft palate is seen. Moebius syndrome (VIth and VIIth nerve palsies) is sometimes associated. Most are sporadic and attributed to vascular disruption.

Oculoauriculovertebral (OAV) spectrum

Also known as Goldenhar syndrome, hemifacial microsomia, first and second arch syndrome, and craniofacial microsomia. OAV spectrum is a heterogeneous condition that affects primarily the development of the ear, oral structures, and mandible. In the majority of children, the disorder is unilateral. When bilateral, there is a difference in severity between the right and left sides. The chin is often small. See 'Facial asymmetry' in Chapter 2, 'Clinical approach', p. 146.

Cerebrocostomandibular syndrome (CCMS)

CCMS, also known as 'rib-gap syndrome', is characterized by Robin sequence, multiple rib defects, and the occasional occurrence of intellectual impairment. Over 60 cases have been reported, nearly half of which are familial. Families suggestive of AR and AD inheritance are both reported and are not distinguishable on the basis of clinical manifestations.

Genetic advice

Recurrence risk

Counsel as for the specific syndrome. When Robin syndrome is truly an isolated defect, the recurrence risk is low.

Carrier detection

TCS is highly variable and on occasion virtually non-penetrant. If a mutation is identified, mutation detection can be offered to the parents to help in determining the risk to future pregnancies.

Prenatal diagnosis

Very severe micrognathia can be visualized on USS from ~12 to 14 weeks' gestation.

Support groups: Cleft Lip and Palate Association (CLAPA), http://www.clapa.com; American Cleft Palate–Craniofacial Association (ACPA), http://www.cleftpalate-craniofacial.org. Many of the individual syndromes have their own support groups. See Contact a Family, http://www.cafamily.org.uk; Pierre Robin Network, http://www.pierrerobin.org.

References

Bengami H, Handley M, *et al*. Clinical and molecular consequences of disease-associated de novo mutations in SATB2. *Genet Med* 2017 (in press).

Bernier FP, Caluseriu O, Ng S, *et al*. Haploinsufficiency of SF3B4, a component of the pre-mRNA spliceosomal complex, causes Nager syndrome. *Am J Hum Genet* 2012; **90**: 925–33.

Dauwerse JG, Dixon J, Seland S, *et al*. Mutations in genes encoding subunits of RNA polymerases I and III cause Treacher Collins syndrome. *Nat Genet* 2011; **43**: 20–2.

Gordon CT, Petit F, Oufadem M, *et al*. EFTUD2 haploinsufficiency leads to syndromic oesophageal atresia. *J Med Genet* 2012; **49**: 737–46.

Hanson JW, Smith DW. U-shaped palatal defect in the Robin anomalad: developmental and clinical relevance. *J Pediatr* 1975; **87**: 30–3.

James PA, Aftimos S. Familial cerebro-costo-mandibular syndrome: a case with unusual prenatal findings and review. *Clin Dysmorphol* 2003; **12**: 63–8.

Lines MA, Huang L, Schwartzentruber J, *et al*. Haploinsufficiency of a spliceosomal GTPase encoded by EFTUD2 causes mandibulofacial dysostosis with microcephaly. *Am J Hum Genet* 2012; **90**: 369–77.

Shprintzen RJ. Robin sequence. In: SB Cassidy, JE Allanson (eds.). *Management of genetic syndromes*, pp. 323–36. Wiley-Liss, New York, 2001.

van den Elzen AP, Semmekrot BA, Bongers EM, Huygen PL, Marres HA. Diagnosis and treatment of the Pierre Robin sequence: results of a retrospective clinical study and review of the literature. *Eur J Pediatr* 2001; **160**: 47–53.

Microphthalmia and anophthalmia

The embryological development of the eye is complex, controlled by many developmental genes, and is very sensitive to teratogens. The lens is derived from the surface ectoderm, the retina from the neural ectoderm, the extraocular muscles from the mesoderm, and the cornea, iris, and connective tissue of the extraocular muscles are neural crest derivatives (see Figure 2.4 for diagram of the anatomy of the eye). It is not surprising that eye anomalies are common and the eye is second only to the brain in its sensitivity to damage. The Scottish study of microphthalmia, anophthalmia, and coloboma over a 16-year period gave a minimum birth prevalence of 14/100 000 for microphthalmia and 3/100 000 for anophthalmia (Morrison et al. 2002).

Microphthalmia is a small eye, and it is usually associated with other ocular malformation. Even when it is thought to be unilateral, there is often mild abnormality in the apparently normal eye. The eye volume is reduced. The normal mean axis length of an eye is 22.5 mm in a child of 2 years, and in microphthalmia this is usually <18.5 mm. There is a spectrum of abnormality from microphthalmos to complete absence of the globe (anophthalmos). The term 'clinical anophthalmos' is a useful term to mean the clinical absence of eyes (there may be rudimentary eye vestiges histopathologically).

A small eye with no structural abnormality is nanophthalmos or simple microphthalmia. The nanophthalmic eye has a proportionately thicker sclera. The lens is usually of normal size that leads to a narrow anterior chamber and glaucoma may develop.

Cryptophthalmos is the presence of microphthalmos with skin covering the globe; the lids are attached to the cornea.

You may be asked to see a baby or child with microphthalmos as part of a more generalized condition or may be asked to counsel recurrence or offspring risks for isolated microphthalmia. Obtain a detailed examination and report from an ophthalmologist prior to genetic counselling.

Clinical approach

History: key points
- Exposure to teratogens, alcohol, and infections during pregnancy.
- Family history. At least three generations. Ask about all visual difficulties. Affected individuals may be minimally affected.
- Consanguinity.
- Growth (most chromosomal conditions show poor growth, association with pituitary abnormalities).
- Abnormalities of renal structure and/or function (Fraser syndrome, PAX2 mutations, del 14q22).
- Developmental progress (allowing for visual difficulties).

Examination: key points
- Growth parameters, including the OFC.
- Eye:
  - measurement and photography of the eye and surrounding structures and USS of the eye to measure the axial length and to exclude retinal detachment

or retinal dysplasia (usually performed by the ophthalmologist);
  - coloboma, in addition to micro- or anophthalmia (colobomatous microphthalmia, CHARGE association);
  - eyelid fusion (Fraser syndrome).
- Face:
  - facial asymmetry, skin tags, external ear anomalies (Goldenhar syndrome);
  - oro-facial clefts (trisomy 13, colobomatous microphthalmia, Fryns 'anophthalmia plus' syndrome);
  - nasal shape and sparse hair (Hallerman–Strieff syndrome);
  - abnormal dentition (Lenz syndrome).
- Limbs:
  - polydactyly (trisomy 13); syndactyly/ectrodactyly/limb reduction defects (Waardenburg anophthalmia);
  - nail hypoplasia (FAS).
- Oesophageal atresia (AEG (anophthalmia–(o)esophageal atresia–genital anomalies) syndrome).
- Patchy skin lesions (Goltz syndrome, del Xp).
- Genital abnormalities (chromosomal abnormalities, Fraser syndrome, AEG syndrome, CHARGE association).

Special investigations
- Genomic analysis in presence of features suggestive of a chromosomal or syndromic diagnosis, e.g. genomic array, gene panel, or WES/WGS as appropriate.
- Sixteen per cent of children with microphthalmia and anophthalmia have a chromosomal anomaly (EUROCAT Registry).
- Save DNA for possible genetic testing. In Fantes et al.'s (2003) study, de novo truncating mutations of SOX2 were found in 4/35 (11%) individuals with anophthalmia and in up to 20% of patients with bilateral anophthalmia (Fitzpatrick, personal communication, 2004). Both eyes were affected in all cases with an identified mutation. Some children with truncating mutations in SOX2 have associated learning difficulties.
- Renal USS in children with genital anomalies.
- MRI scan of the head and orbits is indicated for all children with clinical anophthalmos or severe microphthalmos.
- TORCH screen.
- Consider maternal PKU.
- Examine parents and sibs for subtle colobomata.

Some diagnoses to consider

Chromosomal syndromes
TRISOMY 13. In the neonate. See 'Patau syndrome (trisomy 13)' in Chapter 5, 'Chromosomes', p. 678.

DELETIONS INVOLVING 3q26.3. The observation that deletions in this area cause microphthalmia/anophthalmia led to the identification of truncating heterozygous SOX2 mutations in 4/35 (11%) of individuals with anophthalmia overall (Fantes et al. 2003).

DELETIONS OF 14q22 AND SIX6 HEMIZYGOSITY. Panhypopituitarism and early-onset renal failure.

FEMALES WITH DELETIONS OF XP22. Have microphthalmia and linear skin pigmentary abnormalities of the face.

CAT-EYE SYNDROME (CES). Anal anomalies (imperforate anus, anal atresia, or anteriorly placed anus), preauricular pits/tags, congenital heart defects, iris colobomata, renal anomalies, and variable learning disability. Microphthalmia is a less common feature (Schinzel *et al.* 1981). CES results from a small marker chromosome containing a duplication of 22q11, resulting in tetrasomy 22q11. See 'Coloboma' in Chapter 2, 'Clinical approach', p. 110.

Isolated microphthalmia
A heterogeneous group of disorders of the genes mutated in syndromic microphthalmia, e.g. *SOX2*, *OTX2*. Biallelic mutations in the *ALDH1A3* have recently been found in some patients (Aldahmesh *et al.* 2013).

Neonatal syndromes
FRASER SYNDROME. Not all cases are lethal. Cryptophthalmos, syndactyly, renal and genital abnormalities, laryngeal stenosis. AR. *FRAS 1* and *FRAS 2* genes. See 'Ptosis, blepharophimosis, and other eyelid anomalies' in Chapter 2, 'Clinical approach', p. 292.

CEREBRO-OCULO-FACIO-SKELETAL (COFS) SYNDROME. AR condition with cataract and congenital contractures, see 'DNA repair disorders' in Chapter 3, 'Common Consultations', p. 398.

WALKER WARBURG SYNDROME. AR syndrome with major CNS anomalies, retinal dysplasia, and raised CK. See 'Lissencephaly, polymicrogyria, and neuronal migration disorders' in Chapter 2, 'Clinical Approach', p. 222.

Other recognizable syndromes
GOLDENHAR SYNDROME. Asymmetry of face and ear anomalies. See 'Facial asymmetry' in Chapter 2, 'Clinical approach', p. 146.

CHARGE (COLOBOMA–HEART DEFECTS–ATRESIA CHOANAE–RETARDATION OF GROWTH AND/OR DEVELOPMENT–GENITAL DEFECT–EAR ANOMALIES AND/OR DEAFNESS) SYNDROME. See 'Facial asymmetry' in Chapter 2, 'Clinical approach', p. 146.

COLOBOMATOUS MICROPHTHALMIA AND CLEFTING. This has been reported in families, so consider the possibility of variable AD inheritance.

NON-SYNDROMIC COLOBOMATOUS MICROPHTHALMIA. See 'Coloboma' in Chapter 2, 'Clinical approach', p. 110.

PULMONARY HYPOPLASIA, DIAPHRAGMATIC EVENTRATION/HERNIA, ANOPHTHALMIA/MICROPHTHALMIA, CARDIAC DEFECT (PDAC). Also known as Matthew Wood syndrome. A severe condition with early lethality in some and severe delay in survivors. Caused by biallelic mutation of the *STRA6* gene encoding a component of the retinoic acid signalling pathway (Casey *et al.* 2011) and also by biallelic and *de novo* heterozygous mutations in the retinoic acid receptor beta gene (Srour *et al.* 2013).

GOLTZ SYNDROME. Focal dermal hypoplasia, limb deficiencies. XLD. Caused by heterozygous variant in females in the *PORCN* gene. See 'Coloboma' in Chapter 2, 'Clinical approach', p. 110.

FRYNS 'ANOPHTHALMIA PLUS' SYNDROME. Facial cleft, nasal deformity, NTD. Possibly AR as there was a recurrence in the original report, but a small chromosomal rearrangement would be an alternative mechanism.

BRANCHIO-OCULO-FACIAL (BOF) SYNDROME (HAEMANGIOMATOUS BRANCHIAL CLEFTS). An AD condition with distinctive areas of thin, erythematous, wrinkled skin in the neck or infra-/supra-auricular regions, in addition to craniofacial, auricular, ophthalmologic (coloboma of the iris and/or retina), and oral anomalies. See 'Coloboma' in Chapter 2, 'Clinical approach', p. 110.

ANOPHTHALMIA–(O)ESOPHAGEAL ATRESIA–GENITAL ANOMALIES (AEG) SYNDROME. Anophthalmia with oesophageal atresia and genital abnormalities (cryptorchidism and hypospadias in males). Neuronal migration defects in the CNS are part of the syndrome. Caused by heterozygous mutation of *SOX2*. See 'Genetic syndromes' in 'Oesophageal and intestinal atresia (including tracheo-oesophageal fistula)', Chapter 2, 'Clinical approach', p. 266.

LENZ MICROPHTHALMIA SYNDROME. A very rare XL condition with MR, highly arched or cleft palate, and skeletal anomalies; genetically heterogeneous and caused by heterozygous variants in BCOR on Xp14 and NAA10 on Xq28.

OPHTHALMO-ACROMELIC (WAARDENBURG ANOPHTHALMIA) SYNDROME. Anophthalmia associated with variable limb defects ranging from syndactyly to ectrodactyly. Caused by biallelic mutation in *SMOC1* (Rainger *et al.* 2011).

Environmental effects
FETAL ALCOHOL SYNDROME (FAS). Ask about alcohol intake. Low birthweight, developmental delay, microcephaly, cardiac abnormalities, digital hypoplasia, and craniofacial features.

CONGENITAL INFECTIONS. Rubella and varicella.

MATERNAL PHENYLKETONURIA (PKU). See 'Maternal phenylketonuria (PKU)' in Chapter 6, 'Pregnancy and fertility', p. 758.

Genetic advice

Simple microphthalmia and colobomatous microphthalmia and anophthalmia
This diagnosis is made after excluding syndromal and chromosomal causes of microphthalmia.

The aetiology of unilateral microphthalmia is often unclear and may be due to somatic mutation in some cases; however, germline mutations in microphthalmia genes may be asymmetric in their effect.

Recurrence risk
- Bilateral involvement increases the probability of a genetic or chromosomal aetiology, but inherited microphthalmia may be unilateral, as is very often the case.
- As parents have sometimes been shown to be affected after the birth of a second child, arrange parental ophthalmological assessment of the eye size and structure. In particular, small retinal colobomata may be unrecognized without a specialist examination.
- The Scottish group (Morrison *et al.* 2002) proposed a robust classification of the eye phenotype, based on the absence or presence of a defect in closure of the optic (choroidal) fissure. All recurrences in first-degree relatives occurred in the optic fissure closure defect group. The recurrence risk was between 8% and 13%, depending on the statistical method used. Recurrences occurred with both unilateral and bilateral involvement.
- Sibling risks following the birth of a child with anophthalmia where both parents have normal eyes on detailed ophthalmological assessment may be of the order of 5%, but offspring risks for an affected

individual may be considerably higher (a high proportion of *SOX2* mutations are *de novo* nonsense
mutations).
- Spectrum of normal vision to complete blindness in a
future affected child.
- All forms of Mendelian inheritance have been reported.
- Check the literature for recent gene localizations. At
present, known autosomal genes include *PAX2*, *SOX2*,
and the sine oculis homeobox cluster at 14q22 (AD)
and *CHX10* (AR locus at 14q32) and *SHH* when AD
microphthalmia occurs in association with coloboma. AR mutations in the *RAX* homeobox gene have been
reported in a patient with anophthalmia and sclerocornea (Voronina et al. 2004).

Carrier detection
- By ophthalmological examination.
- Is possible in families where a causative mutation has
been identified.

Prenatal diagnosis
- By genetic testing where there is molecular or chromosomal confirmation of diagnosis.
- USS in mid trimester can visualize the eye and lens
but may not be sensitive enough to detect recurrence
of microphthalmia, although anophthalmia should be
detectable with specialist scanning.

Natural history and further management (preventative measures)

Hornby et al. (2000) describe a classification system
that helps predict the likely visual prognosis. Long-
term ophthalmological follow-up is indicated for children with microphthalmos. Babies with anophthalmos
require insertion of orbital expanders to encourage the
eye socket to grow to enable prostheses to be fitted in
childhood.

Support group: MACS (Microphthalmia, Anophthalmia,
and Coloboma Support), http://www.macs.org.uk, Tel.
0870 600 6227.

Expert adviser: David FitzPatrick, Paediatric Geneticist,
Royal Hospital for Sick Children, Edinburgh, UK.

References

Aldahmesh MA, Khan AO, Hijazi H, Alkuraya FS. Mutations in ALDH1A3 cause microphthalmia. *Clin Genet* 2013; **84**: 128–31.

Casey J, Kawaguchi R, Morrissey M, et al. First implication of STRA6 mutations in isolated anophthalmia, microphthalmia, and coloboma: a new dimension to the STRA6 phenotype. *Hum Mutat* 2011; **32**: 1417–26.

Esmailpour T, Riazifar H, et al. A splice donor mutation in NAA10 results in the dysregulation of the retinoic acid signalling path-way and causes Lenz microphthalmia syndrome. *J Med Genet* 2014; **51**: 185–196.

Fantes J, Ragge NK, Lynch SA, et al. Mutations in SOX2 cause anophthalmia. *Nat Genet* 2003; **33**: 461–3.

Gregory-Evans K. Developmental disorders of the globe. In: A Moore (ed.). *Pediatric ophthalmology*, pp. 53–61. BMJ Books, London, 2000.

Hornby SJ, Adolph S, Gilbert CE, Dandona L, Foster A. Visual acu-ity in children with coloboma: clinical features and a new pheno-typic classification system. *Ophthalmology* 2000; **107**: 511–20.

Morrison D, FitzPatrick D, Hanson I, et al. National study of microphthalmia, anophthalmia and coloboma (MAC) in Scotland: investigation of genetic aetiology. *J Med Genet* 2002; **39**: 16–22.

Rainger J, van Beusekom E, Ramsay JK, et al. Loss of the BMP antag-onist, SMOC-1, causes Ophthalmo-acromelic (Waardenburg Anophthalmia) syndrome in humans and mice. *PLoS Genet* 2011; **7**: e1002114.

Schimmenti LA, de la Cruz J, Lewis RA, et al. Novel mutations in sonic hedgehog in non-syndromic colobomatous microphthal-mia. *Am J Med Genet A* 2003; **116A**: 215–21.

Schinzel A, Schmid W, Fraccaro M, et al. The 'cat eye syn-drome': dicentric small marker chromosome probably derived from a no. 22 (tetrasomy 22pter to q11) associated with a char-acteristic phenotype. Report of 11 patients and delineation of the clinical picture. *Hum Genet* 1981; **57**: 148–58.

Srour M, Chitayat D, Caron V, et al. Recessive and dominant mutations in retinoic acid receptor beta in cases with micro-phthalmia and diaphragmatic hernia. *Am J Hum Genet* 2013; **93**: 765–72.

Voronina VA, Kozhemyakina EA, O'Kernick CM, et al. Mutations in the human *RAX* homeobox gene in a patient with anophthal-mia and sclerocornea. *Hum Mol Genet* 2004; **13**: 315–22.

Minor congenital anomalies

Aase (1990) subdivides phenotypic anomalies into abnormalities and minor variants. Abnormalities are further subdivided into malformations, deformations, disruptions, and dysplasias (see 'Approach to the consultation with a child with dysmorphism, congenital malformation, or developmental delay' in Chapter 1, 'Introduction', p. 4). Minor variants can be subdivided into minor anomalies (prevalence ≤4%) and common variants (prevalence >4%) in the general population.

Ear tags and/or pits
Preauricular skin tags or pits are present in 0.5–1% of newborns. Of these, 20% have associated anomalies, so a careful assessment of the external ear and a search for other dysmorphic features is warranted before the ear tag/pit is regarded as an isolated anomaly.
- Hearing assessment is indicated as 17% of infants with isolated tags/pits have conductive and/or sensorineural hearing impairment.
- Renal USS should be performed in patients with bilateral preauricular pits/tags or isolated preauricular pits/tags accompanied by one or more of the following: other malformations or dysmorphic features; a family history of deafness; auricular and/or renal malformations; maternal diabetes. In the absence of these findings, renal USS is not indicated.

Syndromic diagnoses to consider include OAV (Goldenhar) syndrome, TCS, and BOR syndrome. See 'Ear anomalies' in Chapter 2, 'Clinical approach', p. 142.

Epicanthic folds
Epicanthic folds are seen in only ~3% of the Caucasian population in teenage and young adult life (12–25 years) but are very common in infancy (<6 months) when 73.0% of Caucasian babies have epicanthic folds. Epicanthic folds are lateral extensions of the skin of the nasal bridge that extend down over the inner canthus of the eye, covering the medial angle of the orbital fissure. In young babies, the nasal root is low and hence epicanthic folds are common but become less so with age as the root of the nose becomes less depressed and the nasal bridge becomes more prominent. Epicanthic folds are common in Down's syndrome and other conditions where the nasal bridge remains hypoplastic.

Inverted nipples
Inverted nipples are seen in ~3% of the normal female population. If inverted nipples occur in a child with hypotonia and developmental problems, consider carbohydrate glycoprotein deficiency (transferrin isoelectric focussing) and propionic acidaemia (elevated glycine in blood and urine). Carbohydrate-deficient glycoprotein disorders are AR disorders of glycosylation characterized by a variable degree of MR, liver dysfunction, and intestinal disorder. Propionic acidaemia is an AR organic acidaemia characterized by high ammonia, metabolic acidosis and low platelets and white cell count.

Sacral pits and dimples
Small, blind-ending sacral pits or dimples occur in 2% of neonates. In one study of 75 babies, each with a sacral dimple or pit, none had an abnormality on spinal USS, suggesting that these skin lesions (if blind-ending and not accompanied by skin pigmentation or a hairy patch or subcutaneous lumbosacral mass) do not indicate a high risk for occult spinal dysraphism. In the absence of additional features, regard as a normal variant.

If other features are present, there may be a dorsal dermal sinus connecting the skin surface to the dura or to an intradural dermoid cyst. Arrange imaging and seek input from a paediatric neurologist or neurosurgeon.

Transverse palmar crease
A single palmar crease (simian crease) is present in 4% of the normal population—twice as common in males as females. One per cent of the normal population have bilateral single palmar creases.

2/3 syndactyly of toes
When isolated, this is a common AD condition with variable expressivity.

Y-shaped 2/3 syndactyly of the toes is found in 79.5% of infants with SLO syndrome, an AR syndrome with prenatal and postnatal growth deficiency, developmental delay (almost all), cleft palate (37–52%), cardiac defects (36–38%), hypospadias and/or cryptorchidism (90–100%) in affected males, and PAP (~50%). See 'Hypospadias' in Chapter 2, 'Clinical approach', p. 186.

Expert adviser: Judith Hall, Professor Emerita of Paediatrics and Medical Genetics, UBC & Children's and Women's Health Centre of British Columbia, Department of Medical Genetics, British Columbia's Children's Hospital, Vancouver, Canada.

References
Aase JM. *Diagnostic dysmorphology*. Plenum, New York, 1990.

Elements of Morphology. Special issue. *Am J Med Genet* 2009; **149**: 1–127.

Gibson PJ, Britton J, Hall DM, Hill CR. Lumbosacral skin markers and identification of occult spinal dysraphism in neonates. *Acta Paediatr* 1995; **84**: 208–9.

Kugelman A, Hadad B, Ben-David J, et al. Preauricular tags and pits in the newborn: the role of hearing tests. *Acta Paediatr* 1997; **86**: 170–2.

Merks JH, van Karnebeek CD, Caron HN, Hennekam RC. Phenotypic abnormalities: terminology and classification. *Am J Med Genet A* 2003; **123A**: 211–30.

Park HS, Yoon CH, Kim HJ. The prevalence of congenital inverted nipple. *Aesthetic Plast Surg* 1999; **23**: 144–6.

Wang RY, Earl DL, Ruder RO, Graham JM Jr. Syndromic ear anomalies and renal ultrasounds. *Pediatrics* 2001; **108**: E32.

Nasal anomalies

The nose is a variable structure, but there are times when the shape of the nose may be the feature that is the key to syndrome recognition. This is most likely to be the case when the nasal structures (see Figure 2.24) have an appearance that is not found within normal variation.
- Root of the nose (nasion). The point where the nose meets the forehead.
- Nasal bridge. This forms the profile of the nose and is between the root and the tip. Flatter in infancy, compared to its appearance in adults. In isolation, it is not a good discriminatory feature, except for extreme cases.
- Nasal tip. The most anterior point of the nose.
- Nares. Nostrils.
- Columella. Fleshy inferior border of the nasal septum.
- Ala nasi. The lateral part of the nose forming the outer side of each nostril.
- Nasal choanae. The posterior nasal openings that are used for nasal breathing.

Clinical approach

History: key points
- Three-generation family tree with enquiry for similar features in relatives.
- Pregnancy history. Any drug exposure?
- Low birthweight, other congenital malformations (del 4p).
- Developmental milestones, schooling, and education.
- Expressive speech delay (Floating Harbor syndrome (FHS)).

Examination: key points
- Growth parameters. Short stature (FHS).
- Head:
  - scalp defects (Johanson–Blizzard syndrome (JBS));
  - skull shape asymmetry (craniosynostosis syndromes);
  - sparse hair (trichorhinophalangeal syndrome (TRPS)).
- Nose:
  - root of the nose (nasion). High with a 'Greek helmet' appearance in del 4p;
  - nasal bridge. Flat in many syndromes. Is it bulbous or beaked or wide and built-up;
  - nasal tip. Bifid (frontonasal dysplasia), grossly bifid (acromelic frontonasal dysostosis), bulbous (TRPS).

- nares. Single opening (trisomy 13, holoprosencephaly);
- columella. Is it lower than the alae nasi (RTS);
- ala nasi. Hypoplastic (JBS), OFD-1, frontorhiny. Absent in Bosma arhinia microphthalmia syndrome.
- Mouth:
  - oral frenulae (OFD-1);
  - cleft palate (Stickler syndrome, OFD-1, 22q11, Opitz syndrome).
- Hands:
  - syndactyly (oculodentodigital dysplasia, OFD-1);
  - polydactyly (OFD-1) acromelic frontonasal dysostosis;
  - broad thumbs (RTS, Pfeiffer);
  - progressively bent fingers (TRPS).
- Genitalia:
  - hypospadias (Opitz syndrome);
  - genital hypoplasia (ATRX).

Special investigations
- Genomic analysis in presence of features suggestive of a chromosomal or syndromic diagnosis, e.g. genomic array, gene panel, or WES/WGS as appropriate.
- Skull X-rays and further skeletal films, if indicated from clinical assessment, e.g. left wrist for bone age (FHS).

Some diagnoses to consider

Flat nasal bridge

STICKLER SYNDROME. A dominantly inherited disorder of collagen. In infants, the nose is hypoplastic with a flat nasal bridge. This grows out well during childhood. Ophthalmic complications include a congenital vitreous gel anomaly and myopia. There may be a cleft palate with micrognathia, deafness, and an arthropathy that is due to epiphyseal changes. See 'Stickler syndrome' in Chapter 3, 'Common consultations', p. 528.

WARFARIN EMBRYOPATHY. Warfarin and other coumarin derivatives are vitamin K antagonists that cross the placenta and, after exposure at 6–12 weeks' gestation, can cause an embryopathy (CDP with nasal hypoplasia and/or stippled epiphyses). The nasal hypoplasia may be severe. See 'Chondrodysplasia punctata' in Chapter 2, 'Clinical approach', p. 98.

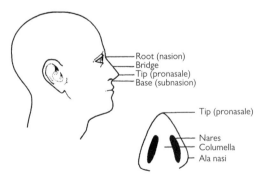

Figure 2.24 Landmarks of the nose.
Reproduced with permission from Judith G. Hall JG, Froster-Iskenius UG, and Allanson JE, *Handbook of Normal Physical Measurements*, Figure 7.63a, page 176, Copyright © 1989 Oxford University Press, New York, USA. www.oup.com.

BINDER SYNDROME (MAXILLONASAL DYSPLASIA). Characterized by maxillary hypoplasia and a flat, vertical nose. The main feature is a hypoplastic nose with flattening of the tip and alae nasi, and absence of the nasal septum/spine. The maxillary hypoplasia creates the impression of relative prognathism. Inheritance is uncertain. There is debate as to whether Binder syndrome is a distinct entity or if it represents the adult phenotype of milder forms of CDP. See 'Chondrodysplasia punctata' in Chapter 2, 'Clinical approach', p. 98.

X-LINKED ALPHA-THALASSAEMIA/MENTAL RETARDATION SYNDROME (ATRX). The key facial features are the characteristic tenting of the upper lip associated with a small triangular-shaped nose and a flat nasal bridge. Abnormalities of the genitalia in males, ranging from hypoplasia of the external genitalia to ambiguous genitalia, are found. Caused by mutations in the ATRX gene. See 'Intellectual disability with apparent X-linked inheritance', in Chapter 2, 'Clinical approach', p. 194.

High nasal root

DEL 4P (WOLF–HIRSCHHORN SYNDROME). Characterized by low birthweight and postnatal failure to thrive, microcephaly, developmental delay, and hypotonia. There is a characteristic facial appearance with sagging everted lower eyelids, a 'Greek helmet' profile, a short nose, and a very short philtrum. Patients may have iris colobomata. Seizures are common. See 'Deletions and duplications (including microdeletions and microduplications)' in Chapter 5, 'Chromosomes', p. 660.

Bulbous nose

TRICHORHINOPHALANGEAL SYNDROME (TRPS). An AD disorder characterized by fine, sparse-growing scalp hair, dystrophic brittle nails, brachyphalangia with cone-shaped epiphyses on X-ray, and a pear-shaped bulbous nose. TRPS1 is on 8q24. TRPS may be caused by intragenic mutations in TRPS1 or be part of a contiguous gene deletion syndrome that includes multiple exostosis that is detectable by genomic array.

FLOATING HARBOR SYNDROME (FHS). Predominantly postnatal short stature with growth −4 to −5 SD. The nose is broad, the mouth is large, and the ears are low-set and posteriorly rotated. The skull is long from front to back and affected children have mild developmental delay, especially of expressive language. The eyes are deep-set. Bone age is markedly delayed. Hypertension common in adults. Caused by DNM in SRCAP (Hood et al. 2012). Some phenotypic overlap with mild RTS.

VELOCARDIOFACIAL SYNDROME (VCFS)/DEL 22Q11. Wide and prominent nasal bridge and root. Other dysmorphic features include: short palpebral fissures with telecanthus, a wide and prominent nasal bridge and root, a small mouth; the ears are round in shape with deficient upper helices. See '22q11 deletion syndrome' in Chapter 5, 'Chromosomes', p. 624.

Beaked nose

RUBINSTEIN–TAYBI SYNDROME (RTS). The facial features vary with age and include a prominent beaked nose, with the columella below the alae nasi, and downslanting eyes. The other striking physical feature is broad, sometimes angulated, thumbs and first toes. Caused by microdeletions and truncating mutations in CREBBP. A milder RTS phenotype can be due mutation in EP300. See 'Broad thumbs' in Chapter 2, 'Clinical approach', p. 82.

CROUZON SYNDROME. Shallow orbits leading to exorbitism and a hooked nose are characteristic features. Molecular testing can help to establish if there is a recurrence risk to parents as the clinical features in an affected parent can be mild. Caused by mutations in FGFR2.

SAETHRE–CHOTZEN SYNDROME (SCS). Asymmetric coronal suture involvement gives facial asymmetry. The nose is prominent and may continue in a straight profile from the sloping forehead. A low frontal hairline, ptosis, and small ears with a prominent crus are other helpful facial features. Examine for evidence of skin syndactyly and broad halluces. The majority of patients with SCS have mutations in the TWIST1 gene. See 'Craniosynostosis' in Chapter 3, 'Common consultations', p. 378.

SECKEL SYNDROME AND MAJEWSKI OSTEODYSPLASTIC PRIMORDIAL DWARFISM II (MOPD II). Severe IUGR with proportionate head size. In MOPD II (Rauch et al. 2008), children become more microcephalic with age. Beaked prominent nose, progressive hyperextensibility and bony dysplasia, high squeaky voice, prominent eyes, small teeth. Both have AR inheritance. See 'Microcephaly' in Chapter 2, 'Clinical approach', p. 228 for more detail on causative genes.

Hypoplastic alae nasi

JOHANSON–BLIZZARD SYNDROME (JBS). There is hypoplasia and notching of the alae nasi. An AR condition with IUGR, scalp defects, and exocrine pancreatic insufficiency, combined with dysmorphic features. CHD and deafness may occur. Faecal elastase is a useful test of pancreatic exocrine function. Caused by mutations in UBR1 on 15q (Zenker et al. 2005).

ORAL-FACIAL-DIGITAL TYPE 1 (OFD-1). An XLD malformation syndrome. The features in the hands are syndactyly, usually skin syndactyly affecting variable digits, brachydactyly, and PAP. Other craniofacial anomalies are clefts, tongue cysts, and excess oral frenulae caused by mutations in the CXORF5 gene on Xp22 (Ferrante et al. 2001).

OCULODENTODIGITAL DYSPLASIA. An AD syndrome with a thin, pinched nose with hypoplastic alae nasi, syndactyly of the third, fourth, and fifth digits, dental anomalies, and neurodegeneration. Caused by mutations in connexin 43, GJA1, at 6q22–23. See 'Syndactyly (other than 2/3 toe syndactyly)' in Chapter 2, 'Clinical approach', p. 328.

Bifid nasal tip

FRONTONASAL DYSPLASIA. Is a malformation. It is usually sporadic and more common in twins. Severely affected infants have a midline facial cleft with encephalocele; those mildly affected have hypertelorism and a bifid nasal tip. This is a sporadic disorder, but take care to distinguish from all the disorders listed below.

CRANIOFRONTONASAL SYNDROME (CFNS). The presence of coronal synostosis and facial asymmetry helps distinguish this condition. Seen from above, the nasal tip is broad with a shallow groove. Longitudinally split nails, syndactyly, sloping shoulders, and cleft lip are other features. XL, but females are more severely affected; caused by mutations in ephrin-B1 (EFNB1) on Xq13.1 (Twigg et al. 2004).

ALX HOMEOBOX-RELATED FRONTONASAL DYSPLASIA/MALFORMATIONS. Recessive mutations in all three ALX genes are rare, but important, causes of frontonasal dysplasia. Mutations of ALX1 are most severe with facial clefting. *ALX3* mutations (frontorhiny syndrome) cause a distinctive facial appearance with splayed nasal bones, a bifid nasal tip, and prominent phitral pillars. *ALX4* mutations are associated with alopecia and defective skull ossification.

ACROMELIC FRONTONASAL DYSOSTOSIS. Specific mutations in *ZSWIM6*, usually *de novo*. Severe hypertelorism, ptosis, median cleft face with nasal bifurcation and widely separated alae nasi, parietal foramina, dysgenesis of the corpus callosum, interhemispheric lipoma, hydrocephalus, pre-axial polydactyly of the feet, tibial aplasia or hypoplasia, talipes equinovarus.

FREM1 PHENOTYPES. A wide range of additional features from apparently isolated hypertelorism to a phenotype similar to Fraser syndrome. The eyebrow configuration is a major clue to the diagnosis. Ensure renal USS for renal agenesis. (Nathanson *et al.* 2013).

OPITZ SYNDROME. Previously known as Opitz G/BBB and named after the initials of the original families. *MID1* on the X chromosome at Xp22 does not account for all cases. Ocular hypertelorism is the most characteristic facial feature, but the nasal tip may be bifid and, in addition, affected individuals may have hypospadias and cleft lip and/or palate and some have a laryngeal cleft that may cause feeding/respiratory problems.

Arhinia

ISOLATED ARHINIA AND BOSMA ARHINIA MICROPHTHALMIA SYNDROME. Arhinia (absence of the nose) is a rare malformation. Heterozygous mutation in the ATPase domain of *SMCHD1* (a gene associated with FSHD) can cause isolated arhinia and Bosma arhinia microphthalmia syndromes.

Choanal atresia

CHARGE SYNDROME. C = coloboma, H = heart defects, A = atresia choanae, R = retardation of growth and/or development, G = genital defect, E = ear anomalies and/or deafness. It is caused by mutation in the gene *CHD7* which acts in early embryonic development by affecting chromatin structure and gene expression (Vissers *et al.* 2004). Some children have a whole gene deletion (detection may require FISH or dosage sensitive analysis). See also 'Coloboma' in Chapter 2, 'Clinical approach', p. 110.

CARBIMAZOLE/METHIMAZOLE EMBRYOPATHY. Choanal atresia, hypoplastic nipples, scalp defects, and developmental delay have been reported in infants exposed to these drugs to treat maternal hyperthyroidism. For choanal atresia, the critical period of exposure is days 35–38.

Acromelic frontonasal dysplasia

Caused by *ZSWIM6* mutation (Twigg 2016). A recurrent (Arg1163Trp) occurs in acromelic frontonasal dysostosis, associated with severe hypertelorism, widely bifid nose, parietal foramina, brain, and limb malformations.

Genetic advice

Carefully examine the parents.

Recurrence risk
Counsel for the individual syndrome, as appropriate.

Carrier detection
May be possible by molecular testing (see above) or by clinical examination.

Prenatal diagnosis
Although USS can provide details of the phenotype from the second trimester onwards, only very significant nasal hypoplasia could be confidently predicted from prenatal scans.

Natural history and further management (preventative measures)
In some conditions, e.g. 22q11 deletion, a hypoplastic nasal bridge in infancy may grow into a high nasal bridge in older children and adults.

Support group: Many of the individual syndromes have their own support groups. See Contact a Family, http://www.cafamily.org.uk.

Expert adviser: Andrew Wilkie, Nuffield Professor of Pathology, Weatherall Institute of Molecular Medicine, University of Oxford, Oxford, UK.

References
Cohen MM, Hennekam RCM (eds.). *Syndromes of the head and neck*, 5th edn. Oxford University Press, Oxford, 2009.

Ferrante ML, Giorgio G, Feather SA, et al. Identification of the gene for oral-facial-digital I syndrome. *Am J Hum Genet* 2001; **68**: 569–76.

Foulds N, Walpole I, Elmslie F, Mansour S. Carbimazole embryopathy: an emerging phenotype. *Am J Med Genet A* 2005; **132A**: 130–5.

Hall JG, Froster-Iskenius UG, Allanson JE. *Handbook of normal physical measurements*. Oxford University Press, Oxford, 1989.

Hood RL, Lines MA, Nikkel SM, et al. Mutations in *SRCAP* encoding SNF2-related CREBBP activator protein, cause Floating Harbor syndrome. *Am J Hum Genet* 2012; **90**: 308–13.

Nathanson J, Swarr DT, Singer A, et al. Novel *FREM1* mutations expand the phenotypic spectrum associated with Manitoba-oculo-tricho-anal (MOTA) syndrome and bifid nose renal agenesis anorectal malformations (BNAR) syndrome. *Am J Med Genet A* 2013; **161A**: 473–8.

Rauch A, Thiel CT, Schindler D, et al. Mutations in the pericentrin (*PCNT*) gene cause primordial dwarfism. *Science* 2008; **319**: 816–19.

Roelfsema JH, Peters DJM. Rubinstein–Taybi syndrome: clinical and molecular overview. *Expert Rev Mol Med* 2007; **9**: 1–16.

Shaw ND, Brand H. SMCHD1 mutations associated with a rare muscular dystrophy can also cause isolated arhinia and Bosma arhinia microphthalmia syndrome. *Nat Genet* 2017; doi: 10.1038/ng.3743. [Epub ahead of print.]

Twigg SR, Kan R, Babbs C, et al. Mutations of ephrin-B1 (*EFNB1*), a marker of tissue boundary formation, cause craniofrontonasal syndrome. *Proc Natl Acad Sci U S A* 2004; **101**: 8652–57.

Twigg SR, Ousager LB, et al. Acromelic frontonasal dysostosis and *ZSWIM6* mutation: phenotypic spectrum and mosaicism. *Clin Gen* 2016; **90**: 270–5.

Vissers L, Ravenswaaij C, Admiraal R, et al. Mutations in a new member of the chromodomain gene family cause CHARGE syndrome. *Nat Genet* 2004; **36**: 955–7.

Zenker M, Mayerle J, Lerch MM, et al. Deficiency of UBR1, a ubiquitin ligase of the N-end rule pathway, causes pancreatic dysfunction, malformations and mental retardation (Johanson–Blizzard syndrome). *Nat Genet* 2005; **37**: 1345–50.

Neonatal encephalopathy and intractable seizures

The main difficulty facing the neonatologist and geneticist in this situation is to differentiate metabolic or genetic causes of neonatal encephalopathy and seizures from those arising as part of HIE. It is important to note that seizures may occur without features of an encephalopathy and that encephalopathy may be present with no seizures.

Usually by the time the geneticist is called, both a basic metabolic screen will have been completed, including blood gases, glucose, electrolytes, calcium, magnesium, lactate, as well as second-line investigations including ammonia, plasma amino acids, urine for amino and organic acids, ketones, and reducing substances, as well as a lumbar puncture.

Persistent hypoglycaemia, metabolic acidosis, and high levels of ammonia are all features of metabolic conditions and require further investigation. In addition, investigations to exclude sepsis and other non-genetic causes will be in progress.

There are many monogenic causes of severe infantile encephalopathy with few distinguishing clinical features, including e.g. KCNQ2, STXBP1, SCN2A, SCN8A, etc. Molecular genetic analysis using a gene panel approach is of proven utility where metabolic and imaging investigations are normal or have not provided diagnostic leads (Epi4k Consortium 2013). See 'Epilepsy in infants and children' in Chapter 3, 'Common consultations', p. 410. Obtaining a molecular genetic diagnosis may, in some conditions, help in the selection of appropriate therapy.

Cowan et al. (2003) studied 261 infants of >36 weeks gestation with neonatal encephalopathy who were referred to a tertiary-referral NICU. The fact that the study was not population-based limits the epidemiological conclusions that can be reached, and the possibility of referral bias is another limitation. In Cowan et al.'s study (2003), cranial MRI scan in 80% showed evidence of acutely evolving lesions that were compatible with a hypoxic–ischaemic insult. These lesions were mostly bilateral abnormalities in the basal ganglia, thalami, cortex, or white matter (see Box 2.7); 16% had normal scans, and the remainder showed either additional findings or had other diagnoses, as well as HIE (e.g. absent corpus callosum in non-ketotic hyperglycinaemia (NKH), basal ganglia cysts in a mitochondrial disorder, cerebellar hypoplasia in WWS, and complex 1 deficiency of the mitochondrial respiratory chain). Box 2.9 outlines the timing of MRI findings in evolving neonatal brain injury, and Figure 2.25 shows typical MRI findings in a cranial MRI from a baby with a severe perinatal insult.

The geneticist should be wary of a diagnosis of HIE if the above features (see Box 2.7) are not present.

Neonatal seizures may be a manifestation of neonatal encephalopathy when they occur in conjunction with abnormal tone, poor feeding, altered alertness plus, in the context of HIE, signs of fetal distress (see Box 2.8). They may be difficult to recognize and may take a variety of forms such as episodes of apnoea, repetitive sucking movements of the lips, episodes of hiccoughing, subtle jerking, or twitching movements of the limbs. If there is frequent seizure activity, the baby may also have been treated with anticonvulsants (e.g. phenobarbitone) and possibly sedated, muscle-relaxed, and ventilated, making it difficult to complete a neurological assessment. The majority of infants with neonatal encephalopathy will have continuous cerebral monitoring with amplitude integrated electroencephalography (aEEG). The aEEG provides a single- or dual-channel assessment of overall cerebral activity. As well as providing information on background activity which may include loss of sleep–wake cycling and moderate or severe (burst) suppression, it is also a sensitive tool for the assessment of neonatal seizures, particularly if there is electroclinical dissociation (electrical seizures in the absence of clinical signs) or if the patient has been sedated or muscle-relaxed. The background activity can be influenced by medication, particularly anticonvulsants.

Cowan et al.'s (2003) study found a high rate of focal infarctions or haemorrhages in infants with seizures who did not meet other criteria for encephalopathy. They studied 90 infants of >36/40 gestation who had seizures within 72 hours of birth, but not neonatal encephalopathy, and who were referred to a tertiary-referral NICU. Cranial MRI scan in most infants (69%) had evidence of an acutely developing region of focal infarction in an arterial territory or in a parasagittal distribution. A substantial proportion (31%) had an identifiable metabolic, neurocutaneous, vascular, or developmental disorder that was clearly of genetic or congenital origin, e.g. TS, IP, Zellweger syndrome, neonatal ALD, non-ketotic hyperglycaemia, cortical dysplasia.

Box 2.7 MRI scan abnormalities suggestive of an acute perinatal insult

- Brain swelling
- Cortical highlighting
- Focal of global loss of grey–white matter differentiation
- Abnormal signal density in the basal ganglia and thalami—typically the posterior putamen and venterolateral nucleus of the thalamus (VLNT) but could include the caudate nucleus and globus pallidus
- Loss of normal signal intensity in the posterior limb of the internal capsule (PLIC) associated with the above cortical, white matter, or basal ganglia and thalami abnormality
- Acute and subacute parenchymal, intraventricular, or extracerebral haemorrhage
- Acutely evolving focal infarction in an arterial territory or in a parasagittal or watershed distribution

Reprinted from The Lancet, Vol 361, Cowan et al., Origin and timing of brain lesions in term infants with neonatal encephalopathy, pp. 736–42, copyright 2003, with permission from Elsevier.

Box 2.8 Features of neonatal encephalopathy

Neonatal encephalopathy in an infant of >36/40 gestation may be defined as:
- Abnormal tone pattern
- Altered alertness (usually sleepiness, not waking for feeds or excessive startle response)
- Weak or absent reflexes (both primitive—suck and moro—and tendon)
- Feeding difficulties
- In addition, for HIE, three of the following features:
  (1) late decelerations on fetal monitoring or meconium staining
  (2) delayed onset of respiration
  (3) arterial cord blood pH <7.1
  (4) Apgar score <7 at 5 min
  (5) multiorgan failure.

Box 2.9 MRI scans in neonatal encephalopathy or seizures

- Within the first 24 hours of life, MRI scans may appear normal and give a false negative result.
- Scan abnormalities apparent very early, i.e. 1–5 days of life, are often suggestive of a severe insult.
- The earliest changes are with diffusion-weighted imaging (DWI) seen within the first 5 days of life. Changes on conventional imaging are best seen within 5–14 days following the insult.
- Atrophy associated with perinatal insults does not usually appear until at least 2 weeks after birth and if present earlier suggests a prenatal cause.

Clinical approach

History: key points

- Three-generation family history with specific enquiry for consanguinity and seizures or illness or infant/neonatal death.

- Were fetal movements normal or reduced? Were there periodic bursts of repetitive fetal activity or hiccoughs *in utero*, suggestive of antenatal seizure activity?
- Is there a history of maternal drug ingestion, making it possible that the infant is suffering from drug withdrawal, e.g. opiates, valproate?

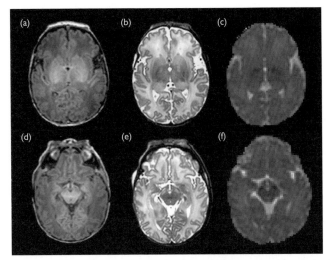

Figure 2.25 T1-weighted images (a and d), T2-weighted images (b and e), and ADC maps (c and f) at the level of the basal ganglia (a–c) and mesencephalon (d–f) in an infant born at 40 weeks' gestational age and imaged 4 days after birth. The infant was bradycardic (100 beats/min) for 30 min before delivery and his Apgar scores were 3 at 1 min, 3 at 5 min, and 7 at 10 min. Abnormal signal intensity can be seen in the basal ganglia and thalami and in the cerebral peduncles. Regions of restricted diffusion can be seen as low signal intensity in the lentiform nuclei (c) and cerebral peduncles (f).
Reprinted from *Seminars in Perinatology*, volume 34, issue 1, Counsell SJ et al., Magnetic Resonance Imaging of Brain Injury in the High-Risk Term Infant, pp. 67–78, Copyright 2010, with permission from Elsevier.

- Detailed account of events in pregnancy—were there any events in the third trimester which may have resulted in neurological damage (e.g. antepartum haemorrhage, death of an identical co-twin)?
- Detailed account of labour and delivery—was there any suggestion of fetal distress?
- What were the Apgar scores at delivery? Was prolonged resuscitation required and what were the cord blood gases?
- Was the baby handling normally and feeding well before the onset of symptoms (babies who appear normal at birth and handle and feed well and subsequently deteriorate are more likely to have a metabolic cause)? Organic acidaemias and urea cycle defects tend to present on days 2–3 (protein load from feeding).
- How old was the infant when the first abnormalities were noted?

Examination: key points
- Is the OFC within normal limits?
- Assess the posture and tone of the infant and note any abnormal movements such as tremor or myoclonic jerks.
- Is the anterior fontanelle large? (Consider Zellweger syndrome.)
- Are there dysmorphic features?
- Does the baby have an unusual odour (e.g. MSUD, isovaleric acidaemia)?
- Hepatomegaly or liver failure (see 'Prolonged neonatal jaundice and jaundice in infants below 6 months' in Chapter 2, 'Clinical approach', p. 288).
- CM (see 'Cardiomyopathy in children under 10 years' in Chapter 2, 'Clinical approach', p. 84).

Special investigations
Note that non-genetic causes of encephalopathy are being concurrently investigated, e.g. infection, meningitis, infarction.
- Cranial USS—to identify structural brain anomalies.
- MRI scans will demonstrate cortical abnormalities better than USS. The hazards of transporting a ventilated neonate to the scanner need to be balanced against the need to make a diagnosis. This is an important investigation which should be considered if initial rapidly available blood tests are normal and there is still no diagnosis in the face of continuing seizures or encephalopathy. Non-contrast CT should only be performed in infants with a history of birth trauma or a high suspicion of intra- or extracranial haemorrhage (falling haematocrit or coagulopathy) due to the radiation involved in CT. If CT findings are inconclusive, MRI should be performed between days 5 and 14 to assess the location and extent of injury. Conventional MRI imaging before day 5 may detect focal infarction or congenital brain anomalies but may underestimate the extent of hypoxic–ischaemic injury. The pattern of injury identified with conventional MRI may provide diagnostic and prognostic information for term infants with evidence of encephalopathy. Acute hypoxic–ischaemic injury is typically associated with lesions in the basal ganglia and thalamus, while changes in the white matter or cortex would suggest a more chronic lesion or a non-hypoxic–ischaemic cause (Rutherford et al. 2010).

- EEG.
- Cardiac echo and ECG.
- Clotting studies (liver dysfunction).
- Magnesium level.
- Plasma amino acids and urine amino and organic acids.
- Two blood spot cards for tandem mass spectrometric analyses. (Diseases diagnosable by these techniques will probably vary between centres.)
- Urine dinitrophenylhydrazine (DPNH) test for the presence of alpha-keto acids (MSUD).
- Sulfitest (sulfite oxidase deficiency).
- 3-hydroxybutyrate and acetoacetate (plasma samples) done at the same time as lactate and pyruvate (respiratory chain disorders).
- Acyl carnitine (can be measured on a dried blood spot, e.g. Guthrie card).
- CSF glycine and lactate (NB. CSF lactate may be high after asphyxia and takes longer to fall than blood lactate; it is also affected by fitting).
- Ophthalmological opinion (looking for cataracts, lens dislocation, optic atrophy).
- Genomic analysis in presence of features suggestive of a chromosomal or syndromic diagnosis, e.g. genomic array, gene panel, or WES/WGS as appropriate/available.
- Consider coagulation studies, e.g. thrombophilia screen if the MRI scan is suggestive of an arterial stroke.
- If the neonate seems likely not to survive, consider arranging for DNA to be saved (ethylenedinitrilotetraacetate (EDTA) sample), two spots of blood on filter paper, plasma (heparinized sample) and urine to be frozen at −20°C, CSF (1 ml) frozen, a skin biopsy for fibroblast culture, a muscle and liver biopsy frozen at −70°C, clinical photographs, and a skeletal and chest X-ray.

In infants with dysmorphic features and/or seizures, consider the following additional investigations:
- biotinidase (plasma);
- VLCFAs;
- transferrin isoelectrophoresis (CGD);
- cholesterol, 7-dehydrocholesterol (SLO);
- enzyme analysis for lysosomal disorders;
- CSF pipecolate and urine amino adipic semialdehyde (AASA) for pyridoxine-dependent seizures and CSF pyridoxal phosphate for pyridoxyl-dependent seizures, followed by a trial of pyridoxine.

Some diagnoses to consider
See Table 2.25 for some diagnoses to consider for the cause of neonatal and early-onset encephalopathy.

Hypoxic–ischaemic encephalopathy (HIE)
The main issue is to determine whether the degree of asphyxia at delivery correlates with the subsequent clinical course. In HIE, fits usually start after 6–12 hours. Therapeutic hypothermia for 72 hours after birth is now the standard of care for all infants with HIE. This must be commenced as soon as possible after birth, but other causes of neonatal encephalopathy must be considered in all infants being cooled, especially if the clinical picture is not typical of HIE. Infants with a metabolic or genetic diagnosis may not tolerate labour and delivery well, and so HIE can coexist. If the diagnosis is clearly not HIE, then it would be reasonable to rewarm the infant before 72 hours; if there is a suggestion that, regardless

Table 2.25 Metabolic diagnoses to consider for the cause of neonatal and early-onset encephalopathy

Disorder	Supporting clinical signs	Test
Neonatal/early onset	Presentation	
Peroxisomal defects of β-oxidation and organelle genesis	Dysmorphism, hypotonia, liver dysfunction	Plasma very long-chain fatty acids
Biotinidase deficiency	Alopecia, skin rashes, hypotonia	Plasma biotinidase
Non-ketotic hyperglycinaemia	Hypotonia, apnoea, burst-suppression EEG	Plasma and CSF glycine
3-phosphoglycerate dehydrogenase deficiency	Microcephaly, psychomotor retardation	Plasma and CSF serine
Molybdenum cofactor deficiency	Lens dislocation	Urine and plasma low urate
		Urine and plasma sulfocysteine
		Undetectable plasma homocysteine
Isolated sulfite oxidase deficiency	Lens dislocation	Urine and plasma sulfocysteine
		Undetectable plasma homocysteine
Glutaric acidaemia type 1	Macrocephaly, dystonia	Urine organic acids and blood spot acylcarnitines are not always positive. It may be necessary to assay the enzyme in cultured fibroblasts
GLUT 1 deficiency	Slow head growth, microcephaly	CSF glucose (low) (ratio to plasma)
Homocystinuria, remethylation defects	Hypotonia, microcephaly	Plasma total homocysteine
γ-aminobutyrate transaminase deficiency	Psychomotor retardation, hypotonia	CSF GABA
Aromatic amino acid decarboxylase deficiency	Mental retardation, movement disorders, hypotonia, recurrent hyperthermia, hypersalivation, bulbar symptoms, temperature instability	Urine vanilylactic acid increased
		CSF neurotransmitters, HVA, HIAA, and dopamine low
Pyridoxine-responsive seizures	Respond to pyridoxine; may take up to 4 weeks	Linked to mutations in the antiquitin gene. Can be diagnosed by measuring urine AASA (alpha amino adipic semi-aldehyde); will also have urine vanillactic acid increased. CSF neurotransmitters, HVA, HIAA, and dopamine low. Incr gly and threo and his
Pyridoxal phosphate-responsive seizures	Pyridoxine-unresponsive but responds to pyridoxal phosphate	Urine vanillactic acid increased. CSF neurotransmitters, HVA, HIAA, and dopamine low. Incr gly and threo and his. Urine AASA not increased
Pterin disorders	Mental retardation, movement disorders, hypotonia, recurrent hyperthermia, hypersalivation, bulbar symptoms	Quantitative plasma phenylalanine
		CSF pterins
		Erythrocyte
		DHPR
		Plasma and urine pterins
Tyrosine hydroxylase deficiency	Oculogyric crises, movement disorders, Parkinsonian symptoms, hypotonia	CSF neurotransmitters
		Low HVA
Menkes syndrome (X-linked)	Kinky hair	Plasma copper and caeruloplasmin
	Hypothermia	
	Developmental delay	

Reproduced with kind permission of MetBioNet. MetBioNew Guidelines, Fits and Seizures, http://www.metbio.net/docs/MetBio-Guideline-NACU622286-23-07-2009.pdf. MetBioNet cannot be held liable for any of the recommendations contained in this table as this guideline is out of its review period.

of the underlying diagnosis, the infant has also suffered a hypoxic–ischaemic insult, then cooling should be continued. There is no evidence that cooling is either beneficial or harmful in non-hypoxic–ischaemic causes of neonatal encephalopathy.

MRI and CT are more sensitive for identifying intraparenchymal haemorrhage than USS. Consider getting an expert opinion as to whether the MRI/CT scan findings are supportive of a diagnosis of HIE.

With neurological deterioration and seizures

NON-KETOTIC HYPERGLYCINAEMIA (NKH). An AR disorder due to abnormality of the glycine cleavage enzyme. The incidence of NKH is 1/50 000–1/100 000, except in Finland where the incidence is higher. Characteristically, fits begin in the first 24 hours of life and are accompanied by bursts of hiccoughing. The baby becomes profoundly floppy and compromised, requiring ventilatory support. CSF glycine levels are typically increased out of

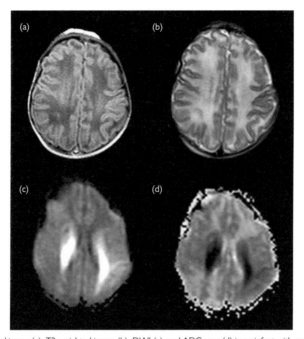

Figure 2.26 T1-weighted image (a), T2-weighted image (b), DWI (c), and ADC map (d) in an infant with maple syrup urine disease. Regions of abnormal signal can clearly be seen on the DWI and ADC map.
Reprinted from *Seminars in Perinatology*, volume 34, issue 1, Counsell SJ *et al.*, Magnetic Resonance Imaging of Brain Injury in the High-Risk Term Infant, pp. 67–78, Copyright 2010, with permission from Elsevier.

proportion to increases in plasma levels. In order to offer PND in a subsequent pregnancy, it is advisable to confirm the glycine cleavage enzyme activity in a liver biopsy. This can be taken immediately post-mortem and snap-frozen in a plain tube without medium and placed in liquid nitrogen. Enzyme activity can be assayed in the liver (100–300 mg tissue) and trophoblast but is not present in fibroblasts. The glycine cleavage enzyme comprises four subunits, each encoded by a different gene. Mutation analysis is complicated by the fact that most mutations are likely to be rare or private, except in Finnish patients where there is a founder effect. Unless the causative mutations are known, PND depends upon an assay of enzyme activity in uncultured chorionic villi.

With predominantly neurological deterioration

MAPLE SYRUP URINE DISEASE (MSUD), ORGANIC ACIDAEMIAS, AND UREA CYCLE DISORDERS. Babies with these conditions rarely have seizures in the absence of encephalopathy or hypoglycaemia. The EEG shows a periodic pattern with bursts of intense activity alternating with almost flat readings. Typical cranial MRI findings are shown in Figure 2.26.

MULTIPLE CARBOXYLASE DEFICIENCY* (MCD). Holocarboxylase synthetase (HLCS) deficiency is a rare AR disorder of biotin metabolism. The diagnosis is made by analysis of urine organic acids. The *HLCS* gene encodes an enzyme which catalyses the biotinylation of the four human biotin-dependent carboxylases. Clinical findings, age of onset, and response to biotin treatment are variable.

With predominantly intractable seizures

PYRIDOXINE-DEPENDENT SEIZURES*. Incidence 1/150 000; an AR disorder. One-third had atypical presentations and one-third had features and/or an initial diagnosis of birth asphyxia and HIE. A trial of pyridoxine is justified in all cases of early-onset intractable seizures, whatever the suspected cause.

BIOTINIDASE DEFICIENCY* (LATE-ONSET MULTIPLE CARBOXYLASE DEFICIENCY). Biotin is an essential water-soluble vitamin and is the coenzyme for four carboxylases necessary for normal metabolism in humans (see 'Multiple carboxylase deficiency (MCD)' above). Biotinidase (BTD) recycles biotin in the body by cleaving biocytin, a normal product of carboxylase degradation, resulting in the regeneration of free biotin. The baby is born with presumably normal stores of free biotin but, once dependent on dietary biotin, becomes deficient, with some delay in the onset of symptoms (as compared to the neonatal onset in MCD). Age of onset usually 1 week to 2 years. Seizures, either alone or with other neurologic or cutaneous findings (skin rash and alopecia), are the most frequent initial symptom. Metabolic ketoacidosis and organic aciduria are also features.

FOLINIC ACID-RESPONSIVE SEIZURES*. Presents with seizures with onset within a few hours of birth to onset in the first week of life. May be responsive initially to phenobarbitone, but later breakthrough seizures occur. Seizures stop within 24 hours of starting folinic acid. Untreated intractable seizures develop. Torres *et al.* (1999) suggests that a trial of folinic acid be considered in neonates with unexplained early-onset intractable seizures. Sibling recurrence has been reported (Torres et al. 1999).

CONGENITAL MAGNESIUM MALABSORPTION*. Primary infantile hypomagnesaemia is an infrequent cause of neonatal hypocalcaemic seizures, but one that responds well to magnesium supplementation.

SULFITE OXIDASE DEFICIENCY. Molybdenum cofactor deficiency and isolated sulfite oxidase deficiency are AR inborn errors of metabolism. The phenotype is severe, with progressive neurological damage leading in most cases to early childhood death, and results primarily from the deficiency of sulfite oxidase. The deficiencies can be diagnosed prenatally by monitoring sulfite oxidase activity in CVS tissue. In those families in which the specific defects have been identified, diagnosis can be achieved by mutation analysis or linkage studies directed at affected genes. These include *MOCS1, MOCS2,* or *GEPH,* in cases of molybdenum cofactor deficiency, or *SUOX* in patients with isolated sulfite oxidase deficiency (Johnson 2003).

CEREBRAL MALFORMATIONS. Refer to appropriate sections.

EARLY INFANTILE EPILEPTIC ENCEPHALOPATHY WITH SUPPRESSION BURST (OHTAHARA SYNDROME). There are characteristic EEG features. Exclude cortical malformations and respiratory chain disorders and then proceed to genetic testing. See 'Epilepsy in infants and children' in Chapter 3, 'Common consultations', p. 410.

EARLY MYOCLONIC ENCEPHALOPATHY. There are characteristic clinical and EEG features. Exclude metabolic disease.

BENIGN NEONATAL CONVULSIONS AND BENIGN FAMILIAL NEONATAL CONVULSIONS. See 'Epilepsy in infants and children' in Chapter 3, 'Common consultations', p. 410.

IN MALES: RARE SEVERE PRESENTATION OF XL DISORDERS. Consider mutation in *ARX, NEMO,* and *MeCP2.*

With dysmorphic features

PEROXISOMAL DISORDERS (E.G. ZELLWEGER SYNDROME). An AR condition characterized by dysmorphic features with a large fontanelle, a high forehead, stippling at the knees on X-ray, and raised VLCFAs. See 'Floppy infant' in Chapter 2, 'Clinical approach', p. 154.

CHOLESTEROL BIOSYNTHETIC DEFECTS (E.G. SLO SYNDROME, DESMOSTEROLOSIS). Prenatal growth deficiency, cleft palate (37–52%), cardiac defects (36–38%), hypospadias, and/or cryptorchidism (90–100%) in affected males. Y-shaped 2/3 toe syndactyly (>95%) and PAP (~50%). See 'Hypospadias' in Chapter 2, 'Clinical approach', p. 186.

CHROMOSOMAL DISORDERS. Consider genomic array or FISH for Miller–Deiker microdeletion 17p13.3.

Genetic advice

Recurrence risk

As for the given diagnosis. If the cause remains undiagnosed, the possibility of a genetic condition needs to be considered with a risk of up to 25% for recurrence.

Thorough testing usually gives a clue to the aetiological group, even if a precise diagnosis is not possible.

If due to HIE, recurrence risk should be low, as long as the diagnosis is secure. Refer to a fetal medicine specialist for expert supervision of future pregnancy and delivery.

Prenatal diagnosis

May be possible if known diagnosis; otherwise not possible.

Natural history and further management

* Denotes treatable disorder. Pyridoxine-dependent seizures, folinic acid-responsive seizures, biotin-responsive multicarboxylase deficiency, and congenital malabsorption of magnesium are *treatable* conditions.

Support group: Climb (Children Living with Inherited Metabolic Diseases), http://www.climb.org.uk.

Expert adviser: Topun Austin, Consultant Neonatologist, Rosie Hospital, Cambridge University Hospitals NHS Foundation Trust, Cambridge, UK.

References

Baxter P. Epidemiology of pyridoxine dependent and pyridoxine responsive seizures in the UK. *Arch Dis Child* 1999; **81**: 431–3.

Blankenberg FG, Loh NN, Bracci P, et al. Sonography, CT, and MR imaging: a prospective comparison of neonates with suspected intracranial ischaemia and haemorrhage. *Am J Neurol* 2000; **21**: 213–18.

Cowan F, Rutherford M, Groenendaal F, et al. Origin and timing of brain lesions in term infants with neonatal encephalopathy. *Lancet* 2003; **361**: 736–42.

Epi4K Consortium; Epilepsy Phenome/Genome Project, Allen AS, Berkovic SF, Cossette P, et al. De novo mutations in epileptic encephalopathies. *Nature* 2013; **501**: 217–21.

Johnson JL. Prenatal diagnosis of molybdenum cofactor deficiency and isolated sulfite oxidase deficiency. *Prenat Diagn* 2003; **23**: 6–8.

Ment LR, Bada HS, Barnes P, et al. Practice parameter: neuroimaging of the neonate: report of the Quality Standards Subcommittee of the American Academy of Neurology and the Practice Committee of the Child Neurology Society. *Neurology* 2002; **58**: 1726–38.

Morrone A, Malvagia Donati MA, et al. Clinical findings and biochemical and molecular analysis of four patients with holocarboxylase synthetase deficiency. *Am J Med Genet* 2002; **111**: 10–18.

National Metabolic Biochemistry Network. http://www.metbio.net/metbioHome.asp.

Rahman S. Mitochondrial disease and epilepsy. *Dev Med Child Neurol* 2012; **54**: 397–404.

Rutherford M, Malamateniou C, McGuinness A, Allsop J, Biarge MM, Counsell S. Magnetic resonance imaging in hypoxic-ischaemic encephalopathy. *Early Hum Dev* 2010; **86**: 351–60.

Saudubray JM, Nassogne MC, de Lonlay P, Touati G. Clinical approach to inherited metabolic disorders in neonates: an overview. *Semin Neonatol* 2002; **7**: 3–15.

Torres OA, Miller VS, Buist NM, Hyland K. Folinic acid-responsive neonatal seizures. *J Child Neurol* 1999; **14**: 529–32.

Trump N, McTague A, Brittain H, et al. Improving diagnosis and broadening the phenotypes in early-onset seizures and severe developmental delay disorders through gene panel analysis. *J Med Genet* 2016; **53**: 310–17.

Nystagmus

Nystagmus is an involuntary continuous oscillatory disorder of eye movement. It is commonly described by parents as 'wobbly eyes'. It is a symptom of disordered oculomotor control. In infancy, it may be an indicator of bilateral visual impairment; later-onset nystagmus is more likely to be secondary to neurological disease. Nystagmus is usually horizontal but can be vertical or rotatory. See Figure 2.34 on p. 302 for a diagrammatic representation of the genetic causes of various forms of retinal dystrophy.

Clinical approach

History: key points
- Three-generation family history, or more if a suggestion of X-linkage.
- Age of onset.
- Photophobia (achromatopsia, aniridia, albinism).
- Eye poking, rubbing.
- Developmental milestones.
- CNS symptoms (especially cerebellar in adults).
- Seizures.
- Ensure adequate documentation of ophthalmic and neurological assessment from hospital notes.

Examination: key points
- Detailed eye examination by an ophthalmologist to include slit-lamp examination for iris translucency (albinism) and fundal examination.
- Neurological examination. Assess hypotonia or dystonia in infants, and cerebellar and long tract signs in an adult.
- Dysmorphic features as a marker for possible intracerebral malformation.
- Skin (albinism).

Special investigations
- Ophthalmic assessment of the eye structure, retina, and disc.
- Electrophysiology of the visual system (ERG and VEPs) to rule out retina dystrophies and albinism.
- All children with acquired nystagmus of onset >6 months of age need a brain MRI scan to rule out chiasmal disease.
- Genomic analysis, e.g. genomic array, gene panel, or WES/WGS as appropriate, e.g. if dysmorphic features or significant unexplained developmental delay.
- Metabolic and/or endocrine screen if there are signs of a progressive condition.
- DNA sample. Specific genetic testing may be available. If not, store DNA for possible future diagnostic use.
- Consider video of nystagmus, if unusual.
- Audiology (peroxisomal disorders).
- Renal USS (Lebers/Joubert).
- Cardiac echo (Alstrom).

Some diagnoses to consider: infants

Optic nerve hypoplasia
Commonly presents with nystagmus, if bilateral. See 'Optic nerve hypoplasia' in Chapter 2, 'Clinical approach', p. 270.

Infantile retinal dystrophies

ROD MONOCHROMATISM OR ACHROMATOPSIA. Total colour blindness is rare. An AR disease characterized by early onset of photophobia, poor visual acuity, and total colour blindness that involves complete absence of all cone function. A number of mutations in the genes encoding the cone-specific alpha- and beta-subunits of the cation channel (*CNGA3* and *CNGB3*) and the alpha-subunit of transducin (*GNAT2*) have been implicated in this disorder.

X-LINKED BLUE CONE MONOCHROMATISM. A rare disorder that involves the absence of red and green cone function. It is caused either by deletion of a critical region that regulates the expression of the red/green gene array or by mutations that inactivate the red and green pigment genes.

CONGENITAL STATIONARY NIGHT BLINDNESS. Normal fundus. Inheritance AR or XL. The AD form of congenital stationary night blindness does *not* have nystagmus.

LEBER CONGENITAL AMAUROSIS (LCA). One of the most common inherited cause of blindness in childhood and is characterized by a severe infantile rod–cone dystrophy which presents in the first few months of life with poor vision and nystagmus or roving eye movements. Highly heterogeneous, and many genes have been identified that together account for just over 50% of all LCA patients. These genes are expressed preferentially in the retina or the retinal pigment epithelium. Their putative functions are quite diverse and include retinal embryonic development (*CRX*), photoreceptor cell structure (*CRB1*), phototransduction (*GUCY2D*), protein trafficking (*AIPL1*, *RPGRIP1*), and vitamin A metabolism (*RPE65*) (Cremers *et al.* 2002). The fundus often appears normal in infancy, but the ERG is very subnormal or, more usually, non-recordable. Later there may be signs of retinal degeneration. Variable neurological involvement and seizures may be present. Mostly AR. Retinal dystrophy similar to LCA is also seen in a number of syndromes, including ciliopathies and peroxisomal disorders.

JOUBERT SYNDROME (JS). See 'Ciliopathies' in Chapter 3, 'Common consultations', p. 366.

ALSTROM SYNDROME. A rare AR syndrome caused by mutations in *ALMS1*. Alstrom syndrome is characterized by childhood obesity with T2D (hyperinsulinism and chronic hyperglycaemia) and neurosensory deficits, e.g. cone–rod retinal dystrophy. A subset of individuals have DCM, hepatic dysfunction, hypothyroidism, male hypogonadism, short stature, and mild/moderate developmental delay.

PEROXISOMAL DISORDERS. Check plasma VLCFAs and phytanic acid.

NEURONAL CEROID LIPOFUSCINOSIS (NCL; BATTENS). In association with seizures and regression.

Ocular and oculocutaneous albinism

OCULAR ALBINISM IS XL. Oculocutaneous albinism is AR.

X-LINKED OCULAR ALBINISM (XLOA) (NETTLESHIP–FALLS). Affects ~1/50 000 males in the population and is due to mutations in *OA1* at Xp22.32. It results in hypopigmentation of the iris and retina, nystagmus, strabismus, foveal hypoplasia, abnormal decussation of optic nerve fibres, and reduced visual acuity. Female carriers of XLOA have a classic pattern of mosaic retinal pigmentation and patchy iris translucency. Carriers also have macromelanosomes on skin biopsy. Approximately 50% of reported mutations in *OA1* are intragenic deletions and the rest are point mutations.

OCULOCUTANEOUS ALBINISM (OCA). See 'Generalized disorders of skin pigmentation (including albinism)' in Chapter 2, 'Clinical approach', p. 162.

Other

OCULAR MOTOR APRAXIA (OMA). A disorder of saccadic initiation and may be congenital or acquired. Although previously considered benign, a structural brain anomaly, particularly of the cerebellum, and neurodevelopmental delay are found in >50% (Marr *et al.* 2005). Many of these are caused by mutations in ciliopathy genes (see 'Ciliopathies' in Chapter 3, 'Common Consultations', p. 366). NB. Congenital fibrosis of the extraocular muscles may cause diagnostic confusion and can be caused by mutations in *TUBB3* (Tischfield *et al.* 2010).

PELIZAEUS–MERZBACHER DISEASE (PMD). Absent myelination on brain MRI scan. XLR. Mutations and duplications in the *PLP* gene.

Some diagnoses to consider: adult onset

Mostly caused by neurological diseases; it is important for a neurologist to evaluate the patient to exclude tumours and other non-genetic causes.

AUTOSOMAL DOMINANT CEREBELLAR ATAXIA (ADCA). Test for *SCA* genes. Assess if retinopathy is a feature (ADCA type 7). See 'Ataxic adult' in Chapter 2, 'Clinical approach', p. 70.

Genetic advice

Recurrence risk

When no other disorder has been identified, and the nystagmus is an isolated feature, the ophthalmologist may consider the possibility of idiopathic or ocular motor nystagmus. *Remain aware of the possibility of coexisting or evolving neurological problems, so counsel with caution.*

Carrier detection

Possible by molecular genetic analysis in those families where the diagnosis is known and in whom a causative mutation has been identified.

Examination of the eye, including fundal examination and electrophysiology, in other family members may help, particularly in XL conditions.

Prenatal diagnosis

Available to those families where there is molecular confirmation of the diagnosis.

Natural history and further management (preventative measures)

Long-term follow-up with an ophthalmologist or a neurologist, or both, depending on the diagnosis.

Support groups: Nystagmus Network, http://nystagmusnetwork.org, Tel. 01392 627 004; Albinism fellowship, http://www.albinism.org.uk, Tel. 01282 771 900.

References

Cideciyan AV, Jacobson SG, Beltran WA, *et al.* Human retinal gene therapy for Leber congenital amaurosis shows advancing retinal degeneration despite enduring visual improvement. *Proc Natl Acad Sci U S A* 2013; **110**: E517–25.

Cremers FP, van den Hurk JA, den Hollander AI. Molecular genetics of Leber congenital amaurosis. *Hum Mol Genet* 2002; **11**: 1169–76.

Deeb SS, Kohl S. Genetics of color vision deficiencies. *Dev Ophthalmol* 2003; **37**: 170–87.

den Hollander AI, Koenekoop RK. Mutations in *LCA5*, encoding the ciliary protein lebercilin, cause Leber congenital amaurosis. *Nat Genet* 2007; **39**: 889–95.

Hearn T, Renforth GL. Mutation of *ALMS1*, a large gene with a tandem repeat encoding 47 amino acids, causes Alstrom syndrome. *Nat Genet* 2002; **31**: 79–83.

Kerrison JB. New genetic, pathophysiologic and therapeutic issues in nystagmus. *Curr Opin Ophthalmol* 1999; **10**: 411–19.

Marr et al.

Oetting WS. New insights into ocular albinism type 1 (OA1): mutations and polymorphisms of the *OA1* gene. *Hum Mutat* 2002; **19**: 85–92.

Tischfield MA, Baris HN, Wu C, Rudolph G, *et al.* Human *TUBB3* mutations perturb microtubule dynamics, kinesin interactions, and axon guidance. *Cell* 2010; **140**: 74–87.

Obesity with and without developmental delay

Obesity that prompts referral to the genetic clinic is usually severe (i.e. weight >99.6th centile, or a major discrepancy between the height and weight, e.g. height on 2nd centile, weight on 90th); sometimes there are accompanying learning difficulties. With currently available investigations, the diagnostic yield is about 10%. See 'Overgrowth' in Chapter 2, 'Clinical approach', p. 272 if all growth parameters are increased.

Body mass index (BMI)
BMI = weight (kg)/height^2 (m^2). This formula is based on the assumption that most variation in weight for persons of the same height is due to differences in fat mass. It provides some objective measure of the degree of obesity. Table 2.26 shows the classification of BMI in adults.

Distribution of fat mass
Truncal obesity (where the extremities can appear normal or even thin) is characteristic of some syndromes.

Clinical approach
History: key points
- Three-generation family tree, noting the height/weight of parents and siblings and birthweight of siblings and consanguinity.
- Pregnancy and perinatal history (birthweight, length, OFC).
- Detailed feeding history in early infancy. Were there feeding difficulties and hypotonia in the first year of life (PWS)?
- When did abnormal weight gain begin? Was it present from early infancy; most genetic obesity syndromes within first few years of life. Albright typically have onset of severe obesity from 6 months, whereas PWS from 18–24 months.
- What is the child's appetite like? Is there food searching/stealing? Is there impaired satiety (wanting additional food soon after a meal)?
- Detailed developmental and behavioural profile—autistic features; aggression; are behaviours triggered by demands for food or other circumstances?
- Is there any indication of visual deficit/night blindness?
- Deafness.

Examination: key points
- Growth parameters (height, weight, OFC).

Table 2.26 The classification of obesity according to BMI in adults

BMI	World Health Organization (WHO) (1995) classification	Popular description
<18.5	Underweight	Thin
18.5–24.9	Normal	
25–29.9	Grade 1 overweight	Overweight
30.0–39.9	Grade 2 overweight	Obese
40.0 or greater	Grade 3 overweight	Morbid obesity

- Distribution of obesity. Truncal obesity is typical of PWS, Bardet–Biedl syndrome (BBS), Alstrom syndrome, and Cohen syndrome.
- Are there dysmorphic features? Children with AHO have a flattened facial profile; those with Cohen syndrome typically have large prominent upper incisors. Red hair in Caucasians (pro-opiomelanocortin (POMC)).
- Are the hands generally small (PWS/SMS); is there brachydactyly (BBS); are the fourth/fifth metacarpals short (ask the child to make a fist and look at the knuckle profile; (AHO); is there syndactyly (usually 2/3 toes) or polydactyly (BBS)?
- Discrete foci of calcification in the skin (AHO).
- Small genitalia are commonly seen in males with PWS and BBS and some patients with leptin deficiency. Female genital tract anomalies common in BBS.
- Is there acanthosis nigricans (thickened hyperpigmentation of axillae and skinfolds indicative of severe insulin resistance; Alstrom, *SH2B1*)?
- Cardiovascular system. Hypertension, murmurs (aortic stenosis/LVH; BBS).
- Eyes should be examined for visual field defects, strabismus, myopia, photophobia, and retinal pigmentation (BBS, Alstrom syndrome, Cohen syndrome, TUB mutations).

Special investigations
- Genomic analysis e.g. array, gene panel, WES/WGS as available.
- PWS methylation studies if history of hypotonia with poor suck.
- Free thyroxine (T4) and TSH.
- Hypothyroidism can present with obesity in childhood; also high incidence of hypothyroidism in AHO, leptin and leptin receptor deficiency.
- Consider 24-hour urine cortisol (if symptoms and signs suggest Cushing's syndrome).
- Consider measuring levels of testosterone, gonadotrophins, GH, fasting glucose, insulin (and proinsulin if considering prohormone convertase-1 (PCSK1); consider glucose tolerance test (PWS, BBS, Alstrom syndrome); serum leptin to exclude leptin deficiency.
- Plasma calcium and PTH (low calcium and high/normal PTH suggestive of AHO, but levels can be normal).
- Consider paediatric neurology referral/brain MRI scan if problems are of recent onset with a short history, to exclude a hypothalamic tumour/head injury.

If associated developmental delay, also include the following.
- Ophthalmology for RP plus ERG if considering BBS, Alstrom, or Cohen syndrome).
- Renal USS if considering BBS.
- Hand X-ray to assess metacarpal length if clinically suspect (AHO).

Some diagnoses to consider
With developmental delay

PRADER–WILLI SYNDROME (PWS). The most common recognized genetic form of obesity affecting 1/10 000–15 000 individuals. Babies have central hypotonia and feeding difficulties, with failure to thrive in infancy. There is rapid weight gain between the ages of 1 and 6 years, characterized by truncal obesity with small hands and feet, small genitalia in males, and short stature. Typically, there is insatiable appetite and food-seeking/hoarding. Most patients have IQs in the 60s to low 70s. Individuals with PWS are often good at jigsaws and word-find puzzles. Behavioural problems can be a major issue. Most adults with PWS will require support/supervision in adult life and few will live independently. Both males and females have hypogonadotrophic hypogonadism. Sexual activity is uncommon and fertility is rare (but note if deletion; girls are at 50% risk for a child with Angelman syndrome (AS)).

Due to imprinting, the maternally inherited genes on 15q11 (in the Prader–Willi/Angelman syndrome critical region (PWACR)) are usually inactivated and normal development is dependent upon paternally inherited genes. Seventy-five per cent of patients with PWS have del 15q11–13; 24% have maternal UPD 15, and only 1% have an imprinting defect (abnormal methylation, but normal FISH and UPD studies). SNRPN methylation analysis detects PWS in 99%. Small deletions encompassing only the HBII-85 family of snoRNAs have been reported in association with the cardinal features of PWS, including obesity, suggesting that these non-coding RNAs and the genes they regulate may be important in the aetiology..

SIM1. A transcription factor involved in hypothalamic development. Chromosomal deletions on 6q14-q21 which encompass *SIM1* and heterozygous point mutations in *SIM1* are associated with hyperphagia, severe obesity, learning difficulties, and autistic-like behaviours which can overlap with phenotypes seen in PWS. However, unlike PWS, patients do not typically have dysmorphic features and hypogonadism and reduced growth are not seen with LOF *SIM1* mutations.

BARDET–BIEDL SYNDROME (BBS). One of a number of disorders arising from disruption of the primary cilia, leading to obesity, retinal dystrophy, and in some cases, skeletal abnormalities. More than 20 BBS genes have been cloned to date. See Table 3.4 in 'Ciliopathies' in Chapter 3, 'Common Consultations', p. 367. BBS is characterized by a pigmentary retinal dystrophy, PAP, obesity, cognitive impairment, and renal defects. For the majority of cases, BBS follows a Mendelian AR pattern of inheritance; however, a few families exhibit triallelic inheritance where three mutations in at least two loci appear to be necessary to manifest the disorder, but occasionally the third mutant allele may modify the severity of the phenotype. Individuals with BBS are at risk for progressive renal insufficiency and creatinine and BP should be monitored at 6-month intervals.

ALSTROM SYNDROME. A rare AR syndrome caused by mutations in *ALMS1*, involved in intraflagellar transport in the primary cilium. Alstrom syndrome is characterized by childhood obesity with T2D (severe insulin resistance) and neurosensory deficits, e.g. cone–rod retinal dystrophy. A subset of individuals have DCM, hepatic dysfunction, hypothyroidism, male hypogonadism, short stature, and mild/moderate developmental delay.

TUB. Early-onset retinal dystrophy and obesity are also seen in patients with homozygous mutations affecting TUB, another protein which localizes to the primary cilia.

ALBRIGHT HEREDITARY OSTEODYSTROPHY (AHO). This term describes a phenotype characterized by short adult stature with generalized obesity and relative microcephaly, brachydactyly particularly involving the distal phalanges (especially of the thumbs) and metacarpals/metatarsals, mild to moderate learning disability, and cutaneous ossifications (subcutaneous or intradermal lumps or flakes) in around 60%. The facial features are subtle, but usually patients have a round face with a short neck, a short nose, and mild midface hypoplasia. The brachydactyly is associated with cone epiphyses and disharmonic bone age. Stature may be normal or above average in childhood, but there is reduced longitudinal growth and early epiphyseal closure. The basis of the AHO phenotype is a 50% reduction in bioactivity of GsA, a subunit of the heterotrimeric G-protein that transduces signals between various cell surface hormone receptors and intracellular adenyl cyclase. It results from heterozygous deactivating mutations in the genes. *GNAS* gene. *GNAS* is subject to tissue-specific imprinting. Mutations on the maternally derived allele are associated with pseudohypoparathyroidism (PHP type Ia) where individuals have variable hypocalcaemia due to end-organ resistance to PTH and abnormal thyroid function due to resistance to TSH and TRH. Mutations of the paternally derived allele are not associated with endocrine abnormalities and these patients with AHO are said to have pseudo-pseudohypoparathyroidism (PPHP).

Where subcutaneous ossifications and/or PHP type Ia (including raised PTH and abnormal thyroid function) are present in association with other features of AHO, the diagnosis is very likely. Random PTH levels are usually very high in association with normal or low calcium and normal or raised inorganic phosphate. TSH levels are often high with triiodothyronine (T3)/T4 levels that may be normal or reduced. Note that PHP can occur in isolation (i.e. with a normal thyroid axis and no features of AHO) when it is known as PHP type Ib. Abnormal methylation of exon 1A, upstream of *GNAS*, has been reported in at least some patients. Screening *GNAS* for sequence changes in the exons and adjacent splice sites detected mutations in around 75% of a cohort with confirmed reductions in GsA bioactivity. Most mutations are family-specific. Some patients may present with severe obesity alone.

SMITH–MAGENIS SYNDROME (SMS). Some patients are short and obese with small hands and feet, as well as square, rather heavy, facies. They may have a history of hypotonia in infancy, developmental delay, behaviour disturbance (especially sleep), and sometimes food-searching behaviour. If PWS testing is negative, consider FISH for SMS (17p) if there is a history of sleep disturbance. Some individuals with SMS have mutations in *RAI1*, a gene encompassed by the common 17p11.2 microdeletion.

COHEN SYNDROME. An AR disorder due to mutations in *COH1*; characteristic craniofacial appearance with prominent upper incisors, global developmental delay, truncal obesity with relatively short stature, severe myopia with visual impairment and choroidal–retinal dystrophy, and benign neutropenia. The myopia usually starts at <5 years and progresses to >−7 SD by the second decade. Young children have a 'bull's eye' maculopathy and, by the age of 10 years, patients have a generalized symptomatic retinopathy. Visual handicap is progressive and significant, with 35% registered partially sighted or blind. The neutropenia does not predispose to infection and does not generally require treatment.

BRAIN-DERIVED NEUROTROPHIC FACTOR (BDNF) AND TROPOMYCIN-RELATED KINASE B (TRKB) DEFICIENCY. Severe hyperphagia and obesity, impaired short-term memory, hyperactivity, and learning disability are seen in patients with chromosomal deletions or point mutations that disrupt BDNF or its tyrosine kinase receptor TrkB. Given the severe developmental phenotype of these patients, it is not surprising that mutations often seem to arise *de novo* and as such should be considered where both parents are of normal weight and IQ.

Without developmental delay

CONGENITAL LEPTIN DEFICIENCY. A rare AR disorder causing extreme obesity from early childhood. Children are born with a normal birthweight, but marked hyperphagia accompanied by weight acceleration begins after weaning. Hypogonadism and hypothalamic hypothyroidism are also features. The disorder is treatable with recombinant human leptin, with dramatic effects on appetite and normalization of weight.

LEPTIN RECEPTOR DEFICIENCY. An AR disorder characterized by severe hyperphagia, hypogonadism, short stature, and hypothyroidism. LOF mutations found in 2–3% of severely obese children.

PRO-OPIOMELANOCORTIN (POMC). An AR disorder characterized by red hair, pale skin, with isolated ACTH deficiency presenting as an adrenal crisis or features of cortisol deficiency (cholestatic jaundice) in neonatal life, and hyperphagia.

PROHORMONE CONVERTASE-1 (PCSK1). Homozygous or compound heterozygous mutations lead to neonatal enteropathy (diarrhoea requiring parenteral nutrition), hypoglycaemia, and impaired processing of several prohormones leading to hypothyroidism, hypogonadism, hypocortisolaemia, and central diabetes insipidus. Abnormally elevated levels of proinsulin (compared to insulin) are characteristic of this condition.

MELANOCORTIN 4 RECEPTOR (MC4R). Disorder characterized by increased growth velocity in childhood, hyperphagia, and severe hyperinsulinaemia. Usually AD inheritance, but homozygotes with *MC4R* mutations have been identified in consanguineous families where heterozygotes have an intermediate phenotype suggesting co-dominant inheritance. Mutations in *MC4R* are found in 1–7% of patients with BMI >40 who become severely obese before the age of 10 years.

SH2B1. CNVs deleting 16p11.2 and heterozygous mutations involving the adapter protein Src homology 2 (SH2) B adapter protein 1 (SH2B1) are associated with hyperphagia, obesity, and disproportionate insulin resistance. Mild speech and language delay and aggressive behaviours are seen. Some patients with larger deletions on 16p11.2 have developmental delay and autistic-type features.

Genetic advice
Recurrence risk
If you are able to make a syndromic diagnosis, counsel appropriately. Targeted sequencing of the genetic obesity syndromes is likely to be available in the near future.

Carrier detection
Not possible, unless a molecular genetic diagnosis has been possible in the proband and the familial mutations are known.

Prenatal diagnosis
Not possible, unless a specific diagnosis has been made with laboratory confirmation.

Natural history and further management (preventative measures)
Consider referral to a paediatric endocrinologist.

Support groups: Prader–Willi Syndrome Association (UK), http://www.pwsa.co.uk, Tel. 01332 365 676; Prader–Willi Syndrome Association (USA), http://www.pwsausa.org, Tel. 1 800 926 4797; Bardet-Biedl Syndrome UK, http://www.lmbbs.org.uk, Tel. 01892 682 680; Cohen Syndrome Support Group, Tel. 0161 653 0867. Additional information and papers at Genetics of Obesity Study (GOOS), http://www.goos.org.uk.

Expert adviser: Sadaf Farooqi, Professor of Metabolism and Medicine, Wellcome Trust–MRC Institute of Metabolic Science, Addenbrooke's Hospital, Cambridge, UK.

References
Ansley SJ, Badano JL, Blacque OE, *et al*. Basal body dysfunction is a likely cause of pleiotropic Bardet–Biedl syndrome. *Nature* 2003; **425**: 628–33.
Doche ME, Bochukova EG, Su HW, *et al*. Human SH2B1 mutations are associated with maladaptive behaviors and obesity. *J Clin Invest* 2012; **122**: 4732–6.
Farooqi IS, Keogh JM, Yeo GS, Lank EJ, Cheetham T, O'Rahilly S. Clinical spectrum of obesity and mutations in the melanocortin 4 receptor gene. *N Engl J Med* 2003; **348**: 1085–95.
Farooqi IS, Matarese G, Lord GM, *et al*. Beneficial effects of leptin on obesity, T cell hyporesponsiveness, and neuroendocrine/metabolic dysfunction of human congenital leptin deficiency. *J Clin Invest* 2002; **110**: 1093–103.
Goldstone AP. Prader–Willi syndrome: advances in genetics, pathophysiology and treatment. *Trends Endocrinol Metab* 2004; **15**: 12–20.
Hearn T, Renforth GL, Spalluto C, *et al*. Mutations of ALMS1, a large gene with a tandem repeat encoding 47 amino acids, causes Alstrom syndrome. *Nat Genet* 2002; **31**: 79–83.
Ramachandrappa S, Raimondo A, Cali AM, *et al*. Rare variants in single-minded 1 (SIM1) are associated with severe obesity. *J Clin Invest* 2013; **123**: 3042–50.
van der Klaauw AA, Farooqi IS. The hunger genes: pathways to obesity. *Cell* 2015; **161**(1): 119–32.
Weinstein LS, Chen M, Liu J. Gs(alpha) mutations and imprinting defects in human disease. *Ann N Y Acad Sci* 2002; **968**: 173–97.

Ocular hypertelorism

Ocular hypertelorism is otherwise known as widely spaced eyes. In clinical practice, measurements are made of the inner and outer canthal distances and the interpupillary distance. In ocular hypertelorism, the interpupillary distance (IPD) is increased. Orbital measurements from X-rays can also be used.

It is important to distinguish true ocular hypertelorism from telecanthus (lateral displacement of the inner canthi and lacrimal puncta, as seen in Waardenburg syndrome type 1) and epicanthic folds (see Figure 2.27).

There is no single mechanism that gives rise to this feature. Isolated hypertelorism is rare; thus it is usually found as part of a syndrome. Chromosomal disorders, single gene disorders, and environmental factors can all give this phenotype. In this section, we will concentrate on those syndromes where ocular hypertelorism is a major diagnostic feature. Many of the syndromes also have a bifid nasal tip. See 'Nasal anomalies' in Chapter 2, 'Clinical approach', p. 242.

Clinical approach

History: key points

- Family history. Syndromes may be AD with variable expressivity, AR, and XL.
- Pregnancy:
- threatened miscarriage and twinning. Frontonasal dysplasia is more common in twins;
- maternal illness and teratogen exposure.
- Neurological problems/developmental delay.
- Laryngeal abnormalities and swallowing difficulties in Opitz syndrome.

Examination: key points

- Stature and proportions (short in Robinow and Aarskog syndromes).
- Cranial shape and size, any asymmetry, or plagiocephaly.

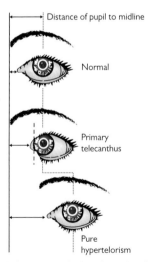

Figure 2.27 Comparison of telecanthus and ocular hypertelorism.

- Frontal encephalocele (frontonasal dysplasia).
- Hairline, widow's peak (Opitz syndrome), temporal hair loss, and abnormal vertical extension of the eyebrow (*FREM1* phenotypes).
- Bifid nose/nasal tip—grooved when viewed from above.
- Cleft lip/palate. Hypertelorism can occur secondary to major facial clefts.
- Prominent philtral pillars (frontorhiny).
- Gum hypertrophy (Robinow syndrome).
- Sloping shoulders and asymmetric nipples (CFNS).
- Cardiac murmur. Sometimes children with Noonan or LEOPARD (lentigines–ECG abnormalities–ocular hypertelorism–pulmonary stenosis–abnormal genitalia–retardation of growth–deafness) syndromes have hypertelorism, but it is usually mild.
- Genitalia (shawl scrotum in Aarskog, small penis in Robinow, hypospadias in Opitz syndrome).
- Polysyndactyly (Greig syndrome).
- Longitudinal nail ridges/splits (CFNS).

Special investigations

- Careful eye measurements and ophthalmological assessment (eye measurements taken in clinic are difficult to do with accuracy, especially IPD). Beware of parallax errors. Eye measurements should be related to the OFC.
- Skull X-ray (craniosynostosis, small defects in the frontal area).
- Brain imaging may be appropriate, especially to determine if there are any midline abnormalities, e.g. lipomas, agenesis of the corpus callosum.
- Skeletal survey (Robinow syndrome).
- Consider referral for laryngoscopy in infants with Opitz syndrome.
- DNA for genomic analysis in presence of features suggestive of a chromosomal or syndromic diagnosis, e.g. genomic array, gene panel, or WES/WGS as available.

Syndromic diagnoses to consider

Frontonasal dysplasia

Is a malformation. It is usually sporadic and more common in twins. Severely affected infants have a midline or an oblique facial cleft with encephalocele; those mildly affected have hypertelorism and a bifid nasal tip. Additional associations include microphthalmia, coloboma, cerebral lipoma, and agenesis of the corpus callosum.

Craniofrontonasal syndrome (CFNS)

The presence of coronal synostosis and facial asymmetry help distinguish this condition. Ridged nails, syndactyly, sloping shoulders, and cleft lip are other features. XL disorder mapping to Xq13 and caused by mutation in the ephrin-B1 gene (*EFNB1*) (Twigg et al. 2004). Females paradoxically are more severely affected than males.

Opitz syndrome

Previously known as Opitz G/BBB and named after the initials of the original families. A gene *MID1* on the X chromosome at Xp22 does not account for all cases. In addition to ocular hypertelorism, affected males may have hypospadias and cleft lip and/or palate, and some have a laryngeal cleft that may cause feeding/respiratory problems.

Greig cephalopolysyndactyly
An AD condition characterized by a high forehead with frontal bossing, macrocephaly, hypertelorism, and a broad base to the nose. Both pre- and PAP. The thumbs and halluces are often broad or bifid. Caused by mutations in *GLI3* on 7p13.

Aarskog syndrome (faciogenital dysplasia)
A genetically heterogeneous developmental disorder characterized by short stature (rhizomelic), ptosis in some, hypertelorism, hypermetropia, shawl scrotum, and brachydactyly with hyperextendable PIP joints. Facial features tend to normalize with age. MR is present in only a minority of affected males and is seldom severe. The XL form is caused by mutations in the *FGD1* gene. Behavioural and learning problems in childhood occur in ~50% of males with the XL form (Orrico *et al.* 2004). Some families appear to show AD inheritance.

Baraitser-Winter syndrome
AD disorder characterized by short stature, hypertelorism, bilateral ptosis, ocular coloboma, prominent metopic suture and neuronal migration disorder. Caused by heterozygous mutation in ACTB or ACTG1.

Robinow syndrome
Both AD and AR types. Skeletal survey to assess mesomelia, costovertebral abnormalities, and distinctive phalangeal changes. There is brachydactyly with abnormal orientation of the thumbs and occasional bifid thumbs. Large mouth and tongue, gingival hypertrophy, micropenis, and congenital heart defects. The AR type is due to homozygous abnormality in the *ROR2* gene. Different heterozygous mutations in *ROR2* cause brachydactyly type B. Some AD Robinow is caused by mutation in *DVL1* or *DVL3*.

Teebi syndrome
Teebi (1987) has reported, separately, patients with features similar to those of craniofrontonasal syndrome and Aarskog syndrome. Some cases are caused by mutation in *SPECC1L*.

ALX homeobox-related frontonasal dysplasia/malformations
Recessive mutations in all three *ALX* genes are rare, but important, causes of frontonasal dysplasia. Mutations of *ALX1* are most severe with facial clefting. *ALX3* mutations (frontorhiny syndrome) cause a distinctive facial appearance with splayed nasal bones, a bifid nasal tip, and prominent phitral pillars. *ALX4* mutations are associated with alopecia and defective skull ossification.

FREM1 phenotypes
From apparently isolated hypertelorism to a phenotype similar to Fraser syndrome. There is a bifid nasal tip. The eyebrow configuration is a major clue to the diagnosis. Ensure renal USS for renal agenesis (Nathanson *et al.* 2013).

Acromelic frontonasal dysplasia
Caused by ZSWIM6 mutation (Twigg *et al.* 2016). A recurrent (Arg1163Trp) occurs in acromelic frontonasal dysostosis, associated with severe hypertelorism, widely bifid nose, parietal foramina, brain, and limb malformations.

Genetic advice
Carefully examine the parents and note ocular measurements before counselling an apparently sporadic case.

Recurrence risk
This is low in cases of frontonasal dysplasia and those syndromes where a DNM has been established by DNA testing. Counsel for the individual syndrome as appropriate.

Carrier detection
May be possible by molecular testing (see above) or by clinical examination.

Prenatal diagnosis
Although USS can provide details of the phenotype from the second trimester onwards, and there are normal ranges for eye spacing at different gestations, only very significant hypertelorism could be confidently predicted from prenatal scans.

Natural history and further management (preventative measures)
Children with significant hypertelorism need multidisciplinary assessment by a specialist craniofacial team, including careful ophthalmological assessment (strabismus).

Support groups: Many of the individual syndromes have their own support groups. See Contact a Family (UK), http://www.cafamily.org.uk; National Organization for Rare Disorders (USA), http://www.rarediseases.org.

Expert adviser: Andrew Wilkie, Nuffield Professor of Pathology, Weatherall Institute of Molecular Medicine, University of Oxford, Oxford, UK.

References
Gorlin RJ, Cohen MM, Hennekam RCM (eds.). *Syndromes of the head and neck*, 4th edn. Oxford University Press, Oxford, 2001.

Nathanson J, Swarr DT, Singer A, et al. Novel *FREM1* mutations expand the phenotypic spectrum associated with Manitoba-oculo-tricho-anal (MOTA) syndrome and bifid nose renal agenesis anorectal malformations (BNAR) syndrome. *Am J Med Genet A* 2013; **161A**: 473–8.

Orrico A, Galli L, Cavaliere ML, et al. Phenotypic and molecular characterisation of the Aarskog–Scott syndrome: a survey of the clinical variability in light of *FGD1* mutation analysis in 46 patients. *Eur J Hum Genet* 2004; **12**: 16–23.

Patton M. Robinow syndrome. *J Med Genet* 2002; **39**: 305–10.

Teebi AS. A new autosomal dominant syndrome resembling craniofrontonasal dysplasia. *Am J Med Genet* 1987; **28**: 581–91.

Trockenbacher A, Suckow V, Foerster J, et al. *MID1*, mutated in Opitz syndrome, encodes an ubiquitin ligase that targets phosphatase 2A for degradation. *Nat Genet* 2001; **29**: 287–94.

Twigg SR, Kan R, Babbs C, et al. Mutations of ephrin-B1 (*EFNB1*), a marker of tissue boundary formation, cause craniofrontonasal syndrome. *Proc Natl Acad Sci U S A* 2004; **101**: 8652–7.

Twigg SR, Ousager LB, et al. Acromelic frontonasal dysostosis and *ZSWIM6* mutation: phenotypic spectrum and mosaicism. *Clin Gen* 2016; **90**: 270–5.

Uz E, Alanay Y, Aktas D, et al. Disruption of *ALX1* causes extreme microphthalmia and severe facial clefting: expanding the phenotype of *ALX*-related frontonasla dysplasia. *Am J Hum Genet* 2010; **86**: 789–96.

Oedema—generalized or puffy extremities

Generalized oedema may occur in any very sick neonate, particularly if there has been inadequate nutritional support. It does not usually have a genetic basis. The causes of generalized oedema in the very preterm infant merge with the causes of fetal hydrops, some of which are genetic (see 'Oedema—increased nuchal translucency, cystic hygroma, and hydrops' in Chapter 6, 'Pregnancy and fertility', p. 768). If the infant is sick, severe anaemia and hypoalbuminaemia will usually have been excluded by the neonatologists before you are asked to review the baby.

Lymphoedema may arise as a consequence of a developmental disorder of the lymphatic system that leads to a disabling and disfiguring swelling of the extremities. Skin changes may be present, including brawny fibrotic skin. Small, flesh-coloured papules (papillomatosis) may occur later due to dilatation and fibrosis of upper dermal lymphatics. Lymph fluid may sometimes leak following minimal trauma. Hereditary lymphoedema generally shows AD inheritance with reduced penetrance, variable expression, and variable age at onset. Swelling may appear in one or all limbs. Swelling varies in degree and distribution and, if untreated, worsens over time. See Table 2.27 for genes involved in lymphatic anomalies.

Clinical approach

History: key points

- Three-generation family history with specific enquiry for consanguinity, oedema, lymphoedema, varicose veins, distichiasis, and congenital heart disease.
- Detailed pregnancy history. Enquire about polyhydramnios and fetal movements.

Examination: key points

- Which limbs are swollen?
- Is it possible to pick up a fold of skin at the base of the second toe (failure to do this is pathognomonic of lymphoedema due to increased thickness of the skin)?
- Is there microcephaly?
- Are the facial features coarse?
- The following queries all relate to markers of intrauterine oedema and are seen in a number of congenital lymphoedema syndromes.
- Are there medial epicanthic folds?
- Are the ears low-set?
- Is the neck broad/webbed? Are there redundant nuchal folds?
- Are the nipples wide-spaced?

Special investigations

- Karyotype (to exclude 45,X and other rare chromosome rearrangements). If clinical features are suggestive of Turner syndrome (TS), ask for a mosaicism screen if routine karyotype normal.
- Genomic analysis in presence of features suggestive of a chromosomal or syndromic diagnosis, e.g. genomic array, gene panel, or WES/WGS as available.
- Echo (to assess for possible Noonan syndrome (NS)—pulmonary stenosis, CM).
- Urinalysis for protein to exclude nephrotic syndrome.

- White-cell enzymes if GM1 gangliosidosis or other lysosomal disorders are a possibility.
- Consider ophthalmological assessment.
- FLT4 (VEGFR3) gene analysis if suggestive of Milroy disease, e.g. congenital pedal oedema.

Some diagnoses to consider
See Figure 2.28.

Presenting in infancy

TURNER SYNDROME (45,X) OR MOSAIC TURNER SYNDROME. Oedema that resolves in utero may present in the newborn as residual puffiness of the hands and feet and redundant nuchal folds. See 'Turner syndrome, 45,X and variants' in Chapter 5, 'Chromosomes', p. 696.

NOONAN SYNDROME (NS). Oedema that resolves in utero is thought to account for many of the dysmorphic features. Babies with NS have thick eyelids with ptosis, epicanthic folds, a webbed neck with low-set, posteriorly rotated ears, and widely spaced nipples. See 'Noonan syndrome and the Ras/MAPK pathway syndromes: neuro-cardio-facial-cutaneous syndromes' in Chapter 3, 'Common consultations', p. 512.

MILROY PRIMARY CONGENITAL LYMPHOEDEMA (MILROY DISEASE). The swelling is present at birth, mainly affecting the dorsal aspects of the feet, with deep interphalangeal creases and small dysplastic 'ski-jump' nails. Inheritance is AD with reduced penetrance (90%) and it is caused by mutations in FLT4 (VEGFR3) on chromosome 5q.

GM1 GANGLIOSIDOSIS (BETA-GALACTOSIDASE DEFICIENCY). A lysosomal disorder following AR inheritance that presents from birth. Coarse features, facial oedema, pitting oedema of the hands and feet, large tongue, thick gums, floppy, poor feeding.

GENERALIZED LYMPHATIC DYSPLASIA/HENNEKAM SYNDROME. An AR condition comprising congenital lymphoedema, facial anomalies (flat face, flat and broad nasal bridge, and hypertelorism), intestinal lymphangiectasia, and developmental delay. The lymphoedema is usually congenital; it can be markedly asymmetrical and is often gradually progressive. Approximately 25% are due to mutations in the CCBE1 gene but can also be caused by biallelic variants in FAT4 and PIEZO1.

CHOLESTASIS—LYMPHOEDEMA SYNDROME (CLS; AAGENAES SYNDROME). Patients with CLS suffer from severe neonatal cholestasis that usually lessens during early childhood and becomes episodic; they also develop chronic severe lymphoedema. The condition maps to 15q. Very rare outside Scandinavia.

KLIPPEL—TRENAUNAY SYNDROME (KTW). Can present with limb swelling at birth with associated cutaneous vascular naevus over the trunk or limbs, varicosities, and asymmetrical hypertrophy of all or part of a limb.

MICROCEPHALY WITH OR WITHOUT CHORIORETINOPATHY LYMPHOEDEMA AND MENTAL RETARDATION (MCLMR). A rare AD condition characterized by microcephaly, lymphoedema, and chorioretinopathy with variable visual deficit and variable expression. It is associated with heterozygous mutations in KIF11.

Table 2.27 Genes involved in lymphatic anomalies

Lymphatic anomalies/additional signs	Gene (protein)	Cases[a]	Penetrance[b]	Mutation type	Inheritance	Animal models[c]
Isolated lymphoedema						
Primary congenital lymphoedema/Nonne–Milroy lymphoedema	FLT4 (VEGFR-3)	>100	High	Inactivating	AD, AR, de novo	**Chy**, Flt4^−/−
Milroy-like disease	VEGFC	1	High	LOF	AD	**Chy-3**, Vegfc^−/−
Syndromic lymphoedema						
Hennekam lymphangiectasia–lymphoedema syndrome/mental retardation	CCBE1	13	High	LOF	AR	**fof**
Lymphoedema–distichiasis and yellow nail syndromes/ptosis	FOXC2	>85	High	LOF	AD	**Foxc2**^−/−
Hereditary lymphoedema II (Meige disease)	GJC2 (CX47)	7	High	Missense	AD	(Gjc2^−/−)
Oculodentodigital dysplasia/lymphoedema	GJA1 (CX43)	1	High	Missense	AD	(Gja1^−/−)
Choanal atresia/lymphoedema	PTPN14	1	High	LOF	AR	Ptpn14^−/−
Hypotrichosis–lymphoedema–telangiectasia syndrome	SOX18	3	High	LOF?/D-N	AR, AD, de novo	**Ragged**, (Sox18^−/−)
Lymphoedema–lymphangiectasia	HGF	4	Medium	LOF?	AD?	(Met^−/−)
MCLMR	KIF11	14	Low	LOF	AD, de novo	(Kif11^−/−)
Noonan syndrome 1 (54% with lymphoedema)	PTPN11 (SHP2)	>100	Medium	GOF	AD	**Shp2**^−/−
Noonan syndrome 1 (63% with lymphoedema)	SOS1	Few with lymphoedema	Medium	GOF	AD	–
Primary lymphoedema, myelodysplasia (Emberger syndrome)	GATA2	13	Low	LOF	AD	(Gata2^−/−)
OLEDAID	IKBKG (NEMO)	5	Low	Hypomorphic	X-linked	(Ikbkg^−/−)
CM-AVM/lymphoedema	RASA1	Few with lymphoedema	Low	LOF	AD	(**Rasa1**^−/−)
Cholestasis–lymphoedema syndrome (Aagenaes syndrome)	Locus in 15q	–	–	–	AR	–

(continued)

Table 2.27 Continued

Lymphatic anomalies/additional signs	Gene (protein)	Cases[a]	Penetrance[b]	Mutation type	Inheritance	Animal models[c]
Syndromic chylothorax/chylous ascites, lymphangiectasia						
Fetal chylothorax	ITGA9	6	High	Missense	AR, de novo	**Itga9**[−/−]
Noonan syndrome, cardiofaciocutaneous syndrome/chylothorax	KRAS	Few with chylothorax	Low	GOF	AD	**Kras**[−/−]
Noonan syndrome 1/lymphangiectasia	RAF1	Few with lymphangiectasia	Low	GOF	AD	**Raf1-KI**
Costello syndrome/chylous ascites, chylothorax	HRAS	Few with chylous ascites/ chylothorax	Low	GOF	AD	**Hras**[−/−]
Syndromes with LMs						
Turner syndrome/nuchal translucency	Monosomy X	>100	Medium	–	Sex-linked	(XO mice)
Proteus syndrome, Pten hamartoma tumour syndrome	PTEN	~10	Medium	LOF	AD, de novo	(Pten[−/−])
CLOVES, Klippel–Trenaunay–Weber syndrome	PIK3CA	3	N/A	GOF	Somatic	**Pa100-KI**
Proteus syndrome	AKT1	40	N/A	GOF	Somatic	**Akt1**[−/−]

[a] Number of index cases reported with a mutation.

[b] Penetrance of lymphatic anomalies when carrying a mutation.

[c] Germline mutants only. Parentheses indicate the absence of lymphatic anomaly, and bolded text indicates that the model partially mimics the human phenotype.

[d] Inactivation in adults.

AD, autosomal dominant; AR, autosomal recessive; D-N, dominant negative; GOF, gain of function; KI, knockin; LOF, loss of function; –, not applicable.

Question marks indicate that mutation type and/or inheritance is unclear.

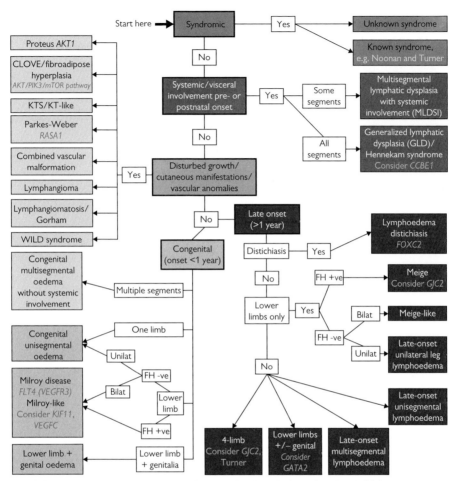

Figure 2.28 The classification and diagnostic algorithm for primary lymphatic dysplasia. bilat., bilateral; FH, family history; unilat., unilateral; +ve, positive; −ve, negative.
Reproduced with permission from FC Connell, K Gordon, G Brice et al., The classification and diagnostic algorithm for primary lymphatic dysplasia: an update from 2010 to include molecular findings, *Clinical Genetics*, Volume 84, Issue 4, pp. 303–314, Copyright © 2013 John Wiley and Sons.

Presenting during childhood or puberty

LYMPHOEDEMA–DISTICHIASIS SYNDROME. An AD syndrome characterized by primary lymphoedema of the lower limbs only, with aberrant eyelashes arising from the inner eyelid (distichiasis is penetrant in 95%) and caused by mutations in the forkhead transcription factor *FOXC2* on 16q24. Associated findings included ptosis (31%), CHD (6.8%), and cleft palate (4%) (Brice et al. 2002). Other than distichiasis, the most commonly occurring anomaly is varicose veins of early onset (49%).

EMBERGER SYNDROME. A rare AD syndrome with variable expression and penetrance. Primary lymphoedema of the lower limbs and genitalia, associated with an increased risk of immunodeficiency, sensorineural deafness, myelodysplasia, and acute myeloid leukaemia (AML). Due to mutations in *GATA2*.

MEIGE DISEASE. An AD condition associated with pubertal onset of primary lymphoedema of the lower limbs, but with no other abnormalities. No specific genes have been identified and it is probably heterogeneous but has been associated with mutations in *GJC2*.

Genetic advice
Counsel for the specific diagnosis.

Recurrence risk
As for the specific diagnosis.

Prenatal diagnosis
Possible only if a chromosomal abnormality or mutation has been defined in the proband.

Natural history and further management (preventative measures)
If there is chronic lymphoedema, refer to a specialist clinic or lymphoedema therapist for management of the lymphoedema.

Support groups: Lymphoedema Support Network, http://www.lymphoedema.org; British Lymphology Society, http://www.thebls.com.

Expert adviser: Sahar Mansour, Consultant and Honorary Professor in Clinical Genetics, St George's Healthcare NHS Trust, London, UK.

References

Alders M, Hogan BM, Gjini E, et al. Mutations in *CCBE1* cause generalized lymph vessel dysplasia in humans. *Nat Genet* 2009; **41**: 1272–4.

Brice G, Child AH, Evans A, et al. Milroy disease and the *VEGFR-3* mutation phenotype. *J Med Genet* 2005; **42**: 98–102.

Brice G, Mansour S, Bell R, et al. Analysis of the phenotypic abnormalities in lymphoedema–distichiasis syndrome in 74 patients with *FOXC2* mutations or linkage to 16q24. *J Med Genet* 2002; **39**: 478–83.

Brouillard P, Boon L, Vikkula M. Genetics of lymphatic anomalies. *J Clin Invest* 2014; **124**: 898–904.

Bull LN, Roche E, Song EJ, et al. Mapping of the locus for cholestasis–lymphedema syndrome (Aagenaes syndrome) to a 6.6cm interval on chromosome 15q. *Am J Hum Genet* 2000; **67**: 994–9.

Connell F, Gordon K, Brice G, et al. The classification and diagnostic algorithm for primary lymphatic dysplasia: an update from 2010 to include molecular findings. *Clin Genet* 2013; **84**: 303–14.

Ferrell RE, Levinson KL, Esman JH, et al. Hereditary lymphoedema: evidence for linkage and genetic heterogeneity. *Hum Mol Genet* 1998; **7**: 2073–8.

Karkkainen MJ, Ferrell RE, Lawrence EC, et al. Missense mutations interfere with VEGFR-3 signalling in primary lymphoedema. *Nat Genet* 2000; **25**: 153–9.

Ostergaard P, Simpson MA, Connell FC, et al. Mutations in *GATA2* cause primary lymphedema associated with a predisposition to acute myeloid leukemia (Emberger syndrome). *Nat Genet* 2011; **43**: 929–31.

Ostergaard P, Simpson MA, Mendola A, et al. Mutations in *KIF11* cause autosomal-dominant microcephaly variably associated with congenital lymphedema and chorioretinopathy. *Am J Hum Genet* 2012; **90**: 356–62.

Oesophageal and intestinal atresia (including tracheo-oesophageal fistula)

For all types of GI obstruction, the birth frequency is around one in 2000. A tracheo-oesophageal fistula (TOF) occurs in ~1/3000 live births (see Figure 2.29); there is a small male preponderance. In >85%, the fistula is associated with oesophageal atresia (OA). Approximately 50% have a major associated malformation (Shaw-Smith 2006). TOF results from an incomplete division of the cranial part of the foregut into respiratory and oesophageal parts during 23–28 days post-conception.

The intestine develops as a hollow tube. The middle of the enteric tube is tethered to the umbilical cord by the vitelline duct. In the embryo, this middle portion of the enteric system grows and rotates within the umbilical cord. By week 10, the intestines are situated within the abdominal cavity.

The mechanisms of occurrence of atresia (Greek 'unpierced') are heterogeneous and include: due to a single gene disorder; fetal teratogens, vascular disruption, and deformation, instanced by duodenal atresia due to constriction by the annular pancreas.

Duodenal atresia is the most common form of intestinal atresia.

The role of the geneticist is to help patients and their families understand the aetiology, whichever of the above described may apply. A clear aetiology is rarely apparent in non-syndromic cases; fortunately the recurrence risk in that scenario is low.

Clinical approach

History: key points
- Family history: previous affected sib or parent, consanguinity.
- Maternal age (Down's syndrome).
- Maternal diabetes, teratogen exposure.
- Prenatal features: polyhydramnios, premature delivery.
- Postnatal presenting features: abdominal distension, excessive gastric aspirates (bile-stained), vomiting.
- Co-twin or a history suggestive of early loss of a co-twin (scan appearance; bleeding). Twinning is associated with an increased risk of congenital malformations, including OA/TOF.

Examination: key points
- If seen preoperatively, features of atresia, as described above.
- Features of Down's syndrome: hypotonia, cardiac murmur, facial features.
- Omphalocele or
- Anorectal anomalies.
- Radial or thumb hypoplasia (VACTERL; see 'Syndromic diagnoses to consider' below).
- Digital: short fifth finger with clinodactyly, and brachymesophalangy of second and fifth fingers; syndactyly of toes (Feingold syndrome).
- Ear anomalies, preauricular skin tags (Goldenhar syndrome), and dysplastic external ears (CHARGE syndrome).
- Eyes: corneal clouding (Fryns syndrome), colobomata (CHARGE), and structural ocular abnormalities in several syndromes discussed below.

Special investigations
- Operation. Note the surgical findings (site of atresia, single or multiple, malrotation, volvulus, 'apple peel atresia', vascular anatomy, structural abnormality of the pancreas).
- X-ray of the spine (structural vertebral anomalies) in children with TOF and OA.
- X-ray of the lower spine and sacrum in infants of diabetic mothers.
- Genomic analysis in presence of features suggestive of a chromosomal or syndromic diagnosis, e.g. genomic array, gene panel, or WES/WGS as appropriate.
- Consider Fanconi testing by chromosome breakage studies in infants with bilateral upper limb anomalies, especially radial aplasia.
- Consider DNA for storage.
- Consider ophthalmology referral (for fundal exam for colobomata, e.g. CHARGE).
- Echo (VACTERL association, CHARGE syndrome).
- Renal USS (for VATER/CHARGE).
- Consider CF in the case of intestinal atresias (see below), e.g. jejuno-ileal atresia and colonic atresia.

Syndromic diagnoses to consider

Tracheo-oesophageal fistula (TOF) or oesophageal atresia (OA)

Isolated TOF presents with a characteristic triad of symptoms: choking and cyanosis on feeding; recurrent lower respiratory tract infection; and abdominal distension. Babies are invariably symptomatic from birth, although the symptoms may be intermittent and may vary in severity. A high index of suspicion is required because the symptoms are not specific. Establishing the diagnosis can be difficult and neither radiology nor bronchoscopy is infallible. Surgical division of the fistula is curative. Only ~45% of TOFs are isolated anomalies, so search carefully for other malformations.

OA presents far less of a diagnostic challenge as it is incompatible with swallowing without surgical intervention.

CHROMOSOMAL ANOMALIES. A wide variety of chromosomal conditions have been reported with OA/TOF, including trisomy 21, trisomy 18, del 22q11, and rarely 17q interstitial deletion.

DEVELOPMENTAL MALFORMATION SYNDROMES (USUALLY SPORADIC).
- **VATER/VACTERL association.** Incidence 1.6/10 000. The individual letters in VATER/VACTERL have the following significance:
  - 'V, vertebral defects, usually upper to mid-thoracic and lumbar regions. Usually hemivertebrae, but dyssegmented and fused vertebrae may occur—may be accompanying rib anomalies;
  - A, anal atresia—may be associated genital defects (hypospadias, bifid scrotum) or fistulae;
  - C, cardiac anomalies—present in ~80%; any type, any severity;

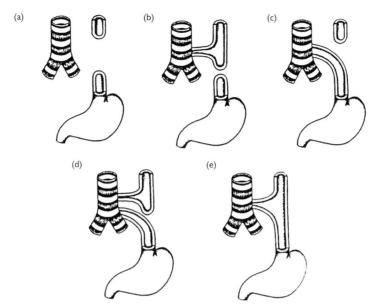

Figure 2.29 Schematics of various types of oesophageal atresia (OA) and tracheo-oesophageal fistula (TOF). (a) OA without TOF. (b) OA with proximal TOF. (c) OA with distal TOF. (d) OA with proximal and distal TOF. (e) TOF without oesophageal atresia. Reproduced with permission from Stevenson RE and Hall JG, *Human Malformations and Related Anomalies*, Second Edition, 2005, Figure 24.7, page 1074, with permission from Oxford University Press, New York, USA. www.oup.com.

- TE, Tracheo-oesophageal fistula or oesophageal atresia;
- R, renal; renal anomalies in 80%, e.g. renal agenesis/dysplasia;
- L, limb (radial defects)—preaxial with underdevelopment or agenesis of thumbs and radial bones; usually bilateral defects but may be asymmetric. Reduced thenar muscle mass is mildest end of spectrum. The lower limbs are not affected. The aetiology of VACTERL association is not understood, and diagnostic criteria are lacking.'

Reprinted from *The Journal of Pediatrics*, Vol 82, Issue 1, Linda Quan, David W. Smith, The VATER association -Vertebral defects, -Anal atresia, -T-Efistula with esophageal atresia, -Radial and -Renal dysplasia: A spectrum of associated defects, pp. 104–107, Copyright 1973 with permission from Elsevier.

- **Goldenhar (facio-auriculo-vertebral) syndrome.** OA/TOF is a recognized, but not common, feature of this syndrome. See 'Ear anomalies' in Chapter 2, 'Clinical approach', p. 142 for additional details.
- **OEIS.** OEIS complex refers to a combination of defects consisting of omphalocele, extrophy of the cloaca, imperforate anus, and spinal defect. Mostly sporadic. See 'Anal anomalies (atresia, stenosis)' in Chapter 2, 'Clinical approach', p. 58.
- **Teratogens.** Carbimazole and methimazole, used to treat thyroid endocrinopathy in pregnancy, are associated with an increased incidence of OA/TOF.

SINGLE GENE DISORDERS.

- **Feingold syndrome.** AD. Also known as MODED (microcephaly–oculo–digito–(o)esophageal–duodenal) syndrome. A clinically variable disorder comprising hand and foot abnormalities (brachydactyly with clinodactyly of fifth fingers and bilateral syndactyly of toes 2/3 and 4/5); microcephaly; short palpebral fissures; learning disabilities; and OA (25%) and/or duodenal atresia (20%). The gene is *MYCN* (von Bokhoven *et al.* 2005).
- **CHARGE syndrome.** OA/TOF is present in 10–20% of individuals with CHARGE syndrome which is caused by mutations in the *CHD7* gene. Mutation analysis of this gene has meant that there is now better appreciation of the differences between CHARGE syndrome and VACTERL association. See 'Ear anomalies' in Chapter 2, 'Clinical approach', p. 142.
- **Opitz syndrome.** Opitz (or G/BBB) syndrome is characterized by hypertelorism, hypospadias, laryngeal cleft, and additional midline defects. This syndrome is heterogeneous with an XL (XLOS) form caused by mutations in *MID1* on Xp22 and an AD (ADOS) form. De Falco *et al.* (2003) found that laryngo-tracheo-(o) esophageal (LTE) defects are also common anomalies in males carrying a *MID1* mutation.
- **Mandibulo-facial dysostosis with microcephaly (MFDM).** A recently described association with OA/TOF (Gordon *et al.* 2012) due to heterozygous mutations in the spliceosomal GTPase *EFTUD2*. Severe microcephaly, malar and mandibular hypoplasia, dysplastic ears/microtia, and cleft palate are typical findings. See

also 'Ear anomalies' in Chapter 2, 'Clinical approach', p. 142.

- **AEG syndrome.** Anophthalmia with oesophageal atresia and genital abnormalities (cryptorchidism and hypospadias in males). Neuronal migration defects in the CNS are probably part of the syndrome. Caused by new dominant mutations of the *SOX2* gene.
- **Martinez–Frias syndrome.** AR. Low birthweight, TOF, duodenal atresia, intra- and extrahepatic biliary atresia, and hypospadias. There is some overlap with Mitchell–Riley syndrome (see below). Neonatal diabetes is a feature of the latter; OA/TOF occurs in the former.
- **Hydrocephalus with features of VATER.** AR. Children have been reported with the cytogenetic features of Fanconi anaemia. XL families with mutations in *FANCB* have been described.
- **Disorders of laterality due to mutations in ZIC3.** An XLR disorder. Atresia of the oesophagus, duodenum, and anus are reported, as well as malformations of the heart, biliary tract, and kidneys. Gut atresias are possibly an underappreciated component of laterality disorders.

Duodenal atresia

NB. Duodenal stenosis may be associated with an annular pancreas.

CHROMOSOMAL ANOMALIES. Down's syndrome (trisomy 21) is the main condition to exclude in babies with duodenal atresia; it accounts for 30–50% of duodenal atresias.

DEVELOPMENTAL MALFORMATION SYNDROMES (USUALLY SPORADIC).

- **Maternal diabetes and caudal regression.** See 'Maternal diabetes mellitus and diabetic embryopathy' in Chapter 6, 'Pregnancy and fertility', p. 756.
- **OEIS.** See previous OEIS section.
- **Vascular disruption.** Direct evidence for a vascular aetiology for intestinal atresias in humans is lacking, although evidence from animal models does exist (e.g. Louw and Bernard 1955).

SINGLE GENE DISORDERS.

- **Feingold syndrome.** See previous Feingold syndrome section.
- **Martinez–Frias syndrome.** See previous Martinez–Frias syndrome section.
- **Mitchell–Riley syndrome.** Recently reported to be due to biallelic mutations in *RFX6*. Neonatal diabetes is a prominent feature. Multiple organs within the GI tract are affected, including the small intestine (intestinal malrotation, duodenal atresia, jejunal atresia), pancreas (annular pancreas, hypoplastic pancreas), and hepatobiliary system (gall bladder agenesis, extra- and intrahepatic biliary atresia).
- **Multiple gastrointestinal atresias (MGIA).** Rare, AR, due to mutations in *TTC7A*. Immunodeficiency is associated. Described in French–Canadian ethnic group.
- **Alveolar capillary dysplasia with misalignment of pulmonary veins.** Very rare, but well-described lethal disorder of alveolar capillarization, incompatible with independent survival. Due to heterozygous mutations in *FOXF1*. GI malformations, including duodenal atresia, anal atresia, and intestinal malrotation are associated. Also cardiac and renal malformations.

- **Disorders of laterality.** See previous disorders of laterality section.
- **Fryns syndrome.** A rare lethal AR condition with nail/digital hypoplasia, corneal clouding, and diaphragmatic hernia as the main features.

Jejuno-ileal atresia

Developmental malformation syndromes. As for duodenal atresia.

SINGLE GENE DISORDERS.

- **CF.** Roberts *et al.* (1998) calculated that the presence of jejuno-ileal atresia gave a 210 times increased risk for CF, as four out of 38 Caucasian babies with jejuno-ileal atresia had CF. A CF workup is routinely recommended for all infants presenting with jejuno-ileal atresia.
- **Stromme syndrome** is characterized by ocular anomalies, 'apple-peel' type jejunal atresia, and microcephaly. It is caused by biallelic variants in the *CENPF* gene. The phenotype is variable. CENPF encodes a component of the ciliary centriole (Filges 2016).

Colonic atresia

May occur in the context of small intestinal atresias due to single gene disorders: CF, Martinez–Frias syndrome, and MGIA. May occur in some disorders of unknown aetiology mentioned above: caudal regression syndrome and OEIS. Vascular aetiologies discussed above may also apply.

DEVELOPMENTAL MALFORMATION SYNDROMES. As for duodenal atresia.

Anal atresia

See 'Anal anomalies (atresia, stenosis)' in Chapter 2, 'Clinical approach', p. 58.

Genetic advice

Recurrence risk

Identify those infants with a syndromic cause and counsel appropriately. Initiate genetic testing where a single gene disorder is suspected.

- Isolated TOF. The recurrence risk for siblings of a child with an isolated TOF is very small at ~1%. The risk to offspring of an individual with an isolated TOF is very small and estimated at ~1% (Warren *et al.* 1979).
- Isolated intestinal atresia. As described above, there have been a small number of reports of familial occurrence of isolated bowel atresia, but the proportion that are recessive remains uncertain. The majority of isolated single-site bowel atresias are usually attributed to vascular disruption and are associated with a low recurrence risk. In a 10-year survey by the American Academy of Pediatricians, the recurrence risk for sibs of infants with duodenal atresia was ~1 in 50. The recurrence risk may be higher than this in infants with multiple atresia or jejuno-ileal atresia.

Carrier detection

Not possible, unless associated with CF or other genetic conditions with a known mutation or chromosomal rearrangement.

Prenatal diagnosis

USS in the second and third trimesters. USS findings suggesting TOF/OA include polyhydramnios and a small or absent stomach. Approximately one-third of babies with gut atresias were prenatally detected (40% of these before 24 weeks) in the Haeusler *et al.* (2002) series.

Natural history and further management (preventative measures)

The primary management is surgical. Delivery should be planned at a hospital with full neonatal intensive care facilities and good links with a specialist paediatric surgical team. For suspected TOF/OA, a senior paediatrician should be present at delivery since expert management of the neonate from the moment of delivery is necessary to minimize the risk of aspiration pneumonia.

Support group: TOFS (Tracheo-Oesophageal Fistula Support), http://www.tofs.org.uk, Tel. 0115 961 3092.

Expert adviser: Charles Shaw-Smith, Consultant Clinical Geneticist, Peninsula Clinical Genetics Service, Royal Devon and Exeter Hospital NHS Trust, Exeter, UK.

References

Boyd PA, Chamberlain P, Gould S, et al. Hereditary multiple intestinal atresia—ultrasound findings and outcome of pregnancy in an affected case. Prenat Diagn 1994: **14**: 61–4.

Buttiker V, Wojtulewicz, Wilson M. Imperforate anus in Feingold syndrome. Am J Med Genet 2000; **92**: 166–9.

Celli J, van Beusekom E, Hennekam RC, et al. Familial syndromic esophageal atresia maps to 2p23–p24. Am J Hum Genet 2000; **66**: 436–44.

De Falco F, Cainarca S, Andolfi G, et al. X-linked Opitz syndrome: novel mutations in the MID1 gene and redefinition of the clinical spectrum. Am J Med Genet A 2003; **120A**: 222–8.

Filges I, Bruder E, et al. Stromme syndrome is a ciliary disorder caused by mutations in CENPF. Hum Mutat 2016; **37**: 359–63.

Fonkalsrud EW, DeLorimier AA, Hays DM. Congenital atresia and stenosis of the duodenum: a review compiled from the members of the surgical section of the American Academy of Pediatrics. Pediatrics 1969; **43**: 79–83.

Gordon CT, Petit F, Oufadem M, et al. EFTUD2 haploinsufficiency leads to syndromic oesophageal atresia. J Med Genet 2012; **49**: 737–46.

Haeusler MC, Berghold A, Stoll C, et al. Prenatal ultrasound detection of gastrointestinal obstruction: results from 18 congenital anomaly registers. Prenat Diagn 2002; **22**: 616–23.

Louw JH, Bernard CN. Congenital intestinal atresia: observations on its origin. Lancet 1955; **2**: 1065–7.

Roberts HE, Cragan JD, Cono J, et al. Increased frequency of CF among infants with jejunoileal atresia. Am J Med Genet 1998; **78**: 446–9.

Shaw-Smith C Oesophageal atresia, tracheooesophageal fistula, and the VACTERL association: review of genetics and epidemiology. J Med Genet 2006; **43**: 545–54.

von Bokhoven H, Celli J, van Reeuwijk J, et al. MYCN haploinsufficiency is associated with reduced brain size and intestinal atresias in Feingold syndrome. Nat Genet 2005; **37**: 465–7.

Warren J, Evans K, Carter CO. Offspring of patients with tracheo-oesophageal fistula. J Med Genet 1979; **16**: 338–40.

Optic nerve hypoplasia

This is a non-progressive congenital anomaly that may be unilateral or bilateral and affect all, or part, of the optic nerve. The optic disc is small and pale and may show a peripapillary ring of pigmentation. The presenting feature is often nystagmus in bilateral cases, and strabismus in unilateral cases. Visual function varies from near normal to complete loss of vision. The prognosis is difficult to predict in small infants. The most important association to exclude in infancy is endocrine abnormalities due to a developmental disorder of the midline brain structures, e.g. septo-optic dysplasia (SOD) or other midline anomalies. For this reason, all infants with unilateral or bilateral optic nerve hypoplasia (ONH) should see a paediatric endocrinologist.

PAX2 and PAX6 are involved in ocular morphogenesis and are expressed in numerous ocular tissues during development.

ONH is associated not only with other anomalies of the CNS (see above) and with teratogenic exposure (alcohol, anticonvulsants, maternal diabetes), but also with signs of general disturbance in fetal development. Risk factors include young maternal age, first parity, maternal smoking, preterm birth, and factors associated with preterm birth (Tornqvist et al. 2002).

Clinical approach

History: key points
- Three-generation family tree with specific enquiry regarding visual problems.
- Pregnancy: alcohol exposure, anticonvulsant use.
- Maternal diabetes mellitus.
- Developmental milestones.
- Visual function.

Examination: key points
- Short stature (pituitary dysfunction, SOD).
- Micropenis (pituitary dysfunction).
- Facial dysmorphic features.

Special investigations
- Ophthalmological assessment to differentiate ONH from optic atrophy and the crowded disc of hypermetropia.
- Refraction.
- Electrophysiology. ERG normal, VERs abnormal.
- Cranial and optic nerve MRI; midline structural lesions.
- Endocrine investigations, particularly pituitary hormones. Refer to a paediatric endocrinologist.
- Genomic analysis in presence of features suggestive of a chromosomal or syndromic diagnosis, e.g. genomic array, gene panel, or WES/WGS as appropriate/available.
- Renal USS (PAX2).

Syndromic diagnoses to consider

Septo-optic dysplasia (SOD)
ONH with absent septum pellucidum and pituitary endocrine abnormalities. Mutations in HESX1 (heterozygous and homozygous) have been found in a few individuals. See 'Structural intracranial anomalies (agenesis of the corpus callosum, septo-optic dysplasia, and arachnoid cysts)' in Chapter 2, 'Clinical approach', p. 320.

Tubulin disorders
Heterozygous mutations in members of the tubulin gene family may have ONH together with severe brain neuronal migration disorders, e.g. lissencephaly.

Papillorenal syndrome (PAX2)
Heterozygous mutations in PAX2 cause papillorenal syndrome, an AD disorder characterized by both ocular anomalies (e.g. optic disc dysplasia or 'morning glory' anomaly) and renal anomalies (small kidneys that may progress to chronic renal failure), and may include VUR, high-frequency hearing loss, CNS anomalies, and/or genital anomalies, consistent with the expression of PAX2 in these tissues during development.

PAX6
Heterozygous PAX6 mutations have been identified in some families with optic nerve malformations, including colobomata, morning glory disc anomaly, optic nerve hypoplasia/aplasia, and persistent hyperplastic primary vitreous (Azuma et al. 2003).

Environmental aetiology
Maternal diabetes, alcohol, or anticonvulsant use. See 'Maternal diabetes mellitus and diabetic embryopathy', p. 756, 'Fetal alcohol syndrome (FAS)', p. 728, and 'Fetal anticonvulsant syndrome (FACS)', p. 732 in Chapter 6, 'Pregnancy and fertility'.

Genetic advice

Recurrence risk
For isolated ONH, the recurrence risk is low, but there are rare reports of dominant inheritance. A recurrence may have more than just ONH, e.g. there may be features of SOD.

Carrier detection
May be available in families for conditions with a known mutation.

Prenatal diagnosis
Genetic testing may be available in families with a known mutation.

Natural history and further management (preventative measures)
A non-progressive developmental disorder. Visual function is difficult to predict in small infants.

Support group: FOCUS Families (ONH/SOD Information, Education and Support), http://www.focusfamilies.org.

References

Azuma N, Yamaguchi Y, Handa H, et al. Mutations of the PAX6 gene detected in patients with a variety of optic-nerve malformations. Am J Hum Genet 2003; **72**: 1565–70.

Fitzpatrick DR, van Heyningen V. Developmental eye disorders. Curr Opin Genet Dev 2005; **15**: 348–53.

Golnik KC. Congenital optic nerve abnormalities. Curr Opin Ophthalmol 1998; **9**: 18–26.

Tornqvist K, Ericsson A, Kallen B. Optic nerve hypoplasia: risk factors and epidemiology. Acta Ophthalmol Scand 2002; **80**: 300–4.

Wall PB, Traboulsi EI. Congenital abnormalities of the optic nerve: from gene mutation to clinical expression. Curr Neurol Neurosci Rep 2013; **13**: 363.

Overgrowth

Overgrowth can be defined as regional or global excess growth, compared either to an equivalent body party or an age-related peer group. Growth is considered excess if >2 SD above the mean (approximates to the 98th centile). In general, an individual with global overgrowth (increased height and head circumference) would be suspected as having an overgrowth syndrome when they additionally have an ID and/or a congenital medical anomaly. Regional overgrowth frequently involves one or more limbs (i.e. leg and arm) and can be static or progressive.

In recent years, the molecular cause of the majority of known overgrowth syndromes has been elucidated and two principal families have emerged: genes that encode epigenetic regulators and genes that encode components of the PI3K/mTOR pathway (see Figure 2.30). Activation of the PI3K/mTOR cascade results in increased growth and, to date, both activating mutations (*AKT1*/*AKT3*/*PI3KCA*/*PIK3R2*) and inactivating mutations within inhibitors of this pathway (e.g. PTEN) have been shown to cause overgrowth disorders. It is likely that, over the coming years, germline/somatic mutations within genes encoding other components of this pathway are shown to cause global/regional overgrowth and new clinical syndromes will be delineated for those individuals currently classified as having 'non-specific' overgrowth.

Clinical approach

History: key points

- Three-generation family tree with specific enquiry regarding parental birthweights, growth, and family history of ID.
- Detailed pregnancy history with specific enquiry about maternal gestational diabetes, assisted conception, growth during pregnancy, and abnormal findings on USS.
- Birth and neonatal history. Birth growth parameters (weight, OFC, and length (if available)) should be requested and gestation of pregnancy. Pregnancy complications are also important, particularly polyhydramnios. Particular note should be made of the presence of an anterior abdominal wall defect or neonatal hypoglycaemia.
- Postnatal growth: a detailed growth history should be obtained, i.e. any periods of accelerated growth, compared to peers, or whether regional overgrowth is static or progressive.
- A detailed developmental history, including early motor milestones and current educational attainment.
- A detailed medical history with particular attention to skeletal, cardiac, renal, and neurological systems. Where there is regional overgrowth, detailed enquiry about cutaneous manifestations is particularly important.

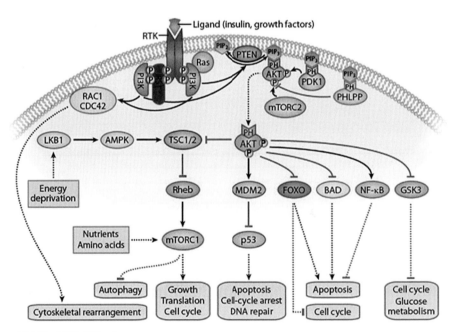

Figure 2.30 The PI3K/mTOR pathway.
Reproduced from Nader Chalhoub and Suzanne J. Baker, *Annual Review of Pathology*, 2009, 4, 1, pp. 12–50. Reproduced with permission of *Annual Review of Pathology* © 2009 by Annual Reviews, http://www.annualreviews.org.

Examination: key points
- Growth parameters (height/length, weight, and OFC), the age at measurement, and the SD above the mean should be calculated and carefully documented. The face should be carefully examined for dysmorphic features.
- Ears for earlobe creases/helical pits (look carefully behind the ear).
- Tongue for macroglossia (BWS) or midline groove (SGB).
- Supernumerary nipples (SGB).
- Hands for polydactyly, brachydactyly, or syndactyly (SGB).
- Hemihypertrophy or areas of regional overgrowth: measure discrepancy (length and circumference using bony landmarks), compared to normally grown limb/ body region (see Figure 2.12 in 'Hemihypertrophy and limb asymmetry' in Chapter 2, 'Clinical approach', p. 164).
- Cutaneous manifestations, including pigmentary abnormalities (penile freckling in PTEN), lipomas, haemangiomas (PTEN), and connective tissue naevi (Proteus): look particularly on the soles of the feet.
- Spinal examination for scoliosis.
- Cardiac auscultation.
- Abdomen for abdominal wall defects (omphalocele, umbilical hernia, diastasis recti (BWS); umbilical hernia (Weaver)).

Special investigations
- Genomic analysis, e.g. by genomic array, gene panel, or WES/WGS as appropriate. Various chromosome

Table 2.28 Genetic basis of overgrowth disorders

Syndrome	Gene/region	Inheritance
Monogenic disorders		
Sotos*	NSD1	AD
Weaver*	EZH2 and EED	AD
Tatton-Brown Rahman*	DNMT3A	AD
Malan and Marshall Smith	NFIX	AD
Simpson-Golabi-Behmel	GPC3	XLR
P13K/mTOR pathway		
PTEN hamartoma	PTEN	AD
Other phenotypes	PPP2R5D, MTOR, AKT3, PIK3R2	AD
Somatic mosaicism disorders		
MCAP	PIK3CA	Sporadic
CLOVE	PIK3CA	Sporadic
Proteus	AKT1	Sporadic
Imprinting disorders		
Beckwith–Wiedemann	11p15	Sporadic (except CDKN1C)
	~50% loss of methylation KvDMR1, IC2	
	~20% paternal UPD11	
	~5% hypermethylation H19, IC1	
	~5% mutation in maternal CDKN1C	
	~1% chromosome rearrangements	
Isolated hemihypertrophy	11p15	Usually sporadic

*Epigenetic regulator

anomalies, e.g. dup 4p, dup 11p15 (BWS), tetrasomy 12p (Pallister–Killian), duplication or triplication at 15qter, del5q35 (Sotos), del19p13.2 (NFIX), and del 22q13, are characterized by overgrowth.
- DNA for *FRAXA* if developmental delay.
- DNA for molecular genetic analysis to investigate specific genetic diagnoses (see Table 2.28). If a mosaic disorder is suspected (some hemihypertrophy cases, Proteus syndrome, CLOVE, M-CM), then DNA extracted from an alternative tissue to blood, e.g. skin, may be required.
- Renal USS for Wilms tumour surveillance (BWS-specific at-risk epigenotypes, SGB) or baseline investigation for associated renal abnormality (particularly Sotos and 15q overgrowth syndrome).
- Echo, baseline, in Sotos syndrome and SGB.
- ECG to look for cardiac dysrhythmias in SGB (the incidence of such dysrhythmias required clarification).

Some diagnoses to consider
Global overgrowth disorders

INFANT OF DIABETIC MOTHER. Fetal macrosomia with risk of neonatal hypoglycaemia and increased risk for congenital malformation, especially CHD, NTDs, and skeletal defects. See 'Maternal diabetes mellitus and diabetic embryopathy' in Chapter 6, 'Pregnancy and fertility', p. 756.

SOTOS SYNDROME. Prevalence ~1/14 000. An AD disorder due to mutations or deletions of *NSD1* (5q35). Most cases are sporadic, caused by DNMs, but familial cases do occur. Sotos syndrome is characterized by pre- and postnatal overgrowth (height and/or head circumference); a variable learning disability (mild to severe) and a distinctive facial appearance (dolicocephaly, downslanting palpebral fissures, fronto-temporal hair sparsity, and malar flushing). The facial appearance is most easily recognized in early childhood and so, where suspected in adulthood, photos at a younger age should be requested. Associated clinical features include cardiac and renal anomalies, seizures, and scoliosis. In the neonatal period, jaundice, hypotonia, and poor feeding are commonly reported. Although bone age is commonly advanced, it is within the normal range in ~15% of individuals. Tumours are rare and screening is not currently recommended.

MALAN SYNDROME. An AD disorder caused by heterozygous mutations within *NFIX* (19p13). Malan syndrome is associated with globally increased growth, advanced bone age, developmental delay, scoliosis and unusual facies: there is considerable overlap in the facial gestalt characteristic of both Malan and Sotos syndrome.

WEAVER SYNDROME. Caused by AD mutations within *EZH2* (7q35). These are predominantly missense mutations, but truncating mutations within the final exon, sparing the critical SET domain, are reported. Weaver syndrome is characterized by tall stature, mild learning disability (rarely a severe ID is reported), and subtle facial dysmorphism most easily recognized between the ages of 1 and 3 years–a round face with frontal bossing, hypertelorism, 'stuck-on' chin, and an associated horizontal crease. Associated clinical features include camptodactyly in the neonatal period; soft, doughy skin; a hoarse, low-pitched cry; and an umbilical hernia. Based upon limited available clinical data, tumour screening is not currently recommended, but, given that somatic mutations within *EZH2* are associated with tumorigenesis, particularly chronic haematological malignancies, this advice may alter as longitudinal data on more cases with germline *EZH2* mutations are obtained. There is considerable phenotypic overlap between Weaver and Sotos syndromes and *EZH2* testing should be considered in *NSD1*-negative Sotos syndrome.

PTEN HAMARTOMA SYNDROME (PREVIOUSLY SUBDIVIDED INTO CHILDHOOD BANNAYAN–RILEY–RUVALCABA (BRR) SYNDROME AND ADULT COWDEN SYNDROME (CS)). An AD disorder due to *PTEN* (10q23) mutations/deletions. Although birthweight is usually >+2 SD, this is a disorder which is predominantly characterized by macrocephaly, rather than macrosomia, with a head circumference above the 99.6th centile. Additional clinical associations include variable learning disability in some, but not all, affected individuals, autistic spectrum disorder, haemangiomas and lipomas, penile freckling, and mucocutaneous lesions (trichilemmomas, acral keratosis, and papillomatous lesions). In adulthood, there is an increased risk of benign and malignant tumours of the thyroid (particularly follicular), breast, and endometrium (Cowden syndrome). However, the long-term risk for those individuals shown to have a *PTEN* mutation/deletion in childhood is not yet delineated.

SIMPSON–GOLABI–BEHMEL (SGB) SYNDROME. An XLR disorder due to *glypican 3* (*GPC3*, Xq26) mutations or deletions. SGB is characterized by pre- and postnatal overgrowth, a distinctive facial appearance (hypertelorism, coarse facial features, macrostomia, and a midline groove in the lower lip and/or a furrow in the middle of the tongue), supernumerary nipples, hand anomalies (brachydactyly, syndactyly, polydactyly), and various congenital anomalies including congenital cardiac defects, renal abnormalities, and diaphragmatic hernia. Variable ID is reported and ranges from normal intellect to severe learning difficulties. Individuals with SGB are at increased risk of developing embryonal tumours and should be enrolled on the Wilms tumour surveillance programme.

TATTON-BROWN RAHMAN SYNDROME. An AD condition due to heterozygous mutation in *DNMT3A* (2p23). The core physical features include tall stature, increased weight—often with rapid weight gain in late childhood—and a characteristic facial appearance with heavy horizontal eyebrows and prominent frontal incisors. Other frequent associations of TBRS include autistic spectrum disorder, scoliosis and short widely spaced toes.

PERLMAN SYNDROME. An extremely rare AR condition caused by germline mutations within *DIS3L2*. It is characterized by pre- and postnatal overgrowth, polyhydramnios, nephromegaly, and dysmorphic features with a broad, flat nasal bridge, an everted V-shaped upper lip, deep-set eyes, and low-set ears. Perlman syndrome is associated with a high incidence of nephroblastomatosis (~75%) and Wilms tumour (~25%). Neonatal mortality, attributable to renal failure, hypoxaemia, and pulmonary hypoplasia, is high.

BECKWITH–WIEDEMANN SYNDROME (BWS). Prevalence of ~1/14 000. Characterized by macrosomia, anterior abdominal wall defects, macroglossia, anterior earlobe creases, and posterior helical pits. BWS is associated with an increased risk of developing embryonal tumours. The degree of risk is influenced by the underlying 11p15 epigenotype—individuals with patUPD11, hypermethylation at H19, and no 11p15 defect should be enrolled on a Wilms tumour surveillance programme (Scott

et al. 2006). BWS is caused by disruption of the normal imprint at the 11p15 growth regulatory region. See 'Beckwith–Wiedemann syndrome (BWS)' in Chapter 3, 'Common consultations', p. 358.

CHROMOSOME ABNORMALITIES ASSOCIATED WITH GLOBAL OVERGROWTH. Various chromosome abnormalities have been associated with overgrowth, including duplication/triplication of 15q (encompassing *IGF1R*), 4p16.3 duplication (encompassing *FGFR3*), tetrasomy of 12p (Pallister–Killian), and terminal deletion of 22q13 (associated with autistic behaviour and severe ID).

Regional overgrowth disorders

ISOLATED HEMIHYPERTROPHY (IH). Where there is regional overgrowth in an individual with no other clinical features, it can be caused by 11p15 imprinting defects, although these are identified in a minority of affected individuals. 11p15 analysis is recommended in all individuals with IH to stratify to Wilms tumour screening—surveillance for Wilms tumour is indicated if paternal UPD11 or hypermethylation at H19 is identified.

M-CM/MCAP (MACROCEPHALY–CAPILLARY MALFORMATION, ALSO KNOWN AS M-CMTC (MACROCEPHALY–CUTIS MARMORATA–TELANGIECTATICA CONGENITA)). Associated with segmental overgrowth and brain malformations, including hemimegalencephaly, pachygyria, and PMG. Hydrocephalus may develop. Additional associations include capillary malformations, 2/3 syndactyly, and variable learning disability. M-CM is a mosaic condition caused by somatic mutations within *PIK3CA*. The phenotype and severity of the presentation therefore reflect which tissues are affected and the degree of mosaicism.

CLOVE SYNDROME (CONGENITAL LIPOMATOUS OVERGROWTH, VASCULAR MALFORMATION, AND EPIDERMAL NAEVI). May also be associated with hemimegalencephaly. CLOVE syndrome is also caused by somatic mutations within *PIK3CA*.

PROTEUS SYNDROME. A severe, complex disorder characterized by progressive, segmental overgrowth of the skin, connective tissue, brain, and skeleton. Also associated are cerebriform connective tissue naevi, linear epidermal naevi, and vascular/lymphatic malformations. Proteus syndrome is caused by a recurrent somatic activating p.Glu17Lys mutation within *AKT1*, a key component of the PI3K/mTOR pathway. See 'Hemihypertrophy and limb asymmetry' in Chapter 2, 'Clinical approach', p. 164.

Genetic advice

Recurrence risk
As for the specific disorder.

Carrier detection
As for the specific disorder.

Prenatal diagnosis
Usually only possible early in pregnancy if a specific mutation or chromosome anomaly has been identified.

Tumour surveillance
Although specific overgrowth disorders are known to be associated with an increased risk of tumours, particularly embryonal tumours, Wilms tumour screening is the only consensus surveillance programme currently undertaken in the UK (Scott *et al*. 2006): 3- to 4-monthly renal USS until the age of 7 years indicated in high-risk BWS and IH epigenotypes, SGB syndrome, and Perlman syndrome. There is not yet a consensus view regarding screening for

other embryonal tumours, including hepatoblastoma, although these recommendations are being developed. In addition, although it is well established that germline *PTEN* mutations confer an increased tumour susceptibility, as exemplified by adult Cowden syndrome, this tumour risk has not yet been quantified for children in whom a germline *PTEN* mutation has been identified.

Treatment

Therapeutic strategies are being devised and evaluated for the management of overgrowth disorders caused by variants in PI3K/AKT/mTOR pathway. Check current status of trials and therapies. (Keppler-Noreuil 2016).

Support groups: Child Growth Foundation, http://www.childgrowthfoundation.org, Tel. 0208 995 0257; Sotos Syndrome Support Association (SSSA), http://sotossyndrome.org.

Expert adviser: Kate Tatton-Brown, Consultant Clinical Geneticist, South Thames Regional Genetics Service, St George's Universities NHS Foundation Trust, London, UK.

References

Astuti D, Morris MR, Cooper WN, *et al.* Germline mutations in *DIS3L2* cause the Perlman syndrome of overgrowth and Wilms tumour susceptibility. *Nat Genet* 2012; **44**: 277–84.

Choufani S, Shuman C, Weksberg R. Molecular findings in Beckwith–Wiedemann syndrome. *Am J Med Genet C Semin Med Genet.* 2013; **163C**: 131–40.

Keppler-Noreuil KM, Parker VE, *et al.* Somatic overgrowth disorders of the PI3K/AKT/mTOR pathway & therapeutic strategies. *Am J Med Genet C Semin Med Genet* 2016; **172**(4): 402–42.

Lindhurst MJ, Sapp JC, Teer JK, *et al.* A mosaic activating mutation in *AKT1* associated with the Proteus syndrome. *N Engl J Med* 2011; **365**: 989–91.

Malan V, Rajan D, Thomas S, *et al.* Distinct effects of allelic *NFIX* mutations on nonsense-mediated mRNA decay engender either a Sotos-like or a Marshall–Smith syndrome. *Am J Hum Genet* 2010; **87**: 189–98.

Riviere JB, Mirzaa GM, O'Roak BJ, *et al.* De novo germline and postzygotic mutations in *AKT3, PIK3R2* and *PIK3CA* cause a spectrum of related megalencephaly syndromes. *Nat Genet* 2012; **44**: 934–40.

Scott RH, Walker L, Olsen ØE, *et al.* Surveillance for Wilms tumour in at-risk children: pragmatic recommendations for best practice. *Arch Dis Child* 2006; **91**: 995–9.

Tatton-Brown K, Douglas J, Coleman K, *et al.* Genotype-phenotype associations in Sotos syndrome: an analysis of 266 individuals with *NSD1* aberrations. *Am J Hum Genet* 2005; **77**: 193–204.

Tatton-Brown K, Hanks S, Ruark E, *et al.* Germline mutations in the oncogene *EZH2* cause Weaver syndrome and increased human height. *Oncotarget* 2011; **2**: 1127–33.

Patchy hypo- or depigmented skin lesions

As with the disorders of patchy increase in pigmentation, the differential diagnosis of these conditions depends on the distribution, shape of the lesions, and the presence of other features. The skin pigments (eumelanin and pheomelanin) are produced in melanosomes by melanocytes, which are large cells found among the basal cells of the epidermis. The melanin is then transferred to keratinocytes. Melanocytes are of neural crest origin.

Depigmentation ('amelanosis') describes the situation where melanocytes are either absent or entirely non-functional; hypopigmentation describes a reduction in colour where melanocytes are either not entirely absent or only partly functional.

Common causes of patchy hypomelanosis without significant genetic implications are the following:

- single hypopigmented macule. Single lesions resembling the hypopigmented macules seen in TSC are found in 6% of normal children and 4% of adults <45 years of age, with <1% having multiple lesions and no non-TSC individual having >3. Multiple hypopigmented macules is suggestive of TSC but can also be found in NF1;
- vitiligo. Common disorder of unknown aetiology in which the melanocytes are selectively destroyed, leading to complete depigmentation in the affected areas. This is usually characterized by symmetrical distribution affecting extensor surfaces and peri-orificial skin;
- naevus anaemicus. Single ill-defined area of hypopigmentation characterized by rubbing the lesion, which leads to intensification of the pallor and failure to redden. Benign, but more common in NF1;
- tinea versicolor. Common fungal infection of the skin which can be various colours, including hypopigmented. Slightly raised, ill-defined edges, characteristically on the anterior chest. Skin scrapes mounted on a microscope slide in potassium hydroxide (KOH) and sent for microscopy or, if clinically typical, trial of treatment with an appropriate antifungal agent.

Clinical approach

History: key points

- Three-generation family tree with specific enquiry regarding family members with pigmentary and other skin lesions.
- Presence, or not, from birth.
- Increasing in number or size?
- Deafness.
- Neurological features, developmental delay, seizures.
- Hirschsprung's disease or chronic constipation from birth.

Examination: key points

- Make a careful clinical and photographic record of the skin.
- Are the margins of the lesions sharply defined or poorly defined?
- Does the pattern of distribution follow Blaschko's lines or other recognizable embryological distribution?
- Document the number of lesions/areas of reduced pigmentation.
- Do they cross the midline of the body?

- Other skin lesions, e.g. of TSC or NF1.
- Areas/streaks of 'atrophic' hypopigmented skin with absence of appendages in the involved areas (last stage of IP and Goltz syndrome).
- Any areas of hyperpigmentation?
- Hair. White forelock; early greying.
- Nervous system (any neurocutaneous disorder?).
- Eye. Retinal hamartoma in TSC; heterochromia (WS).

Special investigations

- Clinical photography.
- Examination under UV (Woods) lamp can be helpful.
- Genomic array of blood *and skin* in the presence of developmental delay (unless the cause is thought to be a single gene disorder) or other structural malformations.
- Genomic analysis e.g. gene panel, WES/WGS as available.

NB. In conditions with a mosaic aetiology, paired blood and skin DNA samples have an important role, although specialist advice should be sought as skin fibroblasts may not be the correct cells to test.

Some diagnoses to consider

Tuberous sclerosis (TSC)

The hypopigmented lesion is described as a hypomelanotic macule or ash leaf patch which may or may not be present from birth. They are usually on the trunk or limbs and are 1–5 cm in size. The number varies, but most affected individuals have fewer than six (see 'Tuberous sclerosis (TSC)' in Chapter 3, 'Common consultations', p. 534). However, there may be fewer in childhood or a confetti appearance can be seen.

Piebaldism

A striking clearly defined congenital disorder of depigmentation of primarily the anterior body surfaces. This often includes the forehead/forelock and is usually symmetrical. The congenital and non-progressive nature differentiates it from vitiligo. AD inheritance due to mutations in *KIT* or *SNAI2*.

Waardenburg syndrome (WS)

WS manifests with variable presence of a white forelock, sometimes with more extensive depigmentation of the skin, sensorineural deafness, dystopia canthorum, heterochromia irides, synophrys, and a high nasal bridge. Some patients have premature greying of the hair. WS typically follows AD inheritance, but see 'Deafness in early childhood' in Chapter 2, 'Clinical approach', p. 122 for exceptions and further details about the four types of WS.

Hypopigmentary mosaicism (previously hypomelanosis of Ito)

Areas of the skin may be affected by hypopigmented streaks or whorls distributed along the lines of Blaschko. It may be particularly striking over the trunk. Individuals can be otherwise healthy; however, associated abnormalities can include neurological, ophthalmological, dental, and skeletal, and appropriate investigations should be performed. A mosaic chromosomal aetiology has been found in ~60% of reported individuals.

Incontinentia pigmenti (IP) type 2
XLD disorder caused by mutations in the *IKBKG* gene. Eighty per cent carry a common deletion. Skin features occur in four stages which are not always all seen.

- Stage 1. First few days or weeks of life: blistering lesions cropping in distribution of Blaschko's lines (vesicular fluid is highly eosinophilic), accompanied by marked peripheral blood eosinophilia. Linear distribution along the limbs, circumferential on the trunk, usually spares the face (from birth to 4 months; there are rare reports of onset as late as 18 months).
- Stage 2. Verrucous lesions (less widespread, often confined to the lower legs; <6 months).
- Stage 3. Streaky lines of hyperpigmentation, especially in the axillae and groin (childhood and teens).
- Stage 4. Pale, atrophic streaks, particularly noticeable on the back of the calves (from childhood to adult). Forty per cent have nail dystrophy; 80% have dental abnormalities affecting deciduous and/or permanent dentition, e.g. missing teeth, small teeth, delayed eruption, conical teeth, accessory cusps. Hair is often sparse in childhood and later is wiry/coarse; there may be patchy alopecia. Thirty per cent have eye findings, but most have normal vision. Seizures in 14%, which are persistent in 6%. Learning disability in 10% of affected females. Affected male pregnancies are usually lost spontaneously in the first or early second trimester.

Adapted by permission from BMJ Publishing Group Limited, *Journal of Medical Genetics*, S J Landy, D Donnai, Incontinentia pigmenti (Bloch-Sulzberger syndrome), volume 30, issue 1, pp. 53–59, copyright 1993, BMJ Publishing Group Ltd.

Microphthalmia with linear skin defects (MLS)
Girls with MLS syndrome have microphthalmia with linear skin defects of the face and neck, which can be hypopigmented, hyperpigmented, or erythematous. There is associated sclerocornea, corpus callosum agenesis, and other brain anomalies. This XLD, male-lethal condition is associated with mutations affecting *HCCS*.

Goltz syndrome
An XLD condition due to mutations in the *PORCN* gene. Areas of focal dermal hypoplasia may be found on the trunk and limbs and there may fat herniation through the skin deficiency. Again lesions can be hypo- or hyperpigmented or erythematous. See 'Coloboma' in Chapter 2, 'Clinical approach', p. 110.

Rothmund–Thomson syndrome
Characterized by poikiloderma congenita, with growth deficiency, alopecia, photosensitivity, dystrophic nails, abnormal teeth, cataracts, and hypogonadism. The skin abnormalities appear before 6 months of age with reticular or diffuse erythema on the face, hands, and extensor surfaces of the limbs. Hypopigmentation can be a feature in the atrophic areas. The trunk is relatively spared. It is caused by mutations in the helicase gene *RECQL4*.

Genetic advice
Recurrence risk
As for specific disorder.

Carrier detection
As for specific disorder.

Prenatal diagnosis
Usually only possible if a specific mutation or chromosome anomaly has been identified.

Support groups: Tuberous Sclerosis Association, http://www.tuberous-sclerosis.org; Incontinentia Pigmenti International Foundation, http://www.ipif.org; Unique (The Rare Chromosome Disorder Support Group), http://www.rarechromo.org.

Expert adviser: Veronica Kinsler, Consultant Paediatric Dermatologist, Great Ormond St Hospital for Children, London, UK.

References
Alper JC, Holmes LB. The incidence and significance of birthmarks in a cohort of 4,641 newborns. *Pediatr Dermatol* 1983; **1**: 58–68.

Flannery DB. Pigmentary dysplasia, hypomelanosis of Ito and genetic mosaicism. *Am J Med Genet* 1990; **35**: 18–21.

Flannery DB. Skin: pigmentary disorders. In: RE Stevenson, JG Hall, RM Goodman (eds.). *Human malformations and related anomalies, Vol. II*, Oxford monographs on medical genetics no. 27, pp. 907–17. Oxford University Press, New York, 1993.

Happle R. Incontinentia pigmenti versus hypomelanosis of Ito: the whys and wherefores of a confusing issue. *Am J Med Genet* 1998; **79**: 64–5.

Prakash SK, Cormier TA, McCall AE, *et al*. Loss of holocytochrome c-type synthetase causes the male lethality of X-linked dominant microphthalmia with linear skin defects (MLS) syndrome. *Hum Mol Genet* 2002; **11**: 3237–48.

Spritz R. Piebaldism, Waardenburg syndrome and related disorders of melanocyte development. *Semin Cutan Med Surg* 1997; **16**: 15–23.

Sybert VP. *Genetic skin disorders, Oxford monographs in medical genetics*. Oxford University Press, New York, 1997.

Vanderhooft SL, Francis JS, Pagon RA, Smith LT, Sybert VP. Prevalence of hypopigmented macules in a healthy population. *J Pediatr* 1996; **129**: 355–61.

Patchy pigmented skin lesions (including café-au-lait spots)

The skin pigments (eumelanin and pheomelanin) are produced in melanosomes by melanocytes, which are large cells found among the basal cells of the epidermis. The melanin is then transferred to keratinocytes. Melanocytes are of neural crest origin.

The differential diagnosis of these conditions depends on the distribution and shape of the lesions and the presence of other features.

Clinical approach

History: key points
- Presence, or not, from birth. Have they changed in character?
- Increasing in number or size?
- Other skin lesions, e.g. plexiform neurofibroma in NF1 or lipomas with *PTEN* mutations.
- Blistering in the neonatal period (IP).
- Family history of similar lesions.
- Neurological features, developmental delay, seizures.

Examination: key points
- Make a careful clinical and photographic record of the skin.
- Are the margins of the lesions sharply defined or irregular?
- Does the pattern of distribution follow Blaschko's lines?
- Are the lesions flat (macular) or raised (papular, verrucous)?
- Document the number of lesions/areas of hyperpigmentation.
- Do they cross the midline of the body?
- How dark is the pigment and are there any darker areas within the area of hyperpigmentation?
- Areas of skin atrophy with loss of pigment and hair (last stage of IP).
- Any areas of hypopigmentation.
- 'Lumps and bumps', e.g. neurofibromas, lipomas.
- Eye and nervous system. These organs are particularly associated with skin disorders (neurocutaneous syndromes).

Special investigations
Some conditions have a presumed, or known, mosaic aetiology, either of a single gene or chromosomal origin.
- Clinical photography.
- Karyotype or array CGH of blood and/or skin DNA if mosaicism is suspected. Molecular genetic analysis is available for many pigmentary conditions.
- Skin biopsy for histology may sometimes be helpful. Consider referral to a paediatric dermatologist.

Some diagnoses to consider

Considering specific patterns of pigmentation narrows the differential diagnosis.

Irregular 'mosaic-patterned' pigmentation

INCONTINENTIA PIGMENTI (IP). (See 'Incontinentia pigmenti (IP) type 2' in 'Patchy hypo- or depigmented skin lesions', Chapter 2, 'Clinical approach', p. 276.) The hyperpigmented phase begins between 3 and 6 months and the distribution follows Blaschko's lines (whorled on the trunk and linear on the limbs.

MCCUNE–ALBRIGHT SYNDROME (MCAS). The pigmentary changes in MCAS are café-au-lait macules (CALM), but they are often more irregular ('coast of Maine') and larger than those associated with 'NF1'. Isolated congenital (previously 'naevoid') CALM pigmentation can, however, have a very similar appearance. The condition is caused by mosaicism for mutations in *GNAS*. Radiological and endocrinological investigations are indicated if MCAS is suspected. Molecular diagnosis is most reliable from affected tissue.

HYPERPIGMENTARY MOSAICISM. (See also 'Hypopigmentary mosaicism (previously hypomelanosis of Ito)' in 'Patchy hypo- or depigmented skin lesions', Chapter 2, 'Clinical approach', p. 276.) Increased pigmentation in a Blaschko-type distribution (whorls on the trunk, linear on the limbs) is indicative of mosaicism and has been described as a sequel of chromosomal mosaicism and functional due to XL disease (as in IP). Point mutations or small copy number changes are the likely cause of the remainder but have not yet been described. Mosaic-like pigmentary changes are also noted in some females with the X-linked ID disorders DDX3X and PHF6 (Di Donato *et al.* 2014, Snijders Blok 2015).

Café-au-lait macules (CALM)

CALM are the colour of milky coffee, though they are darker in individuals who are naturally dark-skinned. They have a sharply defined margin and are usually round or oval and can be any size. Ten to 20% of adults have at least one CALM; however, more than one in a normal neonate is rare.

NEUROFIBROMATOSIS TYPE 1 (NF1). This is the most common cause of multiple CALM. Affected individuals typically have six or more CALM of 1.5 cm or larger in post-pubertal individuals or 0.5 cm or larger in prepubertal individuals. These, however, may develop slowly, and six CALM are often not present until the age of 6 (Nunley *et al.* 2009). See 'Neurofibromatosis type 1 (NF1)' in Chapter 3, 'Common consultations', p. 506.

NEUROFIBROMATOSIS TYPE 2 (NF2). Typically 1–6 CALs. Only 4% of affected individuals in Evans *et al.*'s (1992) study had >3 spots; none had >6. See 'Neurofibromatosis type 2 (NF2)' in Chapter 4, 'Cancer', p. 596.

RING CHROMOSOME PHENOTYPE. CALs indistinguishable from those of NF1 are found in association with ring chromosomal abnormalities. See 'Ring chromosomes' in Chapter 5, 'Chromosomes', p. 682.

BANNAYAN–RILEY–RUVALCABA (BRR; PTEN HAMARTOMATOUS SYNDROME). A highly variable AD disorder consisting of macrocephaly, vascular malformations, lipomas, and pigmented macules on the shaft of the penis. See 'Cowden syndrome (PTEN hamartoma tumour syndrome (PHTS))' in Chapter 4, 'Cancer', p. 564.

SCHIMKE IMMUNO-OSSEOUS DYSPLASIA. A rare AR spondylo-epiphyseal dysplasia. The characteristic features include short stature with hyperpigmented macules and an unusual facies, proteinuria with progressive renal failure, lymphopenia with recurrent infections, and cerebral ischaemia (Boerkoel *et al.* 2000).

URTICARIA PIGMENTOSA (UP). UP is sometimes confused with NF1 because the mast cell infiltrates can resemble CALM, although they are raised. In this condition, rubbing the red/brown spots initiates histamine release from the mast cells, leading to localized urticaria and associated pruritus. Biopsy of these lesions is usually diagnostic.

RECESSIVE MUTATIONS IN MISMATCH REPAIR (MMR) GENES. Recessive mutations in the MMR genes *PMS2* and *MLH1* can cause a phenotype of CALM, axillary freckling, subtle generalized increase in skin pigmentation, primitive neuroectodermal tumours (PNETs), and non-Hodgkin's lymphoma (NHL). This NF1-like condition has a highly malignant phenotype and follows AR inheritance (Sheridan *et al.* 2003).

Patchy macular pigmentation (not typical of CALM)
Areas of pigmented skin that are macular but are not typical CALM can be found in a number of rare genetic syndromes, including syndromes with associated malignancies. Consider the possibility of Fanconi anaemia, AT, Nijmegen breakage syndrome, syndromes with *PTEN* mutations (Bannayan–Zonana, Cowden), and Turcot syndrome. See 'DNA repair disorders' in Chapter 3, 'Common consultations', p. 398.

Lentigines
These are brown to black in colour, with even pigmentation and a sharply defined border. They are darker than freckles and have characteristic histology. They are common and normal when seen on adult skin, but are unusual on mucous membranes or in children where they may be a hallmark of a single gene disorder such as Peutz–Jeghers syndrome (PJS). In these conditions, they often become apparent in early childhood. Lentigines are the cutaneous markers of several genetic disorders (Bauer *et al.* 2005) which include:

PJS. In PJS, lentigines of the lips, buccal mucosa, and genital skin are found in association with intestinal polyps. See 'Peutz–Jeghers syndrome (PJS)' in Chapter 4, 'Cancer', p. 604.

LEOPARD SYNDROME. An association of lentigines–ECG abnormalities–ocular hypertelorism–pulmonary stenosis–abnormal genitalia–retardation of growth–deafness. LEOPARD syndrome is caused by mutations in *PTPN11*;

CARNEY COMPLEX (CNC). An AD condition characterized by skin pigmentary abnormalities, cardiac and cutaneous myxomas, endocrine tumours, and schwannomas. See 'Multiple endocrine neoplasia (MEN)' in Chapter 4, 'Cancer', p. 592.

Congenital melanocytic naevi (CMN)
Single CMN are found in 1% of newborns. Multiple CMN (>1) are a sign of somatic mosaicism for mutations in NRAS (Kinsler et al. 2013). They can be associated with characteristic facial features (broad forehead, eyebrow anomalies, hypertelorism, short nose with a broad tip, long philtrum, and prominent/everted lower lip) (Kinsler et al. 2012). They can also be associated with neurological abnormalities and an increased risk of malignant melanoma. This risk is related to the size and number of the CMN. Neonates should be referred to a paediatric dermatologist for an MRI scan of the CNS and require monitoring for melanoma.

Acquired melanocytic naevi (moles)
Acquired melanocytic naevi are common and the average adult has 15–30. These should be distinguished from dysplastic naevi, which have the potential to develop into a malignant melanoma, and are often larger than 0.5 cm. Children with TS or an atypical mole syndrome may have

an increased number of pigmented or atypical naevi (usually second decade).

Acanthosis nigricans
Raised, thickened areas of darkly pigmented skin, more often seen in the axillae, groin, and neck areas. As the disorder progresses, the skin gets rougher and the affected areas enlarge. Acanthosis nigricans is believed to result from insulin resistance and can be associated with diabetes, obesity, or malignancy.

Syndromic causes of acanthosis nigricans include insulin resistance syndromes such as Donohue syndrome, Berardinelli syndrome, Crouzon syndrome, and Beare–Stevenson syndrome.

Poikiloderma
This condition is usually widespread but is particularly found in sun-exposed areas. Although there is hyperpigmentation, this is accompanied by areas of hypopigmentation, atrophy, and telangiectasia and is dissimilar to CALM and other forms of hyperpigmentation. It is found in Rothmund–Thompson syndrome, XP (see 'DNA repair disorders' in Chapter 3, 'Common consultations', p. 398), progeria, and Majewski osteodysplastic primordial dwarfism (MOPD) and Poikiloderma with neutropaenia (due to biallelic mutation in *USP1*). There are non-genetic conditions with poikiloderma as well.

Support groups: Incontinentia Pigmenti International Foundation, http://www.ipif.org; Unique (The Rare Chromosome Disorder Support Group), http://www.rarechromo.org.

Expert adviser: Veronica Kinsler, Consultant Paediatric Dermatologist, Great Ormond St Hospital for Children, London, UK.

References

Bauer AJ, Stratakis CA. The lentiginoses: cutaneous markers of systemic disease and a window to new aspects of tumourigenesis. *J Med Genet* 2005; **42**: 801–10.

Boerkoel CF, O'Neill S, André JL, et al. Manifestations and treatment of Schimke immuno-osseous dysplasia: 14 new cases and a review of the literature. *Eur J Pediatr* 2000; **159**: 1–7.

Di Donato N, Isidor B, et al. Distinct phenotype of PHF6 deletions in females. *Eur J Med Genet* 2014; **57**(2–3): 85–9.

Evans DGR, Huson SM, Donnai D, et al. A clinical study of type 2 neurofibromatosis. *Q J Med* 1992; **304**: 603–18.

Kinsler V, Shaw AC, Merks JH, Hennekam RC. The face in congenital melanocytic nevus syndrome. *Am J Med Genet A* 2012; **158A**: 1014–19.

Kinsler VA, Thomas AC, Ishida M, et al. Multiple congenital melanocytic nevi and neurocutaneous melanosis are caused by postzygotic mutations in codon 61 of NRAS. *J Invest Dermatol* 2013; **133**: 2229–36.

Legius E, Schrander-Stumpel C, Schollen E, et al. PTPN11 mutations in LEOPARD syndrome. *J Med Genet* 2002; **39**: 571–4.

Nunley KS, Gao F, Albers AC, Bayliss SJ, Gutmann DH. Predictive value of café au lait macules at initial consultation in the diagnosis of neurofibromatosis type 1. *Arch Dermatol* 2009; **145**: 883–7.

Sheridan E, De Vos M, Hayward B, Picton S. Recessive mutations in MMR genes are a cause of an NF-1 like phenotype with a highly malignant phenotype and a high recurrence risk. *J Med Genet* 2003; **40**(Suppl. 1): SP28.

Snijders Blok L, Madsen E, Juusola J, et al. Mutations in DDX3X are a common cause of unexplained intellectual disability with gender-specific effects on Wnt signaling. *Am J Hum Genet* 2015; **97**: 343–52.

Sybert VP. *Genetic skin disorders, Oxford monographs in genetics.* Oxford University Press, New York, 1997.

Plagiocephaly and abnormalities of skull shape

When asked to see a baby or infant who has an abnormality of the shape of the cranium, the aim is to distinguish a postural, deformational cause, which usually resolves with time, from syndromic or non-syndromic craniosynostosis.

Craniosynostosis, or craniostenosis, is premature fusion of one or more of the skull sutures. This fusion prevents or restricts growth perpendicular to the synostosis, but not in the parallel direction. Characteristic skull shapes arise, depending on the suture involved.

Descriptive terms for abnormalities of skull shape

These can be confusing. The skull shape can be described in terms of the length, width, and prominence of parts of the skull.

- Dolicocephaly and scaphocephaly. Increased length, compared to the width of the skull. This can be a postural deformation associated with prematurity and breech presentation but is also a feature of sagittal synostosis.
- Brachycephaly. Flattening of the occiput and forehead with increased width, compared to the length of the skull. This is a common postural deformity, particularly in infants with developmental delay, but also occurs when there is excessive growth in the sagittal suture due to bilateral coronal synostosis.
- Plagiocephaly. Asymmetry of the head shape. Postural deformation needs to be distinguished from unilateral coronal or lambdoid synostosis.
- Trigonocephaly. The forehead assumes a triangular shape and is a feature of metopic synostosis. It should be distinguished from simple ridging over the metopic suture.
- Turricephaly, oxycephaly, and acrocephaly all refer to a high, narrow, 'tower'-shaped skull. This is found in association with severe coronal or multisuture synostosis.
- Kleeblattschädel, or clover leaf skull. Premature fusion of all the cranial sutures. This is a serious, life-threatening condition with considerable morbidity and mortality that requires urgent surgical management.

See Figure 3.7 in 'Craniosynostosis', Chapter 3, 'Common consultations', p. 378.

Deformation

Deformational plagiocephaly may occur if external forces are applied to a skull with normal sutures. Many babies are born with mild asymmetry of the skull due to one of the factors listed below.

- Immediately after a difficult vaginal delivery, the baby's skull shape may have been 'moulded' due to cephalopelvic disproportion. Reassess the baby's skull shape at the 6-week baby check.
- Commonly, there is flattening of the frontal region due to mild compression in the later part of pregnancy. In most babies, this resolves, but babies with hypotonia and developmental delay are at risk of gravitational forces, accentuating the asymmetry if the child is unable to hold his/her head unsupported.
- The 'Back to sleep' campaign, to encourage parents to place babies in a supine sleeping position to reduce the risk of sudden infant death, has led to increasing referrals of infants with an unusually shaped skull (mainly brachycephaly) due to postural deformation.

In an infant with a postural deformation, the entire face and cranium appear to have turned around a central axis, with the forehead, brow, cheek, and ear all moving back and slightly down on the 'affected side' while reciprocal flattening is seen on the opposite side posteriorly. This point is very helpful when trying to distinguish between a postural cause and true craniosynostosis. In a postural deformity of the frontoparietal region, the ear is pushed back on the side of the deformation, whereas in unilateral synostosis of the coronal suture the ear on the affected side is further forward (see Figure 2.31).

If unable to determine if the asymmetry is due to a postural cause or if the deformity is progressing, refer to a craniofacial centre for evaluation.

Craniosynostosis

Premature fusion of one or more cranial sutures is found in one in 2500 live births. It is a heterogeneous condition and about 15% have a recognizable syndromic cause; in a further 10%, a genetic cause is revealed by targeted genetic testing. Molecular testing is indicated in children with syndromic and non-syndromic coronal synostosis. Thirty per cent of children with non-syndromic coronal craniosynostosis have mutations in *FGFR3* (749C>G, Pro250Arg) and a further 10–30% have mutation in *TCF12* (10% unicoronal and 30% bicoronal). An early referral to a specialist craniofacial unit should be arranged to assess whether there is raised intracranial pressure and to discuss the timing of operative treatment. Untreated craniosynostosis may lead to increasing intracranial pressure and asymmetry of the midface and, if craniosynostosis is suspected, expert assessment is mandatory. See 'Craniosynostosis' in Chapter 3, 'Common consultations', p. 378.

Clinical approach

History: key points

- Three-generation family tree. Enquire for family history of craniosynostosis or unusual skull shape.
- Pregnancy. Primiparity, decreased liquor, abnormal fetal presentation, persistent discomfort and sensation of the 'head being stuck', twin pregnancy (deformation), teratogen exposure especially sodium valproate causing metopic synostosis.
- Uterine abnormalities such as bicornuate uterus (deformation).
- Precipitate delivery (deformation). Relevant when assessing a neonate, but not for older infants.
- Obstructed labour (pre-existing synostosis).
- Skull shape unusual at birth.
- Progression of deformity.
- Sleeping position (deformation).
- Delayed motor milestones or prematurity may mean that an infant spends a longer period on his/her back, rather than holding the head unsupported (deformation). Some craniosynostosis syndromes have associated delay and untreated synostosis may lead to developmental problems.

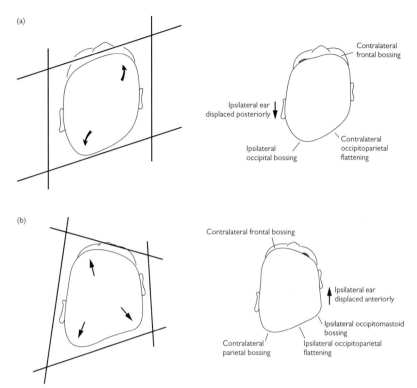

Figure 2.31 Diagram to illustrate useful pointers in the clinical differentiation of positional plagiocephaly and unilateral craniosynostosis. (a) Positional moulding of the L fronto-orbital region (the entire face and cranium are turning around a central axis). (b) Unilateral R-sided craniosynostosis. Note that positional moulding results in a parallelogram-shaped head with the forehead flattening on the opposite side to the forward ear, whereas unilateral coronal craniosynostosis results in a trapezium-shaped head with the ear further forward on the side of the synostosis.

- Seizures (raised intracranial pressure from craniosynostosis).
- Respiratory and feeding difficulties.

Examination: key points
- OFC and other growth parameters.
- Fontanelle. Position, size, and tension.
- Sutures. Palpate for sutural ridging (craniosynostosis).
- Skull shape. Examine the head from both sides, from above, and from the front. Describe the skull shape. Photographs of the head from the front, in profile, and from above (babies and young infants) can be very helpful and are also useful in documenting objectively whether there is progression or improvement in the skull shape over time. Look carefully for compensatory bulging/bossing (craniosynostosis).
- Ear position. Used in conjunction with the skull shape to assess if deformation or craniosynostosis is likely.
- Shape of the face and supraorbital area, asymmetry.
- Eye spacing (measure) and/or exorbitism; check for eyelid closure.
- Hands and feet for evidence of syndactyly. Fusion of digits in Apert syndrome; minor degrees of syndactyly in Pfeiffer and Saethre–Chotzen syndromes.
- Cleft palate (Apert syndrome).

- Broad thumbs and halluces (Pfeiffer syndrome), brachydactyly.
- Assessment of parental head shape, hands, and feet.

Special investigations
- SXR. PA, lateral. Interpretation is difficult in infants and requires good-quality films and expert reporting. The signs of synostosis are partial or total absence of the suture, indistinct zones along the suture, and perisutural sclerosis. Assess for evidence of a Harlequin sign (elevation of the lesser wing of the sphenoid) in coronal synostosis. If your clinical impression is that the child has craniosynostosis, seek expert advice, even if a routinely reported SXR is normal. Expert assessment and CT scanning may be required to resolve matters.
- Chromosome analysis. Routine analysis in the normally developing infant with no features other than plagiocephaly is not indicated. The presence of developmental delay would be sufficient to warrant investigation.
- Genomic analysis in presence of features suggestive of a chromosomal or syndromic diagnosis, e.g. genomic array, gene panel, or WES/WGS as available.
- EDTA sample for molecular genetic analysis in infants with syndromic craniosynostosis or non-syndromic coronal synostosis.

Genetic advice

Recurrence risk

- In infants with developmental delay and hypotonia, investigate and counsel appropriately.
- If there is an identifiable uterine anomaly, the recurrence risk for future pregnancies will be high without treatment of the anomaly.
- For infants with craniosynostosis, see 'Craniosynostosis' in Chapter 3, 'Common consultations', p. 378.

Carrier detection

For infants with craniosynostosis, see 'Craniosynostosis' in Chapter 3, 'Common consultations', p. 378.

Prenatal diagnosis

For infants with craniosynostosis, see 'Craniosynostosis' in Chapter 3, 'Common consultations', p. 378.

Natural history and further management

In plagiocephaly or brachycephaly due to deformation, the prognosis for a normal skull shape is good.

Support group: For craniosynostosis, Headlines Craniofacial Support, info@headlines.org.uk.

Expert adviser: Andrew Wilkie, Nuffield Professor of Pathology, Weatherall Institute of Molecular Medicine, University of Oxford, Oxford, UK.

References

Johnson D, Wilkie AOM. Craniosynostosis. *Eur J Hum Genet* 2011; **191**: 369–76.

Wall SA. Diagnostic features of the major non-syndromic craniosynostoses and the common deformational conditions which may be confused with them. *Curr Paediatr* 1997; **7**: 8–17.

Polydactyly

Post-axial polydactyly (PAP) is defined as an extra digit on the post-axial (radial or fibular) side of the hand or foot. Much is now known about the genes that control and initiate fetal limb development. The digits of the hand and feet are separated by 55 days post-fertilization. The prevalence is between one in 1000 and one in 2000 newborns and PAP is particularly common in Africans. PAP is classified into two types (see Figure 2.32).

- Type A (PAP-A). The digit is well formed and articulates with a metacarpal.
- Type B (PAP-B). The digit may be as small as a skin tag and is attached to the medial border of the fifth finger (pedunculated post-minimus).

PAP can be inherited as an isolated feature (AD with incomplete penetrance and variable expression) or can be a useful marker for a number of relatively common syndromes. It is often found with syndactyly or may be isolated or part of a syndrome.

Mesoaxial polydactyly (central or insertional)

The presence of a supernumerary finger or toe (not a thumb or hallux) involving the third or fourth metacarpal/tarsal with associated osseous syndactyly. X-ray shows a Y-shaped metacarpal bone.

Preaxial polydactyly (PPD) and triphalangeal thumb

In PPD, the extra digit or duplicated digit is on the radial/tibial side of the hand/foot. The thumb and hallux are the most commonly affected. A triphalangeal thumb is a digitalized or finger-like thumb with three phalanges.

There is great variability from broad distal phalanges to complete duplication. It is less common than PAP and, in isolated PPD, males are more frequently affected.

The aim is to establish if the polydactyly is an isolated event or part of a syndrome. Correct classification will aid syndrome diagnosis (see Table 2.29 and Figure 2.33).

Clinical approach

History: key points

- Three-generation family history with enquiry about presence (may be minimal) in other family members.

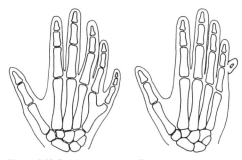

Figure 2.32 Post-axial polydactyly. The schematic shows type A post-axial polydactyly on the left and type B on the right. In type B, the extra digit is usually only a pedunculated tag attached to the fifth digit between the first and second flexion creases. Reproduced with permission from Stevenson RE and Hall JG, *Human Malformations and Related Anomalies*, Second Edition, 2005, Figure 21.3, page 944, with permission from Oxford University Press, New York, USA. www.oup.com.

Table 2.29 Classification of preaxial polydactyly

Type of preaxial polydactyly	Description
Type I	Duplication of the thumb/hallux
Type II	Triphalangeal thumbs/duplication of the hallux
Type III	Absent thumbs: one or two extra preaxial digits
Type IV	Broad thumbs, preaxial polysyndactyly, post-axial polydactyly

Reproduced from Temtamy SA and McKusick VA, *The genetics of hand malformations*, copyright 1978, Alan R. Liss, New York, with permission from Wiley.

- Consanguinity. Ciliopathies, deafness–onychodystrophy–onycholysis–retardation (DOOR) syndrome, Carpenter syndrome, acrocallosal syndrome (ACS)).
- Maternal age (trisomy 13).
- Early pregnancy events/teratogen exposure, maternal diabetes.
- Failure to thrive (marked in SLO syndrome).
- Developmental delay.

Examination: key points

- Hands and feet. Describe the shape and count the total number of digits. A good way to document this in the clinic is to put the hand/foot directly on the paper and draw around it.
- Post-axial digit fully formed of the small minimus/nubbin of tissue.
- Thumb. Document the structure and function:
  - (1) number of phalanges; three phalanges known as 'triphalangeal';
  - (2) if duplicated;
  - (3) if broad;
  - (4) opposition.
- Hallux (great or big toe). Document the structure as above.
- Mesoaxial polydactyly (Pallister–Hall, *LZTFL1* (BBS17).
- Other types of polydactyly, syndactyly, and limb defects.
- Features suggestive of any other skeletal abnormalities or limb shortening.
- Short stature (EVC syndrome).
- Overgrowth (SGB syndrome).
- Obesity (BBS).
- Cranial shape (for craniosynostosis, Pfeiffer and Carpenter syndromes), size (macrocephaly (Greig syndrome) and microcephaly), and skull defects/scalp aplasia.
- Irregular breathing (JS).
- Eyes (microphthalmia, trisomy 13), pigmentary retinopathy (BBS).
- Oral frenulae, tongue hamartomas (ciliopathies).
- Cleft lip and/or cleft palate.
- Bell-shaped chest (EVC syndrome).
- Cardiac defects. (EVC, HOS, and TBS).

(a)   (b)

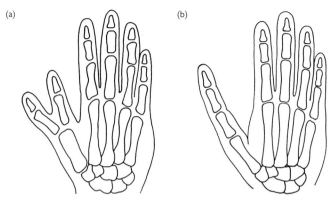

Figure 2.33 Preaxial polydactyly. (a) Preaxial polydactyly type I, showing partial duplication of a biphalangeal thumb. (b) Preaxial polydactyly type II (triphalangeal thumb), showing three phalanges in a thumb that is opposable.
Reproduced with permission from Stevenson RE and Hall JG, *Human Malformations and Related Anomalies*, Second Edition, 2005, Figure 21.4 and 21.5, pages 944–945, with permission from Oxford University Press, New York, USA. www.oup.com.

- Renal anomalies, especially cysts (JS and Meckel syndromes).
- Genital anomalies (Kaufman–McKusick, BBS, and SLO syndromes).

Special investigations
- Photographs and X-rays.
- Chromosome analysis: trisomy 13, del 22q11, and many other abnormalities.
- Brain imaging for structural abnormalities of the CNS; may start with USS in the neonatal period.
- Skeletal survey and SXRs, if indicated from the examination.
- Renal USS if there are other features of a syndrome with known renal anomalies.
- Cardiac echo in the presence of a murmur or the presence of other features of a syndrome with known cardiac defects.
- 7-dehydrocholesterol analysis (SLO syndrome).
- Genomic analysis in presence of features suggestive of a chromosomal or syndromic diagnosis, e.g. genomic array, gene panel, or WES/WGS as appropriate.

Some diagnoses to consider

Isolated polydactyly
Post-axial polydactyly (PAP) is approximately 10 times more common in individuals of black African ancestry, where it is usually inherited as an AD trait with variable expression and incomplete penetrance.

HOXD13 synpolydactyly
Also known as syndactyly type II; is defined as syndactyly between the middle and ring fingers and the fourth and fifth toes; variably associated with PAP in the same digits.

Syndromic polydactyly
The presence of the combination of PAP with pre- or mesoaxial polydactyly and/or syndactyly: the differential diagnosis points towards a syndrome diagnosis.

Chromosomal disorders
The most common example is PAP in trisomy 13. See 'Patau syndrome (trisomy 13)' in Chapter 5, 'Chromosomes', p. 678.

Syndromes
CILIOPATHIES THAT ARE USUALLY LETHAL IN THE NEONATAL PERIOD. See 'Ciliopathies' in Chapter 3, 'Common consultations', p. 366.

- **Meckel–Gruber syndrome.** Lethal AR syndrome with occipital encephalocele, bilaterally large kidneys with multicystic dysplasia and fibrotic changes of the liver, and PAP. The kidneys are typically filled with thin-walled cysts of various sizes. In Fraser and Lytwyn's (1981) study of 38 secondarily ascertained cases of Meckel syndrome, 100% had cystic dysplasia of the kidney, 63% had an occipital meningocele, 55% had polydactyly, and 18% had no brain malformation. Genetically heterogeneous. See 'Ciliopathies' in Chapter 3, 'Common consultations', p. 366.
- **Hydrolethalus syndrome.** An AR condition similar to Meckel–Gruber syndrome, but without cystic dysplasia of the kidneys. A rare disorder, but more common in Finland. PAP occurs in 80%. See 'Short limbs' in Chapter 6, 'Pregnancy and fertility', p. 784 and 'Ciliopathies' in Chapter 3, 'Common consultations', p. 366.
- **Short-rib–polydactyly syndromes.** A group of lethal skeletal dysplasias with AR inheritance, characterized by markedly short ribs, short limbs, usually polydactyly, and multiple anomalies of the major organs. See 'Short limbs' in Chapter 6, 'Pregnancy and fertility', p. 784' and 'Ciliopathies' in Chapter 3, 'Common consultations', p. 366.

NON-LETHAL CILIOPATHIES. See 'Ciliopathies' in Chapter 3, 'Common consultations', p. 366.

- **Bardet–Biedl syndrome (BBS).** Characterized by pigmentary retinal dystrophy, PAP, obesity, mild cognitive impairment, and renal defects. An AR condition that is genetically heterogeneous. *BBS6* and Kaufman–McKusick syndrome are allelic and caused by mutations in *MKKS*. See 'Obesity with and without developmental delay' in Chapter 2, 'Clinical approach', p. 254 and 'Ciliopathies' in Chapter 3, 'Common consultations', p. 366.
- **Ellis–van Creveld syndrome (EVC).** An AR condition characterized by PAP of the hands and occasionally

of the feet. Shortening of the limbs, small deep-set nails, multiple oral frenulae, and sometimes natal teeth. There is often CHD, usually an ASD. The ribs are short and the thorax is long and narrow. Radiologically, the features are difficult to distinguish from those of Jeune syndrome, but Jeune lacks polydactyly. The condition is caused by biallelic mutations in either *EVC* or *EVC2*—two non-homologous genes arranged in a head-to-head configuration on 4p16.

- **Mohr–Majewski syndrome.** An AR condition that is sometimes classified as OFD syndrome type 4 and also as one of the short rib–polydactyly syndromes, although the rib shortening is mild, allowing survival. See 'Ciliopathies' in Chapter 3, 'Common consultations', p. 366. Typically there is a midline cleft or notch in the upper lip, a high-arched or cleft palate, oral frenulae, and fleshy hamartomas on the tongue. PAP of the hands is common, with pre- or post-axial polydactyly of the feet. Complex CHD, e.g. tetralogy of Fallot and TGA may occur.

- **Kaufman–McKusick syndrome** (hydrometacolpos–polydactyly syndrome). An AR condition characterized by PAP, sometimes with syndactyly. Female infants have hydrometacolpos with an imperforate hymen or vaginal atresia. Cyanotic CHD is common. Caused by mutations in the *MKKS* gene and allelic to *BBS6*—see below.

- **Joubert syndrome (JS).** An AR condition usually diagnosed in infancy with hypotonia and cerebellar vermis hypoplasia and a characteristic episodic respiratory pattern. Polydactyly is an occasional feature. Genetically heterogeneous. See 'Ciliopathies' in Chapter 3, 'Common consultations', p. 366.

- **Oro-facial-digital (OFD) syndromes**, especially OFD type 1. OFD type 1 is an XLD malformation syndrome caused by mutation in *CXORF5*. The features in the hands and feet are PPD, syndactyly, usually skin syndactyly affecting variable digits, brachydactyly, and sometimes PAP. Craniofacial anomalies are midline cleft lip, tongue cysts, and excess oral frenulae.

GLI3-RELATED SYNDROMES.

- **Greig cephalopolysyndactyly.** An AD condition characterized by a high forehead with frontal bossing, macrocephaly, hypertelorism, rarely metopic synostosis, and a broad base to the nose. Both pre- and post-axial polydactyly can occur. The thumbs are broad; the halluces are often duplicated. Caused by mutations in *GLI3* on 7p13.

- **Pallister–Hall syndrome (anocerebrodigital syndrome).** Characterized by imperforate anus, post-axial (or often *mesoaxial*) polydactyly, hypopituitarism, and hypothalamic hamartoblastoma. Approximately 50% have a cleft larynx or bifid epiglottis. An AD condition with a very variable expression, caused by mutations in *GLI3* on 7p13.

OTHER SYNDROMES WITH POST-POLYDACTYLY.

- **Simpson–Golabi–Behmel (SGB) syndrome.** An XLR condition characterized by overgrowth and caused by mutations in *glypican 3*. Some have PAP. See 'Overgrowth' in Chapter 2, 'Clinical approach', p. 272.

- **Smith–Lemli–Opitz (SLO) syndrome.** Approximately 50% have PAP. Other features are pre- and postnatal growth deficiency and developmental delay (almost all), cleft palate (37–52%), cardiac defects (36–38%), hypospadias and/or cryptorchidism (90–100%) in affected males, and Y-shaped 2/3 toe syndactyly (>95%). See 'Hypospadias' in Chapter 2, 'Clinical approach', p. 186.

- **Central or mesoaxial polydactyly.** Consider *GLI3* Pallister–Hall syndrome and *LZTFL1* mutations (BBS17).

THUMB ABNORMALITY, BROAD AND TRIPHALANGEAL.

- **Lacrimo-auriculo-dental-digital (LADD) syndrome.** An AD condition characterized by the absence or atresia of the lacrimal punctae causing overflow of tears (epiphora) and recurrent infection, simple, cup-shaped ears with sensorineural or conductive deafness, hypoplastic teeth, and bifid or triphalangeal thumbs with clinodactyly. Heterogeneous: *FGFR2/3* and *FGF10*.

- **Pfeiffer syndrome.** *FGFR1/P252R* mutation. AD. Presents with broad, flattened, and medially deviated halluces, and soft tissue syndactyly of the second and third toes. It is included here because of phenotypic overlap with GLI3/Greig syndrome.

- **Diamond–Blackfan anaemia.** Characteristically presents with hypoplastic macrocytic anaemia in the first year of life; 75% by 3 months of age. There is a 20-fold increased risk of leukaemia. Only ~20% of patients have thumb anomalies (e.g. triphalangeal thumb). Most cases are sporadic, but, when familial, kindreds usually show AD inheritance with variable expressivity (although AR inheritance is reported). Approximately 20% of patients have heterozygous mutations in the ribosomal subunit gene *RPS19* on 19q13.

- **Deafness–onychodystrophy–onycholysis–retardation (DOOR) syndrome.** A rare AR syndrome in which the nails can be absent with hypoplasia of the distal phalanges. There is congenital deafness and there may be triphalangeal thumbs.

- **Holt–Oram syndrome (HOS).** An AD heart–hand syndrome caused by mutations in *TBX5*. Penetrance is 100%. Skeletal defects affect the upper limbs exclusively and are invariably bilateral and usually asymmetrical. They range from clinodactyly, limited supination, and narrow, sloping shoulders to absent, hypoplastic, or triphalangeal thumbs and severe reduction deformities of the upper arm (4.5%).

- **Townes–Brock syndrome (TBS).** An AD condition with imperforate anus, hand anomalies (triphalangeal thumb, hypoplastic thumb), and ear malformations (dysplastic ears and ear tags) with sensorineural hearing loss. Within and between families, the phenotype displays striking variability. *SALL1*, a zinc finger transcription factor, is the disease-causing gene. High incidence of new mutations. Cardiac anomalies are part of the phenotype.

Genetic advice

Recurrence risk

A unilateral polydactyly without other features may be a sporadic event, but bilateral changes affecting the hands and feet are likely to be genetic and most commonly dominantly inherited. Carefully examine the parents and exclude features of syndromes.

- Isolated PAP and isolated triphalangeal thumb usually follows AD inheritance, but the condition is not always fully penetrant.

- Syndromic polydactyly. Counsel, as appropriate, for the underlying syndrome.

Prenatal diagnosis

- Genetic testing for some of these syndromes may be available.
- USS. A well-formed extra digit can be visualized from the second trimester. Other ultrasound markers should be used to confirm a diagnosis.

Support groups: Many of the syndromes have their own support groups. See Contact a Family, http://www.cafamily.org.uk; National Organization for Rare Disorders (USA), http://www.rarediseases.org.

Expert adviser: Stefan Mundlos, Group Leader of the Research Group Development & Disease, Max Planck Institute for Molecular Genetics, Berlin, Germany.

References

Biesecker LG, Aase JM, Clericuzio C, Gurrieri F, Temple IK, Toriello H. Elements of morphology: standard terminology for the hands and feet. *Am J Med Genet A* 2009; **149A**: 93–127.

Biesecker LG. Polydactyly: how many disorders and how many genes? 2010 update. Dev Dyn 2011; **240**: 931–42.

Fraser FC, Lytwyn A. Spectrum of anomalies in the Meckel syndrome, or: 'Maybe there is a malformation syndrome with at least one constant anomaly'. *Am J Med Genet* 1981; **9**: 67–73.

Huber C, Cormier-Daire V. Ciliary disorder of the skeleton. *Am J Med Genet C Semin Med Genet* 2012; **160C**: 165–74.

Malik S, Grzeschik K-H. Synpolydactyly: clinical and molecular advances. *Clin Genet* 2008; **73**: 113–20.

Temtamy SA, McKusick VA. *The genetics of hand malformations.* Alan R Liss, New York, 1978.

Prolonged neonatal jaundice and jaundice in infants below 6 months

Jaundice manifests as yellow discoloration of the skin and sclera of the eye. It is caused by deposition of bile pigments in the deep layers of the skin.

Jaundice (unconjugated or indirect hyperbilirubinaemia) is very common in newborn babies and many normal babies develop jaundice on the second or third day (physiological jaundice). Jaundice requires further investigation when it persists for >2–4 weeks. Cholestatic jaundice (conjugated or direct hyperbilirubinaemia) is always pathological, and early detection and appropriate management could save lives or prevent the need for liver transplantation.

Bilirubin comes from the breakdown of haemoglobin. This form of bilirubin is indirect bilirubin and is toxic to the brain (kernicterus and deafness) and cannot be excreted by the kidneys. Bilirubin is attached to albumin for transport and in the liver it is conjugated with glucuronic acid by the action of the enzyme glucuronyl transferase. Bilirubin can then be excreted in the bile and through the kidneys.

Geneticists may be asked to see children with prolonged jaundice to determine if there is a genetic cause, or contribution, to the problem.

Clinical approach

History: key points

- Three-generation family history with specific enquiry regarding:
  - consanguinity (metabolic conditions, ARC);
  - ethnic origin (glucose-6-phosphate dehydrogenase deficiency (G6PD), Niemann–Pick);
  - prolonged neonatal jaundice in sibling or parent;
  - drug/food reactions (G6PD);
  - other structural anomalies, i.e. CHD (Alagille syndrome);
  - previous affected half-sibling (same mother)—neonatal haemochromatosis.
- Intrahepatic cholestasis of pregnancy (found in some carriers of progressive familial intrahepatic cholestasis (PFIC)).
- Onset of jaundice, pruritus, scratching.
- Any fluctuation in the level of jaundice?
- Treatment given, e.g. phototherapy or exchange transfusion.
- Failure to thrive, steatorrhoea.

Examination: key points

- Confirm jaundice clinically.
- Neurological abnormalities (Zellweger syndrome, Niemann–Pick dsease).
- Large fontanelle (Zellweger).
- Facial dysmorphism (consider metabolic syndromes and Alagille syndrome).
- Cataract (galactosaemia).
- Hepatosplenomegaly (congenital infections, Zellweger syndrome, Niemann–Pick disease, cirrhosis).
- Heart murmur (Alagille syndrome).
- Bruising and bleeding (vitamin K deficiency).
- Contractures (ARC syndrome).
- Colour of urine and stool.

Special investigations

The geneticist is usually involved after the common paediatric causes of jaundice have been excluded. Note the following results:

- bilirubin conjugated/unconjugated—document levels and trends of conjugated and unconjugated bilirubin;
- gamma glutamyltransferase (gamma GT) (low to normal PFIC types 1 and 2, ARC, and bile acid biosynthesis disorders; elevated in most other causes of cholestasis);
- other LFTs and ammonia;
- cholesterol (often raised in Alagille syndrome);
- urine-reducing substances;
- haematological investigations for evidence of haemolysis (Coombs' test, rhesus, and ABO incompatibility, abnormal red cells, e.g. spherocytes);
- congenital infection screen—IgM (herpes, CMV, rubella, Coxsackie) (TORCH screen);
- thyroid function; consider the need for pituitary function tests;
- liver USS (structural lesions, choledochal cysts, biliary atresia), hepatobiliary scintigraphy (to evaluate biliary excretion), and/or liver biopsy.

Next consider the need for more specialized testing for genetic conditions:

- bile acids (defects in bile synthesis);
- alpha-1 antitrypsin level/phenotype;
- VLCFCs (Zellweger syndrome);
- 7-dehydrocholesterol if there are features of SLO syndrome;
- urine: mass spectroscopy of bile acids, organic acids;
- chest and vertebral X-rays (Alagille syndrome);
- echo (Alagille syndrome);
- ophthalmological exam (chorioretinitis seen in intrauterine infections, anterior chamber defects seen in Alagille syndrome);
- Genomic analysis in the presence of features suggestive of a chromosomal or syndromic diagnosis e.g. gene panel, WES/WGS as available.

Some diagnoses to consider

Non-dysmorphic babies

DEVELOPMENTAL ANOMALIES AFFECTING THE BILIARY SYSTEM.

- Biliary atresia. Jaundice gradually develops and is often not apparent for the first 2–3 weeks. It is important to detect the condition prior to irreversible liver damage occurring. The anatomy of the atresia must be defined and this is usually done radiologically. Extrahepatic atresia is the most amenable to surgical correction. Consider Alagille syndrome when there is paucity of the intrahepatic bile ducts. Once genetic causes of bile duct atresia have been excluded, the recurrence risk is low.
- Choledochal cysts. The typical presenting triad is pain, mass, and jaundice. However, they are sometimes detected prenatally on USS and may be an incidental finding later in infancy. Surgery is the treatment of choice. There is an association between congenital

anomalies of the biliary tree and the pancreatic duct with biliary tract malignancy later in life.

ALPHA-1 ANTITRYPSIN DEFICIENCY. A common AR disorder (1/1600–1/1800), characterized by a predisposition to emphysema and cirrhosis. In Sveger's (1984) survey of 127 neonates with ZZ phenotype, virtually all had raised liver enzymes and 14 (11%) had prolonged neonatal jaundice. Most of the infants with neonatal jaundice recovered, but overall three (2.4%) of the ZZ cohort developed cirrhosis in infancy or childhood. It is important to diagnose this condition because cerebral haemorrhage can occur (vitamin K deficiency). See 'Alpha-1 antitrypsin deficiency' in Chapter 3, 'Common consultations', p. 338.

GILBERT'S SYNDROME. Gilbert's syndrome is one of the most common genetic disorders and is characterized by mild fluctuating *unconjugated* hyperbilirubinaemia (normal 85 µmol/l), often precipitated by intercurrent illness. It is found in 4–7% of the general population; penetrance is governed by other factors, e.g. gender (much less common in adult women, possibly due to lower daily bilirubin production) and environmental factors. It is caused by homozygosity for the Gilbert-type promotor insertion (A(TA)$_7$TAA) in the *UGT1A1* gene on 2q37. Approximately 50% of the European and North American population are heterozygous for this promotor insertion and 9% are homozygous.

Prolonged neonatal jaundice is found in babies who are heterozygous or homozygous for Gilbert's syndrome but, in addition, have G6PD, Coombs'-negative ABO disease, spherocytosis, or prolonged breastfeeding.

CRIGLER–NAJJAR (CN) TYPES 1 AND 2. These conditions are also caused by mutations in the *UGT1A1* gene. They are characterized by non-haemolytic unconjugated hyperbilirubinaemia; other hepatic functions are unaffected and the liver is morphologically normal.

• Crigler–Najjar type 1 (CN1) is an AR condition which is rare in the Western hemisphere (prevalence <1/10^6, carrier frequency ~1/1000). It is caused by inactivating mutations in *UGT1A1*, resulting in a virtual absence of hepatic UGT1A1 enzyme activity and severe hyperbilirubinaemia (SB 340–685 µmol/l). Before the institution of phototherapy, CN1 was uniformly lethal due to kernicterus. Treatment with plasmapheresis and/or liver transplantation.

• Crigler–Najjar type 2 (CN2) is associated with intermediate levels of hyperbilirubinaemia (120–340 µmol/l) as a result of incomplete deficiency of hepatic UGT1A1 activity, caused either by compound heterozygosity for partial LOF mutations or compound heterozygosity for a CN mutation together with a Gilbert-type promotor insertion (in *trans*).

Intermediate levels of hyperbilirubinaemia are observed commonly in families of patients with CN.

GLUCOSE-6-PHOSPHATE DEHYDROGENASE DEFICIENCY (G6PD). G6PD is a red cell enzyme. Deficiency of G6PD is found more commonly in populations from Africa, South East Asia, and the Mediterranean. There are several subtypes. Haemolysis occurs after exposure to certain drugs and food (favism). It may contribute to prolonged neonatal jaundice if the child is also affected with Gilbert's syndrome.

GALACTOSAEMIA. Galactosaemia is an AR condition caused by a deficiency of galactose-1-phosphate uridyltransferase (which converts galactose to glucose) encoded by the *GALT* gene. Incidence in the UK is ~1:45 000 live births (estimated carrier frequency ~1/105); most patients are either homozygous or heterozygous for the *Q188R* mutation. Babies with galactosaemia usually present in the first days and weeks of life with feeding difficulties, vomiting, jaundice, failure to thrive, and progressive liver failure. Untreated, the disorder can be fatal due to overwhelming sepsis. Once galactose is removed from the diet, there is rapid improvement in the clinical symptoms. Babies may have cataracts, although many of these are minor and resolve with dietary treatment. Dietary treatment must be lifelong to stop recurrence of acute toxicity (Walter *et al.* 1999), but this does *not* prevent the long-term complications, which occur in the majority of patients (Schweitzer *et al.* 1993; Waggoner *et al.* 1990). These include ovarian failure in most females, speech problems, developmental delay, and specific learning difficulties. Growth may be delayed, but the final height is normal. Girls may require induction of puberty and counselling about fertility. Life expectancy of treated individuals appears normal. However, there are reports of neurological complications such as movement disorders and intention tremor with increasing age. Cognitive function may worsen with age and recent evidence suggests that there is endogenous production of galactose that may be responsible for the emergence of these long-term effects despite early diagnosis and appropriate dietary treatment.

PROGRESSIVE FAMILIAL INTRAHEPATIC CHOLESTASIS (PFIC). Babies present in the first few months. There is failure to thrive due to malabsorption. Loose stools are noted from birth. Liver biopsy is usually required to confirm the diagnosis. PFIC1 is due to mutations in *ATP8B1*, PFIC2 in *ABCB11*, and PFIC3 in *ABCB4*. All PFIC types are AR.

NEONATAL HAEMOCHROMATOSIS. A condition of acute liver damage with iron accumulation. This encompasses severe iron overload in neonates of undefined pathogenesis (not all are genetic) and is not linked to *HFE*. In many patients, an ill-characterized maternofetal alloimmune disorder appears to develop, and in others, diverse genetic defects, including disorders of bile acid formation, have been identified. Antenatal administration of immunoglobulins from 14 weeks' gestation appears to prevent the development of neonatal haemochromatosis in many subsequent pregnancies.

MITOCHONDRIAL RESPIRATORY CHAIN DISORDERS. These may present with prolonged neonatal jaundice. See 'Mitochondrial DNA diseases' in Chapter 3, 'Common consultations', p. 490.

With dysmorphic features

ALAGILLE SYNDROME. An AD multisystem condition characterized by bile duct paucity, cholestasis (abnormal LFTs and raised cholesterol), CHD (especially tetralogy of Fallot and peripheral pulmonary artery stenosis (90%)), vertebral anomalies (e.g. butterfly vertebrae), ophthalmological changes (posterior embryotoxon), and subtle facial dysmorphism (a prominent forehead, deep-set eyes, a straight nose with a flattened tip, and a prominent and, in some cases, pointed chin). Ninety-five per cent of Alagille syndrome is caused by mutations in human *Jagged1* (JAG1) which is a ligand in the Notch signalling pathway and plays a role in early cell fate determination. A small number of patients with Alagille syndrome were found to have mutation in *NOTCH2*. Five to 7% have a 20p12 deletion detectable by FISH with a *JAG1* probe. *JAG1* mutations in Alagille syndrome include gene deletions and protein truncating, splicing, and missense mutations, suggesting that haploinsufficiency is the mechanism of disease causation. There is no clear genotype–phenotype correlation. There is wide variation in expressivity. Investigate the parents of an apparently sporadic case very carefully by:

- LFTs and cholesterol (typically cholestasis with raised cholesterol);
- vertebral X-ray (e.g. butterfly vertebrae);
- echo;
- slit-lamp exam for posterior embryotoxon;
- assessment of facial features;
- molecular genetic studies, if possible.

The new mutation rate is ~60%; a small proportion of parents with mild features may be gonosomal mosaics. However, there is a great deal of clinical variability, even within families, among individuals with *JAG1* mutations. The frequency of cardiac and liver disease is notably lower in secondarily ascertained mutation-positive relatives (Kamath *et al.* 2003).

ZELLWEGER SYNDROME. An AR peroxisomal disorder, often presenting in the neonatal period with central hypotonia ± seizures. The fontanelle is large and the forehead high. There may be stippled epiphyses (especially the knees). See 'Floppy infant' in Chapter 2, 'Clinical approach', p. 154.

NIEMANN–PICK DISEASE. An AR condition that is prevalent in the Jewish population and, due to consanguinity, also seen more frequently in the Pakistani population. Features are hepatomegaly, cholestatic jaundice, and neurological deterioration. There is deficiency of sphingomyelinase and the causative gene is acid sphingomyelinase (*SMPD1*) on 11p15.4. The prognosis is poor for those with type A. Niemann–Pick type B and Niemann–Pick type C have an older age of onset.

SOTOS SYNDROME. An overgrowth disorder in which neonatal jaundice is often seen. It is caused by heterozygous variants in the NSD1 gene. See 'Overgrowth' in Chapter 2, 'Clinical approach', p. 272.

ARTHROGRYPOSIS, RENAL DYSFUNCTION, CHOLESTASIS (ARC) SYNDROME. An AR syndrome characterized by arthrogryposis, neonatal cholestasis with bile duct hypoplasia, and renal dysfunction. Affected infants fail to thrive and usually die in the first year of life. Caused by mutations in the *VPS33B* gene on 15q26.1, involved in the regulation and fusion of membrane-bound organelles (Gissen *et al.* 2004).

Genetic advice

Recurrence risk
As appropriate for the cause of the jaundice.

Carrier detection
- Is possible in families where a causative mutation has been identified.

- May be possible for some biochemical abnormalities.

Prenatal diagnosis
Available to those families where there is molecular or biochemical confirmation of the diagnosis.

Natural history and further management (preventative measures)
Children with chronic liver disease should be under the care of a paediatric hepatologist. After biliary atresia, alpha-1 antitrypsin deficiency is the most frequent reason for liver transplantation in childhood.

Support group: Children's Liver Disease Foundation, http://www.childliverdisease.org, Tel. 0121 212 3839.

Expert adviser: Paul Gissen, Head of Genetics and Genomic Medicine Programme, University College London Institute of Child Health, Great Ormond Street Hospital for Children, London, UK.

References
Gissen P, Johnson CA, Morgan NV, et al. Mutations in *VPS33B*, encoding a regulator of SNARE-dependent membrane fusion, cause arthrogryposis-renal dysfunction-cholestasis (ARC) syndrome. *Nat Genet* 2004; **36**: 400–4.

Hartley JL, Gissen P, Kelly DA. Alagille syndrome and other hereditary causes of cholestasis. *Clin Liver Dis* 2013; **17**: 279–300.

Kadakol A, Sappal BS, Ghosh SS, et al. Interaction of coding region mutations and the Gilbert-type pomoter abnormality of the UGT1A1 gene causes moderate degrees of unconjugated hyperbilirubinaemia and may lead to neonatal kernicterus. *J Med Genet* 2001; **38**: 244–9.

Kamath BM, Bason L, Piccoli DA, Krantz ID, Spinner NB. Consequences of *JAG1* mutations. *J Med Genet* 2003; **40**: 891–5.

Kaplan M. Genetic interactions in the pathogenesis of neonatal hyperbilirubinaemia: Gilberts syndrome and glucose-6-phosphate dehydrogenase deficiency. *J Perinatol* 2001; **21**(Suppl 1): S30–4.

Krantz ID. Alagille syndrome: chipping away at the tip of the iceberg. *Am J Med Genet* 2002; **112**: 160–2.

Krantz ID, Colliton RP, Genin A, et al. Spectrum and frequency of *JAGGED1* (*JAG1*) mutations in Alagille syndrome patients and their families. *Am J Hum Genet* 1998; **62**: 1361–9.

National Metabolic Biochemistry Network. http://www.metbio. net/metbioHome.asp.

Schweitzer S, Shin Y, Jakobs C, Brodehl J. Long-term outcome in 134 patients with galactosaemia. *Eur J Pediatr* 1993; **152**: 36–43.

Shimotake T, Aoi S, Tomiyama H, Iwai N. DPC-4 (Smad-4) and Kras gene mutations in biliary tract epithelium in children with anomalous pancreaticobiliary ductal union. *J Pediatr Surg* 2003; **38**: 694–7.

Sveger T. Prospective study of children with alpha 1-antitrypsin deficiency: eight-year-old follow-up. *J Pediatr* 1984; **104**: 91–4.

Waggoner DD, Buist NR, Donnell GN. Long-term prognosis in galactosaemia: results of a survey of 350 cases. *J Inherit Metab Dis* 1990; **13**: 802–18.

Walter JH, Collins JE, Leonard JV. Recommendations for the management of galactosaemia. UK Galactosaemia Steering Group. *Arch Dis Child* 1999; **80**: 93–6.

Ptosis, blepharophimosis, and other eyelid anomalies

Ptosis (drooping of the eyelids) is an abnormality of eyelid elevation caused by poor function of the levator palpebrae superioris (LPS) muscle. This muscle has unique fibre types and is rich in mitochondria that make it fatigue-resistant. Ptosis is a feature of many neuromuscular conditions and may be due to a primary abnormality of the muscle or due to a disorder of its innervation. Despite the relatively long list of conditions of which ptosis is a feature, simple or congenital ptosis is the most common cause and results from a dysplasia of the levator muscle. It occurs sporadically and is non-progressive and usually unilateral.

Amblyopia may coexist with ptosis as a result of a coexisting squint or refractive error, but is only caused by the ptosis if the visual axis is obstructed (rare). The amblyopia is corrected before the ptosis, unless the pupil is obstructed.

Blepharophimosis is a decrease in palpebral fissure aperture. The distance between the internal and external canthi of each eye is reduced.

Cryptophthalmos is the covering of the globe of the eye by skin. The skin is adherent to the anterior structures of the eye. The main syndromal association is Fraser syndrome.

Clinical approach

History: key points
- Three-generation family tree with specific enquiry about ptosis and neurological problems.
- Congenital/acquired.
- Progressive, fatigability (congenital ptosis is non-progressive).
- Muscle weakness and dysphagia (DM, oculopharyngeal myopathy).
- Surgery to the head and neck and other trauma.
- CNS disease.
- Developmental delay/MR.

Examination: key points
- Eye movement, pupil size, and length of palpebral fissures (distance between the inner and outer canthi).
- Fundus. Pigmentary retinopathy in mitochondrial diseases.
- Muscle strength and myotonia (neurological disorders).
- Non-ocular dysmorphic features.
- Cardiac murmur (NS, Kabuki syndrome).
- Eczema (Dubowitz syndrome).
- Six per cent of ptosis is associated with a Marcus Gunn phenomenon. This is a unilateral ptosis that is reduced or overcompensated when chewing or sucking.

Special investigations
- DNA testing for mitochondrial conditions, DM, blepharophimosis–ptosis–epicanthus inversus syndrome (BPES), and oculopharyngeal dystrophy is possible.
- Anticholinesterase antibodies and Tensilon® test for myasthenia (usually conducted by a neurologist).
- Blood CK to exclude muscle disease.
- Ophthalmological testing as necessary.
- Genomic analysis in presence of features suggestive of a chromosomal or syndromic diagnosis, e.g. genomic array, gene panel, or WES/WGS as available.

Ptosis: some diagnoses to consider

Non-genetic causes
- Congenital ptosis (simple ptosis). The most common cause of ptosis in children. Often unilateral and non-progressive.
- Trauma, Horner's syndrome, IIIrd nerve palsy. Often unilateral and non-progressive.

Muscle disorders associated with ptosis

MITOCHONDRIAL DISORDERS.
- Chronic progressive external ophthalmoplegia (CPEO). Large-scale mitochondrial deletion.
- MELAS. Point mutation.
- KSS. Large-scale mitochondrial deletion.
- AD CPEO.

MYOTONIC DYSTROPHY (DM). Myotonia, cataract, frontal balding in males. AD inheritance with anticipation through maternal inheritance. See 'Myotonic dystrophy (DM1)' in Chapter 3, 'Common consultations', p. 496.

MYASTHENIA GRAVIS. Maternal transmission of antibodies to the fetus can cause arthrogryposis.

OCULOPHARYNGEAL MYOPATHY (OPMD). An AD disorder of late onset that commonly presents with ptosis and dysphagia. The genetic basis of the condition is a stable trinucleotide repeat expansion in exon 1 of the poly(A) binding protein 2 gene (*PABP2*), in which (GCG) (6) is the normal repeat length. The prevalence of OPMD is greatest in patients of French–Canadian origin (Hill *et al.* 2001).

CONGENITAL FIBROSIS OF THE EXTRAOCULAR MUSCLES. AD and AR forms. One gene is *ARIX* (*PHOX2A*) encoding a homeodomain transcription factor protein that has an important role in the formation of the IIIrd and IVth cranial nerve nuclei (Nakano *et al.* 2001).

Dysmorphic syndromes

AARSKOG SYNDROME (FACIOGENITAL DYSPLASIA). A genetically heterogeneous developmental disorder characterized by short stature (rhizomelic), ptosis in some, hypertelorism, hypermetropia, shawl scrotum, and brachydactyly with hyperextendable PIP joints. Facial features tend to normalize with age. MR is present in only a minority of affected males and is seldom severe. The XL form is caused by mutations in the *FGD1* gene. Behavioural and learning problems in childhood occur in ~50% of males with the XL form (Orrico *et al.* 2004). Some families appear to show AD inheritance.

BARAITSER-WINTER SYNDROME. AD disorder characterized by short stature, hypertelorism, bilateral ptosis, ocular coloboma, prominent metopic suture, and neuronal migration disorder. Caused by heterozygous mutation in *ACTB* or *ACTG1*. A recurrent *de novo* variant in *ACTG1* has been detected in isolated coloboma and no features of Baraitser-Winter syndrome (Rainger 2017).

MULTIPLE PTERYGIUM SYNDROME. AD or AR inheritance. May be evidence of myopathy.

NEUROFIBROMATOSIS TYPE 1 (NF1). See 'Neurofibromatosis type 1 (NF1)' in Chapter 3, 'Common consultations', p. 506.

NOONAN SYNDROME (NS). See 'Noonan syndrome and the Ras/MAPK pathway syndromes: neuro-cardio-facial-cutaneous syndromes' in Chapter 3, 'Common consultations' p. 512.

SAETHRE–CHOTZEN SYNDROME. A disorder characterized by craniosynostosis caused by mutations in *TWIST1* on 7p21. Asymmetric coronal suture involvement gives facial asymmetry. A low frontal hairline, ptosis, and small ears with a prominent crus are other helpful facial features. Examine for evidence of skin syndactyly, proximally inserted thumbs, or broad halluces.

SMITH–LEMLI–OPITZ (SLO) SYNDROME. An AR syndrome characterized by microcephaly, prenatal onset growth deficiency, cleft palate, 2/3 syndactyly of toes, small proximally placed thumbs, and sometimes PAP. Males have ambiguous genitalia or hypospadias with hypoplastic scrotum. 7-dehydrocholesterol levels are elevated. Mutations in the *DHCR7* gene on 11q13 lead to deficient activity of 7-dehydrocholesterol reductase (DHCR7), the final enzyme of the cholesterol biosynthetic pathway (Jira et al. 2003).

WIEDEMANN-STEINER SYNDROME (WSS). An AD condition caused by heterozygous variants in KMT2A (MLL) gene. WSS is characterized by excessive growth of terminal hair around the elbows (hypertrichosis cubiti), back, and lower limbs, in association with ID and a distinctive facial appearance.

Blepharophimosis (short palpebral fissures) with/without ptosis: some diagnoses to consider

BLEPHAROPHIMOSIS–PTOSIS–EPICANTHUS INVERSUS SYNDROME (BPES). In this condition, there is a reduced horizontal diameter of the palpebral fissures, droopy eyelids, and a fold of skin that runs from the lower lids inwards and upwards (epicanthus inversus). Mutations in *FOXL2*, a forkhead transcription factor on 3q, are found in ~67% of patients. Intelligence is mostly normal, except where there is microdeletion encompassing the gene. In type I BPES, eyelid abnormalities are associated with POF. Type II has eyelid defects only. For proteins with a truncation before the poly-Ala tract, the risk for development of POF is high (BPES type I). For mutations leading to a truncated or an extended protein containing an intact forkhead and poly-Ala tract, no predictions are possible since some of these mutations lead to both types of BPES, even within the same family. Poly-Ala expansions may lead to BPES type II.

DUBOWITZ SYNDROME. Is an ill-defined AR condition characterized by pre- and postnatal growth retardation, microcephaly, developmental delay/ID, sparse hair, telecanthus, ptosis, blepharophimosis, and prominent epicanthic folds. It likely consists of a number of genetically distinct and phenotypically overlapping conditions (Stewart 2014).

FETAL ALCOHOL SYNDROME (FAS). See 'Fetal alcohol syndrome (FAS)' in Chapter 6, 'Pregnancy and fertility', p. 728.

OHDO SYNDROME. Blepharophimosis is the key feature in the recognition of this syndrome, which is also characterized by ptosis, very small teeth, and mild to moderate learning disability. Affected children are often very floppy at birth and have major feeding problems requiring tube feeding. They have generally decreased movements, particularly facial movements. CHD is common and can be severe. Some have agenesis of the corpus callosum. All reports to date, except the original report by Ohdo et al. (1986) of two affected siblings and the report by Mhanni et al. (1998) of an affected mother and son, are of sporadic cases. A chromosomal

aetiology has been suggested in some cases. However, sporadic mutations have been identified in several cases in the *KAT6B* gene (Clayton-Smith et al. 2011). The same syndrome has been described by Young and Simpson (1987) with severe MR, a bulbous nose, and hypothyroidism.

Cryptophthalmos: some diagnoses to consider

FRASER SYNDROME. A rare AR syndrome, with a birth incidence of ~1 in 250 000. Part of the skin of the forehead may be continuous with the cheek, but the degree of cryptophthalmos is variable. In addition to crytophthalmos, the features are:
• 50–60% of cases, cutaneous syndactyly;
• 40–60% of cases, malformed ears with degrees of conductive deafness;
• 40% of cases, renal agenesis;
• 25% of cases, laryngeal stenosis;
• 20% of cases, abnormal genitalia (ambiguous/vaginal atresia/cryptorchid testes).
There are several proposed loci. Two genes have been identified; the *FRAS1* gene at 4q21 in Pakistani and Lebanese patients and the *FRAS2* gene at 13q13 in two Spanish gypsy families. It is not known whether the variability of the condition is caused by mechanical effects or other genetic factors.

Long palpebral fissures: some diagnoses to consider

KABUKI SYNDROME. Characterized by facial dysmorphism with long palpebral fissures, eversion of the lateral one-third of the lower lid, and arched eyebrows that are more sparse laterally. Postnatal growth retardation, skeletal anomalies with joint laxity, mild to moderate MR, and persistent fetal finger pads are present in most individuals with Kabuki syndrome. A highly arched palate or cleft palate, congenital heart defects, dental anomalies, and recurrent otitis media are very common. Breast development (premature thelarche) in female infants is frequently found. Between 50 and 75% of cases with a secure clinical diagnosis of Kabuki syndrome have been shown to have mutations in the *KMT2D* (MLL2) gene, while mutation of the *KDM6A* gene has been demonstrated in a small number of other cases of Kabuki syndrome (Banka et al. 2012).

Eyelid coloboma: some diagnoses to consider
See 'Coloboma' in Chapter 2, 'Clinical approach', p. 110.

Genetic advice
Recurrence risk
• Most forms of ptosis are non-genetic, especially if unilateral and non-progressive.
• Isolated hereditary ptosis is usually AD and non-progressive.
• Counsel as appropriate for the specific syndrome.

Carrier detection
May be possible if the molecular or biochemical basis of a specific condition is identified.

Prenatal diagnosis
If the molecular or biochemical basis of a specific condition is identified, PND may be possible.

Natural history and further management (preventative measures)
If there is severe ptosis, regular ophthalmological review is appropriate to ensure that the eyelids are not

obstructing the visual axis. Eyelid surgery may be considered for cosmetic reasons in older children.

Support groups: Many of the individual syndromes have their own support groups. See Contact a Family (UK), http://www.cafamily.org.uk; National Organization for Rare Disorders (USA), http://www.rarediseases.org.

Expert adviser: Willie Reardon, Department of Clinical Genetics, Our Lady's Children's Hospital, Dublin, Ireland.

References

Banka S, Veeramachaneni R, Reardon W, et al. How genetically heterogeneous is Kabuki syndrome?: MLL2 testing in 116 patients, review and analyses of mutation and phenotypic spectrum. Eur J Hum Genet 2012; **20**: 381–8.

Clayton-Smith J, O'Sullivan J, Daly S, et al. Whole-exome-sequencing identifies mutations in histone acetyltransferase gene KAT6B in individuals with the Say-Barber-Biesecker variant of Ohdo syndrome. Am J Hum Genet 2011; **89**: 675–81.

De Baere E, Beysen D, Oley C, et al. FOXL2 and BPES: mutational hotspots, phenotypic variability, and revision of the genotype–phenotype correlation. Am J Hum Genet 2003; **72**: 478–87.

Hill ME, Creed GA, McMullan TF, et al. Oculopharyngeal muscular dystrophy: phenotypic and genotypic studies in a UK population. Brain 2001; **124**(Pt 3): 522–6.

Hughes D. Eyelid disorders. In: A Moore (ed.). Paediatric ophthalmology, Fundamentals of clinical ophthalmology series, pp. 154–61. BMJ Books, London, 2000.

Jira PE, Waterham HR, Wanders RJ, Smeitink JA, Sengers RC, Wevers RA. Smith–Lemli–Opitz syndrome and the DHCR7 gene. Ann Hum Genet 2003; **67**(Pt 3): 269–80.

Mhanni AA, Dawson AJ, Chudley AE. Vertical transmission of the Ohdo blepharophimosis syndrome. Am J Med Genet 1998; **77**: 144–8.

Nakano M, Yamada K, Fain J, et al. Homozygous mutations in ARIX (PHOX2A) result in congenital fibrosis of the extraocular muscles type 2. Nat Genet 2001; **29**: 315–20.

Ohdo S, Madokoro H, Sonoda T, Hayakawa K. Mental retardation associated with congenital heart disease, blepharophimosis, blepharoptosis, and hypoplastic teeth. J Med Genet 1986; **23**: 242–4.

Orrico A, Galli L, Cavaliere ML, et al. Phenotypic and molecular characterisation of the Aarskog–Scott syndrome: a survey of the clinical variability in light of FGD1 mutation analysis in 46 patients. Eur J Hum Genet 2004; **12**: 16–23.

Stewart DR, Pemov A, et al. Dubowitz syndrome is a complex comprised of multiple, genetically distinct and phenotypically overlapping disorders. PLoS One 2014; **9**(6):e98686.

Young ID, Simpson K. Unknown syndrome: abnormal facies, congenital heart defects, hypothyroidism, and severe retardation. J Med Genet 1987; **24**: 715–16.

Radial ray defects and thumb hypoplasia

The most severe presentation is that of a radial club hand with a single, often rudimentary, forearm bone and an absent thumb. Milder phenotypes involve only minimal disturbance of thumb development. Non-articulating thumbs attached by a small tissue band (floating thumbs) are also seen. Radial and thumb hypoplasia may be unilateral or bilateral, and about 50% of affected children will have other anomalies that aid diagnosis and understanding of the aetiology. The upper limb bud is formed on days 26–27 after fertilization and limb development is complete by day 55. Environmental factors within this time can lead to varying degrees of limb defects. Some genetic syndromes can affect predominantly radial ray development and these are more likely to lead to bilateral features with less variability between the left and right sides. There is a strong association with haematological and cardiac disorders.

Clinical approach

History: key points

- Three-generation family tree. Ask about mild features that may indicate an affected individual. Note consanguinity.
- Pregnancy. Medication, bleeding or threatened miscarriage, maternal diabetes, drug exposure (e.g. vitamin A, retinoids).
- Birthweight (much reduced in trisomy 18, de Lange syndrome).
- Anaemia or other haematological problem.
- Cardiac murmur or surgery.
- Developmental delay.

Examination: key points

- Carefully describe and photograph the upper limbs and hands.
- Growth parameters. Stature and head circumference and cranial shape.
- Cleft lip/palate (Diamond–Blackfan syndrome, Roberts syndrome, de Lange syndrome).
- Malar hypoplasia and micrognathia (Nager syndrome).
- Duane anomaly, which is a complex type of strabismus (Okihiro syndrome).
- Examine the feet and lower limbs, especially the tibial ray, and exclude terminal transverse defects.
- Examine for evidence of scoliosis and vertebral anomalies (VATER (vertebral defects–anal atresia–tracheo-oesophageal fistula–(o)esophageal atresia–renal anomalies) association).
- Cardiac murmur (HOS).
- Pigmented skin lesions (CALs develop with time in Fanconi anaemia), haemangiomata.

Special investigations

- Genomic analysis if presentation suggestive of a chromosomal or syndromic diagnosis, e.g. genomic array, gene panel, or WES/WGS as available.
- Routine chromosome analysis, e.g. by FISH or QF-PCR (if presenting in pregnancy or neonatal life to exclude trisomy 18 and triploidy).
  - Fanconi anaemia (especially in the presence of bilateral thumb/radial anomalies, consanguinity, or other

supportive features such as CALs and microcephaly. Increased chromosome breaks on exposure to mitomycin C (MMC) and diepoxybutane (DEB).
- Roberts syndrome. Chromosome 'puffing'. Should be seen on careful observation of a routine microscopy-based karyotype.
- Baller–Gerold syndrome. This is a heterogeneous condition, with reports of some patients having the same cytogenetic findings as those of Roberts syndrome and occasional reports of *TWIST1* mutations (the gene for Saethre–Chotzen syndrome) in affected individuals.

- Haematological investigation. FBC and platelet analysis. Referral to a haematologist if abnormalities detected.
- X-ray of the affected limb(s). Consider chest and vertebral X-rays: vertebral abnormalities (VACTERL), cardiac enlargement, shoulder girdle (HOS).
- Cardiac echo and ECG; especially in the presence of a murmur or if there is a possibility of HOS or if there is a TOF).
- Renal USS (VATER and Fanconi anaemia).

Some diagnoses to consider

Fetal/neonatal death

Consider triploidy (see 'Triploidy (69,XXX, 69,XXY, or 69,XYY)' in Chapter 5, 'Chromosomes', p. 694), trisomy 18 (see 'Edwards' syndrome (trisomy 18)' in Chapter 5, 'Chromosomes', p. 670), and de Lange syndrome (see 'Limb reduction defects' in Chapter 2, 'Clinical approach', p. 212).

Haematological abnormalities

FANCONI ANAEMIA. A variety of radial ray anomalies are found in Fanconi anaemia, including absent, hypoplastic, supernumerary, or bifid thumbs and hypoplastic or absent radii. Twenty per cent have other skeletal problems (e.g. vertebral and rib anomalies). PND is not straightforward; consult your laboratory prior to counselling. See 'DNA repair disorders' in Chapter 3, 'Common consultations', p. 398.

THROMBOCYTOPENIA–ABSENT RADIUS (TAR) SYNDROME. Unlike many conditions that feature radial hypoplasia, *the thumb is present*. TAR syndrome is characterized by bilateral absence of the radii and thrombocytopenia. The lower limbs and the GI, cardiovascular, and other systems may also be involved. In a survey of 34 cases, Greenhalgh *et al.* (2002) found that all cases had a documented thrombocytopenia and bilateral radial aplasia, 47% had lower limb anomalies, 47% cows' milk intolerance, 23% renal anomalies, and 15% cardiac anomalies. The inheritance is unclear. TAR syndrome is caused by either a microdeletion at 1q21.1 or null *RBM8A* gene mutation in combination with one of two minor SNP alleles in the *RBM8A* gene 5′ UTR or intron 1 (Albers *et al.* 2013)

DIAMOND–BLACKFAN ANAEMIA. In this condition, red cell anaemia develops and may be treated with corticosteroids. Short stature is almost always found and other features have been well documented. It is likely to be the same condition as Aase or Aase–Smith II syndrome. It is genetically heterogeneous and mutations in ten different ribosomal proteins has been detected in

Diamond–Blackfan anaemia patients (Gazda et al. 2012; Horos et al. 2012).

With dominant inheritance

HOLT–ORAM SYNDROME (HOS). See subsequent Holt–Oram syndrome section.

OKIHIRO SYNDROME. Is the association of forearm malformation with Duane syndrome of eye retraction due to *SALL4* mutations (Kohlhase et al. 2002).

NAGER SYNDROME (ACROFACIAL DYSOSTOSIS). An AD condition with Treacher–Collins-like facies combined with radial ray limb defects, e.g. absent/hypoplastic thumbs and radial hypoplasia. Caused by haploinsufficiency for the *SFB34* gene (Bernier 2012).

With recessive inheritance

Roberts syndrome (pseudothalidomide syndrome). An AR disorder with symmetrical limb defects (severe shortening of the limbs, with radial defects and oligodactyly or syndactyly), together with craniofacial abnormalities. Caused by mutations in *ESCO2* (Vega et al. 2005). See 'Limb reduction defects' in Chapter 2, 'Clinical approach', p. 212.

With cardiac anomalies

VATER/VACTERL ASSOCIATION. Incidence 1.6/10 000. Usually 3–4 features present. Hall (2001) suggests at least one anomaly from the limb, thorax, and pelvis/lower abdomen for a secure diagnosis and at least two anomalies in each of two of those regions for a probable diagnosis. Normal cognitive development expected. Usually sporadic with low recurrence risk. The significance of the letters is as follows.

- V Vertebral defects. Usually upper to mid thoracic and lumbar regions. Usually hemivertebrae, but dyssegmented and fused vertebrae may occur. There may be accompanying rib anomalies.
- A Anal atresia. There may be associated genital defects (hypospadias, bifid scrotum) or fistulae.
- C Cardiac anomalies are present in ~80%—any type, any severity.
- T Tracheo-oesophageal fistula (TOF).
- E (O)esophageal atresia. 80% have an associated TOF.
- R Renal anomalies in 80%, e.g. renal agenesis/dysplasia.
- L Limb (radial defects). Preaxial with underdevelopment or agenesis of thumbs and radial bones, usually bilateral defects, but may be asymmetric. Reduced thenar muscle mass is mildest end of spectrum. Limb anomalies are restricted to the upper limbs.

Reprinted from *The Journal of Pediatrics*, Vol 82, Issue 1, Linda Quan, David W. Smith, The VATER association -Vertebral defects, -Anal atresia, -T-Efistula with esophageal atresia, -Radial and -Renal dysplasia: A spectrum of associated defects, pp. 104–107, Copyright 1973 with permission from Elsevier.

HOLT–ORAM SYNDROME (HOS). An AD heart–hand syndrome caused by mutations in *TBX5*. Penetrance is 100%.

- Skeletal defects affect the upper limbs exclusively and are invariably bilateral and usually asymmetrical. They range from clinodactyly, limited supination, and narrow, sloping shoulders to absent, hypoplastic, or

triphalangeal thumb and severe reduction deformities of the upper arm (4.5%). Hypoplasia of the thenar eminence accompanies thumb hypoplasia. The radial ray is predominantly affected and the left side is usually more severely affected than the right.
- Cardiac defects include ASD (34%), VSD (25%), MVP (7%), with ECG changes only in 39% (long PR interval, bradycardia, and left or right axis deviation being the most frequent). Pectus deformity occurs in 40%. Cardiac defects (including minimal ECG changes) occur in 95%.

The offspring of a parent with HOS who inherits a *TBX5* mutation has a 1:3 chance of having a severe reduction defect of the upper limb, e.g. absent thumb, and a 5% risk of phocomelia. Prenatal USS may be helpful in identifying the more severe skeletal and cardiac defects. Sequence analysis of *TBX5* detects mutations in ~25% of sporadic cases and 53% of familial cases of HOS (Brassington et al. 2003). Microdeletions and duplications of *TBX5* (and *TBX3*) may be detected by genomic array.

Environmental and teratogenic effects

Thalidomide embryopathy is the most well known. Other drugs and agents that have a vasodilatory action can cause radial hypoplasia, e.g. carbamazepine, alcohol. Vitamin A teratogenicity can cause limb defects, especially radial defects. Radial aplasia/hypoplasia is sometimes seen in diabetic embryopathy.

Genetic advice (for apparently isolated radial hypoplasia)

Examine carefully to exclude other features. Document if unilateral or bilateral. Examine the lower limbs. Listen for cardiac murmur.

Recurrence risk

- Apparently isolated and unilateral cases with no family history of limb abnormality. Most are non-genetic. Recurrence risk low and offspring risk low. Explain that there is a small residual risk due to the variability of this feature in dominant conditions.
- Apparently isolated and bilateral cases with no family history. All Mendelian modes of inheritance have been described, but X-linkage is rare. Bilateral features increase the possibility of a genetic aetiology. Carefully exclude syndromic and environmental causes.

Prenatal diagnosis

The radius and ulna can be identified from the beginning of the second trimester. Hypoplasia of the thumb would not be detected, unless there are absent thumbs. Prenatal testing for TAR syndrome can be undertaken by CVS or amniocentesis if radial ray defects detected by USS.

Natural history and further management (preventative measures)

Consider the need for occasional blood counts.

Support groups: Reach (for upper limb defects), http://www.reach.org.uk, Tel. 08451 306 225; Fanconi anaemia, http://www.fanconi-anaemia.co.uk.

Expert adviser: Ruth Newbury-Ecob, Lead Clinician, Department of Clinical Genetics, University Hospitals Bristol NHS Foundation Trust, Bristol, UK.

References

Albers CA, Newbury-Ecob R, Ouwehand WH, Ghevaert C. New insights into the genetic basis of TAR (thrombocytopenia–absent radii) syndrome. *Curr Opin Genet Dev* 2013; **23**: 316–23.

Bernier FP. Haploinsufficiency of SF3B4, a component of the pre-mRNA spliceosomal complex, causes Nager syndrome. *Am J Hum Genet* 2012; **90**: 925–33.

Brassington AM, Sung SS, Toydemir RM, *et al.* Expressivity of Holt–Oram syndrome is not predicted by TBX5 genotype. *Am J Hum Genet* 2003; **73**: 74–85.

Da Costa L, Willig TN, Fixler J, Mohandas N, Tchernia G. Diamond–Blackfan anemia. *Curr Opin Pediatr* 2001; **13**: 10–15.

Gazda et al.

Greenhalgh KL, Howell RT, Bottani A, *et al.* Thrombocytopenia–absent radius syndrome: a clinical genetic study. *J Med Genet* 2002; **39**: 876–81.

Gromp M, D'Andrea A. Fanconi anemia and DNA repair. *Hum Mol Genet* 2001; **10**: 2253–9.

Hall BD. Vater/Vacterl association. In: SB Cassidy, JE Allanson (eds.). *Management of genetic syndromes*, 3rd edn, pp. 871–80. John Wiley & Sons, Inc., Hoboken, 2010.

Horos R, von Lindern M. Molecular mechanisms of pathology and treatment in Diamond Blackfan Anaemia. *Br J Haematol* 2012; **159**: 514–27.

Joenje H, Patel KJ. The emerging genetic and molecular basis of Fanconi anemia. *Nat Rev Genet* 2001; **2**: 446–57.

Kohlhase J, Heinrich M, Schubert L, *et al.* Okihiro syndrome is caused by *SALL4* mutations. *Hum Mol Genet* 2002; **11**: 2979–87.

Newbury-Ecob RA, Leanage R, Raeburn JA, Young ID. Holt–Oram syndrome: a clinical genetic study. *J Med Genet* 1996; **33**: 300–7.

Vega H, Waisfisz Q, Gordilo M, *et al.* Roberts syndrome is caused by mutations in *ESCO2*, a human homolog of yeast ECO1 that is essential for the establishment of sister chromatid cohesion. *Nat Genet* 2005; **37**: 468–70.

Retinal dysplasia

Retinal dysplasia is a bilateral congenital structural abnormality of the retina. It is often associated with malformations of the CNS. Sometimes the description 'retinal folds' is used. In retinal dysplasia, there is failure of retinal and vitreous development, resulting in bilateral retinal detachment that is present at birth. Most cases are seen in males (Norrie disease is the most common cause of retinal dysplasia). The main conditions to exclude are retinoblastoma, severe forms of familial exudative vitreoretinopathy (FEVR), and, in premature infants, retinopathy of prematurity (ROP).

Clinical approach

History: key points

- Three-generation family history; consider X-linkage and consanguinity.
- Prenatal exposure to teratogens, trauma, or other adverse events.
- Gestation (ROP can give a similar picture).
- Neurological abnormality.
- Seizures.
- Bone fracture (osteoporosis pseudoglioma).
- Other eye pathology.

Examination: key points

- Microphthalmos and other structural eye abnormalities.
- OFC (either microcephaly or hydrocephalus may be found with MEB).
- Encephalocele (MEB/WWS).
- Other growth parameters.
- Lymphoedema.
- Polydactyly (trisomy 13, JS).
- Congenital heart defect (trisomy 13).
- Neurological examination, particularly hypotonia and weakness (WWS).

Special investigations

- Full eye examination.
- Brain MRI (migrational abnormalities, hydrocephalus).
- CK (elevated in WWS and cerebro-ocular dysplasia–muscular dystrophy (COD-MD)).
- Muscle biopsy in children with an elevated CK.
- Genomic analysis, e.g. genomic array, gene panel, or WES/WGS as appropriate.

Syndromes to consider

A common cause of retinal dysplasia is Norrie disease (see below), which can be confirmed by molecular genetic diagnosis (mutations in the *NDP* gene).

Isolated ophthalmic disorders

RETINOBLASTOMA. See 'Retinoblastoma' in Chapter 4, 'Cancer', p. 614.

RETINOPATHY OF PREMATURITY (ROP). A vasoproliferative retinopathy that may develop in very premature infants. In most infants, the disease is mild and undergoes spontaneous regression, but in a small minority the disorder progresses to total retinal detachment and blindness. The incidence and severity of ROP is inversely related to birthweight and gestational age. High levels of inspired oxygen are an important risk factor. Severe cicatricial disease is seen almost exclusively in infants weighing <1000 g at birth.

PERSISTENT HYPERPLASTIC PRIMARY VITREOUS. This is always unilateral.

Autosomal dominant conditions

Familial exudative vitreoretinopathy (FEVR). A rare AD condition characterized by abnormal development of the retinal vasculature that may lead to vitreous haemorrhage and traction retinal detachment necessitating surgical intervention. Genetically heterogeneous with four loci (*EVR1–4*) (Toomes et al. 2005).

AD MICROCEPHALY VARIABLY ASSOCIATED WITH CONGENITAL LYMPHOEDEMA AND CHORIORETINOPATHY. Due to heterozygous mutations in KIF11 (Ostergaard et al. 2012). Characteristic retinal changes are seen in some affected individuals.

Autosomal recessive conditions

WALKER–WARBURG SYNDROME (WWS) AND MUSCLE–EYE–BRAIN DISEASE (MEB). Are disorders that share the combination of cerebral neuronal migration defects, ocular abnormalities, and a CMD. The features of WWS are hydrocephalus, agyria, retinal dystrophy, and sometimes an encephalocele, hence its alternate name of HARD ± E. WWS is caused by mutations in the *O*-mannosyltransferase 1 gene (*POMT1*).

OSTEOPOROSIS PSEUDOGLIOMA. A rare AR disorder characterized by severe juvenile-onset osteoporosis and congenital or early-onset blindness. Other features include muscular hypotonia, ligamentous laxity, mild MR, and seizures. Mutation in the *LRP5* gene on 11q11–12.

COATS PLUS DISEASE DUE TO BIALLELIC CTC1 MUTATIONS. Mutations in the gene encoding conserved telomere maintenance component 1 (CTC1) were recently identified as the cause of Coats plus disease. This is a multisystem disorder characterized by: retinal telangiectasia and exudates (Coats disease), ICC with associated leukoencephalopathy and brain cysts, osteopenia with a tendency to fractures and poor bone healing, and a high risk of life-limiting GI bleeding and portal hypertension caused by the development of vascular ectasias in the stomach, small intestine, and liver (see 'Intracranial calcification' in Chapter 2, 'Clinical approach', p. 200).

X-linked disorders

NORRIE DISEASE. Affected infants are blind and have roving eye movements. Ophthalmological examination shows bilateral retrolental masses and USS shows evidence of bilateral retinal detachment without evidence of intraocular calcification. Shallowing of the anterior chamber may cause pupil-block glaucoma, which is treated surgically. About 50% of males with Norrie have learning difficulties and may show poorly characterized behavioural abnormalities or psychotic-like features. At least 40%, and probably the majority, of affected males develop a progressive sensorineural hearing loss starting in early childhood. Some boys also develop epilepsy. The diagnosis of Norrie disease is often difficult. The ability to test for specific mutations permits clarification of the diagnosis in atypical presentations.

Norrie disease follows XLR inheritance and is caused by mutations in the *NDP* gene at Xp11 that encodes 'norrin'. The majority of mutations are unique point mutations, but intragenic and submicroscopic deletions, including NDP and adjacent regions, have been identified in about 15% of patients. There is no genotype–phenotype correlation. Mutations in *NDP* are associated with a spectrum of retinal disorders, ranging from Norrie disease to XL FEVR, including some cases of persistent hyperplastic primary vitreous (PHPV), Coats disease, and advanced ROP. A clinical phenotype in carrier females is rare.

INCONTINENTIA PIGMENTI (IP). An ectodermal multisystem disorder that can affect dental, ocular, cardiac, and neurological structures. The ocular changes of IP can have a very similar appearance to the retinal detachment of XL FEVR, which has been shown to be caused by the mutations in the Norrie disease gene. See 'Unusual hair, teeth, nails, and skin' in Chapter 2, 'Clinical approach', p. 330.

JUVENILE X-LINKED RETINOSCHISIS. An XLR disorder resulting in visual loss in affected males in early life with splitting within the inner retinal membrane. A rare infantile form of juvenile XL retinoschisis may present with large bullous retinoschisis resembling retinal detachment. It is caused by mutations in the *RS1* gene on Xp21.1–22.1, which encodes a soluble secretory protein. There is no obvious genotype–phenotype correlation.

Chromosomal abnormalities

Trisomy 13. See 'Patau syndrome (trisomy 13)' in Chapter 5, 'Chromosomes', p. 678.

Genetic advice

Recurrence risk

As appropriate for the diagnosis. For an isolated retinal dysplasia, the geneticist should consult with ophthalmological colleagues over the likely aetiology.

NORRIE DISEASE. The majority of mothers of an apparently isolated male proband are carriers of an *NDP* disease-causing mutation, even when the family history is negative. Only rarely do affected males have a DNM. Intrafamilial and interfamilial variability in the appearance and expression of the cognitive and behavioural difficulties is common.

Carrier detection

Available in families where there is a known mutation.

Prenatal diagnosis

- Available by genetic testing in families where there is a known mutation.
- If genetic testing is unavailable, USS for signs of associated features, such as hydrocephalus, may be performed.

Natural history and further management (preventative measures)

Dependent on the diagnosis and associated features.

Support group: Royal National Institute for the Blind (RNIB), https://www.rnib.org.uk/eye-health/eye-conditions.

References

Beltrán-Valero de Bernabé D, Currier S, Steinbrecher A, et al. Mutations in the O-mannosyltransferase gene POMT1 give rise to the severe neuronal migration disorder Walker–Warburg syndrome. *Am J Hum Genet* 2002; **71**: 1033–43.

GeneReviews®. https://www.ncbi.nlm.nih.gov/books/NBK1116.

Meindl A, Berger W, Meitinger T, et al. Norrie disease is caused by mutations in an extracellular protein resembling C-terminal globular domain of mucins. *Nat Genet* 1992; **2**: 139–43.

Ostergaard P, Simpson MA, Mendola A, et al. Mutations in KIF11 cause autosomal dominant microcephaly variably associated with congenital lymphedema and chorioretinopathy. *Am J Hum Genet* 2012; **90**: 356–62.

Sabatelli P, Columbaro M, Mura I, et al. Extracellular matrix and nuclear abnormalities in skeletal muscle of a patient with Walker–Warburg syndrome caused by POMT1 mutations. *Biochem Biophys Acta* 2003; **1638**: 57–62.

Toomes C, Downey LM, Bottomley HM, Mintz-Hittner HA, Inglehearn CF. Further evidence of genetic heterogeneity in familial exudative vitreoretinopathy; exclusion of EVR1, EVR3, and EVR4 in a large autosomal dominant pedigree. *Br J Ophthalmol* 2005; **89**: 194–7.

Wang T, Waters CT, Rothman AM, Jakins TJ, Römisch K, Trump D. Intracellular retention of mutant retinoschisin is the pathological mechanism underlying X-linked retinoschisis. *Hum Mol Genet* 2002; **11**: 3097–105.

Retinal receptor dystrophies

The outer receptor cell layer of the retina comprises rods and cones, the light-sensitive photoreceptors. Cones work best in good illumination and are important for detailed visual acuity and colour discrimination. Rods work best at low illumination and, unlike cones, can function at very low light levels and subserve visual field and motion detection. Inherited retinal disorders are categorized by the cell population that is affected—rod, cone, or both—and whether the macula is involved (see Figure 2.34). There are now >200 genes associated with retinal receptor dystrophies. The age of onset of degeneration varies from infancy to adult life, depending on the causative genetic mutations. Most, but not all, of these disorders are progressive.

- Rod dysfunction. Patients with impaired rod function have poor vision in dim illumination (nyctalopia).
- Cone dysfunction. Symptoms of cone dysfunction include reduced central vision, sensitivity to light, and reduced colour vision. Those affected by cone disorders will often function better in dim illumination but will be uncomfortable and severely dazzled in normal lighting.
- Retinitis pigmentosa (RP) is a heterogeneous group of disorders in which there is early loss of rod function, followed by impaired cone function; foveal cones are affected late in the disease. In RP, the loss of rods leads to early symptoms of night blindness and later there is loss of the peripheral visual fields, often starting in the mid periphery. Examination of the fundus in the majority of cases shows pigmentary changes in the mid-peripheral retina. RP may be isolated or occur as part of a systemic disease or syndrome.

Macular dystrophy is a term used to describe central/retinal degeneration and appearances range from mild involvement to bull's eye to central atrophy. Electrophysiology may show that the disorder is confined to the macula; some macular dystrophies have both rod and cone involvement.

Pure cone or rod dystrophies are rare and most have involvement of both photoreceptors, although one type may be predominantly affected. Stationary congenital cone dystrophies are discussed in 'Nystagmus' in Chapter 2, 'Clinical approach', p. 252.

Genetic testing for inherited retinal dystrophies has been widely available in the UK since 2012 and at the present time, the majority is carried out using retinal gene panels. With good phenotyping and a clear family history, there is around a 55% chance of obtaining a genetic diagnosis (O'Sullivan 2012).

The aim of this section is to determine if the retinal dystrophy is part of a syndrome. If isolated, see 'Retinitis pigmentosa (RP)' in Chapter 3, 'Common consultations', p. 518.

Clinical approach

History: key points

- Three-generation family tree. Note if consanguinity is present.
- Age of onset.
- Neurological symptoms (mitochondrial disorders, ADCA, Refsum's disease), cerebello-oculo-renal syndrome (CORS), Batten disease, congenital disorders of glycosylation.

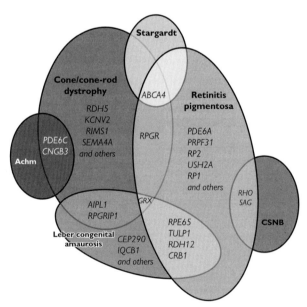

Figure 2.34 Genetic heterogeneity in retinal dystrophies. Diagrammatic representation of overlap between genetic causes of various forms of retinal dystrophy with some example genes shown. Achm, achromatopsia; CSNB, congenital stationary night blindness. Reproduced from Nash et al., Retinal dystrophies, genomic applications in diagnosis and prospects for therapy, *Translational Pediatrics*, Vol 4, No 2 (April 2015). Reused with permission from AME Publishing Company.

- Developmental delay (BBS, peroxisomal disorders).
- Obesity (BBS, Cohen syndrome, Alstrom syndrome).
- Diabetes mellitus (obesity syndromes).
- Deafness (Usher syndrome, Refsum's disease, Alstrom syndrome).
- Malabsorption (abetalipoproteinaemia).
- Renal disease (BBS, nephronophthisis).
- CM (Alstrom syndrome, mitochondrial disorders).

Examination: key points
- Verify eye signs.
- Weight (obesity index), height, and OFC.
- BP (renal disease).
- Facial dysmorphism (peroxisomal disorders).
- Skeletal anomalies: Refsum's.
- PAP (BBS).
- Dysmorphic features (Cohen).
- Prominent incisors (Cohen syndrome).
- Muscle weakness.
- Spasticity.
- Ataxia.
- Cardiac murmur/enlargement (structural defects and CM).
- Acanthosis nigricans (Alstrom and insulin resistance).

Special investigations
- Ophthalmology assessment, including full international standard electrophysiology (ISCEV), visual fields, and retinal imaging).
- Examine other family members (especially the mother in affected males to exclude an XL carrier state).
- Biochemistry. Basic biochemical screen of electrolytes, renal and liver function, and fasting blood sugar to exclude diabetes.
- Phytanic acid (Refsum's syndrome).
- Genomic analysis, e.g. genomic array, gene panel, or WES/WGS as appropriate.

Additional specialist investigation (below) is not usually required in isolated retinal dystrophies following AD or XL inheritance.
- Metabolic investigations, if indicated, for NCL, VLCFAs and phytanic acid (Refsum's), and abetalipoprotein B (abetalipoproteinaemia).
- Plasma amino acids (raised plasma ornithine in gyrate atrophy); vitamin E deficiency, vitamin A to exclude deficiency.
- Haematology. Neutrophil count (low in Cohen syndrome), acanthocytosis (abetalipoproteinaemia), vacuolated lymphocytes (Batten).
- Renal USS, (Senior Loken syndrome, Leber's amaurosis, nephronophthiasis).
- ECG and cardiac echo (Alstrom, BBS, mitochondrial disorders).
- Muscle biopsy (mitochondrial disorders).
- DNA sample. Mitochondrial DNA studies, SCA7, NCL (Batten), BBS, Usher syndrome. Store for future diagnostic purposes.
- Skin biopsy, UV irradiation (Cockayne syndrome).

Some diagnoses to consider

Autosomal recessive syndromes

USHER SYNDROME. Sensorineural deafness. See 'Deafness in early childhood' in Chapter 2, 'Clinical approach', p. 122.

BARDET–BIEDL SYNDROME (BBS). Rod/cone dystrophy, MR, PAP, obesity, renal abnormality (persistent fetal lobulation, dilatation of the collecting system with blind-ending cysts). McKusick–Kaufman syndrome is allelic. See 'Ciliopathies' in Chapter 3, 'Common Consultations', p. 366.

PEROXISOMAL DISORDERS
- **Refsum's syndrome**[*]. A peroxisomal disorder that leads to very high phytanic acid levels, with anosmia, ataxia, deafness, and polyneuropathy. Eye signs can precede neurological signs. So important to carry out phytanic acid testing in simplex and AR cases and look for skeletal anomalies, so that early dietary advice can be given.
- **Infantile Refsum's syndrome.**
- **Neonatal ALD.**
- **Zellweger syndrome.** Presents in the neonatal period with hypotonia and seizures and dysmorphic features, e.g. large fontanelle, high forehead, stippled epiphyses. See 'Floppy infant' in Chapter 2, 'Clinical approach', p. 154.

GYRATE ATROPHY OF THE CHOROID AND RETINA.[*] Rare, but treatable, AR disorder caused by deficiency of the mitochondrial enzyme ornithine aminotransferase encoded by the *OAT* gene. Presents with night blindness and myopia. The ERG becomes abnormal as the disease progresses. Plasma ornithine levels are elevated, and treatment with pyridoxine may, in a small subset of patients, lead to reduced plasma ornithine levels and slowing of the progression of the retinal dystrophy. Most affected individuals need to follow an arginine-restricted diet in order to minimize progressive deterioration of vision.

ABETALIPOPROTEINAEMIA.[*] Failure to thrive with fat malabsorption, acanthosis, ataxia, and absence of LDLs. Progressive pigmentary retinal degeneration accompanied by subnormal ERG changes are seen in patients with abetalipoproteinaemia caused by mutations in the microsomal triglyceride transfer protein (*MTP*) gene. Combined oral vitamin A and E supplementation that is initiated prior to 2 years of age can markedly attenuate severe retinal degeneration.

COCKAYNE SYNDROME. An AR neurodegenerative disorder characterized by low to normal birthweight, aged appearance, postnatal growth failure, brain dysmyelination with calcium deposits, cutaneous photosensitivity, pigmentary retinopathy and/or cataracts and/or optic atrophy, and sensorineural hearing loss. See 'DNA repair disorders' in Chapter 3, 'Common consultations', p. 398.

JOUBERT SYNDROME (JS). An AR developmental brain condition characterized by hypoplasia/dysplasia of the cerebellar vermis and by ataxia, hypotonia, oculomotor apraxia, and neonatal breathing dysregulation. A form of JS that includes retinal dysplasia and cystic dysplastic kidneys has been differentiated from other forms of JS and is designated 'cerebello-oculo-renal syndrome' (CORS). See 'Cerebellar anomalies' in Chapter 2, 'Clinical approach', p. 92 and 'Ciliopathies' in Chapter 3 'Common conditions'.

NEURONAL CEROID LIPOFUSCINOSES (NCLS; BATTEN DISEASE). Lysosomal storage disorders characterized by mental and motor deterioration, seizures, and visual loss. The juvenile form is Batten disease. Until recently, confirmation of these diagnoses depended on EM detection of specific lysosomal storage material in tissue—a rectal or skin biopsy or conjunctival tissue. It is now possible for most neurologists and geneticists to have access to molecular testing for the genes *CLCN 1, 2*, and *3* and enzyme analysis of palmitoyl-protein thioesterase (PPT)-1 and tripeptidyl-peptidase (TPP)-1. See also 'Developmental regression' in Chapter 2, 'Clinical approach', p. 128.

CARBOHYDRATE-DEFICIENT GLYCOPROTEIN SYNDROME. CDG are a group of AR metabolic disorders that are characterized biochemically by defective glycosylation of proteins (abnormal transferrin isoelectrophoresis). The most common type is CDG-Ia, which is a multisystem disorder affecting the nervous system (cerebellar atrophy and encephalopathy), liver, kidney, heart, adipose tissue (lipodystrophy and abnormal fat pads), bone, and genitalia. It is caused by phosphomannomutase (PMM) deficiency, and mutations have been identified in the gene *PMM2*.

COHEN SYNDROME. MR, obesity, prominent incisors, neutropenia—due to mutations in *COH1* on 8q22–23. Most affected children are myopic. See 'Obesity with and without developmental delay' in Chapter 2, 'Clinical approach', p. 254.

ALSTROM SYNDROME. Progressive deafness, obesity, small external genitalia in males, acanthosis nigricans, DCM, renal failure (glomerulosclerosis). Due to mutations in *ALMS1* on 2p13. See 'Obesity with and without developmental delay' in Chapter 2, 'Clinical approach', p. 254. The retinal dystrophy is an early-onset cone–rod dystrophy and photophobia is a prominent early symptom.

Autosomal dominant conditions

Autosomal dominant cerebellar ataxia (ADCA) with retinal pigmentation, *SCA7*. See 'Ataxic adult' in Chapter 2, 'Clinical approach', p. 70.

X-linked conditions

CHOROIDERAEMIA. A diffuse progressive condition that presents in childhood with night blindness. Later there is development of peripheral field loss and usually by the 50s loss of central vision. In the early stages, the fundus appearance may be confused with that of RP (although it is not primarily a photoreceptor dystrophy), but later in the disease there is a characteristic appearance with extensive atrophy of the choriocapillaris and retinal pigment epithelium. Gene *REP-1* at Xq21. Gene therapy has been started for this condition.

X-LINKED RETINITIS PIGMENTOSA (XLRP).

XLRP ASSOCIATED WITH DEAFNESS.

Mitochondrial disorders

May be sporadic, maternal, or autosomal inheritance. See 'Mitochondrial DNA diseases' in Chapter 3, 'Common consultations', p. 490.

KEARNS–SAYRE SYNDROME (KSS). A subtype of CPEO with a poorer prognosis. Onset is <20 years and, in addition to CPEO and pigmentary retinopathy, there is often a cardiac conduction defect and ataxia. Unlike CPEO, the condition is usually life-limiting. See 'Mitochondrial DNA diseases' in Chapter 3, 'Common consultations', p. 490.

Macular dystrophies

Types include Stargardt disease (caused by *ABCA4* mutations which, in some cases, progresses to generalized retinal involvement), dominant drusen (*EFEMP-1* gene mutation), and Sorsby fundus dystrophy. Best disease and pattern dystrophies (both of which are vitelliform dystrophies affecting the retinal pigment epithelium layer).

Genetic advice

Recurrence risk

- For sporadic individuals with RP, cone–rod dystrophy, or macular dystrophy in whom a definitive diagnosis has not been made after thorough investigation, the presence of these often bilateral and symmetrical findings are indicative of a genetic aetiology and a high recurrence risk. AR inheritance is the most likely mode of inheritance, although vitelliform dominant dystrophies are associated with reduced penetrance and variable expressivity.
- XL conditions should be considered if there have been two or more affected boys and/or there is a family history compatible with X-linkage, or if the ophthalmological findings are typical of an XL dystrophy. The mothers of isolated males with RP should have a careful fundus examination and ERG, as they may have carrier signs of the heterozygote. See 'Retinitis pigmentosa (RP)' in Chapter 3, 'Common consultations', p. 518.
- Some families with AD RP may show reduced penetrance. Some of the causative genes have been identified and molecular genetic diagnosis may be helpful in counselling (see splicing factor genes on 1q, 7p, and 19q). See 'Retinitis pigmentosa (RP)' in Chapter 3, 'Common consultations', p. 518.
- Mitochondrial conditions pose difficult counselling problems. See 'Mitochondrial DNA diseases' in Chapter 3, 'Common consultations', p. 490.
- Store DNA and/or fibroblast cell line for future diagnostic use. Check the literature for the availability of genetic testing.

Carrier detection

- Possible in those families in whom a causative mutation has been identified.
- May be possible for some biochemical abnormalities.
- Fundus examination and electrophysiology of other family members may help, particularly in choroideraemia and XLRP, but genetic testing should also be used where available.

Prenatal diagnosis

Available to those families where there is molecular or biochemical confirmation of the diagnosis.

Natural history and further management (preventative measures)

The visual loss is usually progressive. Regular reviews are indicated, as other co-pathologies may emerge, such as macular oedema, cataracts, and new diagnoses, and children may require psychological and educational support, respectively, with multidisciplinary team input.

Support groups: Royal National Institute for the Blind (RNIB), https://www.rnib.org.uk/eye-health/eye-conditions. Macular Society, RP Fighting Blindness UK, Fight for Sight, SENSE as well as local support groups.

Expert adviser: Susan Downes, Consultant Ophthalmologist, Associate Professor University of Oxford, Oxford Eye Hospital, Oxford University Hospital NHS Trust, John Radcliffe Hospital, Oxford, UK.

* Indicates treatable diseases.

References

Chowers I, Banin E, Merin S, Cooper M, Granot E. Long-term assessment of combined vitamin A and E treatment for the prevention of retinal degeneration in abetalipoproteinaemia and hypobetalipoproteinaemia patients. *Eye* 2001; **15**: 525–30.

Michaelides M, Hunt DM, Moore AT. The genetics of inherited macular dystrophies. *J Med Genet* 2003; **40**: 641–50.

Moore AT. Disorders of the vitreous and retina. In: A Moore (ed.). *Paediatric ophthalmology, Fundamentals of clinical ophthalmology* series. BMJ Books, London, 2000.

Nash BM, Wright DC, Grigg JR, Bennetts B, Jamieson RV. Retinal dystrophies, genomic applications in diagnosis and prospects for therapy. *Transl Pediatr* 2015; **4**: 139–63.

Nemeth AH, Downes SM. Disorders of vision. In: TT Warner, SR Hammans (eds.). *Practical guide to neurogenetics*, pp. 49–74. Saunders Elsevier, Philadelphia, 2009.

O'Sullivan J, Mullaney BG, *et al*. A paradigm shift in the delivery of services for diagnosis of inherited retinal disease. *J Med Genet* 2012; **49**: 322–6.

Rivolta C, Sharon D, De Angelis MM, Dryja TP. Retinitis pigmentosa and allied diseases, genes and inheritance patterns. *Hum Mol Genet* 2002; **11**: 1219–27.

Simunovic MP, Moore AT. The cone dystrophies. *Eye* 1998; **12**: 553–65.

Scalp defects

Aplasia cutis congenita.

Rare congenital malformation characterized by a local defect of the epidermis, dermis, and subcutaneous tissue occurring predominantly over the vertex of the scalp. The underlying bone growth is abnormal. There may be a single area with a 'raw' appearance—the skin is a thin, transparent membrane—or several small defects. It may occur as an isolated defect (when it may be familial) or occur as a feature of a chromosome disorder, genetic syndrome, or teratogen exposure. The defects often heal under conservative management. With time, the defect may change into a raised area of scarred granulation tissue.

Clinical approach

History: key points

- Three-generation family history with special note of scalp defects, cardiac abnormalities, and limb defects (including neonatal deaths).
- Pyloric atresia in an affected individual (epidermolysis bullosa with pyloric atresia or Carmi syndrome).
- Pregnancy history with specific enquiry about drug exposure (e.g. methimazole, carbimazole, an antithyroid drug, or misoprostol) or infection (intrauterine varicella or herpes).
- History of delivery (was there a difficult instrumental delivery or any possibility that the defects are traumatic?). Often the lesions are thought to be traumatic when they are, in fact, congenital.
- Visual difficulties (cone–rod dysfunction and myopia).
- Deafness (Johanson–Blizzard syndrome (JBS)).
- Developmental delay (chromosomal anomalies).

Examination: key points

- Position and number of skin defects (bitemporal aplasia in Setleis syndrome and focal facial dermal dysplasia, random distribution in Goltz syndrome).
- Hair growth. Hair does not grow over the affected areas. Unruly hair with cowlicks in JBS; poor hair growth over the temples in Pallister–Killian syndrome.
- Examine very carefully for transverse limb deficiency (looking at all fingernails and toenails is a convenient way to do this).
- Facies. Look carefully at alae nasae for features of JBS.
- Eyes. Structural malformations and epibulbar dermoids.
- Examine for other malformations, e.g. cardiac murmurs, hypospadias.
- Skin abnormalities at other sites, e.g. deficiency, blisters, scarring, pigmentary abnormality.

Special investigations

- Clinical photography.
- Genomic analysis e.g. gene panel, WES/WGS as available. Scalp defects may occur in +13 and 4p− and a variety of rare unbalanced chromosome rearrangements.
- Fibroblast culture for chromosomal mosaicism (Pallister–Killian syndrome).
- FE1 (a screen for pancreatic exocrine sufficiency) and thyroid function if facies suggestive of JBS.
- Consider SXR if the defect is very large (occasionally there are bony defects of the skull underlying cutis aplasia) to check for parietal foramina.

- Cranial USS in infants.

Some diagnoses to consider

Adams–Oliver syndrome (AOS)

An AD or AR condition featuring a combination of scalp defects and terminal transverse limb defects (usually minor reduction defects of fingers/toes and brachydactyly, although severe transverse deficiency can occur). Penetrance is incomplete and expression is highly variable, making this a difficult disorder to counsel. CHD may occur. Examine the parents of affected children. AOS is most usually caused by heterozygous mutation of the *ARHGAP31* gene, but there is genetic heterogeneity with several other genes associated with this condition, e.g. biallelic mutations in *DOCK6* or *EOGT* (Shaheen *et al.* 2013) or heterozygous variants in DLL4 (Meester 2015).

Johanson–Blizzard syndrome (JBS)

An AR condition with IUGR, scalp defects, and exocrine pancreatic insufficiency, combined with dysmorphic features, notably a 'pinched' nose and notching of the alae nasi. CHD and deafness may occur. Faecal elastase is a useful test of pancreatic exocrine function. Caused by biallelic mutation of the *UBR1* gene.

Setleis syndrome

An AD condition in which the scalp defects are bitemporal and resemble 'forceps marks'. There may also be a coarse facial appearance, anomalies of the eyelashes and eyebrows, and periorbital puffiness. The mouth has a typical appearance with large lips, an inverted 'V' contour, and downturned overly defined corners (McGaughran and Aftimos 2002). Patients usually have normal intelligence, but some have developmental delay. It is likely that Setleis syndrome is the same condition as Brauer syndrome and focal facial dermal dysplasia. An AR form of Setleis syndrome may be caused by biallelic mutation of the *TWIST2* gene.

Microphthalmia with linear skin defects (MLS)

Girls with MLS syndrome have microphthalmia with linear skin defects of the face and neck, sclerocornea, corpus callosum agenesis, and other brain anomalies. This XLD male lethal condition is associated with heterozygous deletions of a critical region in Xp22.31. The *HCCS* gene, encoding human holocytochrome c-type synthetase, is the only gene located inside the critical region (Prakash *et al.* 2002).

Goltz syndrome

XLD (due to mutations in, or deletions encompassing, the *PORCN* gene at Xp11.23). Areas of focal dermal hypoplasia may be found on the trunk and limbs and there may be fat herniation through the skin deficiency. See 'Coloboma' in Chapter 2, 'Clinical approach', p. 110.

Delleman syndrome (oculocerebrocutaneous syndrome)

Delleman syndrome is a rare disorder characterized by orbital cysts, micro-/anophthalmia, malformations of the CNS, focal aplasia cutis, and multiple skin appendages (skin tags). The inheritance pattern is uncertain.

Parietal foramina

If the scalp defect is in the parietal area, it may be associated with parietal foramina, but *MSX2* mutation/deletion is not a frequent cause of scalp defects.

Epidermolysis bullosa with pyloric atresia or Carmi syndrome
A lethal AR condition. Mutations have been found in *ITGB2* and *ITGA6*. PND also described by USS and skin biopsy.

Epidermolysis bullosa dystrophica (EBD)
Consider if a skin disorder such as EBD could be the cause of the scalp lesions.

Genetic advice

Recurrence risk
- As for the specific diagnosis.
- Isolated aplasia cutis congenita can follow AD inheritance. It is possible that apparent isolated aplasia cutis congenita could be part of the Adams–Oliver spectrum. Arrange detailed scans of the digits and heart in pregnancy.

Carrier detection
By careful clinical examination.

Prenatal diagnosis
Is possible for some of these conditions by fetal USS for structural abnormalities or by chromosomal or mutation analysis.

Natural history and further management (preventative measures)
Surgical management in a specialist centre because of the risk of associated vascular malformation and bleeding.

Support groups: Many of the individual syndromes have their own support groups. See Contact a Family (UK), http://www.cafamily.org.uk; National Organization for Rare Disorders (USA), http://www.rarediseases.org.

References
Cambiaghi S, Levet PS, Guala G, Baldini D, Gianotti R. Delleman syndrome: report of a case with a mild phenotype. *Eur J Dermatol* 2000; **10**: 623–6.

Casanova D, Amar E, Bardot J, Magalon G. Aplasia cutis congenita. Report on 5 family cases involving the scalp. *Eur J Pediatr Surg* 2001; **11**: 280–4.

Evers ME, Steijlen PM, Hamel BC. Aplasia cutis congenita and associated disorders: an update. *Clin Genet* 1995; **47**: 295–301.

Meester JAN, Southgate L, Stittrich A-B, *et al.* Heterozygous loss-of-function mutations in DLL4 cause Adams–Oliver syndrome. *Am J Hum Genet* 2015; **97**: 475–82.

McGaughran J, Aftimos S. Setleis syndrome: three new cases and a review of the literature. *Am J Med Genet* 2002; **111**: 376–80.

Prager W, Scholz S, Rompel R. Aplasia cutis congenita in two siblings. *Eur J Dermatol* 2002; **12**: 228–30.

Prakash SK, Cormier TA, McCall AE, et al. Loss of holocytochrome c-type synthetase causes the male lethality of X-linked dominant microphthalmia with linear skin defects (MLS) syndrome. *Hum Mol Genet* 2002; **11**: 3237–48.

Shaheen R, Aglan M. Mutations in *EOGT* confirm the genetic heterogeneity of autosomal-recessive Adams–Oliver syndrome. *Am J Hum Genet* 2013; **92**: 598–604.

Tukel T, Sosic D, Al-Gazali LI, et al. Homozygous nonsense mutations in *TWIST2* cause Setleis syndrome. *Am J Hum Genet* 2010; **87**: 289–96.

Verdyck P, Holder-Espinasse M, Hul VW, Wuyts W. Clinical and molecular study of 9 families with Adams–Oliver syndrome. *Eur J Hum Genet* 2003; **11**: 457–63.

Walkowiak J. Faecal elastase-1: clinical value in the assessment of exocrine pancreatic function in children. *Eur J Pediatr* 2000; **159**: 869–70.

Seizures with developmental delay/intellectual disability

This section discusses the approach to the differential diagnosis in children with a seizure disorder and delayed development. For the child with isolated seizures, see 'Epilepsy in infants and children' in Chapter 3, 'Common consultations', p. 410.

The average annual rate of new cases (incidence) of epilepsy in children is 5–7 cases per 100 000; about five in every 1000 children will have epilepsy. Epilepsy may occur as the end point of an acute or acquired process affecting the CNS, but genetic factors and genetically determined syndromes contribute in about 40% of patients.

There are several types of epilepsy syndromes that are unique to children, including infantile spasms (West syndrome), Ohtahara syndrome (early infantile epileptic encephalopathy with burst suppression), Lennox–Gastaut syndrome, and absence seizures.

Isolated epilepsy is usually managed by the paediatrician or paediatric neurologist. The geneticist is involved when there are features that may indicate a syndromic cause or when there is a strong family history that suggests a genetic basis. Genetic counselling for families of children with a severe seizure disorder and ID, in whom no diagnosis has been made, is a common, but difficult, situation where the possibility of an underlying genetic cause has to be considered. The approach here is to highlight which features may indicate a condition with a genetic or chromosomal basis.

Clinical approach

History: key points

- Three-generation family tree with specific enquiry regarding family history of seizures, ID, and skin signs of neurocutaneous disorders. Enquire about consanguinity.
- Onset of the seizures; frequency and type of seizure. Medication.
- Developmental progress before and since the onset of seizures. Try and establish if there is any evidence of developmental regression. This assessment is problematic in children with poorly controlled seizures on high doses of antiepileptic drugs (pseudoregression).
- Pregnancy (evidence of disturbance of brain development by congenital infections, severe bleeding, hypoxia, teratogenic drugs, and alcohol, etc.).
- Perinatal period. Birth trauma, neonatal seizures, blistering rash, neonatal complications, e.g. prematurity, hypoglycaemia.
- OFC at birth and subsequent brain growth.
- Head injury (including NAI).
- Behaviour. Affect, self-harm, unusual movements, stereotypies, tics, hyperventilation.

Examination: key points

- Growth parameters, particularly OFC. Plot serial measurements.
- Dysmorphic features (chromosomal abnormalities and syndromic causes).
- Coarse facial features (metabolic problems), though features can coarsen on antiepileptic medication.
- Hair sparse and brittle in Menkes syndrome. Temporal alopecia in 12p tetrasomy.
- Eyes. Retinal phakoma (TSC), pigmentary retinopathy (mitochondrial disease, NCLs such as Batten disease), cataracts, and corneal clouding, coloboma, and nystagmus
- Skin signs of neurocutaneous disorders: TSC, NF, biotinidase deficiency, Sturge–Weber syndrome, pigmentary anomalies in Blaschko's lines (mosaic disorders, e.g. Schimmelpenning, 12p tetrasomy).
- Neurological examination.
- Abnormal movements, behaviour, or gait (Angelman (AS), Rett, Pitt Hopkins, and Ohtahara syndromes).
- Signs of other organ involvement, e.g. hepatosplenomegaly suggesting a metabolic disorder or abnormalities of liver function suggesting POLG (Alpers syndrome).

Special investigations

- Brain imaging, preferably MRI. An MRI carried out early in life, e.g. <15 months of age, may need to be repeated when the child is older.
- Genomic analysis, e.g. genomic array and gene panel or WES/WGS as appropriate. Microarray analysis should be considered in all children with seizures who have ID, a malformation, or a suggestive family history.
- EEG. To look for specific diagnostic patterns or associations with known conditions, e.g. hypsarrhythmia, burst suppression, high voltage (ring chromosome 20 and AS). If the EEG has the features of AS, full molecular analysis, including *UBEA3* mutation testing, is indicated (see 'Angelman syndrome' in Chapter 3, 'Common consultations', p. 346).
- Biochemical screening. Basic biochemical screening has usually already been performed but should include plasma electrolytes (sodium, calcium, magnesium, and phosphate), LFTs, acid/base status, fasting glucose, pyruvate and lactate, ammonia, amino acids, and congenital infection screen. Urine screen for glucose, ketones, reducing sugars, amino and organic acids, mucopolysaccharides, transferrin isoelectric focussing, phosphate, and alkaline phosphatase.
- Further biochemical testing to consider: biotinidase, white cell enzymes, long-chain fatty acids. Simultaneous measurement of CSF and blood glucose to rule out GLUT1 deficiency.
- UV Woods light to check for abnormalities of skin pigmentation (TSC, IP, and pigmentary mosaicism).
- Consider methylation analysis for AS (*SNRPN*) if there is associated developmental delay with minimal or absent speech, jerky movement disorder, and 2- to 3-Hz large-amplitude slow-wave bursts on EEG. Consider *UBEA3* in children who clinically have AS, but with normal FISH and *SNRPN* methylation studies.
- Consider mitochondrial conditions, e.g. POLG, especially if raised lactate.

Some diagnostic groups to consider

One approach to diagnosing the symptomatic group of epilepsies is to consider the evidence for any of the following groups of disorders.

Cytogenetic abnormalities

Seizures are found in a wide spectrum of chromosomal anomalies. Array all children with non-isolated epilepsy. There may be facial features suggestive of a chromosomal cause, e.g. upslanting palpebral fissures. Epilepsy in

Down's syndrome increases with age and is associated with diffuse abnormalities of the EEG, consistent with dementia. Many chromosomal disorders have a strong association with epilepsy. Several recurrent microdeletions (e.g. 15q11.2, 15q13.3, and 16p13.3) have been identified in 3% of individuals with primary generalized epilepsy and duplications of Xq28 involving *MECP2* cause hypotonia and epilepsy in males. Microarrays may detect chromosomal mosaicism in some cases, but if streaky skin pigmentation is present and array is normal, skin biopsy for fibroblast culture should be considered.

• Ring chromosomes 14 and 20 are best detected on a G-banded karyotype, as they may be present in mosaic form.

Brain malformations with epileptogenic potential

• **Lissencephaly.** See 'Lissencephaly, polymicrogyria, and neuronal migration disorders' in Chapter 2, 'Clinical approach', p. 216, and the XL conditions noted below.

• **TSC.** See 'Tuberous sclerosis (TSC)' in Chapter 3, 'Common consultations', p. 534.

• **Schizencephaly.** Heterozygous mutations in *EMX2* have been reported in some children but are extremely rare.

• *COL4A1* mutations predispose to haemorrhage and porencephaly. Cataracts may also be associated.

• **Focal areas of brain malformation** often cause severe epilepsy, but these may have a mosaic genetic or a non-genetic aetiology.

Single gene disorders

Recent advances in genetic technologies using WES have identified a large number of single genes which are implicated in syndromic epilepsy. Examples of these are:

AD DISORDERS.

• **TSC** is the most common dominant disorder and is caused by mutations in *TSC1* and *TSC2*. See 'Tuberous sclerosis (TSC)' in Chapter 3, 'Common consultations', p. 534.

• **Mowat–Wilson syndrome**, due to mutation of *ZEB2* on chromosome 2q; often presents with microcephaly, seizures, developmental delay, and dysmorphic features. See 'Hypospadias' in Chapter 2, 'Clinical approach', p. 186.

• **Ohtahara syndrome** due to *STXBP1* mutation. Early-onset seizures often resolve and a movement disorder emerges.

• *TCF4* mutations cause **Pitt Hopkins syndrome**, characterized by a wide mouth, hyperventilation, and head shaking.

• Point mutation or deletion of the *MEF2C* gene at 5q14 is associated with seizures and a Rett-like picture.

AR DISORDERS.

• **Metabolic conditions**, e.g. leukodystrophies, Batten disease, PKU, organic acidaemias. See 'Developmental regression' in Chapter 2, 'Clinical approach', p. 128.

• **Congenital disorders of glycosylation** including carbohydrate deficient glycoprotein disorders and GPI deficiencies. Often, but not always, detectable by abnormal transferrin isoelectric focussing and abnormal alkaline phosphatase or phosphate levels. Genomic analysis may be particularly helpful in these conditions. See 'Floppy infant' in Chapter 2, 'Clinical approach', p. 154.

• **Genetically determined brain malformations**, particularly disorders of neuronal migration.

• **Significant microcephaly in association with seizures.** See 'Microcephaly' in Chapter 2, 'Clinical approach', p. 228.

• **Progressive myoclonic** epilepsy (most are recessive; see below).

• **Mitochondrial DNA depletion syndromes (MDDS).** Biallelic mutations in *POLG* (Alpers syndrome) cause a triad of intractable epilepsy, developmental delay often with regression, and abnormal liver function. Defective polymerase gamma is one of the commonest causes of mitochondrial DNA depletion syndrome. Genetically heterogeneous with ~15 genetic causes.

• **PEHO** (progressive encephalopathy–(o)edema–hypsarrhythmia–optic atrophy) syndrome. Originally described in Finland, there are reports from other parts of Europe. Progressive cerebellar atrophy is a key MRI feature. Likely to be genetically heterogenous and may represent the severe end of the infantile epileptic encephalopathy spectrum (Gawlinski 2016).

XL DISORDERS.

• **Menkes syndrome.** Pili torti, abnormal skeletal survey, joint laxity and inguinal herniae, abnormal copper and caeruloplasmin levels. Mutation analysis available.

• **XL isolated lissencephaly sequence** (XLIS; or DCX) mutations, leading to SBH in heterozygous females and predominantly anterior lissencephaly in hemizygous males.

• **Bilateral periventricular nodular heterotopia (BPNH).** Lethal in the perinatal period in males; focal epilepsy in carrier females who have BPNH on MRI scan. Filamin A (*FLNA*) gene at Xq28. See 'Lissencephaly, polymicrogyria, and neuronal migration disorders' in Chapter 2, 'Clinical approach', p. 216, and the XL conditions noted below.

• *ARX* (Aristaless-related homeobox) gene abnormalities. A spectrum of clinical phenotypes have been described with mutations in *ARX*. These include XL lissencephaly, with abnormal genitalia in males and agenesis of the corpus callosum in females. XL infantile spasms (West syndrome) and Partington syndrome (XLMR with dystonia).

• **Rett syndrome.** See 'Rett syndrome' in Chapter 3, 'Common consultations', p. 520.

• Seizures may occasionally occur with **IP** in heterozygous females, but significant MR is rare.

• **Aicardi syndrome** (XLD disorder, epilepsy, agenesis of the corpus callosum, punched-out retinal lesions).

MITOCHONDRIAL DISORDERS: MERRF, MELAS, NARP. MERRF, myoclonic epilepsy with ragged red fibres; MELAS, mitochondrial myopathy–encephalopathy–lactic acidosis–stroke-like episodes; NARP, neuropathy–ataxia–retinitis pigmentosa. See 'Mitochondrial DNA diseases' in Chapter 3, 'Common consultations', p. 490. Lactic acidosis is a good clue to mitochondrial disorders. Muscle biopsy with assay of respiratory chain enzymes is needed for further investigation if common mutations/deletions negative.

Non-genetic causes

Moderate to severe trauma, infections, including congenital infections such as CMV.

Genetic advice

Generalized symptomatic epilepsy, known cause

Symptomatic epilepsies are those where there is a known or suspected disorder of the CNS. Counsel as for the underlying condition.

PROGRESSIVE MYOCLONIC EPILEPSY (PME). This is the triad of stimulus-sensitive myoclonus, grand mal and absence epilepsy, and progressive neurological deterioration/regression. Most causes of PME are rare AR conditions. Exclude ceroid lipofuscinoses such as Batten disease, Unverricht–Lundborg disease, Lafora disease, and sialodosis. Non-AR causes to exclude are MERRF and DPRLA.

Generalized symptomatic epilepsy but no definite cause identified

In this group, there will be some families with a high risk, and features such as true regression and progressive microcephaly are clues to a genetic aetiology with up to 25% recurrence. For more information on the counselling of specific epilepsy syndromes, see 'Epilepsy in infants and children', p. 410 and 'Epilepsy in adults', p. 416 in Chapter 3, 'Common consultations'.

Support groups: Epilepsy Action, http://www. epilepsy.org.uk; Epilepsy Foundation (USA), http://www.epilepsy.com.

Expert adviser: Jill Clayton-Smith, Consultant Clinical Geneticist, Manchester Centre For Genomic Medicine, Central Manchester Hospitals NHS Trust, Manchester, UK.

References

Beaudet AL. The utility of chromosomal microarray analysis in developmental and behavioural pediatrics. *Child Dev* 2013; **84**: 121–32.

Cowan LD. The epidemiology of the epilepsies in children. *Ment Retard Dev Disabil Res Rev* 2002; **8**: 171–81.

Delgado-Escueta AV, Ganesh S, Yamakawa K. Advances in the genetics of progressive myoclonus epilepsy. *Am J Med Genet* 2001; **106**: 129–38.

Engel J Jr; International League Against Epilepsy (ILAE). A proposed diagnostic scheme for people with epileptic seizures and with epilepsy: report of the ILAE task force on classification and terminology. *Epilepsia* 2001; **42**: 769–803.

Gawlinski P, Posmyk R. PEHO syndrome may represent phenotypic expansion at the severe end of the early-onset encephalopathies. *Pediatr Neurol* 2016; **60**: 83–7.

Gould DB, Phalan FC, Breedveld GJ, et al. Mutations in *Col4a1* cause perinatal cerebral hemorrhage and porencephaly. *Science* 2005; **308**: 1167–71.

Guerrini R, Carrozzo R. Epileptogenic brain malformations: clinical presentation, malformative patterns and indications for genetic testing. *Seizure* 2001; **10**: 532–43.

Lemke JR, Riesch E, Scheurenbrand T, et al. Targeted next generation sequencing as a diagnostic tool in epileptic disorders. *Epilepsia* 2012; **53**: 1387–98.

Mastrangelo M, Leuzzi V. Genes of early onset epileptic encephalopathies: from genotype to phenotype. *Pediatr Neurol* 2012; **46**: 24–31.

Milh M, Villeneuve N, Chouchane M, et al. Epileptic and non-epileptic features in patients with early onset epileptic encephalopathy and *STXBP1* mutations. *Epilepsia* 2011; **52**: 1828–34.

Short stature

This is a common problem presenting to paediatricians and is also a feature of many syndromes. This section is a suggested approach to diagnosis in children whose weight and height/length are roughly proportionate (i.e. on similar centiles). If the child's weight is on a considerably lower centile than the height/length, see 'Failure to thrive' in Chapter 2, 'Clinical approach', p. 150.

A length/height of <0.4th centile is used to define short stature. Children with heights below the 0.4th centile or who have sequential heights that cross successive centile bands merit further investigation. The two most common causes of short stature, accounting for 75% of cases, are:

- familial short stature;
- constitutional delay of growth and puberty.

Other causes of short stature (with the approximate prevalence in children with short stature) are: chronic diseases (10%); syndromes (6%); chromosomal anomalies (5%); skeletal dysplasias (1%); GH deficiency and receptor insensitivity (1–2%); and others, including deprivation and psychological problems.

Clinical approach

History: key points

- Three-generation family tree, including parental heights (mid-parental height (MPH)) and consanguinity (rare skeletal dysplasias and inherited endocrine abnormalities).
- Enquire at what age the parents entered puberty and at what age they attained their final adult heights.
- Pregnancy. Maternal illness, medications; ask about alcohol, if appropriate. Did an USS suggest limb shortening or small size?
- Birthweight/length/OFC. Use to determine if the short stature was prenatal (often skeletal dysplasias). Correct for gestation.
- Postnatal growth chart.
- Medical history (chronic diseases).
- Surgical history, particularly orthopaedic procedures such as those to correct talipes, developmental dysplasia of the hip (DDH), scoliosis.
- Developmental history.

Examination: key points

- The skeletal system.
  - Observe for disproportion and measure height/length, weight, and OFC. If they appear disproportionate, measure the arm span and the upper and lower body segments (calculate the ratio). See 'Skeletal dysplasias' in Chapter 2, 'Clinical approach', p. 316.
  - If the limbs are short, assess if this is predominantly affecting the proximal limb, e.g. humerus/femur (rhizomelic shortening), or the forelimb, e.g. radius and ulna/tibia and fibula (mesomelic).
  - Deformity (bowing, talipes, Madelung deformity).
  - Asymmetry.
  - Hands and feet: brachydactyly, broad thumbs, short 4/5 metacarpals and metatarsals, clinodactyly.
- General systems.
  - Signs of poor nutrition.

- Pubertal development. See 'Staging of puberty' in 'Appendix', p. 856.
- Features of renal/cardiac disease.
- Features of hypothyroidism, GH deficiency, and other endocrine disorders.
- Dysmorphic features and malformations.
- Note that overweight children tend to be tall, not short, in childhood, so short stature with obesity is an indication for investigation.

Special investigations

PARENTAL HEIGHTS. If the parents are phenotypically normal, measure their height and calculate the MPH and the target centile range. Children whose projected adult height falls outside the target centile range derived from their parents' heights merit further assessment. NB. This is misleading if one of the parents has a genetic cause of short stature.

- Girls:
  - MPH centile = [(father's height (cm) − 13) + mother's height (cm)]/2;
  - target centile range for girls = MPH centile ± 9 cm.
- Boys:
  - MPH centile = [(mother's height (cm) + 13) + father's height (cm)]/2;
  - target centile range for boys = MPH centile ± 10 cm.

NB. 13 cm is the average difference in height between adult males and females in the UK.

PAEDIATRIC.

- Baseline biochemistry (electrolytes, urea, thyroid function), haematology (FBC and ESR), and urinalysis: to exclude chronic diseases.
- Antigliadin antibodies (coeliac disease).
- Bone age. X-ray the left wrist. Comparing the bone maturation (age) with the chronological age (CA) and height may help diagnostically, e.g. constitutional delay. Difficult to interpret under 4 years, unless bone age advanced.
- Additional endocrine investigations, particularly to exclude GH deficiency, are done under the supervision of a paediatric endocrinologist when the above results are normal but there are persistently subnormal growth rates. Cranial imaging of the pituitary gland may be performed.
- Karyotype/array on all girls (to exclude 45,X) and in the presence of MR/malformation/dysmorphic features in boys.

GENETIC.

- Skeletal survey in children with disproportion, deformities, and joint restrictions/dislocations. See 'Skeletal dysplasias' in Chapter 2, 'Clinical approach', p. 316 for details of which films to request.
- Genomic analysis in presence of features suggestive of a chromosomal or syndromic diagnosis, e.g. genomic array, gene panel, or WES/WGS as available.
- Chromosomal associations with short stature include:
  - TS;
  - deletions/mutations in the SHOX gene (see below);
  - 15q26 deletion (including IGF1R);

- other chromosomal imbalances—most have short stature as a feature but have additional dysmorphic features and MR.
- Consider if mosaicism screen (30 cells) is necessary—mainly applies to girls for investigation of TS (45,X).
- Consider *SHOX* gene testing (for deletions/mutations). If features of Leri–Weill dyschondrosteosis (LWD) (see below) and/or dominant family history of idiopathic short stature.
- Molecular genetic analysis for 11p15 hypomethylation and maternal uniparental disomy of chromosome 7 (mUPD7) in patients with features suggestive of SRS.
- DNA analysis for some endocrine disorders and some skeletal dysplasias. Molecular analysis can help provide carrier detection and prenatal diagnosis.

Some diagnoses to consider

Consider which of the following clinical groupings best fits the child you are assessing:

- short stature;
- short stature/history of low birthweight;
- disproportionate growth;
- short stature with dysmorphic features, mild or no MR;
- short stature with moderate MR.

Then use the headings below to assess suggested diagnoses.

Short stature

Familial short stature and constitutional delay. In familial short stature, the bone maturation is consistent with the chronological age, and the final height may be estimated from the mid-parental target range. Bone maturation in the delayed puberty group is consistent with the height age, and the prognosis for a normal adult height is good.

TURNER SYNDROME (TS). Most of the short stature in TS is due to *SHOX* haploinsufficiency. See 'Turner syndrome, 45,X and variants' in Chapter 5, 'Chromosomes', p. 696.

SHOX-RELATED HAPLOINSUFFICIENCY, INCLUDING LERI–WEILL DYSCHONDROSTEOSIS (LWD). Classic features of LWD are short stature, mesomelia, and Madelung deformity of the forearm. Approximately 70% have identifiable *SHOX* gene deletions/mutations. In addition, 2.4–7% of children with idiopathic short stature have *SHOX*-related haploinsufficiency (Morizio *et al.* 2003; Rappold *et al.* 2002). This prevalence is similar to that of GH deficiency and TS in children with short stature.

SEPTO-OPTIC DYSPLASIA (SOD). Comprises two out of the three features of ONH, absence of the septum pellucidum, and pituitary dysfunction. In one series, 80% had GH deficiency. See 'Structural intracranial anomalies (agenesis of the corpus callosum, septo-optic dysplasia, and arachnoid cysts)' in Chapter 2, 'Clinical approach', p. 320.

OTHER MIDLINE INTRACRANIAL DEFECTS. May be associated with GH deficiency.

Short stature/history of low birthweight

Eighty-eight per cent of low-birthweight babies catch up over the first year of life. However, 'catch-up' may be delayed in preterm infants. Failure to catch up is more common if there has been early growth failure *in utero* and this may be detected by serial USS.

SILVER–RUSSELL SYNDROME (SRS). Pre- and postnatal growth restriction, a proportionately large head, a triangular face, and asymmetry (in around 50%). The majority also have significant feeding difficulties. SRS is genetically heterogeneous. Up to 60% have hypomethylation of the ICR 1 on chromosome 11p15; around 5–10% have maternal UPD7. 11p15 hypomethylation patients are more likely to have classical features of SRS, including asymmetry; mUPD7 is more likely to be associated with mild learning difficulties, particularly speech problems (Wakeling *et al.* 2010). Features vary widely in severity, consensus guidelines for investigation, diagnosis and management of SRS have been published (Wakeling 2016). See 'Failure to thrive' in Chapter 2, 'Clinical approach', p. 150.

3M SYNDROME. Pre- and postnatal growth failure (final height 5–6 SD below the mean), characteristic facies, prominent heels, non-specific findings on X-ray with slender long bones and tall vertebral bodies. AR (*CUL7*, *OBSL1*, *CCDC8* genes).

MUTATIONS IN IGF-1 RECEPTOR GENE (IGF-1R). *IGF-1R* mutations are an uncommon cause of IUGR and postnatal growth failure (Abuzzahab *et al.* 2003). Patients who are haploinsufficient for *IGF-1R* typically have a height of 2.5–3 SD below the mean and delayed bone age. Microcephaly and mild learning difficulties may also be associated.

Disproportionate growth

HYPOCHONDROPLASIA. Disproportion and lumbar lordosis are key features. Features may not be evident on skeletal survey until 2–3 years. *FGFR3* mutations identified in ~70%. See 'Skeletal dysplasias' in Chapter 2, 'Clinical approach', p. 316.

OTHER SKELETAL DYSPLASIAS. See 'Skeletal dysplasias' in Chapter 2, 'Clinical approach', p. 316.

Short stature with dysmorphic features, mild or no mental retardation

AARSKOG SYNDROME. Short stature (rhizomelic), hypertelorism, ptosis in some, shawl scrotum, and brachydactyly with hyperextensible PIP joints. Facial features tend to normalize with age. XL semi-dominant inheritance. Caused by mutations in the *FGD1* gene.

NOONAN SYNDROME (NS). Neck webbing, ptosis, and cardiac defects (especially pulmonary stenosis). See 'Noonan syndrome and the Ras/MAPK pathway syndromes: neuro-cardio-facial-cutaneous syndromes' in Chapter 3, 'Common consultations', p. 512.

ALBRIGHT HEREDITARY OSTEODYSTROPHY (AHO). Short stature, obesity, round face, subcutaneous ossifications, and short fourth/fifth metacarpals. Associated with resistance to PTH and other hormones in some. *GNAS* gene. See 'Obesity with and without developmental delay' in Chapter 2, 'Clinical approach', p. 254.

FLOATING-HARBOR SYNDROME. Predominantly postnatal short stature, with growth around 4–5 SD below the mean. Facial features are characteristic with a broad nose, a large mouth, and low-set and posteriorly rotated ears. Affected children have mild developmental delay, especially of expressive language. Bone age is markedly delayed until later childhood. Heterozygous mutations in *SRCAP*.

DNA REPAIR DEFECTS (FANCONI, BLOOM, NIJMEGEN BREAKAGE SYNDROME (NBS), ETC.). Growth retardation is a feature of most of these conditions. Sun sensitivity, pigmentation changes, including CALs, and microcephaly are clues to the diagnosis. See 'DNA repair disorders' in Chapter 3, 'Common consultations', p. 398.

Short stature with moderate mental retardation

There are many syndromes with short stature and MR, including:

RUBINSTEIN–TAYBI SYNDROME (RTS). Normal birthweight, postnatal short stature and microcephaly, moderate to severe learning difficulties in most, broad thumbs and halluces, prominent fetal finger pads. See 'Broad thumbs' in Chapter 2, 'Clinical approach', p. 82.

CORNELIA DE LANGE SYNDROME (CDLS). Short stature of prenatal onset, microcephaly, hirsuitism, characteristic facial features with synophrys. Upper limb anomalies are common. See 'Limb reduction defects' in Chapter 2, 'Clinical approach', p. 212.

SECKEL SYNDROME AND THE OSTEODYSPLASTIC DWARFISMS. These are characterized by severe prenatal growth restriction and microcephaly. See 'Microcephaly' in Chapter 2, 'Clinical approach', p. 228.

FETAL ALCOHOL SYNDROME (FAS). See 'Fetal alcohol syndrome (FAS)' in Chapter 6, 'Pregnancy and fertility', p. 728.

Genetic advice

Recurrence risk

- For children with apparently isolated constitutional delay with no MR, there may be familial factors that will increase the risk of short stature in other family members.
- For known diagnosis, as appropriate for the condition.

Carrier detection

SHOX testing can detect previously unknown carriers in large families. Complete deficiency of SHOX causes the severe Langer mesomelic dysplasia.

Prenatal diagnosis

- This is possible in families where a causative mutation has been identified.
- Serial scans to monitor fetal growth and look for associated features of the condition.
- See also 'Prenatal diagnosis' in 'Skeletal dysplasias', Chapter 2, 'Clinical approach', p. 316, including the pitfalls of predicting dysplasias at 20 weeks.

Natural history and further management (preventative measures)

- Children with non-syndromic conditions require surveillance of their growth rate by a paediatrician or paediatric endocrinologist.

- GH treatment is licensed in the UK for treatment of TS, GH deficiency, SHOX deficiency, and children who are small-for-gestational age and who fail to show catchup growth by the age of 4 years. There is no clear-cut benefit in most syndromes or in skeletal dysplasias.
- Skeletal dysplasias require a plan of management to prevent complications, to discuss prognosis, and to discuss procedures such as leg lengthening. See 'Skeletal dysplasias' in Chapter 2, 'Clinical approach', p. 316.

Support groups: Child Growth Foundation, http://www.childgrowthfoundation.org; Restricted Growth Association, http://www.restrictedgrowth.co.uk.

Expert adviser: Emma Wakeling, Consultant in Clinical Genetics, North West Thames Regional Genetics Service, London North West Healthcare NHS Trust, Harrow, UK.

References

Abuzzahab MJ, Schneider A, Goddard A, et al. IGF-1 receptor mutations resulting in intrauterine and postnatal growth retardation. N Engl J Med 2003; **349**: 2211–22.

Dattani M, Preece M. Growth hormone deficiency and related disorders: insights into causation, diagnosis and treatment. Lancet 2004; **363**: 1977–87.

Freeman JV, Cole TJ, Chinn S, Jones PRM, White EM, Preece MA. Cross sectional stature and weight reference curves for the UK 1990. Arch Dis Child 1995; **73**: 17–24.

Hanson D, Murray PG, Black GC, Clayton PE. The genetics of 3-M syndrome: unravelling a potential new regulatory growth pathway. Horm Res Paediatr 2011; **76**: 369–78.

Morizio E, Stuppia L, Gatta V, et al. Deletion of the SHOX gene in patients with short stature of unknown cause. Am J Med Genet A 2003; **119A**: 293–6.

Rappold GA, Fukami M, Niesler B, et al. Deletions in the homeobox gene SHOX (short stature homeobox) are an important cause of growth failure in children with short stature. J Clin Endocrinol Metab 2002; **87**: 1402–6.

Wakeling EL, Amero SA, Alders M, et al. Epigenotype-phenotype correlations in Silver–Russell syndrome. J Med Genet 2010; **47**: 760–8.

Wakeling EL, Brionde F, et al. Diagnosis and management of Silver-Russell syndrome: first international consensus statement. Nat Rev Endocrinol 2017; **13**: 105–24.

Skeletal dysplasias

Skeletal dysplasias are a generalized disorders of modelling, growth, or homeostasis of the skeleton. There are a wide variety of >450 conditions and in many the genetic basis is now known. Study of the underlying molecular genetic abnormalities in this group of conditions has enhanced understanding of the gene families and pathways involved in bone development and provided insights into how these conditions may be treated in the future.

Terminology is complex, but many dysplasias are named according to the anatomical region of involvement, so these descriptive terms identify the type of dysplasia.

- Epiphysis. An area of secondary ossification, usually present at each end of long bones (metacarpals and metatarsals only have one epiphysis each). Irregular bones, such as the carpal bones, each have a single ossification centre.
- Metaphysis. The growing area of a long bone immediately adjacent to the epiphyses.
- Diaphysis. The shaft of a long bone enclosed by periosteum.
- Spondylo-. Indicates spinal involvement in the dysplasia.

In clinical practice, an infant or child may be referred with short stature disproportion or limb deformity to establish if he/she has an underlying skeletal dysplasia and to determine the diagnosis.

Clinical approach

History: key points
- Three-generation family tree with enquiry about short stature (document the estimated adult heights) and consanguinity.
- Family history of early osteoarthritis hip replacement (implies there is involvement of epiphyses/articular surfaces, as in MED or pseudoachondroplasia).
- History of the pregnancy. Were short limbs evident on antenatal USS?
- Birth measurements, especially length and head circumference.
- At what age did the short stature become obvious?

- Joint pain, contractures, and limitation of movement (specific problems may arise in particular conditions, e.g. pronation/supination of the forearm in LWD (*SHOX*).
- Pathological fractures resulting from minimal trauma (occur in OI and other dysplasias associated with low bone density).
- Ask if there is developmental delay.

Examination: key points
- Measurement of height/length, arm span, and upper to lower segment ratio:
  - arm span is the distance between the middle fingertips when the arms are held out horizontally from the body;
- upper to lower segment ratio determines the degree of disproportion and is usually around 1.0 (see Figure 2.35). If the limbs are short, it is helpful to establish which segment is most profoundly affected. Some dysplasias are associated with proximal (rhizomelic) shortening, some with short middle segments (mesomelic), and others with distal shortening (acromelic). Dysplasias are often named using these terms to describe them (e.g. rhizomelic chondrodysplasia punctata).
- Head circumference (macrocephaly occurs in achondroplasia).
- Gait. Waddling gait may arise from hip involvement; pain in the lower limbs on walking may indicate spine problems (spinal stenosis in older children with achondroplasia).
- Limb deformity is common; look for:
  - talipes (diastrophic dysplasia, Kniest syndrome);
  - bowing of long bones (OI, hypophosphataemic rickets);
  - asymmetry of limb length (XLD chrondrodysplasia punctata).
- Joints. Look for limitation of movement with pain, contractures, deformity, and swelling.
- Hands and feet:
- brachydactyly (acromelic dysplasias);

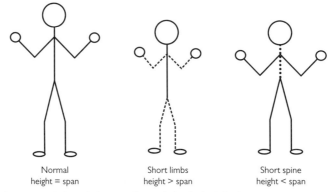

| Normal | Short limbs | Short spine |
| height = span | height > span | height < span |

Figure 2.35 Skeletal proportions limb: trunk. Image kindly provided by Dr Sarah Smithson

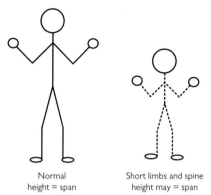

Figure 2.36 Skeletal proportions. Image kindly provided by Dr Sarah Smithson

Normal
height = span

Short limbs and spine
height may = span

- polydactyly (EVC and Jeune syndromes);
  - thumb abnormalities (hitchhiker thumb in diastrophic dysplasia, triphalangeal thumb in radial ray syndromes).
- Eyes. Cataract and myopia, detached retina (occur in collagen II-related dysplasias).
- Palate. Cleft palate also occurs in the collagen II group (Stickler syndrome, Kniest syndrome, and SEDC).
- Teeth (DI, EVC, cleidocranial dysostosis).
- Hair (thin in chondrodysplasia punctata, cartilage–hair hypoplasia, also called metaphyseal dysplasia McKusick type).
- Heart. CHD may occur in some dysplasias (geleophysic dysplasia).
- Neurological signs uncommon, except in specific conditions (cord compression should be considered in dysplasias associated with odontoid hypoplasia such as SEDC and Morquio/MPS type 4; spinal stenosis should be considered in older children with achondroplasia).
- Dysmorphic facial features may occur (midface hypoplasia in the collagen II group, coarse features in metabolic/storage disorders. In the latter group, check for hepatosplenomegaly).

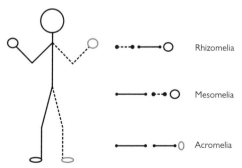

Rhizomelia

Mesomelia

Acromelia

Figure 2.37 Limb proportions. Image kindly provided by Dr Sarah Smithson

Special investigations
Radiological survey for skeletal dysplasia.
- Skull anteroposterior (AP) and lateral.
- Chest PA.
- Spine AP with lateral.
- Pelvis specifically requesting hips.
- One of each limb as follows:
- humerus, radius and ulna, hand, carpal bones, and phalanges;
- femur, tibia and fibula, foot.
Good-quality radiographs and specialist interpretation are essential for all but common, well-known dysplasias. For some skeletal dysplasias, radiological changes may not be obvious in infancy because they are mild (hypochondroplasia) or because the skeleton is not sufficiently developed and many of the findings evolve over time. Children with a normal skeletal survey and delayed bone maturation may require endocrine investigations.
- Radiographs of the cervical spine in flexion or extension may be indicated to assess subluxation in dysplasias where odontoid hypoplasia is a recognized complication. This should be arranged in conjunction with an expert radiologist or orthopaedic/spinal surgeon and is articularly important prior to anaesthesia.
- MRI of the brain with cervical and lower spine scans may be indicated as above or in conditions associated with other spinal complications.
- Exclude metabolic bone disease in children with metaphyseal abnormalities and disorders of bone density.
- Targeted molecular genetic tests can be used to confirm clinical/radiological diagnoses (*FGFR3* in achondroplasia and hypochondroplasia).
- Genomic analysis in presence of features suggestive of a syndromic diagnosis, e.g. genomic array, gene panel, or WES/WGS as available. The genetic causes of the most common dysplasias are listed in 'Appendix', p. 854. In addition, certain disorders may be associated with specific cytogenetic changes (chromosome 17 translocation/SOX 9 disruption in campomelic dysplasia deletions of Xp detectable by FISH analysis in LWD).
- Metabolic investigations as required (urine glycosaminoglycans if an MPS is suspected, VLCFAs for peroxisomal disorders, and sterol analysis (sterol profile) with stippled epiphyses).

Some differential diagnoses to consider
- Differentiate between a skeletal dysplasia and other causes of short stature.
- Exclude the possibility of storage disorders and metabolic bone disease, especially if you find developmental delay.
- Consider whether other family members are affected and whether radiological investigation would help to establish this.
- If a skeletal dysplasia is present, aim to determine which parts of the skeleton are affected, describe the changes, then enlist expert radiological assistance. The UK Skeletal Dysplasia Group has useful publications to help interpret the clinical and radiological findings.

The clinical features can guide the diagnostic groups and help target testing

- Short limbs/trunk less affected:
- achondroplasia, hypochondroplasia, acromesomelic, pseudoachondroplasia.
- Short limbs and trunk:
- diastrophic dysplasia, Kniest dysplasia.
- Epiphyseal disorders:
- delayed, small, irregular epiphyses in MED, stippled epiphyses in various types of chondrodysplasia punctata.
- Short trunk/limbs less affected:
- spondyloepiphyseal and spondylometaphyseal dysplasias.
- Metaphyseal disorders:
- a difficult group to classify and differentiate from metabolic disorders, such as rickets, purely by radiographs.
- Abnormal bone density:
- increased in osteopetrosis and pycnodysostosis; decreased in OI and hypophosphatasia.

Genetic advice

Recurrence risk

- Known diagnosis. Counsel as appropriate.
- Unknown diagnosis. If there is consanguinity, AR is the likely mode of inheritance. An AD or XL mode of inheritance may be established from the family history.

Carrier detection

Possible where there is a causative mutation, biochemical test, or radiological features.

Prenatal diagnosis

If the causative mutation or biochemical defect has been identified, then PND by CVS can be offered, if appropriate.

Often a dysplasia is first suspected when short limbs, with or without a narrow chest, are identified on the 20-week USS. Such findings are non-specific and can be difficult to interpret. There must be additional clinical information or USS evidence before a specific diagnosis is suggested to parents. Testing for *FGFR3*-related dysplasias, e.g. achondroplasia/thanatophoric dysplasia, may be considered and may be available by NIPT/D.

In milder conditions, the scan will often be normal.

Natural history and further management

Children with skeletal dysplasia are ideally managed by a dedicated expert multidisciplinary team, including orthopaedic, rheumatology, ENT, and endocrine specialists, as required. Physiotherapy and psychology input may also be important. Although long-term medical supervision is required for most children and adults, there should be emphasis on living a normal life as far as possible.

- Surgical management, limb alignment for joint preservation and optimal function, may include limb lengthening.
- Medication for specific circumstances, e.g. bisphosphonates for some children with OI.
- GH treatment. May promote rapid growth in the short term but does not have long-term benefit in the majority of children.
- Mobility. Occupational therapy and physiotherapy assessments may also be helpful with activities of daily living.

Support groups: Restricted Growth Association, PO Box 8919, Birmingham B27 6DQ, http://www.restrictedgrowth.co.uk; United Kingdom Coalition of Short People, PO Box 18, Hereford, UK, email: short-peopleleuk@aol.com; Little People of America, http://www.lpaonline.org.

Expert adviser: Sarah Smithson, Consultant, Department of Clinical Genetics, University Hospitals Bristol NHS Foundation Trust, Bristol, UK.

References

Alanay Y, Lachman RS. A review of the principles of radiological assessment of skeletal dysplasias. *J Clin Res Pediatr Endocrinol* 2011; **3**: 163–78.

European Skeletal Dysplasia Network. http://www.esdn.org.

UK Skeletal Dysplasia Group. http://www.skeletaldysplasia-group.org.uk.

Warman ML, Cormier-Daire V, Hall C, et al. Nosology and classification of genetic skeletal disorders: 2010 revision. *Am J Med Genet A* 2010; **155A**: 943–68.

Wynne-Davies R, Hall CM, Wilson LM, UK Skeletal Dysplasia Group. Skeletal dysplasias: a method of diagnosis of the non-lethal skeletal dysplasias. *Skeletal Dysplasia Group Occasional Publication No.* 9a, 2010.

Structural intracranial anomalies (agenesis of the corpus callosum, septo-optic dysplasia, and arachnoid cysts)

Formation of the cerebral commissures begins as early as 6 weeks' gestation when axons destined to cross in the anterior commissure can be seen growing medially within the hemisphere. The most important fibre bundles cross in the lamina terminalis. At 10 weeks' gestation, the first fibres cross to form the anterior commissure. Fibres begin to cross in the corpus callosum from 11 weeks' gestation and over the next few weeks the corpus callosum grows enormously (see Figure 2.38). The growth of the corpus callosum causes the lamina terminalis to become locally thinned and it forms the septum pellucidum. By 18–20 weeks' gestation, the corpus callosum has assumed the adult form, although it continues to thicken and grow caudally for several months.

Agenesis of the corpus callosum (ACC)

ACC is one of the most common brain malformations, with a prevalence of 3–7/1000. Its prevalence in children with developmental disabilities may be as high as 2%. It may occur as an isolated malformation, as one feature of a complex cranial malformation sequence, as part of a syndrome, or as a teratogenic consequence of an inborn error of metabolism.

The corpus callosum is relatively easy to visualize by cranial USS in a neonate; it is also well seen on CT or MRI scans (see Figure 2.39). As such, it is often identified fairly early in the investigations of a neonate with abnormal neurology or a child with developmental delay or seizures. While it contributes to the clinical picture, it is a much less specific finding than is often thought. Occasionally it is an incidental finding in a child with an otherwise normal development.

Clinical approach

History: key points

• Detailed three-generation family tree and enquire about consanguinity.
• Seizures.
• Developmental milestones.

Examination: key points

• Look carefully for dysmorphic features and other congenital malformations.
• Measure the OFC, height, and weight.
• Examine for a gaze palsy (tubulinopathy).

Special investigations

• Genomic analysis, e.g. genomic array, gene panel, or WES/WGS as appropriate/available.
• Ophthalmology assessment for ONH or choreoretinal lacunae (seen in Aicardi syndrome and KIF11).
• Review MRI for other midline anomaly, e.g. agenesis of the septum pellucidum or evidence of a more generalized migration defect, e.g. lissencephaly (tubulin genes), or hydrocephalus (*L1CAM*).
• Urine for amino and organic acids.
• If seizures, CSF glycine (NKH) and lactate (pyruvate dehydrogenase deficiency). In a male infant, consider neonatal ALD (VLCFAs).
• If ONH or absence of the septum pellucidum, need to perform full investigation of hypothalamic–pituitary axis (see below).

Some diagnoses to consider

Tubulinopathies

Heterozygous variants in *TUBA1A, TUBB2A, TUBB2B, TUBB3, TUBB*, or *TUBG1* or biallelic variants in *TUBA8* cause a range of brain malformations. A disordered gyral pattern, in combination with abnormalities of the cerebellum/brainstem and/or corpus callosum and/or basal ganglia anomalies, together with lissencephaly/pachygyria/PMG is characteristic of tubulin disorders. Clinical features include developmental delay and ID, seizures, and a variety of ocular findings.

Coffin–Siris-like conditions

This group of disorders caused by genes in the SWI/SNF complex (e.g. *ARID1B, SMARCA4, SMARCB1*) often have agenesis/hypoplasia of the corpus callosum as a feature.

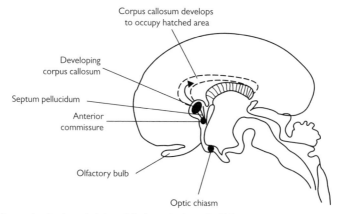

Figure 2.38 Line diagram showing the sagittal view of the brain of a 4-month-old fetus.

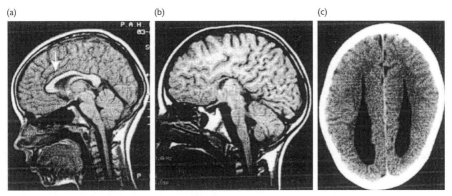

Figure 2.39 (a) Normal brain in a girl aged 2 years. A T1-weighted sagittal MRI scan shows a normal corpus callosum and cingulate gyrus (arrow). (b) Agenesis of the corpus callosum in a girl aged 6 years who has microcephaly and moderate learning difficulties. A T1-weighted sagittal MRI scan shows the absence of the corpus callosum and cingulate gyrus, which normally runs parallel to the corpus callosum. (c) Agenesis of the corpus callosum in the same girl as in (b). Axial CT shows the typical appearance of parallel lateral cerebral ventricles, with divergence of the anterior horns of the ventricles and colpocephaly (dilated posterior part of the lateral ventricles).
Reproduced with permission from Verity CM, Firth H and Ffrench-Constant C, Developmental abnormalities of the central nervous system. In David A. Warrell, Timothy M. Cox, and John D. Firth, *Oxford Textbook of Medicine*, Fourth edition, 2003, Figure 5, page 1208, with permission from Oxford University Press.

Acrocallosal syndrome (ACS; Schinzel syndrome)
A rare recessive disorder characterized by agenesis or hypoplasia of the corpus callosum, craniofacial dysmorphism, duplication of the hallux, PAP, and severe MR. Biallelic mutations in *KIF7*, a key component of the Sonic hedgehog pathway, are responsible for this syndrome in some families (Putoux *et al*. 2011) Intracranial cysts (including arachnoid cysts) were seen in 10/34 published cases of ACS (Koenig *et al*. 2002).

CEDNIK syndrome (cerebral dysgenesis, neuropathy, ichthyosis, and palmoplantar keratoderma syndrome)
Due to biallelic mutation of the *SNAP29* gene. Sometimes one disease allele may be a 22q11 deletion, as the *SNAP29* gene is contained in the typical VCFS deletion.

Greig cephalopolysyndactyly syndrome
This is caused by mutations in *GLI3* and follows AD inheritance with variable expressivity. In particular, large deletions involving *GLI3* may cause an overlap phenotype with ACS.

Mosaic trisomy 8
Deep palmar and plantar creases and small patellae. ACC may also be present (may need a buccal smear/skin biopsy).

Mowat–Wilson syndrome
Characteristic facial appearance (hypertelorism, pointed chin, prominent columella, open-mouthed expression, broad, medial flared eyebrows, and uplifted earlobes), together with severe MR. Microcephaly, seizures, congenital heart defects, aplasia/hypoplasia of the corpus callosum, and urogenital anomalies (especially hypospadias in boys) are frequent findings. Caused by 'de novo' truncating mutations in *ZEB2*.

FOXG1 congenital Rett syndrome
This is caused by heterozygous variants in the FOXG1 gene. Agenesis or hypoplasia of the corpus callosum is commonly seen and a movement disorder is a clue to this diagnosis (Papandreou *et al*. 2016).

ARX syndrome
May present in males with abnormalities of the genitalia, developmental delay, and seizures. ACC is sometimes found on cranial imaging.

Genetic advice
Make every effort to make a specific diagnosis and to substantiate this by appropriate laboratory investigations and then counsel accordingly. If the ACC is isolated, this may be sporadic or follow AD, AR, or XL modes of inheritance.

Septo-optic dysplasia (SOD)
De Morsier's syndrome
This is the association of ONH with agenesis of the septum pellucidum and disturbed hypothalamic/pituitary function. SOD comprises two out of the three features of ONH: unilateral or bilateral absence of the septum pellucidum and pituitary dysfunction. Fifty per cent of patients with this condition have a septum pellucidum present. In one series, 80% had GH deficiency, 60% had ACTH deficiency, 40% had LH/FSH deficiency, and 35% had diabetes insipidus. Visual impairment is extremely variable. Seizures in children with SOD are often secondary to hypoglycaemia (GH deficiency ± cortisol deficiency), rather than secondary to a primary brain abnormality. Overall, approximately half of cases have moderate or severe developmental delay. Children need specialist input from a paediatric endocrinologist and a paediatric ophthalmologist.

SOD is largely thought to be a sporadic disorder with a low recurrence risk. However, in the light of the recent identification of the *HESX1* gene, it is now clear that genetic mutations in this gene may account for some cases of SOD (Dattani *et al*. 1998; Tajima *et al*. 2003). Additionally, there is increasing evidence to suggest that SOD is a multigenic disorder, with other genes being involved, and possible interaction with environmental factors, ultimately leading to a phenotype.

Mutations in the homeobox gene *HESX1*, which is essential for pituitary and forebrain development, have been described in a handful of individuals with phenotypes ranging from severe SOD, relatively mild CPHD, to isolated GH deficiency (Dattani *et al.* 1998; Tajima *et al.* 2003). Very rarely, the characteristic CNS and ocular abnormalities of SOD occur together with limb malformations (digital anomalies) as a distinct entity (Harrison *et al.* 2004).

Special investigations
- Full investigation of the hypothalamic–pituitary axis (including post-pituitary).
- MRI scan, including imaging of the optic chiasm and pituitary.
- Genomic analysis, e.g. genomic array, gene panel, or WES/WGS as appropriate/available.

Arachnoid cysts

Arachnoid cysts are collections of CSF that develop within the arachnoid membrane because of splitting or duplication of the structure. They are developmental anomalies, which are often identified as an incidental finding during cranial imaging by USS, CT, or MRI. Forty per cent are in the midline.

Arachnoid cysts are nearly always sporadic and single. The M:F ratio is >2:1; they are more common on the left side. They are relatively rare, accounting for 71% of intracranial space-occupying lesions. They cause concern when they are identified on a routine antenatal USS. They are usually asymptomatic but can produce symptoms because of expansion or bleeding. Conservative management is usually indicated in the absence of symptoms or signs—but seek neurosurgical advice. Long-standing pressure effects may contribute to maldevelopment of the temporal lobe and may produce obstruction at the level of the third or fourth ventricle, requiring shunting.

With widespread use of imaging, many arachnoid cysts are detected during the antenatal or neonatal period. Some may remain quiescent throughout life; some may resolve, and some may become symptomatic after several years of quiescence. Symptoms depend on size, location, and age. Seizure and headache are the most common symptoms of middle cranial fossa cysts (60%). Ten to 30% are found in the posterior fossa. There is a reported relationship between temporal lobe arachnoid cysts and attention-deficit/hyperactivity disorder (ADHD). Mental impairment and developmental delay have been associated with large arachnoid cysts.

Special investigations
- Bilateral temporal arachnoid cysts occur in glutaric aciduria type 1. If present, do a urine amino and organic acid screen.

Acrocallosal syndrome (Schinzel syndrome)

See above.

Porencephaly

Porencephaly is a neurological disorder characterized by fluid-filled cysts or cavities in the brain that often cause hemiplegia. *De novo* or inherited heterozygous mutations in *COL4A1* and *COL4A2*, which encodes the type IV α1 and α2 collagen chains that are essential for the structural integrity of vascular basement membranes, have been reported in some individuals with porencephaly (Yoneda *et al.* 2012).

Schizencephaly

Schizencephaly is a heterogeneous condition with genetic overlap with holoprosencephaly and porencephaly.

Support group: FOCUS Families (ONH/SOD Information, Education and Support), http://www.focusfamilies.org.

References

Cameron FJ, Khadilkar VV, Stanhope R. Pituitary dysfunction and mortality with congenital midline malformation of the cerebrum. *Eur J Pediatr* 1999; **158**: 97–102.

Dattani MT, Martinez-Barbera JP, Thomas PQ, et al. Mutations in the homeobox gene *HESX1/Hesx1* associated with septo-optic dysplasia in human and mouse. *Nat Genet* 1998; **19**: 125–33.

Dobyns WB. Absence makes the search grow longer. *Am J Hum Genet* 1996; **58**: 7–16.

Gosalakkal JA. Intracranial arachnoid cysts in children: a review of pathogenesis, clinical features and management. *Pediatr Neurol* 2002; **26**: 93–8.

Gupta JK, Lilford RJ. Assessment and management of fetal agenesis of the corpus callosum. *Prenatal Diagn* 1995; **15**: 301–12.

Harrison IM, Brosnahan D, Phelan E, Fitzgerald RJ, Reardon W. Septo-optic dysplasia with digital anomalies—a recurrent pattern syndrome. *Am J Med Genet A* 2004; **131A**: 82–5.

Koenig R, Bach A, Woelki U, et al. Spectrum of the acrocallosal syndrome. *Am J Med Genet* 2002; **108**: 7–11.

Papandreou A, Schneider RB, et al. Delineation of the movement disorders associated with FOXG1 mutations. *Neurology* 2016; **86**(19): 1794–800.

Putoux A, Thomas S, Coene KL, et al. KIF7 mutations cause fetal hydrolethalus and acrocallosal syndromes. *Nat Genet* 2011; **43**: 601–6.

Tajima T, Hattorri T, Nakajima T, et al. Sporadic heterozygous frameshift mutation of *HESX1* causing pituitary and optic nerve hypoplasia and combined pituitary hormone deficiency in a Japanese patient. *J Clin Endocrinol Metab* 2003; **88**: 45–50.

Warrell D (ed.). *Oxford textbook of medicine*, 4th edn. Oxford University Press, Oxford, 2003.

Yoneda Y, Haginoya K, Arai H, et al. De novo and inherited mutations in *COL4A2*, encoding the type IV collagen α2 chain cause porencephaly. *Am J Hum Genet* 2012; **90**: 86–90.

Sudden cardiac death

Sudden cardiac death (SCD) of a young person is a rare event, but in a proportion of such deaths there is an underlying genetic disorder that predisposed to the event. The overall incidence of SCD in individuals <35 years is 1.8/100 000, with 0.48/100 000 due to CM and 0.24/100 000 presumed secondary to a primary arrhythmic aetiology.

Most cases are best assessed with the combined expertise of a cardiologist and a clinical geneticist in a dedicated inherited cardiac conditions (ICC) service. It is essential to obtain as much detail as possible regarding the events leading up to the cardiac arrest, together with the post-mortem findings. Increasingly, DNA samples are being stored from affected individuals, but unfortunately this is not always the case.

The implication of both rare and common variants in sudden cardiac arrhythmia susceptibility may, in part, explain the high phenotype variability encountered in familial forms of the disease. Progress in understanding genetic and environmental modifiers may be helpful in stratifying the risk to family members.

The key contribution of the geneticist is to take a detailed family history, evaluate for features suggestive of a contributory genetic diagnosis, and suggest appropriate genetic investigations. The main aim is to establish a robust genetic diagnosis in the affected individual in order to enable definitive testing for family members at risk. However, due to our incomplete knowledge of the single gene causes of SCD and of the polygenic and environmental factors that influence that risk, it is only possible to establish a molecular genetic diagnosis in about 25% of cases. In such situations, decisions will need to be made about whether there is an appreciable risk to other family members and if so what ongoing cardiac surveillance to recommend.

Clinical approach

History: key points
- Detailed three-generation family history enquiring about any sudden, cardiac, or unexplained deaths.
- History of any fits/faints/funny turns/dizzy spells or seizures in the SCD victim or other family members.
- History of the physical appearance of the affected family member, e.g. height, habitus, arachnodactyly, scarring, bruising, dysmorphic features, muscular weakness.
- Detailed medical history of the affected family member with the circumstances of the death, time of day, and if at rest/sleep or exercise.
- Detailed history of any drug exposure—prescribed, recreational, over-the-counter, and supplements.

Examination: key points
- Cardiovascular examination.
- Where appropriate, examine for features of a connective tissue disorder, e.g. MFS or vascular EDS.

Investigations
- DNA for gene panel/WES/WGS tests. Obtain consent for testing of post-mortem samples, if available; collect DNA from relatives with the phenotype on clinical investigation.
- ECG and rhythm strip.

- 24-hour ECG.
- Exercise test.
- Echo.
- Cardiac MRI may be recommended in some circumstances.
- Sodium channel blocker challenge (e.g. with ajmaline) or other provocation tests.
- Cholesterol and lipid profile in some circumstances.

Diagnoses to consider

Try to categorize the clinical presentation into one of the following groups, and investigate and manage as appropriate:
- primary disorder of cardiac rhythm, e.g. long QT, Brugada (see 'Long QT syndrome and other inherited arrhythmia syndromes' in Chapter 3, 'Common consultations', p. 480), catecholaminergic polymorphic ventricular tachycardia (CPVT);
- primary disorder of cardiac muscle, e.g. HCM (see 'Hypertrophic cardiomyopathy (HCM)' in Chapter 3, 'Common consultations', p. 460), DCM (see 'Dilated cardiomyopathy (DCM)' in Chapter 3, 'Common consultations', p. 394), ARVC;
- aortopathy, e.g. MFS (see 'Marfan's syndrome' in Chapter 3, 'Common consultations', p. 484), Loeys–Dietz syndrome, EDS—vascular type (see 'Ehlers–Danlos syndrome (EDS)' in Chapter 3, 'Common consultations', p. 406);
- premature coronary artery disease due to hyperlipidaemia, e.g. familial hypercholesterolaemia (see 'Hyperlipidaemia' in Chapter 3, 'Common consultations', p. 458);
- non-cardiac cause, e.g. sudden unexpected death in epilepsy (SUDEP).

Genetic advice

Recurrence risk
If it is possible to establish a genetic diagnosis; counsel for that condition (see other chapters referenced above).

Predictive testing and carrier detection
Definitive genetic testing is only possible where a specific genetic diagnosis has been identified. If there is a likely clinical diagnosis, this may provide a basis by which to evaluate, advise, and manage relatives at risk.

Prenatal diagnosis
Not possible, unless a specific genetic cause has been identified. Many diseases have very variable penetrance and expressivity, and therefore even if a genetic diagnosis has been identified, prenatal testing may not be appropriate.

Natural history and further management

- Preventative measures, medication to avoid, advice on exercise participation, and treatment of intercurrent illness.
- At-risk family members should be under the care of a specialist cardiologist.

Support groups: Sudden Arrhythmic Death Syndrome UK (SADS-UK), http://www.sadsuk.org.uk; Cardiac Risk in the Young (CRY), http://www.c-r-y.org.uk; Cardiomyopathy UK, http://www.cardiomyopathy.org.

Expert adviser: Tessa Homfray, Consultant Medical Genetics, St George's University Hospital, Harris Birthright Unit, Kings College Hospital & Royal Brompton Hospital, London, UK.

References

Priori SG, Wilde AA, Horie M, *et al.*; Heart Rhythm Society; European Heart Rhythm Association; Asia Pacific Heart Rhythm Society. Executive summary: HRS/EHRA/APHRS expert consensus statement on the diagnosis and management of patients with inherited primary arrhythmia syndromes. *Europace* 2013; **15**: 1389–406.

Semsarian C, Ingles J, Wilde AA. Sudden cardiac death in the young: the molecular autopsy and a practical approach to surviving relatives. *Eur Heart J* 2015; **36**: 1290–6.

Suspected non-accidental injury

Non-accidental injury (NAI) is suspected by the paediatric team when an infant presents with several fractures of varying ages with no clear history to account for them, or when an infant is found to have subdural haemorrhage (SDH) or when an infant/child presents with recurrent bruising. A genetic opinion may be sought if the diagnosis of NAI is uncertain or if there are clinical pointers suggesting a possible underlying genetic disorder. The paediatric team will usually have a protocol for managing suspected NAI and liaise with appropriate agencies such as the child protection team, social services, and in some circumstances the police and the coroner.

In practice, for an infant or child presenting with fractures, the most important differential diagnosis is OI; for an infant presenting with SDH, it is important to exclude glutaric aciduria and, in males with developmental delay or seizures, Menkes syndrome. In SDH, the paediatric team will investigate for coagulation disorders.

Recurrent fractures or fractures of different ages or occasions where the fracture seems disproportionate to the trauma sustained may all occur in OI. It is important to make a genetic diagnosis accurately and speedily in such circumstances to avoid inappropriate suspicion and investigation of child abuse.

Clinical approach

History: key points

- Three-generation family history, including enquiry for fractures, dental problems, hearing loss, lax joints, short stature, or easy bruising.
- Detailed perinatal history. Was there any birth trauma? (SDH can follow a traumatic delivery and be associated with retinal haemorrhage. SDH at birth may predispose to subsequent SDH in infancy.) Probable increased risk of fracture up to age of 6 months in ex-premature infants born at <1000 g.
- Detailed developmental history. Was the child's development progressing normally prior to this episode?
- Is there any dietary deficiency (scurvy, rickets)?

Examination: key points

- Growth parameters. Height, weight, and OFC.
- Record the size of the anterior fontanelle.
- Eyes. Are the sclerae blue (OI)? This is an age-dependent feature.
- Scalp. Sparse hair (Menkes)?
- Facial features (record with photographs).
- Documentation of bruising/fractures. Record briefly; full documentation will usually be completed by the paediatric team.

Special investigations

- Photographs.
- Full skeletal survey reviewed by a paediatric radiologist (look for wormian bones in OI and Menkes). Survey criteria can be found on the British Paediatric Radiology Society website (http://www.bspr.org.uk).
- Consider a skin biopsy for fibroblast culture.
- Store DNA (EDTA sample).
- FBC with platelet count and coagulopathy screen (if SDH or bruising).

- Urine for organic and amino acids (to exclude glutaric aciduria).
- Samples for copper and caeruloplasmin in a male with subdurals (to exclude Menkes).
- Consider freezing urine, plasma, and serum samples to permit future analysis if the child is likely to die.
- Head CT scan is recommended whenever an NAI is suspected.

Some diagnoses to consider

Osteogenesis imperfecta (OI)

See 'Fractures' in Chapter 2, 'Clinical approach', p. 158. In Marlowe et al.'s (2002) study of biochemical analysis of fibroblasts in 262 children presenting with a suspected NAI, 11 samples had alterations in the amount or structure of type I collagen synthesized, consistent with the diagnosis of OI. In 6/11, the diagnosis of OI was clinically suspected.

Ehlers-Danlos syndrome

See 'Ehlers-Danlos syndrome' in Chapter 3, 'Common consultations', p. 406. In severe forms of EDS, extensive or severe mucocutaneous injuries may occur after minor trauma (Castori 2016).

Glutaric aciduria

Associated with widening of the subdural space that can result in SDH due to stretching and rupture of subdural vessels. Case reports describe associated retinal haemorrhage.

Menkes syndrome

An XLR disorder of copper metabolism. Main features are sparse, steely hair (with pili torti on microscopy) and progressive neurological impairment, often with seizures and spasticity. Wormian bones on SXR. Caused by mutations in ATP7A on Xq13.2–q13.3.

Deficiency disorders

Consider the possibility of scurvy or rickets.

Hypophosphatasia

A rare AR inborn error of metabolism characterized by defective bone mineralization caused by a deficiency of liver-, bone-, or kidney-type alkaline phosphatase due to mutations in the tissue-non-specific alkaline phosphatase (TNSALP) gene. The clinical expression of the disease is highly variable, ranging from stillbirth with a poorly mineralized skeleton to pathological skeletal fractures that develop in late adulthood only. This clinical heterogeneity is due to the strong allelic heterogeneity in the TNSALP gene (Herasse et al. 2002).

Congenital insensitivity to pain

Caused by biallelic mutation in the SCN9A gene; presents with frequent painless fracture, bruises, cuts, and corneal ulceration that may be mistaken for NAI (Cox et al. 2006). Other Mendelian genes causing painlessness include NGF, SCN11A, PRDM12, and CLTC1 (Nahorski 2015).

Congenital insensitivity to pain with anhidrosis (CIPA)

A rare AR sensory autonomic neuropathy caused by mutations in the neurotrophic tyrosine kinase receptor type I (*NTRK1*). Skeletal findings include fractures, joint deformities, joint dislocations, osteomyelitis, avascular necrosis, and acro-osteolysis. MR is common and cranial imaging may show mild loss of brain volume with some ventriculomegaly. Death from hyperpyrexia occurs in almost 20% of patients in the first 3 years of life (Schulman *et al.* 2001).

Brittle cornea syndrome (BCS)

Clinical features include extreme corneal thinning with rupture, high myopia, blue sclerae, deafness of mixed aetiology with hypercompliant tympanic membranes, and variable skeletal manifestations. Corneal rupture may be the presenting feature of BCS, and it is possible that this may be incorrectly attributed to NAI. Caused by biallelic mutation in the *ZNF469* or *PRDM5* genes.

Genetic advice

Recurrence risk

If a genetic disorder is diagnosed, advise as appropriate. Social/environmental issues may generate a risk of recurrence, even in the absence of a genetic risk. If a diagnosis of NAI is made, assessment and management of this risk is the responsibility of the paediatrician and child protection team.

References

Burkitt Wright EM, Porter LF, Spencer HL, *et al.* Brittle cornea syndrome: recognition, molecular diagnosis and management. *Orphanet J Rare Dis* 2013; **8**: 68.

Castori M. Ehlers-Danlos syndrome(s) mimicking child abuse:is there an impact on clinical practice? *Am J Med Genet C*; **169**: 289–92.

Cox JJ, Reimann F, Nicholas AK, *et al.* An *SCN9A* channelopathy causes congenital inability to experience pain. *Nature* 2006; **444**: 894–8.

Herasse M, Spentchian M, Taillandier A, Mornet E. Evidence of a founder effect for the tissue-nonspecific alkaline phosphatase (*TNSALP*) gene E174K mutation in hypophosphatasia patients. *Eur J Hum Genet* 2002; **10**: 666–8.

Kemp AM. Investigating subdural haemorrhage in infants. *Arch Dis Child* 2002; **86**: 98–102.

Marlowe A, Pepin MG, Byers PH. Testing for osteogenesis imperfecta in cases of suspected non-accidental injury. *J Med Genet* 2002; **39**: 382–6.

Nahorski MS, Chen YC, Woods CG. New Mendelian disorders of painlessness trends. *Neurosci* 2015; **38**: 712–24.

Nassogne MC, Sharrard M, Hertz-Pannier L, *et al.* Massive subdural haematomas in Menkes disease mimicking shaken baby syndrome. *Childs Nerv Syst* 2002; **18**: 729–31.

Schulman H, Tsodikow V, Einhorn M, Levy Y, Shorer Z, Hertzanu Y. Congenital insensitivity to pain with anhidrosis (CIPA): the spectrum of radiological findings. *Pediatr Radiol* 2001; **31**: 701–5.

Syndactyly (other than 2/3 toe syndactyly)

For 2/3 toe syndactyly, see 'Minor congenital anomalies' in Chapter 2, 'Clinical approach', p. 240.

Syndactyly occurs when the digits fail to separate during days 52–55 (post-fertilization) or when an external disruptive event occurs during embryonic development. Failure to separate can have a genetic cause, but environmental factors, such as CVS, also need to be considered.

The aim is to distinguish whether the syndactyly is isolated or forms part of a syndrome or is secondary (see below). Correct description of the syndactyly is the first diagnostic step (see Table 2.30).

Clinical approach

History: key points
- At least three-generation pedigree. Explain to parents the minimal signs that could indicate a gene carrier.
- Consanguinity (AR syndromes).
- Increased paternal age (Apert syndrome).
- Early pregnancy events such as CVS, bleeding, teratogen exposure, and fever.
- Neurological/developmental problems.

Examination: key points
- Hands and feet. Describe the shape and count the total number of digits.
- Which fingers and toes are syndactylous?
- Does the syndactyly involve the whole length of the digits, i.e. complete or partial?
- Does the syndactyly appear to involve the bones or just soft tissues?
- Is there any skin webbing between the digits?
- Is there shortening of any of the digits, symbrachydactyly (Poland anomaly)?
- Bilateral or unilateral and symmetry.
- Thumbs and halluces. Are they involved? Document the structure and function.
- Head and skull shape; craniosynostosis (Apert syndrome).
- Microphthalmia (ODD syndrome).
- Hypoplastic alae nasi, 'pinched nose' (ODD).
- Oral region. Cleft palate, oral frenulae, tongue cysts (OFD syndromes).

- Other malformations (chromosomal disorders).
- Skin pigmentary abnormalities (chromosome mosaicism; especially consider diploid/triploid mosaicism).
- Remember to examine the parents.

Special investigations
- Clinical photographs.
- X-rays of the hands and feet are essential to assess the skeletal elements and to detect minor features not seen on clinical examination. The X-ray will assist in the process of definition.
- SXRs and further skeletal films, if indicated from clinical assessment.
- Genomic analysis in presence of features suggestive of a chromosomal or syndromic diagnosis, e.g. genomic array, gene panel, or WES/WGS as available.
- Skin fibroblast if chromosome mosaicism is likely.
- DNA storage and analysis, if available.

Some diagnoses to consider

With asymmetric involvement

MOEBIUS SYNDROME. Congenital cranial nerve palsies affecting VIth (abduction of the eye) and VIIth (facial movement) nerves, in conjunction with terminal transverse defects. See 'Facial asymmetry' in Chapter 2, 'Clinical approach', p. 146. Moebius syndrome may also be a feature of OMLH syndrome and occur with Poland anomaly. See 'Limb reduction defects' in Chapter 2, 'Clinical approach', p. 212.

Be aware of the AR phenocopy Carey–Fineman–Ziter syndrome if talipes and muscle weakness are features.

AMNIOTIC BANDS. Early rupture of the amnion may lead to the production of fibrous mesodermal cords that constrict or cleave parts of the fetus, causing disruption of an otherwise normal development. Another possible causal mechanism is the modification of fetal blood flow—the bands being a secondary phenomenon. Sometimes amniotic bands can be visualized by USS. There may be a clear history that, at delivery, fibrous cords were wrapped tightly round the affected digit(s). Sometimes the syndactyly is terminal and it is possible to pass a probe between the fingers proximally. Recurrence risk is very small at <2%.

Table 2.30 Classification of the syndactylies

Syndactyly type	Fingers	Toes	Comments
Type I (2q34–36)	3–4	2–3	Bilateral in 50%. Syndactyly of toes is four times as common as that of fingers
Type II (also known as synpolydactyly) (HOXD13)	3–4	4–5	Mesoaxial polydactyly frequently present (partial or complete duplication of a digit in the syndactylous web)
Type III (connexin 43, GJA1)	4–5		Found in ODD dysplasia
Type IV	1–5		Rare, polydactyly common, hypoplastic or triphalangeal thumb
Type V	4–5 metacarpals	2–3: 4–5	
Complete syndactyly	2–5	2–5	Thumb may be involved. Mainly seen in Apert syndrome

Reproduced from Temtamy SA and McKusick VA, *The genetics of hand malformations*, copyright 1978, Alan R. Liss, New York, with permission from Wiley.

Malformation syndromes

SYNPOLYDACTYLY. A rare AD disorder characterized by syndactyly between the third and fourth fingers and between the fourth and fifth toes, with a partly or completely duplicated digit in the syndactylous web. Penetrance incomplete and expressivity very variable. Severely affected males may also have hypospadias. Most patients have an expansion of a polyalanine tract in *HOXD13* on 2q31.

APERT SYNDROME (FGFR2). Severe syndactyly, often called a mitten hand. The feet are also affected and there is coronal suture synostosis (see 'Craniosynostosis' in Chapter 3, 'Common consultations', p. 378). Developmental delay is found, even when there has been no evidence of raised intracranial pressure. Two recurrent mutations account for the majority of cases.

CENANI–LENZ SYNDROME. An AR syndrome where the hands and feet are similar to those in Apert syndrome, but there is hypoplasia of the radius and ulna and fusion of the metacarpals caused by biallelic mutation in *LRP4*.

OCULODENTODIGITAL (ODD) DYSPLASIA. An AD syndrome with a characteristic nose, type III syndactyly, and dental anomalies. Approximately 50% of patients develop neurological features, e.g. dysarthria, spastic bladder, or gait disturbance, and cranial MRI may show white matter changes. Caused by mutations in connexin 43, *GJA1*, at 6q22–23 (Paznekas *et al.* 2003). There is a high new mutation rate.

ORO-FACIAL-DIGITAL (OFD) SYNDROMES, ESPECIALLY OFD1. OFD1 is an XLD malformation syndrome caused by mutation in *CXORF5*. The features in the hands are syndactyly (usually skin syndactyly affecting variable digits), brachydactyly, and PAP. Craniofacial anomalies are midline cleft lip, tongue cysts, and excess oral frenulae (Thauvin-Robinet *et al.* 2006).

FILIPPI SYNDROME. Type I syndacyly with microcephaly, MR, and a distinctive nose. The inheritance is AR.

Chromosomal disorders

TRIPLOIDY. Consider this diagnosis in very growth-retarded fetuses with syndactyly. See 'Triploidy (69,XXX, 69,XXY, or 69,XYY)' in Chapter 5, 'Chromosomes', p. 694.

DIPLOID TRIPLOID MOSAIC. Arises from partial 'rescue' of a triploid conception, so the morula is mosaic (3n/2n). The affected fetus may not survive pregnancy or may continue to term and survive. Characteristic findings are syndactyly, especially of fingers 3–4 and toes 2–3, with bulbous ends of the toes and clinodactyly. There may be body asymmetry and streaky skin with hyper- or hypopigmentation. Skin chromosomes are

required to make the diagnosis. Genetic counselling is as for full triploidy. See 'Triploidy (69,XXX, 69,XXY, or 69,XYY)' in Chapter 5, 'Chromosomes', p. 694.

DELETION OF 2Q37. Some patients with syndactyly and brachydactyly type E and developmental delay have a 2q37 deletion.

Genetic advice

Recurrence risk

- Bilateral changes affecting the hands and feet, and fitting into one of the classification groups, are likely to be genetic and dominantly inherited. Carefully examine the parents and exclude features of syndromes in affected individuals.
- In type II (see Table 2.30), the penetrance is 96% in the upper limbs and 70% in the lower limbs. The expression is variable.
- Counsel as appropriate if there is an underlying syndrome.

Prenatal diagnosis

- Genetic testing for some of these syndromes may be available.
- USS. The digits can be visualized from the second trimester. Other USS markers should be used to confirm a diagnosis.

Support groups: Many of the individual syndromes have their own support groups. See Contact a Family (UK), http://www.cafamily.org.uk; National Organization for Rare Disorders (USA), http://www.rarediseases.org.

Expert adviser: Willie Reardon, Department of Clinical Genetics, Our Lady's Children's Hospital, Dublin, Ireland.

References

Goodman FR. Congenital abnormalities of body patterning: embryology revisited. *Lancet* 2003; **362**: 651–62.

Paznekas WA, Boyadjier SA, Shapiro RE, *et al.* Connexin 43 (*GJA1*) mutations cause the pleiotropic phenotype of oculodentodigital dysplasia. *Am J Hum Genet* 2003; **72**: 408–18.

Sharif S, Donnai D. Filippi syndrome: two cases with ectodermal features, expanding the phenotype. *Clin Dysmorphol* 2004; **13**: 221–6.

Stevenson RE, Hall JG, Goodman RM (eds.). *Human malformations and related anomalies, Oxford monographs on medical genetics no.* 27. Oxford University Press, New York, 1993.

Temtamy SA, McKusick VA. *The genetics of hand malformations.* Alan R Liss, New York, 1978.

Thauvin-Robinet C, Cossée M, Cormier-Daire V, *et al.* Clinical, molecular, and genotype-phenotype correlation studies from 25 cases of oral-facial-digital syndrome type 1: a French and Belgian collaborative study. *J Med Genet* 2006; **43**: 54–61.

Unusual hair, teeth, nails, and skin

The hair, teeth, nails, and epidermis are all tissues of ectodermal origin (the dermis of the skin is a mesodermal derivative). Hair follicles, sweat glands, and teeth, three of the ectodermal appendages, are derivatives of both the ectoderm and mesoderm. They arise from an interaction between the two germ layers when the overlying ectoderm extends into the underlying dermis. If an abnormality is noted in one ectodermal appendage, detailed enquiry and examination of the others are appropriate. Some of these disorders affect epithelial–mesenchymal interactions more generally, so that mucus glands of the respiratory and GI tracts may also be affected.

There are many ectodermal dysplasia (ED) syndromes, all sharing in common anomalies of some of these structures—the hair, teeth, nails, and sweat (and other homologous) glands. They are distinguished by the specific pattern of ectodermal structures involved and by associated anomalies, e.g. eyelid adhesion in AEC (ankyloblepharon–ectodermal dysplasia–clefting) syndrome, ectrodactyly in EEC (ectrodactyly–ectodermal dysplasia–clefting) syndrome. It is often not possible to make a specific diagnosis. However, detailed clinical assessment with accurate documentation and good photographs may help to establish a specific diagnosis. Sybert's (1997) excellent monograph is an invaluable tool.

The EDs are highly genetically heterogeneous and classification is in a state of transition as molecular genetic studies lead to a better understanding of the molecular basis of these disorders. Genes causing EDs can be divided into four major functional subgroups—those with products involved in: cell–cell communication and signalling; adhesion; transcription regulation; and development (Lamartine 2003).

Clinical approach

History: key points
- Detailed three-generation family tree with specific enquiry about hair, teeth, nails, skin, infant death, and clefting.
- Hair. Description of the hair as a neonate. Has it ever been cut? Does it break easily? What is the colour?
- Teeth. When did the deciduous and permanent teeth erupt? Are they of normal shape and size? Is there a normal number and are they normally spaced?
- Nails. Description of nails as a neonate. Have they ever been cut? Do they seem to grow at a normal rate?
- Skin. Is the skin unusually dry? Has 'eczema' been diagnosed? Are any treatments used?
- Sweating. Does the individual sweat normally? Is there a history of heat intolerance/hyperpyrexia?
- In females especially, is there any evidence of patchiness in the skin (skin colour, distribution of hair and of sweating)?
- Is the child susceptible to infection? Is there failure to thrive?
- Ankyloblepharon. Any history of eyelid fusion or strands of tissue between the lids at birth?
- Developmental delay/seizures (Coffin–Siris syndrome, sparse hair epilepsy syndromes).

Examination: key points
- Hair. Colour, texture (coarse, thin, unruly), sparse, short with broken ends?

- Teeth. Careful inspection of incisors and canines. Count upper and lower teeth (full complement of deciduous teeth is 20 and of permanent teeth is 32). Are the teeth normal in shape or conical or otherwise misshapen? Effacement of gum ridges in a neonate may indicate absence of teeth.
- Nails:
  - look carefully at each fingernail and each toenail. Nails may be thin, short, thickened, discoloured, and flattened or spoon-shaped (koilonychia);
  - absent nails, hypoplasia of the distal phalanges (DOOR syndrome);
  - greatly thickened nails (pachyonychia congenita);
  - defect down the middle of the nail (EVC syndrome, popliteal pterygium, nail–patella syndrome (NPS)).
- Finger deformities in TRPS develop from mid childhood.
- Skin. If there is dry skin, what is its distribution?
- Orofacial clefts (EEC and other *p63* mutation syndromes).
- Hands and feet. Absence or hypoplasia of digital rays in EEC syndrome.
- Nose (prominent nose in TRPS).
- Eyes. Dry eyes, obstruction or agenesis of the lacrimal duct (especially in EEC syndrome); ankyloblepharon.
- Coarse facial features (Coffin–Siris syndrome).
- If NPS is a possibility (severe nail dysplasia; normal teeth, skin, and hair), palpate the patellae and examine the extension and pronation/supination of the elbow.

Special investigations
- Karyotype is not usually indicated if development is normal and there are no additional malformations, but may be appropriate for an isolated female case with a severe hypohidrotic ED phenotype. Genomic analysis in presence of severe features suggestive of a chromosomal or syndromic diagnosis, e.g. genomic array, gene panel, or WES/WGS as available.
- If a specific diagnosis is made, e.g. hypohidrotic ectodermal dysplasia (HED), IP, NPS, mutation analysis may be possible.
- If NPS is a possibility, radiographs of the hands, elbows, pelvis, and knees, and urine dipstick for proteinuria and measurement of plasma creatinine. Iliac horns (exostoses of the iliac crests) occur in 70% and are pathognomonic for NPS but show age-dependent penetrance (see below).
- Consider referral for expert dermatological/dental opinion.

Some diagnoses to consider

Skin, hair, and nail abnormalities

XL HYPOHIDROTIC ECTODERMAL DYSPLASIA (HED). The most common ED. Males have reduced or absent sweating, dry skin, sparse hair, and missing and abnormally shaped teeth (conical or 'peg'-shaped). If the diagnosis is not recognized, there is a significant infant mortality risk in affected males due to hyperpyrexia with intercurrent infections. Females show very variable expressivity. The gene is known as *EDA*. Stigmatization has a major impact on the lives of males affected with XL HED, although many develop effective strategies for managing this very successfully. There are phenotypically very similar, but rarer, AD and AR disorders; mutation testing is available in *EDAR* and *Wnt10A*. Even rarer are the very few males affected with XL HED and immunodeficiency due to mutations in *NEMO*, the gene mutated in IP (see below).

AD ECTODERMAL DYSPLASIA (ED). There are many families with AD transmission of a relatively mild ED. The classification of some of these disorders is tricky due to overlapping phenotypes and genetic heterogeneity.

- **Witkop syndrome.** Hidrotic ED of hair, teeth, and nails. The hair may be fine, slow-growing, and sparse or may be normal. A variable degree of hypodontia of the permanent dentition is present. Teeth may be widely spaced and conical or peg-shaped. Deciduous teeth may also be conical. Nails are often slow-growing and toenails are more severely affected. Many have small dysplastic nails that are spoon-shaped or concave. Most have normal skin, but some have dry skin. Sweating is normal and heat intolerance is not a feature. AD with variable expression. The nail and hair signs are less noticeable in adults and may normalize. Affected individuals may have minimal signs, e.g. tapering crowns and widely spaced teeth.
- **Clouston syndrome.** An AD hidrotic ED with fine, sparse hair. The nails are dystrophic and there is often dyskeratotic skin that cracks easily and is rough to the touch on the palms and soles. The skin over the knuckles, elbows, knees, and axillae shows hyperpigmentation. Caused by mutations in the connexin 30 gene GJB6 on 13q12 (Fraser and Der Kaloustian 2001).

TP63 DISORDERS: ECTRODACTYLY–ECTODERMAL DYSPLASIA–CLEFTING (EEC) SYNDROME (ALSO ADULT (ACRO-DERMATO-UNGUAL-LACRIMAL-TOOTH), ANKYLOBLEPHARON–ECTODERMAL DYSPLASIA–CLEFTING (AEC OR HAY–WELLS), RAPP–HODGKIN AND LIMB–MAMMARY SYNDROMES). EEC is an AD condition caused by mutations in *TP63* on 7q21–22. Cleft lip and/or palate is common. Dry skin with variable hypohidrosis. Sparse, fair, dry hair, often with absent eyebrows and eyelashes. Anomalies of the tear ducts and Meibomian glands are common and can be important. Patients often have hypodontia. Nails are thin, brittle, and ridged. Mental development is usually normal. The middle rays of the limbs are affected to a variable degree, ranging from no obvious defect to absence of the middle three rays.

Predominantly skin abnormalities

INCONTINENTIA PIGMENTI TYPE 2 (IP; *NEMO*). An XLD disorder caused by mutations in the *NEMO* gene on Xq28. Eighty per cent carry a common deletion. Skin features occur in four stages:

- (1) first few days or weeks of life: blistering lesions cropping in the distribution of Blaschko's lines (vesicular fluid is highly eosinophilic), accompanied by marked peripheral blood eosinophilia. Linear distribution along the limbs, circumferential on the trunk, usually spares the face (birth to 4 months; there are rare reports of onset as late as 18 months);
- (2) verrucous lesions (less widespread, often confined to the lower legs; <6 months);
- (3) streaky lines of hyperpigmentation, especially in the axillae and groin (childhood and teens);
- (4) pale atrophic streaks, particularly noticeable on the back of the calves (childhood to adults).

Forty per cent have nail dystrophy; 80% have dental abnormalities affecting deciduous and/or permanent dentition, e.g. missing teeth, small teeth, delayed eruption, conical teeth, accessory cusps. Hair is often sparse in childhood and later wiry/coarse—there may be patchy alopecia. Thirty per cent have eye findings, but most have normal vision. Seizures in 14%, which are persistent in 6%. Learning disability in 10% of affected females (severe in 3%). Affected male pregnancies are usually lost spontaneously in the first or early second trimester. Hydrops may be seen on USS at 8–13 weeks' gestation.

HYPOMELANOSIS OF ITO. Large areas of the skin may be affected by hypopigmented streaks or whorls distributed along the lines of Blaschko. It may be particularly striking over the trunk. The streaks are mainly present on the limbs and the whorls on the trunk. The lesions are much easier to see under UV light. Swirly hyperpigmentation may also be seen. Seizures and developmental delay are often found. Brain imaging may reveal a migrational abnormality. A mosaic chromosomal aetiology has been found to be the cause in ~60% of reported individuals. The myriad of associated features reflects the extensive variety of aneuploid conditions seen. This pigment pattern can also be seen in otherwise apparently normal individuals. Its cause in them is unknown but presumed to be due to mosaicism for single genes controlling pigment production.

Predominantly nail abnormalities

NAIL–PATELLA SYNDROME (NPS). An AD disorder characterized by dysplasia of the nails, patellae, and elbow joints, exostoses of the iliac crest, and in some cases nephropathy. Fingernails are absent or abnormal (hypoplastic, fragile, split, and longitudinally ridged) from birth in 98%. Triangular or V-shaped lunules are characteristic. Nail abnormalities are most severe on the ulnar side of the thumb, decreasing to the little finger. Toenails are rarely involved. Forty to 60% may develop nephropathy. The first indication is chronic proteinuria, and 15% develop ESRF. The gene is *LMX1B* on 9q34, a transcription factor that regulates the *COL4A3* and *COL4A4* genes. Offer surveillance for nephropathy and glaucoma.

PACHYONYCHIA CONGENITA. A group of AD disorders characterized by symmetrical hypertrophic nail dystrophy, affecting all nails and usually present from birth or developing in the neonatal period. The nails are greatly thickened and have a yellow–brown discoloration. Various subtypes are caused by mutations in keratin K6, K16, or K17.

DOORS SYNDROME (CONGENITAL DEAFNESS, ONYCHODYSTROPHY, ONYCHOLYSIS, RETARDATION, AND SEIZURES). In this disorder caused by biallelic variants in *TBC1D24* gene (Campeau 2014), the nails are small and dystrophic and there may be hypoplasia of the distal phalanges. The thumbs are absent in Yunis–Varon.

YUNIS-VARON SYNDROME. A severe AR disorder, often lethal in infancy, that is characterized by absent/hypoplastic thumbs, hypoplasia of the distal phalanges of the fingers with hypoplastic/absent nails, and absence of the distal phalanx of the great toe. It is caused by biallelic variants in FIG4 gene.

Predominantly hair abnormalities

COFFIN–SIRIS-RELATED DISORDERS. A common, usually *de novo* dominant disorder with sparse hair, coarse facial features, and nail hypoplasia, especially of the fifth finger.

Caused by heterozygous mutations in genes in the SWI/SNF chromatin remodelling complex, especially ARID1B.

NICOLAIDES–BARAITSER SYNDROME. Seizures, sparse hair. X-ray and clinical abnormalities of the phalanges with brachydactyly and swelling of the IP joints. Caused by heterozygous mutation of *SMARCA2*. Other genes in the SWI/SNF complex can cause an overlapping phenotype.

TRICHORHINOPHALANGEAL SYNDROME (TRPS). An AD disorder characterized by fine, sparse-growing scalp hair, dystrophic brittle nails, brachyphalangia with cone-shaped epiphyses on X-ray, and a pear-shaped bulbous nose. *TRPS1* is in 8q24. It may be due to mutation in the gene or be part of a contiguous gene deletion syndrome (Langer–Gideon syndrome). Specific molecular cytogenetic FISH analysis is available for the microdeletion.

MENKES SYNDROME. An XLR disorder of copper metabolism due to mutation in *ATP7A*. Main features are sparse, steely hair (with pili torti on microscopy), progressive neurological impairment, often with seizures and spasticity. Wormian bones on SXR.

Other metabolic disorders
Predominantly dental abnormalities.

AMELOGENESIS IMPERFECTA. A defect of the enamel affecting both deciduous and permanent teeth. The teeth appear yellowed due to thinning of the enamel that allows the yellow colour of the dentine to show through the enamel layer. It is usually AD and due to mutations in the enamelin gene; it can also follow XLR inheritance where it is caused by mutations in the amelogenin gene (female carriers show ridging of the teeth due to irregularity of the enamel covering). A few kindreds show AR inheritance.

DENTINOGENESIS IMPERFECTA (DI). Is sometimes an accompanying symptom of OI, belongs to a group of genetically conditioned dentin dysplasias, and is characterized clinically by an opalescent, amber appearance of the dentin. Although the teeth of DI cases wear more easily and excessively, compared to normal teeth, they do not appear to be more susceptible to dental caries than normal teeth. DI follows AD inheritance.

Predominant abnormality affecting sweating

ANHIDROSIS WITH INSENSITIVITY TO PAIN. An AR disorder of peripheral cholinergic nerves that impacts on sweat gland function (they are structurally normal) and pain sensation (so that distal injuries are common).

Genetic advice

Recurrence risk
- As for the specific disorder.
- IP. New mutation rate is significant; 80% have a common deletion in *NEMO*; 70% of new mutations arise on the paternally inherited X. An adjacent pseudogene facilitates gene conversion events. There is a small chance that parents may be asymptomatic mosaics, so very careful examination of the parents, especially the mother, is important.

Carrier detection
If XL HED is a possibility, any possible female carrier should be examined carefully. Mutation searching in her is useful, even if there is no affected male in whom to identify the family's mutation. If no mutation is found and

doubt remains, it is possible to perform a starch–iodine sweat test, looking for mosaicism, usually on the back (lines of Blaschko). Recognition of female carriers of XL HED is important because of the additional care often required for affected male infants from birth, at a stage when the diagnosis may not otherwise be suspected.

Prenatal diagnosis
May be possible if the mutation is known.

Natural history and further management (preventative measures)

- Hyperpyrexia. Offer advice to prevent hyperpyrexia in infants who are unable to sweat (e.g. avoiding very hot environments, not heating the milk if the infant is fed artificially, removal of items of clothing when the child feels hot, fans, and air conditioning). Precautions must be taken to limit upper respiratory infections. Tepid sponging and antipyretics for fever.
- Dental. Most people with ED have missing or malformed teeth. Dental treatment is necessary, beginning with dentures as early as age of 2, multiple replacements as the child grows, and perhaps dental implants thereafter. Orthodontic treatment may also be necessary. Refer to an orthodontist with specialist expertise.
- Skin. Care must be provided to prevent cracking, bleeding, and infection.
- Eyes may benefit from artificial tears if xerophthalmia is a problem, and review by a specialist is recommended.
- Other. Professional care may minimize the effects of vision or hearing deficits, and surgical and/or cosmetic procedures may lessen facial and other deformities, thus reducing physical disfigurement.

Support groups: Ectodermal Dysplasia Society (UK), http://www.ectodermaldysplasia.org; Incontinentia Pigmenti International Foundation, http://www.ipif.org; National Foundation for Ectodermal Dysplasias (NFED), http://www.nfed.org.

Expert adviser: Angus J. Clarke, Consultant in Clinical Genetics, Institute of Medical Genetics, University Hospital of Wales, Cardiff, UK.

References

Campeau PM, Kasperaviciute D, et al. The genetic basis of DOORS syndrome: an exome-sequencing study. *Lancet Neurol* 2014; **13**: 44–58.

Chitty LS, Dennis N, Baraitser M. Hidrotic ectodermal dysplasia of hair, teeth and nails: case reports and review. *J Med Genet* 1996; **33**: 707–10.

Clarke A, Burn J. Sweat testing to identify female carriers of X-linked hypohidrotic ectodermal dysplasia. *J Med Genet* 1991; **28**: 330–3.

Clarke A, Phillips DIM, Brown R, Harper PS. Clinical aspects of X-linked hypohidrotic ectodermal dysplasia. *Arch Dis Child* 1987; **62**: 989–96.

Donnai D. Incontinentia pigmenti. In: SB Cassidy, JE Allanson (eds.). Management of genetic syndromes, pp. 185–93. Wiley-Liss, New York, 2001.

Fraser FC, Der Kaloustian VM. A man, a syndrome, a gene: Clouston's hidrotic ectodermal dysplasia (HED). *Am J Med Genet* 2001; **100**: 164–8.

Lamartine J. Towards a new classification of ectodermal dysplasias. *Clin Exp Dermatol* 2003; **28**: 351–5.

Sybert VP. *Genetic skin disorders, Oxford monographs in medical genetics.* Oxford University Press, New York, 1997.

Chapter 3

Common consultations

Chapter contents

Achondroplasia

Achondroplasia is the most common cause of dispro-portionate short stature in children and adults. The prevalence at birth is estimated to be ~1/27 000. Individuals with achondroplasia have disproportionate short stature with shortening primarily of the limbs, a relatively normal-sized trunk, and contraction of the base of the skull giving a large-appearing head. There is considerable variation in severity, which is particu-larly apparent in the neonate and early infancy. Severity may range from so mild that there is uncertainty as to whether the clinical impression of rhizomelic limb shortening in a neonate is a real finding to a picture sufficiently severe that a differential diagnosis of than-atophoric dysplasia (TD) is considered. The final adult height in males is 120–145 cm and in females 115–137 cm. The American Academy of Pediatrics Committee on Genetics (1995) have produced guidelines for the management of achondroplasia from birth to adult life. Medical care aims to prevent known complica-tions, especially cervicomedullary compression, sleep apnoea, and spinal stenosis. The mortality in children with achondroplasia is twice normal, with an excess of sudden death under the age of 4 years, of which 50% is due to brainstem compression. Hecht et al. (1987) found a 7.5% risk for death in the first year of life.

Achondroplasia is an AD disorder caused by mutations in the FGFR3 gene on chromosome 4p that potentiate the activity of FGFR3. Eighty per cent of affected individu-als have DNMs. Mutations are almost invariably on the paternal chromosome and there is a marked paternal age effect. Two common mutations G1138A and G1138C account for 98% of mutations in affected individuals. When FGFR3 is mutated at this site, its normal inhibitory function is constitutively activated (i.e. activated even in the absence of bound FGF), resulting in increased inhibi-tion of growth of cartilage cells. There are phase 2 clinical trials of modified recombinant human c-type natriuretic peptide in progress.

Clinical approach

History: key points
- Brief family tree, unless you suspect that one of the parents is affected.
- Document parental heights and assess whether both parents are normal or whether one of them may be affected. Document paternal age if de novo.
- Prenatal measurement of the femur length. Often within normal range until after 22 weeks' gestation.
- Respiratory difficulties and snoring.
- Hypotonia in infants (foramen magnum compression).
- Ability to walk >100 m in older children and adults.

Examination: key points
- Clinical measurement. Height, weight, OFC—plot on achondroplasia-specific charts.
- Limb shortening, predominantly rhizomelic with tibial bowing.
- Wedge-shaped gap between the third and fourth fin-gers ('trident hand').
- Midface hypoplasia with a depressed nasal bridge in infancy, a relatively large jaw, and a prominent forehead.

- Spine: thoracolumbar gibbus in infancy, then lordosis when ambulant.
- Chest shape, respiratory rate, intercostal and subcostal recession (in infants).
- Limitation of elbow extension.
- Evidence of tonsillar or adenoid enlargement and glue ear.
- Dental malocclusion.
- Neurological examination: hypotonia in infants, hyperreflexia and ankle clonus, bowel and bladder disturbance.
- Gait abnormalities due to shape of the pelvis and spinal cord claudication.

Special investigations
- Skeletal X-rays. To confirm the diagnosis.
  - Skull. The vault is large in comparison to the facial bones. The skull base is short.
  - Spine. Short pedicles. Scalloping of the posterior border of the vertebral bodies. Narrowing of the interpedicular distance between L1 and L5.
  - Chest. Short ribs.
  - Pelvis and hips. Horizontal acetabular roof, squared iliac wings, spur at the medial edge of the triradiate cartilage, splaying of the upper femoral metaphysis.
  - Limbs. Rhizomelic shortening, normal epiphyses, splayed metaphyses.
  - Hands. Metacarpals of equal length leading to tri-dent appearance.
- Cranial USS used in neonates and infancy to assess ventricular size.
- MRI scans to assess the brain and cord. There is debate between experts as to whether these should be offered routinely or only if symptoms. Some units offer baseline brain MRI in infancy. Look for:
  - hydrocephalus, usually communicating;
  - cervicomedullary compression: foramen magnum size, displacement of the brainstem;
  - spinal compression due to stenosis or listhesis, often symptomatic.
- Sleep studies should be performed in all children to assess for central apnoea.

Alternative diagnoses/conditions to consider

There is an apparent clinical continuum from TD, achon-droplasia, and hypochondroplasia through to short normal individuals. Skeletal radiographs, together with mutation detection, can be helpful in establishing a secure diagnosis in borderline cases. Many other rarer skeletal dysplasias are often misdiagnosed as 'achondroplasia' in the prenatal or neonatal period until the skeletal surveys have been reported by an expert or until the molecular testing for achondropla-sia is normal, prompting a review of the diagnosis.

Thanatophoric dysplasia (TD)
Is caused by DNMs in FGFR3. TD is a lethal disorder with profound limb shortening, macrocephaly, and a small chest. Infants are stillborn or die in the early neonatal period from respiratory insufficiency or central apnoea. The diagnosis may be evident on USS at 20 weeks' gestation.

Hypochondroplasia
Approximately 60% are heterozygous for the N540K C>A, or the N540K C>G mutations in *FGFR3*. Clinical features resemble achondroplasia but are milder with less involvement of the face, skull, and spine. Diagnostic changes may not be seen on radiographs until 2 years of age. Neurological problems are rare.

Pseudoachondroplasia
Short stature is often not apparent at birth or in infancy but becomes apparent in a toddler. Craniofacial appearance is normal. Limbs are short (as for achondroplasia) and there is joint hypermobility with early arthritis. Mutations in the *COMP* gene on 19p13.1 (allelic with MED).

Homozygous achondroplasia
Early death due to respiratory insufficiency from a small thorax. Radiological changes are more extreme.

Genetic advice
AD, but many cases are new mutations. If a parent is affected, there will be a 50% risk to the offspring of any pregnancy. If *de novo*, the sibling recurrence risk is 0.02% (Mettler and Fraser 2000). Germline mutations are rare.

If both parents have achondroplasia, there is a 25% chance of a child with normal stature, a 50% chance of a child with achondroplasia, and a 25% chance of a child with homozygous achondroplasia (most die in the neonatal period due to respiratory difficulties with features very similar to those of TD).

Variability and penetrance
Penetrance is 100%. Final adult height varies considerably (males 120–145 cm; females 115–137 cm).

Prenatal diagnosis
NIPT may be helpful for PND (except where achondroplasia is maternally inherited) or where achondroplasia is suspected on USS during a pregnancy (see 'Non-invasive prenatal diagnosis/testing (NIPD/T)' in Chapter 6, 'Pregnancy and fertility', p. 764). PND is also possible by CVS at 11 weeks' gestation if the mutation is known. USS is not particularly useful, as the fall-off in the growth of long bones is not observed until after 20 weeks' gestation.

Other family members
Achondroplasia is usually clinically apparent, so testing of other family members is rarely indicated unless there is clinical suspicion that they are affected.

Natural history and management
Cognitive outcome is normal in the great majority. Motor milestones are usually delayed, with independent sitting achieved at 9–20 months and walking at 14–27 months.

Handling in infancy requires special care, with support given to the baby's head. Avoid baby bouncers and swings (risk of cervicomedullary compression and worsening of kyphosis).

Potential long-term complications
- Anaesthetic risks. Expert care of the cervical spine is required to avoid cervical cord compromise during intubation, etc.; increased risk for obstructive apnoea and post-sedation obstruction (Berkowitz *et al.* 1990).
- Cervical spinal stenosis. In infants, compression of the cervicomedullary junction can cause apnoea and sudden death; in children, there is a risk of high cervical myelopathy. Avoid contact sports, e.g. rugby, ice

hockey, or other sports where there is a high risk of impact, e.g. skiing, trampolining, gymnastics.
- Glue ear occurs in the majority and may cause conductive deafness, impairing acquisition of speech and language. Parental vigilance is important, with a low threshold for audiometry and ENT referral.
- Growth. GH administration does lead to a small increase in the final height. The vertebrae are thought to grow more than the limbs, slightly increasing the disproportion. Such treatment should only be considered after a full discussion about the uncertainties and the small gain in height achieved by such therapy. Limb lengthening may give up to 10 extra inches but is complicated and considered expensive. Trials are presently being conducted of drugs aimed at inactivating the mutant gene (Legeai-Mallet 2016).
- Hydrocephalus. Most infants with achondroplasia are macrocephalic. The OFC should be plotted on achondroplasia-specific charts and monitored serially (every 1–2 months) during the first years of life. Some individuals need shunting.
- Pregnancy. Women with achondroplasia can have successful full-term pregnancies. Main risks are respiratory compromise in late pregnancy and the neurological complications of hyperlordosis. Baseline pulmonary function tests early in the third trimester may be helpful. Women should be under specialist obstetric care. Delivery is usually by elective LSCS. Spinal anaesthesia should be avoided in women with achondroplasia.
- Musculoskeletal. Hypermobility is common at all joints, except the elbow where there is restriction of movement. Most infants have a mild lumbar kyphosis, which changes to a marked or severe lumbar lordosis once they are old enough to walk. Their trunks should be supported until sufficient strength is gained to support the trunk independently.
- Respiratory insufficiency. Infants with achondroplasia have smaller than average chests. The respiratory compromise may be sufficient to cause tachypnoea and sweating, particularly with feeding. Such infants are particularly at risk with intercurrent infections, e.g. bronchiolitis.
- Snoring and sleep apnoea. Most individuals with achondroplasia snore loudly. Some suffer with obstructive apnoea, which can be helped by continuous positive airway pressure (CPAP).
- Spinal stenosis. Exercise-induced spinal claudication is present to some extent in most adults with achondroplasia due to stenosis of the lumbar spine. Adults with achondroplasia are also at risk for nerve root or cord compression, which is not exercise-related and may require urgent neurological/neurosurgical assessment (decompressive laminectomy).

Indications for surgery
- Cervical myelopathy with MRI evidence of compression and neurogenic apnoea.
- Thoracolumbar stenosis (inability to walk >100 m, neurological deficits).
- Limb straightening, usually of tibia varum.
- Correction of asymmetry in the tibia/fibula and radius/ulna.
- Limb lengthening procedures are another area of controversy, but the topic should be discussed with all parents. This needs to be performed in specialist centres.

Support groups: Restricted Growth Association, https://www.restrictedgrowth.co.uk; Little People of America, http://www.lpaonline.org.

Expert adviser: Judith Hall, Professor Emerita of Paediatrics and Medical Genetics, UBC & Children's and Women's Health Centre of British Columbia, Department of Medical Genetics, British Columbia's Children's Hospital, Vancouver, Canada.

References

American Academy of Pediatrics Committee on Genetics. Health supervision for children with achondroplasia. *Pediatrics* 1995; **95**: 443–51.

Berkowitz ID, Raja SN, Bender KS, Kopits SE. Dwarfs: pathophysiology and anesthetic implications. *Anesthesiology* 1990; **73**: 739–59.

Hecht JT, Francomano CA, Horton WA, Annegers JF. Mortality in achondroplasia. *Am J Hum Genet* 1987; **41**: 454–64.

Hunter AGW, Bankier A, Rogers JG, Sillence D, Scott CI Jr. Medical complications of children with achondroplasia: a multi-center patient review. *J Med Genet* 1998; **35**: 705–12.

Legeai-Mallet L. C-type natriuretic peptide analog as therapy for achondroplasia. *Endocr Dev* 2016; **30**: 98–105.

Mettler G, Fraser FC. Recurrence risk for sibs of children with 'sporadic' achondroplasia. *Am J Med Genet* 2000; **31**: 250–1.

Pauli RM. Achondroplasia. In: SB Cassidy, JE Allanson (eds.). *Management of genetic syndromes*, pp. 9–32. Wiley-Liss, New York, 2001.

Alpha-1 antitrypsin deficiency

Alpha-1 antitrypsin is a serine proteinase inhibitor that protects the connective tissue of the lungs from the elastase released by leucocytes. Alpha-1 antitrypsin deficiency is a common AR disorder (1/1600–1/1800) characterized by a predisposition to emphysema and cirrhosis. Liver damage arises not from the deficiency of the protease inhibitor, but from pathological polymerization of the variant alpha-1 antitrypsin before its secretion from hepatocytes. Alpha-1 antitrypsin is encoded by the gene *SERPINA1* on 14q32.1.

Mutations in alpha-1 antitrypsin affect the electrophoretic mobility of the protein. Wild-type alpha-1 antitrypsin deficiency is termed M; the S variant (Glu264Val) results in a 40% reduction in plasma alpha-1 antitrypsin levels in homozygotes and the Z variant (Glu342Lys) results in an 85% reduction in homozygotes. Synthesis of the S and Z variants is normal, but intracellular processing and secretion are impaired and the protein is retained in the endoplasmic reticulum. Plasma concentrations in ZZ homozygotes and Z-null and SZ heterozygotes are insufficient to ensure lifelong protection from proteolytic damage, especially in smokers. Resulting lung damage results in the clinical phenotype of predominantly panlobular, basal emphysema. There is also an association with panniculitis, Wegener's granulomatosis, and possibly bronchiectasis. Recent work shows that neutrophils are chemotactically attracted to the polymerized Z protein and so polymerization may also play an important role in lung damage.

In Sveger's (1984) survey of 127 neonates with the ZZ phenotype, virtually all had raised liver enzymes, and 14 (11%) had prolonged neonatal jaundice. Most of the infants with neonatal jaundice recovered, but, overall, three (2.4%) of the ZZ cohort developed cirrhosis in infancy or childhood. The neonatal period is a vulnerable period. One can speculate that, when polymerization of variant alpha-1 antitrypsin occurs, the immature liver is less able to degrade polymerized protein and is more readily overwhelmed, resulting in liver damage. Other factors such as intercurrent infection and fever may facilitate polymerization. Genetic variation in polymer degradation may be another important factor in the enormous variability in hepatic phenotype.

PiM is the normal protein. Ten per cent of the European population are carriers for the S or Z variant (4% (1/25) of North Europeans carry Z, and 6% (1/17) carry S. Common phenotypes are PiMM, PiMS, PiMZ, PiSS, PiSZ, and PiZZ. Null variants are only distinguishable from homozygotes with genotyping.

Clinical approach

History: key points

- Three-generation family tree, with specific enquiry regarding emphysema and liver disease.
- Smoking history.

Investigations

- Clotted sample (serum) for alpha-1 antitrypsin phenotyping. If interpretation of phenotyping is problematic, proceed to genotyping (5 ml of an EDTA sample).

NB. If attempting alpha-1 antitrypsin typing on an individual who has had a liver transplant, the electrophoretic mobility of alpha-1 antitrypsin will reflect the genotype of the donor liver, and you will need to resort to mutation analysis (of DNA from lymphocytes) to determine the genotype of the transplant recipient.

Genetic advice

Inheritance and recurrence risk

AR inheritance. The possibility that apparently healthy parents of a ZZ or SZ child may themselves be ZZ or SZ should be borne in mind when offering phenotyping.

Variability and penetrance

If MZ parents have had a child with a ZZ phenotype and severe neonatal liver disease, it is easy to advise on the 1 in 4 risk for a subsequent ZZ child, but less easy to advise on the probability that subsequent ZZ children will develop severe liver disease. Accurate estimates are very difficult to establish. The risk quoted by Psacharopoulos *et al.* (1983) of 78% is almost certainly an overestimate. Current estimates are closer to 20–30% for significant liver disease in a ZZ sibling (i.e. overall 5–7% risk to a future pregnancy).

Prenatal diagnosis

This is available using CVS. Parents must have been phenotyped first, and subsequently genotyped. PND is by genotyping of DNA from CVS. Consult a specialist lab.

Other family members

- The most important message for family members is not to smoke. Smoking greatly accelerates lung disease in alpha-1 antitrypsin deficiency and markedly reduces life expectancy.
- Because carrier status is so common in the general population (10% (1/10)) and because so few ZZ individuals experience severe neonatal liver disease, cascade screening of the entire family is rarely appropriate. Four per cent (1/25) of North Europeans carry Z and 6% (1/17) carry S.
- Subsequent affected siblings of an alpha-1 antitrypsin-deficient proband should receive intramuscular (IM) vitamin K at birth. On theoretical grounds, it seems appropriate to aim to minimize pyrexia and acute phase inflammation by active treatment of incidental infections in ZZ homozygotes, especially in infancy.

Natural history and management

The frequency of abnormal LFTs in PiZZ individuals with alpha-1 antitrypsin deficiency who do not develop jaundice or hepatomegaly in infancy falls from 60% at 6 months of age to a plateau of ~15% at 12–18 years. Abnormal LFTs may be transient. Most of those with abnormal tests at 16 years were normal at 18 years, and vice versa. PiZZ children may be vulnerable to new or worsening liver dysfunction during intercurrent illness, e.g. appendicitis or pneumonia. PiSZ infants have a better prognosis, with a lower frequency of abnormal LFTs throughout childhood. In Sveger's (1984) study, none of the PiSZ neonates developed prolonged jaundice.

Potential long-term complications

- Emphysema. In healthy non-smokers, forced expiratory volume in 1 s (FEV$_1$) decreases by 35 ml/year; in ZZ non-smokers, the average decrease is 45 ml/year, but in ZZ smokers, the rate can be doubled at 70 ml/year, reflecting the development of panlobar basal emphysema.

- Cirrhosis. The risk of cirrhosis in adult life is difficult to quantify, but ZZ individuals are at increased risk for chronic liver disease. Many have subclinical liver disease at post-mortem.
- Surveillance. Watch for deteriorating LFTs (bilirubin, enzymes, clotting) in an individual with known alpha-1 antitrypsin deficiency. This should prompt assessment for liver transplantation.

Support groups: Alpha-1 Foundation (USA), https://www.alpha1.org; Alpha-1 Awareness UK, http://www.alpha1awareness.org.uk.

Expert adviser: David Lomas, Vice Provost (Health), University College London, London, UK.

References

Carrell RW, Lomas DA. Mechanisms of disease: alpha 1-antitrypsin deficiency—a model for conformational diseases. *N Engl J Med* 2002; **346**: 45–53.

de Serres FJ. Worldwide racial and ethnic distribution of alpha1-antitrypsin deficiency: summary of an analysis of published genetic epidemiologic surveys. *Chest* 2002; **122**: 1818–29.

Eriksson S, Carlson J, Velez R. Risks of cirrhosis and primary liver cancer in alpha 1-antitrypsin deficiency. *N Engl J Med* 1986; **314**: 736–9.

Ibarguen E, Gross CR. Liver disease in alpha-1-antitrypsin deficiency: prognostic indicators. *J Pediatr* 1990; **117**: 864–70.

Miravitlles M, Vila S, Torrella M, *et al.* Influence of deficient alpha1-antitrypsin phenotypes on clinical characteristics and severity of asthma in adults. *Respir Med* 2002; **96**: 186–92.

Primhak RA, Tanner MS. Alpha-1 antitrypsin deficiency. *Arch Dis Child* 2001; **85**: 2–5.

Psacharopoulos HT, Mowat AP, Cook PJ, Carlile PA, Portmann B, Rodeck CH. Outcome of liver disease associated with alpha 1 antitrypsin deficiency (PiZ). Implications for genetic counselling and antenatal diagnosis. *Arch Dis Child* 1983; **58**: 882–7.

Sveger T. Prospective study of children with alpha 1-antitrypsin deficiency: eight-year-old follow-up. *J Pediatr* 1984; **104**: 91–4.

Alport syndrome

Hereditary nephritis and deafness.

Alport syndrome (AS) is characterized by haematuria, proteinuria, progressive renal failure, characteristic pathognomic eye signs, and sensorineural deafness. It is caused by mutations in the genes that code for type IV collagen. Type IV collagen is a major component of the basement membranes of the kidneys, eyes, and cochlea, interweaving with laminins, nidogen, and sulfated proteoglycans.

The most serious complication is progressive renal failure. The glomerular basement membrane (GBM) retains the fetal isoforms of type IV collagen, which appear to be more susceptible to proteolytic attack, and glomerulosclerosis develops.

Histological confirmation of Alport syndrome on renal biopsy may be replaced by molecular testing if pathogenic mutation(s) are identified.

The condition is genetically heterogeneous (see Table 3.1). Approximately 85% is XL (XLAS) with mutations in COL4A5 encoding the alpha-5(IV) collagen chain on Xq22–23.

Most (possibly all) other cases are AR (ARAS) with mutations in COL4A3 or COL4A4 encoding the alpha-3(IV) or alpha-4(IV) chains on 2q35–37. A few families may appear to demonstrate AD inheritance with mutations in COL4A3 or COL4A4, but while carrier status is known to be associated with an increased risk of renal failure (usually later life), the extra-renal manifestations do not occur, and generally there are also other risk factors too, such as diabetes or the incidental co-inheritance of other genetic predisposing factors. Digenic inheritance also occurs, with the inheritance of various combinations of single mutations in more than one COL4 gene, which

can be associated with peculiar segregation (Mencarelli et al. 2015).

The role of the geneticist is to provide genetic advice to families with Alport syndrome and to identify relatives (including carriers) who are at increased risk of renal disease for whom lifelong follow-up, with the early use of ACE inhibitors, is indicated.

XLAS

• Males. Sixty-seven per cent of males present with macroscopic haematuria, usually during an intercurrent infection, at an average age of 3 years (Flinter 2004). Once the macroscopic haematuria clears, there is residual microscopic haematuria. A male who has consistently normal urinalysis at the age of 5 years is very unlikely to develop XLAS. All affected males subsequently develop proteinuria; indeed, some 30% later develop nephrotic syndrome. Proteinuria never precedes haematuria in XLAS. High-tone sensorineural deafness affects 83% of affected males and first becomes apparent at an average age of 11 years. It is progressive and hearing may deteriorate rapidly during the teens, but some residual hearing is retained. Hypertension usually develops in the teens and the average age of reaching ESRF for males with XLAS used to be 21 years; however, the introduction of ACE inhibition significantly prolongs the working life of the native kidneys by an additional 13 years, on average (Gross et al. 2012).

• Females. The clinical course is very variable. One-third present with macroscopic haematuria at an average age of 9 years or present later when microscopic haematuria is detected on routine urinalysis. At the most severe end of the spectrum, a small minority (1–2%) have a similar course to that of affected males. At the other extreme, women may remain asymptomatic into their 80s, despite having microscopic haematuria on careful investigation. One-third develop hypertension (usually in mid-life) and the lifetime risk of ESRF is 8–15%.

ARAS

• The phenotype of affected individuals (male/female) is indistinguishable clinically from males with XLAS.

Clinical approach

History: key points

• Family history. At least three generations. Consider XL and autosomal modes of inheritance; enquire about possible consanguinity.

• Renal failure. Age, treatment, transplantation.

• Obtain copies of renal biopsy findings.

• Hearing problems; review audiograms to establish if hearing loss is sensorineural.

• Visual problems, progressive myopia that is hard to correct, history of lens extraction, dry eyes.

Examination: key points

• Haematuria, proteinuria, hypertension, and impaired renal function.

Table 3.1 Classification of Alport syndrome

Description	Cause
X-linked Alport syndrome (XLAS): • renal failure in early adult life in males; • deafness, usually progressive during later childhood; • classic eye signs in young adults	Mutations in COL4A5
X-linked Alport syndrome and leiomyomatosis: • early onset of renal failure with oesophageal dysfunction; • genital leiomyomas and occasional posterior cataract	Deletions from COL4A5 plus the first two exons of COL4A6
Autosomal recessive Alport syndrome (ARAS): • both males and females affected equally; • renal failure in early adult life; • deafness, usually progressive during later childhood; • classic eye signs in young adults	Homozygous or compound heterozygous mutations in COL4A3 or COL4A4

Data from Hudson et al., Alport's Syndrome, Goodpasture's Syndrome, and Type IV Collagen, New England Journal of Medicine, 2003;348:2543–56.

- Eyes. Examination with a slit-lamp ophthalmoscope is required:
  - dot and fleck retinopathy in 85% of affected adult males;
  - anterior lenticonus 25% (conical protrusion of the central portion of the lens into the anterior chamber may cause progressive myopia, anterior capsular cataract, or spontaneous rupture of the anterior capsule);
  - posterior polymorphous corneal dystrophy (rare);
  - the eye findings are the same in XLAS and ARAS.
- Leiomyomatosis (contiguous gene deletion syndrome with submicroscopic deletion in Xq22 causing loss of a variable portion of COL4A5 plus the first two exons of COL4A6).

Investigations
- Urinalysis. Microscopy (microscopic haematuria) and proteinuria. Send urine to the lab for microscopy for red cells if positive on dipstick.
- Renal function. Creatinine.
- Refer for specialist ophthalmological examination ('dot and fleck' retinopathy, anterior lenticonus, and, rarely, posterior polymorphous corneal dystrophy).
- Audiometry to detect sensorineural hearing loss.
- DNA mutation analysis by single gene panel, WES/WGS as available. In XLAS there is a >90% mutation rate (Hertz et al. 2012).
- Genomic array in the presence of MR or other features (submicroscopic deletion of COL4A5 and FACL4).
- Renal biopsy:
  - may not be necessary if there is a family history of Alport syndrome, in which case renal USS suffices to exclude other causes of haematuria, but may be indicated in an apparently solitary cases if mutation testing is not available;
  - typically shows thickening and splitting of the GBM. Tubules drop out; segmental glomerulosclerosis progresses, and the kidneys eventually fail because of interstitial fibrosis;
  - in XLAS, alpha-3(IV), alpha-4(IV), and alpha-5(IV) collagens are undetectable in most glomeruli, tubules, and the Bowman's capsule by immunostaining. Carrier females may show a mosaic staining pattern. In patients with ARAS, alpha-5(IV) staining is detectable in the Bowman's capsule, but there are no detectable alpha-3(IV) or alpha-4(IV) collagens in glomerular or tubular basement membranes.

Other diagnoses/conditions to consider
Benign familial haematuria
AD, mild haematuria without proteinuria that is usually, but not always, non-progressive. The presence of significant proteinuria suggests the possibility of progressive renal disease. Findings on renal biopsy are relatively normal, except for a thin GBM (also found as a normal variant in 5–10% of the population). In some kindreds, the condition is caused by mutations in the COL4A3 or COL4A4 genes (2q35–37), i.e. patients are carriers of ARAS (Taylor et al. 2013).

Genetic advice
Inheritance and recurrence risk
In large families, the inheritance pattern may be inferred from the family history. If there is only a single affected member, consider the following.

- Eighty-five per cent of Alport syndrome is XL due to mutation in COL4A5.
- The new mutation rate in XL Alport syndrome due to COL4A5 is 15%.
- Germline and gonadal mosaicism in XLAS has been reported (Bruttini et al. 2000).
- ARAS is the next most frequent type, after XLAS. Parental consanguinity and/or affected females may increase the likelihood of this.
- In families with documented male-to-male transmission, the inheritance may be AD, but check the validity of the information–there are many other causes of renal failure.

Variability and penetrance
- In XLAS, the rate of progression of renal disease tends to run true, to some extent, within families. There may be slightly more clinical variability in AR families
- Families vary in the rapidity of onset of organ failure. In XLAS, penetrance is close to 99% if the urine is tested carefully in female carriers (who are heterozygous for COL4A5 mutations), but expressivity is variable. The lifetime risk for ESRF in female patients with XLAS is 8–15%, although risk can be reduced with regular screening and early use of ACE inhibitors.

Prenatal diagnosis and pre-implantation genetic diagnosis
Available if the disease-causing mutation is known or by linkage in suitable pedigrees.

Predictive testing
Possible if the disease-causing mutation is known or by linkage in suitable pedigrees.

Other family members
It is important to identify female carriers in XLAS and male/female carriers of ARAS, as they have a 10–15% risk of renal impairment and should be offered life-long screening of their BP and urinalysis, with the early introduction of ACE inhibitors to protect renal function (Temme et al. 2012). Testing for the familial mutation(s), if known, is the preferred strategy for carrier testing.

Natural history and management
See Savige et al. 2013.

Potential long-term complications
- Renal failure. Progression to renal failure. Renal transplantation is the treatment of choice. One to 5% of individuals with XL Alport syndrome develop anti-GBM nephritis after renal transplantation. The risk is higher for those who carry a mutation resulting in the absence of the non-collagenous (NC) domain.
- Visual problems. Lenticonus can be treated by lens extraction and a replacement lens implant, as for cataracts.
- Deafness. Audiometry at diagnosis and subsequently, with provision of hearing aids as required.

Surveillance
Known mutation carriers and at-risk individuals should be under annual surveillance by a nephrologist.

Support groups: Alport UK, http://www.alportuk.org; Alport Syndrome Foundation (US support group), http://alportsyndrome.org.

Expert adviser: Frances Flinter, Consultant Clinical Geneticist, Department of Clinical Genetics, Guy's and

St Thomas' NHS Foundation Trust, Guy's Hospital, London, UK.

References

Bruttini M, Vitelli F, Melloni I, et al. Mosaicism in Alport syndrome with genetic counselling. *J Med Genet* 2000; **37**: 717–19.

Colville DJ, Savige J. Alport syndrome: a review of the ocular manifestations. *Ophthalmic Genet* 1997; **18**: 161–73.

Flinter F. Alport syndrome. In: F Flinter, E Maher, A Saggar-Malik (eds.). *Genetics of renal disease, Oxford monographs on medical genetics*, pp. 183–201. Oxford University Press, Oxford, 2004.

Gross O, Licht C, Ander HJ, et al. Early angiotensin-converting enzyme inhibition in Alport syndrome delays renal failure and improves life expectancy. *Kidney Int* 2012; **81**: 494–501.

Hertz JM, Thomassen M, Storey H, Flinter F. Clinical utility gene card for: Alport syndrome. *Eur J Hum Genet* 2012, **20**. doi 10.1038/ejhg.2011.237.

Kashtan CE. Alport syndrome. An inherited disorder of renal, ocular, and cochlear basement membranes. *Medicine* 1999; **78**: 338–60.

Lemmink HH, Schröder CH, Monnens LA, Smeets HJ. The clinical spectrum of type IV collagen mutations. *Hum Mut* 1997; **9**: 477–99.

Mencarelli MA, Heidat L, et al. Evidence of digenic inheritance in Alport syndrome. *J Med Genet* 2015: **52**: 163–74.

Savige J, Gregory M, Gross O, Kashtan C, Ding J, Flinter F. Expert guidelines for the management of Alport syndrome and thin basement membrane nephropathy. *J Am Soc Nephrol* 2013; **24**: 364–75.

Taylor J, Flinter F. Familial hematuria: when to consider genetic testing. *Arch Dis Child* 2014; **99**: 857–61.

Temme J, Peters F, Lange K, et al. Incidence of renal failure and nephroprotection by RAAS inhibition in heterozygous carriers of X-chromosomal and autosomal recessive Alport mutations. *Kidney Int* 2012; **81**: 779–83.

Androgen insensitivity syndrome (AIS)

AIS, complete androgen insensitivity (CAIS), testicular feminization syndrome, XY female, partial androgen insensitivity (PAIS).

AIS (1/20 000 live births) is caused by mutations in the androgen receptor gene on Xq11. Primary female sexual differentiation of the human embryo and fetus occurs even if the ovaries are absent and is not apparently under the influence of fetal hormones. Primary male sexual differentiation is dependent on androgens (testosterone and dihydrotestosterone (DHT)) produced by the fetal testes in response to hCG. Thus, an XY embryo carrying a mutation in the androgen receptor gene that prevents androgen binding will develop the external appearances of a female. In addition to testosterone, the fetal testes produce anti-Müllerian hormone (AMH), which causes regression of the structures destined to develop into the Fallopian tubes, uterus, and upper vagina. The female infant with CAIS therefore usually has normal female external genitalia, but a blind-ending vagina.

Girls with CAIS are phenotypically normal females at birth. They present either in infancy/early childhood with bilateral inguinal herniae often containing testes or in young adult life with primary amenorrhoea. The diagnosis is suggested when a karyotype reveals 46,XY.

Girls who do not present in early childhood are often not diagnosed until quite late in their teens. At puberty, the testes produce a large amount of testosterone, which is converted to oestrogen promoting normal breast development. However, usually there is no or scant pubic hair and menarche does not occur.

Clinical approach

Families with a recent diagnosis of AIS are often confused and distressed. Careful, sensitive explanation of the biological basis for AIS is important. Emphasize the basic female pattern of the developing embryo and the normal female development of girls with AIS.

History: key points

- Three-generation family tree. In a family with AIS, a history of maternal female relatives who have been unable to have children raises suspicion.
- Determine how and when the diagnosis was made and obtain confirmation of the karyotype.

Examination: key points

Examination may not be appropriate if the diagnosis is secure. Otherwise:

- in infants and young children, examine for bilateral inguinal herniae;
- in teenagers and adults, examine for lack of axillary and pubic hair;
- consider pelvic USS to confirm absence of the uterus.

Investigations

- Karyotype to support the diagnosis (if not already done).
- DNA for mutation analysis of the androgen receptor gene.

Other diagnoses/conditions to consider

The combination of bilateral inguinal herniae and normal phenotypic female development with a 46,XY karyotype is characteristic of CAIS, but in a girl ascertained coincidentally also consider SRY gene mutations. In PAIS, with ambiguous genitalia, the differential diagnosis is much wider and a diagnosis more difficult.

Partial androgen insensitivity (PAIS)

In this condition, mutations in the androgen receptor gene impair androgen binding and signalling but do not prevent it as in CAIS. The condition usually presents at birth with ambiguous genitalia. Problems with gender identity are often much greater in this group than in patients with CAIS. This may in part be due to the impaired (rather than absent) activity of androgens on the developing brain. Only a minority of females with a PAIS phenotype have a mutation in the gene encoding the androgen receptor; other genes are yet to be identified.

46,XY female due to mutation in SRY

The SRY gene on Yp encodes a testis-determining factor that promotes the indifferent early embryonic gonads to differentiate into testes. Mutations or deletions of this gene will result in female development, but, unlike in CAIS, the testes are dysgenetic or streak gonads and AMH will not be produced so that the uterus and vagina will persist.

Genetic advice

Inheritance and recurrence risk

- XLR. For a woman who is a carrier, there are four possible outcomes to a pregnancy, each equally likely: a normal daughter; a carrier daughter; a daughter with AIS; and a normal boy (i.e. 25% recurrence risk).
- DNMs occur at a high rate within the androgen receptor gene (27% observed by Hiort et al. (1998); actual risk possibly ~33%). Germline and gonosomal mosaicism have been observed in mothers of affected sporadic cases. Hence, as for Duchenne dystrophy, offer carrier detection to sisters of affected individuals, even if the mother is proven on molecular studies not to be a carrier. (The risk is probably small, possibly a few per cent.) Mothers may also wish to consider PND in a future pregnancy because of the small risk of gonadal mosaicism.

Variability and penetrance

For CAIS, the condition is fully penetrant and, apart from variation in time of presentation, there is little variability.

Prenatal diagnosis

If a mutation is identified, PND by CVS at 11 weeks' gestation is technically feasible. Less certain is the decision to undertake PND for a condition whose main impact is infertility.

Carrier testing

Mutation analysis is the gold standard for accurate carrier detection, but note comments above about the risks associated with gonadal mosaicism. If no mutation is known in the family, analysis of the size of the triplet repeat within the androgen receptor gene can be used for intragenic linkage analysis and may enable modification of the risk when combined with pedigree analysis (e.g. a woman who has inherited a different triplet repeat allele to that carried by an affected member of the family will be at low risk of being a carrier). Inability to determine the level in the family at which the mutation originated limits the utility of this approach in confirming the carrier status in families with single affected individuals. A proportion of CAIS carrier females have reduced body hair (axillary and pubic hair).

Other family members
Maternal male relatives are unaffected, with no implications for their offspring. Maternal female relatives may be at risk of being carriers.

Natural history and management
Potential long-term complications
Testes should be removed because of the risk of gonadoblastoma (~30% risk by age 50 years is often quoted but may be an overestimate). Hormone replacement therapy (HRT) should be offered from adolescence to induce puberty and minimize the risk of osteoporosis. During teenage years, consider referral to a gynaecologist with specialist expertise to assess whether the vagina is of sufficient size for sexual intercourse or whether vaginal dilatation or vaginoplasty should be offered.

Many normal adolescent girls feel relatively insecure about their personal and sexual identity. It is perhaps not surprising, therefore, that a diagnosis of AIS in adolescence or young adult life can precipitate severe psychological distress. Referral for ongoing psychological support, psychiatric help, or psychosexual counselling may be appropriate.

Surveillance
Periodic bone mineral density scans may be appropriate in adult life.

Support group: Androgen Insensitivity Syndrome Support Group, http://www.aissg.org.

Expert adviser: Carlo Acerini, University Senior Lecturer, Department of Paediatrics, University of Cambridge, Addenbrooke's Hospital, Cambridge, UK.

References
Boehmer AL, Brinkmann O, Brüggenwirth H, et al. Genotype versus phenotype in families with androgen insensitivity syndrome. J Clin Endocrinol Metab 2001; **86**: 4151–60.

Boehmer AL, Brinkmann AO, Niermeijer MF, Bakker L, Halley DJ, Drop SL. Germ-line and somatic mosaicism in the androgen insensitivity syndrome: implications for genetic counselling. Am J Hum Genet 1997; **60**: 1003–6.

Hiort O, Sinnecker GH, Holterhus PM, Nitsche EM, Kruse K.. Inherited and de novo androgen receptor gene mutations: investigation of single-case families. J Pediatr 1998; **132**: 939–43.

Angelman syndrome

Angelman syndrome (AS) is a distinctive neurobehavioural disorder resulting from disruption to the function of the maternally imprinted *UBE3A* gene on 15q11.13. It affects one in 25 000 children. All individuals with classical AS exhibit:

- severe developmental delay;
- profound speech impairment. Most do not acquire speech or have only 2–3 words. Receptive and non-verbal communication skills are significantly better than expressive skills. Most children with AS use gesture to communicate and some are able to use picture matching (picture exchange communication system (PECS)) or augmented communication systems. A few will master sign language (e.g. Makaton). Rare patients with AS have developed more speech of >200 words;
- a movement and balance disorder: an ataxic, wide-based gait;
- specific behaviour with an excitable personality and sometimes inappropriately happy affect. Hand flapping when excited. Sociable and inquisitive. Love of water and fascination with reflections. Sleep disorder.

Other features include microcephaly, hypopigmentation (in some deletion patients), and seizures. The EEG shows characteristic features and is a good diagnostic pointer.

AS is caused by impaired expression of the *UBE3A* gene on 15q11.13 that can arise in a variety of ways:

- interstitial deletion of 15q11–13mat in 75–80% (may be cytogenetically visible, but now more usually detected on microarray analysis. FISH may also be used for targeted testing);
- paternal UPD of chromosome 15 (2–5%);
- an imprinting defect (2–5%); maternal chromosome 15 carries a paternal imprint;
- point mutation or small deletion of the E3 ubiquitin protein ligase gene *UBE3A* (10%);
- unidentified. The diagnosis most likely lies elsewhere. Mosaicism must be excluded.

Methylation analysis of 15q11-13 is the first-line test for AS. All patients with an interstitial deletion, UPD, or an imprinting defect, i.e. ~80% in total, will have an *SNRPN* (small nuclear ribonuclear protein-associated polypeptide N) methylation abnormality (only unmethylated alleles). Normal individuals will show one methylated (maternal) and one unmethylated (paternal) allele. Patients with *UBE3A* mutations and those who do not have AS fall into the 'unidentified' category will all show normal results on the *SNRPN* methylation assay. Some patients have mosaic imprinting defects where only a faint maternal band is visualized. These individuals often present with hypotonia, hyperphagia, and a larger head size and may have been considered initially to have PWS.

Clinical approach

History: key points

- Three-generation family tree. Are there any other affected individuals? Would this fit with a maternally imprinted phenomenon?
- Feeding difficulties in infancy due to inefficient suckling as a result of oropharyngeal incoordination.
- Developmental milestones. Always delayed. Mean age of sitting 12 months and walking 4 years. Failure to acquire speech.

- Onset of seizure disorder. Usually between the ages of 18 and 24 months. Characteristic EEG with 2–3 Hz large-amplitude slow wave bursts. The EEG may be abnormal, even if there is no history of seizures. However, a normal EEG does not exclude the diagnosis.
- Characteristic behavioural profile with frequent and sometimes inappropriate laughter, a love of water, and sleep disorder.

Examination: key points

- Growth parameters, including OFC (most have OFC <25th centile by 3 years). Severe microcephaly is very unusual. Imprinting mosaics have a larger head size. Do not usually have structural birth defects.
- Happy and sociable affect. Smiling and laughing behaviours do not occur totally inappropriately but are found to increase in social situations and decrease in non-social situations. Hand flapping when excited.
- Wide-based, stiff-legged posture. Axial hypotonia, but increased muscle tone in limbs.
- Jerky and 'lurching' gait, with the arms often held with the elbows bent and the hands uplifted to shoulder level.
- Differences in facial features are subtle and include a wide, smiling mouth, a prominent chin, and deep-set eyes.

Investigations

See Ramsden *et al.* 2010.

- Molecular genetic analysis by *SNPRN* methylation. Eighty per cent will have abnormal methylation. This should be the first-line test. If AS is indicated on methylation analysis, proceed to identify the responsible genetic mechanism by:
  - FISH analysis for AS/PWS critical region or microarray analysis;
  - UPD studies if methylation abnormal, but no evidence of deletion;
  - search for imprinting centre deletion. If the methylation test is positive but no deletion or UPD, an imprinting defect is likely.
- Mutation analysis of *UBE3A* if clinically typical, but methylation studies normal (44% detection rate in one study of methylation-negative sporadic patients) or if family history of AS and pedigree suggestive of an imprinting disorder. *UBE3A* mutations identified in 80% of familial cases and 15% of sporadic cases. Intragenic deletions can occur and should be excluded.
- Genomic analysis for those with negative testing or atypical AS, e.g. genomic array, gene panel, or WES/WGS as available.

Other diagnoses/conditions to consider if investigations are negative

All can be associated with absent speech and seizures.

Rett syndrome (in females)

A proportion of children with a clinical diagnosis of AS, but negative genetic analysis have mutations in *MECP2*. See 'Rett syndrome' in Chapter 3, 'Common consultations', p. 520. Individuals with the congenital variant of

Rett syndrome have *FOXG1* mutations or deletions and microcephaly. The onset of seizures with *CDKL5* mutation Rett syndrome is much earlier than in AS.

Mowat–Wilson syndrome
Recognizable dysmorphic features with upturned ear lobules, hypertelorism, and low columella. Nearly all have microcephaly and seizures. Congenital anomalies include Hirschsprung's disease, CHD, hypospadias and genitourinary anomalies, and ACC. Caused by heterozygous deletions or truncating mutations in the *ZEB2* gene on 2q22.

Pitt–Hopkins syndrome
Severe learning disability with coarsening of facial features over time and appearance of a wide mouth, prominent lips, and deep-set eyes. Start to hyperventilate and breath-hold from mid childhood. ACC frequently present. Associated with *TCF4* mutation or deletion.

SLC9A6 mutations (Christiansen syndrome or XL Angelman syndrome)
Ataxia, seizures, and abnormal EEG. Very similar to AS in young children but is a progressive disorder characterized by dystonia, a slim build, and cerebellar atrophy when older.

X-linked alpha-thalassaemia/mental retardation syndrome (ATRX) in males
The key facial features are tenting of the upper lip associated with a small triangular-shaped nose and a flat nasal bridge and have been confused with those of Coffin–Lowry syndrome. Abnormalities of the genitalia in males, ranging from hypoplasia of the external genitalia to ambiguous genitalia, are found. Search carefully for haemoglobin H (HbH) inclusions in erythrocytes stained with brilliant cresyl. ATRX is caused by mutations in the *XNP* gene on Xq13.

Chromosome abnormalities
These include the 22q13 deletion syndrome (Phelan–McDermid syndrome), deletion of the 5q14 region including the *MEF2C* gene, deletion of 17q21.31 including the *KANSL1* gene, and deletion of *FOXG1* at 14q12 and *TCF4* at 18q21.1. Microarray analysis is recommended in patients presenting with an AS phenotype but no 15q11-13 abnormality.

Genetic advice

Inheritance and recurrence risk
• *De novo* interstitial deletion of the PWS/AS critical region (15q11–q13) on the maternal homologue, with normal parental karyotypes. Risks are very low, probably <1%. Maternal germline mosaicism has been reported (Kokkonen and Leisti 2000).
• UPD15 (pat) arises as a sporadic event, sometimes following rescue of a trisomic conceptus, and so recurrence risks are very low, probably <1/200. Exclude parental Robertsonian translocation.
• *UBE3A* mutation. Women carrying a *UBE3A* mutation have a 50% risk of AS in each pregnancy (when transmitted by a father, development is normal because the gene is silenced). There is a significant risk of gonadal mosaicism in mothers testing negative for a *UBE3A* mutation and PND should still be offered.
• AS without a FISH deletion or UPD. Risks may be high (50%) if there is a *UBE3A* or imprinting centre

mutation. Other imprinting defects are usually sporadic and often mosaic with a low recurrence risk.

Variability and penetrance
Patients with cytogenetic deletions are the most severely affected, while UPD patients are the least affected. Those with imprinting defects may vary greatly, depending on whether they are mosaic. In general, however, all of the phenotypes are severe.

Prenatal diagnosis
If the cytogenetic basis for AS in the proband has been defined using FISH, then this is the method of choice for PND. If there is a known *UBE3A* mutation, deletion, or imprinting centre deletion, then PND by CVS is also possible. If there is no detectable deletion or *UBE3A* mutation, but a methylation abnormality exists in the proband, a small study by Glenn et al. (2000) showed that correct PNDs were obtained in 24/24 samples from amniocentesis and CVS using the *SNRPN* locus. The DNA methylation imprint of *SNRPN* arises in the germline and maintains the imprint in tissues suitable for PND of AS and PWS. (Caution is advised in view of the theoretical possibilities of instability of imprints in the trophoblast in early embryogenesis. Seek specialist advice from a lab with experience in this area.)

Predictive testing
Not usually relevant.

Other family members
Especially important if a *UBE3A* mutation or imprinting mutation is defined, as some relatives may be at high genetic risk.

Natural history and management
Early motor skills are compromised by ataxia, as well as learning disability, and walking is often delayed until 3–4 years. Fewer than 10% fail to achieve independent walking. Portage and other preschool learning programmes have an important role. All children with AS will have special educational needs. Speech is a particular problem and other methods of communication should be pursued. Life expectancy can be normal in the absence of significant medical problems such as severe scoliosis or seizures. Adults with AS need 24-hour supervision but can have a good quality of life. Many live in group homes as adults.

Potential long-term complications
Up to 90% develop seizures (90% with deletion, 20% with UPD). These are worse in early childhood, often disappear in late childhood, and return in adulthood. Forty per cent of adults develop scoliosis. Oesophageal reflux is a prominent symptom in infants and adults. Loss of mobility and development of joint contractures over time. May develop hyperphagia and obesity. There have been some reports of an increased fracture risk in adults with AS. This may be related to lowering of bone density due to immobility.

Surveillance
The child should be under the care of a multidisciplinary child development team.

Support groups: Angelman Syndrome Foundation (USA), https://www.angelman.org, Tel. 800 432 6435;

ASSERT (Angelman Syndrome Support Education and Research Trust), http://angelmanuk.org.

Expert adviser: Jill Clayton-Smith, Consultant Clinical Geneticist, Manchester Centre For Genomic Medicine, Central Manchester Hospitals NHS Trust, Manchester, UK.

References

Clayton-Smith J, Laan L. Angelman syndrome: a review of the clinical and genetic aspects. *J Med Genet* 2003; **40**: 87–95.

Dagli A, Buiting K, Williams CA. Molecular and clinical aspects of Angelman syndrome. *Mol Syndromol* 2012; **2**(3-5): 100–12.

Glenn CC, Deng G, Michaelis RC, *et al*. DNA methylation analysis with respect to prenatal diagnosis of the Angelman and Prader–Willi syndromes and imprinting. *Prenat Diagn* 2000; **20**: 300–6.

Kokkonen H, Leisti J. An unexpected recurrence of Angelman syndrome suggestive of maternal germ-line mosaicism of del (15) (q11q13) in a Finnish family. *Hum Genet* 2000; **107**: 83–5.

Lossie AC, Whitney MM, Amidon D, *et al*. Distinct phenotypes distinguish the molecular classes of Angelman syndrome. *J Med Genet* 2001; **38**: 834–45.

Moncla A, Malzac P, Livet MO, *et al*. Angelman syndrome resulting from *UBE3A* mutations in 14 patients from eight families: clinical manifestations and genetic counselling. *J Med Genet* 1999; **36**: 554–60.

Moncla A, Malzac P, Voelckel MA, *et al*. Phenotype-genotype correlation in 20 deletion and 20 non-deletion Angelman syndrome patients. *Eur J Hum Genet* 1999; **7**: 131–9.

Ramsden SC, Clayton-Smith J, Birch R, Buiting K. Practice guidelines for the molecular analysis of Prader–Willi and Angelman syndromes. *BMC Med Genet* 2010; **11**: 70.

Thibert RL, Larson AM, Hsieh DT, Raby AR, Thiele EA. Neurologic manifestations of Angelman syndrome. *Pediatr Neurol* 2013; **48**: 271–9.

Vendrame M, Loddenkemper T, Zarowski M, *et al*. Analysis of EEG patterns and genotype is patients with Angelman syndrome. *Epilepsy Behav* 2012; **23**: 261–5.

Williams CA, Dagli A. Angelman syndrome. In: SB Cassidy, JE Allanson (eds.). *Management of genetic syndromes*, 3rd edn, pp. 69–80. John Wiley & Sons, Inc., Hoboken, 2010.

Williams CA. Neurological aspects of the Angelman syndrome. *Brain Dev* 2005; **27**: 88–94.

Autism and autism spectrum disorders

Autism is characterized by qualitative impairments in reciprocal social interaction and communication, coupled with restricted and stereotyped patterns of interests and activities. Large-scale genomic studies are gradually revealing some of the genetic factors contributing to autism and autism spectrum disorders (ASD) (see Figure 3.1). The recurrence risk of autism among siblings is many times higher than the rate in the general population. Heritability of autistic disorders is often claimed to be among the highest of all neurodevelopmental conditions, but recent research has suggested that, although concordance in MZ twins is high (60–90%), concordance in DZ twins is moderate too (20–30%), demonstrating the heritable component of autism susceptibility is tempered by shared environmental influences and is probably no greater than 35–40%. Recent research has not supported the validity of the former division of autistic disorders into specific subcategories and instead indicates there are many 'autisms', which are now collectively referred to as ASD (see Figure 3.2).

Only a minority of children with autism have a specific genetic diagnosis. The behavioural phenotype of many rare genetic anomalies indicates a strong association with the autism phenotype. Examples of well-established aetiologies include FRAX, TSC, and Rett syndrome, but there are many more examples, virtually of all which are associated with ID. The use of microarray as a first-line investigation of ID and ASD has confirmed research studies that rare (<1% frequency) CNVs are found at higher frequency (5–10%) in cohorts and individuals with ASD. These CNVs contain genes that particularly affect the neuronal synaptic complex (Devlin and Scherer 2012; Marshall and Scherer 2012). These variants may be inherited from unaffected parents, indicating that there are other coexisting genetic and environmental factors influencing autism and that prenatal testing for these CNVs could not accurately predict the development of ASD. The most commonly found CNV associated with ASD

is the 600-kb deletion/duplication of 16p11.2 in about 0.5% of ASD cohorts. Others include del Xp22.11, del 2p16.3 (including the gene NRXN1), del 7q11.23, del 22q11.2 (di George locus), del 1q21.1, and del 15q13.3. The 16p11.2 deletions appear more penetrant than the duplications, and estimates of penetrance for clinical use for this and other CNVs are now published (Rosenfeld et al. 2013). There are genes within these CNVs that encode synaptic cell adhesion molecules, which suggests that a defect in synaptogenesis may predispose to autism. This is supported by the identification of copy number change in the SHANK genes. This gene family consists of three members implicated by rare CNVs across neurodevelopmental disorders, including schizophrenia, ADHD, and ID. These observations indicate that similar pathways may be involved in phenotypically distinct outcomes (Malhotra and Sebat 2012; Sato 2012). Iossifov et al (2012) performed exome sequencing of 343 families with a single child on the autism spectrum and at least one unaffected sibling. They also suggested a link between autism and synaptic plasticity. There was a paternal age effect, as they showed that de novo small indels and point substitutions come mostly from the paternal line in an age-dependent manner (see 'Timing and origin of new dominant mutations' in Chapter 1, 'Introduction', p. 42 and 'Paternal age' in Chapter 6, 'Pregnancy and fertility', p. 772). De Rubeis (2014) in a large study of the genetic architecture of autistic spectrum showed that many of the genes implicated in ASD encoded for synaptic formation, transcriptional regulation, and chromatin-remodelling pathways.

Prevalence

The distinction between what used to be called 'classical' or 'Kanner-type' autism and other autistic conditions is no longer regarded as meaningful. This may account for some of the increase in prevalence of autism from what just a few years ago was reported

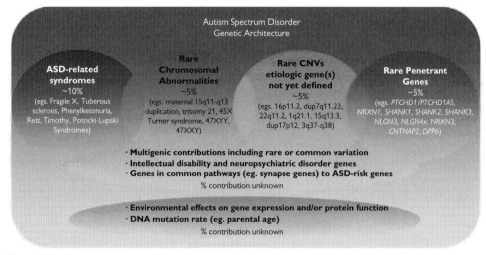

Figure 3.1 Autism spectrum genetic architecture.
Reprinted from *Current Opinion in Genetics & Development*, Volume 22, Issue 3, Bernie Devlin, Stephen W Scherer, Genetic architecture in autism spectrum disorder, pp. 229–237, copyright 2012, with permission from Elsevier.

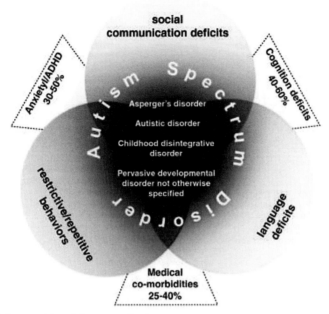

Figure 3.2 The main features of the autistic spectrum disorders.
Reprinted from *Current Opinion in Genetics & Development*, Volume 22, Issue 3, Bernie Devlin, Stephen W Scherer, Genetic architecture in autism spectrum disorder, pp. 229–237, copyright 2012, with permission from Elsevier.

as ~6/1000 (Fombonne 2003) to a generally accepted figure of one in 88 now (Centers for Disease Control and Prevention 2012). The sex ratio, long accepted to reflect a M:F ratio of ~4:1, is also subject to review from recent epidemiological evidence, which suggests this may be an exaggeration—the true figure being nearer 2.5:1 (Kim *et al.* 2011).

Other changes in the conceptualization of autistic disorders concern the former diagnostic requirement for there to have been a delay in onset of language. Recent research indicates that language delay is by no means universal in children who later appear to have typical ASD, especially those with normal-range intelligence. Pragmatic language skills (saying inappropriate or unrelated things during conversations or using unusual language or vocabulary) are, however, universally impaired.

The key features of ASD are impairments of social and behavioural adjustment. Typically, the condition is also associated with an uneven pattern of cognitive defects. A minority of autistic individuals have full-scale IQ scores of <70, but there is no typical cognitive pattern of impairment; verbal skills are as likely to exceed non-verbal skills as they are to be impaired. Some children possess one or more unusual skills, relative to their overall level of ability. The risk of epilepsy developing in adolescence is increased, but recent epidemiological research shows that this outcome is largely confined to those with significant ID (Viscidi *et al.* 2014). The claim that it is typical for infants with ASD to have abnormal patterns of head growth, with early-onset macrocephaly, has also come under increasing scrutiny and is thought now to be unfounded (Raznahan *et al.* 2013).

In 2013, the APA released the final version of the fifth revision of the *Diagnostic and statistical manual for mental disorders* (DSM-5). This introduced some major revisions to the definition of ASD and controversially removed the separate diagnosis of Asperger's syndrome. The link is shown here (http://www.dsm5.org/Documents/Autism%20Spectrum%20Disorder%20Fact%20Sheet.pdf), but we are unable to publish the full guidelines due to copyright restrictions.

The UK National Autistic Society lists the main changes in DSM-5.

• In DSM-5, the terms 'autistic disorder', 'Asperger disorder', 'childhood disintegrative disorder', and 'PDD-NOS' have been replaced by the collective term 'autism spectrum disorder'. For many people, the term 'Asperger's syndrome' is part of their day-to-day vocabulary and their identity, so we understand concerns around the removal of Asperger's syndrome as a distinct category from the manual. All individuals who currently have a diagnosis on the autism spectrum, including those with Asperger's syndrome, will retain their diagnosis. No one will 'lose' their diagnosis because of the changes in DSM-5.
• The previous use of three domains of impairments has been reduced to two domains:
  • social communication and interaction;
  • restricted, repetitive patterns of behaviour, interests, or activities.
• Sensory behaviours are included in the criteria for the first time, under the 'restricted, repetitive patterns of behaviours' descriptors.

- The emphasis during diagnosis will change from giving a name to a condition to identifying all the needs that someone has and how these affect their life.
- DSM-5 has introduced 'dimensional elements' which give an indication of how much someone's condition affects them. This will help to identify how much support an individual needs.
- DSM-5 includes a new condition called 'social communication disorder'.

Clinical approach

History: key points
- Three-generation family tree with specific enquiry about schooling, career choice, hobbies, and sociability of parents and other close relatives.
- Pre-, peri-, and postnatal history.
- Detailed developmental history, especially of language development.
- Specific enquiry regarding regression/loss of skills. Assessment by a child psychiatrist/clinical psychologist.
- Detailed assessment of behaviour, including:
  - social interaction (e.g. eye contact, greeting, turn-taking);
  - repetitive activities (e.g. twirling, spinning);
  - play (e.g. whether it is imaginative);
  - peer relationships;
  - response to close family members and to strangers;
  - response to new situations.

Examination: key points
- Complete physical examination focussed on minor anomalies, neurology, social interaction, and behaviour.
- Careful examination of the skin with Woods light for hypopigmented macules (TSC), if there is a history of seizures.
- Growth parameters. Height, weight, and OFC.

Investigations
- Microarray for children with ID and/or dysmorphic features. WES/WGS currently has an appreciable low detection rate in non-syndromic autism, and an important yield in patients with additional features indicative of an underlying single gene disorder.
- FRAX studies if developmental delay/ID.
- Consider *MECP2* analysis in girls with a history of normal early development and subsequent regression.
- Neuroimaging is not part of routine clinical assessment but is indicated for specific neurological signs. Focus on EEG or the triad of severe learning disability, autism, and epilepsy (Baird et al. 2003).

Diagnoses to consider

Tuberous sclerosis (TSC)
An AD neurocutaneous disorder due to mutations in *TSC1* and *TSC2*. TSC is reported in 1% of children with autism. In TSC, *autism is seen in ~25% of individuals and more broadly defined pervasive developmental disorders are seen in ~50%*. Children who present with seizures, particularly infantile spasms, in the first 2 years of life are more likely to have learning disability and autism or ASD than those who develop seizures later or remain seizure-free. See 'Tuberous sclerosis (TSC)' in Chapter 3, 'Common consultations', p. 534.

Fragile X syndrome (FRAX)
Autistic features are common in FRAX. See 'Fragile X syndrome (FRAX)' in Chapter 3, 'Common consultations', p. 424.

Syndromic conditions where the autistic spectrum is a component of the condition
Autistic spectrum features are a common aspect of many recurrent chromosomal microdeletion/microduplication disorders (see Table 5.5, p. 663) and many Mendelian developmental disorders.

Genetic advice

Inheritance and recurrence risk
Ozonoff et al. (2011) conducted a prospective investigation of ASD sibling recurrence and found a substantially higher rate of ASD in siblings of children with ASD than in earlier studies (which had reported recurrence estimates ranging from 3% to 14%). Better ascertainment procedures may have been responsible for the Ozonoff report that 18.7% of infants with at least one older sibling with ASD went on to develop the disorder. Ozonoff et al. conclude '2 strongest predictors of an ASD diagnosis were the gender of the infant sibling and the number of affected older siblings. Male gender and multiplex family status were independent and significant predictors of an ASD outcome, with a 2.8-fold increase in the risk for ASD for male infants (25.9% of high-risk male infants versus 9.6% of high-risk female infants) and an additional twofold increase in risk if there was more than 1 older affected sibling (13.5% of simplex versus 32.2% of multiplex). The increased risk for male infants replicates previous research. The recurrence rate for multiplex families reported here (32.2%) is similar to that found in an earlier population-based study conducted in Utah. (35.3%)'.

NB. These data were collected prior to the new evidence of CNV changes in ASD and a combined study would further inform genetic counselling.

Variability and penetrance
Variable, even among close family members. See comments elsewhere about the spectrum of disorders within ASD and the estimates of penetrance of CNVs.

Prenatal diagnosis
Not possible, unless there is a specific genetic diagnosis (e.g. TSC, FRAX). Prenatal diagnostic use of CNVs of uncertain significance or fetal sexing for males is not discriminating or accurate enough for use in clinical practice.

Natural history and management
Traditionally autism has been considered to be a lifelong and seriously handicapping disorder, but, now that the condition is being recognized in people with normal-range intelligence, it is becoming appreciated that the outcome may not always be so limited. Educational and behavioural interventions are the mainstay of management. Risperidone shows some promise as a treatment for tantrums, aggression, or self-injurious behaviour in children with these associated features. Depressive and psychotic disorders may develop and require psychopharmacological treatment.

Potential long-term complications

There is considerable uncertainty about the long-term outcome for people with ASD that is associated with normal intellectual abilities, which comprises the majority of cases being diagnosed nowadays in the USA and Western Europe (Centers for Disease Control and Prevention 2012). Although the most seriously affected may not be able to live independently as adults, there is currently little evidence on prognosis. This is likely to improve as supports become available in schools, higher educational establishments, and workplaces. In the most seriously intellectually disabled (a small minority of the total of identified cases of ASD), there is a risk that as many as 20% will develop seizures by adult life (often with an onset in teenage years).

Support group: The National Autistic Society, http://www.nas.org.uk.

Expert adviser: David Skuse, Professor of Behavioural and Brain Sciences, Population, Policy and Practice Program, Institute of Child Health, University College London, London, UK.

References

American Psychiatric Association. *Diagnostic and statistical manual of mental disorders*, 5th edn. American Psychiatric Association, Arlington, 2013.

Baird G, Cass H, Slonims V. Diagnosis of autism [review]. *BMJ* 2003; **327**: 488–93.

Autism and Developmental Disabilities Monitoring Network Surveillance Year 2008 Principal Investigators; Centers for Disease Control and Prevention. Prevalence of autism spectrum disorders-Autism and Developmental Disabilities Monitoring Network, 14 sites, United States, 2008. *MMWR Surveill Summ* 2012; **61**: 1-19.

Cederlund M, Gillberg C. One hundred males with Asperger syndrome: a clinical study of background and associated factors. *Dev Med Child Neurol* 2004; **46**: 652–60.

De Rubeis S, He X, *et al.* Synaptic, transcriptional and chromatin genes disrupted in autism. *Nature* 2014; **515**(7526): 209–15.

Devlin B, Scherer SW. Genetic architecture in autism spectrum disorder. *Curr Opin Genet Dev* 2012; **22**: 229–37.

Fombonne E. The prevalence of autism. *JAMA* 2003; **289**: 87–9.

Iossifov I, Romemus M, Levy D, *et al.* De novo gene disruptions in children on the autistic spectrum. *Neuron* 2012; **74**: 285–99.

Jamain S, Quach H, Betancur C, *et al.* Mutations of the X-linked genes encoding neuroligins NLGN3 and NLGN4 are associated with autism. *Nat Genet* 2003; **34**: 27–8.

Jorde LB, Hasstedt SJ, Ritvo ER, *et al.* Complex segregation analysis of autism. *Am J Hum Genet* 1991; **49**: 932–8.

Kim YS, Leventhal BL, Koh YJ, *et al.* Prevalence of autism spectrum disorders in a total population sample. *Am J Psychiatry* 2011; **168**: 904–12.

Malhotra D, Sebat J. CNVs: harbingers of a rare variant revolution in psychiatric genetics. *Cell* 2012; **148**: 1223–41.

Marshall CR, Scherer SW Detection and characterization of copy number variation in autism spectrum disorder. *Methods Mol Biol* 2012; **838**: 115–35.

Ozonoff S, Young GS, Carter A, *et al.* Recurrence risk for autism spectrum disorders: a Baby Siblings Research Consortium study. *Pediatrics* 2011; **128**: e488–99.

Rapin I. The autistic-spectrum disorders. *N Engl J Med* 2002; **347**: 302–3.

Raznahan A, Wallace GL, Antezana L, *et al.* Compared to what? Early brain overgrowth in autism and the perils of population norms. *Biol Psychiatry* 2013; **74**: 563–75.

Rosenfeld JA, Coe BP, Eichler EE, Cuckle H, Shaffer LG. Estimates of penetrance for recurrent pathogenic copy-number variations. *Genet Med* 2013; **15**: 478–81.

Sato D, Lionel AC, Leblond CS, *et al.* SHANK1 deletions in males with autism spectrum disorder. *Am J Hum Genet* 2012; **90**: 879–87.

Simonoff E, Rutter M. Autism and other behavioural disorders. In: DL Rimoin, JM Connor, RE Pyeritz, BR Korf (eds.). *Emery and Rimoin's principles and practice of medical genetics*, Vol. 3, 4th edn, pp. 2873–93. Churchill Livingstone, London, 2002.

Thomas NS, Sharp AJ, Browne CE, Skuse D, Hardie C, Dennis NR. Xp deletions associated with autism in three females. *Hum Genet* 1999; **104**: 43–8.

Van Den Bossche MJ, Johnstone M, Strazisar M, *et al.* Rare copy number variants in neuropsychiatric disorders: specific phenotype or not? *Am J Med Genet B Neuropsychiatr Genet B* 2012; **159B**: 812–22.

Viscidi EW, Johnson AL, Spence SJ, Buka SL, Morrow EM, Triche EW. The association between epilepsy and autism symptoms and maladaptive behaviors in children with autism spectrum disorder. *Autism* 2014; **18**: 996–1006.

Volkmar FR, Pauls D. Autism [review]. *Lancet* 2003; **362**: 1133–41.

World Health Organization. *The ICD-10 classification of mental and behavioural disorders*. World Health Organization, Geneva, 1992.

Autosomal dominant polycystic kidney disease (ADPKD)

Autosomal dominant polycystic kidney disease (ADPKD) is a common AD disorder, with a prevalence of 1/2000 across all ethnic groups. It is a systemic disorder characterized by:

- age-dependent cysts (see Table 3.2): kidney, liver, pancreas, and spleen;
- cardiovascular abnormalities: hypertension, MVP, intracranial aneurysms (ICAs), and LVH;
- connective tissue abnormalities: hernias, colonic diverticulae;
- age at presentation with renal failure is earlier in polycystic kidney disease (PKD) 1 than PKD2 (54 years versus 74 years, respectively) (Hateboer et al. 1999b).

ADPKD is genetically heterogeneous. Mutations in *PKD1* on chromosome 16 are found in ~77%, while mutations in *PKD2* on chromosome 4 are found in ~14%. Heterozygous mutations in GANAB have also been found to cause ADPKD with a mild phenotype but are rare (Porathetal 2016). PKD2 has a milder phenotype, with most individuals not developing ESRF until their 70s. PKD2 patients are less likely to have hypertension, urinary tract infections (UTIs), or haematuria (Hateboer et al. 1999b).

Many patients with PKD2 will die of another cause. Approximately 6% of patients with ADPKD have an intracranial aneurysm (ICA) with aneurysmal rupture, although uncommon, occurring on average at age 41 years, a decade earlier than in sporadic cases. Patients with PKD2 as well as PKD1 are at risk of ICAs.

Up to 80% have hepatic cysts, but they infrequently cause serious problems. Liver cysts occur more frequently and at a younger age in women than in men. Hypertension is frequent and of early onset.

Each renal and hepatic cyst appears to arise by clonal proliferation following a second-hit somatic mutation.

Clinical approach

History: key points
- Three-generation family tree with specific enquiry about affected relatives, age of diagnosis, reason for diagnosis, age of onset of ESRF, history of subarachnoid haemorrhage (SAH), and cause of death.
- History of loin pain, haematuria, or recurrent UTIs.

Examination: key points
- BP.
- Abdominal examination. Palpable kidneys? Palpable liver?
- Examine the heart. Mid-systolic murmur or MVP?

Investigations
- Consider renal USS after thorough discussion and careful consideration of the optimum age for investigation. Often the first USS is done at 15–25 years (see 'Predictive testing' below). Typical findings are large kidneys containing multiple cysts throughout the renal parenchyma.
- Genomic analysis, gene panel, WES/WGS as available.

Other diagnoses/conditions to consider

Renal cysts and diabetes (RCAD)
An AD disorder characterized by unexplained familial renal cystic disease (renal cysts may be detected *in utero*), early-onset T2D, genital tract malformations, and hyperuricaemia, hypomagnesaemia and early-onset gout. Renal biopsy shows cystic renal dysplasia or glomerulocystic disease. Renal cysts may present before diabetes. It is caused by mutations in *HNF-1β* (hepatocyte nuclear factor-1β).

Tuberous sclerosis (TSC)
A few renal cysts are seen in ~17% of individuals with TSC. They are present from early childhood and do not appear to increase in number with age. Multiple cysts, in conjunction with seizures or ash-leaf macules or other features suggestive of TSC, raise the possibility of a contiguous gene deletion on 16p involving *PKD1* and *TSC2*. See 'Tuberous sclerosis (TSC)' in Chapter 3, 'Common consultations', p. 534.

von Hippel–Lindau (VHL) disease
Renal cysts may be detected from the second decade. Renal cell carcinoma is often, but not invariably, associated with cysts. The kidneys are not usually enlarged and there may be associated pancreatic cysts. See 'von Hippel–Lindau (VHL) disease' in Chapter 4, 'Cancer', p. 618.

Oral–facial–digital (OFD) syndrome type 1 (OFD-1)
A rare XLD condition caused by mutations in *OFD-1* on Xp22, which is lethal in affected males. Characterized in females by highly variable expressivity of polycystic kidneys, midline cleft or notch of the upper lip, multiple oral frenulae, cleft palate, and a lobulated tongue. Limb problems include brachydactyly and skin syndactyly of hands with PPD or bifid halluces. Structural CNS anomalies may occur and some affected females have ID.

Branchio-oto-renal (BOR) syndrome
An AD condition caused by mutations in *EYA1* on 8q11–13. Characterized by preauricular pits/tags and hearing loss in >75% (often with cochlear hypoplasia on MRI).

Table 3.2 Diagnostic criteria for ADPKD as a function of age and genotype

Age (years)	Minimum number of renal cysts for diagnosis	Unknown phenotype	PKD1	PKD2
15–29	≥3 cysts either uni- or bilateral	PPV 100% (sens 82%)	PPV 100% (sens 94%)	PPV 100% (sens 69%)
30–39	≥3 cysts either uni- or bilateral	PPV 100% (sens 95%)	PPV 100% (sens 97%)	PPV 100% (sens 95%)
40–59	≥2 cysts in each kidney	PPV 100% (sens 90%)	PPV 100% (sens 93%)	PPV 100% (sens 89%)
≥60	≥4 cysts in each kidney			

Fewer than two cysts in at-risk individuals ≥40 years is sufficient to exclude the diagnosis.

Data from Pei et al., Unified Criteria for Ultrasonographic Diagnosis of ADPKD, *J Am Soc Nephrol*, 2009 Jan; 20(1): 205–212.

Renal anomalies are very variable and include renal agenesis, duplex kidneys, and renal cysts. Branchial cleft/sinus/cysts occur in some mutation carriers.

Autosomal dominant tubulointestinal kidney disease (ADTID)
An AD disorder, previously called medullary cystic kidney disease type 2, characterized by normal or small kidneys with medullary cysts, hyperuricaemia, and gout. Progressive decline in kidney function occurs with end-stage renal disease (ESRD) typically occurring between the fourth and seventh decades. It is caused by heterozygous mutation in *UMOD* (uromodulin), *MCV1*, *HNF1B*, and *REN*.

Autosomal recessive polycystic kidney disease (ARPKD)
A severe form of PKD that presents primarily in infancy and childhood that is characterized by enlarged kidneys and congenital hepatic fibrosis. The clinical spectrum is widely variable. About 30–50% of affected individuals die in the neonatal period, while others survive into adulthood. See 'Urinary tract and renal anomalies (congenital anomalies of the kidney and urinary tract—CAKUT)' in Chapter 6, 'Pregnancy and fertility', p. 796.

Genetic advice
Inheritance and recurrence risk
AD, with 50% risk to offspring, siblings, and parents of a carrier of a familial mutation. There is usually an extensive family history. DNMs do occur but are uncommon (~10%).

Variability and penetrance
Marked inter- and intrafamilial phenotypic variability occurs. ADPKD is usually regarded as a disease of adult life. However, a small minority may present in childhood with typical symptoms or following abdominal imaging for other indications, e.g. UTI. Rarely (~1%), multiple enlarged echogenic kidneys or intrarenal cysts may be detected during detailed antenatal USS. The phenotype may overlap with infantile PKD but is seen in the context of a family history of ADPKD. Approximately 30% will die in the first few months of life without renal support, and survivors are at high risk for early hypertension and ESRF (MacDermot *et al.* 1998). The severe *in utero* form of ADPKD has a substantial sibling recurrence risk and may be due to the co-inheritance of a hypomorphic mutation from the apparently unaffected parent.
   Familial clustering of ICAs is observed, with the rate of aneurysm detection ~3 times higher in patients with a family history of ruptures of ICAs than in those without. The position of the mutation in *PKD1* is predictive for the development of ICAs—5′ mutations are more commonly associated with vascular disease (Rossetti *et al.* 2003).

Prenatal diagnosis
Technically feasible by CVS if the mutation is known or if the kindred is large enough that clear linkage to chromosome 16 or 4 can be established. In practice, PND is rarely requested. PGD is more frequently requested and is now licensed in the UK.

Predictive testing
Renal USS is the mainstay for predictive testing; mutation analysis is widely available and can be offered. The use of USS for disease exclusion in at-risk individuals aged <30

years may be limited and current genotype-based USS criteria should be used. CT and MRI are more sensitive than USS and may be used following a normal USS if an individual is contemplating donating a kidney to a member of the family with ESRF (living-related transplant). Diagnostic criteria for CT and MRI are now available (Pei *et al.* 2015). With >10 cysts over age 16 years, this gives a sensitivity and specificity of 100%. Linkage may also be desirable in clarifying the status of a potential donor, if mutation analysis is not feasible or does not identify a clearly pathogenic mutation. Genetic testing may identify a pathogenic mutation in ~90% of cases, although careful evaluation of missense variants is required. An international mutation database is available at http://pkdb.mayo.edu.

Other family members
Cascade approach to diagnosis in adult relatives is appropriate because of the benefits of good control of hypertension and the high morbidity and mortality associated with undiagnosed chronic renal failure (CRF).

Natural history and management
Potential long-term complications
- ESRF. Treated by renal transplantation, haemodialysis, or peritoneal dialysis.
- ICA. Asymptomatic 'berry aneurysms' are found in 6% of individuals with ADPKD (population risk is 1–2%). Incidence rises to 16–25% in the presence of a positive family history. The risk of interval rupture in ADPKD is unknown. Management is based on outcome in individuals without ADPKD in whom conservative management is suggested for aneurysms <10 mm in diameter, and surgery considered if aneurysms are >10 mm. (There is a 1% mortality and 3–7% morbidity from surgical intervention.)
- UTI or cyst infection. Prompt treatment of infection is important—if infection becomes established in cysts, it can be very difficult to eradicate.

Surveillance
- Hypertension. BP should be monitored annually from teenage years. Aggressive treatment of hypertension is important in reducing the risk of accelerated cardiovascular and cerebrovascular disease seen in ADPKD and in prolonging renal function. The HALT study (Schrier *et al.* 2014) evaluated the role of BP control in disease progression. In early APKD, rigorous control of blood pressure may be beneficial in disease progression. Dietary sodium restriction is beneficial in the management of ADPKD (Torres *et al.* 2017).
- Renal function. All patients with ADPKD should have their serum creatinine measured once per year. If eGFR falls to <45 ml/min (CKD 3B), referral to renal services is advised if this has not been required previously.
- ICA screening by magnetic resonance angiography (MRA) may be considered if there is a family history of ICA from adulthood. If scans are negative, they may be repeated at 5-yearly intervals; if an aneurysm is present or there has been a previous intracranial bleed, repeat MRA at 2-yearly intervals. Screening should only be arranged in conjunction with neurosurgical colleagues, so that an agreed management plan is in place before imaging is undertaken.
- Pregnancy. Women with ADPKD usually tolerate pregnancy well. They should be under specialist supervision

for monitoring of hypertension (which may worsen in pregnancy) and they are at some increased risk for pre-eclampsia (PET). Renal function usually remains stable throughout pregnancy.

- Drugs. Avoid non-steroidal anti-inflammatory drugs (NSAIDs), e.g. ibuprofen, if renal function is abnormal. Prescribe all drugs with care if renal function is impaired.
- Tolvaptan (vasopressin 2 receptor antagonist) slowed the increase in total kidney volume and the decline in kidney function over a 3-year period in patients with ADPKD, but was associated with a high discontinuation rate due to adverse events (Torres 2012).

Support groups: Polycystic Kidney Disease Charity, http://www.pkdcharity.org.uk, Tel. 0300 111 1234; PKD International, http://www.pkdinternational.org; PKD Foundation, http://www.pkdcure.org.

Expert adviser: Richard Sandford, University Reader in Renal Genetics, Academic Department of Medical Genetics, University of Cambridge, Cambridge, UK.

References

Ferrante MI, Giorgio G, Feather SA, et al. Identification of the gene for oral-facial-digital type 1 syndrome. Am J Hum Genet 2001; **68**: 569–76.

Harris PC, Rossetti S. Determinants of renal disease variability in ADPKD. Adv Chronic Kidney Dis 2010; **17**: 131–9.

Hateboer N, Lazarou LP, Williams AJ, Holmans P, Ravine D. Familial phenotype differences in PKD1. Kidney Int 1999a; **56**: 34–40.

Hateboer N, v Dijk MA, Bogdanova N, et al. Comparison of phenotypes of polycystic kidney disease types 1 and 2. European PKD1–PKD2 Study Group. Lancet 1999b; **353**: 103–7.

MacDermot KD, Saggar-Malik AK, Economides DL, Jeffery S. Prenatal diagnosis of autosomal dominant polycystic kidney disease (PKD1) presenting in utero and prognosis for very early onset disease. J Med Genet 1998; **35**: 13–16.

Magistroni R, He N, Wang K, et al. Genotype–renal function correlation in type 2 autosomal dominant polycystic kidney disease. J Am Soc Nephr 2003; **14**: 1164–74.

Pei Y, Obaji J, Dupuis A, et al. Unified criteria for ultrasonographic diagnosis of ADPKD. J Am Soc Nephrol 2009; **20**: 205–12.

Pei Y, Hwang YH, et al. Imaging-based diagnosis of autosomal dominant polycystic kidney disease. J Soc Nephrol 2015; **26**: 746–53.

Pirson Y, Chauveau D, Torres V. Management of cerebral aneurysms in autosomal dominant polycystic kidney disease. J Am Soc Nephrol 2002; **13**: 269–76.

Porath B, Gainullin VG, et al. Mutations in GANAB, encoding the glucosidase 11α subunit cause autosomal dominant polycystic kidney disease. Am J Hum Genet 2016; **98**: 1193–1207.

Rossetti S, Chauveau D, Kubly V, et al. Association of mutation position in polycystic kidney disease 1 (PKD1) gene and development of a vascular phenotype. Lancet 2003; **361**: 2196–201.

Schrier RW, Abebe KZ, Perrone RD, et al. Blood pressure in early autosomal dominant polycystic kidney disease. N Engl J Med 2014; **371**: 2255–66.

Torres VE, Grantham JJ, Chapman AB, et al. Potentially modifiable factors affecting the progression of autosomal dominant polycystic kidney disease. Clin J Am Soc Nephrol 2011; **6**: 640–7.

Torres VE, Chapman AB, et al. Tolvaptan in patients with autosomal dominant polycystic kidney disease. N Engl J Med 2012; **367**(25): 2407–18.

Torres VE, Abebek Z, et al. Dietary salt restriction is beneficial in the management of autosomal dominant polycystic kidney disease. Kidney Int 2017; **91**: 493–500.

Beckwith–Wiedemann syndrome (BWS)

Wiedemann–Beckwith syndrome, EMG syndrome (exomphalos, macroglossia, and gigantism).

BWS is a somatic overgrowth and cancer predisposition syndrome estimated to affect about 1/13 700 individuals (see Box 3.1 for suggested diagnostic criteria). Eighty-five per cent of cases are sporadic and 15% the result of vertical transmission. The overall risk for tumour development in children with BWS is 7.5%. Tumours are predominantly of embryonal origin, e.g. Wilms, hepatoblastoma, and most of the increased tumour risk is in the first 5–8 years of life.

The genetic basis of BWS is complex. 11p15 encodes a 1-Mb cluster of genes involved in growth regulation, many of which are imprinted. These include *IGF2* (a paternally expressed embryonic growth factor), *H19* (a maternally expressed growth suppressor gene), *CDKN1C* (also known as *p57KIP2*), which negatively regulates cell proliferation and is preferentially expressed from the maternal allele, and *KCNQ1OT1* (*LIT1*), an antisense transcript (encoded within the *KCNQ1* gene and normally expressed from the maternal allele), among others. Disturbance to the balance of gene expression, finely tuned by both growth-promoting and growth-suppressing genes and imprinting (with some genes preferentially expressed from the maternal chromosome and others from the paternal homologue), can result in the BWS phenotype. Paternal UPD 11p15 causes increased expression of paternally expressed growth promoter genes (e.g. *IGF2*) and absence of maternally expressed growth suppressor genes (e.g. *H19*) and is found in 20% of BWS cases. Mosaic paternal UPD 11p15 is thought to arise as a consequence of somatic recombination. Mutations in *CDKN1C* are found in 5–10% and are more commonly found in familial cases. The most common molecular mechanisms are epimutations at the IC1 and IC2 imprinting centres (5–10% and 50% of cases, respectively). A subset of patients with IC2 epimutations will also have epimutations at other imprinted loci, but the clinical consequences of this are not well defined.

There appears to be a 4.2-fold increase in the risk of BWS after assisted reproductive technology, e.g. IVF and intracytoplasmic sperm injection (ICSI) (Maher *et al.* 2003).

Clinical approach

History: key points

- Three-generation family tree with parental and sibling birthweights and family history of overgrowth and exomphalos/omphalocele/umbilical hernia. Were the parents unusually large/tall as the children? Document current parental height. Particular attention should be paid to the maternal family history.
- Pregnancy history, including enquiry about IVF or assisted reproductive technology, details of USS growth parameters. Polyhydramnios, prematurity (~50%)? Placental size (often placental weight is twice normal)?
- Birthweight and neonatal problems (e.g. hypoglycaemia).

Examination: key points

- Growth parameters (height, weight, and OFC).
- Ears for creases of the earlobe and helical pits (look along the rim of the outer helix).
- Forehead for naevus flammeus.
- Tongue for macroglossia.
- Face for dysmorphic features.
- Face and limbs for hemihyperplasia.
- Abdomen for omphalocele, umbilical hernia, and diastasis recti.

Investigations

- Monitor neonates for hypoglycaemia (30–50%) due to hyperinsulinaemia and islet cell hyperplasia.

Box 3.1 Suggested diagnostic criteria for Beckwith–Wiedemann syndrome (BWS)*

Presence of *at least* three of the following features (two major and one minor).

- Major:
  - positive family history (one or more family members with a clinical diagnosis of BWS, or a suggestive history and features);
  - macrosomia (height and weight >97th centile);
  - anterior linear earlobe creases/posterior helical ear pits;
  - macroglossia;
  - omphalocele (exomphalos)/umbilical hernia;
  - visceromegaly involving one or more of liver, spleen, kidneys, adrenal glands, and pancreas;
  - embryonal tumour (e.g. Wilms tumour, hepatoblastoma, rhabdomyosarcoma) in childhood;
  - hemihyperplasia (asymmetric overgrowth of region(s) of the body);
  - adrenocortical cytomegaly;
  - renal abnormalities, including structural abnormalities, nephromegaly, and nephrocalcinosis;
  - cleft palate (rare).
- Minor:
  - polyhydramnios;
  - prematurity;
  - neonatal hypoglycaemia;
  - facial naevus flammeus;
  - haemangioma;
  - characteristic facies, including midface hypoplasia and infraorbital creases;
  - cardiomegaly/structural cardiac anomalies/rarely CM;
  - diastasis recti;
  - advanced bone age;
  - MZ twinning discordance.

* No consensus criteria have yet been agreed upon.

NB. Since children with milder phenotypes have developed tumours, tumour surveillance should be considered in individuals presenting with fewer than three features, e.g. macroglossia and umbilical hernia or hemihyperplasia only.

- Karyotype, looking carefully for 11p15 duplication (<1%).
- DNA sample for UPD studies of 11p15. The microsatellite marker TH that maps to the tyrosine hydroxylase locus is used to detect evidence of mosaic paternal isodisomy seen in 10–20% of sporadic cases of BWS.
- 11p15.5 methylation assays will detect methylation abnormalities at IC1 and IC2 and also indicate UPD.
- Consider *CDKN1C* mutation analysis (5–10%) if the above are negative and a clinical diagnosis of BWS is strong. Most likely to be positive if there is a family history and exomphalos.
- Consider abdominal USS. USS surveillance (renal, adrenal, and hepatic) for nephroblastoma (Wilms), hepatoblastoma, and adrenal cortical tumours.
- Consider echo and ECG. Cardiomegaly of early infancy usually resolves. CM is very rare but can be severe. Other structural cardiac malformations occur in ~5–15%. May be important if surgery is planned.

Other diagnoses/conditions to consider

See 'Overgrowth' in Chapter 2, 'Clinical approach', p. 272.
- Infant of a diabetic mother.
- SGB syndrome.
- Perlman syndrome.
- Costello syndrome.

Genetic advice

Inheritance and recurrence risk
- Eighty-five per cent are sporadic and 15% due to AD transmission (but risks may be modified by the parent of origin).
- Paternal UPD (10–20%). Sporadic; very low recurrence risk.
- 11p15 chromosome rearrangements, e.g. translocation/inversion/duplication (rare). Individual assessment required. Consult with cytogeneticists, but recurrence risk could be substantial.
- *p57KIP2* mutation (5–10%); 50% risk if carried by the mother.
- Affected parent (10–15%). Recurrence risk may be up to 50%, with preferential maternal transmission.
- Karyotype and UPD analysis normal and negative family history. Recurrence risk ~5% and can be further refined by MLPA analysis to detect copy number abnormalities at IC1 and IC2.

Variability and penetrance
Expressivity ameliorates with age. Very obvious features in infancy, e.g. macroglossia and macrosomia, may resolve by late childhood/early adult life. This makes it particularly important, when assessing parents of an apparently sporadic case, to obtain detailed information regarding parental birthweights and any neonatal complications the parents may have suffered, e.g. umbilical hernia and hypoglycaemia, and to examine the parents for earlobe creases and helical pits as the diagnosis may be easy to miss in an adult and has major implications for the assessment of recurrence.

Prenatal diagnosis
- In the uncommon situation that a familial mutation (e.g. *CDKN1C*) or chromosome rearrangement predisposing to BWS has been identified, PND by CVS may be considered.
- Serial USS and growth parameters beginning with dating USS at 8–10 weeks' gestation and including detailed fetal anomaly USS at 19 weeks' gestation and subsequently (looking for macrosomia, macroglossia, anterior abdominal wall defect, nephromegaly, enlarged placenta, and polyhydramnios). Macrosomia does not usually become evident until late in the second trimester.
- Maternal serum AFP at 15 weeks' gestation as a marker for exomphalos (AFP is raised in anterior abdominal wall defects).

Natural history and management

If BWS is suspected antenatally, referral to a specialist in fetomaternal medicine is indicated in view of the obstetric risks of prematurity, polyhydramnios, pre-eclampsia, and fetal macrosomia. Neonates require surveillance for hypoglycaemia for the first few days of life and, if an omphalocele is present, may require surgery in the immediate neonatal period. Macroglossia may make intubation difficult.

Birthweights of babies with BWS are usually ~97th centile and length and weight are also ~+2 SD, although overgrowth is not invariably present. This trend continues through early childhood (bone age typically at the upper limit of normal) and then excessive size becomes less dramatic with increasing age. Growth rate typically decreases from mid childhood through puberty. Adult heights cluster between the 50th and 97th centile (i.e. within the top half of the normal range).

Weng et al.'s (1995) longitudinal survey of 15 children showed normal mental and social development in comparison with unaffected siblings and cousins. (The only exception is 11p15 duplication, which is associated with developmental delay, or if there have been major neonatal complications, e.g. severe prematurity, prolonged symptomatic hypoglycaemia.)

Potential long-term complications
- Tumours. Overall risk for tumour development estimated at 7.5%. Risk is greatest in preschool children, and 96% of all tumours in Beckwith's series of 121 BWS cases presented by 8 years. The risk of Wilms tumour is highest in those with UPD or IC1 epimutations and is very low/absent with *CDKN1C* mutations or IC2 epimutations.
- Tongue. Macroglossia, if present, can cause difficulties in intubation for anaesthesia and occasionally cause serious feeding/respiratory problems and speech problems. Mild to moderate macroglossia tends to improve with time as the mandible grows to accommodate the tongue; severe macroglossia may require surgical intervention by a specialist team, with surgery usually undertaken at age 1–4 years.

Surveillance
- USS of the kidneys, liver, and adrenals at 3-monthly intervals until 7–8 years. In patients with a molecular diagnosis, Wilms tumour screening can be targeted to those at high risk (see above).
- Consider 3- to 4-monthly AFP up to the age of 3 years. Note normal neonates have very high AFP levels (often several thousand kU/l; this declines with a half-life of 5.5 days, so that by 4 months of age the mean is 70

kU/l (SD 56). Adult levels are reached by 7–9 months. Normal adult range is <10 kU/l.

Support group: The Beckwith–Wiedemann Syndrome Support Group, http://www.bws-support.org.uk.

Expert adviser: Eamonn R. Maher, Professor and Honorary Consultant, Department of Medical Genetics, University of Cambridge, Cambridge University Hospitals, Cambridge, UK.

References

Choufani S, Shuman C, Weksberg R. Molecular findings in Beckwith–Wiedemann syndrome. *Am J Med Genet C Semin Med Genet* 2013; **163C**: 131–40.

Choyke PL, Siegel MJ, Craft AW, Green DM, DeBaun MR. Screening for Wilms tumor in children with Beckwith–Wiedemann syndrome or idiopathic hemihypertrophy. *Med Pediatr Oncol* 1999; **32**: 196–200.

Demars J, Rossignol S, Netchine I, et al. New insights into the pathogenesis of Beckwith–Wiedemann and Silver–Russell syndromes: contribution of small copy number variations to 11p15 imprinting defects. *Hum Mutat* 2011; **32**: 1171–82.

Lim D, Bowdin SC, Tee L, et al. Clinical and molecular genetic features of Beckwith–Wiedemann syndrome associated with assisted reproductive technologies. *Hum Reprod* 2009; **24**: 741–7.

Lim DH, Maher ER. Human imprinting syndromes. *Epigenomics* 2009; **1**: 347–69.

Maher ER, Brueton LA, Bowdin SC, et al. Beckwith–Wiedemann syndrome and assisted reproduction technology (ART). *J Med Genet* 2003; **40**: 62–4.

McNeil DE, Brown M, Ching A, DeBaun MR. Screening for Wilms tumour and hepatoblastoma in children with Beckwith–Wiedemann syndrome: a cost-effective model. *Med Pediatr Oncol* 2001; **37**: 349–56.

Weng EY, Moeschler JB, Graham JM Jr. Longitudinal observations on 15 children with Wiedemann–Beckwith syndrome. *Am J Med Genet* 1995; **56**: 366–73.]

Charcot–Marie–Tooth disease (CMT)

Hereditary motor and sensory neuropathy (HMSN), peroneal muscular atrophy.

Usually presents between the ages of 5 and 15 years with difficulty walking due to problems picking up the feet ('foot drop'), progressive foot deformity, high instep, and claw toes. Gradual loss of muscle bulk in the lower calves leads to an 'inverted champagne bottle' appearance with weakness of dorsiflexion and eversion of the foot and high-arched feet (pes cavus). Weakness of the hands may occur later and is rarely symptomatic before adult life. The weakness is very slowly progressive. Affected individuals usually have a loss of sensation in the hands and feet. Sometimes does not present until much later, even into middle age. Severe disease can also present in infancy and early childhood. Tremor can also be present (previously known as Roussy–Levy syndrome).

There is a wide range of severity. A few gene carriers may be asymptomatic in adult life and a few may have severely impaired mobility and become wheelchair-dependent. For the majority, CMT causes problems with sporting activities and footwear in childhood and adolescence and some impairment of mobility by middle life. CMT is the commonest inherited neuromuscular disorder, with an estimated prevalence of one in 2500.

CMT represents a clinically and genetically heterogeneous group of inherited neuropathies characterized by progressive degeneration of the peripheral nerves (see Table 3.3). Classification has relied upon clinical and neurophysiological criteria, pointing towards underlying demyelination or axonal degeneration as the main pathological processes in Schwann cells and axons, respectively. This information can be used to tailor the identification of causative genes. Advances in gene sequencing have led to the identification of over 60 different genes associated with CMT and related inherited neuropathies. Many of the genes play important roles in myelin structure, gene transcription, mitochondrial function, and intracellular membrane transport.

The most common molecular defect leading to CMT is a 1.5-Mb duplication at 17p11.2 arising from unequal crossing over of homologous chromosomes at regions of low copy repeats flanking the duplicated region. This region contains the gene encoding the myelin protein PMP22, resulting in overproduction and demyelination (CMT1A). Deletion of the same region causes the distinct neuropathic syndrome hereditary neuropathy with liability to pressure palsies (HNPP) (see below).

Clinical approach

History: key points

- Three-generation family tree (or more if affected members are known in previous generations), with detailed enquiry for high arches, unusual gait, impaired mobility, e.g. use of sticks, wheelchair.
- Developmental milestones. Difficulty running, walking, participation in sport at school.
- Enquire about difficulty undoing buttons, clumsiness, or frequent falls.
- Document the current level of disability.
- Enquire about vision and hearing.

Examination: key points

- Observe the gait. Is there foot drop with slapping or a high-stepping gait?
- Test walking on heels (usually difficult due to weakness of foot dorsiflexion) and abduction of fingers.
- Examine for wasting of calf muscles, high instep, clawing of toes, and enlargement of peripheral nerves. Examine for wasting of interossei muscles in the hands. Is weakness of thumb abduction disproportionate to weakness of the first dorsal interosseus, indicative of CMT1X?
- Test for loss of vibration sense in the feet and hands. Are the sensory signs more prominent than the symptoms (indicative of a long-standing progressive neuropathy)?
- Test reflexes. Ankle jerks are usually lost early, with progressive loss of other reflexes. (NB. Sometimes the ankle jerks remain present, even in some people with substantial weakness.)
- Palpate the greater auricular nerve (running behind the earlobe near the mastoid bone) for enlargement. Often present in CMT1A.
- If sporadic, look for RP, indicative of Refsum's disease.
- If accompanying learning difficulty, consider genomic array (e.g. Smith Magenis syndrome).

Special investigations

Neurophysiological examination should be arranged to determine the median nerve motor conduction velocity.

If there is a known family history, it may be appropriate to proceed directly to molecular genetic investigation. Even if not, if the clinical picture is that of typical CMT and the neurophysiological findings indicate slowing of motor conduction velocities, it may be reasonable to do DNA testing for a *PMP22* duplication before proceeding to nerve conduction studies to clarify the diagnosis.

- Molecular genetic investigations (DNA):
  - if family history shows AD inheritance, look for duplication 17p11.2–12 (*PMP22*) (CMT1A);
  - if no male-to-male transmission, i.e. family history consistent with XL inheritance, look for connexin 32 (*GJB1*) mutations. (NB. Females are often symptomatic, but usually later than males, so that the family history may appear to be 'AD', but closer scrutiny shows the absence of male-to-male transmission.)
- CMT is highly genetically heterogeneous, so proceed to gene panel analysis/WES/WGS as appropriate.
- NCVs:
  - motor conduction velocities in full-term infants are ~50% of those in adults and approach adult values by ~3 years. HMSN1 motor NCVs are usually in the range of 10–38 m/s;
  - in adults, normal NCV studies show a velocity of >40–45 m/s.
- Additional investigations to consider for sporadic cases in early childhood:
  - NCVs in both parents to detect asymptomatic gene carrier for HMSN;
  - testing for FRDA (triplet repeat expansion in the *frataxin* gene). It can be difficult to distinguish cases of HMSN2 with unsteadiness from early stages of FRDA;
  - ophthalmology assessment for pigmentary retinopathy or optic atrophy;

Table 3.3 Classification of HMSN/CMT

Inheritance and proportion of HMSN	Genetic basis*	Pathology	Clinical features[A0]
HMSN1 (CMT1) AD, ~70–80%	PMP22 in 70–80% (1A). Most are gene duplications. Some are point mutations (which tend to give a more severe phenotype) MPZ in 5–10% (1B) LITAF uncommon (1C) EGR2 uncommon (1D)	Abnormal myelin Slow NCVs typically 10–30 m/s	Distal muscle weakness and atrophy associated with mild/moderate glove-and-stocking sensory loss, depressed reflexes, and pes cavus. A few people with HMSN have a tremor (Roussy–Levy syndrome)
HMSN1 X (CMTX) XL semi-dominant, ~10–20%	Connexin 32 (also known as GJB1) (1X)	Most have a predominantly demyelinating picture, but some have a relatively axonal form that may be confused with HMSN2	Affected males are clinically very similar to HMSN1, but males are consistently more severely affected than females
HMSN2 (CMT2) AD, ~10%	KIF1B-MFN2 (2A) RAB-7 (2B) 6ARS (2C) Neurofilament triplet L protein (2E)	Axonopathy. NCVs usually normal or mildly slowed (38–48 m/s), but amplitude is reduced	Clinically similar to HMSN1, but in general less disabling and with less sensory loss
HMSN3 (CMT3), congenital HMSN, 'Dejerine–Sottas'[E0] AD for CMT1A, 1B, and 1D; and AR for CMT4. Most are de novo AD mutations, MPZ (CMT1B), i.e. reclassified as HMSN1	PMP22 (CMT1A) EGR2 (CMT1D and CMT4)	Usually abnormal myelin with very slow NCVs	Severe demyelinating neuropathy of infancy and childhood with marked clinical weakness and hypertrophy of nerves
HMSN4 (CMT4) AR, rare	Genetically heterogeneous with seven loci. including: EGR2 (CMT4E) PRX (CMT4F)	Either abnormal myelin or axonopathy	Often early childhood onset
Complex forms of HMSN[A4] Rare	Genetically heterogeneous. Some may possibly represent contiguous gene deletions		Neuropathy may be combined with other features, e.g. deafness, retinitis pigmentosa, vocal cord paralysis

* 6ARS, glycyl-tRNA synthetase; EGR2, early growth response protein 2; GJB1, connexin 32; KIF1B, kinesin-like protein KIF1B; LITAF, lipopolysaccharide-induced TNF factor; MFN2, mitochondrial GTPase mitofusin 2; MPZ, myelin protein zero; NEFL, neurofilament triplet L protein; PMP22, peripheral myelin protein 22; RAB7, Ras-related protein Rab-7.

[A0] Subtypes related to the different genes are clinically indistinguishable.

[E0] This clinical category is genetically heterogeneous and has been reclassified on the basis of the genetic pathology, usually as HMSN1.

[A4] Consider the possibility of an alternative diagnosis, especially in a sporadic case.

- phytanic acid (Refsum's may resemble other demyelinating neuropathies, e.g. HMSN2 and HMSN3, but, in addition, children develop night blindness and pigmentary retinopathy);
- MRI scan if any hint of regression, history of seizures, or other CNS abnormality;
- sural nerve biopsy if DNA studies are non-contributory.

Other diagnoses/conditions to consider

Hereditary neuropathy with liability to pressure palsies (HNPP)
The history is of recurrent nerve palsies, often with an AD history of similar problems. Caused by deletion of the PMP22 gene (the same region that is duplicated in CMT1A).

Hereditary neuralgic amyotrophy (familial brachial plexus neuropathy)
An AD disorder characterized by sudden onset of pain and weakness in the shoulder or upper arm associated with weakness. Typically asymmetric, recurring on the same or opposite side. Some recovery of function is usual, particularly early in the course of the disease.

Distal spinal muscular atrophy (SMA)
A heterogeneous group of neuromuscular disorders caused by progressive anterior horn cell degeneration and characterized by progressive motor weakness and muscular atrophy, predominantly in the distal parts of the limbs. One AR variety maps to 11q13. Mutations in HSP22 and HSP27 encoding small heat shock proteins have been found in some families with AD distal hereditary motor neuropathy (Evgrafor et al. 2004; Irobi et al. 2004).

Friedreich's ataxia (FRDA)
Mean onset 15.5 ± 8 years, with a range of 2–51 years. The most common inherited ataxia. AR and caused by mutations in frataxin on 9q. Frataxin is a nuclear-encoded mitochondrial protein. It is characterized by a dying back from the periphery of the longest and largest myelinated fibres (e.g. large fibres arising in dorsal root ganglia). Carrier frequency in Caucasian population is ~1:85, with a disease prevalence of 1/29 000; it is rare in Africans

and Asians. Ninety-eight per cent of mutations are triplet repeat expansions of $(GAA)_n$ in intron 1 and 2% are point mutations or deletions. Normal triplet repeat allele size is 6–34; mutations have 67–1700 repeats. Repeat size is unstable, with a tendency to decrease in size when paternally transmitted and increase or decrease when maternally transmitted. The disease is slowly, but relentlessly, progressive, with loss of walking ~15 years after onset and mean age of death at ~37.5 years (usual cause is CM). Late-onset FRDA (onset >25 years) has been recognized since the onset of molecular testing. See 'Ataxic child' in Chapter 2, 'Clinical approach', p. 74 for more details.

Genetic advice

Inheritance and recurrence risk
Discuss AD inheritance or XL or AR as appropriate.

Variability and penetrance
Variability is often displayed within the extended family and gives parents an idea of the range of possible severity. Approximately 10% of affected individuals are asymptomatic and detected either by careful clinical assessment or NCVs.

Prenatal diagnosis
Technically possible by CVS if the familial mutation is known, but not usually requested.

Predictive testing
Possible for at-risk adult members of the family if the familial mutation has been defined. Genetic testing is usually undertaken in children if they are symptomatic.

Other family members
PND is theoretically possible if a mutation has been identified, but is seldom requested or desired.

Natural history and management

Management
- Ankle–foot orthosis (AFO) if foot drop.
- Referral to an orthopaedic surgeon if severe foot deformity.
- Care of feet if sensory deficit to prevent development of ulcers, etc.
- Monitor adolescents for development of scoliosis.

- Mobility aids, e.g. walking sticks, handrails; wheelchairs, may be required by some over time.
- If adults are drivers, they should inform the Driver and Vehicle Licensing Agency (DVLA).
- Avoid neurotoxic drugs, e.g. vincristine, taxol, cisplatin (chemotherapy), isoniazid (tuberculosis), and nitrofurantoin (antimicrobial used in the treatment of UTIs).

Potential long-term complications
- Pes cavus. Daily stretching exercises to prevent Achilles tendon shortening may be helpful. Careful choice of footwear which has good ankle support. Severe cases may benefit from orthopaedic surgery.
- Loss of mobility. With time, some patients may need aids, such as walking sticks, but <5% need wheelchairs.
- Scoliosis is more common in those with early onset of symptoms. It is rarely severe.

Support group: CMT UK, http://cmt.org.uk.

Expert adviser: Rhys C. Roberts, Consultant Neurologist, Department of Neurology, Cambridge University Hospitals NHS Foundation Trust, Addenbrooke's Hospital, Cambridge, UK.

References
Boerkoel CF, Takashima H, Lupski JR. The genetic convergence of Charcot–Marie–Tooth disease types 1 and 2 and the role of genetics in sporadic neuropathy. *Curr Neurol Neurosci Rep* 2002; **2**: 70–7.

Evgrafor OV, Mersiyanova I, Irobi J, *et al.* Mutant small heat-shock protein 27 causes axonal Charcot–Marie–Tooth disease and distal hereditary motor neuropathy. *Nat Genet* 2004; **36**: 602–6.

Irobi J, Van Impe K, Seeman P, *et al.* Hot-spot residue in small heat-shock protein 22 causes distal motor neuropathy. *Nat Genet* 2004; **36**: 597–601.

Kijima K, Numakura C, Izumino H, *et al.* Mitochondrial GTPase mitofusin 2 mutation in Charcot–Marie–Tooth neuropathy type 2A. *Hum Genet* 2005; **116**: 23–7.

Ouvrier RA, McLeod JG, Pollard JD. Peripheral neuropathy in childhood, 2nd edn. MacKeith Press, London, 1999.

Shy ME. Charcot–Marie–Tooth disease: an update. *Curr Opin Neurol* 2004; **17**: 579–85.

Wilmshurst JM, Pollard JD, Nicholson G, Antony J, Ouvrier R. Peripheral neuropathies of infancy. *Dev Med Child Neurol* 2003; **45**: 408–14.

Ciliopathies

The ciliopathies are a group of genetic disorders caused by mutation in genes that affect ciliary function. The core clinical features of a ciliopathy are retinal degeneration, renal and respiratory disease, brain malformation, situs inversus, and infertility, with congenital fibrocystic diseases of the liver, diabetes, polydactyly, obesity, and skeletal dysplasias as additional features in many of the conditions (Waters and Beales 2011) (see Table 3.4).

There are two types of cilia—motile cilia and non-motile, or primary cilia. In contrast to motile cilia, there is usually only one primary cilium per cell. These are sensory organelles acting as cellular 'antennae' of the cell that coordinate a large number of cellular signalling pathways which are important for cell motility, cytoskeletal integrity, and even cell division and differentiation. Cilia play a vital role in breaking early embryonic symmetry. They are of importance in developmental pathways such as sonic hedgehog (SHH) and Wnt, and mutations may disrupt gradients of signal transduction, explaining why ciliopathies affect the development of many organs, though a pattern of more common ciliopathy features is emerging. Alteration of SHH signalling is associated with a variety of human tumours; thus, cilia may also have roles in cancer as well as development.

A hallmark of ciliary disorders in the brain is the distinctive and easily recognized 'molar tooth sign'. The molar tooth sign is seen on transverse CT and MRI images obtained at the level of the midbrain (see Figure 3.3). The term *molar tooth* refers to the characteristic appearance of an enlarged and horizontally directed tubular structure on each side of the midline emerging from the midbrain. It is caused by a lack of normal decussation of superior cerebellar peduncular tracts.

Clinical approach

History: key points
- Three-generation family tree, noting consanguinity, male infertility.

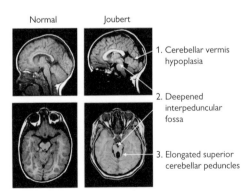

Normal   Joubert

1. Cerebellar vermis hypoplasia

2. Deepened interpeduncular fossa

3. Elongated superior cerebellar peduncles

Figure 3.3 Brain MRI to demonstrate the molar tooth sign. Reproduced with thanks to Doherty and colleagues, University of Washington, http://depst.washington.edu/joubert/joubertsyndrome.php.

- Pregnancy and perinatal history. History of neonatal death and stillbirth (Meckel (Gruber) syndrome (MGS)), echodense 'bright' kidneys (renal cystic disease, BBS), occipital encephalocele (MGS), cerebral ventriculomegaly and 'Dandy–Walker variant' (JS, MGS), polydactyly (BBS, OFD-1, MGS), short limbs and ribs (Jeune).
- Detailed developmental and behavioural profile.
- Apnoea and respiratory difficulties (CNS aetiology in JS, small chest/ribcage in Jeune and EVC).
- Renal disease (all ciliopathies).
- Congenital blindness (LCA).
- Is there any indication of progressive visual deficit/night blindness (BBS/MORM/Alström)?
- Deafness (Alström/Usher).
- Cardiac malformation (EVC), DCM (Alström).

Examination: key points
- Growth parameters (height, weight, OFC). Obesity develops early in BBS and Alström.
- Mouth, tongue, and palate. Tongue cysts (JS), clefts, abnormal frenulae, tongue cysts (OFD-1).
- Encephalocele (MGS).
- Enlarged abdomen due to large cystic kidneys.
- Bell-shaped chest (Jeune and EVC).
- Polydactyly. Typically post-axial in BBS/MGS/Jeune/JS, preaxial in OFD, insertional in McKusick–Kaufman syndrome (MKKS), but overlap between syndromes.
- Eyes should be examined for eye movement disorder, visual field defects, photophobia, colobomata (Biemond I), and retinal pigmentation (RP/BBS/MORM/Alström).
- Small genitalia are commonly seen in males with BBS/MORM. Female genital tract anomalies common in BBS and MKKS.
- In older children, is there acanthosis nigrigans (thickened hyperpigmentation of the axillae and skinfolds, indicative of insulin resistance) (Alström)?
- Cardiovascular system—hypertension, murmurs, situs inversus (BBS, PCD).

Special investigations
- Renal and liver function tests. Glucose (fasting) and HbA1c in older children/adults (BBS/Alström syndrome).
- Renal USS (structural and cystic changes). Consult if further imaging required.
- Brain USS/MRI (cerebellar vermis hypoplasia, molar tooth sign).
- Skeletal survey if evidence of short ribs/limbs (Jeune).
- Ophthalmology for colobomata and RP, and ERG (if possible, age-dependent) and to examine for evidence of an eye movement disorder.
- Genomic analysis e.g. genomic array, gene panel, WES/WGS as available.

Other diagnoses/conditions to consider
Ciliopathy syndromes
See also Table 3.4.

Table 3.4 Ciliary proteins associated with human genetic disease

Disease name	Inheritance	Clinical features	Gene(s)
Primary ciliary dyskinesia (PCD) (Kartagener's syndrome)	AR	Respiratory infections, anosmia, male infertility, otitis media, and situs inversus	*DNAI1, DNAH5, DNAH11, DNA12, TXNDC3, RSPH9, RSPH4A*
Leber congenital amaurosis (LCA)	AR	Retinal degeneration	*CEP290, LCA5, RPGRIP1, TULP1.* Very heterogeneous, ciliary gene mutations not the only cause(s) of LCA
Retinitis pigmentosa (RP)	AR	Retinal degeneration	*RP1, TULP1, ARL6, TTC8*
RP	XLR		*RPGR** Note that Moore and colleagues found mutations in the *RPGR* gene in patients affected by both PCD and RP, indicating an XL transmission of PCD
Autosomal dominant polycystic kidney disease (APKD)	AD	Polycystic kidneys	*PKD1, PKD2*
Autosomal recessive polycystic kidney disease (ARPKD)	AR	Polycystic kidney	*PKHD1*
Nephronophthisis (type 1 juvenile, type 2 infantile, type 3 adolescent)	AR	Kidney cysts, liver fibrosis, retinal dysplasia	*NPHP1, NPHP2, INV, NPHP3, NPHP4, NPHP5/IQCB1I, NPHP6/CEP290, NPHP7, GLIS2 NPHP8, RPGRIP1L, NPHP9, NEK8*
Renal-hepatic–pancreatic dysplasia	AR	Renal dysplasia and cysts, liver fibrosis, pancreatic cysts, situs inversus	*NPHP3*
Senior–Løken syndrome	AR	Renal dysplasia and retinal degeneration	*NPHP1, NPHP4, NPHP5/IQCB1, NPHP6/CEP290*
Meckel (Gruber) syndrome	AR	Brain malformations, post-axial polydactyly, kidney and liver cysts	*MKS1, BBS13, MKS3, TMEM, JBTS6, MKS4, CEP290, JBTS5, MKS5, RPGRIP1L, JBTS7, MKS6, CC2D2A*
Joubert syndrome (JS) COACH syndrome	AR	CNS abnormalities, kidney cysts, brain and retinal malformations	*AHI1, NPHP1, NPHP6/CEP290, MKS3, TMEM, JBTS6, MSK5, RPGRIP1L, JBTS7, INPP5E*
Oral–facial–digital syndrome type I (OFD-1)	XLD	Malformations of the face, oral cavity, and digits (polydactyly), kidney cysts	*OFD1*
Simpson–Golabi–Behmel (SGB) type 2	XLR		
JS	XLR	Features of JS including molar tooth sign	
Bardet–Biedl syndrome (BBS)	AR	Developmental delay, post-axial polydactyly, obesity, anosmia, renal malformation, retinal dystrophy, male infertility, situs inversus, diabetes	*BBS1, BBS2, BBS3, ARL6, BBS4, BBS5, BBS6, MKKS, BBS7,BBS8, TTC8 BBS9, PTHB1,BBS10, BBS11,TRIM32,BBS12, BBS13, MKS1,BBS14, CEP290, CCDC28B, C2orf86*
McKusick–Kaufman syndrome	AR	Polydactyly, cardiac malformation, genital anomalies (hypospadias in males and hydrometrocolpos females)	*MKKS* (same as *BBS6*)
MORM syndrome	AR	Mental retardation, truncal obesity, retinal dystrophy, micropenis	*INPP5E*
Alström syndrome	AR	RP, deafness, obesity, and diabetes mellitus	*ALMS1*
Skeletal dysplasias			
Jeune, asphyxiating thoracic dystrophy	AR	Short ribs and limbs, post-axial polydactyly, renal dysplasia, hepatic fibrosis ± retinal degeneration	*IFT80, DYNC2H1, WDR60, WDR35, TTC21B, WDR19*
Short rib polydactyly type II/III	AR	Lethal dysplasia	*IFT80, DYNC2H1, WDR60, NEK1*
Ellis–van Creveld syndrome (EVC)	AR	Skeletal features as Jeune with cardiac malformation (typically AVSD), polydactyly, and small nails	*EVC* and *EVC2*
Cranioectodermal syndrome (Sensenbrenner)	AR	Phenotype overlaps with Jeune and EvC, but with craniosynostosis	*IFT122, WDR35, WDR19, IFT43*

Joubert syndrome (JS)

AR, often severe developmental, but very variable.

- Hypotonia—present in all patients, moderately severe in infancy with frog-leg posture and lack of spontaneous movement.
- Ataxia—75% learn to sit (average 19 months) and 50% to walk (average 4 years). Gait is unstable and tandem walking is poor.
- Neuroradiology—shows cerebellar vermis hypoplasia and molar tooth sign. PMG common.
- Associated anomalies include episodic hyperpnoea and/or apnoea in 50–75%, especially in infancy, irregular tongue protrusion, eye anomalies (retinal dysplasia, colobomas, nystagmus, strabismus, and ptosis), oculomotor apraxia, microcystic renal disease, occasionally polydactyly, and a variety of other features. May develop renal failure later in childhood.

COACH syndrome (cerebellar vermis hypoplasia, oligophrenia, congenital ataxia, ocular coloboma, hepatic fibrosis)

This is an intermediate phenotype between MGS and JS and is essentially JS with liver fibrosis.

Meckel (Meckel–Gruber) syndrome

A lethal AR syndrome with occipital encephalocele, bilaterally large kidneys with multicystic dysplasia, fibrotic changes of the liver, and PAP. The kidneys are typically filled with thin-walled cysts of various sizes. The condition has been subdivided into several types and there is genetic and phenotypic overlap with other ciliopathies (see Table 3.4).

Bardet–Biedl syndrome (BBS)

Is characterized by a pigmentary retinal dystrophy, PAP, obesity, cognitive impairment, and renal defects. For the majority of cases, BBS follows an AR pattern of inheritance; however, a few families exhibit 'triallelic inheritance'. In these families, three mutations in at least two loci appear to be necessary to manifest the disorder, but occasionally the third mutant allele may modify the severity of the phenotype. The incidence in the UK is <1/100 000, but higher in some ethnic groups. Individuals with BBS are at risk for progressive renal insufficiency, and creatinine and BP should be monitored 6-monthly.

Alström syndrome (AS)

Is characterized by childhood obesity with T2D (hyperinsulinism and acanthosis nigricans) and cone retinal dystrophy (photophobia). A subset of individuals have DCM, hepatic dysfunction, hypothyroidism, male hypogonadism, short stature, and mild/moderate developmental delay.

Skeletal dysplasias

Jeune syndrome. Recent work suggests that genotype can help predict the likelihood of progression to renal failure and the severity of respiratory insufficiency.

Primary ciliary dyskinesia (PCD; Kartagener's syndrome or immotile cilia syndrome)

Is a clinical entity caused by abnormal cilial structure and function resulting in retention of mucus and bacteria in the respiratory tract, leading to chronic respiratory disease and sinusitis, sometimes accompanied by situs anomalies (heterotaxy in ~6%). Approximately 50% of males with PCD are infertile due to abnormal sperm motility. PCD is genetically heterogeneous (17 genes currently identified) and all are AR. The *DNAI1* gene accounts for ~2–9% and *DNAH5* for 15–21% of cases of PCD.

Support group: Ciliopathy Alliance, http://www.ciliopathyalliance.org.

Expert adviser: Phil Beales, Professor of Medical and Molecular Genetics, Genetics and Genomic Medicine Programme, University College London, Institute of Child Health, London, UK.

References

Arts HH, Knoers NV. Current insights into renal ciliopathies: what can genetics teach us? *Pediatr Nephrol* 2013; **28**: 863–74.

Coene KL, Roepman R, Doherty D, et al. OFD1 is mutated in X-linked Joubert syndrome and interacts with LCA5-encoded lebercilin. *Am J Hum Genet* 2009; **85**: 465–81.

D'Angelo A, Franco B. The dynamic cilium in human diseases. *Pathogenetics* 2009; **2**: 3.

Doherty D. Joubert syndrome: insights into brain development, cilium biology, and complex disease. *Semin Pediatr Neurol* 2009; **1**: 143–54.

Ferkol TW, Leigh MW. Ciliopathies: the central role of cilia in a spectrum of pediatric disorders. *J Pediatr* 2012; **160**: 366–71.

Hildebrandt F, Benzing T, Katsanis N. Ciliopathies. *N Engl J Med* 2011; **364**: 1533–43.

Huber C, Cormier-Daire V. Ciliary disorder of the skeleton. *Am J Med Genet C Semin Med Genet* 2012; **160C**: 165–74.

Lancaster MA, Gleeson JG. The primary cilium as a cellular signaling center: lessons from disease. *Curr Opin Genet Dev* 2009; **19**: 220–9.

Lee JE, Gleeson JG. A systems-biology approach to understanding the ciliopathy disorders. *Genome Med* 2011; **3**: 59.

Oh EC, Katsanis N. Context-dependent regulation of Wnt signaling through the primary cilium. *Am Soc Nephrol* 2013; **24**: 10–18.

Quinlan RJ, Tobin JL, Beales PL. Modeling ciliopathies: primary cilia in development and disease. *Curr Top Dev Biol* 2008; **84**: 249–310.

Tobin JL, Beales PL. The nonmotile ciliopathies. *Genet Med* 2009; **11**: 386–402.

Waters AM, Beales PL. Ciliopathies: an expanding disease spectrum. *Pediatr Nephrol* 2011; **26**: 1039–56.

Wong SY, Reiter JF. The primary cilium at the crossroads of mammalian hedgehog signaling. *Curr Top Dev Biol* 2008; **85**: 225–60.

Congenital adrenal hyperplasia (CAH)

An AR condition with a prevalence of 1/12 000–1/15 000, resulting from a deficiency of one of the five enzymes required for synthesis of cortisol in the adrenal cortex.

- 21-hydroxylase deficiency (21-OHase). Carrier frequency 1/50. CYP21 on 6p accounts for >90% of cases.
- 11-beta-hydroxylase (11β-OHase) deficiency. Uncommon.
- 3-beta-hydroxysteroid dehydrogenase deficiency (3β-HSD) deficiency. Rare.

21-OHase is involved in the conversion of 17-OH-progesterone (17-OHP) to 11-deoxycortisol; it is also required for aldosterone biosynthesis. Accumulation of 17-OHP leads to increased androstenedione which is converted in the liver to testosterone. Hence the affected female fetus is exposed to increased fetal androgens from as early as 8 weeks' gestation.

The clinical presentation of CAH is summarized in Table 3.5.

- Girls with classic CAH may be virilized to a variable degree (usually enlarged clitoris; often with labial fusion) due to testosterone production by the adrenals in early pregnancy. The vaginal opening may be normally sited or may open more anteriorly towards the back of the urethra, or even into the back of the urethra at a higher level. Females with classic CAH are likely to be identified at birth due to virilization (ambiguous genitalia).
- Boys with classic CAH usually present in the neonatal period at around 7–10 days old with poor feeding, failure to regain birthweight, dehydration, and collapse (low plasma Na, high K, acidosis, and elevated OHP, sometimes with hypoglycaemia).

- If recognized at birth, the disorder is treatable by steroid therapy (hydrocortisone ± fludrocortisone and salt), and the subsequent physical and mental development of an affected infant should be normal (with expert supervision).
- Non-classic CAH may be asymptomatic or associated with signs of postnatal androgen excess. It occurs in ~0.2% of the white population but is more frequent (1–2%) in some ethnic groups, e.g. Jews of Eastern European origin.

Clinical approach

Review results of the biochemical investigations undertaken when the diagnosis of CAH was made to ensure the diagnosis is secure. In 21-OHase deficiency, these should show raised 17-OHP, raised testosterone, and elevated renin (if salt-losing). Take expert advice regarding the diagnosis of 11β-OHase or 3β-HSD deficiency.

History: key points

- Three-generation family tree with specific enquiry about consanguinity and neonatal and infant deaths.

Examination: key points

- Growth parameters.
- Depending on age, examine for features listed in Table 3.5 giving the clinical presentation.

Investigations

- DNA sample (EDTA) to check for CYP21 mutation in the affected child and parents (if 21-OHase deficiency).

Other diagnoses/conditions to consider

Congenital adrenal hypoplasia

Can present very similarly to CAH with salt-losing crisis (low Na, high K, acidosis, and elevated ACTH) in a male in the first month of life. The presence of normal or low serum 17-OHP strongly suggests XL adrenal hypoplasia congenita. One-third have a contiguous gene defect involving DAX1, glycerol kinase, and DMD (may be a loss of terminal 3′ exons that are not in routine multiplex screen or deletion may extend more proximally or encompass the whole gene). One-third have other affected male relatives (nearly all have mutations in DAX1). One-third have isolated congenital adrenal hypoplasia with no family history (50–70% likelihood of finding a mutation in DAX1). Occasionally may present with adrenal failure later in infancy, and rarely with delayed puberty associated with mild or subclinical adrenal insufficiency.

Check CK.

Pseudohypoaldosteronism

Condition manifesting as a lack of response to aldosterone at the receptor level in the kidney. Presents very similarly to CAH with salt-wasting in the neonatal period (poor feeding, failure to regain birthweight, dehydration, and collapse), but there is no virilization in females and investigations show low Na, high K, normal glucose, and normal 17-OHP and normal testosterone levels. Affected individuals require salt replacement but, unlike in CAH, do not require hydrocortisone. The AR form is caused by mutations in the alpha-subunit (SCNN1A), beta-subunit (SCNN1B), or gamma-subunit (SCNN1C)

Table 3.5 Clinical presentation of congenital adrenal hyperplasias

Type	Female	Male
Classic CAH		
At birth	Ambiguous genitalia	
Neonatal to infancy	Salt loss in 70%	Salt loss in 70%, pigmented scrotum (occasionally)
Early childhood		Penile growth, pubic hair, rapid linear growth, increased musculature
Non-classic CAH		
Late infancy	Clitoromegaly	
Childhood	Pubic hair, increased growth rate	Pubic hair, tall stature
Adolescence	Abnormal menses, hirsutism, acne	Not known
Adult	Hirsutism, oligomenorrhoea, infertility	Not known

Reprinted from *The Lancet*, vol 352, issue 9130, Hughes, Congenital adrenal hyperlasia - a continuum of disorders, pp. 752–4, copyright 1998, with permission from Elsevier.

Table 3.6 Classes of congenital adrenal hyperplasia mutations

Class of CAH mutations	Enzyme activity	Phenotype
Deletions or nonsense mutations	Total loss of enzyme activity	Salt-wasting disease
I172N (missense mutation)	Enzyme activity 1–2% of normal	Simple virilizing disease
	Permits adequate aldosterone synthesis	
V281L, P30L	Enzymes retain 20–60% of normal activity	Non-classic disorder

of the epithelial sodium channel (ENaC). The AD renal form is caused by mutations in the mineralocorticoid receptor gene (NRJC2) and tends to show some improvement with age.

Other causes of ambiguous genitalia
See 'Ambiguous genitalia (including sex reversal)' in Chapter 2, 'Clinical approach', p. 54.

Genetic advice
About ten mutations have been described in the vast majority of patients with CAH, both classic and non-classic (see Table 3.6). Homozygosity for deletion of CYP21 causes classic CAH. In classic CAH, ~20–25% have a gene deletion and ~30% have an intron 2 splice site mutation. The missense mutation V281L is the most common mutation in non-classic CAH. Compound heterozygosity is one of the factors underlying phenotypic variation. An individual with non-classic CAH may be at risk of having a child with classic CAH if their partner carries a CYP21 deletion, and, vice versa, an individual with classic CAH could have a child with non-classic CAH if their partner carried a 'mild' mutation.

One to 2% of mutations are spontaneous mutations not carried by either parent (Speiser and White 2003).

Inheritance and recurrence risk
• Following the diagnosis of an affected infant, the parents have a 1 in 4 risk for an affected pregnancy (1 in 8 risk for a virilized female).
• For an individual with CAH due to 21-OHase deficiency with an unrelated unaffected partner with no family history, the risk to a pregnancy is $1 \times 1/50 \times 1/2 = 1/100$ for an affected infant (1 in 200 for a virilized female).
• For the sibling of an individual with CAH due to 21-OHase deficiency with an unrelated unaffected partner with no family history, the risk to a pregnancy is $2/3 \times 1/50 \times 1/4 = 1/300$ for an affected infant (1 in 600 for a virilized female).

Variability and penetrance
There is some phenotypic variability among relatives carrying the same mutations (modifier genes?).

Prenatal diagnosis
Possible by CVS at 11 weeks' gestation if the familial mutation is known or if there is certainty over the diagnosis of 21-OH deficiency, in which case markers linked to CYP21 can be used.

Discuss management of a future pregnancy and the options of:
(1) no investigations and accepting 1 in 4 risk of an affected

infant, in which case make careful arrangements for expert review of the at-risk baby after delivery;
(2) NIPT to determine fetal sex (see 'Non-invasive prenatal diagnosis/testing (NIPD/T)' in Chapter 6, 'Pregnancy and fertility', p. 764);
(3) PND by CVS, and termination of pregnancy (TOP) in the case of an affected female pregnancy;
(4) post-conception maternal steroid therapy to minimize virilization in an affected female pregnancy. Long-term effects on the developing child are still being evaluated (see below).

Management of a high-risk pregnancy electing for prenatal therapy
• Prior to pregnancy, establish the causative CYP21 mutations and confirm that these are present in the parents. Alternatively, consider the possibility of linkage-based PND, but possibly some genetic heterogeneity with not all 21-OHase families linked to CYP21.
• Pregnancy test as soon as possible after a late period for very early confirmation of pregnancy.
• NIPT as early in the pregnancy as fetal sex can be reliably determined.
• If pregnant, some experts have recommended starting dexamethasone immediately (20 µg/kg/day three times a day; tds; *ter die sumendus*) regimen). If following this regimen, it should be started early, preferably by 6/40 gestation and certainly by 8/40. Treatment started later than 8 weeks is not likely to completely prevent virilization of the external genitalia. However, this approach is controversial as there is incomplete evidence regarding the balance of risks and harms associated with prenatal dexamethasone exposure and further investigation is needed. In the meantime, the decision about initiating treatment should be based on parents' values and preferences (Merce Fernandez-Balsells et al. 2013). Controversy continues in 2016 (Heland et al. 2016).
• CVS at 11 weeks' gestation in a female fetus at high risk.
• If unaffected pregnancy or affected male pregnancy, stop dexamethasone by tailing the dose off over 2 weeks.
• If affected female pregnancy, continue dexamethasone until term (careful antenatal monitoring required).

Management of an at-risk neonate
• Careful assessment for signs of virilization in a female.
• Plasma 17-OHP on day 3 (after first 48 hours) for *urgent* analysis.
• U & Es and blood glucose also on day 3 (look for low Na and high K; may have hypoglycaemia due to cortisol deficiency).

Other family members
Consider whether apparently unaffected siblings should be investigated with U & Es and plasma 17-OHP, possibly repeated following Synacthen® stimulation.

Natural history and management
Management of a woman with CAH during pregnancy
Women with CAH should be under the joint care of an obstetrician and endocrinologist during pregnancy. Careful endocrine monitoring is required particularly to advise about the endocrine management of the stress of labour and delivery. Maternal circulating androgens have a low risk of causing virilization of a female fetus

as placental aromatase efficiently converts testosterone to oestrogens.

Support group: CLIMB Congenital Adrenal Hyperplasia Support Group, http://www.livingwithcah.com.

Expert adviser: Carlo Acerini, University Senior Lecturer, Department of Paediatrics, University of Cambridge, Addenbrooke's Hospital, Cambridge, UK.

References

British Society for Paediatric Endocrinology and Diabetes (BSPED). BSPED Statement on the Use of Prenatal Dexamethasone in Congenital Adrenal Hyperplasia, 2015. https://www.bsped. org.uk/clinical/ docs/UseOfPrenatalDexamethasone InCongenitalAdrenal Hyperplasia.pdf.

Heland S, Hewitt JK, et al. Preventing female virilisation in congenital adrenal hyperplasia: The controversial role of antenatal dexamethasone. Aust N Z J Obstet Gynaecol 2016; **56**(3): 225–32.

Hughes IA. Congenital adrenal hyperplasia—a continuum of disorders [commentary]. Lancet 1998; **352**: 752–4.

Merce Fernandez-Balsells M, Muthusamy K, Smushkin G, et al. Prenatal dexamethasone use for the prevention of virilization in pregnancies at risk for classical congenital adrenal hyperplasia because of 21-hydroxylase (CYP21A2) deficiency: a systematic review and meta-analysis. Clin Endocrinol 2010; **73**: 436–44.

Speiser PW, White PC. Congenital adrenal hyperplasia [review]. N Engl J Med 2003; **349**: 776–88.

Consanguinity

See also 'Developmental delay in the child with consanguineous parents' in Chapter 2, 'Clinical approach', p. 126 and 'Incest' in Chapter 3, 'Common consultations', p. 472.

A consanguineous relationship is one between individuals who are second cousins or closer. Consanguineous marriage is customary in the Middle East, parts of South Asia including Pakistan, some Jewish communities, and among Irish travellers. Although the custom is often perceived to be associated with Islam, in fact, it is (usually) independent of religion. Consanguineous marriage increases the birth prevalence of individuals with recessive disorders. In the Birmingham birth study among Northern European children (0.4% of parents related), the prevalence of recessive disorders was 0.28%, compared with British Pakistani children (69% of parents related) in whom the prevalence of recessive disorders was 3.0–3.3%. The effect is particularly marked for rare recessive disorders. The proportion of nuclear genes shared for a given degree of relationship is given in Table 3.7.

There is no measurable increase in the rate of spontaneous abortion or infertility in populations with a high incidence of customary consanguineous marriage.

The terminology for relationships is given here and illustrated in Figure 3.4.

- First cousin. Individuals are first cousins if one of each set of parents are siblings (A and B in Figure 3.4).
- Double first cousin. Individuals are double first cousins if both of each set of parents, respectively, are siblings (E and F in Figure 3.4).
- First cousin once removed. 'Removed' indicates a difference in generations, e.g. a first cousin once removed is the child of a first cousin (A and D in Figure 3.4; also B and C).
- Second cousins. Individuals are second cousins if a paternal grandparent is sibling to a maternal grandparent, i.e. the offspring of first cousins are second cousins (C and D in Figure 3.4).

Clinical approach

History: key points
- Detailed three-generation family tree, including details of younger generations, i.e. cousins, nephews, and nieces. May be necessary to draw a more extensive family tree. Extend the family tree sufficiently far back that the common ancestors are shown.

Table 3.7 Proportion of nuclear genes shared as a function of degree of relationship

Relationship	Proportion of nuclear genes shared
Monozygotic twins	1 (100%)
First-degree relatives (siblings, parent: CAchild, dizygotic twins)	1/2 (50%)
Second-degree relatives (half-sibs, double CAfirst cousins, uncle/aunt:nephew/niece)	1/4 (25%)
Third-degree relatives (first cousins CAhalf-uncle/aunt:niece/nephew)	1/8 (12.5%)

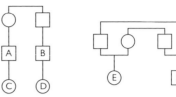

Figure 3.4 Diagram illustrating the terminology of relationships. A and B are first cousins. A and D and also B and C are first cousins once removed. E and F are double first cousins. C and D are second cousins.

- Where there is multiple consanguinity, it may be helpful in clinic to document *in words* the stated relationships in the family, so that you can return to the family tree later (and if necessary redraw it!) to ensure that it accurately reflects the stated relationships in the family.
- If there is a family member with a known recessive disorder or a potentially recessive disorder (e.g. microcephaly), highlight that individual as the proband in the family tree.

Examination: key points
Usually not relevant.

Special investigations
These are determined by the ethnic origin of the family and the recessive disorders with known high carrier rates in that ethnic group. See Table A8 for carrier rates for different ethnicities in 'Appendix', p. 812.
- Northern European/Caucasian. Offer CF carrier testing.
- Mediterranean. Offer haemoglobinopathy screen (thalassaemia and sickle-cell disorders) and CF carrier testing.
- Ashkenazi Jewish. Offer Tay–Sachs carrier testing (carrier risk ~1/30 in Ashkenazim) by plasma levels of hexosaminidase A and mutation analysis for the six common *HEXA* mutations (identifies ~98% of mutations in Jewish and 46% of mutations in non-Jewish carriers). Also offer CF carrier testing (including W1282X).
  - For Ashkenazim, DNA testing is the preferred method to ascertain Tay–Sachs carriers.
  - For Tay–Sachs carrier testing in non-Jewish individuals, enzyme assay should be done initially and positive or indeterminate results should be confirmed by DNA mutation analysis. If only one partner is descended from a high-risk group, that person should be tested first; only if he/she is a carrier, should the other partner be tested. If the couple is pregnant at the time carrier testing is requested, both partners should have enzyme testing (leukocyte assay for the pregnant woman and serum assay for the father) and DNA testing sent concomitantly to expedite counselling (Sutton 2002).
- African-American/African-Caribbean/African. Offer haemoglobinopathy screen (sickle) and CF carrier testing. NB. Approximately 50% of the genes of African-Americans and African-Caribbeans are of Northern European origin.

- Indian/South East Asian. Offer haemoglobinopathy screen (thalassaemia and sickle-cell disorders) and CF carrier testing. The birth prevalence of children with CF is approximately the same among British Pakistanis as among Northern Europeans (although the gene frequency is less) as a result of common consanguineous marriage.
- Other. Offer CF carrier testing.

Genetic advice—*no* autosomal recessive (AR) disorder in extended family

Two alternative approaches exist—the first is to rely on empiric (observed) data, the second to estimate the risk based on the assumption that each of the common grandparents carries one deleterious recessive gene.

First cousins

- Empiric data. Birth prevalence of serious congenital and genetic disorders diagnosed by 1 year for children of unrelated parents is 2.0–2.5%. For children of first-cousin parents, the risk is doubled at 4.0–4.5%. Longer-term studies that include conditions diagnosed later in childhood (neurological disorders, thalassaemia, etc.) give an overall 4.0% risk for children of unrelated parents, with an approximate doubling of this risk to 8.0% in offspring of first cousins.
- Estimated risk. The probability that both first cousins will carry their grandfather's recessive gene is (1/4 × 1/4). The chance that they would have an affected child in each pregnancy is (1/4 × 1/4 × 1/4), i.e. 1/64. Similarly, the probability that both first cousins will carry their grandmother's recessive gene is (1/4 × 1/4). The combined probability for a pregnancy homozygous for a recessive disorder is 1/64 + 1/64 = 1/32 (3%).

Second cousins

- Empiric data. The birth prevalence of serious congenital and genetic disorders diagnosed by 1 year for children of unrelated parents is 2.0–2.5%. For children of first cousins once removed or second cousins, the risk is increased by 1.0% to 3.0–3.5%.
- Estimated risk. The probability that both second cousins will carry their grandfather's recessive gene and that they would have an affected child is (1/8 × 1/8 × 1/4, i.e. 1/256). The probability that both second cousins will carry their grandmother's recessive gene is the same. The combined probability for a pregnancy homozygous for a recessive disorder is 1/128 (<1%).

Other relationships

See Table 3.8.

Multiple consanguinity

The key step is to identify the common ancestors on the family tree. In the case of double first cousins, this is the four grandparents or, with double second cousins the four common great-grandparents. This can be tricky, especially if marriages have occurred between different generations. Once the common ancestors have been identified, then calculate the chance that a pregnancy will be homozygous by descent for each common ancestor and sum them to obtain the overall risk.

Carrier detection

See above under 'Special investigations'.

Prenatal diagnosis

Detailed fetal anomaly USS will detect structural anomalies that occur in a small percentage of pregnancies affected by severe recessive disorders (e.g. polydactyly, cystic kidneys, CHD, structural anomalies of the brain). Most severe recessive disorders will remain undetected as the great majority of metabolic disorders and neurodevelopmental disorders (leukodystrophies, etc.) will not be detectable by fetal USS. Detailed fetal anomaly USS should be offered to first-cousin relationships and closer, but the couple must recognize its limitations. Routine obstetric USS is appropriate for relationships less close than first cousins.

Genetic advice—known AR or possible AR disorder in extended family

If there is a known or possible recessive disorder in the family, other consanguineous relationships within the extended family are at *high* genetic risk for that disorder. The risks are summarized in Figures 3.5 and 3.6.

Method

Working from the nuclear family of the proband, assign the carrier status to the unaffected siblings (2/3) and the parents (1). Each parent will have inherited their carrier status from one or other of their parents, so assign carrier risk to each grandparent (1/2), and each of the parent's sibs will be at 50% risk (1/2). Continue in this manner until you reach each member of the couple seeking advice. The chance that they will have a child homozygous by descent for the disorder in any pregnancy is (carrier risk of father) × (carrier risk of mother) × 1/4.

Carrier detection

Carrier detection for many metabolic disorders by conventional biochemical methods is problematical due to an overlap in values between heterozygotes and normals. Where accurate carrier detection is not feasible by DNA mutation analysis or linkage studies, it may be preferable to rely on the calculated risk from the pedigree combined with the offer of PND.

Table 3.8 Probability for a pregnancy homozygous by descent for an AR disorder in relationships other than first and second cousins

Relationship	Probability
Double first cousins (fathers are sibs, CAmothers are sibs)	1/16
Uncle/aunt:niece/nephew	1/16
First cousins once removed	1/64
Double second cousins	1/64

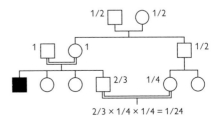

$$2/3 \times 1/4 \times 1/4 = 1/24$$

Figure 3.5 Risk to the offspring of an individual who has a sibling with an AR disorder who marries a first cousin.

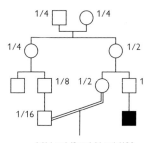

$$1/16 \times 1/2 \times 1/4 = 1/128$$

Figure 3.6 Risk to the offspring of an individual who has a nephew with an AR disorder who marries a first cousin once removed.

Prenatal diagnosis
As for the specific diagnosis in the family. PND is available for most metabolic disorders, but check with the lab providing the analysis regarding the type of sample required (cultured/uncultured CVS cells, amniotic fluid, amniocytes, DNA).

Expert adviser: Eamonn Sheridan, Professor of Clinical Genetics, University of Leeds, Leeds, UK.

References

Bundey S, Aslam H. A five-year prospective study of the health of children in different ethnic groups, with particular reference to the effect of inbreeding. *Eur J Hum Genet* 1993; **1**: 206–19.

Harper P. Practical genetic counselling, 5th edn. Butterworth-Heinmann, London, 1998.

Kaback MM, Desnick RJ. Hexosaminidase A deficiency. In: RA Pagon, MP Adam, HH Ardinger, *et al.* (eds.). GeneReviews®, 2011. http://www.ncbi.nlm.nih.gov/books/NBK1218.

Lazarin GA, Haque IS, Nazareth S, *et al.* An empirical estimate of carrier frequencies for 400+ causal Mendelian variants: results from an ethnically diverse clinical sample of 23,453 individuals. *Genet Med* 2012; **15**: 178–86.

Modell B, Darr A. Genetic counselling and customary consanguineous marriage. *Nat Rev Genet* 2002; **3**: 225–9.

Sutton VR. Tay–Sachs disease screening and counseling families at risk for metabolic disease. *Obstet Gynecol Clin North Am* 2002; **29**: 287–96.

Young ID. *Introduction to risk calculation in genetic counselling*, 2nd edn. Oxford University Press, Oxford, 1999.

Craniosynostosis

Craniosynostosis is defined as premature fusion of the cranial sutures. It has a prevalence of one in 2500 children; 15% of cases have a recognizable syndrome and a further 10% an identifiable genetic cause. Children with craniosynostosis present with an abnormally shaped head (see also 'Plagiocephaly and abnormalities of skull shape', in Chapter 2, 'Clinical approach', p. 280). The aetiology remains unknown in the majority of children with isolated craniosynostosis; environmental factors are likely to be important determinants. The substantial genetic heterogeneity, with at least 57 genes implicated, means that gene panel/WES/WGS approaches are beneficial (Miller *et al.* 2017).

Craniosynostosis can be suspected clinically and confirmed by SXRs that show loss of the affected suture line(s). CT scanning (with bone windows and 3D reconstruction) gives greater precision in borderline cases. Copper beating is evidence of long-standing increased intracranial pressure, although normal markings on the inner vault are at their greatest at 3–4 years of age. Once diagnosed, the condition should be managed by a specialist surgical and medical team.

The sutures between the bones of the skull vault are the main sites of growth, which occurs at right angles to the line of the suture. Growth is controlled by a signalling system that includes ephrins which mark the suture boundaries, FGF receptors, and the transcription factor TWIST1. The five major sutures are coronal, lambdoid, and squamosal, all of which are paired, and the sagittal and metopic which are single. Fontanelles are found where sutures meet.

Premature fusion leads to an abnormality in the shape of the vault and also affects the growth of the face. Brain growth may be restricted and an increasing intracranial pressure can indicate that this is occurring.

Types of craniosynostosis and their effects on skull shape

- Unilateral coronal synostosis (10–15%): causes a wide skull with orbital asymmetry.
- Bicoronal synostosis (5–10%): the skull is short with a compensatory increase in width and height. Most are syndromic. The two sutures may be variably involved, so an asymmetric appearance is possible.
- Lambdoid synostosis (1%): very rare.
- Sagittal synostosis (50%): progressive elongation of the skull, often with a palpable midline ridge.
- Metopic synostosis 15%): triangular appearance of the frontal area.
- Multiple suture involvement: can occur; many are syndromic.
See Figure 3.7.

Clinical approach

It is assumed that craniosynostosis has been proven. The aim is to determine whether the condition is isolated or part of a syndrome and to determine if there are any other affected family members.

History: key points
- Three-generation family history (consider variable penetrance of a dominant condition); enquire about consanguinity.

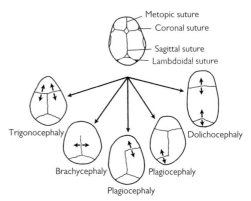

Figure 3.7 Skull shape resulting from abnormal patterns of suture fusion.
Adapted with permission from M.M Cohen, and R. Maclean, *Craniosynostosis: Diagnosis, Evaluations, and Management*, Second Edition, Oxford University Press USA, Copyright © 2000. By permission of Oxford University Press, USA. www.oup.com. Data from S. Pruzansky, Clinical investigations of the experiments of nature. In, Orofacial Anomalies: Clinical and Research Implications, ASHA Report, 8, 1973, American Speech-Language-Hearing Association.

- Pregnancy, breech presentation, multiple pregnancy, reduced liquor volume, persistent discomfort and history of the head 'feeling stuck', uterine constraint. History of maternal hyperthyroidism. History of maternal drug ingestion, e.g. valproate (metopic synostosis), fluconazole (Antley–Bixler syndrome).
- Paternal age. Increased in association with *de novo* FGF receptor mutations.
- Age of presentation and progression of features.
- Neurodevelopmental abnormalities, including seizures and delayed developmental milestones.

Examination: key points
- Head. Measure the OFC and describe the shape of the head (view from above). Look for asymmetry. Palpate for ridging of the sutures; document the presence and shape of the fontanelles.
- Eyes. Measure the spacing and check for exorbitism and proptosis.
- Face. Midface hypoplasia and a beaked nose, in combination with exorbitism, gives rise to the 'Crouzonoid' facies, which is important to recognize.
- Cleft palate.
- Ears. Small with prominent crus helices in Saethre–Chotzen syndrome.
- Hands, feet, and limbs. Mild cutaneous syndactyly in Saethre–Chotzen and Pfeiffer syndrome (occurs in <50%). Syndactylous bony fusion is diagnostic in Apert syndrome. Broad thumbs and/or halluces are diagnostic in Pfeiffer, with medial/radial deviation in more severe cases. The hallux may be broad in Saethre–Chotzen syndrome, but the facial appearance is different. Muenke syndrome is associated with minor degrees of brachydactyly, but this is not diagnostic.

Polydactyly is present in Carpenter syndrome. Limited elbow movement is a feature of *FGFR2* mutations.

- Skin. Acne, acanthosis nigricans, cutis gyratum (Beare–Stevenson).
- Examine both parents for the above features and review family photographs of the parents as children.

Special investigations
To be done in association with a specialist craniofacial team.

- Clinical photography.
- Molecular DNA analysis (EDTA sample). Not indicated for non-syndromic simple metopic and sagittal synostosis. Approximately 40% of children with non-syndromic coronal craniosynostosis have mutations in either *FGFR3* (749C>G, Pro250Arg) (Muenke syndrome) or *TCF12*. For syndromes, see 'The *FGFR* craniosynostosis syndromes' below.
- Genomic array. Cytogenetic abnormalities are rarely found in a normally developing child with a single suture involved. Children with coronal synostosis, developmental delay, and other malformations require analysis. Consider genomic array or MLPA for the microdeletion at 7p21.1 involving the *TWIST1* gene and for 22q11. Craniosynostosis occurs in ~1% of individuals with del 22q11.
- Genomic analysis in presence of features suggestive of a chromosomal or syndromic diagnosis, e.g. genomic array, gene panel, or WES/WGS as appropriate/available.
- Further radiological investigations and intracranial pressure monitoring may be necessary.

Syndromic diagnoses to consider
Mutations in the genes for FGF receptors *FGFR1*, *2*, and *3*, *TWIST1*, and *MSX2* have been identified in syndromic craniosynostosis. The *FGFR* and *MSX2* mutations act by gain of function, but *TWIST1* by haploinsufficiency.

The FGFR craniosynostosis syndromes
These all have AD inheritance, but new mutations are common.

- Apert syndrome *FGFR2* 101200*. Severe syndactyly, often called a mitten hand, distinguishes this syndrome. Developmental delay is found, even when there has been no evidence of raised intracranial pressure. Two recurrent mutations account for the majority of cases (*FGFR2* p.S252W and p.P253R).
- Beare–Stevenson syndrome *FGFR2* 123790*. Cutis gyrata are the key physical feature. AD. Often lethal in the newborn period.
- Crouzon syndrome *FGFR2* 123500*. Shallow orbits, leading to exorbitism, and a hooked nose are characteristic features. Molecular testing can help to establish if there is a recurrence risk to parents, as the clinical features in an affected parent can be mild.
- Crouzon syndrome with acanthosis nigricans *FGFR3* pAla391Gln 134934*. Coronal synostosis; hydrocephalus is frequent.
- Muenke syndrome *FGFR3* 602849*. Has a rather non-specific phenotype with coronal synostosis and occasionally brachydactyly and deafness. It is essential to exclude this diagnosis in every child with coronal synostosis (unilateral or bilateral). This can only be accomplished by molecular genetic testing.

- Pfeiffer syndrome *FGFR1* (rarely) and *FGFR2* 101600*. The face is similar to Crouzon syndrome, but clover leaf skull is a more frequent complication. Sometimes the thumbs and halluces are broad and there may be a degree of skin syndactyly. *FGFR2* mutations may lead to a more severe craniofacial phenotype.

ERF-related craniosynostosis
Heterozygous mutations in *ERF* cause a complex craniosynostosis with Crouzon-like facial features that typically presents later than Crouzon syndrome (which is often apparent at birth) and may affect sagittal and lambdoid sutures as well as coronal sutures. As a result of multisuture involvement, children are at significant risk of raised intracranial pressure and Chiari malformation (Twigg et al. 2013b).

*Saethre-Chotzen syndrome TWIST1 101400**
Asymmetric coronal suture involvement gives facial asymmetry. A low frontal hairline, ptosis, and small ears with a prominent crus are other helpful features. Examine for evidence of skin syndactyly and broad halluces. The majority of patients with Saethre–Chotzen syndrome have mutations in the *TWIST1* gene, which codes for a basic helix–loop–helix transcription factor. The presence of learning difficulties and developmental delay suggest a microdeletion of 7p21, rather than an intragenic *TWIST1* mutation (10–20% of patients with Saethre–Chotzen have a large deletion involving *TWIST1*). The clinical features show variability within families. Use molecular results to aid counselling.

TCF12 coronal synostosis
Heterozygous mutation of *TCF12*, a basic helix–loop–helix transcription factor acting synergistically with *TWIST1*, causes bilateral or unilateral synostosis, accounting for ~32% and 10% of subjects with undiagnosed coronal synostosis in one series (Sharma et al. 2013). The phenotype overlaps with Saethre–Chotzen and non-syndromic coronal craniosynostosis.

*Craniofrontonasal syndrome 304110**
An XLD disorder that has paradoxically mild manifestations in males (Twigg et al. 2013a). The classical presentation is a female with gross hypertelorism, a midline nasal groove, coronal synostosis, sloping shoulders, characteristic longitudinal splits or ridges in the nails, and occasional syndactyly or polydactyly. Caused by diverse mutations in the *EFNB1* gene encoding ephrin-B1.

*IL11RA cranopsynostosis 614188**
An AR form of craniosynostosis resembling Crouzon syndrome but with additional dental anomalies. Caused by biallelic variants in *IL11RA*.

*Boston craniosynostosis. Heterozygous mutation in MSX2 604757**
A rare cause of genetic craniosynostosis. AD inheritance.

Carpenter syndrome (acrocephalopolysyndactyly type II) 201000
A rare AR syndrome with preaxial polysyndactyly and caused by biallelic mutation in the *RAB23* gene. See 'Polydactyly' in Chapter 2, 'Clinical approach', p. 284.

Antley–Bixler syndrome
This syndrome is characterized by skeletal defects, including craniosynostosis, bowed femora, joint ankylosis, especially radiohumeral synostosis, and genital anomalies.

* denotes OMIM number

Biallelic mutations in cytochrome P450 oxidoreductase (POR) have been reported. Patients with POR mutations have a unique urinary steroid profile (Shackleton et al. 2004). A few cases are due to the teratogenic effects of maternal fluconazole, an antifungal drug (Fluck et al. 2004). Individuals with craniosynostosis and radiohumeral synostosis, but without the additional features, often have FGFR2 mutations.

Genetic advice—syndromic craniosynostosis

Recurrence risk
Test the parents when a mutation is known. In the case of a de novo FGFR mutation, the recurrence risk is substantially <1% and the majority of these mutations represent true sporadic events, often associated with increased paternal age. The recurrence risk in the case of a de novo TWIST1 mutation is unknown and the possibility of germline mosaicism should be considered.

Variability and penetrance
Muenke and Saethre–Chotzen syndromes and ERF- and TCF-related craniosynostosis show marked variability; very careful assessment of parents (supported by molecular genetic testing) is needed.

Prenatal diagnosis
Theoretically possible by CVS if a mutation is known. Severity is difficult to predict. Unless definitive PND is possible and the fetus is known not to be affected, arrange for USS at 36/40 to ensure that there is no cephalopelvic disproportion prior to delivery.

Other family members
In familial cases, evaluation of the extended family is indicated.

Genetic advice—isolated craniosynostosis
Sagittal synostosis is the most commonly found (~50%). Bilateral involvement of the coronal sutures suggests a strong possibility of a genetic cause and careful examination to exclude syndromal causes and the presence of features in other members of the family, as well molecular genetic testing for Muenke syndrome mutation and TCF12, is advised. The observation of a significant environmental factor will help explain the aetiology. In many children, the aetiology will be unknown.

Inheritance and recurrence risk
The majority will be sporadic events, but a sib recurrence risk of 5% for coronal synostosis and 3–4% for other synostoses, e.g. sagittal synostosis, covers the possibility of a genetic predisposition. Offspring risks have not been well documented in the literature.

Variability and penetrance
Carefully examine both parents and ask for early childhood photographs.

Prenatal diagnosis
Single suture involvement is unlikely to be detected on prenatal scans. The cranial sutures do not develop until after 16 weeks' gestation. Arrange for fetal USS at 36/40 to ensure that there is no cephalopelvic disproportion prior to delivery.

Other family members
Risks to more distantly related individuals are very low.

Natural history and management of children with craniosynostosis

Potential long-term complications
Restenosis of a surgically opened suture, raised intracranial pressure, poor growth of the midface, sleep apnoea, exposure keratitis, hearing loss, dental malocclusion, and rarely syringomyelia.

Surveillance
Remain under the care of a craniofacial team until facial and cranial growth complete.

Support group: Headlines Craniofacial Support Group, info@headlines.org.uk.

Expert adviser: Andrew Wilkie, Nuffield Professor of Pathology, Weatherall Institute of Molecular Medicine, University of Oxford, Oxford, UK.

References
Fitzpatrick DR. Filling in the gaps in cranial suture biology. Nat Genet 2013; **45**: 231–2.

Fluck CE, Tajima T, Pandey AV, et al. Mutant P450 oxidoreductase causes disordered steroidogenesis with and without Antley–Bixler syndrome. Nat Genet 2004; **36**: 228–30.

Miller KA, Twigg SR, et al. Diagnostic value of exome and whole genome sequencing in craniosynostosis. J Med Genet 2017; **54**: 260–8.

Muenke M, Wilkie AOM. Craniosynostosis syndromes. In: CR Scriver, AL Beaudet, WS Sly, D Valle (eds.). The metabolic and molecular bases of inherited disease, 8th edn, pp. 6117–46. McGraw-Hill, New York, 2001.

Shackleton C, Marcos J, Malunowicz EM, et al. Biochemical diagnosis of Antley–Bixler syndrome by steroid analysis. Am J Med Genet A 2004; **128A**: 223–31.

Sharma VP, Fenwick AL, Brockop MS, et al. Mutations in TCF12, encoding a basic helix-loop-helix partner of TWIST1 are a frequent cause of coronal craniosynostosis. Nat Genet 2013; **45**: 304–7.

Twigg SR, Babbs C, van den Elzen ME, et al. Cellular interference in craniofrontonasal syndrome: males mosaic for mutations in the X-linked EFNB1 gene are more severely affected than true hemizygotes. Hum Mol Genet 2013a; **22**: 1654–62.

Twigg SR, Vorgia E, McGowan SJ, et al. Reduced dosage of ERF causes complex craniosynostosis in humans and mice and links ERK1/2 signalling to regulation of osteogenesis. Nat Genet 2013b; **45**: 308–13.

Wilkie AO, Byren JC, Hurst JA, et al. Prevalence and complications of single-gene and chromosomal disorders in craniosynostosis. Pediatrics 2010; **126**: 391–400.

Cystic fibrosis (CF)

CF is the most common life-limiting AR disorder in the white population. Three clinical phenotypes are associated with mutations in the CF transmembrane conductance regulator (CFTR) gene on 7q31–32. A normal sweat chloride is regarded as <30 mM. A sweat chloride of 30–60 mM is regarded as borderline and is seen in patients with atypical CF and the so-called mild mutations (De Boeck et al. 2006; Ooi et al. 2012).

(1) Classical CF. Obstructive lung disease, bronchiectasis, exocrine pancreatic insufficiency, elevation of sweat chloride concentration (>60 mM), and infertility in males due to congenital bilateral absence of the vas deferens (CBAVD).

(2) Atypical or non-classical CF. Chronic pulmonary disease ± pancreatic exocrine disease ± elevated sweat chloride (30–60 mM) ± CBAVD.

(3) CBAVD. See 'Male infertility: genetic aspects' in Chapter 6, 'Pregnancy and fertility', p. 750.

The incidence of CF in Caucasians of European extraction is 1/2000–1/4000 newborns (1/2500 in the UK). CF is rare in native Africans and Asians. The mutation spectrum and frequency are highly dependent on the ethnic background. See Box 3.2 for the diagnostic criteria for CF.

More than 1000 mutations in CFTR have been identified (see Table 3.9), of which the most common by far is delta F508 (ΔF508). ΔF508 encodes a three-nucleotide deletion resulting in a CFTR protein lacking phenylalanine (F) at position 508 in the protein. This causes misfolding of the newly synthesized mutant CFTR, so that it does not integrate into the cell membrane but remains in the cytoplasm where it is degraded by the ubiquitin–proteosome pathway. ΔF508 accounts for ~70% of CF alleles, but the exact proportion varies depending on the ethnic origin. The next most common mutations are G542X, G551D, Δ1507, W1282X, and N1303K, each accounting for only 1–2.5% of known CF alleles. W1282X is common in the Ashkenazi Jewish population. Standard commercial kits for DNA diagnosis usually identify ~29 mutations. In the English population, this accounts for ~87% of CF alleles. Thus, using a standard screen, 76% of English patients with CF will have two identifiable CFTR mutations, 22% will have a single identifiable CF mutation, and 2% of patients with CF will have no identifiable mutation. Specialist labs may offer rare mutation screens.

Polythymidine (Poly-T) tracts in intron 8 affect the splicing efficiency of a CFTR allele. The most efficient polymorphism is 9T; 7T has reduced efficiency, and 5T has significantly reduced efficiency. R117H in cis with 5T, with ΔF508 as the other allele, usually results in non-classical CF (pancreatic-sufficient), whereas R117H in cis with 9T, with ΔF508 as the other allele, typically causes the much milder phenotype of CBAVD without respiratory symptoms.

Box 3.2 Criteria for the diagnosis of CF

Diagnosis requires at least one criterion from each group

Group 1
- One or more characteristic phenotypic features (see below), e.g. chronic sinopulmonary disease, GI and nutritional abnormalities, salt loss syndromes, and male urogenital abnormalities, e.g. CBAVD
- Sibling with CF
- Positive neonatal IRT (immunoreactive trypsinogen test)

Group 2
- Sweat chloride >60 mM on two occasions (B 375 mg of sweat is critical to reliability). Some laboratories assay sweat osmolality which is increased in CF (normal range is 62–196 mOsm/kg)
- Identification of two CF mutations
- Abnormal nasal potential difference (measure of CFTR-mediated ion transport)

Reprinted from The Journal of Paediatrics, vol 132, issue 4, Rosenstein and Cutting, The Diagnosis of cystic fibroses: a consensus statement, pp. 589–95, copyright 1998, with permission from Elsevier.

Phenotypic features consistent with diagnosis of CF
- Chronic sinopulmonary disease. Persistent colonization with typical CF pathogens (Staphylococcus aureus, Haemophilus influenzae, Pseudomonas aeruginosa, Burkholderia cepacia), chronic cough and sputum production, persistent chest X-ray abnormalities (bronchiectasis, atelectasis, infiltrates, hyperinflation), airway obstruction (wheezing and air trapping), nasal polyps, X-ray or CT abnormalities of paranasal sinuses, clubbing
- GI and nutritional abnormalities. Meconium ileus (10–20%), rectal prolapse (20%), distal intestinal obstruction, pancreatic insufficiency, recurrent pancreatitis, focal biliary cirrhosis or multilobular cirrhosis, failure to thrive (protein–calorie malnutrition), hypoproteinaemia and oedema, complications secondary to lack of fat-soluble vitamins
- Salt loss syndromes. Acute salt depletion, chronic metabolic acidosis
- Male urogenital abnormalities resulting in obstructive azoospermia. CBAVD

Reprinted from The Lancet, Volume 351, Beryl J Rosenstein, Pamela L Zeitlin, Cystic fibrosis, pp. 277–282, copyright 1988, with permission from Elsevier.

Table 3.9 Functional classification of *CFTR* alleles

Class	Functional effect of mutation	Allele
I	Defective protein production	G542X, R553X, W1282X, R11162X, 621–1G → T, 1717–1G → A, 1078 ΔT, 3659 ΔC
II	Defective protein processing	ΔF508, Δ1507, N1303K, S549N
III	Defective protein regulation	G551D, R560T
IV*	Defective protein conductance	**R117H, R334W, G85E, R347P
V*	Reduced amounts of functioning CFTR protein	3849 + 10 kbC → T,2789 + 5G → A, A455E
		711 + 1G → T, 2184DA, 1898 + 1G → A
	Unknown	

* Compared with class II (including ΔF508 homozygotes); classes IV and V have a significantly lower mortality rate and milder clinical phenotype.

** See note in main text regarding R117H.

Reprinted from *The Lancet*, vol 361, issue 9370, McKone *et al*, Effect of genotype on phenotype and mortality in cystic fibrosis: a retrospective cohort study, pp. 1671–6, copyright 2003 with permission from Elsevier.

Thauvin-Robinet *et al.* (2009) undertook a population study to assess the penetrance of the R117H + F508del genotype. Clinical details were documented for 184 individuals and showed that the phenotype was predominantly mild; one child had classical CF and three adults severe pulmonary symptoms. The penetrance of classical CF for R117H;7T + F508del was estimated at 0.03% and that of severe CF in adulthood at 0.06%.

See http://www.genet.sickkids.on.ca/cftr/app for the Cystic Fibrosis Mutation Database by the Cystic Fibrosis Genetic Analysis Consortium.

Clinical approach

History: key points
- Three-generation family tree.
- Genotype of the affected individual, if known.

Examination: key points
Usually not relevant if the affected individual is under the care of a CF paediatrician/physician or you are seeing another family member.

Investigations
DNA sample for mutation analysis of *CFTR*.

Genetic advice

Inheritance and recurrence risk
- AR and so the recurrence risk to parents of an affected child is 1/4. The following recurrence risks are based on pedigree analysis and assuming no consanguinity, no family history of CF in a partner, and a CF carrier rate of 1/23 (see Table 3.10 for carrier rates in different ethnic groups). This risk estimate can be substantially modified by CF mutation analysis in the relative and his/her partner (see below).
  - Risk to offspring of a healthy sib of an affected child is $2/3 \times 1/23 \times 1/4 = 1/138$.
  - Risk to offspring of aunt/uncle or half-sib of an affected child is $1/2 \times 1/23 \times 1/4 = 1/184$.
  - Risk to offspring of an affected individual is $1 \times 1/23 \times 1/2 = 1/46$.

Table 3.10 Carrier rates and mutation detection rates in different ethnic populations

Population	Carrier frequency	Mutation detection rate with panel appropriate to ethnic group (%)
Ashkenazi Jewish	1 in 23	97
Northern European	1 in 23	90
Hispanic	1 in 46	57
African-American	1 in 65	75
Asian	1 in 90	3

Variability and penetrance
Homozygosity for ΔF508 and compound heterozygosity or homozygosity for other non-functional alleles are associated with the classical form of CF. Even in classical CF, the age of onset and rate and progression of pulmonary disease are very variable (influenced by modifier genes, infection, nutrition, therapy, smoking, etc.). ΔF508 homozygotes vary considerably in their manifestation of GI, hepatobiliary, and pulmonary disease. Monozygotic CF twins are more concordant than dizygotic CF twins. The CF phenotype may be modified by loci in the partially imprinted region on 7q 3′ of *CFTR* that determine stature, food intake, and energy homeostasis. All classical cases of CF (ΔF508 homozygotes) have pancreatic insufficiency, but there is considerable variability in pulmonary disease. Decline in lung function in CF is associated with colonization by *Pseudomonas aeruginosa* and *Burkholderia cepacia*.

A partially functional allele in combination with a non-functional allele (e.g. ΔF508) is a typical picture in non-classical CF. However, since the standard screening panel comprises mainly non-functional alleles, many patients with non-classical CF will have only one identifiable CF allele, i.e. those patients in whom a clinical diagnosis is most challenging are often those most difficult to diagnose genetically.

In comparison with ΔF508 homozygotes, ΔF508/R117H, ΔF508/A455E, ΔF508/3849+10kb C → T, and ΔF508/2789+5G → A are associated with mild clinical manifestations (McKone *et al.* 2003).

Prenatal diagnosis
Possible by CVS at 11 weeks' gestation if both mutations are known. If a single or neither mutation is known, the diagnosis of CF is secure, and paternity is certain, it is possible to offer linkage studies to capture unidentified allele(s) and enable PND. PGD for ΔF508 homozygotes is available in some centres.

NIPT for the paternal allele, where available, may halve the need for CVS.

Predictive testing
This may be applicable in younger siblings of a child recently diagnosed with CF, in view of the benefits of treatment with prophylactic antibiotics and pancreatic and vitamin supplements.

Other family members
When an individual is diagnosed with CF and mutation analysis is performed, it is routine practice to offer carrier testing to both parents. Cascade screening of the extended family for the mutation identified in their relative can then be offered. Where an individual is shown

to be a CF carrier, population-based screening (see Table 3.10) can be offered to his/her partner to determine the risk to their offspring. Carrier testing of children is usually deferred until 16 years when they are of an age to be involved in decision-making and old enough to understand the implications of the result.

Natural history and management

Potential long-term complications

- Respiratory failure. Pulmonary disease is the main cause of morbidity and mortality in patients with CF. Heart–lung transplantation may be considered for end-stage disease.
- Diabetes. Twenty-five to 50% have an abnormal glucose tolerance test (GTT) by their 20s and 5% require insulin.
- Liver disease. Five per cent of adults have cirrhosis and portal hypertension.
- Male infertility. Ninety-seven per cent of males with CF have CBAVD with obstructive azoospermia. Pregnancy may be possible with assisted reproductive technology (see 'Male infertility: genetic aspects' in Chapter 6, 'Pregnancy and fertility', p. 750), in which case offer mutation analysis to the partner.

Surveillance and therapy

Evidence is emerging that management of CF in paediatric and adult CF centres results in a better clinical outcome. In the USA, median survival has reached 31.1 years for men and 28.3 years for women. Survival to the 30s and 40s is no longer rare. Median survival for patients with pancreatic sufficiency (non-classical CF) is 56 years.

Disease-modifying therapies e.g. lumacaftor and ivacaftor have shown promising benefits in some patients with cystic fibrosis (Konstan 2016).

Pregnancy in women with CF

Despite theoretical reasons, i.e. abnormal cervical mucus, CF women appear to have normal fertility. In Thorpe-Beeston et al.'s (2013) study of 48 pregnancies in 41 women, there were two miscarriages, 44 singleton pregnancies, and two sets of abnormalities or TOPs. The median birthweight centile was 31.9. Twenty-five (52.1%) of the women had pancreatic insufficiency and 17 (35.4%) required insulin. Women with FEV_1 of <60% were more likely to deliver earlier and by Caesarean section, compared with women with FEV_1 of >60%. Three of the seven women with an FEV_1 of <40% died within 18 months of delivery. Four of the eight women with FEV_1 of 40–50% died between 2 and 8 years after delivery. Pregnancy for women with CF is possible, but the incidence of preterm delivery and Caesarean section is increased. Women with pre-existing poor lung function should be counselled antenatally to ensure that they understand the implications of their shortened life expectancy and parenthood (Thorpe-Beeston et al. 2013).

- Offer mutation analysis to the partner (offer CVS if the partner is a CF carrier).
- Refer to a CF physician for assessment of the likely impact of pregnancy on the respiratory reserve.
- Increased risk of gestational diabetes due to pancreatic insufficiency in women with classical CF.
- Consider the drug regimen of your patient and whether any of the drugs have teratogenic potential.

- Pregnancy should be jointly managed by an obstetrician with special expertise in maternal and fetal medicine and a CF specialist.

Neonatal screening

Most neonatal screening programmes for CF combine the assay of immunoreactive trypsinogen (IRT) on a dried blood spot (Guthrie card), with the analysis for common CF mutations, e.g. ΔF508. An IRT of 60–70 µg/l is equivocal and >70 µg/l is positive. This approach has been well studied but misses some children with CF and detects more ΔF508 carriers than expected. The excess of ΔF508 heterozygotes is associated with the presence of a second mutation or the 5T allele in some infants. In one study of 57 subjects with positive IRT who were ΔF508 heterozygotes, three had clinical CF at 1 year.

Support group: Cystic Fibrosis Trust, https://www.cysticfibrosis.org.uk.

Expert adviser: Di Bilton, Honorary Consultant in Respiratory Medicine, Royal Brompton Hospital, London, UK.

References

Dankert-Roelse JE, te Meerman GJ. Screening for cystic fibrosis—time to change our position? [editorial]. *N Engl J Med* 1997; **337**: 997–8.

De Boeck K, Wilschanski M, Castellani C, et al. Cystic fibrosis. Terminology and diagnostic algorithms. *Thorax* 2006; **61**: 627–35.

Durie PR. Pancreatitis and mutations of the cystic fibrosis gene [editorial]. *N Engl J Med* 1998; **339**: 687–8.

Konstan MW, McKone EF. Assessment of safety and efficacy of long-term treatment with combination lumacaftor and ivacaftor therapy in patients with cystic fibrosis homozygous for the F508del-CFTR mutation (PROGRESS): a phase 3, extension study. *Lancet Respir Med* 2016; pii: S2213–2600(16)30427–1.

Mahadeva R, Webb K, Westerbeek RC, et al. Clinical outcome in relation to care in centres specialising in cystic fibrosis: cross sectional study. *BMJ* 1998; **316**: 1771–7.

Massie RJ, Wilcken B, Van Asperen P, et al. Pancreatic function and extended mutation analysis in DeltaF508 heterozygous infants with an elevated immunoreactive trypsinogen but normal sweat electrolyte levels. *J Pediatr* 2000; **137**: 214–20.

McKone EF, Emerson SS, Edwards KL, Aitken ML. Effect of genotype on phenotype and mortality in cystic fibrosis: a retrospective cohort study. *Lancet* 2003; **361**: 1671–6.

Mekus F, Laabs U, Veeze H, Tümmler B. Genes in the vicinity of CFTR modulate the cystic fibrosis phenotype in highly concordant or discordant F508del homozygous sib pairs. *Hum Genet* 2003; **112**: 1–11.

Neill AM, Nelson-Piercy C. Hazards of assisted conception in women with severe medical disease. *Hum Fertil* 2001; **4**: 239–45.

Ooi CY, Dupuis A, Ellis L, et al. Comparing the American and European diagnostic guideline for cystic fibrosis: same disease, different language? *Thorax* 2012; **67**: 618–24.

Rosenstein BJ, Cutting GR. The diagnosis of cystic fibrosis: a consensus statement. *J Pediatr* 1998; **132**: 589–95.

Rosenstein BJ, Zeitlin PL. Cystic fibrosis. *Lancet* 1998; **351**: 277–82.

Thauvin-Robinet C, Munck A, Huet F, et al. The very low penetrance of cystic fibrosis for the R117H mutation: a reappraisal for genetic counselling and newborn screening. *J Med Genet* 2009; **46**: 752–58.

Thorpe-Beeston JG, Madge S, Gyi K, Hodson M, Bilton D. The outcome of pregnancies in women with cystic fibrosis—single centre experience 1998–2011. *BJOG* 2013; **120**: 354–61.

Dementia—early onset and familial forms

The WHO defines dementia as 'An impairment in cognitive function commonly accompanied by, and occasionally preceded by, deterioration in emotional control, social behaviour, or motivation'. Dementia is usually irreversible and progressive; it is important to identify potentially treatable causes early in the diagnostic pathway.

Clinically, dementia affects memory, speech, perception, and mood. The risk of developing dementia increases with age. Alzheimer's disease is the most common neurodegenerative condition affecting older people. Alzheimer's disease has a prevalence of 1–2% among those aged 65–69 years, increasing to 40–50% among those 95 years of age and over. Dementia is a feature of many progressive disorders affecting the CNS, but the most common dementia over the age of 40 years is Alzheimer's disease. Other common causes include vascular dementia, Lewy body dementia, frontotemporal dementia, and Parkinson's disease.

Pathologically, Alzheimer's disease and many other neurodegenerative disorders are characterized by neuronal loss and intracellular and/or extracellular aggregates of proteinaceous fibrils. In Alzheimer's disease, these are intracytoplasmic neurofibrillary tangles (hyperphosphorylated forms of the microtubular protein tau) and extracellular amyloid or senile plaques. The amyloid in senile plaques is a cleavage product of the beta-amyloid precursor protein formed by the action of the beta- and gamma-secretases. Another group of dementing disorders are known as tauopathies (e.g. some frontotemporal dementia) where the tangles are 'tau'-rich and another group are called synucleinopathies (e.g. Parkinson's disease, Lewy body dementia, multisystem atrophy) where the filamentous lesions comprise alpha-synuclein. There is not, however, a simple relationship between disease, mutation, and pathology as, for example, there is accumulation of 'tau' protein in Alzheimer's disease. The references address these complex issues in more detail.

Early-onset Alzheimer's disease can be defined as onset at age <65 years. Campion et al. (1999) undertook a prevalence study based on the population of Rouen and (using a very strict definition of early-onset Alzheimer's disease with age of onset <61 years) found a prevalence of early-onset Alzheimer's disease of 41.2/100 000 persons at risk and of familial Alzheimer's disease (defined as early-onset Alzheimer's disease in three generations) of 5.3/100 000 persons at risk.

Late-onset Alzheimer's disease has a more complex genomic architecture than early-onset forms and genome-wide and rare variant association studies have identified ~20 genes with common variants contributing to the risk (Naj 2017).

Clinical approach

Affected individuals need a full systems interview, examination, and diagnostic evaluation by an appropriate specialist (e.g. neurologist or old age psychiatrist) in order to identify potentially treatable causes of cognitive impairment or dementia.

History: key points
- Three-generation family history, with specific enquiry regarding affected relatives, age of onset, rate of progression, age at death. Is the progression of the memory loss gradual (Alzheimer's disease) or stepwise (vascular dementia)?
- Past medical history and social history (association of dementia with trauma, infection, alcohol excess, seizures).
- Is there an associated movement disorder (HD, Parkinson's disease)?
- Is there a history of stroke or transient ischaemic attacks (TIAs) (cerebral autosomal dominant arteriopathy with subcortical infarcts and leukoencephalopathy (CADASIL), multi-infarct dementia)?

Examination: key points
- Not usually indicated if you are seeing an asymptomatic relative.
- If you are concerned that the consultand is affected, then refer to a neurologist for specialist evaluation and diagnosis.
- There are no clinical differences between sporadic Alzheimer's disease and early-onset AD types other than the age of onset.

Investigations
- Affected individuals may require diagnostic evaluation before genetic counselling is given to related individuals.
- Consider DNA storage on affected individuals when a genetic aetiology is possible, after obtaining appropriate consent.
- Consider targeted genetic testing or gene panel analysis for β-APP, PSEN1, and PSEN2 mutation analysis in an affected member of the family if they have early-onset disease (onset at <61 years) or a family history of the disease (e.g. an affected relative in three generations with at least one having early-onset disease).

Other diagnoses/conditions to consider
Genetic dementia
ALZHEIMER'S DISEASE. See 'Family history of Alzheimer's disease' below.

AD FRONTAL AND TEMPORAL LOBAR DEGENERATION (INCLUDING PICK'S DISEASE). The second most common presenile dementia after Alzheimer's disease. AD and caused by mutation in the tau gene (MAPT) on 17q21 which encodes the microtubule-associated protein tau, the primary component of neurofibrillary tangles found in Alzheimer's disease and some other neurodegenerative disorders.

LEWY BODY DEMENTIA. One of the three most common causes of dementia in older people (with Alzheimer's disease and vascular dementia). Clinical presentation is typically with fluctuating cognitive impairment, visuospatial dysfunction, marked attentional deficits, psychiatric symptoms (especially complex visual hallucinations), and mild extrapyramidal features (Wilcock 2003).

CADASIL. Associated with NOTCH gene mutation.

HD is characterized by an involuntary movement disorder (chorea), psychiatric disturbance, and cognitive impairment leading eventually to dementia. AD and caused by a triplet repeat expansion (CAG) in the huntingtin gene on 4p. See 'Huntington disease (HD)' in Chapter 3, 'Common consultations', p. 454.

PRION DISEASES. (Gerstmann–Straussler–Shencker syndrome and Creutzfeldt–Jakob disease (CJD).) AD and caused by mutations in the *PRNP* gene on 20p. Prion diseases may also be sporadic or have infectious aetiologies (e.g. new-variant CJD).

FRONTOTEMPORAL DEMENTIA AND/OR AMYOTROPHIC LATERAL SCLEROSIS. AD neurodegenerative disorder with variable expressivity. Patients can have ALS/FTD or both. Onset in adult life. Caused by an expanded hexanucleotide repeat (GGGGCC)n in *C9orf72*.

LATE-ONSET METABOLIC DISORDERS. E.g. ALD (XL), and other rare, mainly AR, disorders.

Multifactorial dementia
- Sporadic Alzheimer's disease.
- Vascular dementia due to repeated infarcts (excluding CADASIL).

Other causes
- Acquired immune deficiency syndrome (AIDS)-related. The most prevalent dementing disease in the USA among those aged <40 years.
- Treatable conditions, such as drug toxicity in the elderly, nutritional deficiency, hypothyroidism.
- Alcohol-related.
- Tumour.
- Vasculitis.
- Head injury.
- Transmitted CJD.

Genetic advice
Family history of Alzheimer's disease
Alzheimer's disease may be caused by monogenic, high penetrance mutations, but Alzheimer's disease risk can also be influenced by complex predisposition alleles, e.g. apolipoprotein E (APOE). As stated above, there is no clinical or pathological way of distinguishing genetic from sporadic Alzheimer's disease in an individual. Family history and age of onset are used to initially determine the likelihood of an inherited Alzheimer's disease.

Linkage analysis of familial Alzheimer's disease has identified three causative genes: beta-amyloid precursor protein (*β-APP*) on chromosome 21; presenilin 1 (*PSEN1*) on chromosome 14; and presenilin 2 (*PSEN2*) on chromosome 1. The presenilin and *β-APP* mutations found in familial early-onset Alzheimer's disease appear to result in the increased production of $A\beta_{42}$, which is probably the principal neurotoxin in these forms of Alzheimer's disease.

The inheritance of different *APOE* genotypes affects the age of onset and apparent risk of Alzheimer's disease. Three variants *APOEε2*, *ε3*, and *ε4* exist. Carrying one *APOEε4* allele doubles the lifetime risk of Alzheimer's disease from 15% to 29%, adjusted for average life expectancy, whereas not carrying an *APOEε4* allele cuts the risk by 40% (Campion et al. 1999). Nevertheless, the rate of disease-free survival in individuals homozygous for *APOEε4* is high. The main effect of the *APOEε4* allele seems to be to shift the age of onset an average of 5–10 years earlier in the presence of one allele and 10–20 years earlier in homozygotes in those with an underlying susceptibility to Alzheimer's disease (Meyer et al. 1998). The usefulness of *APOE* testing is controversial—50% of those with a pathological diagnosis of Alzheimer's made at post-mortem do not carry an *APOEε4* allele.

APOE testing is generally not indicated in a clinical setting, e.g. for clinical diagnosis/prediction. However, it may be useful in research contexts.

Mutation testing for the other three genes is offered by some centres, usually as part of a research facility. Using a very strict definition of AD Alzheimer's disease (early-onset disease in three generations), Campion et al. (1999) found *PSEN1* mutations in ~50% and *β-APP* mutations in 15%.

Inheritance and recurrence risk
EARLY-ONSET DEMENTIA. For families with a known mutation, or clearly dominant family history, Mendelian risks may be used.

LATER-ONSET DEMENTIA. For most families, empiric risks are all that can be given. These are discussed by Breitner (1991) who gives a 3- to 4-fold risk of developing Alzheimer's disease in the first-degree relatives of individuals with Alzheimer's disease, compared to controls (19% against 5%).

Variability and penetrance
In families with genetic Alzheimer's disease, there is age-dependent penetrance, with variability caused by other genetic and environmental factors.

Prenatal diagnosis
Theoretically possible by CVS in families with a known mutation.

Predictive testing
Has been reported in families with known Alzheimer's disease mutations using a protocol similar to that used in HD.

Other family members
LATER-ONSET DISEASE. See Breitner (1991). Risks for second-degree relatives are about twice that for controls (i.e. ~10%).

Natural history and management
Individuals affected by early-onset dementia should be referred to a neurologist or psychiatrist with special expertise in dementia for comprehensive evaluation, investigation, and care. Cholinesterase inhibitors, e.g. Aricept®, may be of limited benefit. Drug therapy for vascular dementia is under development.

Potential long-term complications
Progressive loss of higher mental functions with loss of independence.

Surveillance
At-risk individuals are advised to avoid deleterious environmental factors such as alcohol excess. Folic acid supplementation may have some protective value.

Support group: Alzheimer's Society, https://www.alzheimers.org.uk.

Expert adviser: David Craufurd, Senior Lecturer and Honorary Consultant in Neuropsychiatric Genetics, Manchester Centre for Genomic Medicine, University of Manchester and Central Manchester University Hospitals NHS Foundation Trust, St. Mary's Hospital, Manchester, UK.

References
Breitner JC. Clinical genetics and genetic counselling in Alzheimer disease. *Ann Intern Med* 1991; **115**: 601–6.

Campion D, Dumanchin C, Hannequin D, *et al*. Early-onset dominant Alzheimer disease: prevalence, genetic heterogeneity and mutation spectrum. *Am J Hum Genet* 1999; **65**: 664–70.

Meyer MR, Tschanz JT, Norton MC, *et al*. APOE genotype predicts when—not whether—one is predisposed to develop Alzheimer disease. *Nat Genet* 1998; **19**: 321–2.

Morishima-Kawashima M, Ihara Y. Alzheimer's disease: beta-amyloid protein and tau. *J Neurosci Res* 2002; **70**: 392–401.

Naj AC, Schellenberg GD. Alzheimer's Disease Genetics Consortium (ADGC). Genomic variants, genes, and pathways of Alzheimer's disease: An overview. *Am J Med Genet B Neuropsychiatr Genet* 2017; **174**(1): 5–26.

Nussbaum RL, Ellis CE. Alzheimer's disease and Parkinson's disease. *N Engl J Med* 2003; **348**: 1356–64.

Roses AD, Pericak-Vance MA, Saunders A. Alzheimer disease and other dementias. In: DL Rimoin, JM Connor, RE Pyeritz, BR Korf (eds.). *Rimoin's principles and practice of medical genetics*, 4th edn, pp. 2894–916. Churchill Livingstone, London, 2002.

Royal College of Physicians Committee on Geriatrics. Organic mental impairment in the elderly. Implications for research, education and the provision of services. *J R Coll Physicians Lond* 1981; **15**: 141–67.

Selkoe DJ, Podlisny MB. Deciphering the genetic basis of Alzheimer's disease. *Annu Rev Genomics Hum Genet* 2001; **3**: 67–99.

Tobin SL, Chun N, Powell TM, McConnell LM. The genetics of Alzheimer disease and the application of molecular tests. *Genet Test* 1999; **3**: 37–45.

Trojanowski JQ. Tauists, Baptists, Syners, apostates, and new data. *Ann Neurol* 2002; **52**: 263–5.

Wilcock GK. Dementia with Lewy bodies [commentary]. *Lancet* 2003; **362**: 1689–90.

Yip AG, Brayne C, Easton D, *et al*. Apolipoprotein E4 is only a weak predictor of dementia and cognitive decline in the general population. *J Med Genet* 2002; **39**: 639–43.

Diabetes mellitus

Diabetes mellitus is a common and rapidly growing medical problem arising from a combination of environmental and genetic risk factors. There are multiple subtypes of diabetes, including a growing classification of monogenic diabetes where there is either isolated diabetes or diabetes as part of a multisystem genetic disorder. These need to be differentiated from the more common type 1 and type 2 diabetes.
- Type 1 diabetes mellitus (T1D), formerly known as insulin-dependent diabetes mellitus (IDDM).
- Type 2 diabetes (T2D), formerly known as non-insulin-dependent diabetes mellitus (NIDDM), although often insulin treatment is required to control hyperglycaemia.

T1D affects about 0.3% of Caucasians, with the highest rates in northern Europe (1–1.5% in Finland). The condition becomes less frequent moving south in Europe to Africa. It is ten times less common in Japan than in the USA. The condition is caused by selective destruction of the pancreatic beta-cells as a result of an autoimmune process. Insulin deficiency leads to symptomatic hyperglycaemia. Treatment of T1D is insulin replacement therapy by percutaneous injection. The aetiology is complex and the condition arises from the action of many genes and environmental factors. The diagnosis is strongly suggested by the presence of autoantibodies (glutamic acid decarboxylase (GAD) and/or IA2 present in 80% at diagnosis and remain high for the first 5–10 years after diagnosis) or measurement of C-peptide of <200 pmol/l showing absolute insulin deficiency (this may not be seen in the first 5 years after diagnosis because endogenous insulin production can continue in the honeymoon period).

T2D is becoming more common as the population becomes older and more obese. It is estimated that one in ten of European and US individuals will develop T2D.

T2D is pathologically heterogeneous but is most commonly the result of defects in both the action of insulin (insulin resistance) and insulin production. Treatment is by dietary and lifestyle manipulation and oral hypoglycaemic medication in the early stages, with many progressing to insulin therapy within a few years. There are no specific tests for T2D, but it is rarely diagnosed before the age of 40 years in the absence of obesity, except in high-prevalence populations like South East Asians.

Monogenic diabetes subtypes

Monogenic disorders of the beta-cell
The monogenic disorders of the beta-cell are concisely reviewed by Murphy et al. (2008). The main clinical subgroups are neonatal diabetes, maturity-onset diabetes of the young (MODY), and as part of a multisystem genetic syndrome.

NEONATAL DIABETES
- Neonatal diabetes can readily be identified as it usually is diagnosed in the first 6 months of life while T1D is almost never diagnosed before 6 months. The prevalence of neonatal diabetes is around one in 200 000 births. Most are isolated cases due to *de novo* or recessive mutations and a genetic diagnosis can usually be made in ~80% of patients. All patients diagnosed before 9 months should be referred for genetic testing (available without charge through http://www.

diabetesgenes.org), as it can dramatically alter treatment in up to half of cases. This is well reviewed in Aguilar-Bryan and Bryan (2008).
- Transient neonatal diabetes mellitus (TNDM) is a rare, but distinct, type of diabetes. Classically, neonates present with growth retardation and diabetes in the first week of life. Remission of the diabetes occurs by 3–12 months, but many children subsequently relapse to develop non-insulin dependent diabetes in later life. The most common cause is overexpression of an imprinted and paternally expressed gene/s within the TNDM critical region at 6q24 (Temple and Shield 2002). Three genetic mechanisms have been shown to result in TNDM: paternal uniparental isodisomy of chromosome 6; paternally inherited duplication of 6q24; or a methylation defect that, in some cases, is due to biallelic inactivation of *ZFP57*. Other causes include activating mutations in the *KCNJ11* and *ABCC8* genes.
- Permanent neonatal diabetes mellitus (PNDM). The majority of patients diagnosed in the first 6 months of life will have persistent diabetes and are classified as PNDM. Forty to 50% of patients will have a defect in the beta-cell KATP channel as a result of mutations in *KCNJ11* or *ABCC8* that encode the Kir6.2 and SUR1 subunits, respectively (Gloyn et al. 2004). An early genetic diagnosis is vital as patients with mutations in the KATP channel can, in 90% of cases, be treated with sulfonylurea tablets, rather than insulin. Glucose control is better and fluctuates less, so transfer to sulfonylureas should be made as soon as the diagnosis is made. There are 16 known genetic causes of PNDM and the different subtypes have different associated features. Increasingly a genetic diagnosis is made before the other features are recognized.

MATURITY-ONSET DIABETES OF THE YOUNG (MODY). The major cause of familial monogenic diabetes is MODY. This is a group of AD conditions which typically present with diabetes or hyperglycaemia before 25 years (although it is often later in older generations). While multiple genes have been described, the main three are glucokinase, *HNF1A*, and *HNF4A*. *HNF1B* typically presents with developmental renal disease and other developmental disorders, rather than familial diabetes. Patients with MODY are not insulin-dependent but may often be insulin-treated, as *HNF1A* and *HNF4A* present with marked symptomatic hyperglycaemia in slim, young adults and are mistaken for T1D.

Clinical approach

History: key points
- Features of the diabetes, e.g. age of diagnosis (<6 months neonatal diabetes), features at presentation, initial and subsequent treatment, glycaemic control.
- Family history. Other members of the family with diabetes (particularly parents and grandparents, as dominant inheritance in MODY). For other family members, take details of their diabetes. Any evidence of mitochondrial inheritance?
- Birthweight and gestational age (markedly reduced in neonatal diabetes 1.8–2.5 kg), reduced in HNF1B

(median 2.6 kg), slightly reduced in GCK (median 3 kg), and increased in HNF4A (median 4.3 kg). Note birthweight will be increased in mothers with diabetes or gestational diabetes.

- Autoimmune diseases, e.g. hypo- or hyperthyroidism, vitiligo, Addison's disease, SLE, rheumatoid arthritis.
- Deafness, muscle weakness, stroke-like episodes, ophthalmoplegia, pigmentary retinopathy (mitochondrial disorders).

Examination: key points
- Height and weight. BMI.
- Skin. Acanthosis nigricans (insulin resistance), vitiligo (autoimmune disease).
- Body fat distribution. Look carefully for features of lipodystrophy—inherited lipodystrophy is usually either total or predominantly limb/gluteal. Acquired lipodystrophy has patchy areas of loss of subcutaneous fat, e.g. typically on the face, also on the shoulders and upper arms.
- Pseudoacromegaly in severe insulin resistance; large jaw and hands.
- Insulin resistance may be associated with hyperandrogenism (hirsutism, acne, polycystic ovary syndrome).
- Features of mitochondrial disease (e.g. ptosis).
- Evidence of diabetic complications in affected individuals.
- Syndromic features characteristic of specific monogenic diabetes subtypes, e.g. renal cysts.

Investigations
- If insulin-treated, consider measuring C-peptide as a sign of having endogenous insulin production and so not being insulin-dependent.
- Fasting insulin level if there are signs of insulin resistance and the patient is not obese.
- Autoantibodies are positive in 80% of northern Europeans at the time of diagnosis of T1D but are less common, especially after >5 years of diagnosis (most helpfully anti-GAD, and IA2. Islet cell antibodies are based on the rat pancreas, are not sensitive, and have little value).
- Mutation analysis is available for: (1) all subtypes of neonatal diabetes, (2) all common subtypes of MODY, (3) common subtypes of partial and total lipodystrophy, (4) insulin receptor mutations, and (5) selected multisystem syndromes, including diabetes, e.g. renal cysts and diabetes (RCAD), Wolfram syndrome.
- Mitochondrial DNA testing. 3243-bp mitochondrial deletion commonly found in MELAS in families with a maternal mitochondrial mode of inheritance (consider if there is another affected family member in the matrilineal line or if associated with deafness or other features of MELAS).

If you are seeing an 'at-risk' family member, consider:
- HbA1c. An HbA1c value ≥48 mmol/mol or 6.5% = diabetes mellitus (American Diabetic Association diagnostic criteria), while an intermediate value of 43–47 mmol/mol = impaired glycaemia (i.e. needs follow-up by the general practitioner (GP)/physician).
- Individuals with mutations in GCK (see 'Maturity-onset diabetes of the young (MODY)' below) have stable, mild fasting hyperglycaemia throughout life, with fasting glucose between 5.5 and 8 mmol/l and an HbA1c

38–56 mmol/mol (5.6–7.3%) if aged ≤40 years; 41–60 mmol/mol (5.9–7.6%) if >40 years.

Diagnoses/conditions to consider

Type 1 diabetes
The diagnosis of this is usually on the basis of clinical features and investigations showing either insulin dependence with very low C-peptide or the presence of GAD or IA2 antibodies.

Type 2 diabetes
There are no specific tests for T2D. There are major environmental risk factors for the development of T2D and variants in >60 genes are associated with an increased risk of developing T2D. These variants account for only ~10% of the heritability and as a geneticist it is most important to recognize the monogenic forms of diabetes described below.

MATURITY-ONSET DIABETES OF THE YOUNG (MODY). Shows AD inheritance, non-obese body habitus, and is often diagnosed before 25 years. It accounts for 1–2% of people with diabetes. Mutations in four genes account for most UK MODY.
- GCK mutations cause mild, stable fasting hyperglycaemia from birth (5.5–8 mmol/l). No pharmacological treatment is required outside pregnancy.
- HNF1A and HNF4A transcription factor mutations cause a progressive form of diabetes mostly diagnosed in adolescence or early adulthood. Low-dose sulfonylureas are the first recommended pharmacological treatment (Pearson et al. 2003). HNF4A mutations also cause increased birthweight (mean 800 g) and neonatal hypoglycaemia in ~10% (Pearson et al. 2007)
- HNF1B mutations cause the RCAD syndrome. The renal cysts are often detected *in utero* and cause progressive renal dysfunction. Other features include female genital tract malformations, hyperuricaemia, hypomagnesaemia, and abnormal liver function. Pancreas atrophy is common (Bellanne-Chantelot et al. 2004). Diabetes can present in the neonatal period (usually transient), during childhood, or during adulthood (mean age at onset 26 years). Large genomic deletions of >1 Mb account for ~50% of cases and overall ~50% of mutations have arisen *de novo*.

MITOCHONDRIAL MUTATIONS. The most common symptom other than the diabetes is deafness and this usually precedes the diabetes. Other signs of mitochondrial disease may be present and should be considered in all affected members of the family. The most common mutation found is the m.3243A>G mutation, which is also found in MELAS. For more details about genetic advice, see 'Mitochondrial DNA diseases' in Chapter 3, 'Common consultations', p. 490.

INSULIN RECEPTOR (INSR) MUTATIONS.

(1) When two mutations are present, there is severe insulin resistance and extremely high insulin levels.
- Donohue syndrome (leprechaunism). This is the most severe form, presenting in infancy with pre- and postnatal failure to thrive, hirsutism, an aged face with thick lips and prominent ears, and enlargement of the breasts and genitalia. Inheritance is AR.
- Rabson–Mendenhall syndrome (acanthosis nigricans, polycystic ovaries, virilization of females) is a less severe form, presenting later. Inheritance is AR.

(2) AD inheritance of a single dominant-negative mutation may cause type A insulin resistance ± diabetes mellitus.

Lipodystrophy

Lipodystrophy syndromes are characterized in broad terms by loss of subcutaneous adipose tissue and have similar metabolic attributes, including insulin resistance, hyperlipidaemia, and diabetes.

FAMILIAL PARTIAL LIPODYSTROPHY (DUNNIGAN VARIETY). An AD disorder caused by missense mutations in the lamin A/C gene (*LMNA*). It is characterized by loss of subcutaneous fat from the extremities and trunk and accumulation of fat in the head and neck regions. Congenital generalized lipodystrophy is an AR disorder caused by mutations in the *BSCL2* or *AGPAT2* genes.

Other syndromes that include diabetes
See Table 3.11.

WOLFRAM SYNDROME (DIABETES INSIPIDUS–DIABETES MELLITUS–OPTIC ATROPHY–DEAFNESS (DIDMOAD)). An AR condition. It is caused by mutations in *WFS1* on 4p16.1. Patients often have renal tract anomalies, e.g. hydronephrosis.

Genetic advice

Inheritance and recurrence risk
- T1D shows:
  - 30–50% concordance in MZ twins;
  - sibling risk 6% (up to 10% in some studies with a higher background rate), with human leucocyte antigen (HLA) identical sibs having a greatly increased risk of developing T1D;
  - offspring risks show some differences between affected fathers and mothers; a greater proportion of fathers (~4%) than mothers (~2%) of children with IDDM have the disease themselves.
- Neonatal diabetes is most caused by de novo heterozygous mutations in non-consanguineous families. Germline mosaicism has been reported. AR inheritance is most common in consanguineous pedigrees. XLR inheritance is also possible (immunodysregulation–polyendocrinopathy–enteropathy, X-linked (IPEX) syndrome).
- MODY follows AD inheritance.
- Insulin receptor mutations. Both Donohue and Rabson–Mendenhall syndrome follow AR inheritance.
- Type A insulin resistance (less severe) may also be AD.
- Lipodystrophies can be AD (partial lipodystrophy due to *LMNA* or *PPARG* mutations) or AR (congenital generalized lipodystrophy).

Variability and penetrance
- T1D. Although thought of as a disease of childhood, the onset is after 20 years in 50%.
- Neonatal diabetes. Penetrance is high, ~95%.
- MODY. Penetrance is high, ~95%. Environmental factors influence the age of onset.

Prenatal diagnosis
- T1D. Not available.
- Neonatal diabetes. Mostly undertaken for syndromic forms, e.g. Wolcott–Rallison or IPEX syndromes which can be fatal during childhood.
- MODY. Not usually requested.
- Donohue syndrome. Available by CVS if mutations are known.

Predictive testing
- T1D. HLA testing of sibs has been used, but half of HLA-compatible sibs will never develop the condition. There is no pre-symptomatic treatment to alter the disease process. Consider the ethical position and issues of informed consent. Autoantibodies (anti-islet cell, anti-GAD, etc.) have been used predictively to assess risk in sibs in research, but not in routine clinical practice.
- MODY. Possible in those with a known mutation, but issues of consent and autonomy regarding testing in childhood.

Other family members
- T1D. Individuals who are at high genetic risk should know the symptoms of diabetes mellitus and attend for prompt assessment if they develop these features.
- MODY. Mutation testing is recommended for other affected family members in order to confirm the aetiology of their diabetes. Asymptomatic individuals who are at high risk of inheriting an *HNF1A/4A/1B* mutation can undergo predictive molecular genetic testing. For those who have inherited the mutation, annual testing for diabetes by measuring HbA1c is recommended. *HNF1A* mutations cause glycosuria which can be detected by urine testing.

Natural history and management

Potential long-term complications
The long-term complications of diabetes are well documented, but it is important to remind patients and their doctors of the risks in pregnancy to the fetus if the diabetes is poorly controlled. See 'Maternal diabetes mellitus and diabetic embryopathy' in Chapter 6, 'Pregnancy and fertility', p. 756.

Table 3.11 Associations between syndromes and diabetes

Deafness	Eye signs*	Renal disease	Severe obesity	Severe insulin resistance
MELAS[AO]	Prader–Willi (RP)	Renal cysts and diabetes	Prader–Willi[BF]	Donohue
Wolfram[BF]	Alstrom (RP)	Wolfram	Alstrom	Rabson–Mendenhall
	Bardet–Biedl (RP)	Bardet–Biedl[BF]	Bardet–Biedl	Partial lipodystrophy
	Wolfram (OA)			

* OA, optic atrophy; RP, retinitis pigmentosa.

[BF] See 'Mitochondrial DNA diseases' in Chapter 3, 'Common consultations', p. 490.

[AO] See 'Obesity with and without developmental delay' in Chapter 2, 'Clinical approach', p. 254.

Fetal macrosomia

The inheritance of *GCK* and *HNF4A* mutations by the fetus influences birthweight. Any fetus inheriting an *HNF4A* mutation (from their mother or father) will produce increased insulin *in utero*, leading to increased insulin-mediated growth and be on average 800 g heavier than a fetus without an *HNF4A* mutation. Many will be macrosomic and hence at risk of complications during delivery. In addition, some babies will have hypoglycaemia at or soon after birth, which may require treatment. Macrosomia is also a risk for the babies of women with *GCK* mutations who *do not* inherit the mutation, who on average have a 700-g increased birthweight. This is because the mother's blood glucose is regulated at a higher level, compared to the fetus, which results in increased fetal production of insulin. Until non-invasive PND becomes routinely available, serial USS is used to predict fetal size and guide management of delivery.

Surveillance

Individuals with all types of diabetes require regular medical and nursing supervision to ensure accurate control of the disease in order to help prevent long-term complications. Assessment of cardiovascular risk is probably the most important part of the management of T2D in terms of prognosis due to the constellation of associated metabolic risk factors for atherosclerosis.

Support groups: Diabetes UK, https://www. diabetes.org.uk; Diabetes Genes (information on genetic testing), http://www.diabetesgenes.org.

Expert advisers: Andrew Hattersley, Professor of Molecular Medicine, University of Exeter Medical School, Exeter, UK and Sian Ellard, Consultant Clinical Scientist, University of Exeter Medical School, Exeter, UK.

References

Aguilar-Bryan L, Bryan J. Neonatal diabetes mellitus. *Endocr Rev* 2008; **29**: 265–91.

American Diabetes Association (ADA). Diabetes and classification of diabetes mellitus [ADA position statement—detailed discussion of classification, terminology, and diagnostic criteria]. *Diabetes Care* 2014; **37**(Suppl 1): S81–90. http://care.diabetesjournals.org/content/37/Supplement_1/S81.full.

Bellanné-Chantelot C, Chauveau D, Gautier JF, et al. Clinical spectrum associated with hepatocyte nuclear factor-1 beta mutations. *Am Intern Med* 2004; **140**: 510–17.

Diabetes Genes. http://www.diabetesgenes.org.

Edghill EL, Bingham C, Ellard S, Hattersley AT. Mutations in hepatocyte nuclear factor-1beta and their related phenotypes. *J Med Genet* 2006; **43**: 84–90.

Fajans SS, Bell GI, Polanky KS. Molecular mechanisms and clinical pathophysiology of maturity-onset diabetes of the young. *N Engl J Med* 2001; **345**: 971–80.

Gloyn AL, Pearson ER, Antcliff JF, et al. Activating mutations in the gene encoding the ATP-sensitive potassium-channel subunit Kir6.2 and permanent neonatal diabetes. *N Engl J Med* 2004; **350**: 1838–49.

Mein CA, Esposito L, Dunn MG, et al. A search for type 1 diabetes susceptibility genes in families from the United Kingdom. *Nat Genet* 1998; **19**: 297–300.

Murphy R, Ellard S, Hattersley AT. Clinical implications of a molecular genetic classification of monogenic beta-cell diabetes. *Nat Clin Pract Endocrinol Metab* 2008; **4**: 200–13.

Onengut-Gumuscu S, Concannon P. Mapping genes for autoimmunity in humans: type 1 diabetes as model. *Immunol Rev* 2002; **190**: 182–94.

Owen KR, Stride A, Ellard S, Hattersley AT. Etiological investigation of diabetes in young adults presenting with apparent type 2 diabetes. *Diabetes Care* 2003; **26**: 2088–93.

Pearson ER, Boj SF, Steele AM, et al. Macrosomia and hyperinsulinaemic hypoglycaemia in patients with heterozygous mutations in the *HNF4A* gene. *PLoS Med* 2007; **4**: e118.

Pearson ER, Starkely BJ, Powell RJ, Gribble FM, Clark PM, Hattersley AT. Genetic causes of hyperglycaemia and response to treatment in diabetes. *Lancet* 2003; **362**: 1275–81.

Pociot F, McDermott MF. Genetics of type 1 diabetes mellitus. *Genes Immunol* 2002; **3**: 235–49.

Seminars in Medical Genetics. The genetics of diabetes mellitus. *Am J Med Genet* 2002; **115C** (Issue 1).

Temple IK, Shield JP. Transient neonatal diabetes, a disorder of imprinting. *J Med Genet* 2002; **39**: 872–5.

Dilated cardiomyopathy (DCM)

DCM is a disease of the myocardium, characterized by dilatation and impaired contraction of the left ventricle (LV) (or both ventricles), causing progressive heart failure and ventricular arrhythmia. Impaired LV function is most commonly due to coronary artery disease, and this must be excluded to make a diagnosis of DCM. DCM can be associated with hypertension, alcohol excess, viral myocarditis, metabolic disorders (e.g. haemochromatosis), systemic disorders (hypothyroidism, hypocalcaemia), late pregnancy, and the puerperium. In an individual without a family history, take care to ensure that other causes have been adequately excluded before assuming a genetic basis, as only about one-half of cases appear to be hereditary.

DCM is sometimes inherited as an isolated trait, but familial DCM may be associated with other features (see below). Familial DCM has a prevalence of >2/10 000. Currently there are over 30 nuclear-encoded genes cloned for familial DCM and a number of mitochondrial genes. However, mutations in these genes appear to account for <20% of familial DCM. This appears to be likely to change with the usage of next-generation sequencing techniques identifying titin as an important gene in the pathogenesis of DCM. Nonetheless it is likely to remain a multifactorial and oligogenic disease, and clear monogenic aetiologies will underlie a minority of cases.

Cardiomyopathy mutations are notable for substantial variation in clinical presentation. Both genetic heterogeneity and allelic variation contribute to variable morphological phenotypes and disease severity (Burke 2016). Note that the Exome Sequencing Project identified an average of one rare TTN missense variant per individual *without* cardiomyopathy (Herman *et al.* 2012).

There are four broad categories of clinical presentation:

(1) DCM without additional features. Likely to follow AD inheritance. Mutations have been identified in three cardiac sarcomere genes that are also critical genes in hypertrophic cardiomyopathy (HCM): troponin T, beta-myosin heavy chain (MHC), and cardiac actin. Mutations in delta-sarcoglycan, which is implicated in one form of limb–girdle dystrophy, can also cause familial DCM with no/subclinical skeletal muscle involvement.

(2) DCM with premature conduction disease and/or ventricular arrhythmias. Likely to follow AD inheritance. Mutations have been identified in lamin A/C (mutations in this gene also cause AD Emery–Dreifuss) and desmin (mutations in this gene usually cause a severe skeletal myopathy), as well as *SCN5A*, the sodium channel gene. There is an increased risk of atrial fibrillation, ventricular arrhythmias, and sudden death. Arrhythmogenic right ventricular cardiomyopathy (ARVC) can be associated with LV involvement and a late-stage presentation of a biventricular CM indistinguishable clinically from DCM. This is usually associated with a high risk of ventricular arrhythmias and sudden death. ARVC is encoded for by desmosome-associated gene products (plakoglobin, plakohyllin, desmoplakin, desmocollin, etc.).

(3) DCM with rapid progression in young men. Likely to be XL with mutation in dystrophin (Xp21). (Mutations in tafazzin (Xq28) usually cause a CM that is fatal in infancy (Barth syndrome), but patients can survive to adult life.)

(4) DCM with sensorineural hearing loss. One autosomal locus (6q23–24) and one mitochondrial-encoded gene (tRNA–Lys).

Clinical approach

History: key points

- Three-generation family history, with specific enquiry about:
  - heart failure;
  - sudden death, conduction disorders (palpitations, dizzy spells, 'faints', pacemakers), atrial fibrillation;
  - stroke (embolic from thrombus forming in dilated cardiac chambers);
  - 'muscular dystrophy', muscle weakness (ability to climb stairs or get up from a chair), abnormal gait, wheelchair use, contractures;
  - sensorineural deafness.
- Fits, faints, or funny turns.
- Exercise tolerance and breathlessness.
- Enquire about muscle weakness. Difficulty rising from chairs implies hip girdle involvement; difficulty lifting the arms above the head, e.g. brushing hair, hanging out washing, implies shoulder girdle involvement.
- Current level of mobility. Rising from chairs, walking on flat, use of aids.

Examination: key points

- If not already seen by a cardiologist, basic cardiovascular assessment, e.g. pulse, BP, jugular venous pressure (JVP), palpation of the apex, auscultation of the heart.
- Muscle bulk (e.g. calf hypertrophy in BMD) and limb–girdle muscle power (Gower's manoeuvre and lifting the arms above the head).
- Look for contractures, especially at the elbows and ankles (Emery–Dreifuss).

Investigations

Basic investigations should include the following:

- echo;
- 12-lead ECG with rhythm strip;
- 24-hour tape;
- CK (total CK and isoenzyme CK-MB);
- cardiac MRI.

Genetic investigations should be focussed on a single clearly affected family member:

- gene panel/WES/WGS as appropriate;
- dystrophin deletion/duplication screen (if family history consistent with XLR inheritance, i.e. no male-to-male transmission and CK elevated);
- if young males only affected, no accompanying muscle weakness, and family history compatible with XLR inheritance, check for promoter mutations in dystrophin and for exon 29 deletions (deletion of exon 29 from the mid-rod regions disrupts sarcoglycan assembly in cardiac muscle, but not in skeletal muscle);
- consider lamin A/C mutation analysis if family tree consistent with AD Emery–Dreifuss or AD DCM,

especially if there are early atrial fibrillation and conduction disease. (Mutations in lamin A (*LMNA*) are a rare cause of isolated DCM.)

- consider lamin A/C, *SCN5A*, and desmosomal gene testing if there is a family history of sudden death or if ventricular arrhythmias and cardiac arrest have been present.

All first-degree relatives should be offered investigation with an ECG and echo for initial screening, unless a pathogenic mutation has been identified and predictive testing offered. In the absence of such a test and with a high likelihood of age-related penetrance, follow-up screening must be considered, depending on the likelihood of familial disease and the age of relatives.

Other diagnoses to consider

Becker muscular dystrophy (BMD)
Is caused by in-frame mutations in *dystrophin* on Xp21. Cardiac complications (DCM) are a major cause of morbidity and mortality in BMD. BMD patients should be under regular review by a cardiologist, with regular surveillance from the teens onwards (annual ECG and echo in the first instance). See 'Duchenne and Becker muscular dystrophy (DMD and BMD)' in Chapter 3, 'Common consultations', p. 402.

Emery–Dreifuss muscular dystrophy
Usually XLR due to mutations in *emerin* on Xq28, but some AD forms exist, e.g. lamin A/C (*LMNA*). Variable muscular dystrophy with development of contractures (especially elbows and knees) from teens. Cardiac conduction defects are a prominent feature. See 'Limb–girdle muscular dystrophies' in Chapter 3, 'Common consultations', p. 476.

Genetic advice

Inheritance and recurrence risk
The great majority of familial DCM follows AD inheritance. AR inheritance is less common, accounting for ~15% of affected families. Homozygous mutation in cardiac troponin 1 has been identified in one such family (Murphy *et al*. 2004). XL inheritance is particularly important for families presenting with rapidly progressive DCM affecting young males. DCM is a significant cause of death in men with BMD; female carriers for BMD and DMD may develop CM, but this is usually mild and subclinical. DCM is a feature of some mitochondrial disorders (both matrilineal and nuclear), usually with additional abnormalities.

Variability and penetrance
Clinical features can be quite variable, even among family members carrying the same mutation. Penetrance is age-dependent and overall (for categories 2 and 3 above) is estimated at 10% in those <20 years, 34% in young adults of 20–30 years, 60% in adults of 30–40 years, and 90% in those >40 years.

Prenatal diagnosis
In a family with a known mutation (the minority), this is technically possible.

Predictive testing
In a family with a known mutation (the minority), this could be offered so that cardiac surveillance could be targeted more appropriately. Otherwise screening of at-risk relatives should be offered.

Box 3.3 Major and minor criteria for the diagnosis of familial dilated cardiomyopathy in adult members of affected families

Major criteria
- A reduced ejection fraction of the LV (<45%) and/or fractional shortening (<25%), as assessed by echo cardiography, radionuclide scanning, or angiography
- An increased LV end-diastolic diameter corresponding to >117% of the predicted value corrected for age and body surface area

Minor criteria
- Unexplained supraventricular or ventricular arrhythmia
- Ventricular dilatation (>112% of the predicted value)
- An intermediate impairment of LV dysfunction
- Conduction defects
- Segmental wall motion abnormalities in the absence of intraventricular conduction defect or ischaemic heart disease
- Unexplained sudden death of a first-degree relative or stroke at <50 years

Reproduced from David A. Warrell, Timothy M. Cox, John D. Firth, and Jeremy Dwight, *Oxford Textbook of Medicine: Cardiovascular Disorders*, 2016, Box 7.2.2, page 265, with permission from Oxford University Press.

Other family members
See Box 3.3.

Natural history and management
Beta-blockers have an important role in reducing overall mortality and hospitalization rates for heart failure. ACE inhibitors have a role in the management of heart failure due to DCM. Pacemakers should be considered in families with conduction disorders. Amiodarone may be of value in patients with ventricular arrhythmia, but there is little evidence of long-term benefit. An implantable cardioverter–defibrillator (ICD) may be useful in patients with a high risk of sudden death from ventricular arrhythmia: prior cardiac arrest; haemodynamically compromising ventricular arrhythmias; unexplained syncope; and severe LV impairment, especially with conduction disease where cardiac resynchronization therapy may be appropriate. The presence of lamin A/C, SCN5A, and ARVC-associated mutations may lower the threshold for ICD implantation. Cardiac transplantation or LV assist devices have a role in the management of some individuals with end-stage heart failure due to DCM.

Potential long-term complications
Systemic and pulmonary emboli are common, and anticoagulation with warfarin may be advised for patients in atrial fibrillation, with intracardiac thrombus, a history of stroke, or severe ventricular dilatation and dysfunction.

Surveillance
Affected individuals should be under regular long-term surveillance by a cardiologist. It is difficult to know how long cardiac surveillance should be continued in

an apparently unaffected individual, but infrequent surveillance is probably advisable at least until the age of 45 years (see 'Variability and penetrance' above).

Support group: Cardiomyopathy UK, http://www.cardiomyopathy.org.

Expert adviser: Elijah Behr, Reader in Cardiovascular Medicine, Consultant Cardiologist, Cardiology Clinical Academic Group, St George's University of London, St George's University Hospitals NHS Foundation Trust, London, UK.

References

Burke MA, Cook SA. Clinical and mechanistic insights into the genetics of cardiomyopathy. *J Am Coll Cardiol* 2016; **68**(25): 2871–86.

Franz W-M, Muller OJ, Katus A. Cardiomyopathies: from genetics to the prospect of treatment [review article]. *Lancet* 2001; **358**: 1627–37.

Herman DS, Lam L et al. Truncations of titin causing dilated cardiomyopathy. *N Engl J Med* 2012; **366**(7): 619–28.

McKenna WJ. The cardiomyopathies: hypertrophic, dilated, restrictive and right ventricular. In: DA Warrell, TM Cox, JD Firth (eds.). *The Oxford textbook of medicine*, 4th edn, pp. 1021–34. Oxford University Press, Oxford, 2003.

Murphy ET, Mogensen J, Shaw A, Kubo T, Hughes S, McKenna WJ. Novel mutation in cardiac troponin 1 in recessive idiopathic dilated cardiomyopathy. *Lancet* 2004; **363**: 371–2.

Sebillon P, Bouchier C, Bidot LD, et al. Expanding the phenotype of *LMNA* mutations in dilated cardiomyopathy and functional consequences of these mutations. *J Med Genet* 2003; **40**: 560–7.

Sweet M, Taylor MRG, Mestroni L. Diagnosis, prevalence, and screening of familial dilated cardiomyopathy. *Expert Opin on Orphan Drugs* 2015; **3**(8): 869–76.

DNA repair disorders

These disorders all share defects in the DNA repair mechanisms of the cell. They are caused by mutations in 'caretaker genes' that encode the proteins that function to protect the genome against acquired alterations. Typically, DNA damage is generated by UV radiation, ionizing radiation, free radicals, and exogenous chemicals. The impaired capacity to maintain genomic integrity results in the accelerated accumulation of key genetic changes that promote cellular transformation and neoplasia. DNA repair proteins also have a role in joining the double-stranded breaks between the variable (V), diversity (D), and joining (J) gene segments of the lymphocyte immunoglobulin and antigen receptor genes to generate immunological diversity. Deficiency of this repair process may contribute to the immunodeficiency characteristic of these disorders. Other features found in several of these disorders are neurological abnormalities and premature ageing. Some have distinctive features, e.g. radial hypoplasia in Fanconi anaemia (FA), but for others there is considerable phenotypic overlap. As a group, they are probably significantly underdiagnosed.

- Nucleotide excision repair (NER) is a DNA repair pathway that removes DNA damage (such as UV light-induced pyrimidine dimers) by excising the region of DNA that contains the damaged base(s). Defective in XP and trichothiodystrophy (TTD).
- Transcription-coupled repair is a specialized NER pathway that facilitates the repair of damaged DNA during transcription. The transcribed strand of active genes is preferentially repaired. Defective in Cockayne syndrome (CS), COFS, and UV-sensitive syndrome (UVSS).
- Cross-linking agent repair. Agents such as MMC and DEB and a variety of cytotoxic agents (e.g. cisplatin, cyclophosphamide) form covalent cross-links in double-stranded DNA (either between the two strands (interstrand) or between adjacent bases (intrastrand)) that obstruct DNA replication. Specific repair pathways are required to detect interstrand crosslinks and facilitate its repair. Defective in FA.
- Double-strand break repair (DSBR) can occur via two pathways—non-homologous end-joining (NHEJ) in which a complex of proteins enables the cell to join the break directly, and homologous recombination which is available during the S and G2 phases when a sister chromatid is available to facilitate repair of the break by recombination. Defective in severe combined immunodeficiency (SCID) (caused by ligase IV, Artemis, or DNA-PKcs deficiency) and in immunodeficiency caused by Cernunnos deficiency. All radiosensitive. Defects in recognition and signalling of damage in the DSB pathway in AT, ataxia telangiectasia-like disorder (ATLD), NBS, Nijmegen breakage syndrome-like disorder (NBSLD), and RIDDLE syndrome, again all radiosensitive.
- Cohesinopathies. Caused by mutations in cohesin subunits enabling chromosome cohesion. DDX11 defective in Warsaw breakage syndrome. MMC and ionizing radiation sensitivity.

Clinical approach

History: key points
- Three-generation family history with specific enquiry for consanguinity.
- Pregnancy history with birthweight.

- Developmental milestones and postnatal growth.
- Sun sensitivity.

Examination: key points
- Growth parameters. Height, weight, OFC; short stature is common.
- Face. Deep-set eyes, pinched nose, premature ageing (CS), microcephaly with prominent midface (NBS), freckling (XP and NBS), solar keratoses (XP), butterfly rash (Bloom syndrome).
- Skin. CALs and areas of increased pigmentation (FA), excessive sunlight-induced skin injury (XP), especially pigmentation changes (XP), skin cancers (XP) and sunburn (XP, CS, TTD, UVSS).
- Eyes. Telangiectasiae (AT), cataract (CS).
- Neurology. Balance (AT), spasticity (CS).
- Brittle, sulfur-deficient hair (TTD).

Investigations
- Genomic analysis e.g. genomic array, gene panel, WES/WGS as available may be very helpful given the genetic heterogeneity of DNA repair disorders.
- AT:
  - Serum AFP. Usually unmeasurable levels in childhood, but high levels in AT;
  - FBC for white cell counts;
  - EDTA sample (3–5 ml) for immunoglobulin subclasses (IgA and IgG2 deficiency is common) and lymphocyte subsets;
  - 5 ml of blood in LiHeparin (LiHep) for radiosensitivity assay (up to 10-fold increased chromosome breakage after irradiation in the lab). Also present in peripheral T cells is a high frequency of chromosome translocations involving chromosomes 7 and 14. A lymphoblastoid cell line can be made from the heparin sample and tested for reduced level/absence of ATM protein by western blotting and activity of any residual ATM protein (6 weeks). Identification of the *ATM* mutations can then follow using the same cell line.
- Bloom syndrome. Measurement of sister chromatid exchanges (SCEs) in blood sample.
- CS and COFS. Skin biopsy for fibroblast culture for the study of RNA synthesis following exposure to UV light. Reduced RNA synthesis recovery is seen on exposure of cells to UV light. Unlike in XP, excision repair after UV damage is grossly normal, but there is a slow recovery of DNA and RNA synthesis. Mutation analysis of *CSA/ERCC8* and *CSB/ERCC6*.
- FA:
  - FBC for haematological indices;
  - AFP is often elevated;
  - spontaneous and DEB-induced chromosome breakage analysis in LiHep blood sample. In FA, both measures of chromosome breakage are increased. Exact levels are lab-dependent, but in the Guy's Hospital lab, spontaneous breaks/cell in control samples are 0.00–0.20 and in Fanconi samples 0.08–2.03, and DEB-induced breaks/cell in control samples are 0.00–0.23, and in Fanconi samples 0.48–18.40.
- NBS:
  - FBC for white cell counts;

- EDTA sample (3–5 ml) for immunoglobulin subclasses and lymphocyte subsets;
- 5 ml of blood in LiHep for radiosensitivity assay. Increased breakage of chromosomes, as for AT. In unirradiated peripheral T cells, there is an increased frequency of chromosome translocations involving chromosomes 7 and 14, again as for AT. A lymphoblastoid cell line can be made from heparin sample and tested for the absence of NBS1 protein by western blotting, 6 weeks. If suggestive, proceed to mutation analysis of *NBS1* (EDTA sample). A common 5-bp deletion is present in homozygous or compound heterozygous form in the majority of patients.
- TTD:
  - skin biopsy for fibroblast culture for study of NER following UV irradiation (as for XP);
  - blood sample for FBC and Hb electrophoresis (TTD patients show the beta-thalassaemia triad: decreased mean corpuscular volume (MCV); decreased mean corpuscular haemoglobin (MCH); increased HbA_2).
- XP:
  - skin biopsy for fibroblast culture for analysis of NER using unscheduled DNA synthesis (UDS) assay following UV irradiation—defective in 80% of XP cases. Levels of UDS are 0–50% of normal;
  - in the variant form (20%), UDS is normal. Defect is in specialized DNA polymerase eta. The assay involves UV irradiation, incubating for 2 days in caffeine, then measuring replicative DNA synthesis as a measure of survival—defective in XP variants. Mutation analysis of *POLH*.

Diagnoses/conditions to consider

Ataxia with oculomotor apraxia type 1 (AOA-1)
Early-onset cerebellar ataxia, peripheral neuropathy, and oculomotor apraxia. Caused by mutations in the *APTX* gene encoding aprataxin, which removes abortive ligation intermediates during repair of single-strand breaks. *APTX* is small and can be sequenced readily. Prevalence unknown, but probably the least common of AT, AOA-2, and AOA-1.

Ataxia with oculomotor apraxia type 2 (AOA-2)
Teenage-onset cerebellar ataxia, peripheral neuropathy, and oculomotor apraxia, caused by mutation of the large *SETX* gene encoding senataxin, with roles in transcription control and DNA damage response. Prevalence unknown, but possibly similar to AT.

Ataxia with oculomotor apraxia type 4 (AOA-4)
A progressive condition that includes hyperkinetic movement disorder, eye movement abnormalities, polyneuropathy, variable ID and obesity is caused by alleleic mutation in PNKP (Paucer *et al.* 2016).

Ataxia with oculomotor apraxia and axonal polyneuropathy (XRCC1)
Biallelic mutations in *XRCC1* causes a progressive cerebellar ataxia with OMA and axonal neuropathy (Hoch *et al.* 2017).

Ataxia telangiectasia (AT)
Prevalence ~1/300 000. A child with AT usually appears normal until he/she begins to walk and ataxia becomes evident. Characteristics include:

- neurological problems, e.g. unsteady (wobbly) gait, difficulty standing without swaying. Progressive difficulty with eye movements (oculomotor apraxia), and squint, slurred speech (dysarthria), and drooling may be evident from early years; involuntary movements (fidgety movement of the hands) can make skilled movements difficult in late childhood; dysfunctional swallowing can be problematic in teens;
- telangiectasiae usually visible on sclerae by 4–8 years. Sun sensitivity and premature ageing of the skin with dark spots and occasional grey hairs;
- immunodeficiency in 80%—variable, typically sinusitis and/or bronchitis/pneumonia;
- impaired growth and delayed/incomplete puberty;
- predisposition to cancer, especially lymphoma and leukaemia; 10–30% of AT patients, including 15% of those <16 years.

AT is an AR disorder caused by mutations in *ATM* (A-T mutated) on chromosome 11. Mutations occur throughout the gene (66 exons) and are usually truncating. The ATM protein activates cellular responses to DNA damage caused by radiation, certain chemicals, or normal cellular metabolism. It is also required for repair of double-strand breaks in heterochromatin. Chromosome instability in lymphocytes from AT patients takes the form of non-random translocations and inversions that preferentially involve the T- and B-cell receptor gene involving chromosomes 7 and 14. Avoid therapeutic doses of ionizing radiation (seek advice); avoid diagnostic X-rays where possible. Life-limiting condition, but life expectancy varies. Female AT patients have a large increased risk of breast cancer at an early age.

Approximately 1/200 individuals are carriers for AT. Hence, there is a low risk to the extended family, unless there is consanguinity, e.g. risk for a sibling having an AT child is $2/3 \times 1/200 \times 1/4 = 1/1200$ or an aunt/uncle having an AT child is $1/2 \times 1/200 \times 1/4 = 1/1600$. Determining the AT carrier status for someone from the general population not generally feasible. PND usually possible for parents of an affected child.

Heterozygous carriers for AT are at a 3.6-fold risk of breast cancer. Current advice is to avoid regular mammographic screening because of potential radiation risk and consider breast awareness or clinical evaluation from 50 years in lieu of mammographic screening. AT carriers should minimize exposure to diagnostic X-rays, e.g. restrict exposure to situations where X-rays would significantly alter management.

An AT-like disorder (ATLD) that is neurologically indistinguishable from AT has been described. At the cellular level, there is also an increased sensitivity to ionizing radiation. The patients do not have mutations in the *ATM* gene, but in the *hMRE11* gene.

RIDDLE syndrome (Radiosensitivity, ImmunoDeficiency, Dysmorphic features and Learning difficulty)
Very rare. Small increased cellular radiosensitivity, a likely class switch defect, and biallelic mutation of the *RNF168* gene.

Bloom syndrome
A very rare AR disorder caused by mutations in *BLM* on 15q26.1, which encodes a RecQ DNA helicase involved in the maintenance of DNA integrity. Children with Bloom syndrome are small and usually have an erythematous 'butterfly rash' that is sensitive to sunlight,

excessive hyper- and hypopigmented skin lesions located anywhere on the body, and a high rate of bacterial infections due to immunodeficiency. They are prone to cancer, chronic lung disease, and diabetes. Bloom syndrome is more common among Ashkenazi Jews.

Cerebro-oculo-facial-skeletal syndrome (COFS)

AR, rapidly progressive neurological disorder leading to brain atrophy with calcifications, cataracts, microcornea, optic atrophy, progressive joint contractures, and growth failure. Usually presents in fetal or neonatal life. COFS is part of the spectrum of NER disorders, which includes XP, CS, TTD, and UVSS, and is probably a variant of CS.

Cockayne syndrome (CS)

An AR neurodegenerative disorder characterized by low to normal birthweight, postnatal growth failure, brain dysmyelination with calcium deposits, cutaneous photosensitivity, pigmentary retinopathy and/or cataracts and/or optic atrophy, and sensorineural hearing loss. The facies are characteristic with a prematurely aged appearance with deep-set eyes and a pinched appearance to the nose (loss of subcutaneous fat). There is progressive microcephaly with developmental delay, spasticity, and often ataxia. Patients usually have sun sensitivity. A more severe form (sometimes called type II) shows features from birth. Prevalence in Western Europe ~2 per million live births.

CS is caused by mutations in the genes CSA or CSB. Cultured CS cells are hypersensitive to UV radiation, because of impaired NER of UV-induced damage in transcribed strands of actively transcribed DNA (global genome NER is unaffected).

Fanconi anaemia (FA)

An AR disorder caused by mutations in 16 FA genes: FANCA, B, C, D1 (BRCA2), D2, E, F, G, I, J (BRIP1), L, M, N (PALB2), O (RAD51C), P (SLX4), and Q (XPF) (FANCA accounts for 60%, with FANCC most common among Ashkenazi Jews). The clinical phenotype of all FA complementation groups is similar and is characterized by:

- pre- and postnatal growth retardation; 50% of FA patients are <3rd centile for height;
- pancytopenia, aplastic anaemia; median age of onset of marrow failure is 7 years (usual range 3–12 years). BMT is sometimes offered;
- radial ray anomalies: absent, hypoplastic, supernumerary, or bifid thumbs and hypoplastic or absent radii. Twenty per cent have other skeletal problems (e.g. vertebral and rib anomalies);
- structural renal malformations: 25% have unilateral renal agenesis, and rotated, misshapen, or fused kidneys;
- pigmentary skin changes: many FA patients develop CALs. In some, the entire body or large areas of the body may have a suntanned appearance (hyperpigmentation);
- other features may include: microcephaly; microphthalmos; CHD (e.g. ASD, VSD); and learning disability;
- increased risk for myelodysplasia, AML, and other cancers, especially squamous carcinomas of the head, neck, and oesophagus and cancers of the female reproductive tract;
- Cells from patients with biallelic mutations in BRCA2, PALB2, BRCA1, RAD51C and the RAD51 dominant mutations, designated FA-D1, FA-N, FA-R, and FA-S receptively are invariably unusually sensitive to both DNA crosslinking agents as well as ionising radiation consistent with a defect in homologous recombination.

The chromosomal aberrations that occur spontaneously and randomly in dividing FA cells affect the newly replicated DNA. They are microscopically visible at metaphase as broken chromatids. Cells show increased sensitivity to cross-linking agents such as MMC and DEB. This forms the basis of diagnostic testing (see 'Investigations' above). Misrepair leads to quadriradial formation. Overall life expectancy is reduced to an average of 20 years (range 0–50 years). PND is not straightforward but is usually possible by CVS—consult your laboratory prior to counselling.

Nijmegen breakage syndrome (NBS)

NBS is extremely rare. Affected children have microcephaly, IUGR, short stature, prominent midface, growth retardation, mild learning difficulties, susceptibility to infections with panhypogammaglobulinaemia, and susceptibility to lymphoma and other tumours. AR due to mutations in NBS1 on 8q, which encodes 'nibrin', a novel protein involved in DNA DSBR and DNA damage signalling. Cells show increased sensitivity to ionizing radiation. A common 5-bp deletion is present in the homozygous or compound heterozygous form in the majority of patients.

Nijmegen breakage syndrome-like disorder (NBSLD)

Single patient with microcephaly, growth retardation, increased cellular radiosensitivity, and biallelic mutation of the RAD50 gene.

Rothmund–Thomson syndrome

Characterized by poikiloderma congenita, with growth deficiency, alopecia, photosensitivity, dystrophic nails, abnormal teeth, cataracts, and hypogonadism. Twenty per cent have radial ray defects. The skin abnormalities appear before 6 months of age with reticular or diffuse erythema on the face, hands, and extensor surfaces of the limbs. The trunk is relatively spared. It is caused by mutations in the helicase gene RECQL4 on 8q24.

Seckel syndrome

A microcephalic primordial dwarfism with profound growth delay, severe disproportionate microcephaly, and skeletal abnormalities. Mutations have been found in several genes, including ATR and ATRIP. These proteins form the apex of a DNA damage-signalling pathway, similar to that of the ATM protein, but in response to different lesions.

Severe combined immunodeficiency (SCID)

Some forms of SCID are caused by defects in DSBR, resulting from mutations in genes encoding components of the NHEJ pathway. These conditions are denoted as radiosensitive SCID to distinguish them from RAG1/2- or ADA-deficient SCID. Mutations have been found in DNA ligase IV, Artemis, Cernunnos, and DNA-dependent protein kinase, all components of the NHEJ pathway. Some of these patients have associated developmental abnormalities.

Spinocerebellar ataxia with axonal neuropathy-1 (SCAN-1)

A rare peripheral neuropathy characterized by moderate progressive ataxia, dysarthria, and cerebellar atrophy. It results from mutations in the TDP-1 gene, which encodes the enzyme tyrosyl-DNA phosphodiesterase1. TDP1 removes covalent complexes between topoisomerase 1 and DNA. Deficiencies in TDP1 results in the accumulation of these protein–DNA complexes, which lead to unrepaired single-strand breaks.

Trichothiodystrophy (TTD)

A rare condition characterized by brittle sulfur-deficient hair (trichorrhexis nodosa on microscopy), short stature,

MR, unusual facies, and sometimes ichthyosis. About 50% are sun-sensitive. These can be caused by mutations in *XPB*, *XPD* (most common), and *TTDA*. Patients with *XPD* mutations have reduced expression of beta-globin genes, resulting in the beta-thalassaemia trait. Non-photosensitive TTDs do not appear to be deficient in DNA repair, and other than *TTDN1* in a few patients and *GTF2E2* mutations in two patients, the defective gene has not been identified.

UV-sensitive syndrome (UVSS)
Individuals with this rare disorder have photosensitivity without associated development defects or skin cancer. Mutations can occur in the *CSA* or *CSB* genes or the recently identified *UVSSA1* gene. Despite a cellular defect in response to UV that is indistinguishable from that in CS, these patients show none of the multisystem features characteristic of the latter. It is likely that UVSS is underdiagnosed.

Werner syndrome
A progeroid syndrome characterized by premature greying and thinning of the hair, a prematurely aged appearance, short stature, T2D, hypogonadism, osteoporosis, premature atherosclerosis, a weak or hoarse voice, and cataracts. It is caused by mutations in *WRN*, which is a member of the *RECQ* family of DNA helicases. The mean age of diagnosis is 39 years (SD 7.7 years), with the mean age of initial symptoms being 13 years. Some patients with atypical Werner syndrome have mutations in the lamin A/C gene *LMNA*.

Xeroderma pigmentosum (XP)
An AR disorder characterized by extreme sensitivity of the skin to sunlight-induced changes. Prevalence in Western Europe ~2–3 per million. About 50% of people with XP will get unusually severe sunburn after a short sun exposure. The sunburn will last much longer than expected—perhaps for several weeks—and usually occurs during a child's first sun exposure. Some people with XP will not get sunburnt more easily and the disease is then recognized by unusually early freckling in sun-exposed areas. Without early diagnosis and sun protection, multiple skin cancers (BCC, squamous cell carcinoma, and melanoma) will result at an early age. Individuals with XP have a 1000-fold or more increase in incidence of sunlight-induced skin cancers. Most patients with XP develop dense freckling at an early age. Other skin changes, such as irregular dark spots, thinning of the skin, excessive dryness, and solar keratoses typical of those usually seen in the elderly, begin in infancy and are almost always present by age of 20 years. The eyes are often painfully sensitive to the sun. Corneal clouding and cancerous and non-cancerous growths on the eyes may occur. Approximately 20% develop neurological problems, e.g. deafness, impaired coordination, spasticity, and developmental delay. Neurological problems are progressive. Note that early diagnosis followed by strict and complete protection from sunlight with UV-resistant face masks, gloves, and UV-resistant film on windows can completely prevent all skin symptoms.

Genetically, XP is complex, with features in the majority of patients resulting from a defect in one of seven genes (*XPA*, *XPB*, ..., *XPG*) controlling NER. Approximately 20% of XP patients have normal levels of NER and are known as XP variant (XP-V) and have mutations in the gene encoding DNA polymerase eta, causing a reduced ability to replicate DNA after UV irradiation. Even though some patients with XP-V have a high incidence of tumours, many of them survive

to a relatively old age, compared with NER-defective patients with XP.

Genetic advice
Inheritance and recurrence risk
All are AR, with 1 in 4 risk to future pregnancies.

Variability and penetrance
All are 100% penetrant in the homozygous or compound heterozygous state, but especially for XP and CS, features are very variable.

In AT, approximately a third of patients have a milder presentation, with occasional patients still independently walking at age of 40+. The majority of adults with AT probably have a milder presentation.

Prenatal diagnosis
Usually possible by CVS at 11 weeks' gestation, but liaise carefully with an expert laboratory as these are highly specialized investigations. If the mutation is identified, PND can be done using standard molecular procedures.

Other family members
In FA, careful consideration should be given to testing apparently healthy siblings. Occasionally chromosome breakage tests demonstrate FA in an apparently healthy sibling with no congenital anomalies and normal FBC.

Natural history and management
Potential long-term complications
These are life-limiting disorders. See individual disease entries.

Surveillance
Refer to a specialist centre for advice.

Support groups: AT Society, http://www.atsociety. org.uk; Fanconi Hope, http://www.fanconi.org. uk; XP Family Support Group (USA), http://www. xpfamilysupportgroup.org.

Expert advisers: Malcolm Taylor, Professor of Cancer Genetics, Institute of Cancer and Genomic Sciences, University of Birmingham, Birmingham, UK and Alan R. Lehmann, Research Professor, Genome Damage and Stability Centre, School of Life Sciences, University of Sussex, Brighton, UK.

References

Ambrose M, Gatti RA. Pathogenesis of ataxia-telangiectasia: the next generation of ATM functions. *Blood* 2013; **121**: 4036–45.

Auerbach AD. Fanconi anemia and its diagnosis. *Mutat Res* 2009; **668**: 4–10.

Fassihi H, Sethi M, et al. Deep phenotyping of 89 xeroderma pigmentosum patients reveals unexpected heterogeneity dependent on the precise molecular defect. PNAS 2016; **113**: E1236–45.

Hoch NC, Hanzlikova H, et al. XRCC1 mutation is associated with PARP1 hyperactivationand cerebellar ataxia. *Nature* 2017; **541**: 87–91.

International Nijmegen Breakage Syndrome Study Group. Nijmegen breakage syndrome. *Arch Dis Child* 2000; **82**: 400–6.

Lehmann AR, McGibbon D, Stefanini, M. Xeroderma pigmentosum. *Orphanet J Rare Dis* 2011; **6**: 70.

Nakazawa Y, Sasaki K, Mitsutake N, et al. Mutations in UVSSA cause UV-sensitive syndrome and impair RNA polymerase IIo processing in transcription-coupled nucleotide-excision repair. *Nat Genet* 2012; **44**: 586–92.

Paucar M, Malmgren H, et al. Expanding the ataxia with oculomotor ataxia phenotype. *Neurol Genet* 2016; **2**: e49.

Duchenne and Becker muscular dystrophy (DMD and BMD)

Meryon disease.

Duchenne muscular dystrophy (DMD) affects >1 in 3000–4000 male births. It is the most common and severe form of childhood muscular dystrophy. The natural history of the disease is that it results in early loss of ambulation between the ages of 7 and 13 years (mean age 9 years) and death in the late teens or early twenties. DMD is an XLR disorder caused by mutations in the dystrophin gene (*DMD*) on Xp21. Dystrophin is a protein localized to the inner side of the plasma membrane that interacts with a group of proteins linking into the extracellular matrix and also on the intracellular surface with actin. Immunolabelling of a muscle biopsy from a boy with DMD using antibodies to dystrophin shows a complete or almost complete absence of the protein with secondary loss of the dystrophin-associated proteins in the muscle fibre membrane.

Sixty to 65% of DMD is caused by large out-of-frame deletions that remove one or more exons. At least a further 5% result from exon duplication. There are two hotspot regions for deletions: at the 5' end, affecting exons 3–8, and towards the 3' end, affecting exons 44–60, but deletions may occur anywhere in the gene. The remaining cases of DMD are mostly nonsense or frameshift mutations that cause chain termination. Loss of the 3' end of the gene, as in the contiguous gene deletion syndrome involving DAX1 and glycerol kinase, also results in DMD.

Approximately 30% of boys with DMD have a mild learning disability that is not progressive. They may present with developmental delay, especially with speech delay and late walking.

Lifespan is markedly reduced in DMD. For boys receiving specialist care and nocturnal ventilation, the mean age of death is around 30 years (Eagle *et al.* 2002). CM is almost universal but usually asymptomatic; surveillance is indicated as early detection may allow appropriate and timely treatment; severe symptomatic CM is usually a poor prognostic indicator. National Institute of Care and Health Excellence (NICE) process-accredited guidelines for the diagnosis and management of DMD are published and family guides to these guidelines are available (Bushby *et al.* 2010a, b; TREAT-NMD website).

Becker muscular dystrophy (BMD) is clinically similar to DMD, but milder, with a mean age of onset of 11 years. Loss of the ability to walk may occur late (e.g. 40s or 50s) and many individuals with BMD survive into middle age and beyond. Often cramps on exercise are the only problem initially, but some affected boys are late in learning to walk and are unable to run fast. Later in the teens and 20s, muscle weakness becomes evident, causing difficulty in rapid walking, running, and climbing stairs. It may become difficult to lift objects above waist height. Cognitive impairment is not a major feature of BMD. BMD is caused by 'in-frame' mutations in dystrophin that result in reduced dystrophin being produced. Immunolabelling of muscle biopsy from a man with BMD shows a reduction in the intensity of staining which may vary within and between fibres.

Some patients present with an *intermediate dystrophin phenotype*, i.e. a clinical picture intermediate between those of DMD and BMD. See Figure 3.8 for an illustration of the predominant muscle weaknesses in DMD and BMD.

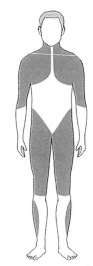

Figure 3.8 Distribution of predominant muscle weakness in Duchenne and Becker muscular dystrophy.
Reproduced from *The BMJ*, Alan E H Emery, The muscular dystrophies, volume 317, p. 992, copyright 1998, with permission from BMJ Publishing Group Ltd.

Manifesting female carriers

In Hoogerwaard *et al.*'s (1999a) survey of 129 carriers of muscular dystrophy, 75% had myalgia/cramps and 17% had mild/moderate muscle weakness on testing (but only ~10% were aware of symptoms prior to testing). None had severe weakness, and severe disabling muscle weakness among carriers is probably rare but can be seen and may be as severe as in boys. Onset of symptoms in this study did not occur at <16 years and the average age of onset was 33 years. Seventy per cent of women who complained of myalgia, cramps, or muscle weakness were weak on testing. Weakness was primarily proximal and asymmetric, and in 40% only the shoulder girdle or upper arm was affected. Severe disabling muscle weakness among carriers is probably rare but can occur. Carriers of BMD are less frequently and less severely affected than carriers of DMD. Serum CK was raised in 53% of carriers of DMD and 30% of carriers of BMD. Mean serum CK was 306 U/l (range 48–1860). Surprisingly, there was no significant difference in mean CK activity between carriers with and carriers without muscle weakness. IHC of muscle biopsy from a manifesting DMD carrier using labelled antibodies shows some reduction in the intensity of staining which varies both between and within fibres.

- Approximately 20% of carriers have evidence of cardiac involvement on investigation.
- Females with early-onset or severe muscle weakness should have a karyotype (X-autosome translocations, AIS, etc.).

Clinical approach

History: key points

- Detailed three-generation family tree, with careful enquiry for other affected males (e.g. maternal brother,

uncles, and great-uncles). Extend the family tree as far as possible on the affected side of the family.
- Detailed developmental history. Boys with DMD usually have mild delay of motor milestones, e.g. late walking and tiptoe and unsteady gait.
- Difficulty rising from the floor (leading to Gower's manoeuvre where the child pushes up on his thighs with his hands to get up off the floor) and difficulties going upstairs (e.g. needing to get both feet on to the step before tackling the next step). Ungainly and slow running are common in the first 2–3 years of life. Boys with DMD can rarely jump with both feet together.

Examination: key points
- Observe the child's gait. You may need more space to observe this than is available in the consulting room. Abnormalities of gait become much more evident when a child tries to hurry.
- Boys with DMD never achieve a normal run; very few of them ever learn to jump with both feet together.
- Proximal limb weakness.
- Calf hypertrophy occurs in most children in the early phase of the disease.

Investigations
- CK: usually several 1000s. Children with DMD invariably have serum or plasma levels >10 times normal. See 'Predictive testing' below.
- DNA for dystrophin deletion/duplication analysis and sequencing.
- Muscle biopsy may be a useful adjunct to the diagnostic process if no dystrophin mutation is identified and a clinical picture indicative of a dystrophic process meriting invasive diagnostic investigations. Examination of dystrophin in the muscle biopsy gives a quantitative idea of the effect of the mutations and can provide further prognostic information, though it needs to be interpreted in the context of the clinical and genetic findings. Muscle biopsy may also give evidence for one of the conditions that may be considered in the differential diagnosis such as some forms of AR LGMD.
- Echo and ECG at diagnosis.

Other diagnoses/conditions to consider
See 'Limb–girdle muscular dystrophies' in Chapter 3, 'Common consultations', p. 476.

Genetic advice
Inheritance and recurrence risk
XLR. In any pregnancy of a carrier female, there are four possible outcomes, each equally likely: normal male; normal female; affected male; carrier female. Carrier rate is similar across different ethnic groups.

Variability and penetrance
Penetrance is complete in males inheriting a pathogenic dystrophin mutation. A small percentage of women are manifesting carriers with raised CK and a variable degree of muscle weakness (see above).

Prenatal diagnosis
- Available to carriers of a known dystrophin mutation by CVS at 11 weeks' gestation.
- Available to mothers of an apparently *de novo* Duchenne mutation because of the significant risk arising from germline mosaicism (see below).

- Available in families where a mutation has not been found, but where a 'high-risk X' can be identified by linkage studies, though this option should be needed much less frequently due to the wider availability of direct mutation testing in suspected carriers. If the pregnancy is found to carry the high-risk X and a TOP is requested, consider dystrophin staining of fetal muscle tissue to gain additional information for future pregnancies.
- The first step is fetal sexing (e.g. amelogenin probe). Molecular genetic analysis is usually only pursued if the pregnancy is male. Fetal sexing using ffDNA in maternal serum late in the first trimester is usually the first step in PND. See 'Non-invasive prenatal diagnosis/testing (NIPD/T)' in Chapter 6, 'Pregnancy and fertility', p. 764.
- PGD may be available for those with a familial causative mutation where DNA from an affected relative or a proven carrier is available in order to identify the high-risk haplotype in the dystrophin gene. PGD with selection of female pregnancies may also be a possibility for carriers in a family where the causative mutation is unknown (but beware that one reason for an elusive mutation is wrong diagnosis).
- Patients with a known dystrophin mutation should be given information about their relevant national patient registry (see TREAT-NMD website) which facilitates access to up-to-date information and access to trials and other clinical studies.
- Access to patient support groups should be provided at diagnosis.

Predictive testing
- Newborn males. Women at risk of being carriers who decline prenatal testing and who give birth to a son may wish their infant son to be tested before embarking on another pregnancy. CK is often elevated in cord blood or in blood samples taken within the first week after delivery. CK may also be elevated following IM injections (e.g. infant immunizations). Affected males, even as neonates, will usually have a CK of several thousands. A value in the normal range excludes DMD. CK levels in cord blood are fine if they are very high or in the normal range; CK values in the hundreds or just outwith the normal range should be repeated at 6 weeks of age. If arranging CK estimation in cord blood, ensure that the family understands that if the result is equivocal, they may need to wait until the boy is 6 weeks old for a repeat test; otherwise defer testing until the infant is 6 weeks old.
- BMD. CK levels in BMD can be as high as in DMD but usually are not. CK levels in BMD fall with disease progression, so you may get almost normal levels in very elderly people. It is difficult to be dogmatic about levels in early infancy.

Other family members—carrier testing and assessment of risk of carrier status in female relatives
Assemble the maximum information available using:
- a family tree—include accurate information about unaffected males and symptomatic enquiry about muscle weakness, muscle cramps, CM, etc. in 'at-risk' females;
- confirmation of diagnosis in the proband (dystrophin mutation analysis).

MUTATION KNOWN. If the mutation in the affected individual is known, determination of the carrier status is straightforward by direct analysis of the consultand's DNA for the known dystrophin mutation in the family—but note risks arising from germline mosaicism. The precise incidence of germline mosaicism in DMD is not clear. The following is based on an estimated risk.

- For the mother of an affected boy with a known mutation that is not present in the mother's genomic DNA, there is a suggested 1 in 5 (20%) risk to a future son who inherits the same X chromosome as his affected brother (i.e. there is an overall 5% risk to future pregnancies).
- In families with a single affected boy with a known mutation, not present in his mother's genomic DNA, it is important that sisters of the affected boy are offered mutation-based carrier testing. Sisters inheriting the same maternal X as the affected boy will have a 20% risk of being carriers as a result of maternal germline mosaicism.

MUTATION UNKNOWN. If the mutation in the affected individual is unknown, assessment of carrier status in female relatives is more complex.

- Families with a single affected male—unknown mutation.
  (1) Identify the closest female relative from whom both the consultand and proband are descended—this is the 'dummy consultand'.
  (2) Use Bayes's theorem to calculate the risk that the 'dummy consultand' is a carrier for DMD/BMD—include the mother of the affected boy in the risk calculation (see worked examples in 'Appendix', p. 807); include conditional information about unaffected sons of the 'dummy consultand', the mother of the affected boy, the mother of the consultand, and the consultand herself.
  (3) Use linkage, where possible, to determine whether or not the consultand is carrying the 'high-risk X'. Samples from maternal grandparents and from unaffected males may be helpful here.
  (4) Use serial CKs from the consultand as conditional information in the Bayes analysis.
- Families with more than one affected male—unknown mutation.
  (1) If the affected males are in different generations, all intervening female relatives are obligate carriers (e.g. a woman with an affected maternal uncle and an affected son is an obligate carrier, as is her mother, and the maternal grandmother has a two-thirds chance of being a carrier).
  (2) As above, identify the closest female relative from whom both the consultand and the nearest affected male relative are descended—the 'dummy consultand'.
  (3) Use Bayes's theorem to derive the carrier risk, unless this is immediately apparent, i.e. the daughter of an obligate carrier will have a 50% carrier risk (unless she has had unaffected male pregnancies which can be included as conditional information and will lower her risk).
  (4) Use linkage, where possible, to determine whether or not the consultand is carrying the 'high-risk X'. Samples from maternal grandparents and from unaffected males may be helpful here.

(5) Use three serial CKs from the consultand as conditional information in the Bayes analysis.

Natural history and management

Gene therapy remains a hope for the future. Possibilities currently under development include upregulation of utrophin and targeted exon skipping to restore the reading frame. Meanwhile, comprehensive guidelines exist for the management of the potential complications of DMD (Bushby *et al.* 2010a, b). Moderate-quality evidence from RCTs indicates that corticosteroid therapy in DMD improves muscle strength and function in the short term (12 months), and strength up to 2 years. On the basis of the evidence available for strength and function outcomes, our confidence in the effect estimate for the efficacy of a 0.75-mg/kg/day dose of prednisone or above is fairly secure. There is no evidence other than from non-randomized trials to establish the effect of corticosteroids on prolongation of walking. In the short term, adverse effects were significantly more common with corticosteroids than placebo, but not clinically severe. A weekend-only prednisone regimen is as effective as daily prednisone in the short term (12 months), according to low-to-moderate-quality evidence from a single trial, with no clear difference in BMI (low-quality evidence) (Matthews *et al.* 2016). There are several disease-modifying trials at present recruiting and evaluating, such as exon skipping therapies. Please consult locally for up to date information.

Potential long-term complications in DMD

- Loss of ambulation. Muscle weakness is progressive and children with DMD will lose ambulation between 7 and 13 years (mean age 9 years) and become wheelchair-dependent. This is due to a combination of weakness and contractures affecting the ankles, knees, and hips. Ankle splints to prevent contracture of the tendo-achilles are important in maintaining ambulation for as long as possible. Steroid treatment is well documented to prolong the period of independent ambulation and prevent complications such as scoliosis. It also has a beneficial effect on forced vital capacity (FVC) and delays the requirement for nocturnal ventilation. As with any group of patients on long-term steroids, management of the side effects of the drugs is very important and is described in the care guidelines.
- Scoliosis. Affected children confined to a wheelchair are at high risk of developing a scoliosis. More than 90% of boys with DMD will eventually develop a significant scoliosis. Bracing may reduce the rate of progression of the scoliosis, but often major surgery is required to stop the progression. Surgery is high-risk and should be undertaken in specialist centres that have the facility to undertake a comprehensive cardiac assessment prior to intervention. Corticosteroid use reduces the risk of scoliosis and has dramatically reduced the rate of surgery.
- Nocturnal hypoventilation. Respiratory muscles are also affected and this becomes a clinical problem usually in the late teens. Respiratory failure causing nocturnal hypoventilation is common at this age and can be treated with night-time facial or nasal mask ventilation. Without treatment, death often ensues within a few months. Proactive surveillance and management for respiratory complications are described in the care guidelines.

- Cardiac problems. Because of their immobility, patients with DMD rarely develop signs of cardiac failure; however, on investigation, signs of CM are almost universal. Patients are at a significantly increased risk of arrhythmia and other cardiac problems perioperatively. Guidelines exist for cardiovascular investigations and management (see below) (Bushby et al. 2003; 2010a, b).
- Cognitive impairment may be a significant part of the condition and may particularly have an effect on verbal, rather than performance, IQ. This deficit is non-progressive. There is a frequent association with behavioural problems and autism spectrum disorder.

Potential long-term complications in BMD
- Impaired mobility. Some men with BMD retain ambulation throughout their lives, but others will become dependent on aids (sticks/walking frames) and eventually become wheelchair-dependent.
- Cardiac complications (e.g. DCM) are a major cause of morbidity and mortality in BMD. BMD patients should be under regular review by a cardiologist, with regular surveillance from their teens onwards (annual ECG and echo in the first instance). As for DMD, BMD patients are at increased risk perioperatively and an anaesthetist should always be made aware of the diagnosis. Guidelines exist for cardiovascular investigations and management (see below) (Bushby et al. 2003).

Potential long-term complications in carriers for DMD or BMD
There is unequivocal evidence that ~10% of female carriers of dystrophin mutations (DMD or BMD) may develop overt cardiac failure in later life, even in the absence of skeletal muscle involvement (Bushby et al. 2003; Hoogerwaard et al. 1999b).

Surveillance
Access to a neuromuscular centre is crucial to provide coordination of the many specialized areas of care needed by patients with DMD to maintain optimum function and quality of life and to have access to novel therapies and trials. One model of care is for the local community paediatric team to share care with a specialist centre with expertise in paediatric neuromuscular disorders.
- DMD. Cardiac investigations (echo and ECG) every 2 years to age of 10 years and annually thereafter. Echo and ECG should be repeated before any surgery. Respiratory surveillance with FVC and overnight oximetry, as per guidelines.
- BMD. Cardiac investigations (echo and ECG) every 5 years.
- Carriers. All carriers of DMD or BMD should have an echo and ECG at diagnosis or after the age of 16 years

and at least every 5 years thereafter. Carriers manifesting severe skeletal muscle symptoms or cardiac symptoms require more frequent investigation (Bushby et al. 2003).

Support groups: Muscular Dystrophy UK, http://www.musculardystrophyuk.org; Duchenne Family Support Group, http://dfsg.org.uk; Parent Project Muscular dystrophy, http://www.parentprojectmd.org.

Expert adviser: Katie Bushby, Act. Res. Chair of Neuromuscular Genetics, Institute of Genetic Medicine, Newcastle University, Newcastle, UK.

References
Abbs S, Tuffery-Giraud S, Bakker E, Ferlini A, Sejersen T, Mueller CR. Best practice guidelines on molecular diagnostics in Duchenne/Becker muscular dystrophies. *Neuromuscul Disord* 2010; **20**: 422–7.

Bundey S. Calculation of genetic risks in Duchenne muscular dystrophy by geneticists in the United Kingdom. *J Med Genet* 1978; **15**: 249–53.

Bushby K, Finkel R, Birnkrant DJ, et al. Diagnosis and management of Duchenne muscular dystrophy, part 1: diagnosis, and pharmacological and psychosocial management. *Lancet Neurol* 2010a; **9**: 77–93.

Bushby K, Finkel R, Birnkrant DJ, et al. Diagnosis and management of Duchenne muscular dystrophy, part 2: implementation of multidisciplinary care. *Lancet Neurol* 2010b; **9**: 177–89.

Bushby K, Muntoni F, Bourke JP. 107th ENMC International Workshop: the management of cardiac involvement in muscular dystrophy and myotonic dystrophy. 7th–9th June 2002, Naarden, the Netherlands. *Neuromuscul Disord* 2003; **13**: 166–72.

Connolly AM, Schierbecker J, Renna R, Florence J. High dose weekly oral prednisone improves strength in boys with Duchenne muscular dystrophy. *Neuromuscul Disord* 2002; **12**: 917–25.

Eagle M, Baudouin SV, Chandler C, Giddings DR, Bullock R, Bushby K. Survival in Duchenne muscular dystrophy: improvements in life expectancy since 1967 and the impact of home nocturnal ventilation. *Neuromuscul Disord* 2002; **12**: 926–9.

Emery AE. The muscular dystrophies. *BMJ* 1998; **317**: 991–5.

Hoogerwaard EM, Bakker E, Ippel PF, et al. Signs and symptoms of Duchenne muscular dystrophy and Becker muscular dystrophy among carriers in the Netherlands: a cohort study. *Lancet* 1999a; **353**: 2116–19.

Hoogerwaard EM, van der Wouw PA, Wilde AA, et al. Cardiac involvement in carriers of Duchenne and Becker muscular dystrophy. *Neuromuscul Disord* 1999b; **9**: 347–51.

Matthews E, Brassington R, Kuntzer T, Jichi F, Manzur AY. Corticosteroids for the treatment of Duchenne muscular dystrophy. *Cochrane Database Syst Rev* 2016; **5**: CD003725.

TREAT-NMD Neuromuscular Network. http://www.treat-nmd.eu/care/dmd/diagnosis-management-DMD.

Wong BL, Christopher C. Corticosteroids in Duchenne muscular dystrophy: a reappraisal. *J Child Neurol* 2002; **17**: 183–90.

Young ID. *Introduction to risk calculation in genetic counselling*, 2nd edn. Oxford University Press, Oxford 1999.

Ehlers–Danlos syndrome (EDS)

All forms of EDS cause clinical problems, such as skin fragility, unsightly bruising and scarring, musculoskeletal discomfort, and, in some, a susceptibility to osteoarthritis (see Tables 3.12 and 3.13). Approximately 1/5000 people are affected by EDS. The hypermobility type of EDS is far more prevalent than all the other forms of EDS combined, many of which are very rare. A diagnostic checklist for hEDS can be downloaded from www.ehlers-danlos.com/heds-diagnostic-checklist.

Vascular EDS

AD due to mutations in COL3A1, encoding type III collagen. Affected individuals are prone to arterial rupture, intestinal perforation (usually colon), and uterine rupture.

Table 3.12 The main features of EDS (numbers in brackets show 2017 International classification—see Table 3.13). Please note that the major and minor criteria have now been revised for some types (see Malfait 2017 for further details)

Type	Major criteria	Minor criteria	Inheritance	Protein	Gene
Classical cEDS (1)	• Skin hyperextensibility • Widened atrophic scarring • Joint hypermobility	• Easy bruising • Smooth and velvety skin • Molluscoid pseudotumours • Subcutaneous spheroids • Muscular hypotonia • Surgical complications • Positive family history	AD	Type V procollagen (~90%) Type I collagen	COL5A1 COL5A2 COL1A1 C.934C>T
Hypermobility hEDS (5)	• Generalized joint hypermobility • Mild skin involvement	• Recurrent joint dislocations • Chronic joint pain • Positive family history	AD		
Vascular vEDS (4)	• Excessive bruising • Thin, translucent skin • Arterial/intestinal/uterine fragility or rupture • Characteristic facial appearance	• Acrogeria • Early-onset varicose veins • Hypermobility of small joints • Tendon and muscle rupture • Arteriovenous or carotid-cavernous sinus fistula • Pneumo-(haemo-)thorax • Positive family history, sudden death in close relative(s)	AD	Type III procollagen Rare Type I collagen	COL3A1 COL1A1 (see Table 3.13)
Kyphoscoliotic kEDS (8)	• Floppy baby (severe neonatal muscular hypotonia) • Congenital or early kyphoscoliosis • Premature rupture of fetal membranes • Joint dislocations	• Tissue fragility, including atrophic scars • Easy bruising • Osteopenia • Myopathy • Hearing loss • Scleral fragility and rupture of the globe (PLOD1)	AR	Type VIA: lysyl hydroxylase A FKBP22	PLOD1 FKBP14
Musculo-contractural mcEDS (11)	• Contractures, e.g. adducted thumbs, club foot • Joint and skin laxity • Wrinkled palms • Atrophic scarring	• Muscular hypotonia • Thin skin • Blue sclerae • Myopia • Retinal detachment	AR	D4ST1 DSE	CHST14 DSE
Arthrochalasia aEDS (6)	• Severe generalized joint hypermobility with recurrent subluxations • Congenital bilateral hip dislocation	• Skin hyperextensibility • Tissue fragility, including atrophic scars • Easy bruising • Muscular hypotonia • Kyphoscoliosis • Mild osteopenia	AD	Type 1 procollagen	COL1A1 COL1A2

Table 3.12 Continued

Type	Major criteria	Minor criteria	Inheritance	Protein	Gene
Dermatosparaxis dEDS (7)	• Severe skin fragility • Sagging, redundant skin • Excessive bruising	• Soft, doughy skin texture • Premature rupture of membranes • Large herniae	AR	Procollagen-N-proteinase	ADAMTS-2
EDS with pre-tibial scarring and periodontal disease pEDS (13)	• Pre-tibial scarring • Periodontal disease with premature loss of secondary dentition	• Easy bruising • Mild joint hypermobility	AD	C1r C1s	C1R C1S
EDS with short stature and limb anomalies spEDS (10)	• Short stature • Limb anomalies • Radioulnar synostosis	• Wrinkled palms and soles	AR	β4GalT7	B4GALT7
Progeroid type spEDS (10)	• Premature aged appearance • Club feet • Cutis laxa	• Blue sclerae • Kyphoscoliosis with platyspondyly	AR	β3GalT6	B3GALT6
Brittle cornea syndrome (9)	• Brittle cornea • Scleral fragility and rupture of the globe • Moderate joint laxity • Severe myopia (e.g. −12D)	• Blue sclerae • Osteopenia	AR	ZNF469 PRDM5	ZNF469 PRDM5
Spondylodysplastic spEDS (10)	• Short stature • Skeletal dysplasia with spinal involvement • Abnormal teeth	• Lax skin • Joint laxity	AR	ZIP13 (zinc transporter)	SLC39A13

Adapted with permission from Beighton *et al.*, Ehlers-Danlos syndromes: Revised nosology, Villefranche, 1997, *American Journal of Medical Genetics Part A*, Volume 77, Issue 1, pp. 31–37, Copyright © 1998 John Wiley and Sons.

Table 3.13 Clinical classification of the Ehlers–Danlos syndromes, inheritance pattern, and genetic basis

	Clinical EDS subtype	Abbreviation	IP	Genetic basis	Protein
1	Classical EDS	cEDS	AD	Major: COL5A1, COL5A1	Type V collagen
				Rare: COL1A1	Type I collagen
				c.934C>T, p.(Arg312Cys)	
2	Classical-like EDS	clEDS	AR	TNXB	Tenascin XB
3	Cardiac-valvular	cvEDS	AR	COL1A2 (biallelic mutations that lead to COL1A2 NMD and absence of pro α2(I) collagen chains)	Type I collagen
4	Vascular EDS	vEDS	AD	Major: COL3A1	Type III collagen
				Rare: COL1A1	Type I collagen
				c.934C>T, p.(Arg312Cys)	
				c.1720C>T, p.(Arg574Cys)	
				c.3227C>T, p.(Arg1093Cys)	
5	Hypermobile EDS	hEDS	AD	Unknown	Unknown
6	Arthrochalasia EDS	aEDS	AD	COL1A1, COL1A2	Type I collagen
7	Dermatosparaxis EDS	dEDS	AR	ADAMTS2	ADAMTS-2
8	Kyphoscoliotic EDS	kEDS	AR	PLOD1	LH1
				FKBP14	FKBP22
9	Brittle Cornea syndrome	BCS	AR	ZNF469	ZNF469
				PRDM5	PRDM5

(Continued)

Table 3.13 Continued

	Clinical EDS subtype	Abbreviation	IP	Genetic basis	Protein
10	Spondylodysplastic EDS	spEDS	AR	B4GALT7	β4GalT7
				B3GALT6	β3GalT6
				SLC39A13	ZIP13
11	Musculocontractural EDS	mcEDS	AR	CHST14	D4ST1
				DSE	DSE
12	Myopathic EDS	mEDS	AD or AR	COL12A1	Type XII collagen
13	Periodontal EDS	pEDS	AD	C1R	C1r
				C1S	C1s

IP, inheritance pattern; AD, autosomal dominant; AR, autosomal recessive, NMD, nonsense-mediated mRNA decay.

Reproduced from F Malfait *et al.*, The 2017 International Classification of the Ehlers–Danlos Syndromes, *American Journal of Medical Genetics Part C*, 175, 1, pp. 8–26, copyright 2017, Wiley.

Complications are rare in infancy but occur in up to 25% before 20 years, and 80% before 40 years. Median life expectancy is 51 years, with arterial rupture accounting for most deaths (Pepin *et al.* 2014). Arterial repairs are technically challenging because the vessels are extremely friable.

Diagnosis is based on specific facial features, thin translucent skin, propensity to bleeding (bruising), and rupture of vessels. There may be increased joint mobility of the hands. Diagnosis is confirmed by finding abnormalities in type III collagen and/or a mutation in *COL3A1*. Although arterial tears are the hallmarks of vascular EDS, 25% of all complications affect the GI tract.

In Pepin *et al.*'s (2000) study, most deaths resulted from arterial dissection or rupture. Approximately 80% of these deaths involved thoracic or abdominal vessels and <10% resulted from intracranial haemorrhage. Most of the bowel complications affected the colon, especially the sigmoid. Perforation of the small bowel and gastric perforation were uncommon. Vascular EDS should be suspected in any young person presenting with an unexplained arterial rupture or visceral rupture, carotid dissection, or colonic perforation.

- Molecular pathogenesis. The majority of mutations in *COL3A1* have a 'dominant-negative' effect. Patients who are heterozygous for mutations in *COL3A1* that do not cause premature chain termination produce about equal amounts of normal and abnormal type III procollagen polypeptides. These interact to form the homotripolymer type III procollagen protein. However, only $(1/2 \times 1/2 \times 1/2)$, i.e. 1/8 of the proteins, will contain three normal polypeptides, whereas the other 7/8 will contain at least one mutant polypeptide and will function abnormally.

Clinical approach

History: key points

- Three-generation family tree, with specific enquiry regarding joint hypermobility, easy bruising, or abnormal scarring. (For vascular EDS, enquire about arterial or intestinal rupture.)
- Enquire about dislocation/subluxation of joints (especially shoulders, patellae, temporomandibular joints, and digits).

Examination: key points

- Assess the Beighton score (see 'Hypermobile joints' in Chapter 2, 'Clinical approach', p. 176).
- Ask the patient whether they have any 'party tricks' to demonstrate their joint hypermobility.

- Enquire about symptoms relating to dysautonomia (postural hypotension, GI motility disorder, etc.), particularly prevalent in the hypermobility type.
- Assess the skin. Is it soft and velvety? Is it hyperextensible (pick up a small fold of skin over the dorsal forearm and gently draw it away from the underlying muscle)? Extension beyond 1.5 cm at this site is considered significant. Extension of 3 cm is considered significant at elbows, knees or neck.
- Examine the skin over the elbows and knees for abnormal scarring (e.g. thin atrophic ('cigarette paper' scars); also examine any scars from surgery for abnormal widening and thinning.
- Examine for bruising.

Investigations

- Consider DNA for mutation analysis in one family member (not feasible in families with hypermobile EDS). Molecular testing is available for classical (I, II) vascular (IV), kyphoscoliosis (VI), and arthrochalasia (VII) types and tenascin-X deficiency.
- Consider echo for MVP and aortic root diameter in patients with classical EDS, vascular EDS, and kyphoscoliotic EDS.
- Consider MRI/MRA of the thoracic and abdominal aorta and iliac arteries in individuals with vascular EDS. (Endovascular repair may be a helpful strategy in vascular EDS patients with significant aortic dilatation.)
- Consider skin biopsy for EM for ultrastructural analysis and for fibroblast culture for collagen studies—this is very much a second-line investigation due to the increased role of genetic testing in diagnosis.

Other diagnoses/conditions to consider

Joint hypermobility spectrum disorders

This term is sometimes used synonymously with EDS, hypermobility type. See 'Hypermobile joints' in Chapter 2, 'Clinical approach', p. 176. (Castori 2017).

Cutis laxa

Inherited cutis laxa is a connective tissue disorder characterized by loose skin and variable internal organ involvement, resulting from paucity of elastic fibres. Developmental delay may be present. Mutations in the elastin gene have been reported in three families with AD inheritance, and a family with AR cutis laxa was recently reported to have a homozygous missense mutation in the fibulin-5 (*FBLN5*) gene. Markova *et al.* (2003) reported a patient with a heterozygous tandem duplication within *FBLN5*. At least 10 genes have now been identified in cutis laxa.

Marfan's syndrome (MFS)
See 'Marfan's syndrome' in Chapter 3, 'Common consultations', p. 484.

Genetic advice
Inheritance and recurrence risk
Most are AD (see Table 3.12).

Variability and penetrance
Some inter- and intrafamilial variability is seen. Significant variability is uncommon, but mild phenotypic variability is commonly seen.

Prenatal diagnosis
Technically possible if the familial mutation is known, but rarely indicated (with the possible exception of vascular EDS).

Predictive testing
Recent evidence suggests beta-blockade can reduce catastrophic consequences in vascular EDS patients (Ong et al. 2010). Knowledge of the diagnosis may influence the management of surgery, pregnancy, and major complications. Patients should avoid any activity that leads to a sudden increase in BP.

Natural history and management
Potential long-term complications
- Pregnancy. There is an increased risk for preterm delivery in fetuses affected by classical EDS. Overall, post-partum haemorrhage (PPH) and complicated perineal wounds are more common in women with EDS than without (19% versus 7% and 8% versus <1%, respectively).

Women with vascular EDS have a risk of uterine rupture (as well as arterial and bowel rupture). In Pepin et al.'s (2000) study, 81 women with EDS-vascular type had a total of 183 pregnancies, with 167 deliveries of live-born infants at term, three stillbirths, ten spontaneous abortions, and three voluntary terminations. Twelve women died during the peripartum period or within 2 weeks after delivery (five of uterine rupture during labour, two of vessel rupture at delivery, and five in the post-partum period after vessel rupture). Although several women died of uterine rupture at term, it is uncertain whether the use of elective LSCS would decrease mortality (uterine rupture may occur before the onset of labour).

- Early arthritis. Joint hypermobility can predispose to premature onset of osteoarthritis in early or mid-adult life. Referral to a management service for high-risk pregnancies is advised (ideally for counselling pre-pregnancy).
- Aortic root dilatation although present is rarely clinically significant. In Wenstrup et al.'s (2002) study of 71 individuals with EDS, 14/42 (33%) individuals with classical EDS and 6/29 (20%) with hypermobile EDS had aortic root dilatation. The risk of aortic root rupture appears to be significantly less than in MFS, but nevertheless, occasional cases have been reported in both classical and hypermobile types.

Support groups: The Ehlers–Danlos Society, http://ehlers-danlos.com; Ehlers–Danlos Support UK, http://www.ehlers-danlos.org.

Expert adviser: Nigel P. Burrows, Consultant Dermatologist, Addenbrooke's Hospital, Cambridge University Hospitals NHS Foundation Trust, Cambridge, UK.

References
Baumann M, Giunta C, Krabichler B, et al. Mutations in *FKBP14* cause a variant of Ehlers–Danlos syndrome with progressive kyphoscoliosis, myopathy, and hearing loss. *Am J Hum Genet* 2012; **90**: 201–16.

Beighton P, De Paepe A, Steinmann B, Tsipouras P, Wenstrup RJ. Ehlers–Danlos syndromes: revised nosology, Villefranche 1997. Ehlers–Danlos National Foundation (USA) and Ehlers–Danlos Support Group (UK). *Am J Med Genet* 1998; **77**: 31–7.

Bowen JM, Sobey GT, Burrows NP, et al. Ehlers Danlos syndrome classical type. *Am J Med Genet* C 2017; **175**: 27–39.

Castori M, Tinkle B, et al. A framework for the clarification of joint hypermobility and related disorders. *Am J Med Genet* 2017; **175C**: 148–57.

Germain DP. Clinical and genetic features of vascular Ehlers–Danlos syndrome. *Ann Vasc Surg* 2002; **16**: 391–7.

Lind J, Wallenburg HC. Pregnancy and the Ehlers–Danlos syndrome: a retrospective study in a Dutch population. *Acta Obstet Gynecol Scand* 2002; **81**: 293–300.

Malfait F, Coucke P, Symoens S, Loeys B, Nuytinck L, De Paepe A. The molecular basis of classic Ehlers–Danlos syndrome: a comprehensive study of biochemical and molecular findings in 48 unrelated patients. *Hum Mutat* 2005; **25**: 28–37.

Malfait F, Francomano C, Byers P, et al. The 2017 international classification of the Ehlers-Danlos syndromes. *Am J Med Genet* 2017; **175**: 8–26.

Markova D, Zou Y, Ringpfeil F, et al. Genetic heterogeneity of cutis laxa: a heterozygous tandem duplication within the fibulin-5 (*FBLN5*) gene. *Am J Hum Genet* 2003; **72**: 998–1004.

Mohamed M, Voet M, Gardeitchik T, Morava E. Cutis laxa. *Adv Exp Med Biol* 2014; **802**: 161–84.

Ong KT, Perdu J, De Backer J, et al. Effect of celiprolol on prevention of cardiovascular events in vascular Ehlers–Danlos syndrome: a prospective randomised, open, blinded-endpoints trial. *Lancet* 2010; **376**: 1476–84.

Pepin MG, Schwarze U, Rice KM, Liu M, Leistritz D, Byers PH. Survival is affected by mutation type and molecular mechanism in vascular Ehlers–Danlos syndrome (EDS type IV). *Genet Med* 2014; **16**: 881–8.

Pepin M, Schwarze U, Superti-Furga A, Byers PH. Clinical and genetic features of Ehlers–Danlos syndrome type IV, the vascular type. *N Engl J Med* 2000; **342**: 673–80.

Pyeritz RE. Ehlers–Danlos syndrome [editorial]. *N Engl J Med* 2000; **342**: 730–2.

Schalkwijk J, Zweers MC, Steijlen PM, et al. A recessive form of the Ehlers–Danlos syndrome caused by tenascin-X deficiency. *N Engl J Med* 2001; **345**: 1167–75.

Symoens S, Syx D, Malfait F, et al. Comprehensive molecular analysis demonstrate type V collagen mutations in over 90% of patients with classical EDS and allows to refine diagnostic criteria. *Hum Mutat* 2012; **33**: 1485–93.

Wenstrup RJ, Hoechstetter LB. The Ehlers–Danlos syndromes. In: SB Cassidy, JE Allanson (eds.). *Management of genetic syndromes*, pp. 131–49. Wiley-Liss, New York, 2001.

Wenstrup RJ, Meyer RA, Lyle JS, et al. Prevalence of aortic root dilation in the Ehlers–Danlos syndrome. *Genet Med* 2002; **4**: 112–17.

Epilepsy in infants and children

For the classification and terminology of epilepsies, see Figure 3.11 in 'Epilepsy in adults', in Chapter 3, 'Common consultations', p. 416, from the ILAE Proposal for Revised Terminology for Organization of Seizures and Epilepsies 2010.

These conditions are often difficult to control and associated with developmental delay, and families ask for genetic advice about recurrence risk and PND.

The conditions discussed in this section are primarily monogenic causes of infantile epilepsy in infants with a structurally normal brain. See 'Lissencephaly, polymicrogia, and neuronal migration disorders' in Chapter 2, 'Clinical approach', p. 216 for the evaluation of infants with structural brain anomalies. If there is associated developmental delay/ID, see 'Seizures with developmental delay/intellectual disability' in Chapter 2, 'Clinical approach', p. 308.

Large multicentre reviews of infants and children with epilepsy have established a framework for genetic analysis and shown that severe early-onset epilepsy can be caused by mutation in the same genes (predominantly channelopathies) that were previously considered to cause 'benign' familial seizures. As there is considerable phenotypic and genetic overlap between the epilepsy syndromes, there is diagnostic utility in a gene panel approach.

Ion channels provide the basis for the regulation of excitability in the CNS, and many of the childhood epilepsies with a known molecular basis are channelopathies. Ion channel mutations (*SCN1A, SCN2A, SCN8A, KCNQ2, KCNT1*, etc.) are a common cause of rare monogenic idiopathic epilepsies, but a rare cause of common epilepsies. In addition to channelopathies, there are a number of molecular mechanisms and a large number of genes contributing to childhood epilepsy. e.g. *CDKL5, MECP2, PCDH19* (epilepsy limited to females), *STXBP1* (see Figure 3.9). Using a gene panel approach, the diagnostic rate is highest in those with onset of seizures at <2 months at ~40% (Trump *et al.* 2016). Figure 3.10 illustrates the genetic heterogeneity of infantile and early-childhood epilepsies.

Clinical approach

History: key points

- Three-generation family history for epilepsy, including febrile convulsions (may indicate a dominant, recessive, or XL pattern of inheritance).
- Parental consanguinity and previous affected sibling; increases the probability of a recessive disorder.
- Pregnancy (congenital infections, severe bleeding, hypoxia, teratogenic drugs, and alcohol by disturbance to brain development). Abnormal movements *in utero*, e.g. recurrent 'hiccuping'.
- Perinatal period: birth trauma, neonatal seizures, blistering rash (IP).
- OFC at birth and subsequent brain growth.
- Onset of seizures, frequency and type of seizure. Medication. Any associated movement disorder, e.g. dyskinesia, dystonia, ataxia.
- Developmental progress before and since the onset of seizures. Try and establish if there is any evidence of developmental regression. This assessment is problematic in children with poorly controlled seizures on high doses of antiepileptic drugs (pseudoregression).

Examination: key points

- OFC; beware OFC falling down the centiles.
- Neurological signs (pyramidal features, ataxia).
- Eyes and fundus.
- Dysmorphic features/other system involvement may indicate a possible syndromic cause.
- Teeth for dental hypoplasia or enamel hypoplasia.
- Neurocutaneous signs, Woods light examination.

Investigations

- Review biochemical and metabolic investigations. See 'Neonatal encephalopathy and intractable seizures', p. 246 and 'Seizures with developmental delay/intellectual disability', p. 308 in Chapter 2, 'Clinical approach'.
- Brain MRI scan (with epilepsy protocol to identify subtle cortical dysplasias) to exclude structural malformation.
- EEG for specific diagnostic changes. Consider if repeats are required. The 'gold standard' would be video-EEG capturing ictal episodes and with a period of sleep.
- Genomic array in children with complex seizure disorders or with developmental delay. See 'Seizures with developmental delay/intellectual disability' in Chapter 2, 'Clinical approach', p. 308.
- Consider gene panel/WES/WGS as appropriate. Due to the high genetic heterogeneity of early infantile epilepsies, these approaches should be implemented early in the diagnostic process (Myers 2015).
- Consider mitochondrial DNA analysis.

Epilepsy syndromes in infants and children (in approximate order of presentation by age)

Self-limited familial neonatal epilepsy (also known as benign neonatal epilepsy)
Seizures occur repeatedly in the first days of life and remit by ~4 months of age. Heterogeneous (*KCNQ2/KCNQ3*), though note mutations in *KCNQ2* may also cause early infantile epileptic encephalopathy (EIEE) (see below).

Self-limited familial neonatal–infantile epilepsy (also known as benign familial neonatal–infantile seizures, BFNIS)
An AD disorder presenting in the first year of life, caused by mutations in the sodium channel subunit gene *SCN2A* or *KCNQ2*. This may be a benign familial epilepsy syndrome beginning in early infancy, but the phenotype includes later developmental difficulties.

Self-limited familial infantile epilepsy (also known as benign infantile epilepsy)
Heterozygous *PRRT2* mutations (predominantly LOF mutations) are found in the majority of patients with benign familial infantile epilepsy and infantile convulsions. They are also found in choreoathetosis and paroxysmal kinesigenic dyskinesia, confirming a common disease spectrum for these paroxysmal conditions (Ebrahimi-Fahkari *et al.* 2015). A positive family history is present in nearly 90% of cases and *PRRT2* mutations are familial in a high proportion (87%).

Biallelic mutation in the *SLC13A5* gene (a citrate transporter) can cause a rare form of neonatal epilepsy, with multiple seizures occurring in the first few days of life and

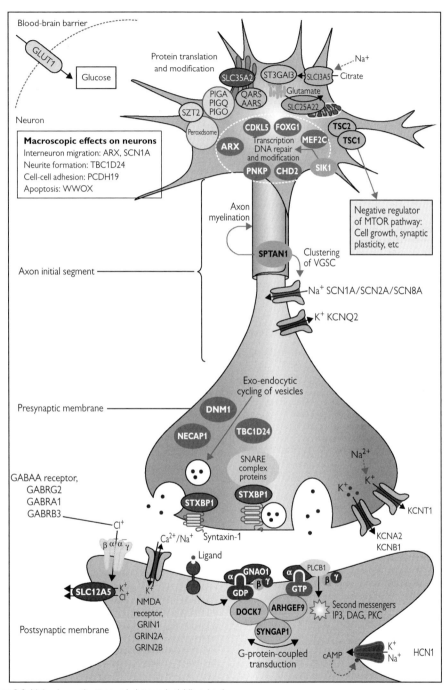

Figure 3.9 Molecular mechanisms underlying early childhood epilepsy.
Reprinted from *The Lancet Neurology*, Volume 15, Issue 3, Amy McTague, Katherine B Howell, J Helen Cross, Manju A Kurian, Ingrid E Scheffer, The genetic landscape of the epileptic encephalopathies of infancy and childhood, pp. 304–316, copyright 2016, with permission from Elsevier.

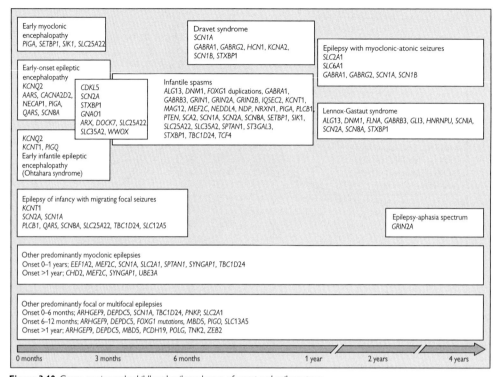

Figure 3.10 Genes causing early-childhood epilepsy by age of onset and epilepsy type.
Reprinted from *The Lancet Neurology*, Volume 15, Issue 3, Amy McTague, Katherine B Howell, J Helen Cross, Manju A Kurian, Ingrid E Scheffer, The genetic landscape of the epileptic encephalopathies of infancy and childhood, pp. 304–316, copyright 2016, with permission from Elsevier.

persisting and evolving into multiple seizure types associated with developmental delay and teeth hypoplasia.

Severe neonatal epilepsies with suppression burst pattern
Epileptic syndromes with either neonatal onset or onset during the first months of life. These disorders are characterized by suppression burst on the EEG, in which higher-voltage bursts of slow waves mixed with multifocal spikes alternate with isoelectric suppression phases and may be caused by biallelic mutation in the *SLC25A22* gene (Molinari et al. 2005).

Ohtahara syndrome or early infantile epileptic encephalopathy (EIEE)
One of the early syndromes associated with burst suppression on EEG. This is the earliest type of age-dependent epileptic encephalopathy with frequent tonic spasms. It is a heterogeneous condition and while it is mostly sporadic, there are familial cases. Exclude structural abnormalities of the brain by MRI and defects in energy metabolism/mitochondrial disorders. Poor prognosis with severe handicap likely. DNM in *STXBP1*, *KCNQ2*, *SCN2A*, and *ARX* are the most frequently reported genetic causes of EIEE.

Early myoclonic epileptic encephalopathy (EMEE)
Also associated with burst suppression, but unlike EIEE this is non-continuous but more marked in sleep. Frequent myoclonic and focal seizures are seen. This may be a presenting feature of an underlying metabolic disorder such as NKH, so a thorough metabolic workup is important. More rarely, mutations in genes, such as *ErbB4*, *PIGA*, *SETBP1*, *SIK1*, *SLC25A22*, have been identified.

Epilepsy of infancy with migrating focal seizures (EIMFS)
A clinical term for a severe form of infantile epileptic encephalopathy with seizure onset between 1 day and 6 months. The seizures are focal and may be clinically migratory and associated with autonomic features such as flushing or apnoea. There is a characteristic ictal EEG with migration of the ictal focus. Heterozygous, largely *de novo*, mutations in *KCNT1* are found in 30–50% of cases. *SCN2A* is also emerging as an important cause.

Infantile spasms and West syndrome
West syndrome is the triad of infantile spasms, hypsarrhythmia, and developmental delay. An infantile spasm is a sudden bilateral and symmetrical contraction of the muscles. The prevalence is 0.4 per 100 000 and is more common in boys.

The symptomatic group accounts for >85% of children with infantile spasms; in these children, there is an underlying abnormality affecting brain development. All children with infantile spasms should have brain imaging.

Before counselling the family of a child with infantile spasms, check particularly that the following conditions have been excluded:

- structural brain anomalies such as lissencephaly, periventricular nodular heterotopia;
- TSC—accounts for 25% of cases (see 'Tuberous sclerosis (TSC)' in Chapter 3, 'Common consultations', p. 534);
- metabolic disorders;
- mitochondrial or other defects of energy metabolism;
- XL infantile spasms in males (*ARX*) and in females (*CDKL5*);
- early-onset infantile spasms with severe neurodevelopmental retardation in females due to 'de novo' mutations in *CDKL5*;
- rarer causes include *FOXG1* duplications, *STXBP1*, *GNA01*, and a number of others;
- non-genetic causes include trauma and infections.

Dravet syndrome or severe myoclonic epilepsy in infancy (SMEI)
An epileptic encephalopathy with febrile hemiclonic seizures or prolonged febrile generalized tonic–clonic seizures in the first year of life, along with slowing of developmental progress and regression. The onset of seizures is often attributed to post-vaccination effect. Focal, absence, and myoclonic seizures appear with motor impairment and ataxia. The major genetic cause is DNM in *SCN1A*.

Landau–Kleffner syndrome (LKS)
Affects previously normal children who develop focal seizures and loss of language. Males are more frequently affected. The EEG characteristically shows centrotemporal spike-wave discharges. Clinically variable in severity. Mutation in *GRIN2A* in some.

Alpers syndrome (POLG)
A triad of severe epilepsy, hepatic dysfunction, and regression affecting infants and young children (<3 years of age). *POLG* is a nuclear gene involved in mitochondrial DNA replication; biallelic mutation of this gene leads to mitochondrial depletion.

Epilepsy with myoclonic atonic seizures (also known as myoclonic astatic epilepsy or Doose syndrome)
Has a peak onset between 2 and 4 years and occurs in previously developmentally normal children. Frequent myoclonic astatic seizures where there is a jerk followed by a loss of tone are the hallmark, and onset is associated with developmental regression. Absences and periods of non-convulsive status epilepticus are also seen. It is important to exclude glucose transporter 1 deficiency (*SLC2A1* mutations in 5% of epilepsy with myoclonic absences (epilepsy with myoclonic absences). Other genetic causes include mutations in the gamma aminobutyric acid (GABA) transporter *SLC6A1* in 4%, *KCNA2*, and *CHD2*.

Lennox–Gastaut syndrome (LGS)
Has a peak age of onset of 3–5 years and is characterized by multiple seizure types, including drop attacks, atypical absences, tonic seizures, and a characteristic EEG. Both EIEE/Ohtahara syndrome and West syndrome may evolve into LGS. There is marked developmental delay.

As in West syndrome, LGS may be symptomatic of cerebral malformations or the sequelae of infection or birth injury. In addition, a small number of patients with genetic causes such as *DNM1* or *IQSEC2* have been identified.

Genetic epilepsy with febrile seizures (GEFS (+))
A familial epilepsy where febrile convulsions persist past early childhood and/or afebrile fits occur. Genetically heterogeneous, mutations have been identified in three sodium channel subunit genes and a GABA(A) subunit gene (*SCN1A*, *SCN1B*, *SCN2A*, *GABRG2*).

Juvenile myoclonic epilepsy (JME)
This accounts for 5–10% of seizures. It is the most frequent cause of hereditary generalized tonic–clonic seizures. The peak age of onset is in adolescence but presents from childhood onwards. Ninety per cent have tonic–clonic seizures and 30% absence seizures, in addition to myoclonic seizures. AD JME in some families is a channelopathy associated with mutations in the gene encoding a GABA(A) receptor alpha-1 subunit (*GABRA1*). Mutations in *EFHC1* on 6p11-12 have been found to segregate with epilepsy or EEG polyspike wave in some other families.

Benign childhood epilepsy with centrotemporal spikes (BCECTS)
Includes benign rolandic epilepsy and benign focal epilepsy.

Other diagnoses/conditions to consider
Syndromic causes of epilepsy
See 'Seizures with developmental delay/intellectual disability' in Chapter 2, 'Clinical approach', p. 308.

Chromosome microdeletion syndromes
Recurrent microdeletions at 15q13.3, 15q11.2, and 16p13.11 are associated with seizures and ID.

Hyperekplexia (exaggerated startle response/stiff baby syndrome)
Can be confused with a neonatal seizure disorder and is important to recognize, as there is a small risk of sudden infant death during the episodes. The condition resolves during the first year. Mostly AR and due to mutation in *GLRA*.

Ring chromosome 20
See 'Seizures with developmental delay/intellectual disability' in Chapter 2, 'Clinical approach', p. 308.

Genetic advice
As per individual condition. Note that many, but not all, of the epileptic encephalopathies arise as a consequence of DNM. While typically this is a DNM that is not detected in the parents and has a low recurrence risk (~1.3%), parental mosaicism may occur (see 'Timing and origin of new dominant mutations' in Chapter 1, 'Introduction', p. 42). If parental mosaicism is identified, risk figures will need to be adjusted accordingly, in view of the higher chance of sibling recurrence.

Prenatal diagnosis
Potentially available when a causative mutation has been identified in the proband, but note variability in phenotypes where a mutation is inherited from an apparently normal parent or a parent with minimal features—a particularly frequent problem in *SCN1A*.

NIPD may be appropriate for *de novo* dominant mutations.

Natural history and further management

Surveillance

Requires long-term management by a paediatric neurologist.

Support groups: Epilepsy Action, http://www. epilepsy.org.uk; Epilepsy Foundation (USA), http://www.epilepsy.com.

Expert adviser: Amy McTague, Research Fellow, Developmental Neurosciences Programme, University College London, Great Ormond Street Institute of Child Health, London, UK.

References

Ebrahimi-Fakhari D, Saffari A, Westenberger A, Klein C. The evolving spectrum of PRRT2-associated paroxysmal diseases. *Brain* 2015; **138**(Pt 12): 3476–95.

Epi4K Consortium; Epilepsy Phenome/Genome Project, Allen AS, Berkovic SF, Cossette P, *et al. De novo* mutations in epileptic encephalopathies. *Nature* 2013; **501**: 217–21.

Guerrini R. Epilepsy in children. *Lancet* 2006; **367**: 499–524.

Hardies K, de Kovel CG, Weckhuysen S, *et al.*; autosomal recessive working group of the EuroEPINOMICS RES Consortium. Recessive mutations in *SLC13A5* result in a loss of citrate transport and cause neonatal epilepsy, developmental delay and teeth hypoplasia. *Brain* 2015; **138**(Pt 11): 3238–50.

McTague A, Howell KB, Cross JH, Kurian MA, Scheffer IE. The genetic landscape of the epileptic encephalopathies of infancy and childhood. *Lancet Neurol* 2016; **15**: 304–16.

Molinari F, Raas-Rothschild A, Rio M, *et al.* Impaired mitochondrial glutamate transport in autosomal recessive neonatal myoclonic epilepsy. *Am J Hum Genet* 2005; **76**: 334–9.

Mullen SA, Carvill GL, Bellows S, *et al.* Copy number variants are frequent in genetic generalized epilepsy with intellectual disability. *Neurology* 2013; **81**: 1507–14.

Myers CT, Mefford HC. Advancing epilepsy genetics in the genomic era. *Genome Med* 2015; **7**: 91.

Trump N, McTague A, Brittain H, *et al.* Improving diagnosis and broadening the phenotypes in early-onset seizures and severe developmental delay disorders through gene panel analysis. *J Med Genet* 2016; **53**: 310–17.

Weckhuysen S, Ivanovic V, Hendrickx R, *et al.*; KCNQ2 Study Group. Extending the KCNQ2 encephalopathy spectrum: clinical and neuroimaging findings in 17 patients. *Neurology* 2013; **81**: 1697–703.

Epilepsy in adults

See also 'Epilepsy in infants and children' in Chapter 3, 'Common consultations', p. 410, 'Seizures with developmental delay/intellectual disability' in Chapter 2, 'Clinical approach', p. 308, and 'Neonatal encephalopathy and intractable seizures' in Chapter 2, 'Clinical approach', p. 246.

Epilepsy is a disorder of the brain. Genetic factors and genetically determined syndromes contribute in many patients. Epilepsy and seizures are common medical problems. In the general population, the cumulative incidence for developing epilepsy to the age of 40 years is just under 2%.

Bianchi et al. (2003), in a huge epidemiological survey of >10 000 patients with epilepsy, found that the prevalence of epilepsy in first-degree relatives of patients with idiopathic generalized epilepsies was 5.3%. Peljto et al. (2014) in a similar study established that the cumulative risk of epilepsy in first degree relatives to age 40 years was 4.7%. Probands with idiopathic generalized epilepsies were highly concordant with respect to their relative's type of epilepsy. Risks to relatives were higher when the epilepsy in the proband began at <14 years of age. Berkovic et al. (1998) studied twin pairs with seizures and found that concordance was higher in MZ twin pairs than in DZ twin pairs (case-wise concordance of 0.62 and 0.18, respectively). In 94% of concordant MZ pairs and 71% of concordant DZ pairs, both twins had the same major epilepsy syndrome. This strongly suggests the presence of syndrome-specific genetic determinants, together with a broad genetic predisposition to seizures.

Most genetic epilepsies have a complex mode of inheritance and genes identified so far account only for a minority of families and sporadic cases (Epi4K 2017). Genes associated with idiopathic generalized epilepsy are typically within the ion channel family. Mutations in non-ion channel genes are implicated in AD lateral temporal lobe epilepsy, malformations of cortical development, and XLMR syndromes in which seizures are a component.

To understand the epilepsy literature, it is helpful to review the current definitions and classification. See Figure 3.11.

Neurologists manage and investigate the patient with epilepsy. Correct classification of the epilepsy is required prior to treatment choice.

Clinical approach

History: key points

- Family history. Three-generation family tree, with specific enquiry about seizures.
- Perinatal history, past medical history. Is there evidence of an acquired cause for the epilepsy such as head injury, meningitis?
- Developmental milestones. Delay/MR.
- Natural history of the seizures. Age of onset, e.g. neonatal, change in seizure type with age, seizure types, frequency, precipitating factors, medication. An eyewitness account is often invaluable in determining the seizure type. Are there seizures from sleep?

Examination: key points

Consider examination of affected individuals when the aetiology is unknown.

- Focal neurological signs.

- Skin examination for signs of a neurocutaneous syndrome. Consider Woods light to exclude depigmented lesions of TSC, IP, and hypomelanosis of Ito.
- Eye and fundal examination.
- Dysmorphic features: storage, metabolic, or chromosomal conditions.
- Cardiological examination at least is also required and there should be a complete physical exam in all new patients.

Investigations

- EEG. Note if specific diagnostic features have been seen.
- Brain imaging. If this has not already been performed, MRI may be required prior to counselling to exclude genetically determined structural malformations of the brain.
- ECG. Arrhythmias, long QT interval leading to syncope and an erroneous diagnosis of epilepsy.
- Genomic array if dysmorphic features and/or MR. See 'Seizures with developmental delay/intellectual disability' in Chapter 2, 'Clinical approach', p. 308.
- DNA analysis is available for some epilepsy syndromes; consider gene panel analysis/WES/WGS where there is a high clinical suspicion of a monogenic cause.
- Consider if mitochondrial DNA analysis is necessary (MERFF, MELAS).

Other diagnoses/conditions to consider

Long QT syndromes

See 'Long QT syndrome and other inherited arrhythmia syndromes' in Chapter 3, 'Common consultations', p. 480.

Non-epileptic causes

For example, syncope, psychogenic non-epileptic attacks, Munchausen syndrome (by proxy in children). These diagnoses should be evaluated by a neurologist.

Genetic advice

Idiopathic epilepsy

Define the epileptic syndrome as far as possible (see 'Appendix', p. 833, for the classification of epilepsies based on Berg et al. 2010). Analyse the family tree to determine the evidence for a Mendelian pattern of inheritance. Ensure that a structural brain lesion has been excluded in the proband (by cranial imaging) (see Table 3.14).

Some known AD syndromes:

- AD nocturnal frontal lobe epilepsy (mutations in neuronal nicotinic AChR genes CHRNA4, CHRNB4, and others);
- benign familial neonatal convulsions (potassium channel genes KCNQ2, KCNQ3);
- DEPDC5, part of the mTOR pathway, is an important gene in AD focal epilepsies (Ishida et al. 2013);
- generalized epilepsy with febrile seizures (GEFS (+); voltage-gated sodium channel genes SCN1B, SCN1A, and the GABA(A) receptor GABRG2. In most families, GEFS (+) is not AD;
- remember to exclude TSC;
- there are many other AD syndromes, some with known genes, e.g. AD partial epilepsy with auditory features (LG11) and benign familial infantile

Table 3.14 Genetic risks in idiopathic epilepsy

Individual affected	Cumulative risk of clinical epilepsy to age 20 years (%)*
Monozygotic twins	~60
Dizygotic twins	~10
Sibling with onset <10 years	6
Sibling with onset >25 years	1–2
Overall sibling risk	2.5
Parent	4 (1.5–7.5)
Parent and sibling	~10
Both parents	~15
General population	~1

* Excluding febrile convulsions.

From *Practical Genetic Counselling*, Seventh Edition, Harper PS, Copyright © 2010 Taylor and Francis. Reproduced with permission of Taylor & Francis Books UK.

seizures mapped to chromosomes 16 and 19 (genes unknown).

Locus and allelic heterogeneity make DNA analysis problematic in idiopathic AD epilepsies which are mainly caused by ion channel gene mutations. Approximately 15% of 'epilepsy plus' cases will have a pathogenic or possibly pathogenic CNV and a similar percentage with epilepsy and developmental delay/epileptic encephalopathy have a de novo mutation in a good candidate gene.

Inheritance and recurrence risk
Where possible, use figures that are specific for the type of epilepsy; these may be found by consulting the references listed below.

For isolated/idiopathic epilepsy with no clear familial inheritance, multifactorial inheritance is assumed and empiric risk figures used. The offspring risk for epilepsy is between 1.5% and 7.5%.

Variability and penetrance
Most of the familial epilepsy syndromes show intra- and interfamilial variability, with some mutation carriers unaffected with epilepsy.

Prenatal diagnosis
Only available in conditions with a known mutation or cytogenetic abnormality. Be alert to the teratogenic effects of antiepileptic medications. See 'Fetal anticonvulsant syndrome (FACS)' in Chapter 6, 'Pregnancy and fertility', p. 732.

Other family members
For AD families, pedigree analysis may refine carrier risks. Multifactorial inheritance for other idiopathic types means that risks for second-degree relatives are not much higher than population risks.

Natural history and management
Potential long-term complications
• Fetal antiepileptic drug effects and increased risk of NTDs. See 'Fetal anticonvulsant syndrome (FACS)' in Chapter 6, 'Pregnancy and fertility', p. 732. Possible

neurodevelopmental consequences for the fetus with frequent maternal tonic–clonic seizures in pregnancy (Adab et al. 2004).
• Increased risk of sudden death in patients with epilepsy (mainly attributable to the underlying disease, accidents, or suicide), especially in certain groups (e.g. young people and those with frequent generalized seizures and MR).
• Restrictions on driving; possible discrimination; long-term effects of the epilepsy, seizures, and medication.

Surveillance
By a neurologist.

Support group: Epilepsy Society, https://www.epilepsysociety.org.uk; Epilepsy Foundation (USA), http://www.epilepsy.com.

Expert adviser: Sanjay M. Sisodiya, Professor of Neurology, Department of Clinical and Experimental Epilepsy, University College London, London, UK.

References
Adab N, Kini U, Vinten J, et al. The longer term outcome of children born to mothers with epilepsy. J Neurol Neurosurg Psychiatry 2004; **75**: 1575–83.
Berg AT, Berkovic SF, Brodie MJ, et al. Revised terminology and concepts for organization of seizures and epilepsies: report of the ILAE Commission on Classification and Terminology, 2005–2009. Epilepsia 2010; **51**: 676–85.
Berkovic SF, Howell RA, Hay DA, Hopper JL. Epilepsies in twins: genetics of the major epilepsy syndromes. Ann Neurol 1998; **43**: 435–45.
Bianchi A, Viaggi S, Chiossi E. Family study of epilepsy in first degree relatives: data from the Italian Episcreen Study. Seizure 2003; **12**: 203–10.
Callenbach PM, Geerts AT, Arts WF, et al. Familial occurrence of epilepsy in children with newly diagnosed multiple seizures; Dutch Study of Epilepsy in Childhood. Epilepsia 1998; **39**: 331–6.
Chang BS, Lowenstein DH. Epilepsy [review]. N Engl J Med 2003; **349**: 1257–66.
Engel J Jr; International League Against Epilepsy (ILAE). A proposed diagnostic scheme for people with epileptic seizures and with epilepsy: report of the ILAE task force on classification and terminology. Epilepsia 2001; **42**: 769–803.
Epi4K Consortium. Ultra-rare genetic variation in common epilepsies: a case-control study. Lancet Neurol 2017; **16**: 135–43.
Gutierrez-Delicado E, Serratosa JM. Genetics of the epilepsies [review]. Curr Opin Neurol 2004; **17**: 47–53.
Harper PS. Practical genetic counselling, 6th edn. Arnold, London, 2004.
Hirose S, Scheffer IE, Marini C, et al. SCN1A testing for epilepsy: application in clinical practice. Epilepsia 2013; **54**: 946–52.
Ishida S, Picard F, Rudolf G, et al. Mutations of DEPDC5 cause autosomal dominant focal epilepsies. Nat Genet 2013; **45**: 552–5.
Kjeldsen MJ, Kyvik KO, Christensen K, Friis ML. Genetic and environmental factors in epilepsy: a population-based study of 11900 Danish twin pairs. Epilepsy Res 2001; **44**: 167–78.
Lerche H, Jerkat-Rott K, Lehmann-Horn F. Ion channels and epilepsy. Am J Med Genet 2001; **106**: 146–59.
Peljto AL, Barker-Cummings C, et al. Familial risk of epilepsy: a population-based study. Brain 2014; **137**(Pt 3): 795–805.
Seminars in Medical Genetics. The genetics of epilepsy. Am J Med Genet C 2001; **106C** (Issue 2).

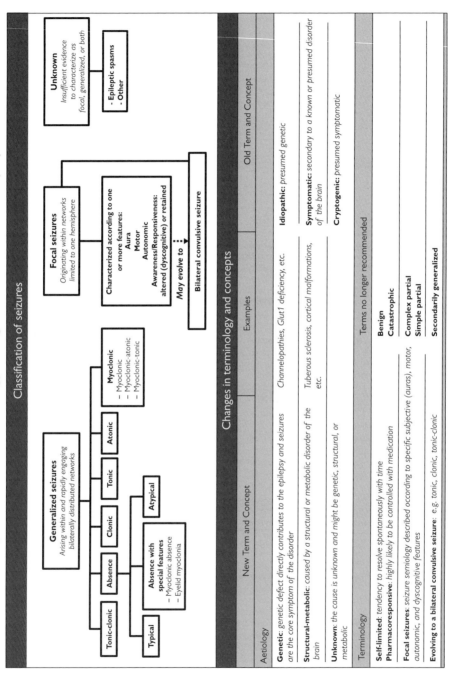

ILAE Proposal for Revised Terminology for Organization of Seizures and Epilepsies 2010

Classification of seizures

Generalized seizures
Arising within and rapidly engaging bilaterally distributed networks

- Tonic-clonic
- Absence
  - Typical
  - Atypical
  - Absence with special features
    - Myoclonic absence
    - Eyelid myoclonia
- Clonic
- Tonic
- Atonic
- Myoclonic
  - Myoclonic
  - Myoclonic-atonic
  - Myoclonic-tonic

Focal seizures
Originating within networks limited to one hemisphere

Characterized according to one or more features:
Aura
Motor
Autonomic
Awareness/Responsiveness: altered (dyscognitive) or retained

May evolve to → Bilateral convulsive seizure

Unknown
Insufficient evidence to characterize as focal, generalized, or both

- Epileptic spasms
- Other

Changes in terminology and concepts

New Term and Concept	Examples	Old Term and Concept
Aetiology		
Genetic: genetic defect directly contributes to the epilepsy and seizures are the core symptom of the disorder	Channelopathies, Glut1 deficiency, etc.	**Idiopathic:** presumed genetic
Structural-metabolic: caused by a structural or metabolic disorder of the brain	Tuberous sclerosis, cortical malformations, etc.	**Symptomatic:** secondary to a known or presumed disorder of the brain
Unknown: the cause is unknown and might be genetic, structural, or metabolic		**Cryptogenic:** presumed symptomatic
Terminology		Terms no longer recommended
Self-limited: tendency to resolve spontaneously with time		**Benign**
Pharmacoresponsive: highly likely to be controlled with medication		**Catastrophic**
Focal seizures: seizure semiology described according to specific subjective (auras), motor, autonomic, and dyscognitive features		**Complex partial**
		Simple partial
Evolving to a bilateral convulsive seizure: e.g. tonic, clonic, tonic-clonic		**Secondarily generalized**

Figure 3.11 Classification of epilepsy.
Reproduced with permission from the International League Against Epilepsy (ILAE). Data from: Berg AT *et al.* Revised terminology and concepts for organization of seizures and epilepsies: report of the ILAE Commission on Classification and Terminology, 2005–2009. *Epilepsia* 2010;51:676–685. Berg AT, Cross JH. *Lancet* 2010:9;459–61. Blume WT *et al.* Glossary of descriptive terminology for ictal semiology: Report of the ILAE task force on classification and terminology. *Epilepsia* 2001;42;1212–1218.

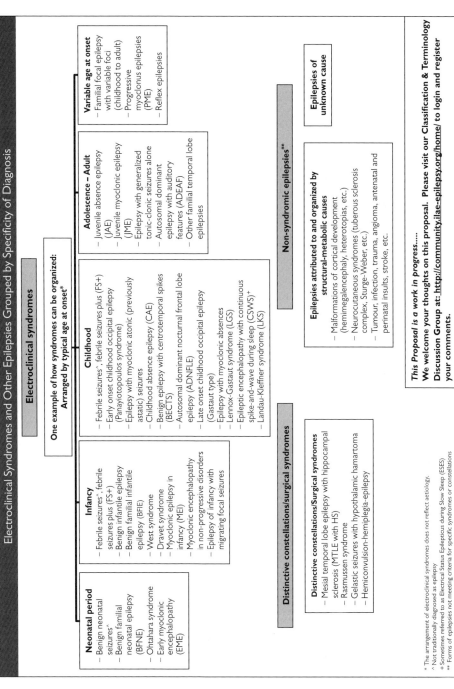

Figure 3.11 Continued

Facioscapulohumeral muscular dystrophy (FSHD)

Landouzy–Dejerine muscular dystrophy, facioscapulop-eroneal muscular dystrophy.

FSHD typically presents before the age of 20 years with weakness of the facial muscles and the stabilizers of the scapula (see Figure 3.12). The legs are affected to some degree in ~50%, with weakness of the dorsiflexors of the foot often being an early feature. Hearing impairment may be associated (Brouwer *et al*. 1991; Rogers *et al*. 2002), as also may an asymptomatic retinal vasculopathy comprising telangiectasia and microaneurysms visible with fluorescein angiography (Fitzsimmons *et al*. 1987). Early childhood-onset cases are often 'de novo'.

FSHD is an AD disorder caused by deletion of an integral number of tandem 3.3-kb repeats, termed *D4Z4*, on 4q35. Prevalence is estimated at ~1/20 000 in the UK (Lunt *et al*. 1995). Deletion of *D4Z4* may lead to the inappropriate transcriptional de-repression of genes on 4q35 in muscle, the overexpression of which leads to FSHD (Gabellini *et al*. 2002) (see Figure 3.13). Contraction in the polymorphic *D4Z4* repeat array is associated solely with the 4qA allele, and not with the 4qB allele (Lemmers *et al*. 2002). Recent studies have provided a plausible disease mechanism for FSHD, in which FSHD results from inappropriate expression of the germline transcription factor *DUX4* (van der Maarel *et al*. 2012).

Clinical approach

History: key points

- Three-generation family tree, with specific enquiry regarding:
- facial weakness (reduced facial expression, especially when smiling; sleeping with eyes slightly open; unable to whistle or blow up balloons);
- weakness of shoulders (difficulty lifting the arms above the head, e.g. combing hair, pegging out washing);
- weakness of the ankles ('foot drop').

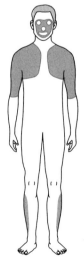

Figure 3.12 Distribution of predominant muscle weakness in facioscapulohumeral muscular dystrophy.
Reproduced from *The British Medical Journal*, Alan EH Emery, 'The muscular dystrophies', vol 317, fig 1d, p. 992, copyright 1998, with permission from BMJ Publishing Group Ltd.

- Developmental milestones and participation in sports and physical education at school.
- Document the age at which weakness was first noted. A baby or child may show little facial expression. Later excessive aching around the shoulders with 'rounded' or 'dropped' shoulders may be noted. Shoulder symptoms often begin unilaterally, usually being noted first in the dominant arm in the second or third decade.

Examination: key points

- Facial weakness. More in the lower facial muscles than the upper (inability to bury the eyelashes, puff the cheeks, purse the lips, or whistle).
- Scapular winging (ask the patient to face the wall with their arms bent and hands at shoulder height and to place their palms on the wall and lean with their weight on their palms). Observe from behind to detect winging.
- Observe for stepping of the shoulders on elevation of the arms.
- Thin upper arms with wasting of the biceps and triceps. Asymmetry is common.
- Examine for weakness of ankle dorsiflexors (may cause foot drop).
- Severely affected patients may have some hip girdle weakness—difficulty rising from a chair or from the floor.
- Reflexes are often reduced.

Investigations

- CK. Usually normal or mildly elevated. Rarely >3–5 times the upper limit of normal.
- DNA for analysis of deletion of the *D4Z4* motif. Disease alleles are typically 34 kb or smaller; normal alleles are usually >42 kb. In ~5%, the typical deletion may be obscured by the testing method; whether 4q35 FSHD can occur without a typical deletion is not known. (Alleles between 34 and 42 kb represent an overlap region between normal and mild FSHD (usually presenting with mild scapulohumeral weakness), probably with an increasing likelihood of clinical symptoms with reducing fragment size.)
- Muscle biopsy. With the advent of molecular genetic diagnosis, it is usually possible to avoid a muscle biopsy for diagnostic purposes. If performed, it typically shows non-specific chronic myopathic changes, often including small angular fibres, and sometimes with a mononuclear inflammatory reaction.

Other diagnoses/conditions to consider

Myotonic dystrophy

An AD muscle disorder characterized by myotonia with facial weakness, weakness of sternomastoid muscles with weakness, and wasting of forearm and hand muscles in the early stages. See 'Myotonic dystrophy (DM1)' in Chapter 3, 'Common consultations', p. 496.

Limb–girdle muscular dystrophies

Especially LGMD2A with shoulder girdle onset prior to pelvic girdle. See 'Limb–girdle muscular dystrophies' in Chapter 3, 'Common consultations', p. 476.

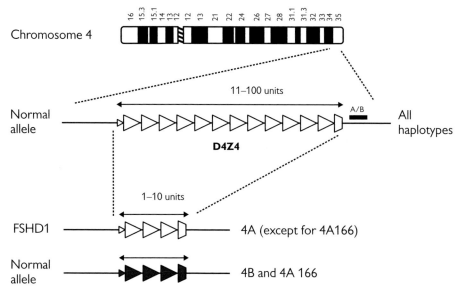

Chromosome 4

Normal
allele

D4Z4

11–100 units

A/B

All
haplotypes

FSHD1

1–10 units

4A (except for 4A166)

Normal
allele

4B and 4A 166

Figure 3.13 Schematic comparison of the structure of the normal *D4Z4* allele and the contracted mutant *D4Z4* allele that causes FSHD. The normal *D4Z4* allele has between 11 and 100 units of the 3.3-kb repeat sequence (depicted by triangles), whereas the contracted mutant FSHD-causing *D4Z4* allele has a contracted *D4Z4* repeat array of between one and ten units on a permissive chromosome 4A haplotype.
Reproduced with permission from *Gene Reviews*, Pagon *et al.*, www.ncbi.nlm.nih.gov/books/NBK1116/ copyright University of Washington, Seattle.

Nemaline myopathy
Is a diagnosis made by the identification of nemaline bodies ('rods') on histological analysis of a muscle biopsy. It is caused by mutations in one of at least six different genes. The clinical picture varies widely, in terms of the grade and distribution of muscle weakness. Muscle weakness is usually most severe in the face, neck flexors, and proximal limb muscles. In familial cases, AR inheritance is more common than AD inheritance, and in some patients the disorder is caused by new dominant mutations. Because of the genetic heterogeneity and the large size of 'nebulin', one of the genes commonly involved, no routine molecular genetic testing is yet available, with the exception of the actin gene (*ACTA1*) which accounts for 15–25% of cases. Diagnosis often rests on clinical and histological criteria. Management of patients with nemaline myopathy requires regular monitoring of respiratory capacity to detect the onset of insidious hypoventilation (Wallgren-Pettersson 2002).

Mitochondrial myopathy
See 'Mitochondrial DNA diseases' in Chapter 3, 'Common consultations', p. 490.

Becker muscular dystrophy (BMD)
Clinically similar to DMD, but milder, with a mean age of onset of 11 years. Loss of the ability to walk may occur late (e.g. 40s or 50s) and many individuals with BMD survive into middle age and beyond. Often, cramps on exercise are the only problem initially, but some affected boys are late in learning to walk and are unable to run fast. Later in the teens and 20s, muscle weakness becomes evident, causing difficulty in rapid walking, running, and climbing stairs. It may become difficult to lift objects above waist height. See 'Duchenne and Becker muscular dystrophy (DMD and BMD)' in Chapter 3, 'Common consultations', p. 402.

Emery–Dreifuss muscular dystrophy
See 'Limb–girdle muscular dystrophies' in Chapter 3, 'Common consultations', p. 476.

Genetic advice
The great majority of families are linked to 4q35, but a small group of families do not map to this locus.

Inheritance and recurrence risk
AD with 50% risk to offspring of an affected individual. In view of the wide variability and incomplete penetrance, testing of asymptomatic adult family members should be considered before giving advice about risks to their offspring. High DNM rate of 10–30%. In general, patients with de novo disease have shorter 4q35 fragments than those with familial disease and tend to be symptomatic earlier with more severe disease. At least 40% of new mutations for FSHD arise in mitosis (presumably in the early blastocyst), giving somatic and germline mosaicism (van der Maarel *et al.* 2000). This should be checked for in parents of an apparently isolated case, as the recurrence risk in sibs would be significant. Even in molecularly apparent DNMs, there is a small theoretical risk of sibling recurrence due to parental germline mosaicism.

Variability and penetrance
Penetrance is fairly high. Zatz *et al.* (1998) found a penetrance of 83% by 30 years that was higher in males than females. Signs of muscle weakness (particularly in the face) are evident by 12 years in at least 50% of mutation carriers. The disease shows high interfamilial

variability—some patients with severe infantile FSHD have muscle weakness at birth, whereas other mutation carriers can remain asymptomatic throughout life. Non-penetrance may be more likely with larger alleles. Within a family, the severity tends to follow a similar trend. It is unusual to find siblings who are affected to very different degrees. There is some genotype–phenotype correlation, with earlier age of onset, earlier age of loss of ambulation, and muscle weakness all correlated with shorter 4q35 fragments.

Prenatal diagnosis

Possible by CVS, but tends to be requested only in the context of the more severe presentations because otherwise FSHD is usually a condition of adult life with normal cognition and fairly normal life expectancy.

Predictive testing

FSHD is usually penetrant by early adult life. For those adults wishing to clarify their status, perhaps before starting a family, this is feasible if the proband has a short 4q35 fragment.

Other family members

If 'at-risk' children are symptomatic, testing has an important role in diagnosis. Testing of unaffected 'at-risk' children is generally discouraged, so that testing can be deferred until the individual is mature enough to give their own consent (usually as an adult).

Natural history and management

Potential long-term complications

- Loss of mobility. Up to 20% of sufferers eventually require a wheelchair. The earlier in life the weakness appears, the greater its eventual severity. Foot splints may be helpful for patients with 'foot drop'.
- Impaired use of arms in severe disease. The operation of scapula fixation (attaching the scapula to the ribs) may help some patients to regain useful arm function; however, if an individual has rapidly progressive disease, the benefits may be short-lived.
- Hearing impairment. High-tone sensorineural hearing loss can be a feature, although there is no good agreement between different studies on a figure for the proportion of FSHD patients who have an abnormal audiogram (Brouwer et al. 1991; Rogers et al. 2002).

Surveillance

No specific surveillance is currently advised. An increased incidence of atrial tachyarrhythmias has been noted (Laforet et al. 1998), but these are rarely symptomatic and cardiac surveillance is not routinely indicated.

Support group: Muscular Dystrophy UK, http://www.musculardystrophyuk.org.

References

Brouwer OF, Padberg GW, Ruys CJ, Brand R, de Laat JA, Grote JJ. Hearing loss in facioscapulohumeral muscular dystrophy. *Neurology* 1991; **41**: 1878–81.

Emery AE. The muscular dystrophies. *BMJ* 1998; **317**: 991–5.

Fitzsimmons RB, Gurwin EB, Bird AC. Retinal vascular abnormalities in facioscapulohumeral muscular dystrophy. A general association with genetic and therapeutic implications. *Brain* 1987; **110**(Pt 3): 631–48.

Gabellini D, Gren MR, Tupler R. Inappropriate gene activation in FSHS: a repressor complex binds a chromosomal repeat deleted in dystrophic muscle. *Cell* 2002; **110**: 339–48.

Laforet P, de Toma C, Eymard B, et al. Cardiac involvement in genetically confirmed facioscapulohumeral muscular dystrophy. *Neurology* 1998; **51**: 1454–6.

Lemmers RJ, de Kievit P, Sandkuijl L, et al. Facioscapulohumeral muscular dystrophy is uniquely associated with one of the two variants of the 4q subtelomere. *Nat Genet* 2002; **32**: 235–6.

Lunt PW, Jardine PE, Koch M, et al. Phenotypic–genotypic correlation will assist genetic counselling in 4q35-facioscapulohumeral muscular dystrophy. *Muscle Nerve* 1995; **2**: S103–9.

Rogers MT, Zhao F, Harper PS, Stephens D. Absence of hearing impairment in adult onset facioscapulohumeral muscular dystrophy. *Neuromuscul Disord* 2002; **12**: 358–65.

Van der Maarel SM, Deidda G, Lemmers RJ, et al. De novo facioscapulohumeral muscular dystrophy: frequent somatic mosaicism, sex-dependent phenotype, and the role of mitotic transchromosomal repeat interaction between chromosomes 4 and 10. *Am J Hum Genet* 2000; **66**: 26–35.

van der Maarel SM, Miller DG, Tawil R, Filippova GN, Tapscott SJ. Facioscapulohumeral muscular dystrophy: consequences of chromatin relaxation. *Curr Opin Neurol* 2012; **25**: 614–20.

Wallgren-Pettersson C. Nemaline and myotubular myopathies. *Semin Pediatr Neurol* 2002; **9**: 132–44.

Zatz M. Marie SK, Cerqueira A, et al. The facioscapulohumeral muscular dystrophy (FSHD1) gene affects males more severely and more frequently than females. *Am J Med Genet* 1998; **77**: 155–61.

Fragile X syndrome (FRAX)

FMR1, Martin–Bell syndrome.

FRAXA is the most common inherited cause of MR with ~1 in 5500 males carrying a full mutation. *FMR1* at Xq27.3 contains a triplet repeat $(CGG)_n$ in the 5′ untranslated region of the gene. Allele sizes outside the normal range are unstable in meiosis. The risk of expansion of FMR1 alleles increases with size and there is a continuum of risk as one moves from the intermediate allele range to the premutation range. There is no 'step change'. Nevertheless, it is useful for practical purposes to triage alleles into these ranges in order to manage this risk clinically. The triplet repeat expansion in FRAXA is a dynamic mutation. Several studies have shown strong somatic stability of the expansion size after the initial period of expansion, during which one or more different allele sizes may be generated (see Table 3.15).

In the presence of a full mutation, the *FMR1* gene is methylated and, although mRNA may be produced, no FMR protein (FMRP) is produced. Polysomal association of *FMR1* mRNA, which is high in normal cells, becomes progressively lower with increasing (CGG) repeat expansion. Impairment of *FMR1* mRNA translation may be the cause of the lower FMRP levels that lead to clinical involvement. The level of FMRP correlates with the degree of cognitive involvement in both males and females (Tassone et al. 2000).

FRAXE is rare with ~1 in 23 000 males carrying a full mutation. It is caused by a triplet repeat $(GCC)_n$ in *FMR2* on Xq28. The phenotype is poorly defined with milder developmental delay than seen in FRAXA.

Full mutation in males (fragile X syndrome)

* Developmental delay. Hypotonia and mild motor delay are relatively common.
* Speech and language. Variable, ranging from no speech through to mild communication problems. Speech is often not very fluent. The speech of affected individuals tends to be characterized by the use of many incomplete sentences, repetition, and echolalia.
* IQ. Males with a full mutation that is methylated have an average IQ of 41. Males mosaic for a full and premutation have an average IQ of 60. Males with a full mutation with >50% of cells unmethylated have an average IQ of 88.

Table 3.15 Full, premutation, intermediate, and normal allele sizes in FRAXA*

Category	Allele size
Normal individuals	<45 repeats
Intermediate allele	45–58 repeats
Premutation carrier females and normal-transmitting males	59–200 repeats unmethylated
Affected individuals and full-mutation carrier females	>200 repeats methylated

* In FRAXA, as in the other repeat disorders, there are no distinct boundaries separating the different repeat size categories. Individuals with intermediate-size alleles have ~45 to ~60 repeats, whereas males and females with premutation alleles have ~55 to ~200 repeats. The distinction between intermediate and premutation alleles is made by family history and repeat instability. Categories vary considerably in different publications.

* Behaviour. Overactivity and impulsiveness with marked concentration problems, fidgetiness, and distractability. Affected individuals are easily overwhelmed by a variety of sensory stimuli. Autistic features with gaze avoidance, stereotyped repetitive behaviours such as hand flapping, resistance to change of routines or environment, and strong preoccupations or fascinations are common. Perseveration with an affected individual becoming fixated on a particular activity or asking questions about the same issue over and over again is quite common. Most children with FRAXA are affectionate and have an interest in relating socially but have difficulty in social interaction and tend to be shy and anxious in group situations.
* Adult life. Adults with full mutations often show strengths in skills of daily living, relative to their communication and socialization abilities. Nevertheless, a degree of supported living is needed by most full mutation males (Hartley et al. 2011).

Full mutation in females

Females are less affected by fragile X than males, because the normal X produces variable amounts of FMRP. Up to 50% of females with a full FMR1 mutation demonstrate learning difficulties that are similar to, but usually less severe than, those seen in affected males. Behavioural problems tend to be more social withdrawal than overactivity. However, more subtle problems with learning, behavioural, and emotional difficulties are common, even in females with a full mutation who have a normal IQ. As is the case for affected males, verbal abilities tend to be better than performance skills, and special needs in arithmetic, visuospatial abilities, and visual and auditory memory are common.

Premutation alleles

Premutation alleles appear more common in the population than would be predicted from full mutation individuals. This is because the risk of expansion to a full mutation is likely to be modified by other factors such as AGG interspersions. Approximately 0.5% of the population carries a premutation-sized allele (Nolin et al. 2011). On rare occasions, individuals with a premutation may be clinically affected with learning disabilities or cognitive deficits, although the vast majority of individuals with the premutation have an IQ in the normal range (Hagerman et al. 1996; Tassone et al. 2000). When a child with learning difficulties is found to have a premutation, this should not be assumed to be the cause and other investigations should be considered. There is accumulation evidence in the literature about subtle neuropsychological changes in premutation carriers (Hunter et al. 2012; Turk 2011).

Intermediate alleles

Youings et al. (2000) tested 2932 mother-to-boy transmissions and found only five changes in transmission in the common and intermediate range. Transmissions from females with common or intermediate repeats are remarkably stable (in the absence of a family history of FRAX), although instabilities are ~90 times more frequent for alleles in the size range of 40–59 repeats than for alleles of <40 repeats. Instability was related to the absence of AGG interspersions by Nolin et al. (2011). Intermediate alleles are potential precursors of a full mutation in future generations. By definition, only premutation alleles have the potential to expand to full mutations in one generation, and so any potential small risk is to more distant generations, with grandchildren being the closest possible generation at risk.

Some intermediate alleles are stably transmitted within families, while others show allele instability and may be the potential precursors of a premutation in a subsequent generation. The differences are likely due, at least in part, to differences in AGG interruptions within the FMR1 repeat. In the normal population, the CGG repeat is interrupted by AGG trinucleotides, most often at positions 10 and 20. In contrast, premutation alleles are distinguished by the absence of AGG or the presence of only one AGG interruption at the 5′ end of the repeat and long tracts of uninterrupted CGG repeats at the 3′ end.

Clinical approach

History: key points
- Three-generation family tree that may need to be extended to further generations in the maternal line to facilitate cascade carrier testing.
- Pregnancy and perinatal history.
- Developmental milestones, including language development and schooling.
- Behaviour.

Examination: key points
- Height, weight, OFC; relative macrocephaly is common.
- Face and ears. Classically, individuals with FRAX have a long face and mildly prominent ears with cupping of the upper pinnae, but this is rarely striking and usually only evident in older boys. Many young children look entirely normal.
- Joints. Joint hypermobility is common.
- Large testes in post-pubertal individuals.
- Heart. Examine for a mid-systolic click or murmur (MVP).
- Behaviour. Eye contact, hyperactivity, motor incoordination.

Investigations
- DNA for FRAXA $(CGG)_n$ repeat size. The initial step is PCR. If two different normal-sized alleles are detected, no further analysis is usually done. If no normal allele is detected in a male or only one allele is detected in a female, a triplet-primed PCR method (Amplidex) is used next to determine whether there is an expanded allele present. (Note some females are homozygous for a normal-sized allele; FRAX carriers will have one normal and one expanded allele.)
- Assessment of methylation status. Use of a methylation-sensitive enzyme (EagI) that cuts non-methylated DNA at the CpG island but leaves methylated DNA uncut, allowing analysis of the methylation status of *FMR1*.

Other diagnoses/conditions to consider

See 'Intellectual disability with apparent X-linked inheritance' in Chapter 2, 'Clinical approach', p. 194.

Genetic advice

Inheritance and recurrence risk
FEMALES. Expansion of a triplet repeat may not occur with every pregnancy in a woman carrying a premutation,

Table 3.16 Risk of maternal premutation expansion to full mutation

Maternal CGG premutation	Risk of expansion to >200 CGG repeats (%)
55–59	3.7
60–69	5.3
70–79	31.1
80–89	57.8
90–99	80.1
100–139	>94
>140	100

This table was published in *American Journal of Human Genetics*, Vol 59, Issue 6, Nolin SL, Lewis FA, Ye LL, *et al.*, Familial transmission of the FMR1 CGG repeat, pp. 1252–61, Copyright Elsevier (1996).

but huge expansion into the full mutation range is a potential risk with all premutation alleles. Women with a FRAX premutation face four possible outcomes to each pregnancy—each equally likely. These are: a normal male; a normal female; a male with a FRAX premutation or a full mutation; and a female with a FRAX premutation or a full mutation.

In Nolin *et al.*'s (2011) study of the offspring of 1112 premutation females (see Table 3.16), the risks of expansion observed prospectively in pregnancy are presented. Shown here are those for women with a family history of fragile X; the risks are lower in women without such a history. The smallest allele to increase to a full mutation in a single generation is 56 (Fernandez-Carvajal *et al.* 2009).

MALES. Males with the premutation will pass this on to all of their daughters and none of their sons. The repeat size is likely to remain fairly stable (although small expansions and contractions are possible). Males with the full mutation are unlikely to form mature sexual relationships as adults. Several studies have found that adult FMR1 males who carry a full mutation in their somatic tissues have only premutation size repeats in their sperm/gonadal tissue.

Variability and penetrance
- Males with a full mutation that is methylated have an average IQ of 41.
- Males mosaic for a full and premutation have an average IQ of 60.
- Males with a full mutation with >50% of cells unmethylated have an average IQ of 88.
- Females. Approximately one-half of females with a full mutation have learning and behavioural difficulties that are similar to, but usually less severe than, those seen in males with a full mutation. As for affected males, verbal abilities tend to be better than performance skills; special needs in arithmetic and difficulties with visuospatial skills and abstract concepts are common.

Prenatal diagnosis
Feasible by CVS (adequate sample size needed), but note difficulty of predicting the phenotype in females carrying a full mutation. Exclude maternal cell contamination. Backup confirmation by linkage is also often used and can usually be available quickly, as there can sometimes be technical problems and delay with the Southern blot analysis.

Daughters of mothers carrying a full or premutation
Testing of sisters of affected boys who have no schooling problems is generally deferred until 16 years of age or later when they may wish to discover their carrier status before planning a family. Sisters who experience mild difficulties at school should be offered a vision and hearing check and, for younger girls, a paediatric developmental assessment or, for older girls, an assessment by an educational psychologist. Once these are complete and if there is evidence for a learning difficulty and no obvious alternative cause (e.g. poor hearing due to glue ear), then it may be helpful to pursue diagnostic testing for FRAX.

Other family members
Cascade screening of adult family members is indicated. A premutation in a female may have been inherited from her mother or her father, but a full mutation can only be maternally inherited. Remember that, if the familial mutation is maternally inherited, normal brothers may be premutation carriers (normal transmitting males) and should be offered testing because of the potential risk to their daughters' offspring and advice about FXTAS.

Natural history and management
Refer to a developmental paediatrician who will arrange preschool learning support and liaise with community paediatric services. Individuals with FRAX have special educational needs. Most can manage in mainstream primary school with appropriate support, although behavioural difficulties can make special education appropriate earlier than for other children with similar levels of cognitive difficulty. Children with FRAX are readily overwhelmed by noisy and busy environments, e.g. supermarkets, leading to tantrums, overactivity, withdrawal, repetitive behaviour, etc. Careful thought needs to be given to this in planning educational support. Children often learn best when auditory and visual distraction is minimized and work is packaged into short (maximum 15 minutes) blocks and presented in side-by-side interactions, rather than face-to-face. See Fragile X Society for further information on educational needs.

Potential long-term complications in affected individuals
- Recurrent otitis media occurs in 60–80%, causing conductive hearing loss. Consider grommets and/or prophylactic antibiotics if this is troublesome.
- Seizures occur in ~20%. They usually resolve by adolescence.
- MVP is rare in childhood but may occur in ~50% of adults.

Potential long-term complications in premutation carriers
- Males. Some adult males with FRAX premutations may develop a progressive neurological syndrome—fragile X tremor ataxia syndrome (FXTAS), with cerebellar tremor/ataxia, cognitive decline, and generalized brain atrophy characterized by intranuclear inclusions and characteristic, but not specific, MRI findings (Greco et al. 2002).The origin of the inclusions is unknown, although elevated FMR1 mRNA levels in these premutation carriers may lead to the neuropathological changes. Penetrance is age-related; it affects 17% of male premutation carriers aged 50–59 years, rising to 75% in patients aged 80 years. Most premutations found in FXTAS patients are of >70 repeats. It is reported in women premutation carriers but appears to be less common (Hagerman and Hagerman 2013).
- Females. Approximately 20% of female premutation carriers will undergo premature menopause (cessation

of menses at <40 years), compared to 1% of the general population. The risk appears to be greater for premutations in the 80–100 CGG repeat range. This information may be helpful to carrier women for reproductive planning (e.g. if considering PGD). See 'Premature ovarian failure (POF)' in Chapter 6, 'Pregnancy and fertility', p. 778.

Treatment
Recent years have seen an increasing understanding of the molecular mechanism of fragile X syndrome and evidence that altering the metabotropic glutamate receptor (mGluR-5)-dependent protein synthesis may directly affect the synaptic alterations underlying the phenotype, with promising results in animal models. However, recent clinical trials with two different mGlu5 inhibitors showed no therapeutic benefit in fragile X patients (Scharf et al. 2015).

Support group: The Fragile X Society, http://www.fragilex.org.uk, Tel. 01424 813 147; National Fragile X Foundation (USA), https://fragilex.org.

Expert adviser: Angela Barnicoat, Consultant Clinical Geneticist, Department of Clinical Genetics, Great Ormond Street Hospital NHS Foundation Trust, London, UK.

References
Association for Clinical Genetic Science. *Practice guidelines for molecular diagnosis of fragile X syndrome*, 2012. http://www.acgs.uk.com/media/908997/frx_bpg_final_nov_2014.pdf.

de Graaff E, Willemsen R, Zhong N, et al. Instability of the CGG repeat and expression of the FMR1 protein in a male fragile X patient with a lung tumour. *Am J Hum Genet* 1995; **57**: 609–18.

Fernandez-Carvajal I, Lopez Posadas B, Pan R, Raske C, Hagerman PJ, Tassone F. Expansion of an FMR1 grey-zone allele to a full mutation in two generations. *J Mol Diagn* 2009; **11**: 306–10.

Greco CM, Hagerman RJ, Tassone F, et al. Neuronal intranuclear inclusions in a new cerebellar tremor/ataxia syndrome among fragile X carriers. *Brain* 2002; **125**: 1760–71.

Hagerman R, Hagerman P. Advances in clinical and molecular understanding of the FMR1 premutation and fragile X-associated tremor/ataxia syndrome. *Lancet Neurol* 2013; **12**: 786–98.

Hagerman RJ, Staley LW, O'Conner R, et al. Learning disabled males with a fragile X CGG expansion in the upper premutation size range. *Pediatrics* 1996; **97**: 122–6.

Hartley SL, Seltzer MM, Raspa M, Olmstead M, Bishop E, Bailey DB. Exploring the adult life of men and women with fragile X syndrome: results from a national survey. *Am J Intellect Dev Disabil* 2011; **116**: 16–35.

Heitz D, Devys D, Imbert G, Kretz C, Mandel JL. Inheritance of the fragile X syndrome: size of the fragile X premutation is a major determinant of the transition to full mutation. *J Med Genet* 1992; **29**: 794–801.

Hunter et al. 2012

Nolin SL, Glicksman A, Ding X, et al. Fragile X analysis of 1112 prenatal samples from 1991 to 2010. *Prenat Diagn* 2011; **31**: 925–31.

Nolin SL, Lewis FA 3rd, Ye LL, et al. Familial transmission of the FMR1 CGG repeat. *Am J Hum Genet* 1996; **59**: 1252–61.

Scharf SH, Jaeschke G, Wettstein JG, Lindemann L. Metabotropic glutamate receptor 5 as drug target for Fragile X syndrome. *Curr Opin Pharmacol* 2015; **20**: 124–34.

Tassone F, Hagerman RJ, Taylor AK, et al. Clinical involvement and protein expression in individuals with FMR1 premutation. *Am J Med Genet* 2000; **91**: 144–52.

Turk 2011

Youings SA, Murray A, Dennis N, et al. FRAXA and FRAXE: the results of a five year survey. *J Med Genet* 2000; **37**: 415–21.

Glaucoma

Glaucoma is an optic neuropathy with characteristic field loss that may or may not be associated with increased intraocular pressure. It is classified according to the mechanism causing glaucoma into the following:

(1) primary open-angle glaucoma (POAG) is due to an intrinsic disorder of the trabecular meshwork;

(2) closed-angle glaucoma (acute and chronic);

(3) secondary glaucomas arise as a consequence of disease or abnormality either elsewhere in the eye or in other systems.

Most adult-onset glaucoma is a complex disease showing multifactorial inheritance, and family history is an important risk factor (Tielsch et al. 1994).

Glaucoma in infancy and childhood may form part of a wider condition but is usually an isolated occurrence. Primary congenital glaucoma is also known as buphthalmos and has a birth incidence of ~3/100 000 (Bermejo and Martinez-Frias 1998).

The aim is to determine whether the glaucoma is a purely ocular condition or if there are non-ocular features that suggest a syndrome diagnosis. 'Anterior segment eye malformations' in Chapter 2, 'Clinical approach', p. 62 may also be useful. Approximately 50% of patients with anterior segment dysgenesis will develop glaucoma (Ito and Water 2014).

Clinical approach

History: key points

- Family history. At least three-generation family tree. Enquire for consanguinity.
- Growth. Most chromosomal conditions show poor growth. Rieger syndrome is associated with pituitary abnormalities.
- Developmental progress, allowing for visual difficulties.
- Vision, photophobia.

Examination: key points

- Ophthalmology opinion to confirm diagnosis by measuring the intraocular pressure (may require general anaesthesia in infants), examination of optic discs, and visual testing in adults and older children.
- Exclude other structural abnormalities of the eye such as iris hypoplasia, aniridia, sclerocornea, megalocornea, microphthalmia, and lens abnormality.
- Uni- or bilateral?
- Growth parameters (short stature in Peter's plus syndrome, Rieger syndrome).
- Orofacial clefts (Peter's plus syndrome, Kivlin syndrome).
- Abnormal dentition (Rieger syndrome).
- Hypospadias (Rieger syndrome).
- Redundant periumbilical skin (Rieger syndrome).
- Olfaction (abnormalities may be found with *PAX6* mutations).

Special investigations

- Examine the parents to exclude minor signs of anterior segment dysgenesis.
- Genomic array in children with malformation syndromes and/or developmental delay. Exclude deletion 11p13 in children with aniridia (FISH 11p13) if genomic array not available.
- Consider gene panel/WES/WGS as appropriate in patients where there is a high clinical suspicion of a monogenic cause.
- Echo if there is dislocation/subluxation of the ocular lens or if there are other features of MFS.

Syndromic diagnoses to consider

Secondary causes of childhood glaucoma

ANTERIOR SEGMENT DISORDERS. See 'Anterior segment eye malformations' in Chapter 2, 'Clinical approach', p. 62 for more details.

- Aniridia (*PAX6* gene).
- Axenfeld–Rieger syndromes.
- Peter's anomaly.

NEUROFIBROMATOSIS TYPE 1 (NF1). Typically six or more CALs. Glaucoma is really only seen in a rare form of NF1 with extensive ipsilateral plexiform neuroma. See 'Neurofibromatosis type 1 (NF1)' in Chapter 3, 'Common consultations', p. 506.

STURGE–WEBER SYNDROME. Association of facial capillary haemangioma (port-wine stain) involving the ophthalmic division of the Vth cranial nerve with meningeal angiomata. Seizures and MR may be complications. Most cases are sporadic.

Secondary causes of juvenile and adult glaucoma

As above plus the following.

NAIL–PATELLA SYNDROME. An AD disorder characterized by dysplasia of the nails, patellae, and elbow joints, exostoses of the iliac crest, and in some cases nephropathy. Fingernails are absent or abnormal in 98%. Gene is *LMX1B* on 9q34, a transcription factor that regulates the *COL4A3* and *COL4A4* genes. Offer surveillance for nephropathy. See 'Unusual hair, teeth, nails, and skin' in Chapter 2, 'Clinical approach', p. 330.

NANOPHTHALMOS OR SIMPLE MICROPHTHALMIA. The nanophthalmic eye has a proportionately thicker sclera, but the lens is of normal size, which leads to a narrow anterior chamber, and glaucoma may develop. See 'Microphthalmia and anophthalmia' in Chapter 2, 'Clinical approach', p. 236.

MARFAN'S SYNDROME (MFS) AND ECTOPIA LENTIS. An AD condition characterized by tall stature, long limbs, pectus deformity, and aortic root enlargement. Caused by mutations in fibrillin (*FBN1*) on 15q. Acute glaucoma secondary to lens dislocation may develop. See 'Marfan's syndrome' in Chapter 3, 'Common consultations', p. 484.

HOMOCYSTINURIA. An AR condition caused by deficiency of cystathionine synthetase encoded on 21q22 and characterized by lens dislocation (typically downward displacement) and thrombophilia. Most thrombotic events are cerebrovascular. Acute glaucoma secondary to lens dislocation may develop.

NORRIE DISEASE. Secondary angle-closure glaucoma may occur as a result of lens dislocation and may complicate retinal dysplasia in Norrie disease. See 'Retinal dysplasia' in Chapter 2, 'Clinical approach', p. 300.

Genetic advice

Inheritance and recurrence risk

BUPHTHALMOS/PRIMARY CONGENITAL GLAUCOMA. Corneal opacification, photophobia.

- Exclude other anterior segment anomalies.
- Exclude secondary causes of glaucoma (see above).

Recessive inheritance possible. Genetic heterogeneity with at least three loci. One is *CYP1B1* on 2p21. Another, the forkhead transcription factor gene *FKHL7* on 6p25, is responsible for a spectrum of glaucoma phenotypes, including primary congenital glaucoma, Rieger anomaly, Axenfeld anomaly, and iris hypoplasia (Nishimura *et al.* 1998). In the absence of consanguinity, recurrence risks are about 5%.

JUVENILE AND ADULT PRIMARY GLAUCOMA. AD inheritance; many loci. Mutations in the myocilin gene (*MYOC*) are found in a proportion (~6–8%) of families with POAG and juvenile glaucoma (Bruttini *et al.* 2003; Williams-Lyn *et al.* 2000). The phenotype associated with mutation in *MYOC* is highly variable, even within the same kindred, ranging from normal through ocular hypertension to severe open-angle glaucoma (OAG) (Cobb *et al.* 2002). Compared with adult-onset POAG, there is a higher incidence of affected family members in juvenile-onset disease. Nevertheless, many cases of juvenile glaucoma do not have a family history. Most adult glaucoma is a complex (multifactorial) disease.

Tielsch *et al.* (1994) in a population-based study found age-adjusted associations of POAG with a history of glaucoma were higher in siblings (OR = 3.69) than in parents (OR = 2.17) or children (OR = 1.12).

SECONDARY CAUSES OF GLAUCOMA. Counsel for the specific syndrome diagnosed.

Prenatal diagnosis

Most glaucoma is treatable if appropriate surveillance is offered and it is identified early. Parents may desire PND for congenital glaucoma where the visual results may be poor despite treatment, but this will only be feasible if the mutation(s) are known.

Predictive testing

Possible in the few families in which molecular genetic testing has been done which has identified the causative mutation. Note that mutations in *MYOC* may have variable expressivity and penetrance. Predictive testing could be used to target surveillance.

Other family members

Offer ophthalmological surveillance to first-degree relatives. The age at which to begin screening will depend on the family history. Seek guidance from your ophthalmological colleagues.

Natural history and management

Potential long-term complications

Untreated glaucoma can lead to irreversible constriction of the visual fields.

Surveillance

Ensure ophthalmological surveillance for affected individuals and arrange ophthalmological follow-up for 'at-risk' family members.

Support group: International Glaucoma Association (IGA), http://www.glaucoma-association.com, Tel. 0207 737 3265.

References

Alward WLM. *Glaucoma genetics 1999.* Presented at 9th Robert J Gorlin Conference on Dysmorphology, October 1999.

Bermejo E, Martinez-Frias ML. Congenital eye malformations: clinical–epidemiological analysis of 1,124,654 consecutive births in Spain. *Am J Med Genet* 1998; **75**: 497–504.

Bruttini M, Longo I, Frezzotti P, *et al.* Mutations in the myocilin gene in families with primary open-angle glaucoma and juvenile open-angle glaucoma. *Arch Ophthalmol* 2003; **121**: 1034–8.

Cobb CJ, Scott G, Swingler RJ, *et al.* Rapid mutation detection by the transgenomic wave analyser DHPLC identifies *MYOC* mutations in patients with ocular hypertension and/or open angle glaucoma. *Br J Ophthalmol* 2002; **86**: 191–5.

Ito YA, Water MA. Genomics and anterior segment dysgenesis: a review. *Clin Exp Ophthalmol* 2014; **52**: 13–24.

Nishimura DY, Swiderski RE, Alward WL, *et al.* The forkhead transcription factor gene *FKHL7* is responsible for glaucoma phenotypes which map to 6p25. *Nat Genet* 1998; **19**: 140–7.

Tielsch JM, Katz J, Sommer A, Quigley HA, Javitt JC. Family history and risk of primary open angle glaucoma. The Baltimore Eye Survey. *Arch Ophthalmol* 1994; **112**: 69–73.

Weinrab RN, Khaw PT. Primary open-angle glaucoma. *Lancet* 2004; **363**: 1711–20.

Williams-Lyn D, Flanagan J, Buys Y, *et al.* The genetic aspects of adult-onset glaucoma: a perspective from the Greater Toronto area. *Can J Ophthalmol* 2000; **35**: 12–17.

Haemochromatosis

Hereditary haemochromatosis (HH), genetic haemochromatosis (HC).

HFE (HH type 1) is an AR disorder of iron metabolism of low penetrance. It is characterized by progressive iron overload and caused by mutations in the *HFE* gene (HLA-H) on chromosome 6. *HFE* is expressed in the intestinal crypt cells and is likely to play a key role in coupling the iron-sensing mechanism of the crypt cells to iron absorption by the mature enterocyte. The predominant feature of HFE is excessive absorption of dietary iron and once incorporated, the body has limited means for the excretion of iron. With the increasing identification of genes implicated in the control of iron homeostasis and a greater understanding of the pathophysiology of haemochromatosis, a schema for the interaction of these gene products is emerging. Patients with haemochromatosis who undergo successful allotransplantation of the liver no longer develop iron overload. Eventually, deposition of iron in parenchymal tissues results in skin pigmentation and cirrhosis of the liver, arthropathy, and endocrine failure, including diabetes mellitus and hypogonadotrophic hypogonadism; rarely CM occurs. Genetically predisposed homozygous individuals occur with an estimated frequency ranging from 1/2000 (Finland) to 1/200 (Utah); the prevalence of homozygosity for the C282Y *HFE* allele is highest in the Irish population (1%). Dietary factors and gender interact with hereditary disposition; given losses of iron incurred through menstruation and pregnancy, full-blown haemochromatosis is unusual in women; moreover, clinical expression of iron storage disease, as well as cirrhosis, is enhanced markedly in patients who consume alcohol. In evolutionary terms, heterozygotes, and even homozygotes, for mutations in *HFE* may have been at a selective advantage when diets lacked iron and infestation with gut parasites was common; enhanced retention of dietary iron may also compensate for malabsorption, blood loss, and epithelial exfoliation in coeliac disease, which is also frequent in populations of North European and Celtic origin.

There are two common mutations C282Y and H63D. Approximately 90% of patients with HH are homozygous for C282Y; a further 4% are compound heterozygotes for C282Y/H63D. H63D homozygotes do not develop HH. HH due to C282Y is common in populations associated with Celtic migrations, e.g. the UK, especially Northern Ireland, Brittany, and Australia. It is rare in Asia, the Middle East, and most of Africa. Penetrance of clinical haemochromatosis among individuals homozygous for C282Y is age-dependent and incomplete. In the UK, the S65C mutation may be implicated in ~1% of cases of haemochromatosis but appears to be associated with a mild form of HH. A few patients with other disabling mutations in the *HFE* gene have been identified.

In *HFE* C282Y homozygotes, tissue injury from iron overload is unusual before the age of 20 years, unless there has been co-segregation of mutant alleles of other genes implicated in the regulation of iron homeostasis—'digenic inheritance' (see below). If HH is recognized early, before irreversible liver damage, treatment by serial phlebotomy is both straightforward and effective and many of the manifestations of the disease, including fatigue and other non-specific symptoms, are reversible (except arthropathy). It is presumed that when iron depletion is initiated before cirrhosis develops, life expectancy will be near normal. If a late diagnosis is made and irreversible organ damage has resulted, life expectancy is reduced and hepatocellular carcinoma of the liver is a common cause of death.

Haemochromatosis is genetically heterogeneous and, although *HFE* is the most common cause among the Caucasian population, haemochromatosis can also occur due to mutations in the transferrin receptor 2 gene on 7q22 (AR) (type 3); mutations in transferrin receptor 2 occur frequently in certain regions of Italy. Mutations occur in the ferroportin 1 gene (*SLC11A3*) on 2q32 (AD) (type 4). This latter type of haemochromatosis is less frequently associated with visceral injury and excess iron is principally deposited in the mononuclear phagocyte system, and thus prominent in the spleen and bone marrow, rather than the parenchymal cells of the liver, endocrine glands, or the heart. Some of the molecular interactions important in iron homeostasis are shown in Figures 3.14 and 3.15.

- Juvenile haemochromatosis (type 2) is an AR condition of high penetrance in which there is clinical onset between 10 and 30 years of age. Most juvenile-onset cases are caused by homozygous mutation in hemojuvelin (*HJV*) on 1q21. Rare cases of juvenile haemochromatosis are caused by homozygous mutation in the *HAMP* gene on 19q13.1 which encodes hepcidin, a peptide which plays a key role in regulating iron distribution in the body, as well as absorption by the small intestine. Juvenile haemochromatosis is characterized by rapidly progressive CM and hypogonadotrophic hypogonadism; diabetes mellitus and liver disease are often present, but hypogonadism, adrenocortical failure, hypoparathyroidism, and cardiac disease are more prominent than in adult-onset HH and should be evaluated. Digenic inheritance of mutations in *HFE* and *HAMP* can result in either juvenile haemochromatosis or HH, depending upon the severity of the mutation in *HAMP* (Robson *et al.* 2004).
- Neonatal haemochromatosis is largely a gestational alloimmune disorder with fetal liver disease due to activation of the classical complement pathway by maternal antibody and fetal antigen complexes. There are rarer causes such as maternal Parvo, CMV and HSV infection, alloimmunisation due to red blood cell antigens, mitochondrial disease and other rare disorders. Antenatal administration of immunoglobulins from 14 weeks' gestation appears to prevent the development of neonatal haemochromatosis in many subsequent pregnancies (Lopriore 2013).

Clinical approach

Before the consultation, try to confirm the diagnosis in the affected relative and, if possible, determine whether genotyping has been done. Increasingly, genetic testing for haemochromatosis is managed in primary care with guidance from regional genetics services.

History: key points

- Family tree. Estimate the relationship to the proband and the genetic risk, based on a crude carrier rate of 10% (1 in 4 for siblings, 1 in 20 for offspring).
- For siblings, enquire for symptoms of HH. Late features of the disease are well known, e.g. bronzed or slate-grey skin pigmentation, cirrhosis, impotence, lack

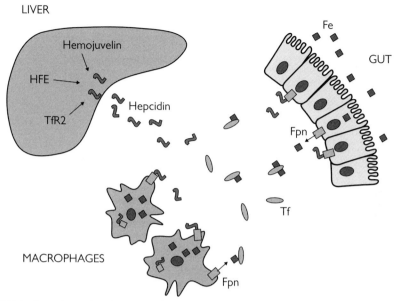

Figure 3.14 Molecular regulation of iron homeostasis. This is maintained by hepcidin, a peptide released by hepatocytes into the circulation under stimulatory control of a common pathway involving HFE, hemojuvelin, and transferrin receptor 2. Hepcidin normally inhibits iron export from enterocytes and macrophages via its interaction with ferroportin. Mutations in haemochromatosis genes reduce hepcidin expression and allow excess iron to enter the plasma compartment and bind to transferrin, with consequent tissue iron loading.
Reproduced with permission from Griffiths WJH and Cox TM. Hereditary haemochromatosis, In Warrell, Cox and Firth, *Oxford Textbook of Medicine*, Fifth Edition, 2010, Figure 12.7.1.4, page 1670, with permission from Oxford University Press.

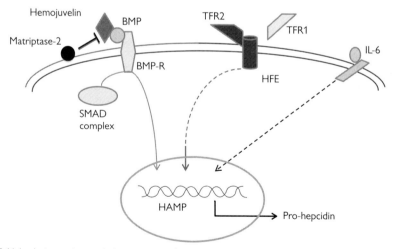

Figure 3.15 Molecular interactions on the hepatocyte membrane in response to iron that coordinate downstream synthesis of hepcidin. Hemojuvelin binds to a bone morphogenetic protein (BMP) receptor complex and signals via SMAD phosphorylation. HFE binds to transferrin receptors as part of an additional signalling mechanism. Mutations in *HJV*, *HFE*, or *TFR2* disrupt hepcidin expression to cause iron overload. Interleukin 6 (IL-6) mediates increased hepcidin production during inflammatory states; iron export from macrophages is reduced via internalization of ferroportin, and anaemia of chronic disease ensues. The serine protease matriptase-2 normally inhibits hemojuvelin binding—recessive mutations in the *TMPRSS6* gene encoding matriptase-2 have been described in humans with iron-refractory iron deficiency anaemia (IRIDA), whereby inappropriately high concentrations of hepcidin are observed.
Reproduced with permission from Griffiths WJH and Cox TM. Hereditary haemochromatosis, In Warrell, Cox and Firth, *Oxford Textbook of Medicine*, Fifth Edition, 2010, Figure 12.7.1.5, with permission from Oxford University Press. Adapted from *Medicine*, 39, W. J. H. Griffiths, 'Haemochromatosis', pp. 597–601. Copyright (2011) with permission from Elsevier.

of libido, premature menopause, and diabetes mellitus, but early features in adults are characteristically non-specific, with fatigue as a prominent symptom:
* weakness and lethargy;
* arthralgia with signs of arthritis, especially IP and MCP joints of hands (especially digits II and III), as well as premature disease of large joints (hip, knee, and shoulder); chondrocalcinosis and crystal arthropathy due to calcium pyrophosphate (pseudogout) are common;
* diabetes mellitus;
* impotence, lack of libido, premature menopause (iron is deposited in the gonadotrophs of the anterior pituitary, as well as other endocrine sites, including the zona glomerulosa of the adrenal and parathyroid glands);
* cardiac arrhythmia (usually atrial fibrillation) and symptomatic of cardiac failure (CM).

Examination: key points
* Hands for arthropathy of small joints.
* Pigmentation (especially shins; note that stigmata of liver disease and coexisting overconsumption of alcohol may also be present).
* Cardiac arrhythmia.
* Signs of hypogonadism with loss of body hair, testicular atrophy, and prominent gynaecomastia in males.
* Signs of cirrhosis—hepatomegaly is frequent and hepatocellular carcinoma may be present at the time of diagnosis.
* Splenomegaly (this is unusual but indicates cirrhosis complicated by portal hypertension).

Special investigations
* DNA sample for genotype for C282Y and H63D mutations in HFE, unless juvenile onset in which case consider mutation analysis of HJV and HAMP.
* Iron studies, including serum iron, ferritin (reflects total body iron stores), and transferrin saturation (best screening test).
* Ferritin. In normal subjects, ferritin concentrations of >200 µg/l for men and post-menopausal women and >200 µg/l for premenopausal women indicate elevated iron stores (levels may vary between different labs). Serum ferritin is an acute phase reactant and so may be raised in intercurrent illness or inflammation; persistent hyperferritinaemia may indicate latent malignancy, including Hodgkin's disease and other lymphomas.
* Transferrin saturation. If transferrin saturation >50%, repeat on a fasting morning sample; serum iron concentrations undergo marked diurnal variation and are highest in the morning. Fasting transferrin saturation >55% (men) and >50% (women) is abnormal and is a surrogate biomarker of haemochromatosis but does not reflect iron deposition. Normal values are 20–40%; carriers may have intermediate levels and genotyping may be helpful in determining the significance. (In exceptional cases, significant tissue iron storage can occur in the absence of an elevated serum ferritin, although in most cases serum transferrin and iron saturation will be elevated.)
* If symptomatic, include measurement of LFTs and glucose, serum vitamin B12, and AFP for primary hepatocellular carcinoma, LH/FSH if impotence/

amenorrhoea, and ECG for patients with a history of palpitations or signs of arrhythmia and echo if there are symptoms of cardiac disease, including heart failure. Refer to the appropriate physician.
* A liver biopsy may be considered for any patient with a raised transferrin saturation, a serum ferritin concentration of >1000 µg/l, and/or evidence of liver damage (hepatomegaly or raised aspartate transaminase (AST) activity). For patients with a raised transferrin saturation, ferritin of <1000 µg/l, no hepatomegaly, and normal AST activity, a biopsy is usually not necessary because the likelihood of hepatic fibrosis or cirrhosis is low. Histological examination of liver tissue obtained by biopsy may have prognostic value.

Genetic advice for HFE
Compound heterozygotes for C282Y/H63D may accumulate iron, but the risk of clinical haemochromatosis is much less than that for C282Y homozygotes.

Inheritance and recurrence risk
AR. The general population allele frequencies for both mutations are high, e.g. 8% for C282Y and 15.7% for H63D in a survey in north-east Scotland. Frequency of heterozygosity for C282Y is 9.6% in whites from the USA, 17.3% in Northern Ireland, 13.2% in New Zealand, 9.6% in northern Germany, and 13.3% in Denmark—overall an approximate 1/10 risk for carrier status in the general population.

Genetic risk to sibs is 1 in 4, to offspring is $(1 \times 1/10 \times 1/2) = 1/20$, to grandchildren is $(1 \times 1/10 \times 1/4) = 1/40$, and to nephews/nieces is $(2/3 \times 1/10 \times 1/4) = 1/60$.

Variability and penetrance
Although HFE is often underdiagnosed, penetrance is incomplete and disease expression is variable, so many of those with genetic predisposition to HFE will never manifest serious clinical features. Males are more often affected than females with a ratio of ~10M:1F. In Beutler et al.'s (2002) large population-based study, the penetrance of haemochromatosis in individuals (average age ~50 years) homozygous for C282Y was <1%. The validity of this study and the population base from which it is drawn is controversial; the real value in Caucasian populations is probably rather higher, say a few per cent. What the comparable penetrance figure is for family members who may share important genetic modifiers is unknown, but it is likely that homozygotes ascertained through cascade screening of families will have a higher penetrance than individuals in the general population. Nevertheless, the penetrance is likely to remain fairly low, even among close family members. Mura et al. (2001) found a lack of correlation of the iron marker status between pairs of sibs homozygous by descent for C282Y, indicating a variable phenotypic expression of iron loading, independent of the HFE genotype.

Prenatal diagnosis
Technically feasible, but rarely requested since this is a treatable condition in which complications are largely preventable and lifespan should be normal with careful monitoring of iron torage and venesection where indicated.

Predictive testing
Appropriate in adult life (see below) to identify which members of a family require regular monitoring of iron status.

Other family members

Offer testing by *HFE* genotyping, transferrin saturation, and serum ferritin concentration to:

- siblings (1 in 4 risk for HH genotype; lower risk for symptomatic disease);
- parents.

In addition, testing should be offered in the following situations.

- If the proband has children, the partner could be offered testing to determine the risk to offspring. There is a 1/10 chance that the partner will carry C282Y and a 1/5 chance that the H63D mutation will be present. If the partner is not a carrier of C282Y or H63D, offspring can be reassured that they are obligate carriers, but not at risk of disease.
- If the proband's partner is not available or declines testing, offer testing to offspring from the age of 15 years (if in their teens or 20s, they may choose to have iron studies only, rather than risk a 'genetic' diagnosis of HH with implications for life insurance, pensions, etc., or since the risk of diagnosis is fairly low at 1/20, they may choose to have genetic testing in an attempt to avoid the need for future screening and evaluation). Some, but not all, insurance companies take the view that HH properly diagnosed and managed does not justify refusal of cover or increased premiums.

The low penetrance of *HFE* makes cascade screening of extended families inappropriate. Risks to second-degree relatives, e.g. grandchildren (1/40 × penetrance of say 5% = 1/800) and nephews/nieces (1/60 × penetrance of say 5% ≤ 1/1000), and third-degree relatives, e.g. cousins, become sufficiently small that systematic iron studies and genetic testing are not indicated.

Natural history and management

For C282Y homozygotes diagnosed with haemochromatosis, the mean age of onset is 44.1 years in males and 49.8 years in females (Mura *et al.* 2001). In homozygotes, serum ferritin rises progressively with age. If patients are diagnosed in the pre-cirrhotic, pre-diabetic stage and treated with venesection to remove excess iron, then life expectancy is normal.

Our practice is to advise all individuals with C282Y/C282Y or C282Y/H63D against taking over-the-counter preparations containing iron, such as multivitamin and mineral supplements, and to avoid a very high dietary intake of iron (red meat, red wine, etc.).

Potential long-term complications

- Liver cirrhosis —with greatly increased risk for hepatocellular carcinoma—irreversible.
- Hepatocellular carcinoma and cholangiocarcinoma are responsible for one-third of deaths from HH. Most of these cancers arise in cirrhotic livers, but they have been reported in non-cirrhotic livers.
- Arthritis is irreversible.
- Congestive CM. Early cardiac changes on echo may improve with venesection or after iron chelation therapy, which may be indicated in severe cases.
- Diabetes mellitus. Non-insulin-dependent diabetes or impaired glucose tolerance may be improved in a small proportion of patients by venesection; insulin-dependent diabetics will remain insulin-dependent.

- Loss of libido and impotence. Hypogonadotrophic hypogonadism may, in its early stages, improve or resolve after iron depletion; androgen augmentation treatment is usually effective Androgen therapy is used by men who have offspring or do not wish to induce pregnancy. While testosterone reverses the symptoms and signs of hypogonadism, at the same time, gonadotrophin-releasing hormone (GnRH) or gonadotrophin therapies are preferred options for men who wish to procreate.

Note there is a strong relationship between porphyria cutanea tarda and HFE, and this is compounded by 'environmental' factors such as oestrogen therapy, alcohol, and hepatitis C and human immunodeficiency viral infections.

Surveillance

- Repeat normal iron studies in homozygotes every 3 years in males, and every 5 years in females and compound heterozygotes (C282Y/H63D), with referral for specialist assessment if results indicate iron overload.
- Proven heterozygotes do not require repeated measures of iron status if initial studies are normal.

Treatment

For individuals with HH who have already accumulated excess iron, the usual treatment is weekly venesection. Once excess iron has been removed, the transferrin saturation should be maintained below 50% and the serum ferritin at <40 μg/l, which can usually be achieved on a programme of venesection in which one unit (568 ml) of whole blood is removed 2–4 times per year; this is the equivalent of an annual total of ~0.55–1.14 g of elemental iron, but venesection induces a state of enhanced compensatory absorption of iron from dietary sources, so that continued monitoring of serum parameters of iron status and end-organ function is advisable. In the long-term management of patients with haemochromatosis, clinical and radiological evaluation of liver structure and function with endocrine status is advisable; since only small hepatocellular carcinomas and cholangiocarcinomas are suitable for operative treatment; regular hepatic imaging studies by USS and, if necessary, MRI (which can detect increased ferromagnetic signals) are useful for assessing any clinical deterioration, especially in patients with known cirrhosis. Where relevant, patients with established haemochromatosis should be advised to restrict their consumption of alcohol and preferably abstain. To reduce re-accumulation of toxic iron, frequent consumption of dark meats and gratuitous supplementation of vitamin/mineral preparations containing iron and vitamin C is best avoided.

Support groups: The Haemochromatosis Society, http://haemochromatosis.org.uk, Hollybush House, Hadley Green Road, Barnet, EN5 5PR, Fax: 44 (0) 208 449 1363, email: info@haemochromatosis.org.uk; Hemochromatosis.org, http://www.hemochromatosis.org.

Expert adviser: Timothy M. Cox, Director of Research and Professor of Medicine Emeritus,

University of Cambridge, Addenbrooke's Hospital, Cambridge, UK.

References

Andrews NC. Forging a field: the golden age of iron biology. *Blood* 2008; **112**: 219–30.

Beutler E, Felitti VJ, Koziol JA, Ho NJ, Gelbart T. Penetrance of 845GIA (C282Y) HFE hereditary haematomatosis mutation in the USA. *Lancet* 2002; **359**: 211–18.

British Committee on Standards in Haematology. *Guideline on haemochromatosis*, 2000. http://www.bcshguidelines.com.

Camaschella C. Treating iron overload. *N Engl J Med* 2013; **368**: 2325–7.

Camaschella C, Roetto A, Gobbi M. Genetic haemochromatosis: genes and mutations associated with iron loading. *Best Pract Res Clin Haematol* 2002; **15**: 261–76.

D'Alessio F, Hentze MW, Muckenthaler MU. The hemochromatosis proteins HFE, TfR2, and HJV form a membrane-associated protein complex for hepcidin regulation. *J Hepatol* 2012; **57**: 1052–60.

Dooley JS, Walker AP, Macfarlane B, Worwood M. Genetic haemochromatosis. Report of a meeting of physicians and scientists at the Royal Free Hospital School of Medicine. *Lancet* 1997; **347**: 1688–93.

Dooley J, Wowood M. *Genetic haemochromatosis. British Committee for Standards in Haematology. Guideline on diagnosis and therapy*. British Society for Haematology, London, 2000.

Haddow JE, Bradley LA. Hereditary haemochromatosis: to screen or not. Conditions for screening are not yet fulfilled. *BMJ* 1999; **319**: 531–2.

Kanwar P, Kowdley KV. Diagnosis and treatment of hereditary hemochromatosis: an update. *Expert Rev Gastroenterol Hepatol* 2013; **7**: 517–30.

Kelly AL, Lunt PW, et al. Classification and genetic features of neonatal haemochromatosis: a study of 27 affected pedigrees and molecular analysis of genes implicated in iron metabolism. *J Med Genet* 2001; **38**(9): 599–610.

Lopriore E, Mearin ML et al. Neonatal hemochromatosis: management, outcome, and prevention. *Prenat Diagn* 2013; **33**: 1221–5.

Miedzybrodzka Z, Loughlin S, Baty D, et al. Haemochromatosis mutation in North-East Scotland. *Br J Haematol* 1999; **106**: 385–7.

Mura C, Le Gac G, Scotet V, Raguenes O, Mercier AY, Férec C. Variation of iron loading expression in C282Y homozygous haemochromatosis probands and sib pairs. *J Med Genet* 2001; **38**: 632–6.

Pietrangelo A. Medical progress: hereditary haemochromatosis—a new look at an old disease [review]. *N Engl J Med* 2004; **350**: 2383–97.

Robson KJ, Merryweather-Clarke AT, Cadet E, et al. Recent advances in understanding haemochromatosis: a transition state. *J Med Genet* 2004; **41**: 721–30.

Worwood M. Inherited iron loading: genetic testing in diagnosis and management. *Blood Rev* 2005; **19**: 69–88.

Haemoglobinopathies

Haemoglobinopathies are the most common single gene disorders in the world population, with ~7% of the population being carriers. An estimated 300 000 babies are born each year with a severe inherited disease of haemoglobin and >80% of these births occur in low- or middle-income countries (Weatherall 2011). The incidence of the various haemoglobinopathies varies enormously in different population groups, so that detailed knowledge of your patient's ethnic background is often extremely helpful.

Haemoglobin (Hb) is a tetramer composed of two different pairs of globin chains. Adult Hbs are HbA ($\alpha_2\beta_2$), HbA$_2$ ($\alpha_2\delta_2$), and HbF ($\alpha_2\gamma_2$). The α-globin chains are present in both fetal and adult Hb, so severe homozygous forms of α-thalassaemia cause IUD or neonatal death. β-chain abnormalities do not become clinically significant until Hb synthesis switches from HbF to HbA in early infancy. There are two α-globin genes in tandem array on chromosome 16 (normal genotype: $\alpha\alpha/\alpha\alpha$). The β-like globin cluster is on chromosome 11 and contains one β-, two γ-, and one δ-globin gene (normal β-genotype: β/β). Therefore α-globin gene defects can be co-inherited with β-globin gene defects.

There are two main types of haemoglobinopathy: (1) disorders caused by structural variant Hbs, e.g. sickle-cell anaemia; and (2) disorders in which there is a reduced rate of production of one or more of the globin chains, e.g. thalassaemia. Heterozygotes are often referred to as 'trait' and homozygotes as 'disease'. Several disorders result from the inheritance of the sickle-cell gene, together with different forms of thalassaemia (β- and $\delta\beta-$) or other structural variants.

Structural variants

Structural variants are named after letters of the alphabet (e.g. S, C, D, E) or places where they were discovered (e.g. Zurich, Constant Spring). More than 750 abnormal Hbs have been characterized, the majority comprising α- and β-chain variants. The majority are clinically silent and do not cause any disease. However, a number have altered properties, either being unstable, having a higher oxygen affinity (resulting in polycythaemia), a lower oxygen affinity (resulting in cyanosis in some cases), reduced synthesis (resulting in thalassaemia), or altered solubility, e.g. HbS.

Most variants have a single amino acid replacement due to a point mutation. For example, HbS differs from HbA due to a missense mutation in the β-globin gene E6V (glutamic acid at amino acid 6 is changed to valine). This substitution alters the solubility of the Hb molecule in the deoxygenated state, resulting in aggregation, with consequent sickling of the red cell. Sickled red cells have increased fragility and shortened survival, leading to chronic haemolytic anaemia. The sickled red cells can themselves aggregate in the microvasculature, leading to a thrombotic crisis.

HEREDITARY PERSISTENCE OF FETAL HEMOGLOBIN (HPFH). In this AD condition, expression of the γ-globin gene of HbF persists at high levels in adult erythroid cells. Increased levels of fetal hemoglobin (HbF) ameliorate the clinical course of inherited disorders of β-globin gene expression such as β-thalassemia and sickle-cell anaemia. In vitro research is exploring the potential for induction of HbF genes in postnatal life as a potential therapy for β-globin disorders.

Hb electrophoresis

See Table 3.17 for normal red cell indices and those for some haemoglobinopathies.

- In normal adults, ~97% of Hb is HbA, 0–3.5% HbA$_2$, and 0–1% HbF.
- In α-thalassaemia, Hb electrophoresis is normal. DNA analysis is required to make the diagnosis.
- In β-thalassaemia trait, HbA$_2$ is >3.5% (usually 4–6%; but not in the presence of iron deficiency), with a slight elevation of HbF to 1–3% in some. A few mutations are associated with borderline normal HbA$_2$ values of 3.3–3.8% (normal HbA$_2$ β-thalassaemia) and a few very rare ones with borderline normal HbA$_2$ values and normal red cell indices (silent β-thalassaemia). In homozygous $\beta°$-thalassaemia, there is no HbA—only HbF and HbA$_2$. In homozygous $\beta°$-thalassaemia, HbF is almost 100% and HbA$_2$ is usually normal.
- Most Hb variants have been detected by electrophoretic methods due to the variant having a change in electric charge. For example, HbS migrates differently from HbA and appears as a distinct band (heterozygotes have both HbA and HbS; those with sickle-cell disease have HbS and no HbA and a variable amount of HbF).
- In HbSC disease, HbS and HbC are present in approximately equal proportions.
- In HbC disease, HbC is present with small amounts of HbF and no HbA.

Clinical approach

History: key points
- Three-generation family tree, with specific enquiry about ethnic origin and consanguinity. Specific detail about the country of origin of relatives can be very helpful.
- Enquire about previous pregnancies and miscarriages.

Investigations
- FBC with red cell indices.
- Hb electrophoresis.
- Sickle test if indicated by ethnic background.
- DNA for molecular studies where indicated, e.g. diagnosis of α-thalassaemia carrier status, or to permit future PND for α- or β-thalassaemia or structural variants, e.g. HbS, HbC.

Specific diagnoses/conditions to consider

Sickling disorders
Frequent in African black populations and commonly throughout the Mediterranean and Middle East. Occur in some parts of India, but *not* in South East Asia. The heterozygous state for sickle cell may confer resistance to malaria. It should be noted that the term 'sickle-cell disease' is often used to describe a similar phenotype that is seen with any of several genotypes (SS, SC, S/β-thalassaemia, S/D Punjab, or S/O Arab).

SICKLE-CELL ANAEMIA (GENOTYPE β^S/β^S). The clinical course is extremely variable, ranging from crippling haemolytic anaemia with frequent crises to mild disorder.

Table 3.17 Normal red cell indices and red cell indices for some haemoglobinopathies*

	Hb (g/dl)	MCH (pg)	MCV (fl)	HbA₂ (%)	HbF (%)
Normal red cell indices					
Male	13–17	27–32	82–102	0–3.5	0–1
Female	12–16	27–32	82–102	0–3.5	0–1
Typical red cell indices for some haemoglobinopathies					
α⁺-thalassaemia trait	11–16	24–28	75–90	1.5–3.0	0–1
Homozygous α⁺-thalassaemia	11–16	21–24	68–76	1.5–3.0	0–1
α°-thalassaemia trait	11–15	20–23	65–75	1.5–3.0	0–1
HbH disease	8–11	17–21	55–70	1–2	0–1
β-thalassaemia trait	8–16	18–25	63–80	3.5–7	0–8
Normal α₂β-thalassaemia	12–16	23–26	67–79	3.3–3.8	0–2
Silent β-thalassaemia	12–16	27–29	80–90	3.3–3.8	0–2
Thalassaemia intermedia	5–13	14–22	50–85	1–7	5–100
Thalassaemia major	2–7	12–18	50–60	1–7	15–100
HbE/β-thalassaemia	5–10	16–23	61–75	3.5–8	5–85
AS	12–16	26–32	80–95	3.0–5.0	0.5–1.5
SS (African)	6–10	26–32	80–95	1.5–3.5	5–10
SS (Arab–Indian)	8–10	26–32	80–95	1.5–5	10–25
S/β°	7–11	18–25	60–80	3.5–6	5–15
S/β°	9–11	20–25	65–80	3.5–6	5–15
S/δβ°	10–12	20–25	65–80	1.5–2.5	10–25
S/HPFH	12–16	24–30	68–88	1–2	20–35

* HPFH, hereditary persistence of fetal haemoglobin; MCH, mean corpuscular haemoglobin; MCV, mean corpuscular volume.

It usually presents in infancy with jaundice and anaemia from about 3 months of age. Hb is typically 6–8 g/dl; transfusion is not usually required. Crises due to blockage of vessels by sickled erythrocytes may cause infarction of bone and bone marrow, abdominal pain, chest syndrome (shortness of breath, pleuritic chest pain, and fever), and neurological syndrome (TIAs and strokes). Crises may be precipitated by infection or dehydration, but often no precipitant is identified. Repeated splenic infarction in early childhood makes children vulnerable to infection, and prophylactic penicillin reduces early mortality. In the long term, avascular necrosis of the hip, renal impairment, and ischaemia of the retinal vasculature may occur. A study based on survival of >3000 patients attending a Jamaican clinic estimated median survival for men at 53 years and for women at 58.5 years. Patients from the Eastern Province of Saudi Arabia and central India have higher HbF levels and a milder clinical course than patients of African origin.

SICKLE-CELL TRAIT (βˢ/β). Normal FBC. Diagnose by positive sickling test and Hb electrophoresis demonstrating HbA and HbS (34–40%). NB. The co-inheritance of alpha-thalassaemia causes reduced red cell indices and lowers the percentage of HbS to 29–34% for αα/α– and to 24–28% for α–/α– genotypes. Asymptomatic, except in conditions of extreme anoxia. It is possible for heterozygotes to suffer from vaso-occlusive episodes if they become unusually hypoxic during anaesthesia. Apart from advice about anaesthaesia and avoidance of unpressurized aircraft or deep-sea diving, individuals with sickle trait require no treatment.

HAEMOGLOBIN SC DISEASE (βˢ/βᶜ). Relatively common in West Africa, e.g. Ghana. Characterized by a milder anaemia than sickle-cell anaemia (SS) and may be undiagnosed until adult life when patients present with one of the complications. Aseptic necrosis of the femoral head and unexplained haematuria are common complications. Widespread thrombosis may occur in pregnancy/puerperium or during an intercurrent infection. Infarction of the retinal vasculature may lead to retinitis proliferans with retinal detachment and loss of vision.

HAEMOGLOBIN C DISEASE (βᶜ/βᶜ). The homozygous state for HbC is characterized by mild haemolytic anaemia with splenomegaly. Film shows 100% target cells. This is a mild disorder for which no treatment is required.

β-thalassaemias

These produce severe anaemia in their homozygous and compound heterozygous states. They occur widely in a broad belt stretching from the Mediterranean and parts of North and West Africa through the Middle East and India to South East Asia including the Balkans and southern parts of Russia and southern China (see Figure 3.16). Some mutations are inactivating (β°) and others cause reduced levels of β-globin synthesis (β⁺).

HOMOZYGOUS β-THALASSAEMIA (β°/β°, β°/β⁺, β⁺/β⁺). Most homozygous β°-thalassaemia presents in the first year with failure to thrive and intermittent bouts of fever. Hb at presentation ranges from 2 to 8 g/dl. If regular transfusion is instigated, development progresses reasonably normally until puberty when side effects of secondary haemochromatosis become apparent with

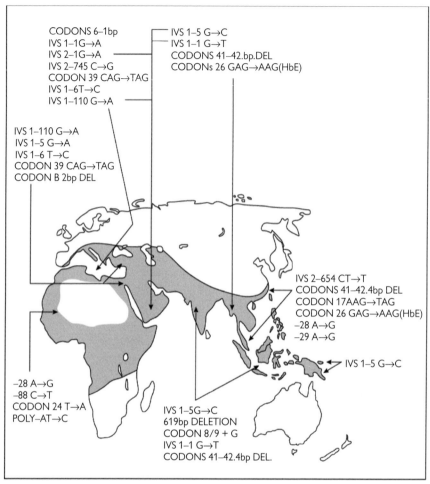

CODONS 6–1bp
IVS 1–1G→A
IVS 2–1G→A
IVS 2–745 C→G
CODON 39 CAG→TAG
IVS 1–6T→C
IVS 1–110 G→A

IVS 1–5 G→C
IVS 1–1 G→T
CODONS 41–42.bp.DEL
CODONs 26 GAG→AAG(HbE)

IVS 1–110 G→A
IVS 1–5 G→A
IVS 1–6 T→C
CODON 39 CAG→TAG
CODON B 2bp DEL

IVS 2–654 CT→T
CODONS 41–42.4bp DEL
CODON 17AAG→TAG
CODON 26 GAG→AAG(HbE)
–28 A→G
–29 A→G

IVS 1–5 G→C

–28 A→G
–88 C→T
CODON 24 T→A
POLY–AT→C

IVS 1–5G→C
619bp DELETION
CODON 8/9 + G
IVS 1–1 G→T
CODONS 41–42.4bp DEL.

Figure 3.16 Map showing the distribution of the different β-thalassaemia mutations.
Reproduced with permission from Weatherall DJ. Disorders of the synthesis or function of haemoglobin, In David A. Warrell, Timothy M. Cox, and John D. Firth, *Oxford Textbook of Medicine*, Fifth edition, 2010, Figure 22.5.7.4, page 4425, with permission from Oxford University Press.

lack of secondary sexual characteristics and short stature. In the absence of intensive iron chelation therapy, death usually occurs in the late teens or 20s due to progressive cardiac damage from iron overload. However, with regular transfusion and compliance with optimal iron chelation therapy, life expectancy improves considerably and patients can survive to their third or fourth decade with a good quality of life.

A few β+-thalassaemia mutations have a milder phenotype than the majority of β° and β+ mutations. Homozygotes for these mutations have a milder condition called *thalassaemia intermedia*. Patients have an Hb of 6–9 g/dl, splenomegaly, and some bone deformities, but are not dependent on regular transfusions for survival. Thalassaemia intermedia is caused by a wide range of different genotypes, e.g. homozygous delta β-thalassaemia, and by the co-inheritance of ameliorating factors, e.g. homozygous β-thalassaemia with co-inherited α-thalassaemia.

HETEROZYGOUS β°-THALASSAEMIA (β/β°) AND HETEROZYGOUS BETA+-THALASSAEMIA (β/β+). Carriers for β-thalassaemia are usually asymptomatic, except in periods of stress such as pregnancy when they may become anaemic. Life expectancy is normal. Hb is 9–11 g/dl with hypochromia and microcytosis and low MCV and MCH. A heterozygous state for β-thalassaemia may mask a coexistent carrier state for α-thalassaemia (the latter is usually characterized by microcytosis and reduced MCH, which may be attributed to the β-thalassaemia trait).

α-thalassaemias
These are more common than the β-thalassaemias but pose less of a health problem, as the homozygous forms of the severe types (α°-thalassaemias) are lethal. They occur widely throughout the Mediterranean, parts of West Africa, the Middle East, parts of India, and throughout South East Asia. The most serious forms of α-thalassaemia are restricted to some of the Mediterranean

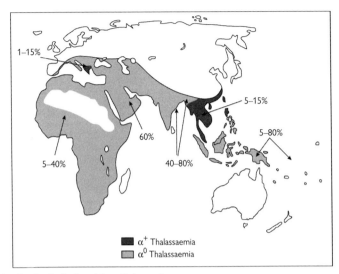

Figure 3.17 Map showing the distribution of the α-thalassaemias.
Reproduced with permission from Weatherall DJ. Disorders of the synthesis or function of haemoglobin, In David A. Warrell, Timothy M. Cox, and John D. Firth, *Oxford Textbook of Medicine*, Fifth edition, 2010, Figure 22.5.7.14, page 4431, with permission from Oxford University Press, Oxford.

island populations (e.g. Cyprus) and South East Asia (see Figure 3.17).

Heterozygotes are of two main types: α° in which both α genes on one chromosome 16 are deleted (αα/− −) and α⁺ in which there is a deletion or mutation in only one of the two tandem α-globin genes (αα/α− or αα/αᵀα). (See Figure 3.18 for the genetics of α-thalassaemia.)

HOMOZYGOUS α°-THALASSAEMIA (HAEMOGLOBIN BART'S HYDROPS FETALIS SYNDROME) (− −/− −). Common cause of fetal loss throughout South East Asia and also in Greece and Cyprus. Affected infants produce no α chains and so are unable to make HbA or HbF. Usually stillborn in the third trimester (their fetal blood is 80% Hb Bart's, i.e. β-globin tetramers and 20% embryonic Hb). High risk of pre-eclampsia (PET) and other obstetric problems due to an enlarged placenta.

HBH DISEASE (α−/− −). Usually compound heterozygotes for α° and α⁺. Absence of three α genes leads to formation of β-globin tetramers. Microcytic anaemia with Hb 7–10 g/dl. Splenomegaly is common and haemolytic crises may occur in response to infection. Most patients survive to adulthood, but life expectancy is shortened.

α-THALASSAEMIA HOMOZYGOTE (α−/α−); α HETEROZYGOTE (αα/− −); α⁺-THALASSAEMIA HETEROZYGOTE (αα/α−). α⁺ homozygotes and α° heterozygotes are well, with a mild microcytic hypochromic anaemia; α⁺ heterozygotes are well with a normal Hb level, but mild microcytosis and hypochromia.

Thalassaemias with variant haemoglobins

SICKLE-CELL β°-THALASSAEMIA (β^s/β°) OR SICKLE-CELL β⁺-THALASSAEMIA (β^s/β⁺). Variable phenotype. In Mediterranean populations where one parent may have β° and the other β^s, the picture is one of sickle-cell disease. In African blacks, several mild forms of β⁺-thalassaemia are commonly found that, when they interact with β^s, produce a condition with mild anaemia and few sickling crises and normal life expectancy.

HbS also interacts with delta β-thalassaemia to produce sickle-cell disease, in contrast to the interaction of HbS with HPFH where patients are clinically normal.

HAEMOGLOBIN C β-THALASSAEMIA (β^c/β° OR β^c/β⁺). Found in West Africans and some North African and Southern Mediterranean populations. Mild haemolytic anaemia associated with splenomegaly. Hb electrophoresis shows mainly HbC.

HAEMOGLOBIN E β-THALASSAEMIA (β^E/β° OR β^E/β⁺). The most common severe form of thalassaemia in South East Asia and India. The majority of the β-thalassaemia alleles commonly found with HbE are the β° or the severe β⁺ type. HbE is inefficiently synthesized and, when co-inherited with a β°-thalassaemia allele, there is marked deficiency in β-chain production and a picture that can be similar to that of homozygous β°-thalassaemia.

Genetic advice

Inheritance and recurrence risk

• Sickle-cell disease and other structural variants. AR, with 25% sibling recurrence risk.
• Thalassaemias. AR, with 25% sibling recurrence risk.
• Beware the possibility of interaction of thalassaemia with variant Hbs.
• Beware the possibility that the β-thalassaemia trait may mask a coexistent α-thalassaemia trait.

Variability and penetrance
See text concerning individual conditions.

Prenatal diagnosis
Always test both parents to define their genotype before embarking on PND. PND by CVS at 11 weeks' gestation is available if mutations have been identified in both parents. PGD is available in some centres for sickle-cell anaemia and thalassaemia and should be discussed where available. See 'Assisted reproductive technology:

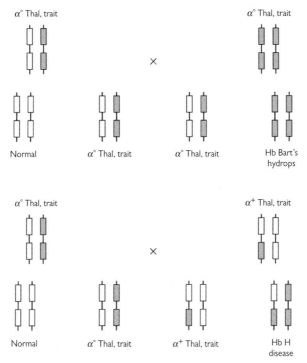

Figure 3.18 The genetics of α-thalassaemia. The black α genes represent gene deletions or otherwise inactivated genes. The open α genes represent normal genes. α°-thalassaemia and α⁺-thalassaemia are defined in the text.
Reproduced with permission from Weatherall DJ. Disorders of the synthesis or function of haemoglobin, In David A. Warrell, Timothy M. Cox, and John D. Firth, *Oxford Textbook of Medicine*, Fifth edition, 2010, Figure 22.5.7.16, page 4432, with permission from Oxford University Press.

in vitro fertilization (IVF), intracytoplasmic sperm injection (ICSI), and pre-implantation genetic diagnosis (PGD)' in Chapter 6, 'Pregnancy and fertility', p. 706.

Carrier testing
Carrier testing is appropriate in the following circumstances:
- if there is a significant incidence of haemoglobinopathy in individuals of a given ethnic group;
- if a partner has a known haemoglobinopathy, the other partner should be tested, even if they are from a low-risk group (since haemoglobinopathies can occur at a very low incidence in most populations).

Other family members
Cascade testing of families and partners should be offered.

Natural history and management

Potential long-term complications
See individual conditions.

Surveillance
Refer affected individuals to a haematologist.

New therapies
Stem cell or bone marrow transplantation may be a potential option for some children with thalassaemia major or sickle cell disease (Angelucci *et al.* 2014).

Support groups: UK Thalassaemia Society, http://www.ukts.org; Sickle Cell Society, http://sicklecellsociety.org; Advice for carriers, http://www.chime.ucl.ac.uk/APoGI/menu.htm.

Expert adviser: Swee-Lay Thein, Senior Investigator, Sickle Cell Branch, National Heart, Lung and Blood Institute, NIH, Bethesda, MD, USA.

References

Angelucci E, Matthes-Martin S, *et al.* Hematopoietic stem cell transplantation in thalassemia major and sickle cell disease: indications and management recommendations from an international expert panel. *Haematologica* 2014; **99**(5): 811–20.

Forger BG. Molecular basis of hereditary persistence of fetal hemoglobin. *Ann N Y Acad Sci* 1998; **850**: 38–44.

Higgs DR. The molecular basis of α-thalassemia. *Cold Spring Harb Perspect Med* 2013; **3**: a011718.

Stuart MJ, Nagel RL. Sickle-cell disease. *Lancet* 2004; **364**: 1343–60.

Weatherall D. The inherited disorders of haemoglobin: an increasingly neglected global health burden. *Indian J Med Res* 2011; **134**: 493–97.

Weatherall DJ. Disorders of the synthesis or function of haemoglobin. In: DA Warrell, TM Cox, JD Firth (eds.). Oxford textbook of medicine, 4th edn, pp. 676–95. Oxford University Press, Oxford, 2003.

Wierenga KJ, Hambleton IR, Lewis NA. Survival estimates for patients with homozygous sickle-cell disease in Jamaica: a clinic-based population study. *Lancet* 2001; **357**: 680–3.

Haemophilia and other inherited coagulation disorders

The geneticist's main role is to clarify the nature of the bleeding disorder in the family, to determine its severity, and to assess the level of risk to the consultand. Of the families we have encountered in clinic who were referred with a family history of 'haemophilia', only ~50% actually had a relative with factor VIII or factor IX deficiency. Other diagnoses that have emerged during further investigation included von Willebrand disease (vWD) and factor XI deficiency. Consultands or their families may have links with one or more haemophilia centres; it is important for geneticists to collaborate closely with haemophilia centre staff.

Haemophilia A (factor VIII deficiency) and haemophilia B (factor IX deficiency or Christmas disease) are clinically indistinguishable. The incidence of haemophilia A is one in 5000 male births and that of haemophilia B is one in 30 000 male births. Females with disadvantageous X-inactivation may have mild haemophilia, but severe disease is rare in females unless there is extreme skewing of X-inactivation or the girl has TS or the child has a father who is a haemophiliac and a mother who is a carrier. Bleeding occurs in haemophilia owing to failure of secondary haemostasis. Primary haemostasis (formation of a platelet plug) occurs normally, but stabilization of the plug by fibrin is defective because inadequate amounts of thrombin are generated. The type and severity of haemophilia run true in families. There is no known family history in approximately one-third of haemophiliacs. The classification of haemophilia is outlined in Table 3.18.

Factor VIII—haemophilia A

The factor VIII gene is located on Xq28 and consists of 26 exons. Forty-five per cent of patients with severe haemophilia A have an inversion in intron 22 that disrupts the factor VIII gene. This mutation arises almost exclusively in the male germline. Other mutations are predominantly point mutations (85% missense, 15% nonsense), with about 5% being large or small deletions and insertions. Approximately 2% of patients with severe haemophilia A do not have a detectable mutation on sequencing of the factor VIII gene.

A proportion of patients who make no, or virtually no, native factor VIII protein will produce antibodies in response to treatment with exogenous factor (inhibitors), currently estimated at about 25% of people with severe haemophilia A. This can significantly complicate treatment. Haemophilia A patients carrying the intron 22 inversion, large deletions, or nonsense mutations have an ~35% incidence of inhibitors (antibodies that inactivate factor VIII), whereas those with missense mutations and small deletions have an ~5% risk. Overall, ~10% of patients with haemophilia A develop inhibitors.

Factor IX—haemophilia B

The factor IX gene is located on Xq27 and consists of eight exons. The vast majority of mutations are point mutations ~67% missense, with ~7% short insertions or deletions and 3% large-scale gene deletions or complex rearrangements. Mutations in the promoter region cause the unusual factor IX Leiden phenotype. Usually endogenous factor IX (and factor VIII) levels do not change significantly with age, but, in those with a factor IX Leiden mutation, the factor IX concentration rises with hormonal changes at puberty. Severe haemophiliacs become mild, and mild haemophiliacs may produce normal or near normal amounts of factor IX.

In haemophilia B, patients with gene deletions or rearrangements have a risk of inhibitor development (see above) of ~50%, whereas for frameshift, premature stop, or splice site mutations, the risk is ~20%. Those with missense mutations almost never develop inhibitors. In general, inhibitors are much less common in haemophilia B than in haemophilia A.

Clinical approach

History: key points

- Three-generation family history, with specific enquiry regarding bleeding disorders; ask about joint bleeding and injury-related bleeding. For milder disorders, it is particularly helpful to ask if anyone has bled after surgery, e.g. dental extractions or tonsillectomy. Extend the family tree further if other affected relatives are known.
- Detailed history of the proband. Try to clarify the type of bleeding disorder (factor VIII, factor IX, vWD, etc.). Try to assess the level of severity. Factor VIII injections? Joint injury from haemarthroses, etc.? Try to establish which haemophilia centre the affected individual attends.

Examination: key points

Usually not relevant (joint arthropathy in severe haemophilia).

Investigations

When the diagnosis in the proband is certain:

- specific factor level, e.g. factor VIII level if the family history is of haemophilia A, factor IX level for a family history of haemophilia B (but note that some family members do not know which type of haemophilia it is);
- DNA (EDTA sample) for molecular diagnosis if a familial mutation known or for linkage.

When the diagnosis in the proband is uncertain (involve a haematologist):

- FBC for platelet count;

Table 3.18 Classification of haemophilia

Severity of haemophilia	Concentration of factor VIIIC or IXC	Clinical features
Mild	5–40% (>0.05–0.40 iu/ml)	Spontaneous bleeding does not occur; excessive bleeding after surgery, dental extractions, and accidents
Moderate	1–5% (0.01–0.05 iu/ml)	Bleeding into joints and muscles after minor injuries; excessive bleeding after surgery and dental extractions
Severe	<1% (<0.01 iu/ml)	Spontaneous joint and muscle bleeding; bleeding after injuries, accidents, and surgery

- coagulation screen (prothrombin time (PT), activated partial thromboplastin time (APTT)). Note that a normal screen does not rule out vWD or some other disorders;
- von Willebrand factor antigen (VWF:Ag);
- ristocetin cofactor (vWF:RiCof)—a functional assessment of vWF;
- specific factor levels, e.g. factor VIII or IX;
- consider DNA storage (EDTA sample) for future studies.

Other diagnoses/conditions to consider

von Willebrand disease (vWD)
Deficiency or dysfunction of the adhesive glycoprotein von Willebrand factor (vWF). vWF protects factor VIII from premature proteolytic degradation and concentrates it at sites of vascular injury. vWD is common, with incidence figures varying between 0.1% and 1%. There are several different subtypes of vWD, but the phenotype is usually relatively mild. Mucosal bleeding predominates, but it is also an important cause of menorrhagia in affected families. vWD is not clearly AD; the inheritance is more variable and there is a strong school of opinion that the common mild type I may be related to genetic or environmental influences, independent of the vWF (e.g. blood group).

Factor VII deficiency
An AR disorder affecting 1/500 000, located on chromosome 13.

Factor X deficiency
An AR disorder affecting 1/100 000, located on chromosome 13.

Factor XI deficiency (previously called haemophilia C)
An autosomally inherited disorder affecting 1/1 000 000. The gene for factor XI is located on chromosome 4. In most cases, a mild bleeding disorder. Heterozygotes may have a bleeding tendency that is poorly related to the factor XI level. Factor XI deficiency is particularly common in Ashkenazi where 1/190 have a severe deficiency and 8% (~1/12) of the population are carriers.

Other coagulation factor deficiencies
Congenital deficiencies can occur in any of the coagulation factors, but all are rare. Inheritance is autosomal, with these disorders being more common in racial groups where cousin marriages occur. This includes type III vWD. Such disorders should be discussed with a haemophilia specialist.

Genetic advice
Inheritance and recurrence risk
XLR.

FACTOR VIII DEFICIENCY. Mutations originate ~3 times more often in males than in females. This implies that 80% of mothers of an isolated patient are expected to be haemophilia carriers.

Variability and penetrance
Haemophilia is fully penetrant. It runs true in families, so if one relative has 'mild' disease, other affected relatives will also be likely to be mildly affected. Similarly for severe disease.

Prenatal diagnosis
This is usually only considered for severe haemophilia. Most patients with mild haemophilia enjoy a normal lifestyle, with appropriate advice about management of trauma or major surgery. Possible by CVS at 11 weeks'

gestation if a familial mutation known or by linkage. PGD with selection of female embryos may be another option to consider.

Predictive testing
Testing of cord blood of 'at-risk' males is indicated to guide future management.

Other family members
Carrier testing of female relatives is often problematic, unless the familial mutation is known. Only a proportion of carriers, about a third, have factor levels below the normal range. A reproducibly normal result does not exclude carrier status. Linked markers may be helpful in excluding carrier status or in identifying the 'high-risk' X. Some carrier females have low concentrations of factor VIIIC or IXC that can predispose to excessive bleeding, with levels in the mild haemophilia range. Factor concentrations should therefore be measured in girls and women who are definite or possible carriers. Mutation testing to determine carrier status is usually deferred until the mid teens when a girl is able to engage actively in the testing process.

Natural history and management
People with bleeding disorders should be referred to a haemophilia centre for registration, advice, and management of bleeding episodes. Haemophilia care in the UK is provided by a network of specialist centres and coordinated by the UK Haemophilia Centre Doctor's Organisation (UKHCDO) which provides relevant protocols and guidelines for management.

- Factor concentrates are the treatment of choice for people with severe and moderate haemophilia A or B.
- Plasma-derived factors. During the 1980s, production of factor concentrates from pooled plasma resulted in a large number of haemophiliacs acquiring one or more of hepatitis B, hepatitis C, and HIV. Virus inactivation procedures are currently used in product manufacture, but concerns remain about prions (e.g. new variant CJD). Hepatitis B can be prevented by immunization.
- Recombinant products are the treatment of choice. In the UK, all patients have been transferred to recombinant products, although some patients with severe factor IX deficiency prefer a plasma-derived product. New recombinant products are likely to have longer half-lives.
- DDAVP (1-deamino-8-D-arginine vasopressin). In mildly affected patients with haemophilia A and mild vWD (some subtypes), it is often possible to use DDAVP, instead of factor VIII concentrate. Patients with severe vWD require factor concentrates containing vWF; these are plasma-derived.

Potential long-term complications
- Complications of the disorder. Recurrent joint bleeding with inadequate treatment in severe haemophilia leads to chronic arthropathy, pain, and loss of function which may lead to crippling. Death from bleeding (e.g. intracranial haemorrhage) may occur.
- Complications related to treatment:
  - transfusion-transmitted infections, e.g. hepatitis B, hepatitis C, HIV (risk is very much reduced with virally inactivated concentrates; risk thought to be eliminated with recombinant products);
  - development of antibodies (inhibitors).

Surveillance

Guidelines for the management of pregnancy in carriers for haemophilia (from Chalmers *et al.* 2011 and Lee *et al.* 2006) are as follows.

- All patients should have a written management plan shared between the obstetrician, midwives, GP, haematologist, paediatrician, and the mother.
- Baseline factor VIII or IX level should be checked at booking and at 28 and 34 weeks' gestation.
- Fetal sex should be determined e.g. by NIPT and/or USS and the obstetrician informed prior to delivery. In many centres, fetal sexing can be performed by testing maternal blood for Y chromosome-specific sequences (NIPD).
- The mode of delivery should be informed by both obstetric and haemostatic factors; haemophilia carrier status itself is not a contraindication to vaginal delivery, but this is a controversial area.
- If required, a Caesarean section may be carried out without haemostatic support if the maternal factor level is >50 iu/dl or 50% of normal.
- Epidural anaesthaesia is permitted if the factor level is >50 iu/dl or 40% of normal.
- The use of invasive fetal monitoring techniques, such as fetal scalp electrodes or the collection of fetal scalp vein samples, should be avoided during the delivery of affected males (or if the status of a male infant is unknown).
- Vacuum extraction (ventouse delivery) *should be avoided*. Use of forceps is not contraindicated, but particular care is required, and if the child proves to be affected, coagulation factor treatment will be required after delivery.
- A cord blood sample should be taken immediately after delivery for testing for haemophilia.
- Vitamin K should *not* be given by IM injection until the result is known (can be given orally).
- The use of coagulation factor concentrates to a haemophiliac neonate after a normal vaginal delivery

is controversial but is recommended if there is any increased risk of bleeding (e.g. following traumatic delivery). Recombinant coagulation factor concentrate should be used for the treatment of neonates if treatment is needed after delivery for any reason (e.g. after forceps delivery).

- Special observations after delivery may be warranted. Risk of intracranial bleeding after a normal vaginal delivery is very low (1–4% in severe haemophiliacs), but it is a recognized complication. It is most likely within the first week and UK guidelines recommend cranial USS prior to discharge.

Support groups: The Haemophilia Society (UK), http://www.haemophilia.org.uk; National Hemophilia Foundation (USA), https://www.hemophilia.org.

Further information:

The Haemophilia Society, http://www.haemophilia.org.uk (a national partnership whose aim is to advance and promote high levels of care for people with haemophilia and related disorders).

Expert adviser: Paula Bolton-Maggs, Consultant Haematologist, Serious Hazards of Transfusion UK National Haemovigilance Scheme, Manchester Blood Centre, Manchester, UK.

References

Bolton-Maggs PHB, Pasi KJ. Haemophilias A and B. *Lancet* 2003; **361**: 1801–9.

Chalmers E, Williams M, Brennand J, *et al.* Guideline on the management of haemophilia in the fetus and newborn. *Br J Haematol* 2011; **154**: 208–15.

Lee CA, Chi C, Pavord SR, *et al.* The obstetric and gynaecological management of women with inherited bleeding disorders—review with guidelines produced by a taskforce of UK Haemophilia Centre Doctors' Organization. *Haemophilia* 2006; **12**: 301–36.

Mannucci PM, Tuddenham EGD. The haemophilias—from royal genes to gene therapy. *N Engl J Med* 2001; **344**: 1773–9.

Hereditary haemorrhagic telangiectasia (HHT)

Rendu–Osler–Weber syndrome.

HHT is an AD vascular dysplasia, with a prevalence of ~1/10 000. There is locus heterogeneity with two loci—endoglin (*ENG*) on chromosome 9 and activin-like receptor kinase (*ALK-1, ACVRL1*) on 12q13, responsible for the majority of cases of HHT. A small number of cases of HHT with juvenile polyposis are caused by mutations in the *SMAD4* gene. Analysis of the coding regions of these genes will identify mutations in ~85% of affected individuals. Both *ENG* and *ALK-1* encode proteins involved in serine–threonine kinase signalling in the endothelial cell. The proteins form a homodimeric integral membrane glycoprotein that is the surface receptor for members of the transforming growth factor beta (TGF-β) superfamily, including BMP-9 that mediate vascular remodelling through effects on extracellular matrix production (Fuchizaki *et al.* 2003).

The characteristic lesions of HHT are cutaneous and mucosal telangiectasia (that consist of focal dilatations of post-capillary venules), as well as visceral AVMs. Pulmonary AVMs (PAVMs), create clinically significant right–left shunts and are much more common in families with endoglin mutations (Berg *et al.* 2003). Primary pulmonary hypertension is a rare complication in some families with *ALK-1* mutations (Trembath *et al.* 2001). Most patients with familial primary pulmonary hypertension have defects in the gene for BMP receptor II (*BMPR2*), which, like *ENG* and *ALK-1*, is a member of the TGF-β superfamily of receptors. Although mutation analysis can support the diagnosis of HHT, the diagnosis is usually made on clinical grounds. Criteria for the diagnosis of HHT are given in Box 3.4.

Clinical approach

History: key points

- Detailed three-generation family tree, with specific enquiry about nosebleeds, telangiectasia, stroke, etc.

Box 3.4 The Curacao criteria for the diagnosis of HHT

Criteria

(1) *Epistaxis*: spontaneous, recurrent nosebleeds[*]
(2) *Telangiectasia*: multiple, at characteristic sites: lips, oral cavity, fingers, nose
(3) *Visceral lesions* such as: GI telangiectasia, PAVM, hepatic AVM, CAVM, spinal AVM
(4) *Family history*: a first-degree relative with HHT according to these criteria.

The diagnosis of HHT is:

definite if three criteria are present[†];
possible or suspected if two criteria are present;
unlikely if fewer than two criteria are present.

[*] Epistaxis should occur spontaneously on more than one occasion.

[†] Within HHT families, a firm diagnosis can be made on the basis of two separate visceral manifestations.

Reproduced from Shovlin and Guttmacher *et al.* Diagnostic criteria for hereditary haemorrhagic telangiectasia (Rendu–Osler–Weber syndrome), *The American Journal of Medical Genetics Part A*, 91: 66–87, Copyright © 2000 Wiley-Liss Ltd.

- Nosebleeds. Do they occur spontaneously? Age of onset, frequency? Night-time bleeds are particularly suspicious.
- Previous unexplained anaemia or GI bleeding.
- History of headache, epilepsy, intracranial haemorrhage due to cerebral AVMs (CAVMs) or TIA, stroke, or cerebral abscess as a complication of PAVMs (paradoxical embolization).
- History of exertional dyspnoea; rarely, haemoptysis or haemothorax due to PAVMs.

Examination: key points

- Look carefully at the lips, mouth, and tongue for characteristic telangiectasia. These may be very subtle and only apparent on close inspection.
- Look carefully at the finger pulps and nail beds for telangiectasia, which again may not be apparent without close inspection.
- Examine for clubbing and cyanosis.
- Examine for liver size and listen for a hepatic bruit.

Special investigations

If there is a clinical diagnosis or a strong suspicion of HHT, the following are appropriate.

- Screen for a PAVM using transthoracic contrast echocardiography (TTCE), if available or as an alternative high-resolution CT scanning of the chest.
- Consider DNA for mutation analysis of endoglin (especially in families with PAVMs), *ACVRL1*, and *SMAD4*.

Genetic advice

Inheritance and recurrence risk

AD inheritance. Fifty per cent risk to offspring of an affected individual.

Variability and penetrance

Age-dependent penetrance. Sixty-two per cent symptomatic by 16 years, 83% by 26 years, and 97% by 35 years. Fully penetrant by 40 years.

Epistaxis (from telangiectasia in the nasal septum and inferior turbinate) is usually the first symptom with onset around puberty. Mucocutaneous telangiectasia appear 5–20 years after the onset of epistaxis and increase in number with age.

Prenatal diagnosis and pregnancy

PND is technically feasible if there is a known familial mutation. Pregnancy is a risk period for progression of PAVMs. *Women with PAVMs in association with HHT are at high risk in pregnancy* when up to 50% experience complications (intrapulmonary bleeding, worsening shunt, etc.). Some women experience a reduction or cessation in nosebleeds during pregnancy, but for others the frequency of nosebleeds increases and they may develop new telangiectasia.

Other family members

Cascade screening of the extended family is important because of the potential for serious avoidable complications. Complications of PAVMs do not usually occur before mid to late teenage years and so screening is usually offered after puberty, and only to those with recurrent nosebleeds (or other bleeding site), clinically evident telangiectasia, or a known mutation in a causative gene.

Natural history and management

Telangiectasia and AVMs tend to increase both in size and number with age.

- GI AVMs (11–40%) can result in iron-deficient anaemia or GI haemorrhage.
- PAVMs (up to 50%, depending on the locus involved) can cause paradoxical embolism, leading to stroke and cerebral abscesses. Less commonly, they can cause hypoxaemia, leading to respiratory failure and polycythaemia. Screening should be offered as discussed below. Patients with PAVMs, even if previously embolized, should receive prophylactic antibiotics for dental and surgical procedures, e.g. co-amoxiclav 375 mg pre- and post-dental visits.
- Hepatic AVMs, although frequently present asymptomatically (11–40%), can rarely cause high-output cardiac failure or port–caval shunting and may cause an unusual appearance on hepatic imaging. Treatment is arranged through specialist units.
- CNS, brain, spinal cord (5–11%). Brain AVMs (BAVMs) can bleed, although numerically more neurological events occur secondary to PAVMs than BAVMs. There is little evidence of benefit in screening for asymptomatic BAVMs in adults or children. In the recently concluded ARUBA trial in adults with unruptured BAVMs, conservative management was superior to surgical intervention over a 3-year follow-up, suggesting no benefit to detection of asymptomatic BAVMs in adults.
- Skin telangiectasia (13–89%) may occur on the oral mucosa, face, conjunctivae, trunk, extremities, nail beds, and finger pads. Laser treatment of these can be effective.
- Nasal telangiectasia (>90%). Management of nosebleeds is difficult and there is no wholly satisfactory approach. Most nosebleeds are self-limiting and patients learn to manage them independently.
  - Routine treatment with packing and humidification, iron and transfusion when necessary.
  - Laser treatment may be successful and is preferable to cautery.
  - Surgery (septal dermoplasty) may be successful in expert hands—but vessels regrow. Lund's procedure may also be effective.
  - Medical treatment with tamoxifen may be helpful in reducing the frequency and severity of nosebleeds.

Treatment with bevacizumab is under investigation for hepatic, GI, and nasal symptoms.

Surveillance

Patients should be screened after puberty for a PAVM using a reliable methodology. Where available, TTCE is currently suggested as the best method, with follow-up of suspected lesions by high-resolution CT of the chest. Chest CT may be indicated in the first line if TTCE is unavailable.

Since pregnancy is a time when PAVMs may develop/progress, repeat screening should be considered between pregnancies.

There is no published evidence to support screening for PAVMs in children, although there are rare case reports of symptomatic lesions presenting in childhood. A simple screening methodology such as clinical examination for cyanosis and clubbing, in addition to pulse oximetry, may be appropriate.

Screening for asymptomatic BAVMs is discussed above, but there is little clinical evidence for benefit.

Patients with SMAD4 mutations may be at risk of aortic root dilatation and should be screened for this, in addition to screening for juvenile polyps.

Monitoring of Hb in those with nosebleeds or possible GI haemorrhage. Patients may need regular iron supplementation or more aggressive treatment of anaemia.

Support groups: Telangiectasia Self Help Group, http://www.telangiectasia.co.uk; HHT Foundation International, http://curehht.org (useful site for clinicians too).

Expert adviser: Jonathan Berg, Senior Lecturer and Honorary Consultant in Clinical Genetics, University of Dundee, Ninewells Hospital and Medical School, Dundee, UK.

References

Berg J, Porteous M, Reinhardt D, et al. Hereditary haemorrhagic telangiectasia: a questionnaire based study to delineate the different phenotypes caused by endoglin and ALK1 mutations. *J Med Genet* 2003; **40**: 585–90.

Fuchizaki U, Miyamori H, Kitagawa S, Kaneko S, Kobayashi K. Hereditary haemorrhagic telangiectasia (Rendu–Osler–Weber disease)—eponym. *Lancet* 2003; **362**: 1490–4.

Shovlin CL, Guttmacher AE, Buscarini E, et al. Diagnostic criteria for hereditary haemorrhagic telangiectasia (Rendu–Osler–Weber syndrome). *Am J Med Genet* 2000; **91**: 66–87.

Shovlin CL, Letarte M. Hereditary haemorrhagic telangiectasia and pulmonary arteriovenous malformations: issues in clinical management and review of pathogenic mechanisms. *Thorax* 1999; **54**: 714–29.

Teekakirikul P, Milewicz DM, Miller DT, et al. Thoracic aortic disease in two patients with juvenile polyposis syndrome and SMAD4 mutations. *Am J Med Genet A* 2013; **161A**: 185–91.

Trembath RC, Thomson JR, Machado RD, et al. Clinical and molecular genetic features of pulmonary hypertension in patients with hereditary haemorrhagic telangiectasia. *N Engl J Med* 2001; **345**: 325–34.

van Gent MW, Post MC, Snijder RJ, Westermann CJ, Plokker HW, Mager JJ. Real prevalence of pulmonary right-to-left shunt according to genotype in patients with hereditary hemorrhagic telangiectasia: a transthoracic contrast echocardiography study. *Chest* 2010; **138**: 833–9.

Velthuis S, Vorselaars VM, van Gent MW, et al. Role of transthoracic contrast echocardiography in the clinical diagnosis of hereditary hemorrhagic telangiectasia. *Chest* 2013; **144**: 1876–82.

Yaniv E, Preis M, Shevro J, Nageris B, Hadar T. Anti-estrogen therapy for hereditary hemorrhagic telangiectasia—a long-term clinical trial. *Rhinology* 2011; **49**: 214–16.

Hereditary spastic paraplegias (HSP)

Hereditary spastic paraparesis.

The HSPs are single gene disorders in which the axons of the corticospinal tract either fail to develop normally or show progressive degeneration after initially normal development. The principal clinical feature in all HSPs is the presence of a bilaterally symmetrical, slowly progressive lower limb spastic paralysis. This occurs in relative isolation in the pure HSPs (PHSPs) or with other neurological or extra-neurological features in the complex HSPs (CHSPs). AD, AR, and XLR inheritance patterns have been described for both PHSPs and CHSPs, with AD PHSP the most common form (70–80% of families) in northern Europe and North America. XLR inheritance is rare. Most HSPs, including probably all of the AD PHSPs, are associated with neurodegeneration, rather than abnormal neurodevelopment. Histopathological studies in PHSP have characterized this neurodegeneration as a length-dependent 'dying back' of the terminal ends of the corticospinal tract and dorsal column axons.

At least 70 HSP loci are recognized and >30 associated genes have been cloned (see OMIM for the current gene list). Mutations in spastin (SPG4) on chromosome 2p21–22 are found in ~40% of families with AD PHSP. A significant proportion of these mutations are whole exon deletions that can be missed with sequence-based mutation screening strategies; typically additional screening by MLPA is required to detect these. Mutations in atlastin (SPG3A; 14q12–21) are responsible in ~10% of families. Mutations in these genes are less frequent in sporadic cases or in cases with an uncertain family history, although consideration should be given to spastin testing in these circumstances, as the pickup rate of mutations may be higher than 10%. The spastin and atlastin proteins interact with each other and with several other HSP proteins and are involved in intracellular membrane shaping and trafficking functions. SPG11 and SPG15 mutations are an important cause of the AR complex 'HSP with thin corpus callosum'. The majority of patients with this disorder have corpus callosum abnormalities on MRI. Among other complicating neurological features, this condition is associated with learning difficulties and progressive cognitive impairment. These features can be present before the onset of paraplegia, which typically begins in the second decade. CYP7B1 (SPG5A) mutations are found in 5–10% of AR PHSP cases, while paraplegin (SPG7) mutations are another cause of AR PHSP or CHSP (by optic, cortical, or cerebellar atrophy). They are associated with defects in mitochondrial oxidative phosphorylation, often with characteristic structural and functional abnormalities on muscle biopsy.

Diagnosis in a family with AD PHSP is often known, and the role of the geneticist lies in advising about inheritance and assessing 'at-risk' family members. Beware misdiagnosis in other family members, e.g. 'multiple sclerosis'. Penetrance is age-dependent and this, together with the striking disease variability within families, makes giving accurate genetic advice a considerable challenge in the absence of an identified mutation.

Clinical approach

History: key points

- Three-generation family history, with special attention to gait disturbance and mobility.
- Age of onset. Paraplegia may begin in early childhood, presenting with delayed motor milestones and clumsiness (25% of cases in AD families are symptomatic by 5 years). Difficulty with physical education at school.
- Gait disturbance (shoe scuffing), history of trips and falls. Enquire about the maximum distance of walking on flat ground and whether aids, e.g. walking stick(s), are used.
- Spasticity affects the lower limbs, and symptomatic involvement of the upper limbs is rare.
- Severity. Spectrum varies from asymptomatic (10–20%) to requiring a wheelchair (10–20%) and very rarely bed-restricted. Insidiously progressive.
- Aggravating features. Tiredness, cold, alcohol.
- Associated features. Bladder or bowel dysfunction.
- Complicating features, e.g. muscle wasting (e.g. Silver syndrome), cerebellar signs, dystonia, dementia, epilepsy, sensory neuropathy, optic atrophy, central retinal degeneration (Kjellin syndrome), ichthyosis (Sjögren–Larsson syndrome), disordered skin pigmentation, adducted thumbs plus MR (MASA (mental retardation–aphasia– shuffling gait–adducted thumbs) syndrome).

Examination: key points

- Observe the gait and examine footwear for toe scuffing.
- Examine for foot deformity (65%). Pes cavus.
- Increased tone is disproportionately severe in comparison to weakness.
- DTRs increased, especially in lower limbs (99%); 7% have decreased power and increased reflexes in upper limbs.
- Clonus. Examine for sustained clonus (>4 beats; 45%).
- Extensor plantar reflexes (80%).

Signs in HSP are predominantly confined to the motor system. However, abnormal vibration sense is found in 40% of patients and other sensory modalities may be involved less frequently (involvement of dorsal columns). Mild distal muscle wasting may be found in long-standing cases.

Special investigations

In the absence of a causative mutation in a family, HSP is a diagnosis of exclusion. Investigations to be considered are the following.

- DNA for gene panel/WES/WGS as appropriate, in view of the extensive genetic heterogeneity.
- VLCFAs for ALD, if inheritance is compatible with XLR, i.e. no male-to-male transmission.
- In cases lacking sensory symptoms, consider a trial of L-dopa to exclude DRD.
- MRI of the brain and spinal cord in one member of an affected family, and particularly in sporadic or complex cases. In AD PHSP, this may show spinal cord atrophy, especially in the cervical and thoracic regions, while some recessive HSPs are associated with thinning of the corpus callosum.
- Consider white cell enzymes if atypical features present, e.g. significant peripheral neuropathy.

A firm diagnosis of HSP should only be made where at least two family members have definitive clinical features (a progressive spastic gait disturbance with frank corticospinal tract signs in the lower limbs, i.e. hyperreflexia with either bilaterally extensor plantar reflexes or bilateral sustained (5+ beats) clonus) or if a proven pathogenic mutation has been identified.

Other diagnoses/conditions to consider

PHSP is a distinctive clinical entity, and diagnosis is usually straightforward. Occasional confusion may occur with the following.

Hereditary motor and sensory neuropathy (HMSN)
Reflexes usually depressed in this condition (rather than increased). Peripheral NCVs are usually normal in HSP, and abnormal in HMSN. See 'Charcot–Marie–Tooth disease (CMT)' in Chapter 3, 'Common consultations', p. 362.

Friedreich's ataxia (FRDA) or spinocerebellar ataxias (SCAs)
Consider atypical FRDA (with preservation of reflexes) if inheritance compatible with AR (DNA for frataxin mutation analysis). See 'Ataxic child' in Chapter 2, 'Clinical approach', p. 74. Spasticity can be a feature of some AD SCAs.

Dopa-responsive dystonia (DRD; Segawa syndrome)
This may rarely present with a spastic paraplegia. Response to a trial of L-dopa is dramatic and sustained and should be considered in any case where sensory signs are not present. See 'Dystonia' in Chapter 2, 'Clinical approach', p. 138.

X-linked adrenoleukodystrophy (X-ALD)
The adrenomyeloneuropathy phenotype may mimic HSP and should be considered in families lacking male-to-male transmission. A normal brain MRI does not exclude this condition. See 'X-linked adrenoleukodystrophy (X-ALD)' in Chapter 3, 'Common consultations', p. 538.

A diagnosis of primary lateral sclerosis may become apparent if the phenotype progresses to involve the upper limbs and bulbar muscles. Eventual lower motor neuron involvement may point to classical amyotrophic lateral sclerosis/motor neuron disease.

Consideration should also be given to non-genetic conditions, such as space-occupying lesions, vitamin B12, vitamin E, or copper deficiency, and infective causes such as syphilis, human T-lymphocytic virus 1 (HTLV-1) infection, or the myelopathy of AIDS.

Table 3.19 Risk of having inherited disease gene for clinically normal offspring of affected individuals (for families with AD disease and age of onset predominantly <35 years)

Age (years)	Residual risk of having disease gene (%)
20	24
25	22
30	19
35	13
40	11
45	9

Genetic advice

Inheritance and recurrence risk
Most PHSP follows AD inheritance (70–80%; see Table 3.19), but AR inheritance (10–20%) and XLR inheritance (<5%) both occur. Most CHSPs are inherited in an AR pattern, although AD and XLR (notably the *L1-CAM* associated disorders) forms exist.

The frequency of asymptomatic gene carriers means that every effort should be made to examine parents of apparently sporadic or recessive PHSP cases. If parents are both normal, recessive inheritance is most likely, but not certain. If both parents of affected siblings cannot be examined, empiric figures indicate a 1/6 chance that one parent was affected, giving a risk to offspring of affected siblings of 1/12. No empiric figures are available for risks to offspring of apparently sporadic cases where the possibility of AR inheritance, a non-penetrant AD parent, and a DNM must all be considered.

Variability and penetrance
For AD families, because 10–20% of gene carriers are asymptomatic, the risk of symptomatic disease in offspring of a gene carrier is 40–45%.

Prenatal diagnosis
Technically possible by CVS if a familial mutation is known or if the family is large enough for linkage analysis.

Predictive testing
Theoretically possible if a familial mutation is known or if the family is large enough for linkage analysis, but restrict to adults who are able to engage fully in the decision-making process and approach as for other adult-onset neurodegenerative conditions.

Other family members
Anxiety may complicate the assessment of 'at-risk' family members by causing a mildly increased tone, hyperreflexia, and a non-sustained clonus. (Do not overinterpret soft physical signs.)

Natural history and management

Surveillance
Because the disorder progresses so insidiously, it may be several years since diagnosis and the patient's disability may have progressed substantially since last reviewed. It may be appropriate to arrange for evaluation of the following.

- Driving. HSP may impair the ability to use pedals in the car. Patients should notify the DVLA of their diagnosis and may need conversion of the car to hand controls.
- Home may need bathroom alterations (e.g. walk-in-shower, rails), stairlift, or downstairs bedroom.
- Urinary symptoms. Less than 50% of patients with HSP have urinary frequency, urgency, or hesitancy. If symptomatic or recurrent infections, consider referral to a urologist. Males may suffer erectile impotence.
- Physiotherapy. No therapy is currently available that slows disease progression. Treatment is aimed at maximizing functional ability and preventing contractures.
- Antispasmodic medication may benefit some patients and should be prescribed under the supervision of a neurologist.

Support group: Familial Spastic Paraplegia Group, Tel. 01702 218 184.

Expert adviser: Evan Reid, University Lecturer and Honorary Consultant in Clinical Genetics, Department of Medical Genetics, University of Cambridge, Cambridge, UK.

References

Blackstone C, O'Kane CJ, Reid E. Hereditary spastic paraplegias: membrane traffic and the motor pathway. *Nat Rev Neurosci* 2011; **12**: 31–42.

Finsterer J, Löscher W, Quasthoff S, Wanschitz J, Auer-Grumbach M, Stevanin G. Hereditary spastic paraplegias with autosomal dominant, recessive, X-linked, or maternal trait of inheritance. *J Neurol Sci* 2012; **318**: 1–18.

Harding AE. Hereditary 'pure' spastic paraplegia: a clinical and genetic study of 22 families. *J Neurol Neurosurg Psychiatry* 1981; **44**: 871–83.

Reid E, Rugarli E. Hereditary spastic paraplegias. In: AL Beaudet, B Vogelstein, KW Kinzler, SE Antonarakis, A Ballabio (eds.). *The online molecular and metabolic basis of inherited diseases (OMMBID)*, pp. 1–65. McGraw Hill, New York, 2010. http://ommbid.mhmedical.com.

Hirschsprung's disease

Congenital intestinal aganglionosis, HSCR, aganglionic megacolon.

Hirschsprung's disease is an important genetic cause of functional intestinal obstruction. It is characterized by the absence of neural crest-derived enteric neural ganglia along a variable length of the intestine. The critical period in embryonic life for cranial–caudal migration of vagal neural crest cells and invasion of the neural crest-derived ganglion cells into the intestinal wall is 5–12 weeks' gestation. Ultrashort-segment Hirschsprung's disease (uncommon and even questionable) involves only the very distal rectum. Short-segment Hirschsprung's disease (60–85%) is characterized by the absence of intestinal ganglion cells from the wall of the rectum through to the upper sigmoid colon. Long-segment Hirschsprung's disease (15–25%) involves the rectum through to a short section of the ascending colon. Total colonic aganglionosis (3–5%) involves the rectum and entire colon and variable parts of the ileum. HSCR is sporadic in about 80% of cases and familial in 20% with incomplete penetrance and variable expressivity. Indeed, the length of aganglionic colon may vary within the same family.

Hirschsprung's disease affects 1/5000 neonates, a figure that varies according to ethnicity, with a higher prevalence in Asians, medium in Caucasians, and lower in African-Americans. Males are much more susceptible than females (M:F 4.5:1 for short-segment and 1.75:1 for long-segment Hirschsprung's disease). Most patients present in the neonatal period with failure to pass meconium in the first 48 hours and/or abdominal distension, and vomiting. Rectal biopsy is needed to confirm the diagnosis. Treatment is surgical with excision of the aganglionic bowel.

Seventy per cent occur as an isolated finding; 20% are syndromic or have another congenital anomaly, and 10% are chromosomal (especially Down's syndrome). Isolated Hirschsprung's disease appears to be an oligogenic malformation with a high heritability. RET is regarded as the major locus in multigenic Hirschsprung's disease.

The oligogenic model for Hirschsprung's disease is complex, not only involving the allelic repertoire at RET (with differential contributions of rare loss of function coding mutations and common non-coding variants to disease liability), but also genetic heterogeneity, with eight genes known to be involved (mainly in the RET and endothelin signalling pathways).

Clinical approach

History: key points

- Careful three-generation family tree, with particular attention to Hirschsprung's disease or unexplained neonatal or early infant deaths, deafness and pigmentary anomalies, neurological features, thyroid cancer, phaeochromocytoma, or parathyroid hyperplasia.
- Determine the extent of gut involved, e.g. short-segment/long-segment/total colonic aganglionosis.
- Confirm the diagnosis from the histology report (if available).

Examination: key points

- Examine for pigmentary anomalies (white forelock, heterochromia, skin streaking).
- Examine for dysmorphic features and features of Down's syndrome.

- Careful cardiac assessment (5% of patients with Hirschsprung's disease have a cardiac lesion, mostly ASD or VSD, respectively).
- Examine for distal limb and more generally skeletal anomalies. There are a series of rare syndromes with Hirschsprung's disease and polydactyly, brachydactyly, or hypoplasia of the distal phalanges and nails.

Investigations

- Genomic analysis in presence of features suggestive of a chromosomal or syndromic diagnosis, e.g. genomic array, gene panel, or WES/WGS as appropriate.
- Consider echo and renal USS in view of the significant incidence of additional anomalies.
- Consider RET mutation analysis. Forty to 50% of familial cases and 15–20% of sporadic cases have RET mutations, with a penetrance of 50–70% in familial cases. Because of poor genotype–phenotype correlation, as well as low and gender-dependent penetrance, the benefit of mutation screening for non-syndromic Hirschsprung's appears low. In addition, mutations are scattered all along the gene-coding sequence with no hotspot, and the role of non-coding polymorphism is still difficult to predict. The distribution of RET variants in diverse HSCR patients suggests a 'cellular recessive' genetic model where the function of both RET alleles is compromised (Emison et al. 2010).
- Consider ZEB2 (ZFHX1B) mutation analysis in patients with Hirschsprung's disease, microcephaly, MR, and typical dysmorphic features with upturned ear lobules, in view of the diagnosis of Mowat–Wilson syndrome (see 'Other diagnoses/conditions to consider' below).
- Consider 7-dehydrocholesterol for SLO if associated features are involved such as IUGR, microcephaly, distal limb anomalies, etc.

Other diagnoses/conditions to consider

Waardenburg syndrome (WS) and related pigmentary anomalies

WS causes pigmentary anomalies and sensorineural deafness due to absence of melanocytes in the skin and stria vascularis in the cochlea. The combination of Waardenburg plus Hirschsprung's disease is termed Shah–Waardenburg, or WS4, and is genetically heterogeneous, including homozygous endothelin pathway mutations (EDN3 or EDNRB genes) and heterozygous SOX10 mutations. In the latter case, various neurological symptoms with demyelinization might occur with a progressive pattern. See 'Deafness in early childhood' in Chapter 2, 'Clinical approach', p. 122.

Multiple endocrine neoplasia type 2A (MEN2A) and familial medullary thyroid cancer (MTC)

Both MEN2A (age-related predisposition to MTC, phaeochromocytoma, and parathyroid hyperplasia) and familial MTC can be associated with Hirschsprung's disease in some families. Screen for mutations in RET exons 10 and 11. See 'Multiple endocrine neoplasia (MEN)' in Chapter 4, 'Cancer', p. 592.

Mowat–Wilson syndrome

All patients have a facial gestalt with a prominent chin, upturned ear lobules, deep-set eyes, and flared eyebrows, in association with severe ID, and nearly all have microcephaly and seizures. Congenital anomalies include Hirschsprung's disease, CHD, hypospadias and genitourinary anomalies, and ACC. Short stature is common. Caused by heterozygous deletions or truncating mutations at the *ZEB2* (*ZFHX1B*) locus on 2q22.

Haddad syndrome—associating congenital central hypoventilation syndrome (CCHS, Ondine's curse) and Hirschsprung's disease
Nearly all patients have a heterozygous *PHOX2B* gene mutation. Clinical and radiological survey of a possible neuroblastoma should be advised whenever the mutation is not a polyalanine expansion.

Goldberg–Shprintzen megacolon syndrome
Caused by biallelic mutations in *KIAA1279*. In addition to Hirschsprung's disease, children have microcephaly with neuronal migration disorders (pachygyria/PMG/ACC) and occasionally iris coloboma and ptosis.

Additional isolated congenital anomaly
A variety of additional anomalies are described: cardiac defects (5%); renal dysplasia/agenesis (4%); genital anomalies, e.g. hypospadias (2–3%).

Genetic advice

Inheritance and recurrence risk in isolated (non-syndromic) Hirschsprung's disease
Make sure that Hirschsprung's disease is non-syndromic and that there is no discernible Mendelian inheritance pattern. Assess the length of the aganglionic segment in the index case, his gender, the sex of the child to be born whenever possible, and the family tree. If you are dealing with a sporadic case for whom the *RET* gene has not been investigated, the overall recurrence risk in sibs of a proband is 4%, and use Table 3.20 to refine the risk. If there are several affected family members, counsel for higher risk, incorporating advice about low penetrance.

Variability and penetrance
In families carrying a mutation in *RET*, penetrance is 50–72% in gene carriers, mostly depending on the gender of the carrier individual. But penetrance is variable and seems not only gene- but also family-specific.

Prenatal diagnosis
PND for Hirschsprung's disease per se is not possible. Bowel dilatation has been exceptionally reported in total colonic aganglionosis cases. If the mutation is known, it would be theoretically possible but may not be desired in view of the incomplete penetrance and variable expressivity of most mutations and the availability of curative surgical treatment.

Table 3.20 Empiric risk for non-syndromic Hirschsprung's disease

Sex of proband	Risk (%) to	
	Male sib	Female sib
Male short segment	5	1
Male long segment	17	13
Female short segment	5	3
Female long segment	33	9

This table was published in *American Journal of Human Genetics*, Vol 46, Issue 3, Badner JA, Sieber WK, Garver KL et al., A genetic study of Hirschsprung disease, p. 568, Copyright Elsevier (1990).

Natural history and management

Potential long-term complications
Chronic constipation and soiling (10–15%).

Support group: Hirschsprung's & Motility Disorders Support Network (HMDSN), http://www.hirschsprungs.info.

Expert adviser: Stan Lyonnet, Clinical Geneticist, Department of Medical Genetics, Hôpital Necker-Enfants Malades, Paris, France.

References

Amiel J, Epinosa-Parilla Y, Steffann J, et al. Large-scale deletions and *SMADIP1* truncating mutations in syndromic Hirschsprung disease with involvement of midline structures. *Am J Hum Genet* 2001; **69**: 1370–7.

Amiel J, Sproat-Emison E, Garcia-Barcelo M, et al. Hirschsprung disease, associated syndromes, and genetics: a review. *J Med Genet* 2008; **45**: 1–14.

Badner JA, Sieber WK, Garver KL, Chakravarti A. A genetic study of Hirschsprung disease. *Am J Hum Genet* 1990; **46**: 568–80.

Emison ES, Garcia-Barcelo M, Grice EA, et al. Differential contribution of rare and common, coding and noncoding *RET* mutations, to multifactorial Hirschsprung disease liability. *Am J Hum Genet* 2010; **87**: 60–74.

Huntington disease (HD)

Previously known as Huntington's chorea.

HD is a progressive neurodegenerative disorder. The features are a triad of involuntary movement disorder, psychiatric disturbance, and dementia. In the early stages of the condition, chorea may be prominent (especially with onset >40 years), but as the disorder progresses, dystonia, bradykinesia, and decreased voluntary movements are the predominant motor features. Rigidity, rather than chorea, is found in juvenile HD and the Westphal variant; psychiatric problems and behavioural problems are common presenting features in young adults. The clinical diagnosis is made after recognition of the symptoms described in the history, physical signs on examination, and family history. Macroscopic examination of the brain at autopsy in advanced disease shows striking degeneration of the basal ganglia structures. The caudate nucleus is particularly atrophied, though the putamen and globus pallidus are also affected. The brain is generally smaller, especially the frontal lobes. A diagnosis of HD is confirmed by specific molecular testing.

The prevalence of HD in the UK is ~1 in 10 000. The birth incidence is about 2.5 times the prevalence, or to express it differently there are several asymptomatic gene carriers for every affected individual. The peak age of onset is between 40 and 45 years. The South Wales study showed 4.5% with onset under 20 years (juvenile HD) and 8% over 60 years (HD in the elderly).

HD is caused by an increased (CAG) trinucleotide repeat number within the huntingtin gene (*HD*) on 4p16 (see Table 3.21). The expanded (CAG) repeat is the underlying mutation in all populations studied. The trinucleotide repeat is unstable during meiosis, which gives rise to the term 'dynamic mutation'. Epidemiological studies have shown evidence for an earlier age of onset through the generations (anticipation) due to expansion of the (CAG) repeat. Large expansions of >60 repeats are usually paternally inherited and almost always have a juvenile presentation (<18 years). The relationship between an increased number of (CAG) repeats and a younger age of onset shows strongest correlation for juvenile onset; however, caution is advised in using the number of repeats to predict age of onset in the clinical setting.

Intermediate alleles are rare in the general population. They may be found in the parent (usually the father) of an apparently new mutation for HD. Intermediate alleles are not likely to cause clinical features of HD but can be unstable during transmission, and a mutation rate of 10% in each generation has been suggested. Approximately 8% of HD patients have no family history of the disease.

Juvenile HD

This is uncommon. It is usually paternally inherited and associated with repeat sizes in excess of ~60. Presentation is different to the adult disorder, often with problems with schoolwork and paucity of facial movement. Diagnosis and progression of HD in a parent can itself account for difficulties at school among younger members of the family, so the clinical presentation may be challenging to evaluate. Assessment by a paediatric neurologist and formal psychometric testing repeated at an interval of 4–6 months may be helpful in determining whether there is progression and an organic basis to the difficulties. MRI should also be performed (looking for basal ganglia changes) to establish a clinical diagnosis before embarking on diagnostic testing to determine the HD repeat size. (Otherwise if the young person does not have juvenile HD, there is a 50% risk that an inadvertent predictive test is performed.)

Clinical approach

History: key points

- Three-generation family tree; extend further, if possible, to include all known affected family members. Note the maiden name of females and addresses of long-term care institutions.
- Age of onset of affected family members and age of death.
- Psychiatric disease, suicide, or dementia in apparently unaffected family members (may actually have been HD).

Examination: key points

- Individuals with pre-symptomatic or early HD have few signs on general examination, but there is evidence of subtle motor, cognitive, and imaging changes up to 15 years before the predicted disease onset.
- Clinical examination is not usually performed on the first meeting with an apparently unaffected individual at risk of HD, unless specifically requested. This meeting is to give information about HD and an explanation of the role of the geneticist in such issues as predictive testing.
- *Close observation during the consultation may be informative.* Fidgety movements of the legs or facial grimacing may increase suspicion. Many patients consulting about HD are very anxious, which may manifest as restlessness or facial twitching, so be wary of overinterpretation.

Investigations: clinically unaffected 'at-risk' individual

- Accurate confirmation of diagnosis (preferably with molecular confirmation) is required from at least one affected member of the family. *Written informed consent will be required before predictive testing is undertaken* (see below).

Investigations: genetic conditions to consider in an individual with suspected HD but no family history or no documentation of family history

- Diagnostic molecular testing for HD.
- Thick wet blood film for acanthocytes (neuroacanthosis).
- Diagnostic molecular testing for DRPLA.
- Diagnostic molecular testing for hereditary SCAs.
- Copper studies for Wilson's disease with a juvenile or rigid presentation.
- DNA storage for future diagnostic studies.

Table 3.21 Allele classification

Allele classification	(CAG)n repeat range
Normal allele	≤26 repeats
Intermediate allele	27–35 repeats
HD allele—reduced penetrance	36–39 repeats
HD allele	≤39 repeats

In children, the issues surrounding genetic testing need special consideration.

Other conditions/diagnoses to consider

Conditions associated with chorea

HUNTINGTON DISEASE-LIKE 1 (HDL-1). A progressive inherited prion disease which is a phenocopy of HD. An AD condition caused by an expanded octapeptide repeat in the prion protein gene.

HUNTINGTON DISEASE-LIKE 2 (HDL-2). Also often indistinguishable from HD. It is an AD condition caused by an expanded CTG repeat in the junctophilin 3 (*JPH3*) gene. Most individuals with HDL-2 have African ancestry.

DENTATORUBROPALLIDOLUYSIAN ATROPHY (DRPLA). AD. This is rare, but features are very similar, in particular in juvenile HD. Ataxia, choreoathetosis, dementia, myoclonus, and epilepsy are features. The neuropathology is diagnostic. DRPLA is also a triple repeat condition with an expansion of CAG in the gene, found on chromosome 12. It is more common in Japan but is increasingly recognized throughout the world since diagnostic molecular testing.

NEUROACANTHOSIS. AR (*CHAC*) gene. Mostly described in the Japanese. Onset in early adult life with a movement disorder involving the muscles of the face and mouth. Chorea and dystonic movements, as well as cognitive, affective problems and an axonal neuropathy, are common.

BENIGN FAMILIAL CHOREA. AD. Onset in early childhood with no progression, dementia, or psychiatric features.

DRUG-INDUCED. Including amiodarone, dopaminergic agents, neuroleptics, carbamazepine, and anticholinergics.

Disorders of the basal ganglia

PARKINSON'S DISEASE. Diagnostically there is not usually any confusion, except in the juvenile rigid form of HD. Some affected individuals with HD have an erroneous diagnosis of Parkinson's disease.

TARDIVE DYSKINESIA. Problems arise when an at-risk individual is treated with phenothiazines for a psychosis.

WILSON'S DISEASE. AR. Is in the differential for the juvenile and rigid forms of HD.

SPINOCEREBELLAR ATAXIA (SCA). SCA17 is associated with chorea, ataxia, dementia, and psychiatric disturbance. SCA3 also has a pronounced movement disorder. See 'Ataxic adult' in Chapter 2, 'Clinical approach', p. 70.

Conditions associated with dementia

- Chorea, rather than dementia, is the presenting feature in early HD.
- See 'Dementia—early onset and familial forms' in Chapter 3, 'Common consultations', p. 386.

Psychiatric conditions

HD has often been misdiagnosed as schizophrenia or paranoid psychosis, but it is also important to note that both conditions are more common in patients with HD.

Genetic advice: unaffected individual at risk of HD

Inheritance and recurrence risk

AD. As HD is due to an unstable triplet repeat, both anticipation and the parental origin may influence the age of onset and presentation.

Families appreciate help and advice in how to talk about the condition in the family and how and when to go about telling the children about HD. This and other issues may be helped by contact with HD support groups.

Variability and penetrance

The main considerations are the age of the person concerned and the presence of juvenile HD in the family. Age of onset curves and risks of an unaffected individual at 50% risk of HD, carrying the HD gene at a particular age, are shown in Table 3.22. Table 3.22 is *not* intended for use in advising individual patients because the risks for an individual are heavily governed by: (i) the age of onset in the family, (ii) whether the mutation is maternally or paternally inherited, and (iii) the expansion size (see Table 3.23). These figures are included here simply to remind the clinician that the risks for an apparently healthy individual remain quite high, even into later life.

Predictive testing

Predictive testing for HD has been the model upon which much of the predictive testing for other genetic conditions have been based. There are usually a series of three or more meetings between the 'at-risk' individual and a genetic counsellor to explore the reasons that they wish to have the test and to discuss possible outcomes and future management.

Fewer than 20% of first-degree relatives opt for predictive testing. Follow-up is offered to at-risk relatives either to keep them informed of new developments and, if they wish, for a clinical assessment for signs of HD. See 'Testing for genetic status' in Chapter 1, 'Introduction', p. 38.

Other family members

Predictive testing for those at <50% risk has a number of difficulties, particularly ethical, that require thought and discussion before testing and results are offered. A predictive test for the intervening relative has effectively been performed if an individual at 25% genetic risk is found to carry the (CAG) expansion.

Prenatal and pre-implantation genetic diagnosis

Both direct gene analysis and exclusion testing are available. PGD is available and PND is also an option where the parental genetic status is known. NIPD may also become available; seek up-to-date advice before counselling.

Prenatal exclusion testing is the procedure whereby an at-risk individual can avoid the birth of a child carrying

Table 3.22 Risk for a healthy individual at 50% prior risk of HD carrying a pathological HD gene expansion at different ages[*]

Age (years)	Risk (%)	Age (years)	Risk (%)	Age (years)	Risk (%)
20	49.6	40	42.5	60	18.7
25	49	45	37.8	65	12.8
30	47.6	50	31.5	70	6.2
35	45.5	55	24.8	72.5	4.6

[*] This table is *not* intended for use in advising individual patients because the risks for an individual are heavily governed by: (1) the age of onset in the family, (2) whether the mutation is maternally or paternally inherited, and (3) the expansion size. These figures are included here simply to remind the clinician that the risks for an apparently healthy individual remain quite high, even into later life.

Reproduced from *Journal of Medical Genetics*, Harper and Newcombe, Age at onset and life table risks in genetic counselling for Huntington's disease, vol 29, issue 4, p. 239, copyright 1992, with permission from BMJ Publishing Group Ltd.

Table 3.23 Influence of expansion size on age at onset

CAG repeat size	Median age at onset (years)[†]	95% CI for median age at onset (years)[‡]
39	66	72–59
40	59	61–56
41	54	56–52
42	49	50–48
43	44	45–42
44	42	43–40
45	37	39–36
46	36	37–35
47	33	35–31
48	32	34–30
49	28	32–25
50	27	30–24

This table is *not* intended for use in advising individual patients. These figures reflect the median onset for a group of individuals with a known expansion size. Hence, the age of onset for an *individual* cannot be estimated with the precision that this table implies. Nevertheless, these data give the clinician a useful 'feel' for the important influence of expansion size in determining age of onset.

[†] Age by which 50% of individuals will be affected.

[‡] CI, confidence interval.

This table was published in *American Journal of Human Genetics*, Volume 60, issue 5, R. R. Brinkman, M. M. Mezei, J. Theilman, E. Almqvist, and M. R. Hayden, The Likelihood of Being Affected with Huntington Disease by a Particular Age, for a Specific CAG Size, pp. 1202–1210, Copyright Elsevier 1997.

the HD gene, but without him/herself having a diagnostic test. Linked markers are used to define a haplotype around the HD gene. The 'at-risk' parent will have inherited one chromosome 4 from the affected grandparent and one from the unaffected grandparent. The haplotype from the affected grandparent carries a 50% risk. The fetus is at 50% risk if it inherits this grandparental haplotype, but at population risk if it inherits the haplotype from the unaffected grandparent. Couples choosing an exclusion test need to weigh the benefits of ensuring that their offspring will not inherit HD (while choosing not to disclose their own status) against the prospect in the event of a 'high-risk' result of terminating a pregnancy which has a 50% chance of being unaffected. 'Non-disclosure' PGD or exclusion PGD is offered in some centres.

Natural history and management (of at-risk individuals and known gene carriers)

Potential long-term complications
Onset of signs and symptoms of HD. Psychological, social, and family problems that can arise from this knowledge.

Surveillance
Follow-up is offered to all gene carriers and those at risk who have declined testing. They may wish to be informed if there are any signs of HD. There is also an obligation for the counsellor to disclose such information to the individual if they are considered unsafe to drive a car or to be a danger to themselves or other people as a result of HD.

Close liaison with HD workers in the community helps to ensure that appropriate supportive help is given. Participation in an HD registry or other research studies may be helpful to some patients.

Treatment
Multidisciplinary management is key with input from neurologists and neuropsychiatrists, as appropriate, as well as physiotherapy, speech and language therapy, and occupational therapy.

Symptomatic treatment of HD is available for the movement disorder and psychiatric complications.

For pre-symptomatic individuals, new research into treatment offers real hope. 'Gene silencing' using small interfering RNA (siRNA) and antisense oligonucleotides (ASOs) has been shown to decrease huntingtin expression and improve symptoms in mouse and primate models of HD and is moving closer to human trials.

Inducible pluripotent stem cells (iPSCs) have shown some promise in mouse models of HD.

Other potential therapeutic options include HDAC inhibitors and sirtuin inhibitors. A selective inhibitor of SIRT1 has entered phase 2 trials in Europe.

Support groups: Huntington's Disease Society of America, http://hdsa.org; Huntington's Disease Association (UK), http://www.hda.org.uk; Huntington's Disease Youth Organization, http://en.hdyo.org; HD Buzz, http://www.hdbuzz.net.

Expert adviser: Nayana Lahiri, Consultant Clinical Geneticist, SW Thames Regional Genetics Service, St George's University Hospitals NHS Foundation Trust, St George's Hospital, London, UK.

References
Bates G, Harper PS, Jones A (eds.). *Huntington's disease*, 3rd edn. Oxford University Press, Oxford, 2002.

Brinkman RR, Mezel MM. The likelihood of being affected with Huntington disease by a particular age, for a specific CAG size. *Am J Hum Genet* 1997; **60**: 1202–10.

Clarke A. The genetic testing of children. Working Party of the Clinical Genetics Society (UK). *J Med Genet* 1994; **31**: 785–97.

Harper PS, Newcombe RG. Age at onset and life table risks in genetic counselling for Huntington's disease. *J Med Genet* 1992; **29**: 239–42.

Macleod R, Tibben A, Frontali M, et al. Recommendations for the predictive genetic test in Huntington's disease. *Clin Genet* 2013; **83**: 221–31.

Novak MJ, Tabrizi SJ. Huntington's disease. *BMJ* 2010; **340**: c3109.

Reilmann R, Leavitt BR, Ross CA. Diagnostic criteria for Huntington's disease based on natural history. *Mov Disord* 2014; **29**: 1335–41.

The Huntington's Disease Collaborative Research Group. A novel gene containing a trinucleotide repeat that is expanded and unstable on Huntington's disease chromosomes. *Cell* 1993; **72**: 971–83.

Hyperlipidaemia

The level of serum cholesterol increases in an individual with advancing age and is the result of the interplay between a number of genetic and environmental factors; hypercholesterolaemia in the population has a multifactorial basis. Hydroxymethyl glutaryl coenzyme (HMG-CoA) reductase inhibitors ('statins') have revolutionized the treatment of hypercholesterolaemia. This section deals primarily with some of the most common monogenic forms of hyperlipidaemia.

The following are considered healthy measurements for most people (Heart UK):
- a total cholesterol of 5 mmol/l or less;
- a non-high-density lipoprotein (HDL)-cholesterol of 4 mmol/l or less;
- an LDL-cholesterol of 3 mmol/l or less;
- a fasting triglyceride should be 2 mmol/l or less;
- a non-fasting triglyceride should be <4 mmol/l.

Clinical approach

History: key points
- Three-generation family tree, with enquiry about relatives with hypercholesterolaemia, heart attacks (document the age), angina (document the age of onset), and cause of death (document the age).
- History of Achilles 'tenosynovitis'.

Examination: key points
- Examine carefully for tendon xanthomata over the Achilles tendons (often there is fibrous swelling overlying cholesterol accumulation deep within the tendon, so the xanthoma may feel hard) and over the tendons overlying the knuckles with the fingers outstretched.
- Look for an arcus senilis.

Investigations
- Lipid profile.
- DNA for molecular genetic testing in an affected member of the family.

Diagnoses/conditions to consider

Familial hypercholesterolaemia (FH)
Although historically the prevalence of FH in the UK was thought to be 1/500, several recent molecular genetic studies have found a prevalence closer to 1/250 (Walter 2015 and Wald 2017) confirming reports from other European countries (Benn 2016). The majority of these patients have a mutation in the gene coding for the Low Density Lipoprotein Receptor (LDLR). There is a much higher incidence of FH in certain populations, such as the Afrikaaners (1/80), Christian Lebanese, Finns, and French-Canadians, due to founder effects. Serum cholesterol concentrations are elevated from birth and generally approximately twice normal values. By adult life, serum cholesterol in heterozygotes is typically 9.0–14.0 mmol/l. Heterozygotes develop xanthomata over tendons, especially the Achilles tendons and the tendons overlying the knuckles of the hand. Corneal arcus and xanthelasma also tend to develop at a younger age than in the general population. Heterozygotes are at high risk of coronary heart disease, and without treatment the elevated serum cholesterol concentrations lead to a

>50% risk of fatal or non-fatal coronary heart disease by age of 50 years in men and at least 30% in women aged 60 years (Marks *et al.* 2003). The clinical diagnosis of FH is based on a family history of hypercholesterolaemia and premature coronary atherosclerosis, the lipid profile, and the presence of xanthomata (Marks *et al.* 2003). Treatment is with statins, which the 2008 NICE guidelines (NICE CG71; (Wierzbicki *et al.* 2008) and recent reviews (Vuorio *et al.* 2013) recommend should be considered by the age of 10 years in both girls and boys, with the presence of additional risk factors, such as early age of onset of CHD in relatives and actual level of LDL-cholesterol, being taken into account. Lifestyle modifications, such as a healthy diet and especially avoidance of smoking, are important adjuncts to drug therapy.

Homozygotes and compound heterozygotes have very severe hypercholesterolaemia and develop xanthomata in childhood over tendons, the skin of the popliteal and antecubital fossae, and the buttocks, and in the webs between the fingers. Statins have only a minor effect on cholesterol levels, and LDL apheresis is the mainstay of treatment. Life expectancy is severely curtailed and most die by the age of 20 years due to supravalvular aortic stenosis and coronary heart disease.

Familial defective apoB-100 (FDB)
Approximately 1/1000 of the European population are heterozygous for a mutation in apolipoprotein B (*APOB*) on 2p23–24. There is a common mutation p.R3527Q that occurs in the LDLR-binding domain of apoB-100 (Rader *et al.* 2003) that is found in ~5% of UK FH patients. In FDB heterozygotes, plasma levels of LDL-cholesterol overlap with the upper end of the normal range. Clinically, FDB is indistinguishable from FH, although there are fewer tendon xanthomata. Treatment is with statins and lifestyle modification.

FDB homozygotes have levels of plasma LDL-cholesterol comparable to those in FH heterozygotes, rather than those in FH homozygotes.

Finally, proprotein convertase subtilisin kexin type 9 (*PCSK9*) was shown in 2003 to be a third gene for FH (Abifadel *et al.* 2003). The gene encodes an enzyme belonging to the proteinase K family of subtilases which is predominantly expressed in the liver and intestine. It is synthesized as a zymogen that undergoes autocatalytic processing in the endoplasmic reticulum (Abifadel *et al.* 2003) and secreted PCSK9 functions in the post-translational regulation of the LDLR during intracellular recycling, thus controlling the number of LDLRs on the cell surface. In the UK, ~2% of FH patients have one gain-of-function mutation p.D374Y in the gene for *PCSK9* (Humphries *et al.* 2006).

Autosomal recessive (AR) hypercholesterolaemia (ARH)
AR hypercholesterolaemia is caused by mutations in the *ARH* gene that encodes a novel adaptor protein involved in the intracellular trafficking of the LDLR (Rader *et al.* 2003). Plasma levels of LDL-cholesterol in ARH patients tend to be intermediate between those in FH heterozygotes and homozygotes. The onset of coronary heart disease is later in ARH patients than in patients with homozygous FH. Despite having lower plasma levels of cholesterol than FH homozygotes, patients with ARH often have large, bulky xanthomata (Rader *et al.* 2003). Treatment is with statins, but LDL apheresis is necessary

to maintain optimal cholesterol levels in most affected patients.

Sitosterolaemia (also known as phytosterolaemia)
A rare AR disorder characterized by the presence of tendon and tuberous xanthomata, accelerated atherosclerosis, and premature coronary artery disease. In normal individuals, cholesterol constitutes >99% of circulating sterols; non-cholesterol sterols, such as sitosterol, are present in only trace amounts. In sitosterolaemia, plasma levels of cholesterol are normal, but sitosterol levels are elevated >50-fold. The disorder is caused by mutations in either the *ABCG8* or *ABCA5* genes, which encode ABC half transporters expressed in the intestine (Rader *et al.* 2003).

Genetic advice
Mutations are detected in 70–80% of patients with the strongest clinical suspicion of FH (Simon Broome definition of FH), but only in 25–30% of those with 'possible' FH (Futema *et al.* 2013). In the majority of those where no mutation can be detected, it is likely that there is a polygenic aetiology to their hypercholesterolaemia (Talmud *et al.* 2013).

Inheritance and recurrence risk
As for the individual condition.

Variability and penetrance
Some families with FH are more susceptible to coronary heart disease than others and, in a few, coronary heart disease occurs at a strikingly young age, e.g. affecting men in their 20s.

Prenatal diagnosis
May be considered for the homozygous form of FH but is not generally indicated for the heterozygous form for which treatment is available.

Predictive testing
Is possible by analysis of lipid profiles or more definitively by molecular genetic analysis if the familial mutation has been defined.

Other family members
Cascade screening of family members is indicated, but in FH and since treatment is recommended to be considered from the age of 10 years, it is not appropriate to defer genetic testing until individuals are in their mid teens and able to participate in the testing process (National Institute for Health and Care Excellence 2008; Wierzbicki *et al.* 2008).

Guidelines for a diagnosis of FH (Scientific Steering Committee on behalf of the Simon Broome Register Group 1999) are a serum cholesterol >6.7 mmol/l in children <16 years, or >7.5 mmol/l in adults plus tendon xanthomata in the patient or a first- or second-degree relative of the patient.

Natural history and management
The prognosis for patients with heterozygous FH has improved with the introduction of more effective treatment, with recent studies showing a decline in the relative risk of coronary mortality in patients aged 20–59 years from an 8-fold risk prior to 1992 and the introduction of statin therapy to 3.7-fold thereafter (Neil *et al.* 2008).

Surveillance
Affected patients should be under the care of a lipid clinic.

Support group: Heart UK, https://heartuk.org.uk, Tel. 01628 628 638.

Expert adviser: Steve E. Humphries, Emeritus Professor Cardiovascular Genetics, Institute Cardiovascular Science, University College London, London, UK.

References
Abifadel M, Varret M, Rabès JP, *et al.* Mutations in *PCSK9* cause autosomal dominant hypercholesterolemia. *Nat Genet* 2003; **34**: 154–6.

Benn M, Watts GF, *et al.* Mutations causative of familial hypercholesterolaemia: screening of 98 098 individuals from the Copenhagen General Population Study estimated a prevalence of 1 in 217. *Eur Heart J* 2016; **37**(17): 1384–94.

Futema M, Whittall RA, Kiley A, *et al.* Analysis of the frequency and spectrum of mutations recognised to cause familial hypercholesterolaemia in routine clinical practice in a UK specialist hospital lipid clinic. *Atherosclerosis* 2013; **229**: 161–8.

Heart UK. *Cholesterol tests—know your number.* https://heartuk.org.uk/health-and-high-cholesterol/cholesterol-tests---know-your-number.

Humphries SE, Whittall RA, Hubbart CS, *et al.* Genetic causes of familial hypercholesterolaemia in UK patients: relation to plasma lipid levels and coronary heart disease risk. *J Med Genet* 2006; **43**: 943–9.

Lee MH, Gordon D, Ott J, *et al.* Fine mapping of a gene responsible for regulating dietary cholesterol absorption; founder effects underlie cases of phytosterolaemia in multiple communities. *Eur J Hum Genet* 2001; **9**: 375–84.

Marks D, Thorogood M, Neil HA, Humphries SE. A review on the diagnosis, natural history, and treatment of familial hypercholesterolaemia. *Atherosclerosis* 2003; **168**: 1–14.

National Institute for Health and Care Excellence. *Familial hypercholesterolaemia: identification and management.* Clinical Guideline CG71, 2008. https://www.nice.org.uk/guidance/cg71.

Neil A, Cooper J, Betteridge J, *et al.* Reductions in all-cause, cancer, and coronary mortality in statin-treated patients with heterozygous familial hypercholesterolaemia: a prospective registry study. *Eur Heart J* 2008; **29**: 2625–33.

Rader DJ, Cohen J, Hobbs HH. Monogenic hypercholesterolemia: new insights in pathogenesis and treatment. *J Clin Invest* 2003; **111**: 1795–803.

Scientific Steering Committee on behalf of the Simon Broome Register Group. Mortality in treated heterozygous familial hypercholesterolaemia: implications for clinical management. *Atherosclerosis* 1999; **142**: 105–12.

Talmud PJ, Shah S, Whittall R, *et al.* Use of low-density lipoprotein cholesterol gene score to distinguish patients with polygenic and monogenic familial hypercholesterolaemia: a case-control study. *Lancet* 2013; **381**: 1293–301.

UK10K Consortium. Walter K, Min JL, *et al.* The UK10K project identifies rare variants in health and disease. *Nature* 2015; **526**(7571): 82–90.

Vuorio A, Docherty KF, Humphries SE, Kuoppala J, Kovanen PT. Statin treatment of children with familial hypercholesterolemia—trying to balance incomplete evidence of long-term safety and clinical accountability: are we approaching a consensus? *Atherosclerosis* 2013; **226**: 315–20.

Wald DS, Bestwick JP, *et al.* Child-parent familial hypercholesterolemia screening in primary care. *N Engl J Med* 2017; **376**(5): 499–500.

Wierzbicki AS, Humphries SE, Minhas R; Guideline Development Group. Familial hypercholesterolaemia: summary of NICE guidance. *BMJ* 2008; **337**: a1095.

Hypertrophic cardiomyopathy (HCM)

Hypertrophic obstructive cardiomyopathy (HOCM).

HCM is a disease of the myocardium characterized by ventricular hypertrophy (usually asymmetric LVH, with preferential hypertrophy of the septum and anterior LV wall). Individuals with HCM are at risk for arrhythmia (which may cause sudden death), myocardial ischaemia, and heart failure. Cardiac hypertrophy can also be secondary to hypertension and valvular or supravalvular aortic stenosis; in the absence of a family history, these need to be excluded before a diagnosis of HCM is made. It can also occur in NS, FRDA, and some mitochondrial disorders.

Familial HCM affects up to 1/500 adults. It follows an AD mode of inheritance and currently there are >10 identified genes (see Table 3.24). The majority of these encode cardiac sarcomere proteins. About 20% of familial HCM can be attributed to mutations in beta-myosin heavy chain, 20% to myosin-binding protein C, 5% to troponin T, and 5% to troponin I. Overall, mutations in one of these genes are found in 50–60% of families with HCM. DNMs do occur but account for <10% of cases. Most mutations are 'private' missense mutations (all mutations in *MYH7* are missense mutations). LVH tends to develop during childhood and adolescence, although myosin-binding protein C can produce later-onset disease. Hypertrophy is variable in pattern and extent, and only a minority of patients have obstruction.

Cardiomyopathy mutations are notable for substantial variation in clinical presentation. Both genetic heterogeneity and allelic variation contribute to variable morphological phenotypes and disease severity (Burke *et al.* 2016). Note that the Exome Sequencing Project identified an average of one rare TTN missense variant per individual *without* cardiomyopathy (Herman *et al.* 2012).

Clinical approach

History: key points

Three-generation family history, with specific enquiry about the following.

- Deaths attributed to heart problems.
- Sudden unexplained deaths.
- Shortness of breath, chest pain/discomfort, palpitation, light-headedness, and blackouts.
- Try to obtain the death certificate/the post-mortem report/a copy of the echo report to verify the diagnosis in an affected family member and to establish whether hypertrophy was obvious or subtle.

Examination: key points

- If not already seen by a cardiologist, basic cardiovascular assessment, e.g. pulse (jerky?), BP, JVP; palpate the apex (forceful?); auscultation of the heart (ejection systolic murmur due to LV outflow tract obstruction?).
- Are there any features of NS (may be subtle in an adult)? Coexisting pulmonary stenosis or short stature would make this a likely diagnosis.
- Are there any features to suggest a neuromuscular condition, a mitochondrial disorder, or Fabry disease?

Investigations

- 12-lead ECG.
- Echo. Assess the thickness of the ventricular wall and interventricular septum; observe for systolic anterior motion (SAM) of the mitral valve. Maximum wall thickness used in risk stratification.
- If abnormalities on echo/ECG, consider 24-hour tape and exercise test for risk stratification.
- Cardiac MRI (CMR) may be considered for further definition of the disease phenotype if the diagnosis is uncertain. CMR may be useful for detection of apical hypertrophy or aneurysm if echo is inconclusive. Late gadolinium enhancement, as seen in contrast MRI, may have an emerging role in risk stratification. CMR may also be used to help differentiate HCM from disease phenocopies such as Fabry disease and amyloidosis.
- Mutation analysis in one affected member of family: *use a gene panel approach*, where available, unless the familial mutation is known. Samples from other affected members may be helpful to confirm segregation of a potential mutation with disease in the family.
- If late-onset disease, consider mutation analysis for myosin-binding protein C.
- If multiple sudden deaths in children and adolescents, or if the deceased had only mild hypertrophy, prioritize mutation analysis for cardiac troponin T.
- If mutation analysis is not available, consider storing DNA from an affected family member.
- If no antecedent family history in a young patient, consider DNM (<10%), but also consider the possibility of FRDA (a frataxin triplet repeat disorder), as cardiac manifestations may precede neurological symptoms in some.
- If fatigue and exercise limitation are disproportionate to the echo findings, and the family history is consistent with maternal inheritance or is sporadic, consider a mitochondrial disorder (see 'Mitochondrial DNA diseases' in Chapter 3, 'Common consultations', p. 490).

Left ventricular non-compaction cardiomyopathy (LVNC) can mimic HCM on echo. CMR is increasingly employed in a clinical diagnostic setting, allowing the

Table 3.24 Gene defects associated with HCM

% of gene product	Chromosome	Familial HCM	Comment
Beta-myosin heavy chain	14q11.2–12	~30	Degree of hypertrophy and risk of sudden death variable. Some mutations (L908V, G256E, and V606M) associated with benign course; others (R403Q, R453C, and R719W) with high risk of sudden death. However, these correlations are not absolute
Myosin-binding protein C	11p11.2	~20	Hypertrophy with later onset reported
Troponin T	1q3	~5	High risk of sudden death, mild or absent hypertrophy
Troponin I, cardiac	19q13.4	~5	

differentiation of these two conditions. Clinical management of HCM and LVNC differ with regard to stroke prophylaxis. Sarcomeric protein gene mutations can cause both phenotypes and they can occur in different members of the same family.

Other diagnoses/conditions to consider

Noonan syndrome (NS)
Typically, pulmonary valve stenosis, peripheral pulmonary artery stenosis, or HCM with short stature and characteristic facies (*PTPN11* mutations are found in ~40%). A stenotic, and often dysplastic, pulmonary valve is found in 20–50% of affected individuals. See 'Noonan syndrome and the Ras/MAPK pathway syndromes: neuro-cardio-facial-cutaneous syndromes' in Chapter 3, 'Common consultations', p. 512.

LEOPARD (lentigines–ECG abnormalities–ocular hypertelorism–pulmonary stenosis–abnormal genitalia–retardation of growth–deafness)
An AD condition. The lentigines are small (<5 mm) numerous dark brown spots, mainly over the face and trunk. Deafness (sensorineural) is variable, ranging from normal to severe.

Friedreich's ataxia (FRDA)
Mean onset 15.5 ± 8 years, with a range of 2–51 years. The most common inherited ataxia. AR and caused by mutations in frataxin on 9q. Frataxin is a nuclear-encoded mitochondrial protein. It is characterized by a dying-back from the periphery of the longest and largest myelinated fibres (e.g. large fibres arising in dorsal root ganglia). The disease is slowly, but relentlessly, progressive with loss of walking ~15 years after onset and mean age of death of ~37.5 years (usual cause is CM). See 'Ataxic child' in Chapter 2, 'Clinical approach', p. 74 for more details.

Fabry disease
An XL semi-dominant disorder caused by deficiency of alpha-galactosidase on Xq. Characterized by angiokeratoma (small, raised, red vascular lesions around the buttocks and genital region), episodes of neuropathic pain (burning sensation in the extremities worsened by exercise and extremes of temperature), and cardiac hypertrophy (especially LV) with conduction defects leading to a shortened PR interval and prolonged QRS complex. Stroke and renal failure are the most common causes of death. Median age of death in untreated males is 48–49 years; life expectancy in heterozygous women is also shortened. See 'Corneal clouding' in Chapter 2, 'Clinical approach', p. 120.

Arrhythmogenic right ventricular dysplasia (ARVD) or cardiomyopathy (ARVC)
An AD heart muscle disorder that causes arrhythmia, heart failure, and sudden death. It is characterized by replacement of the RV myocardium by adipose and fibrous tissue. A total of 14.5% of cases have cardiac hypertrophy, assessed by an increase in heart weight and/or LV wall thickness. See 'Long QT syndrome and other inherited arrhythmia syndromes' in Chapter 3, 'Common consultations', p. 480.

Genetic advice

Inheritance and recurrence risk
AD with 50% risk to offspring of affected individuals.

Variability and penetrance
Variable expression of the disease is common, even among family members carrying the same mutation.

Penetrance is age-dependent and incomplete. Finding of a normal ECG and echo in a child or adolescent reduces the probability of developing HCM but does not exclude it (see 'Surveillance' below).

Prenatal diagnosis
In a family with a known mutation, this is technically possible. It is usually only considered by families with mutations carrying a high risk of sudden death.

Predictive testing
In a family with a known mutation, this could be offered so that cardiac surveillance could be targeted more appropriately. Otherwise, screening of at-risk relatives should be offered. See 'Testing for genetic status' in Chapter 1, 'Introduction', p. 38 for a discussion of the issues relating to genetic testing in children.

Other family members
See Box 3.5.

Natural history and management

Progression of symptoms due to LV dysfunction is usually slow, but about 10% develop a dilated end-stage CM. Beta-blockers, calcium channel antagonists, and disopyramide may improve symptoms. Surgery or catheter intervention is an option for patients with obstruction that has not responded to medical therapy. LV outflow tract obstruction at rest is a predictor of progression to severe symptoms of heart failure and of death.

Potential long-term complications
- Sudden death. Some genetic defects, e.g. cardiac troponin T, may cause sudden death in the absence of symptoms or hypertrophy. Most patients who die from HCM have only mild (15–20 mm) or moderate (20–25 mm) LVH. Annual cardiovascular mortality is 0.7–1.4%. The greatest risk is in young patients with recurrent syncope or with a strong family history of sudden death. Intense physical exertion may trigger sudden death and should be avoided in high-risk patients. Amiodarone reduces the risk of sudden death and ICDs have a role in some high-risk patients.
- Arrhythmia. Ventricular arrhythmias during 48-hour ambulatory ECG monitoring are a predictor of risk in adults. Atrial fibrillation poses a risk of embolism and anticoagulation is advised.
- Subacute bacterial endocarditis (SBE). Patients with outflow obstruction and/or mitral regurgitation need antibiotic prophylaxis, e.g. for dental work.

Surveillance
Affected individuals should be under regular long-term surveillance by a cardiologist. In 'at-risk' relatives, it is difficult to know how early cardiac surveillance should be started or for how long it should be continued. The family history is a very important factor in informing these decisions. Presentation in preschool children is rare (and raises suspicion of a disorder such as NS) and presentation is unusual in children of primary school age.

In most circumstances, children should be screened clinically every 2 years from around 8–10 years of age and then annually through puberty. Except in families where affected adults have minimal hypertrophy or clearly late-onset hypertrophy (as distinct from late presentation), an entirely normal ECG and echo by late teens are sufficient to discontinue surveillance.

Box 3.5 Major and minor criteria for the diagnosis of HCM in adult members of affected families*

Major criteria

Echocardiographic features
LV wall thickness ≥13 mm in the anterior septum or posterior wall or ≥15 mm in the posterior septum or free wall
Severe systolic anterior motion (SAM) of the mitral valve (septal–leaflet contact)

Electrocardiographic (ECG) features
LVH + repolarization changes
T-wave inversion in leads I and aVL (≥3 mm; with QRS–T-wave axis difference ≥30°), V3–V6 (≥3 mm), or II and III and aVF (≥5 mm)
Abnormal Q (>40 ms or >25% R-wave) in at least two leads from II, III, aVF (in absence of left anterior hemiblock), V1–V4; or I, aVL, V5–V6

Minor criteria

Echocardiographic features
LV wall thickness of 12 mm in the anterior septum or posterior wall or 14 mm in the posterior septum or free wall
Moderate systolic anterior motion (SAM) of the mitral valve (no leaflet–septal contact)
Redundant mitral valve leaflets

Electrocardiographic (ECG) features
Complete bundle branch block (BBB) or (minor) interventricular conduction defect (in LV leads)
Minor repolarization changes in LV leads
Deep S V2 (>25 mm)

Clinical features
Unexplained chest pain, dyspnoea, or syncope
Diagnosis of HCM in a first-degree relative of a patient with HCM is fulfilled by:

• One major criterion, *or*
• Two minor echocardiographic criteria, *or*
• One minor echocardiographic plus two minor ECG criteria

*NB. Diagnosis of HCM in the presence of other potential causes of LVH (athletic training, hypertension, obesity) is problematical. Diagnostic criteria in those <10 years old requires a body surface area-corrected LV wall thickness of >10 mm. HCM may not be expressed until after adolescent growth is complete.

Reproduced from *Heart*, McKenna *et al*, Experience from clinical genetics in hypertrophic cardiomyopathy: proposal for new diagnostic criteria in adult members of affected families, vol 77, issue 22, pp. 130–2, copyright 1997, with permission from BMJ Publishing Group Ltd.

Where the familial mutation is known, definitive genetic testing may be possible to determine who needs surveillance.

Support group: Cardiomyopathy UK, http://www.cardiomyopathy.org.

Expert adviser: Edward Blair, Consultant Clinical Geneticist, Oxford University Hospitals NHS Foundation Trust, Churchill Hospital, Oxford, UK.

References

Burke MA, Cook SA, Seidman JG, et al. Clinical and mechanistic insights into the genetics of cardiomyopathy. *J Am Coll Cardiol* 2016; **68**(25): 2871–86.

Cannon RO 3rd. Assessing risks in hypertrophic cardiomyopathy. *N Engl J Med* 2003; **349**: 1016–18.

Elliott P, McKenna WJ. Hypertrophic cardiomyopathy. *Lancet* 2004; **363**: 1881–91.

Gersh BJ, Maron BJ, Bonow RO, et al. 2011 ACCF/AHA guideline for the diagnosis and treatment of hypertrophic cardiomyopathy: executive summary: a report of the American College of Cardiology Foundation/American Heart Association Task Force on Practice Guidelines. *Circulation* 2011; **124**: 2761–96.

Herman DS, Lam L, et al. Truncations of titin causing dilated cardiomyopathy. *N Engl J Med* 2012; **366**(7): 619–28.

Maron BJ, Olivotto I, Spirito P, et al. Epidemiology of hypertrophic cardiomyopathy-related death: revisited in a large non-referral based patient population. *Circulation* 2000a; **102**: 858–64.

Maron BJ, Shen WK, Link MS, et al. Efficacy of implantable defibrillators for the prevention of sudden death in patients with hypertrophic cardiomyopathy. *N Engl J Med* 2000b; **342**: 365–73.

Martin MS, Olivotto I, Betocchi S, et al. Effect of left ventricular outflow tract obstruction on clinical outcome in hypertrophic cardiomyopathy. *N Engl J Med* 2003; **348**: 295–303.

McKenna WJ, Spirito P, Desnos M, Dubourg O, Komajda M. Experience from clinical genetics in hypertrophic cardiomyopathy: proposal for new diagnostic criteria in adult members of affected families. *Heart* 1997; **77**: 130–2.

Watkins H, McKenna WJ, Thierfelder L, et al. Mutations in the genes for cardiac troponin T and alpha-tropomyosin in hypertrophic cardiomyopathy. *N Engl J Med* 1995; **332**: 1058–64.

Immunodeficiency and recurrent infection

Congenital, or primary, immunodeficiency disorders (PIDs) are genetically heterogeneous and result from mutations in the many genes involved in the development of the immune system and the immune response. More than 180 single gene defects causing primary immunodeficiency are currently known. The current International Union of Immunological Societies classification of PID disorders divides them into eight groups, as follows:

  I combined immunodeficiencies (e.g. SCID);

  II well-defined syndromes with immunodeficiency (e.g. Wiskott–Aldrich syndrome);

  III predominantly antibody deficiency syndromes (e.g. XL agammaglobulinaemia (XLA));

  IV diseases of immune dysregulation (e.g. XL lymphoproliferative syndrome);

  V congenital defects of phagocyte number, function, or both (e.g. chronic granulomatous disease (CGD));

  VI defects in innate immunity (e.g. NEMO defects);

  VII autoinflammatory disorders (e.g. familial Mediterranean fever (FMF));

  VIII complement deficiencies.

Many families will come to the genetic clinic with a clinical diagnosis already established by an immunologist or a haematologist. In some families, the molecular diagnosis may have been established, but, despite recent advances, some familial disorders remain uncharacterized. Immunodeficiency can also be acquired, e.g. in critically ill children with overwhelming infection. Discussion with an immunologist will usually enable you to determine whether the immunodeficiency was a component of the underlying condition (i.e. a useful diagnostic handle) or an acquired feature.

Most PIDs are caused by single gene defects and present in infancy or preschool years.

Clinical approach

History: key points

• Three-generation family tree, extended further on the maternal side, if possible, with specific enquiry about immunodeficiency, infant or childhood death, either unexplained or due to infection, malignancy, and haematological disorders.

• Document the postnatal history of the proband, including the types of infections they have experienced, the ages at which they occurred, and the nature of the pathogens. Is the child prone to bacterial or viral infections, or both? Have there been any opportunistic or fungal infections? Vaccination history, including bacille Calmette–Guérin (BCG).

Examination: key points

• Growth parameters. Height, weight, OFC. Failure to thrive is common.

• Examine the skin (eczema, erythroderma, skin virus infections, e.g. warts).

• Examine for lymphadenopathy, presence or absence of tonsils, hepatosplenomegaly.

Investigations

• Blood for molecular genetic analysis for the specific disorder (if available); for those that are molecularly undefined, screening of a panel of immunodeficiency genes by next-generation sequencing, or WES/WGS, may be appropriate. Otherwise store a DNA sample for future use.

• For certain disorders, specific protein analysis is appropriate (and may already have been performed) before embarking on mutation screening.

In addition, if the child has not been diagnosed or comprehensively evaluated by a clinical immunologist and the process of investigation is just beginning, it is important to refer to an immunologist for appropriate Immunology investigations. In most cases, the following investigations will be included.

• FBC (in EDTA) for white cell count, differential count, and in some cases examination of a blood film.

• Immunoglobulins: clotted sample.

• T-cell subsets (EDTA). This will need to be discussed beforehand with the immunology laboratory.

• Antibody response to prior immunization, e.g. tetanus, diphtheria: clotted sample.

• Neutrophil function tests and analysis of innate immune pathways in some cases.

Specific diagnoses/conditions to consider

I Combined immunodeficiencies

A large number of combined immunodeficiencies disorders are now known, but it is beyond the scope of this chapter to discuss all of them. Those encountered most frequently in clinical practice are included.

SEVERE COMBINED IMMUNODEFICIENCIES (SCID). Affects ~1/30 000 live births and is genetically heterogeneous, being caused by mutations that influence the maturation of lymphocytes, particularly T-cells. Symptoms usually start at <7 months with failure to thrive and diarrhoea, oral candidiasis, and opportunistic infections such as *Pneumocystis jiroveci* pneumonia (PJP). Other infections include viral infections, systemic aspergillosis, and systemic candidiasis. Most patients die within 2 years if they do not receive a successful stem cell transplant or, in highly selected cases, gene therapy. The tonsils are usually absent, as is the thymic shadow on chest X-ray. Most affected infants are lymphopenic, with absent or low T-cells. Subtypes of SCID are defined by lymphocyte phenotyping for CD3, CD4, CD8, CD19, and CD16/56. Inheritance is either XL or AR. The underlying genetic defect can be defined in ~70% of cases. Most cases are treated by stem cell transplantation (SCT).

X-LINKED SCID (T−, B+, NATURAL KILLER (NK)−) Is caused by mutations in the common γ-chain (γ_c) gene (also known as interleukin-2 receptor γ-chain). The γ_c chain is an essential component of five cytokine receptors, all of which are necessary for the development of T-cells and NK cells. The causative mutation is identifiable in most families. Affected males become unwell in the first few months and fail to thrive because of frequent infections. Most infants are treated by SCT, and in selected cases gene therapy has been successful. Female carriers show unilateral X-inactivation in purified T-cells.

AUTOSOMAL RECESSIVE SCID

• Defects in VDJ recombination (T−, B−, NK+). Molecular defects in the recombinase-activating genes *RAG1* or *RAG2*, or *Artemis*, lead to a variable phenotype, depending on the amount of residual protein activity.

In complete *RAG* or *Artemis* deficiency, severe SCID results from the failure to express functional T⁻ and B-cell receptors. Partial deficiency may result in a SCID variant known as Omenn syndrome, characterized by severe failure to thrive, erythrodermic skin rash, lymphadenopathy, hepatosplenomegaly, and severe infections. Complete SCID and Omenn syndrome may occur within the same pedigree.

- Adenosine deaminase (ADA) deficiency (T⁻, B⁻, NK⁻). A defect in purine metabolism that leads to accumulation of metabolites that are toxic to lymphocytes. ADA has an important role in the intermediate pathways of purine metabolism in all tissues, and deficiency may also cause a variety of other abnormalities, including skeletal, renal, and neurodevelopmental abnormalities. This condition was the first disorder to be treated by ERT in clinical medicine and also the first disease to be treated by gene therapy. Most cases are still treated by SCT.

- Purine nucleoside phosphorylase (PNP) deficiency (T^{low}, B^{low}, NK^{low}). Another defect in purine metabolism, but much rarer than ADA deficiency, with only a few cases reported worldwide. The immunodeficiency in PNP deficiency often presents later, and neurodevelopmental problems are frequent.

- Interleukin-7 receptor α (IL-7Rα) deficiency (T⁻, B⁺, NK⁺). A rare form of SCID caused by defects in the IL-7Rα gene, which is essential for normal development of T-cells.

- Janus-associated kinase 3 (Jak-3) deficiency (T⁻, B⁺, NK⁻). An AR form of SCID, immunologically indistinguishable from the XL form. Jak-3 is part of the same T-cell signalling pathway as common γc.

OTHER COMBINED IMMUNODEFICIENCIES

- MHC (major histocompatibility complex) class 2 deficiency (bare lymphocyte syndrome). Defects in several regulatory genes essential for expression of MHC class 2 (*DR*) molecules cause a severe immunodeficiency characterized by a clinical syndrome similar to SCID, with low CD4⁺ T-cells, hypogammaglobulinaemia, and absence of *DR* expression. Survival beyond the first decade is unusual without BMT.

- CD40 ligand deficiency (XL hyper-IgM syndrome). Mutations in the CD40 ligand gene cause absence or defective function of the CD40 ligand on the surface of activated T-cells, resulting in failure of the T-cell/B-cell interaction required for immunoglobulin isotype switching, as well as a functional T-cell defect. Affected boys usually present with recurrent bacterial infections or PCP. There is a high incidence of liver disease. Supportive treatment is with immunoglobulin replacement and anti-infective prophylaxis, but increasingly BMT is performed because of the poor long-term survival.

II Well-defined syndromes with immunodeficiency

WISKOTT—ALDRICH SYNDROME. An XL disorder characterized by thrombocytopenia (with small platelets), atypical eczema, and immunodeficiency, with susceptibility to opportunistic and pyogenic infections and lymphoproliferative disease or lymphoid malignancy, often associated with Epstein–Barr virus (EBV). Supportive treatment is with immunoglobulin, anti-infectives, platelet transfusions, and sometimes splenectomy, but BMT is usually recommended. Caused by mutations in *WASP* which is involved in the regulation of the actin cytoskeleton and

is found only in blood cells. Female carriers have non-random X chromosome inactivation in whole blood.

DNA REPAIR DEFECTS (OTHER THAN THOSE INCLUDED IN I). Immunodeficiency is a feature of many of the DNA repair syndromes, especially AT and NBS and occasionally Fanconi syndrome. See 'DNA repair disorders' in Chapter 3, 'Common consultations', p. 398.

THYMIC DEFECTS: DI GEORGE SYNDROME (DGS)/VELOCARDIOFACIAL (DEL 22Q11 SYNDROME). There is a wide spectrum of immunological abnormalities in 22q11 microdeletion syndrome. A small percentage (<2%) of infants have complete DGS with absent T-cells and may require corrective therapy (thymic transplant or BMT), but most have only a moderate T-cell lymphopenia, mainly affecting CD8 T-cells, which improves over the first few years of life. Some affected individuals have a variable degree of humoral immunodeficiency. See '22q11 deletion syndrome' in Chapter 5, 'Chromosomes', p. 624.

CHARGE SYNDROME (CHD7). Patients with CHARGE syndrome (due to heterozygous mutation of *CHD7*) can have a moderate or severe T-cell lymphopenia. See 'Ear anomalies' in Chapter 2, 'Clinical approach', p. 142.

IMMUNO-OSSEOUS DYSPLASIAS. Cartilage–hair hypoplasia is caused by mutations in *RMRP* and is manifest by short-limbed skeletal dysplasia, sparse hair, a variable degree of combined immunodeficiency, and susceptibility to malignancy. The immunodeficiency may be severe enough to warrant SCT.

HYPER-IGE SYNDROMES (AD HYPER-IGE SYNDROME (JOB'S SYNDROME)). Characterized by distinctive facial features, eczema, osteoporosis and fractures, dental abnormalities, and severe skin and pulmonary bacterial (particularly staphylococcal) infections with pneumatocele formation. It is caused by dominant negative heterozygous mutations in *STAT-3*. AR hyper-IgE syndrome caused by mutations in *DOCK-8* results in recurrent respiratory infections and severe cutaneous viral infections (warts, molluscum contagiosum, herpes simplex).

III Predominantly antibody deficiency syndromes

X-LINKED AGAMMAGLOBULINAEMIA (XLA; BRUTON DISEASE). XLA is characterized by early-onset bacterial infections (recurrent otitis media, pneumonitis, sinusitis, and conjunctivitis), marked reduction in all classes of serum immunoglobulins, and very low or absent B-cells (CD19⁺ cells). Babies are usually well in the first few months of life (until transplacentally acquired maternal immunoglobulins wane). Treatment is with lifelong immunoglobulin replacement and early intervention with antibiotics for infection. The long-term outlook is good, although there is a risk of chronic lung disease and enteroviral meningoencephalitis. XLA is caused by mutations in *BTK* on Xq21.3–22. Fifty per cent of males with newly diagnosed XLA have no family history. In this instance, 15–20% have *de novo BTK* mutations, and in 80–85% the mother is a carrier (with the mutation usually arising in her father).

AR IMMUNOGLOBULIN DEFICIENCIES. Clinically and immunologically indistinguishable from XLA, resulting from mutations in other genes that are required for normal B-cell development including μ heavy chain, Igα, λ5, or *BLNK*.

COMMON VARIABLE IMMUNODEFICIENCY (CVID). The most common form of antibody deficiency. CVID most frequently presents in young adulthood but can present at any age. It is characterized by low immunoglobulin levels, variable abnormalities of T- and B-cell numbers and function, and an increased incidence of autoimmunity, granulomatous disease, and malignancy. There is often a family history of IgA deficiency. Variable patterns of inheritance, with some families showing an AD pattern. Exclusion of molecularly defined forms of immunodeficiency is required. In most individuals with CVID, the molecular defect is not known, although rare families have been described with a defect in *BAFF-R*, *CD19*, *CD20*, or *ICOS* gene.

IV Diseases of immune dysregulation

IMMUNODEFICIENCY WITH HYPOPIGMENTATION: CHEDIAK–HIGASHI SYNDROME (CHS). An AR disorder characterized by partial albinism, abnormal leucocytes containing giant granules, easy bruising, and neurological abnormalities. Most affected individuals progress to an 'accelerated' lymphoproliferative or haemophagocytic lymphohistiocytosis-like phase that is fatal without BMT. Caused by defects in *LYST* (*CHS1*), which plays an important role in lysosomal protein trafficking. Griscelli syndrome (defects in *RAB27A*) and Hermansky–Pudlak syndrome (mutations in *AP3B1*) also cause partial albinism and variable degrees of immunodeficiency.

FAMILIAL HAEMOPHAGOCYTIC LYMPHOHISTIOCYTOSIS (FHL) SYNDROMES. AR disorders caused by mutations in perforin, Munc13-4, syntaxin 11, or Munc18-2, and resulting in a severe inflammatory condition with fever, hepatosplenomegaly, pancytopenia, and haemophagocytosis. Requires aggressive treatment with chemotherapy and usually SCT.

LYMPHOPROLIFERATIVE SYNDROMES. XL lymphoproliferative (XLP) syndrome type 1 (Duncan syndrome) is a rare disorder characterized by the inability to effectively handle EBV infection. Manifestations include severe (often fatal) infectious mononucleosis, acquired hypogammaglobulinaemia, lymphoproliferative disease or lymphoma, haemophagocytic lymphohistiocytosis-like syndromes, and aplastic anaemia. XLP1 is caused by defects in the *SH2D1A* gene encoding SAP (SLAM-associated protein). XLP type 2 also manifests as haemophagocytic syndrome, which may be triggered by EBV infection, but can also present with inflammatory bowel disease or splenomegaly. XLP2 is caused by mutations in XIAP (X-linked inhibitor of apoptosis).

SYNDROMES WITH AUTOIMMUNITY. (1) Autoimmune lymphoproliferative syndromes: defects of apoptosis result in chronic lymphadenopathy, hepatosplenomegaly, autoimmune cytopenias, and an increased risk of lymphoma. These are characterized by an increased percentage of CD4$^-$/CD8$^-$ double-negative T-cells and abnormal lymphocyte apoptosis. Causes include mutations in Fas, Fas-ligand, caspase-10, caspase-8, NRAS, and FADD. (2) Autoimmune polyendocrinopathy with candidiasis and ectodermal dystrophy (APECED), caused by mutations in *AIRE* (autoimmune regulator), results in a syndrome with multiple organ-specific autoimmune manifestations and chronic mucocutaneous candidiasis. (3) IPEX (immune dysregulation, polyendocrinopathy, enteropathy, X-linked) syndrome is characterized by severe enteropathy, early-onset IDDM, and other autoimmune disorders and is caused by defects in *FOXP3*.

V Congenital defects of phagocyte number, function, or both

DEFECTS OF NEUTROPHIL DIFFERENTIATION: SEVERE CONGENITAL NEUTROPENIA OR CONGENITAL AGRANULOCYTOSIS (KOSTMANN SYNDROME). A rare disorder characterized by severe persistent neutropenia. AD forms caused by mutations in *ELANE* or *GFI1*, and AR forms by mutations in *HAX1* or *G6PC3*. Treatment with granulocyte colony-stimulating factor (G-CSF) may increase absolute neutrophil counts and reduce vulnerability to overwhelming infection. However, patients are at increased risk of developing AML and myelodysplastic syndromes. Cyclic neutropenia is also caused by mutations in the gene encoding neutrophil elastase (*ELANE*). Cyclic dips in neutrophil counts approximately every 21 days and lasting 3–7 days. Along with neutropenia, there are also cyclic drops in the reticulocyte and monocyte counts. Episodes of neutropenia may be severe, e.g. <200 × 10^6/ml, sometimes with fever, pharyngitis, and bacterial infections. Can also be treated with G-CSF.

DEFECTS OF MOTILITY: LEUCOCYTE ADHESION DEFICIENCIES. AR disorders caused by genes that encode components of the three integrin complexes on the neutrophil cell surface, causing impaired adhesion of leucocytes to the endothelium, impaired chemotaxis, and impaired phagocytosis. The condition can be caused by defects in CD18 (INTGB2), FUCT1, and KINDLIN3. Typically presents in infancy with delayed separation of the umbilical cord, severe superficial infections, and high circulating neutrophil count. Foci of infection show a lack of neutrophils. Severely affected patients often die in infancy or early childhood without BMT.

DEFECTS OF RESPIRATORY BURST: CHRONIC GRANULOMATOUS DISEASE (CGD). Characterized by recurrent severe catalase-positive bacterial and fungal infections, e.g. pneumonia, lymphadenitis, cutaneous infections, hepatic abscesses, osteomyelitis. It is a genetically heterogeneous disorder characterized by defective production of superoxide (O$_2^-$) by neutrophils, monocytes, and eosinophils, as a result of defects in components of the membrane-linked NADPH (reduced nicotinamide–adenine dinucleotide phosphate) oxidase. One XL and three autosomal genes encode protein components of the respiratory burst oxidase. The XL form of CGD accounts for the majority of cases; the other forms are AR. The diagnosis is confirmed by the nitroblue tetrazolium (NBT) slide test confirming abnormal neutrophil O$_2^-$ or peroxide production. Treatment includes antibiotic and antifungal prophylaxis, and interferon γ (IFNγ) may be helpful during severe infective episodes. BMT may be recommended. Female carriers of the XL type show intermediate levels of NBT reduction as a result of lyonization. The molecular type can be confirmed by western blotting prior to mutation screening.

MSMD (MENDELIAN SUSCEPTIBILITY TO MYCOBACTERIAL DISEASE). AR defects in the IFNγ receptor/interleukin-12 (IL-12) pathway result in increased susceptibility to intracellular organisms, including mycobacterial and salmonella infections. The severity varies, and some patients can be managed with antimicrobial prophylaxis and/or IFNγ replacement. BMT has been performed in a few patients, with variable results.

VI Defects in innate immunity

ANHIDROTIC ECTODERMAL DYSPLASIA WITH IMMUNODE-
FICIENCY (EDA-ID). The XL form is caused by NEMO
deficiency and results in a variable degree of immunodeficiency with defective polysaccharide antibody responses,
mycobacterial susceptibility, and inflammatory complications including arthritis and enteropathy. Gain-of-function
mutations in *IKBA* cause AD ectodermal dysplasia and a
variable T-cell immunodeficiency.

DEFECTS OF TLR PATHWAYS. Various TLR defects have
been defined that lead to specific phenotypes, including IRAK-4 deficiency (recurrent pyogenic infections
with low inflammatory markers), TLR3 (herpes simplex
encephalitis), and others.

VII Autoinflammatory disorders
The 2014 classification defines these as disorders marked
by abnormally increased inflammation, mediated predominantly by the cells and molecules of the innate
immune system.
• FMF, caused by heterozygous mutation in *MEFV*
(encoding the protein pyrin), is an AR disorder characterized by recurrent episodes of fever that may be
associated with abdominal pain, joint pain, or chest
pain. FMF usually begins in childhood and is characterized by attacks lasting 1–3 days. It is more common
in people of Mediterranean origin, e.g. Jews, Arabs,
Greeks, Italians, Armenians, and Turks. FMF predisposes to amyloidosis; it may respond well to prophylaxis with colchicine.
• Muckle–Wells syndrome (AD), neonatal-onset multisystem inflammatory disease (NOMID), chronic
infantile neurologic cutaneous and articular syndrome
(CINCA) with mutation in *CIAS1*, and familial cold
inflammatory syndrome (*CIAS1* and *NLRP12*): fevers,
urticarial, rashes, arthropathy, and amyloidosis
in MWS.
• Majeed syndrome: chronic multifocal osteomyelitis and
dyserythropoietic anaemia. Caused by biallelic mutations in *LPIN2*.

VIII Complement disorders
• SLE-like disorders. The most commonly seen due to
heterozygous mutation in *C1Q*.

• Also includes the 3MC syndrome group of conditions
where children have significant facial dysmorphology
(clefts, hypertelorism, etc.).

Other defects
• Asplenia, isolated congenital. A rare cause of primary
immunodeficiency. Affected individuals may die of
overwhelming bacterial infection in early childhood,
but the condition shows incomplete penetrance.
Affected individuals require antibiotic prophylaxis and
immunization against *Pneumococcus*. Caused by heterozygous mutation in *RPSA* (Bolze et al. 2013).
An increasing number of molecular defects are being
defined, and more will emerge. Tables 3.25 and 3.26
provide a summary of the current major known defects.
There are many other complex syndromes that include
immunodeficiency as a component.

Genetic advice
Inheritance and recurrence risk
• Counsel for the specific diagnosis in question.
• XLA. XLR; 80–85% of mothers of isolated cases are
carriers. Most DNMs arise in the maternal grandfather; maternal grandmothers are carriers in <20% of
isolated cases. The risk of carrier status in a woman
whose sister has a son with XLA where there is no
other family history is therefore <10%. More than 90%
of affected boys have detectable mutations in *BTK*. The
causative mutation provides a cornerstone for advising family members about their carrier status. Even if
the mother is not a carrier, there is a small possibility
(<5%) of recurrence due to germline mosaicism.

Prenatal diagnosis
• Mutation analysis is usually possible by CVS, but only if
the causative mutation in the proband has been identi-
fied. Prenatal testing by mutation screening is routinely
available in the UK for a number of genes, including:
  • XLA;
  • SCID: XL SCID (common γ-chain (γc) deficiency)
    and some AR types;
  • XL hyper-IgM syndrome (CD40 ligand deficiency);
  • Wiskott–Aldrich syndrome;
  • XLP syndrome (Duncan syndrome).

Table 3.25 X-linked immunodeficiencies

Disorder	Gene	Chromosome
X-linked severe combined immunodeficiency (SCID)	Common γ chain (γc)	Xq13
X-linked hyper-IgM syndrome (CD40 ligand def)	Common γ chain (γc)	Xq13
Dyskeratosis congenita (variable immunodeficiency) Hoyeraal–Hreidarsson syndrome SCID (T⁺B⁻NK⁻ SCID)	*Dyskerin (DKCI)*	Xq28
Wiskott–Aldrich syndrome	*WASP*	Xp11
X-linked agammaglobulinaemia (Bruton's disease; XLA)	*BTK*	Xq22
X-linked lymphoproliferative (XLP1; Duncan) syndrome	*SAP*	Xq25
X-linked inactivator of apoptosis (XLP2)	*XIAP*	Xq25
X-linked chronic granulomatous disease (CGD)	*gp91phox*	Xp21
IPEX (immunodysregulation, polyendocrinopathy, enteropathy, X-linked)	*FoxP3*	Xp11
NEMO (EDA-ID)	*NEMO*	Xq28
Properdin deficiency	*Properdin*	Xp21

Table 3.26 Autosomal recessive immunodeficiencies

Disorder	Gene	Chromosome
Adenosine deaminase (ADA) deficiency	*ADA*	20q12–13
Purine nucleoside phosphorylase (PNP) deficiency	*PNP*	14q11
Recombinase-activating gene deficiency	*RAG1/RAG2*	11p13
Ommen syndrome		
DNA repair defects	*DNA ligase IV*	13q22
	Artemis	10p
	DNA ligase IV	13q22-q34
	DNA PKc	15q25-26
T-cell receptor deficiencies	*CD3γ/CD3αβ*	11q23
	CD3δ	11q23
	CD3ε	11q23
	CD3γ	11q23
Zap70 deficiency	*ZAP70*	2q12
JAK3 deficiency (T⁻, B⁺, NK⁻ SCID)	*JAK3*	19p13
IL-7 receptor deficiency	IL-7 receptor α	5p13
Coronin 1A deficiency	Coronin 1A	12q24
Reticular dysgenesis	Adenylate kinase 2	1p34
	TAP1	6p21
MHC class II deficiency	*CIITA (MHC2TA)*	16p13
	RFXANK	19p12
	RFX5	1q21
	RFXAP	13q13
MHC class I deficiency	TAP2	6p21
Cernunnos/NHEJ defect	*Cernunnos*	2q35
Zap70 deficiency	*Zap70*	2q12
Stat5b deficiency	*Stat5b*	17q21.2
ITK deficiency	*ITK*	5q33.3
DOCK8 deficiency	*DOCK8*	9p24.3
Ataxia telangiectasia (AT)	*ATM*	11q22
Nijmegen breakage syndrome	*Nibrin (NBS1)*	8q21.3
ICF syndrome	*DNMT3B (ICF1)*	20q11.21
	ZBT2B4 (ICF2)	6q21
di George syndrome	22q11 microdeletion	22q11
Cartilage hair hypoplasia	*RMRP*	9p13.3
AD hyper-IgE (Job's syndrome)	*STAT3*	17q21.2
AR agammaglobulinaemia	*μ heavy chain*	14q32.33
	Igα	19q13.2
	λ5	22q11.2
	Igβ	17q23.3
	BLNK	10q23
Common variable immunodeficiency (CVID)*	*ICOS*	2q33
	CD19	16p11.2
	CD20	11q12.2
	CD81	11p15.5
	BAFF-R	22q13
	TACI	17p11.2

Table 3.26 Continued

Disorder	Gene	Chromosome
AR hyper-IgM syndrome	*CD40*	20q13.12
	AID	12p13.31
	UNG	12q24.11
Chediak–Higashi syndrome	*LYST*	1q42
Griscelli syndrome	*RAB27A*	15q21.3
Hermansky–Pudlak syndrome type 2	*AP3B1*	5q14.1
Familial HLH	*Perforin*	16q22.2
	Munc13-4 (UNC13D)	17q25.1
	Syntaxin 11	6q24.2
	Munc18-2 (STXBP2)	19p13.2
Autoimmune lymphoproliferative syndrome	*FAS (TNFRSF6)*	10q23.3
	Fas-L (TNFSF6)	1q24.3
	Caspase 8	2q33.1
	Caspase 10	2q33.1
	NRAS (activating)	1p13.2
	FADD	11q13.3
APECED	*AIRE*	21q22.3
Congenital neutropenia	*Elastase (ELANE)*	19p13.3
	HAX1	1q21.3
	G6PC3	17q21.31
Cyclical neutropenia	*ELANE*	19p13.3
Leucocyte adhesion deficiency	*CD18 (INTGB2)*	21q22
Type 1	*FUCT*	11p11.2
Type 2	*-1*	11q13.1
Type 3	*KINDLIN3*	
AR chronic granulomatous disease (CGD)	*p47phox*	7q11
	p67phox	1q25
	p22phox	16p24
	p40phox	22q12.3
Inherited mycobacterial susceptibility (MSMD)	*Interferon γ receptor*	6q23
	IL-12 p40	5q31
	IL-12 receptor β1	19p13
	IFNGR2	21q22,1
	STAT1	2q32.2
GATA-2 deficiency (Mono-Mac syndrome)	*GATA2*	3q21.3
AD EDA-ID	*IKBA*	14q13.2
IRAK-4 deficiency	*IRAK-4*	12q12
MyD88 deficiency	*MyD88*	3p22.2
WHIM syndrome	*CXCR4*	2q22.1
Herpes simplex encephalitis	*TLR3*	4q35.1
	UNC93B1	11q13.2
	TRAF3	14q32.32
Chronic mucocutaneous candidiasis	*IL17RA*	22q11.1
	IL17F	6p12.2

- For other defined molecular defects, mutation screening and PND may be available in research or other laboratories worldwide.
- Linkage analysis. If the diagnosis is secure, but the mutation cannot be defined, PND may be possible by linkage analysis.
- Enzyme analysis. Prenatal testing for ADA and PNP deficiency is reliably performed by enzyme analysis of CVS tissue.
- Fetal blood sampling (FBS). For families affected by SCID where the molecular defect cannot be defined, but the phenotype is clear-cut, second-trimester PND by lymphocyte subpopulation analysis of fetal blood can be offered.

Other family members
- Carrier testing for XL disorders where the causative mutation has been defined is feasible. Carrier testing is also possible by biochemical methods for AR SCID due to ADA or PNP deficiency.
- Cord blood analysis and storage. For all severe immunodeficiencies where SCT may be required, it is appropriate to consider umbilical cord blood stem cell banking at the time of delivery of new siblings. Cord blood from unaffected infants is a potential source of stem cells for affected siblings, while cord blood from infants who are affected by the disorder may be used for future gene therapy. For pregnancies where PND has not been possible, or families have chosen not to have predictive testing, umbilical cord blood should be sent for immunophenotyping or other testing, as appropriate to the disorder. Ideally, this should be arranged in advance with the obstetric unit and the immunology laboratory.

Natural history and management

The natural history in PIDs is highly variable, and the severity of individual disorders can also vary within families. For primary antibody deficiency syndromes, the long-term outlook should be good, provided that the diagnosis is made without delay and that treatment and monitoring are optimal. The mainstay of management is long-term immunoglobulin replacement therapy.

Infants affected by SCID are unlikely to survive beyond the first 2 years of life in the absence of corrective treatment. For many of the other disorders, the long-term outlook is also less favourable, and BMT, other forms of SCT, or gene therapy are increasingly recommended.

BMT and gene therapy
For infants affected by all forms of SCID, BMT from an HLA-identical sibling is the best treatment, with a >90% chance of success. Transplantation from an HLA-matched unrelated donor, a phenotypically identical family member, or a haplo-identical parent has a variable success rate of between 60% and 80%, depending on the nature of the underlying disorder, complications at the time of transplant, and the closeness of the match. Early successes with gene therapy have been reported in X-SCID and ADA deficiency, and this may be an appropriate approach in the absence of a matched sibling donor.

Gene therapy trials are also in progress for X-CGD and Wiskott–Aldrich syndrome and are in development for other severe forms of immunodeficiency.

Potential long-term complications
Complications of primary immunodeficiency may arise either as a result of damage caused by infection or as a result of the immune dysregulation that occurs in many immune disorders.
- Organ damage caused by infection is most frequently chronic lung disease—bronchiectasis—which still occurs in patients with primary antibody deficiency, particularly if the diagnosis is delayed, or immunoglobulin replacement is inadequate, or intercurrent infection is not treated aggressively.
- Enteroviral meningoencephalitis occurs with increased frequency in XLA and CVID, although this complication has become more unusual in recent years with use of higher doses of immunoglobulin.
- Autoimmunity and granulomatous disease are common in CVID and other undefined combined immunodeficiencies.
- Liver disease (especially sclerosing cholangitis) is a particular risk in CD40 ligand deficiency and also occurs in other combined immunodeficiencies.
- Lymphoproliferative disease and malignancy are risks in many immunodeficiency disorders, the latter most particularly in the chromosome breakage disorders.

Surveillance
Affected individuals should be under the care of a clinical immunologist.

Support groups: PID UK, http://www.piduk.org, Tel. 0800 987 8986; CGD Society, http://www.cgdsociety.org, Tel. 0800 987 8988; AT Society, http://www.atsociety.org.uk, Tel. 01582 760 733.

Expert adviser: Alison Jones, Consultant Paediatric Immunologist, Department of Immunology, Great Ormond Street Hospital, London, UK.

References

Al-Herz W, Bousfiha A, Casanova JL, et al. Primary immunodeficiency diseases: an update on the classification from the international union of immunological societies expert committee for primary immunodeficiency. *Front Immunol* 2011; **2**: 54.

Al-Herz W, Bousfiha A, Casanova JL, et al. Primary immunodeficiency diseases: an update on the classification from the international union of immunological societies expert committee for primary immunodeficiency. *Front Immunol* 2014; **5**: 162.

Bolze A, Mahlaoui N, Byun M, et al. Ribosomal protein SA haploinsufficiency in humans with isolated congenital asplenia. *Science* 2013; **340**: 976–78.

Bousfiha AA, Jeddane L, Ailal F, et al. A phenotypic approach for IUIS PID classification and diagnosis: guidelines for clinicians at the bedside. *J Clin Immunol* 2013; **33**: 1078–87.

Ochs HD, Hitzig WH. History of primary immunodeficiency diseases. *Curr Opin Allergy Clin Immunol* 2012; **12**: 577–87.

Ochs HD, Smith CIE, Puck JM (eds.). *Primary immunodeficiency diseases: a molecular and genetic approach*, 3rd edn. Oxford University Press, Oxford, 2013.

Incest

Incest is defined as sexual intercourse between close relatives. In English law, it is the crime of sexual intercourse between parent and child or grandchild, or between siblings or half-siblings (*Shorter Oxford English Dictionary*). Incest has major genetic implications because of the greatly increased risk of AR disorders or multiple recessive disorders occurring in the offspring. Incest also has major social implications because it is illegal in many communities, and the offspring (if they survive) may be offered for adoption/fostering.

There is a high chance that the offspring will be homozygous for a recessive disorder, or possibly multiple recessive disorders. There is also an increased risk for disorders that follow multifactorial inheritance.

Incest may now be detected as an additional finding using genome-wide diagnostic analysis such as SNP array/WES/WGS where unusually high levels of loss of heterozygosity/large numbers of rare homozygous variants may be detected.

Clinical approach

History: key points

- Detailed family tree documenting the precise relationship between the parents of the pregnancy/child in question. Include a full three-generation family tree, taking particular care to identify if there are any known/possible recessive disorders in the extended family.
- Routine history of pregnancy, birth, and development.

Examination: key points

- Measurement of weight, length, and OFC.
- Detailed assessment for dysmorphic features and congenital anomalies.
- Detailed neurological examination, with particular emphasis on hearing and vision.

Special investigations

- DNA from parents and child (after suitable consent).
- Detailed metabolic workup, including urine amino and organic acids and plasma amino acids. If associated developmental delay, see 'Developmental delay in the child with consanguineous parents' in Chapter 2, 'Clinical approach', p. 126.
- Consider testing for common recessive disorders, depending on the ethnic background, e.g. CF in northern Europeans. See 'Consanguinity' in Chapter 3, 'Common consultations', p. 374 and 'Carrier frequency and carrier testing for autosomal recessive disorders' in 'Appendix', p. 810.

Genetic advice

For offspring of first-degree relationships (parent:child, sib:sib)

- Empiric risk. There is an observed increase of 30% in severe abnormalities and mortality, giving an overall risk of ~1/3 for death in childhood or severe abnormality. In addition, there is an increased risk for MR without physical anomaly, bringing the overall risk close to 1/2 (50%).
- Estimated risk. The probability that a pregnancy will be homozygous by descent in a relationship between parent:child or siblings is 1/8 (12.5%); this

Table 3.27 Probability that a pregnancy will be homozygous by descent for a recessive disorder for second-degree relationships

Relationship	Probability
Half-siblings	1/16 (6%)
Uncle/aunt:niece/nephew	1/16 (6%)

is considerably less than the observed excess, and so empiric data are preferable over estimated data.

For offspring of second-degree relationships (half-sibs, uncle/aunt:niece/nephew)

See Table 3.27.

- Empiric risk. The excess risk for MR without physical anomaly recognized for offspring of first-degree relationships is less frequently noted in offspring of first-cousin relationships, but an intermediate risk may exist for offspring of second-degree relationships.
- Estimated risk. The calculations for half-sibs, and uncle/aunt:niece/nephew relationships probably considerably underestimate the risk (see above).

Adults who themselves are the product of an incestuous relationship

Children born as the product of an incestuous relationship who develop normally are not at increased genetic risk when they have children of their own.

Prenatal diagnosis

Detailed fetal anomaly USS, but note limitations as only a small minority of recessive diseases have structural anomalies.

Adoption

Harper (2001) estimates that around 75% of severe recessive disorders will manifest in the first 6 months of life.

Natural history and management

Surveillance

- Children who are born as the product of an incestuous relationship require careful neurological and developmental follow-up.
- The mother who has been involved in an incestuous relationship may require support and protection from social services.

Expert adviser: Eamonn Sheridan, Professor of Clinical Genetics, University of Leeds, Leeds, UK.

References

Grote L, Myers M, Lovell A, Saal H, Sund KL. Variable approaches to genetic counseling for microarray regions of homozygosity associated with parental relatedness. *Am J Med Genet A* 2014; **164A**: 87–98.

Harper PS. *Practical genetic counselling*, 5th edn, revised reprint. Arnold, London, 2001.

Lazarin GA, Haque IS, Nazareth S, *et al.* An empirical estimate of carrier frequencies for 400+ causal Mendelian variants: results from an ethnically diverse clinical sample of 23,453 individuals. *Genet Med* 2012; **15**: 178–86.

Young ID. *Introduction to risk calculation in genetic counselling*, 2nd edn. Oxford University Press, Oxford, 1999.

Leigh encephalopathy

Subacute necrotizing encephalomyelopathy, Leigh's disease, Leigh syndrome.

Leigh encephalopathy presents one of the most challenging clinical problems encountered in the genetics clinic. The diagnosis is often rather difficult to establish; the affected members of the family may have died, and the recurrence risks are potentially high. The varied inheritance patterns (AR, mitochondrial, and XL) encountered in Leigh encephalopathy add to the difficulty. The extreme genetic heterogeneity in AR Leigh complicates matters even further. The first priority is to establish a clear clinical diagnosis and determine whether the proband really does/did have features consistent with a diagnosis of Leigh encephalopathy.

Leigh encephalopathy is a neurodegenerative disorder. The prevalence is ~1/32 000–1/40 000, with a slight male preponderance. The condition presents in infancy with non-specific features such as feeding difficulties, vomiting, regurgitation, growth faltering, hypotonia, seizures, and developmental delay. Later, psychomotor regression, spasticity, ataxia, optic atrophy, CPEO, and signs of brainstem dysfunction (dysphagia, apnoea, cranial nerve palsies) may develop. Episodes of developmental regression may be sporadic or secondary to intercurrent illness and patients often recover some of these skills prior to the next episode of regression. Blood lactate is usually elevated, particularly at times of infection, but blood gas analysis during periods of acute deterioration may reveal a mixed respiratory–metabolic acidosis due to central hypopnoea. CSF lactate is often significantly elevated. Cranial MRI shows bilateral, usually symmetrical, changes in the basal ganglia, brainstem, and subthalamic nuclei. The prognosis for patients presenting in infancy is poor, with few surviving beyond early childhood.

Despite genetic heterogeneity, all of the known defects affect intracellular energy production. A subset of patients carry mitochondrial (mt)DNA point mutations, e.g. m.13513G>A, m.10191T>C, m.10158T>C, and m.8993T>G/C. The heteroplasmy level (proportion of mutated to wild-type mtDNA) of mtDNA mutations is important in determining clinical phenotype and patients carrying lower-level heteroplasmy of these mutations can also present in adult life with quite different clinical features. One of the best examples of this genotype–phenotype variation is seen with the m.8993T>G/C mutations which causes Leigh syndrome in young children and NARP (neuropathy–ataxia–retinitis pigmentosa) in adults. Mutations in a variety of nuclear genes encoding structural subunits and assembly factors for the mitochondrial respiratory chain complexes or components of the pyruvate dehydrogenase (PDH) complex are also associated with Leigh encephalopathy (Lake et al. 2016). Mutations in SURF1, an assembly factor for complex IV, underlie 75% of cytochrome-oxidase-deficient Leigh encephalopathy (i.e. 10–20% of all Leigh syndrome) and follow AR inheritance (Wedatilake et al. 2013).

Clinical approach

History: key points
- Three-generation family tree, with specific enquiry about consanguinity. Extend on the maternal line as far as possible.
- Details of affected family members. Age of onset, clinical features, progression, whether tissue or DNA is stored.

- Age of onset of signs and symptoms. Regression? Seizures? Acidosis? Hypopnoea? Dysphagia?
- Careful documentation of development and loss/recovery of skills.

Examination: key points
- Growth parameters: height, weight, and OFC. Note if any deceleration in head growth.
- Neurological features. Hypotonia, dystonia, spasticity, ataxia.
- Neuromuscular features. Muscle wasting and weakness.
- Ptosis, strabismus, external ophthalmoplegia, optic atrophy.
- Cardiac examination (CM).

Investigations
- Blood and CSF lactate.
- DNA for investigation and storage. A genomic array may be useful, especially in consanguineous families if it incorporates SNP genotyping to identify or exclude candidate loci, given the high genetic heterogeneity.
- Gene panel for Leigh encephalopathy or WES/WGS as appropriate; due to the high genetic heterogeneity in Leigh's, the potential to analyse multiple genes in parallel improves the potential for diagnosis.
- mtDNA investigations; point mutations, and depletion. NB. Markedly skewed segregation of mtDNA mutation to different tissues and loss of mtDNA mutations from rapidly dividing tissues, such as blood, may be misleading, unless appropriate tissues are chosen for investigation. Skeletal muscle provides the most reliable source of mtDNA for sequencing, but some mtDNA mutations can be reliably detected in urine samples.
- Skin biopsy for fibroblast culture for investigation and storage.
- Consider a muscle biopsy, as this may confirm a biochemical diagnosis and help in the evaluation of variants.
- Brain MRI scan. Typical features of Leigh encephalopathy are symmetrical lesions in the basal ganglia, subthalamic nuclei, and brainstem. Leukoencephalopathy can be a consequence of mutations in SURF1 (Farina et al. 2002) and is also observed in patients with complex I-deficient Leigh syndrome (Lebre et al. 2011).
- Ophthalmological assessment of the retina and optic disc, looking for evidence of optic atrophy and/or pigmentary retinopathy.

Other diagnoses/conditions to consider

Biotinidase deficiency
This is treatable with large doses of biotin and should be excluded in all cases of Leigh encephalopathy.

Aicardi–Goutières spectrum (AGS) of disorders, including mutations in the ADAR1 gene
This form of AGS presents with acute onset of dystonia in the context of a febrile illness, with subsequent step-wise deterioration. It is associated with ICC and bilateral striatal necrosis.

A few of the hypomyelinating leukodystrophies can present quite acutely with some overlap with the clinical picture seen in Leigh syndrome, e.g. RARS and SARS.

Other neurogenerative conditions
See 'Developmental regression' in Chapter 2, 'Clinical approach', p. 128.

Genetic advice
The following are the most common causes of Leigh encephalopathy.
- PDH deficiency. XL or AR. Some mutations in the E1-alpha subunit are thiamine-responsive (Naito et al. 2002).
- Cytochrome oxidase (COX) deficiency (itself very heterogeneous—many nuclear genes, including *SURF1*, are involved in COX assembly).
- NADH (reduced nicotinamide–adenine dinucleotide) dehydrogenase (complex I) deficiency (both nuclear and mitochondrial genes).
- mtDNA mutations such as m.8993T>G, m.10158T>C, m.13513G>A, m.10191T>C, and others more often associated with later-onset mitochondrial disease (e.g. m.3243A>G and m.8344A>G).

Inheritance and recurrence risk
Even where there is good clinical and MRI evidence of Leigh disease, it is currently possible to make a genetic diagnosis in <40% of patients, despite thorough investigation in a specialist research laboratory. However, this situation is likely to improve with more widespread use of new-generation sequencing technology.

An *empiric risk* of 33% was estimated by van Erven et al. (1987)—this may be an overestimate since the calculation was not corrected for unascertained sibships. See White et al. (1999) for an estimate of the risk for patients carrying m.8993T>G or m.8993T>C. Recurrence risk for Leigh disease due to *SURF1* mutations is 25%. Recurrence risk for PDH deficiency is very low when occurring as a new mutation.

Variability and penetrance
Variation in presentation is very great overall but may be more consistent in siblings with *SURF1* mutations or other AR nuclear gene defects.

Prenatal diagnosis and reproductive options
Once a genetic diagnosis is established, this should be relatively straightforward by CVS in families with *SURF1* and *PDH* mutations, also with nuclear gene causes of complex I deficiency (but not as widely available). PND of mtDNA mutations appears relatively robust (Nesbitt et al. 2014). See also 'Mitochondrial DNA diseases' in Chapter 3, 'Common consultations', p. 490. PGD is available for many of the common nuclear and mtDNA mutations.

Predictive testing
Technically feasible once the genetic defect in the proband has been identified.

Other family members
Once the genetic defect in the proband has been identified, other family members should be offered testing. For mtDNA mutations, it is particularly important that the mother is tested as potentially all offspring could be affected. Information on the level of mtDNA mutation heteroplasmy will be important in assessing risk of disease and transmission. See also 'Mitochondrial DNA diseases' in Chapter 3, 'Common consultations', p. 490.

Natural history and management
Leigh encephalopathy is a progressive neurodegenerative disorder punctuated by episodes of developmental regression. Brainstem dysfunction (dysphagia, aspiration pneumonia, and hypopnoea), dystonia, seizures, and recurrent metabolic acidosis present a significant disease burden and greatly foreshortened life. Cardiac involvement (arrhythmia and/or CM) is not uncommon in Leigh encephalopathy and should be identified early. Treatment of early CM with a beta-blocker and/or an ACE inhibitor may prevent progression and cardiac arrhythmias can be managed conventionally.

Potential long-term complications
Progressive accumulation of neurological damage, especially following intercurrent illnesses. Common outcome is respiratory failure.

Support groups: The Lily Foundation, http://www.thelilyfoundation.org.uk; Climb (Children Living with Inherited Metabolic Diseases), http://www.climb.org.uk, Tel. 0870 770 0326; NORD (National Organization for Rare Disorders), http://rarediseases.org.

Expert adviser: Robert Mcfarland, Clinical Senior Lecturer in Paediatric Neurology, Wellcome Trust Centre for Mitochondrial Research, Institute of Neuroscience, Newcastle University, Newcastle upon Tyne, UK.

References
Darin N, Oldfors A, Moslemi AR, Holme E, Tulinius M. The incidence of mitochondrial encephalomyopathies in childhood: clinical features and morphological, biochemical, and DNA abnormalities. *Ann Neurol* 2001; **49**: 377–83.

Farina L, Chiapparini L, Uziel G, Bugiani M, Zeviani M, Savoiardo M. MR findings in Leigh syndrome with COX deficiency and *SURF-1* mutations. *AJNR Am J Neuroradiol* 2002; **23**: 1095–100.

Lake NJ, Compton AG, Rahman S, Thorburn DR. Leigh syndrome: one disorder, more than 75 monogenic causes. *Ann Neurol* 2016; **79**: 190–203.

Lebre AS, Rio M, Faivre d'Arcier L, et al. A common pattern of brain MRI imaging in mitochondrial diseases with complex I deficiency. *J Med Genet* 2011; **48**: 16–23.

Montpetit VJA, Andermann F, Carpenter S, Fawcett JS, Zborowska-Sluis D, Giberson HR. Subacute necrotizing encephalomyelopathy: a review and study of two families. *Brain* 1971; **94**: 1–30.

Naito E, Ito M, Yokota I, et al. Thiamine-responsive pyruvate dehydrogenase deficiency in two patients caused by a point mutation (F205L and L216F) within the thiamine pyrophosphate binding region. *Biochim Biophys Acta* 2002; **1588**: 79–84.

Nesbitt V, Alston CL, Blakely EL, et al. A national perspective on prenatal testing for mitochondrial disease. *Eur J Hum Genet* 2014; **22**: 1255–9.

Rahman S, Blok RB, Dahl HH, et al. Leigh syndrome: clinical features and biochemical and DNA abnormalities. *Ann Neurol* 1996; **39**: 343–51.

van Erven PM, Cillessen JP, Eekhoff EM, et al. Leigh syndrome, a mitochondrial encephalo(myo)pathy. A review of the literature. *Clin Neurol Neurosurg* 1987; **89**: 217–30.

Wedatilake Y, Brown RM, McFarland R, et al. SURF1 deficiency: a multi-centre natural history study. *Orphanet J Rare Dis* 2013; **8**: 96.

White S, Collins V, Wolfe R, et al. Genetic counselling and prenatal diagnosis for the mitochondrial DNA mutations at nucleotide 8993. *Am J Hum Genet* 1999; **65**: 474–82.

Zhu Z, Yao J, Johns T, et al. SURF1, encoding a factor involved in the biogenesis of cytochrome c oxidase, is mutated in Leigh syndrome. *Nat Genet* 1998; **20**: 337–43.

Limb–girdle muscular dystrophies

The limb–girdle muscular dystrophies (LGMD) are a heterogeneous group of genetically determined progressive muscular dystrophies that are defined by predominant involvement of the pelvic girdle and shoulder girdle musculatures (see Figure 3.19). LGMD used to be very much a diagnosis of exclusion, but, as the molecular basis of many types of LGMD can now be delineated, an attempt should be made in all patients to achieve a precise diagnosis. This may necessitate specialized referral and investigation. The different types of LGMD (see Table 3.28) together probably still only represent in most populations about one-third the frequency of BMD and, within the LGMD classification, some of the subgroups are extremely rare indeed. It is important to recognize therefore that, on empirical grounds, in a patient presenting with a 'limb–girdle' pattern of muscular dystrophy, dystrophinopathy is a more likely diagnosis than LGMD and should be excluded by gene and protein analysis. This is particularly important from a genetic counselling perspective because of the risk to female relatives in the dystrophinopathies.

In addition to the genetic counselling implications for patients with LGMD, there may be significant management points in the various subtypes, e.g. in terms of cardiac and respiratory surveillance.

For the clinical diagnosis of LGMD, a comprehensive approach is needed which may include evaluation by a clinician, serum CK, genetic testing, and muscle biopsy (Mitsuhashi and Kand 2012). Diagnosis and management of patients with limb–girdle dystrophies is a highly specialized area and the patient should be under the care of a neurologist with expertise in muscle disease. As expertise with next-generation sequencing panels grows, genetic testing may pre-empt the need for muscle biopsy in some instances.

Clinical approach

History: key points

- Three-generation (or more) family tree, with specific enquiry regarding muscle weakness, premature cardiac death, and cardiac failure.
- Onset of muscle weakness. Obtain a history of early motor milestones, participation in physical education at school, etc.
- Muscle groups affected. Difficulty rising from chairs implies hip girdle involvement; difficulty lifting the arms above the head, e.g. brushing hair, hanging out the washing, implies shoulder girdle involvement.
- Current level of mobility. Rising from chairs, walking on flat, use of aids.
- Fits, faints, or funny turns.
- Exercise tolerance and breathlessness.
- Sleep history. Difficulty breathing when lying flat may indicate diaphragmatic weakness; difficulty rising in the morning may indicate nocturnal hypoventilation.

Examination: key points

It is often necessary to seek advice from an expert to facilitate diagnosis in LGMD. Photography may be a useful adjunct to clinical assessment for this purpose and also to document progression.

- Is there evidence of muscle wasting?
- Which muscle groups are weak? (Humeroperoneal weakness is suggestive of Emery–Dreifuss.) Involvement of distal muscle groups, facial muscles (suggests FSHD), or extraocular muscles (suggests a mitochondrial disorder) is not a feature of LGMD.
- Is there facial involvement? (Consider FSHD.)
- Are DTRs present?
- Are there any contractures, e.g. at elbows (inability to fully extend the elbows), Achilles tendons (inability to plantar flex the foot), and spine (restricted neck flexion)? These would indicate a need to consider laminopathy or XL Emery–Dreifuss, or Bethlem myopathy.

Special investigations

- CK. Usually elevated <10× normal in dominant disease, though LGMD1C may be higher than this; often elevated >10× normal or up to 100× normal in recessive disease.
- DNA for mutation analysis or storage. Gene panel/WEG/WGS as appropriate; given the high genetic heterogeneity in LGMD, the ability to analyse multiple genes in parallel using next-generation sequencing improves the potential for diagnosis. A dystrophin deletion/duplication screen is appropriate in patients without contractures, unless a muscle biopsy excludes a dystrophinopathy.
- Cardiac assessment. ECG and echo.
- Muscle biopsy with multiple stains if the diagnosis remains unknown (a biopsy may need to be sent to a specialist centre since LGMD is such a genetically heterogeneous condition).
- If LGMD, refer to a neurologist with expertise in muscle disorders (if not already involved).

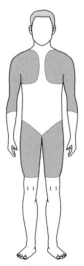

Figure 3.19 Distribution of predominant muscle weakness in limb–girdle muscular dystrophy.
Reproduced from *The BMJ*, Alan EH Emery, The muscular dystrophies, volume 317, Fig 1a, p. 992, copyright 1998, with permission from BMJ Publishing Group Ltd.

Table 3.28 Classification and genetic basis of some of the more common types of limb–girdle muscular dystrophies

Nomenclature	Locus	Gene product	Muscle biopsy	Clinical features
LGMD1B	1q21	Lamin A/C*	Absent/reduced lamin A/C	Invariable cardiac conduction defects, and in some patients also DCM
LGMD1C	3	Calveolin 3	Absent/reduced caveolin 3	Variable, may also present with hyperCKaemia or rippling muscle disease
LGMD2A	15q	Calpain 3	Normal sarcoglycan; absent/reduced calpain 3	Onset 8–15 years. Progression variable
LGMD2B	2p	Dysferlin	Normal sarcoglycans and calpain 3	Onset 16–25 years. Progression often slow. Some variability—may present with proximal or distal disease
LGMD2C	13q	γ-sarcoglycan	Absent/reduced γ-sarcoglycan; reduced α- and β-sarcoglycan	Extremely variable severity with onset from childhood to adult life. All sarcoglycanopathies are at risk of cardiac and respiratory complications
LGMD2D	17q	α-sarcoglycan	Absent/reduced α-sarcoglycan; reduced β- and γ-sarcoglycan	
LGMD2E	4q	β-sarcoglycan	Absent/reduced β-sarcoglycan; reduced α- and γ-sarcoglycan	
LGMD2I	19	Fukutin-related protein (FKRP)	May be secondary reduction in laminin α2, variable reduction of α-dystroglycan expression	Very variable severity, cardiac and respiratory disease common

*Laminopathies. Several diseases share mutations at the lamin A/C gene *LMNA*. These include AD Emery–Dreifuss muscular dystrophy, DCM type 1A, LGMD type 1B, familial partial lipodystrophy, CMT disease type 2, mandibuloacral dysplasia, atypical Werner syndrome, and a rare childhood syndrome of premature ageing Hutchinson–Gilford syndrome. Overlapping phenotypes may exist. In all patients with muscle disease due to laminopathy, there is a major risk of cardiac conduction defects and sudden death.

Adapted from Bushby, The limb-girdle muscular dystrophies—multiple genes, multiple mechanisms, *Human Molecular Genetics*, 1999; 8, 10: 1875–82, by permission of Oxford University Press.

Other diagnoses/conditions to consider

Becker muscular dystrophy (BMD)
BMD is clinically similar to DMD, but milder, with a mean age of onset of 11 years. Loss of the ability to walk may occur late (e.g. 40s or 50s) and many individuals with BMD survive into middle age and beyond. Often cramps on exercise are the only problem initially, but some affected boys are late in learning to walk and are unable to run fast. Later in the teens and 20s, muscle weakness becomes evident, causing difficulty in rapid walking, running, and climbing stairs. It may become difficult to lift objects above waist height. Cognitive impairment is not a major feature of BMD. BMD is caused by 'in-frame' mutations in dystrophin that result in reduced dystrophin being produced. Immunolabelling of muscle biopsy from a man with BMD shows a reduction in the intensity of staining, which may vary within and between fibres. See 'Duchenne and Becker muscular dystrophy (DMD and BMD)' in Chapter 3, 'Common consultations', p. 402.

X-linked Emery–Dreifuss muscular dystrophy (XLEDMD)
Emery–Dreifuss muscular dystrophy is characterized by early contractures of the Achilles tendons, elbows, and spine, slowly progressive muscle wasting and weakness with a distinctive humeroperoneal distribution (upper arms and lower legs; see Figure 3.20), and cardiac conduction defects leading to DCM. Onset is usually in childhood; onset after 20 years is rare. Contractures usually develop *before* there is significant weakness. These involve the elbows (arms carried in a flexed position), Achilles tendon (toe-walking), and spine (limitation of flexion, especially neck flexion). There may be extensor contractures of the wrist and/or flexion contractures of the fingers. Caused by mutations in *STA* on Xq28. The gene product emerin associates with the nuclear envelope.

AD Emery–Dreifuss muscular dystrophy
There is a broad phenotypic spectrum from those with predominant features of DCM and little or no apparent involvement of skeletal muscle to those in whom a progressive LGMD, very similar to that seen in XLEDMD,

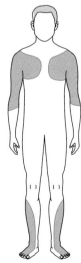

Figure 3.20 Distribution of predominant muscle weakness in Emery–Dreifuss muscular dystrophy.
Reproduced from *The BMJ*, Alan EH Emery, The muscular dystrophies, volume 317, Fig 1a, p. 992, copyright 1998, with permission from BMJ Publishing Group Ltd.

dominates the clinical picture. There is marked intrafamilial variability, often with different family members exhibiting different aspects of the phenotype. Early-onset conduction disease is an important clinical prompt to this diagnosis. It is caused by mutations in the lamin A/C gene (*LMNA*) on 1q21. As for XLEDMD, the gene product is known to associate with the nuclear envelope.

Facioscapulohumeral muscular dystrophy (FSHD)

Often clinically easily recognizable, and the diagnosis can be confirmed in 95% of cases by molecular genetic analysis for the disease-associated deletion on chromosome 4q35. However, there are some patients in whom facial weakness may be very minor and in these patients LGMD may be suggested as the diagnosis. Careful examination for the other characteristic signs of FSHD (prominent scapular winging, stepping of the shoulders on elevation of the arms, foot drop, frequent asymmetry) should suggest the diagnosis. FSHD is important to diagnose as it is an AD condition, though with a high rate of new mutations and germline mosaicism. See 'Facioscapulohumeral muscular dystrophy (FSHD)' in Chapter 3, 'Common consultations', p. 420.

Bethlem myopathy

An AD disease that causes proximal muscle weakness associated with frequent contractures, typically of the elbows, finger flexors, and Achilles tendons, but, as these contractures may be relatively subtle, patients may be misdiagnosed as LGMD. An additional clinical clue may be the presence of keloid scarring and follicular hyperkeratosis. Bethlem myopathy is caused by mutations in one of the genes encoding collagen VIA1, VIA2, or VIA3 (the same genes as those implicated in Ullrich CMD). Collagen VIA2 has also been recently implicated in an AD muscular dystrophy phenotype and AR myosclerosis (Bushby *et al*. 2014).

Clinical diagnostic clues to the different forms of LGMD

Genotype–phenotype correlations in this highly heterogeneous group may be difficult (Zatz *et al*. 2003), but there are some useful clinical correlates.

- LGMD2I, which is probably the most common type of LGMD in the European population, is phenotypically the most similar to dystrophinopathy, with frequent calf hypertrophy and CM.
- The sarcoglycanopathies also share these clinical similarities to dystrophinopathy.
- LGMD2A, or calpainopathy, is relatively rarely associated with muscle hypertrophy and is usually a very atrophic disease with predominant weakness and wasting of the posterior musculature of the lower limbs and frequent scapular winging.
- LGMD2B, or dysferlinopathy, can present with either predominantly proximal or distal disease and the first clinical problem may be standing on the toes. These patients often present with a very clear onset at the end of the second decade.
- Contractures, cardiac conduction disease, and lipodystrophy may be a clue to the diagnosis of laminopathy.
- LGMD1C may be suggested by calf and other hypertrophy and a history of rippling muscle disease.
- For AR LGMD, unlike most AR disorders, a discordant phenotype, ranging from a relatively severe course to mildly affected or asymptomatic carriers, may be seen in patients carrying the same mutation, even within the same family. Careful clinical assessment is used in combination with pedigree analysis and immunohistochemical staining of the muscle biopsy to obtain a precise genetic diagnosis. Molecular analysis for the disease-causing mutations may then be possible.

Genetic advice

Recurrence risk

This is dependent on the specific diagnosis. After excluding BMD and XLEDMD, undiagnosed LGMD may follow an AR or AD pattern of inheritance. If both parents are normal, the mode of inheritance is most likely to be AR, but ~10% of individuals probably have a *de novo* AD mutation.

Carrier detection

Possible if the familial mutation is known.

Prenatal diagnosis

Possible by CVS if the familial mutation is known.

Natural history and further management (preventative measures)

Cardiac surveillance

- XLEDMD. Annual ECG with interpretation by a cardiologist (ECG changes may be subtle and difficult to interpret). Annual 24-hour ECG (Holter monitor). Periodic echo. Consider permanent pacemaker in asymptomatic patients when ECG begins to show signs of sinus node or AV node disease. Carrier females should be offered periodic ECG surveillance (Bushby *et al*. 2003).
- Laminopathy. Except for the partial lipodystrophy and CMT phenotypes, there is strong evidence for cardiac involvement that is progressive with age. DCM may develop, as well as conduction defects. Management should be in a specialist centre with expertise in cardiac electrophysiology and may include consideration of an implantable defibrillator. If atrial fibrillation/flutter or atrial standstill occur frequently, consider anticoagulation with warfarin (Bushby *et al*. 2003).
- Sarcoglycanopathy (LGMD2C–F). Screen for the development of CM (echo and ECG) every 5 years. Routine surveillance is not needed in LGMD2A, 2B, 2G, 2H, 1A, and 1C (Bushby *et al*. 2003).
- LGMD2I. Screen for the development of CM by annual echo and ECG. There is a high risk of CM, especially in patients who are not homozygous for the common *CA26A* mutation (Poppe *et al*. 2004).

Respiratory surveillance

All of these groups are at risk of respiratory failure with increasing disease. Diaphragmatic weakness may be an additional feature in LGMD2I especially. All patients should be followed with regular FVC in sitting and lying positions and additional investigations (e.g. overnight pulse oximetry) as indicated.

Support group: Muscular Dystrophy UK, http://www.musculardystrophyuk.org.

Expert adviser: Katie Bushby, Act. Res. Chair of Neuromuscular Genetics, Institute of Genetic Medicine, Newcastle University, Newcastle, UK.

References

Bione S, Maestrini E, Rivella S, et al. Identification of a novel X-linked gene responsible for Emery–Dreifuss muscular dystrophy. *Nat Genet* 1994; **8**: 323–7.

Brockington M, Yuva Y, Prandini P, et al. Mutations in the fukutin-related protein gene (FKRP) identify limb girdle muscular dystrophy 2I as a milder allelic variant of congenital muscular dystrophy MDC1C. *Hum Mol Genet* 2001; **10**: 2851–9.

Bushby KM. The limb-girdle muscular dystrophies—multiple genes, multiple mechanisms. *Hum Mol Genet* 1999a; **8**: 1875–82.

Bushby KM. Making sense of the limb-girdle muscular dystrophies. *Brain* 1999b; **122**(pt 8): 1403–20.

Bushby KM, Collins J, Hicks D. Collagen type VI myopathies. *Adv Exp Med Biol* 2014; **802**: 185–99.

Bushby K, Muntoni F, Bourke JP. 107th ENMC International Workshop: the management of cardiac involvement in muscular dystrophy and myotonic dystrophy. 7th–9th June 2002, Naarden, the Netherlands. *Neuromuscul Disord* 2003; **13**: 166–72.

Emery AE. The muscular dystrophies. *BMJ* 1998; **317**: 991–5.

Helbling-Leclerc A, Bonne G, Schwartz K. Emery–Dreifuss muscular dystrophy. *Eur J Hum Genet* 2002; **10**: 157–61.

Mitsuhashi S, Kand PB. Update on the genetics of limb girdle muscular dystrophy. *Semin Pediatr Neurol* 2012; **19**: 211–18.

Poppe M, Bourke J, Eagle M, *et al*. Cardiac and respiratory failure in limb-girdle muscular dystrophy 2I. *Ann Neurol* 2004; **56**: 738–41.

Poppe M, Cree L, Bourke J, *et al*. The phenotype of limb-girdle muscular dystrophy type 2I. *Neurology* 2003; **60**: 1246–51.

Zatz M, de Paula F, Starling A, Vainzof M. The 10 autosomal recessive limb-girdle muscular dystrophies. *Neuromuscul Disord* 2003; **13**(7–8): 532–44.

Long QT syndrome and other inherited arrhythmia syndromes

Romano–Ward syndrome (AD), Jervell and Lange–Nielsen syndrome (AR).

Long QT syndromes, usually AD, are characterized by prolonged ventricular repolarization that predisposes carriers to life-threatening arrhythmia, most specifically *torsades de pointes*, a type of ventricular tachycardia that may cause syncope but may also degenerate to VF and cardiac arrest (Grace and Roden 2012; Schwartz and Dagradi 2016). LOF mutations in the potassium channel genes *KCNQ1* (LQT1) and *KCNH2* (LQT2), or gain-of-function mutations in the sodium channel gene *SCN5A* (LQT3) (Wilde 2016), are the most common causes of long QT syndrome, having been estimated to be responsible for, respectively, 76%, 35%, and 5% of families with identifiable mutations (Gray 2016). Mutations in the other potassium channel genes *KCNE1* (LQT5), *KCNE2* (LQT6), and *KCNJ2* (LQT7) are also implicated, with up to 16 genes in total felt to be responsible in many of the remaining families. However, even following a full and detailed genetic analysis, up to 20% of families do not have detectable mutations in any of these genes, with other genes clearly still to be identified (Bezzina 2015).

Birth incidence is unknown but has been estimated at up to 1/2000 (Gray 2016). Typically, syncope occurring during physical activity or emotional upset begins in the pre-teen or teenage years, but the condition may present at any age. First cardiac events are, however, less common after 30–40 years. Importantly, it is estimated that in excess of 30–50% of carriers of mutations associated with the syndrome never have symptoms. Syncope most typically occurs without warning and may help to differentiate from other causes, e.g. vasovagal syncope in which patients may feel dizzy or faint prior to collapse. Long QT syndrome is, however, often incorrectly diagnosed, as e.g. epilepsy, especially in children, and the possibility of the diagnosis always needs careful attention. Sudden cardiac death is thought to occur currently in about 4% of affected individuals (Schwartz and Dagradi 2016).

Known triggers for long QT-related arrhythmias are relatively gene-specific and include:

- swimming, running (may suggest LQT1);
- startle: alarm clock, loud horn, ringing phone (may suggest LQT2);
- emotions: anger, crying, test taking, or other stressful situations.

NB. Sudden death may also occur during sleep.

Diagnosis of long QT syndrome

This is often a difficult diagnosis, relying on careful evaluation of the patient's history, his/her non-invasive test results, especially the 12-lead ECG, his/her family history, and ideally genetic analysis. The criteria for the assignment of phenotype have evolved (Gray 2016), consisting essentially of a prolonged QT interval corrected for heart rate (QT_c) on the ECG (>470 ms in men or >480 ms in women).

If there is a definite diagnosis of long QT in the family, then QT_c >450 ms in men or QT_c >460 ms in women is highly suggestive of affected status (Bezzina 2015). The QT must be measured when the patient is not otherwise affected by systemic illness and drug therapy must also be accounted for (Behr *et al.* 2013; Schwartz and Woosley 2016). The presence of a pathogenic mutation in, e.g.

KCNQ1, KCNH2, SCN5A, may also be of critical importance in the assignment of clinical phenotype.

The QT interval is influenced by the genetic locus, but in general, those patients with QT_c >500 ms are at an increased risk for cardiac events, compared to those with a shorter QT_c. If the QT_c is <400 ms, long QT gene carriage is less likely as <1% of gene carriers have a QT_c in this range, but >50% of gene carriers have QT_c intervals appearing in the range of 400–460 ms, which overlaps with the normal range, and 'at-risk' family members with a QT_c in this range have uncertain status. The 'Schwartz' scoring system that assigns different weights to the characteristics of the individual patient and their family history may need to be applied to achieve a reasonably robust phenotypic assignment (Gray 2016; Schwartz and Dagradi 2016).

Clinical approach

History: key points

- Three-generation family tree, with specific inquiry regarding a history of fainting, 'epilepsy', sudden death, and congenital deafness.

Investigations

- ECG with calculation of QT_c using conventional formulae, e.g. Bazett, to calculate.
- DNA sample for molecular genetic analysis using gene panel/WES/WGS as appropriate.

Other diagnoses/conditions to consider

Jervell and Lange–Nielsen syndrome

Homozygous form of long QT characterized by profound congenital deafness and long QT. AR with 1 in 4 sibling recurrence risk. Parents will both be carriers for long QT and sibs will be at two-thirds carrier risk status for long QT.

Timothy syndrome

A rare condition characterized by long QT syndrome and syndactyly due to mutations in CACNA1C (Cav 1.2, the L-type calcium channel) (Bezzina 2015). Additional features that may be present include mild facial dysmorphism, CHD, intermittent hypoglycaemia, cognitive abnormalities, and autism.

Brugada syndrome

A rare (1/5000–7000) AD condition, caused in ~15% by LOF mutations in the cardiac sodium channel gene *SCN5A* that predisposes to a variety of arrhythmias, including bradycardia, AV conduction delay, and VF (Bezzina 2015; Andorin 2016). The genetic basis in the remaining 85% is currently unknown although may relate to variants affecting some aspect of sodium channel function (Bezzina *et al.* 2015).

Catecholaminergic polymorphic ventricular tachycardia (CPVT)

A severe arrhythmic disease characterized by salvoes of exercise-induced bidirectional and polymorphic tachycardias (Bezzina 2015). It usually follows AD inheritance. Mutations in the gene encoding the ryanodine receptor 2 (*RyR2*) are typically observed. There is also a very rare AR variant due, in some, to variants in the calsequestrin (*CASQ2*) gene. The resting ECG would usually look entirely normal in affected individuals and an exercise

ECG or adrenaline infusion may be needed to demonstrate clinical evidence.

Hypertrophic cardiomyopathy (HCM)

May predispose affected individuals to life-threatening arrhythmia. Post-mortem examination should indicate if this is the cause of sudden death in a family. See 'Hypertrophic cardiomyopathy (HCM)' in Chapter 3, 'Common consultations', p. 460.

Arrhythmogenic cardiomyopathy (formerly, arrhythmogenic right ventricular cardiomyopathy/dysplasia (ARVC/D))

An AD heart muscle disorder that causes arrhythmia, heart failure, and sudden death. It is characterized by replacement of the RV myocardium by adipose and fibrous tissue (Corrado 2017). This disorder has a prevalence in the range of 1:1000–1:5000. Males and females are equally affected and nearly one-third of all deaths occur during the fourth decade, often during everyday circumstances. Five causative desmosomal genes are associated with this disease (Corrado 2017). Heterozygous mutations in genes encoding desmoplakin (*DSP*) and plakoglobin (*JUP*) suggest that altered integrity at cardiac myocyte cell–cell junctions may promote myocyte degeneration and death, with the repair process consisting of replacement of the myocardium by adipose and fibrous tissue. Mutations in the gene encoding plakophilin-2 (*PKP2*) may account for 25–30% of cases.

Naxos disease

Is the triad of AR ARVC with biventricular DCM, palmoplantar keratoderma, and woolly hair caused by mutations in the junctional plakoglobin gene (*JUP*) on chromosome 17q21 (Corrado 2017).

Genetic advice

Inheritance and recurrence risk
AD with low DNM rate.

Variability and penetrance
The disease exhibits both inter- and intrafamilial variability. Penetrance is incomplete, with ~50% of gene carriers remaining asymptomatic.

Prenatal diagnosis
Technically feasible by CVS if the familial mutation is known.

Predictive testing
Cascade screening of family members can be used to clarify the status if the familial mutation is known. In asymptomatic 'at-risk' family members with the QT$_c$ in the equivocal range, molecular genetic analysis may be the only way to definitively assign status.

Natural history and management

- Lifestyle modification. Patients should be advised to approach activities associated with intense physical activity and/or emotional stress, e.g. competitive

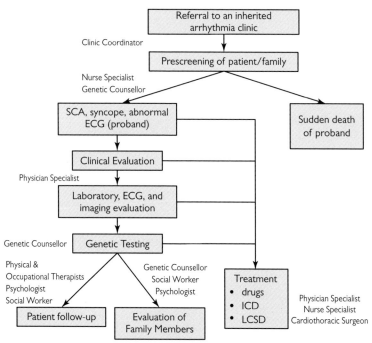

Figure 3.21 Workflow and personnel in the evaluation of patients and families with inherited arrhythmias.
Reprinted from *Heart Rhythm*, Volume 10, Issue 12, Priori *et al.*, HRS/EHRA/APHRS Expert Consensus Statement on the Diagnosis and Management of Patients with Inherited Primary Arrhythmia Syndromes Document endorsed by HRS, EHRA, and APHRS in May 2013 and by ACCF, AHA, PACES, and AEPC in June 2013, pp. 1932–1963, Copyright 2013, with permission from the Heart Rhythm Society and the Cardiac Electrophysiology Society.

sports, amusement park rides, scary movies, jumping into cold water, with caution.

- Avoidance of drugs that prolong the QT interval. See https://crediblemeds.org for a list (Behr et al. 2013).
- Beta-blockers. The first-choice therapy in patients with long QT. Effective in most LQT1 patients and 70% of patients with LQT2 and potential for cardiac events to continue in the remaining 30%. Patients should be strongly advised to pay attention to diligent use.
- ICD. May be necessary for those with symptoms despite beta-blockade or for those with a history of cardiac arrest (John et al. 2012; (Schwartz and Dagradi 2016)).

Potential long-term complications
Sudden death continues to be a risk in mutation carriers, especially if prior evidence of syncope.

Surveillance
A dedicated team that includes specialist cardiologists, clinical geneticists, genetic counsellors, and other support staff should review at-risk family members (see Figure 3.21).

Support groups: SADS UK (The Sudden Arrhythmic Death Syndrome UK), http://www.sadsuk.org.uk; Arrhythmia Alliance, http://www.heartrhythmalliance. org/aa/uk.

Expert adviser: Andrew Grace, Consultant Cardiologist, Papworth Hospital, Cambridge University Health Partners, Cambridge, UK.

References

Andorin A, Behr ER, Denjoy I, et al. Impact of clinical and genetic findings on the management of young patients with Brugada syndrome. *Heart Rhythm* 2016; **6**: 1274–82.

Behr ER, January C, Schulze-Bahr E, et al. The International Serious Adverse Events Consortium (iSAEC) phenotype standardization project for drug-induced torsades de pointes. *Eur Heart J* 2013; **34**: 1958–63.

Bezzina CR, Lahrouchi N, Priori SG. Genetics of sudden cardiac death. *Circ Res* 2015; **116**: 1919–36.

Corrado D, Link MS, Calkins H. Arrhythmogenic right ventricular cardiomyopathy. *N Engl J Med* 2017; **376**:61–72.

Grace AA, Roden DM. Systems biology and cardiac arrhythmias. *Lancet* 2012; **380**: 1498–508.

Gray B, Behr ER. New insights into the genetic basis of inherited arrhythmia syndromes. *Circ Cardiovasc Genet* 2016; **9**: 569–77.

John RM, Tedrow UB, Koplan BA, et al. Ventricular arrhythmias and sudden cardiac death. *Lancet* 2012; **380**: 1520–9.

Priori SG, Wilde AA, Horie M, et al. HRS/EHRA/APHRS expert consensus statement on the diagnosis and management of patients with inherited primary arrhythmia syndromes. *Heart Rhythm* 2013; **12**: 1932–63.

Schwartz PJ, Dagradi F. Management of survivors of cardiac arrest - the importance of genetic investigation. *Nat Rev Cardiol* 2016; **9**: 560–6.

Schwartz PJ, Woosley RL. Predicting the unpredictable: drug-induced QT prolongation and torsades de pointes. *J Am Coll Cardiol* 2016; **67**: 1639–50.

Wilde AA, Moss AJ, Kaufman ES, et al. Clinical aspects of type 3 long-QT syndrome: an international multicenter study. *Circulation* 2016; **134**: 872–82.

Marfan's syndrome

Marfan's syndrome (MFS) is a heritable disorder of connective tissue caused by mutations in *FBN1* (chromosome 15q21) (Loeys *et al.* 2004; OMIM 2013). *FBN1* encodes fibrillin, a protein component of microfibrils. The microfibrillar meshwork in the extracellular matrix is essential in maintaining the integrity of connective tissue. Various components of the extracellular matrix collagens, elastin, and fibrillin are present in varying proportions in different tissues and contribute to the elasticity, tensile strength, and durability of various types of connective tissue. Fibrillin is particularly rich in the wall of the proximal aorta and zonules of the ocular lens.

Cardiovascular complications are the primary cause of major morbidity and mortality in MFS. In untreated MFS, life expectancy is reduced, with an average age at death of 32 years (Murdoch *et al.* 1972). Over the last several decades, increased life expectancy in MFS has been attributed to improved life expectancy in the overall population, advances in aortic aneurysm resection/graft replacement, earlier diagnosis that includes mild cases, and medical therapy (Gott *et al.* 1999; Silverman *et al.* 1995). Severe aortic or mitral valve regurgitation can result in heart failure, whereas death usually results from complications of aortic root dissection or rupture. Clinical manifestations occur along a continuum, whereby individuals at the mild end of the spectrum show subtle clinical manifestations and those at the severe end show rapidly progressive clinical manifestations that begin in infancy. *FBN1* mutation analysis has become more accessible (GeneTests website). A diagnosis of MFS relies on careful clinical evaluation and is supported by the family history and genetic findings (see Box 3.6).

Classification of aortic dissection

Aortic dissection is classified as: type A—proximal or ascending aortic dissection; and type B—distal or descending aortic dissection.

Clinical approach

History: key points

- Family history. Three-generation family tree, with specific inquiry about:
  - skeletal features: parental height, chest wall deformity, scoliosis;
  - ocular and visual acuity problems: lens dislocation, myopia, early-onset cataract and/or glaucoma, and retinal detachment;
  - cardiovascular abnormalities: history and location of aortic aneurysm/dissection; mitral valve disease; history of valvular repair/replacement (mitral, aortic), sudden unexplained death, particularly at a young age.
- Joint hypermobility, subluxation, dislocation, discomfort.
- Dental crowding, highly arched palate/orthodontic treatment.
- Hernia: inguinal, abdominal, incisional, recurrent.
- Easy bruising/bleeding, abnormal scarring, skin translucency, skin striae.
- Spontaneous pneumothorax, lung blebs, emphysema, asthma, haemoptysis.

Examination: key points

- Height, weight, arm span (AS) and lower segment (LS), body surface area (BSA).

Box 3.6 Clinical diagnosis: revised Ghent criteria for diagnosis of Marfan's syndrome and related conditions

Index case, absence of family history of MFS:
- Aortic root dilation (Z score >2) AND ectopia lentis
- Aortic root dilation (Z score >2) AND *FBN1* mutation
- Aortic root dilation (Z score >2) AND systemic score >7 points
- Ectopia lentis AND *FBN1* mutation previously associated with aortic root dilation

Index case, presence of family history of MFS:
- Ectopia lentis with family history of MFS (defined above)
- Systemic score >7 with family history of MFS
- Aortic dilation (Z >2 above 20 years old, >3 below 20 years) with family history of MFS.

Ectopia lentis syndrome = ectopia lentis with or without systemic features with *FBN1* mutation not known to associate with aortic dilation or no *FBN1* mutation

MASS = aortic diameter (Z score <2) AND systemic score <5 with at least one skeletal feature) without ectopia lentis

Mitral valve prolapse syndrome = mitral valve prolapse without aortic root dilation (Z <2), systemic score <5, no ectopia lentis

Caveat: without discriminating features of Shprintzen–Goldberg syndrome, Loeys–Dietz syndrome, or vascular Ehlers–Danlos syndrome AND after *TGFBR1/2*, *SMAD3*, *TGFB2*, collagen biochemistry, *COL3A1* testing if indicated. Other conditions/genes will emerge with time.

Reproduced from *Journal of Medical Genetics*, Loeys *et al.*, The revised Ghent nosology for the Marfan syndrome, volume 47, issue 7, pp. 476–485, copyright 2010, With permission from BMJ Publishing Group Ltd.

- Sclera (white, dusky, blue); inner canthal, interpupillary, and outer canthal distance.
- Head and face shape, palate and uvula anomalies, dental crowding.
- Arachnodactyly, positive wrist and thumb signs, contractures.
- Joint hypermobility (Beighton hypermobility score).
- Chest wall asymmetry/deformity; scoliosis, kyphosis.
- Skin striae, unusual scars, translucency, soft velvety texture, hyperextensibility.
- Pes planus, inward collapse of the medial malleolus.

Investigations
- Echo using age-specific nomograms for normalizing aortic root diameter.
- Ophthalmologic examination with slit-lamp examination.
- Molecular testing: *FBN1* mutation analysis (sequencing and dosage analysis for exon duplication/deletion) or thoracic aortopathy panel/WES/WGS as available.
- Serum homocystinuria, if appropriate (see below).
- Chest MRA or computed tomographic angiography (CTA) to assess proximal and distal thoracic aortic size and morphology (adults with MFS; younger patients with ambiguous diagnosis; or suspicion of a disorder associated with diffuse vascular disease).

Other diagnoses/conditions to consider

Loeys–Dietz syndrome (LDS)
Although there can be considerable overlap in the phenotypic features in MFS and LDS, ectopia lentis does not occur in LDS. LDS is an AD aortic aneurysm syndrome with widespread systemic and variably expressed clinical manifestations (Loeys et al. 2005, 2006). Molecular analyses in patients showing clinical evidence of LDS have revealed mutations in four genes involved in TGF-β signalling: *TGFBR1*, *TGFBR2*, *SMAD3*, and TGFB2. Subclassification of LDS has emerged and is based on genotype: LDS1 (*TGFBR1*); LDS2 (*TGFBR2*); LDS3 (*SMAD3*); LDS4 (*TGFB2*) and LDS5 (*TGFB3*).

While patients with severe craniofacial features of LDS (designated subtype A) may show a somewhat more aggressive vascular disease, mutation carriers with mild or absent craniofacial features (subtype B) commonly show widespread arterial tortuosity and a risk of aneurysm and dissection throughout the arterial tree. Both groups are at risk for pregnancy-associated complications and arterial dissection or rupture at younger ages and smaller arterial dimensions, when compared to MFS. Both subtypes can be seen in members of the same family with identical mutation.

A particular predisposition for early-onset osteoarthritis may distinguish patients with LDS3. Spine osteoarthritis, intervertebral disc degeneration, osteochondritis dissecans, and painful joints have been reported (Regalado et al. 2011; van de Laar et al. 2011, 2012). Patients with MFS and all aetiologies of LDS, as with other connective tissue disorders associated with joint laxity, are at risk for earlier and more severe osteoarthritis. Because mutations in *TGFB2* (LDS4) have been more recently identified, the spectrum of clinical manifestations in LDS4 is limited (Boileau et al. 2012; Lindsay et al. 2012).

X-linked thoracic aortic aneurysm and dissection (X-linked TAAD)
X-linked TAAD is rare but can be caused by variants in the FLNA gene, which is associated with the periventricular nodular heterotopia type of EDS, or by variants in the biglycan gene (BGN). The latter disorder is characterized by hypertelorism, chest deformity, joint hypermobility and contractures, and mild skeletal dysplasia with early onset of TAAD (Meester et al. 2016).

MASS phenotype
Refers to a condition with mild and non-specific features of MFS (myopia, MVP, borderline and non-progressive aortic root measurements (<2 SD), skeletal, and skin anomalies). Not all of these features need to be present to consider this diagnosis. Significant aortic root enlargement or ectopia lentis exclude this diagnosis. This condition can be inherited as an AD trait and some cases are attributable to mutations in *FBN1*. If the specific mutation has been previously associated with significant aortic root enlargement, then the diagnosis of MFS should be made. Patients with this condition should be followed intermittently with echo to exclude emerging MFS (Dietz et al. 1993; Glesby et al. 1989).

Congenital contractural arachnodactyly (CCA; FBN2)
Beal syndrome. Typically there is a history of neonatal contractures that improve during childhood. Ears may appear crumpled at birth. Scoliosis may be severe and cardiovascular involvement is generally mild and typically does not include progressive aortic root enlargement. Significant CHD can be seen but is rare. AD inheritance, caused by mutations in *FBN2* (5q23.3) (Lee et al. 1991; Putnam et al. 1995).

Ehlers–Danlos syndrome (EDS), hypermobility type (previously type III)
An AD disorder that is common and usually mild. Soft skin with hypermobility of large and small joints (Beighton score 5/9 or greater). There can be considerable diagnostic overlap with MFS. See 'Ehlers–Danlos syndrome (EDS)' in Chapter 3, 'Common consultations', p. 406.

Ehlers–Danlos syndrome (EDS), vascular type (previously type IV)
An uncommon, but serious, AD disorder caused by mutations in the *COL3A1* gene encoding type III collagen. The facial features are subtle and include prominent eyes due to decreased adipose tissue below the eyes and thin, slightly 'pinched' nose, thin lips, and hollow cheeks. Thin, translucent skin with visible veins and easy bruising are typical. No significant large joint hypermobility (Beighton score <5/9). Risk of arterial rupture and rupture of the bowel, bladder, and uterus leads to reduced life expectancy. See 'Ehlers–Danlos syndrome (EDS)' in Chapter 3, 'Common consultations', p. 406.

Stickler syndrome
An AD disorder of collagen, resulting in congenital vitreous gel anomaly, myopia, variable orofacial features including cleft palate, sensorineural deafness, and arthropathy. Joint hypermobility and habitus characterized by slender extremities with long fingers confer diagnostic overlap with MFS (although height is normal). Characteristic vitreoretinal changes observed during ophthalmological evaluation should alert the clinical team to Stickler syndrome. Sensorineural deafness and cleft palate are additional clinical features. See 'Stickler syndrome' in Chapter 3, 'Common consultations', p. 528. Mutations in *COL2A1* or *COL11A1* (with ocular findings) and *COL11A2* (without ocular manifestations) confirm Stickler syndrome.

Homocystinuria

An AR condition caused by deficiency of cystathionine beta-synthase (chromosome 21q22), characterized by lens dislocation, typically downward displacement, and thrombophilia. Most thrombotic events are cerebrovascular. The course is variable and often unpredictable. Lens dislocation is rarely present before 3 years. Glaucoma, cataracts, myopia, and retinal detachment may also occur. Patients are usually tall and thin; chest wall deformity is common. Learning disability can occur. If the diagnosis is strongly suspected despite normal urine amino acids, plasma amino acids should be performed, along with metabolic specialty consultation, since methionine load may be necessary to demonstrate biochemical defect.

Sex chromosome anomalies (e.g. XXX, XXY, XYY)

Tall stature can result in phenotypic overlap with MFS, although major features of MFS are absent on careful scrutiny.

Marfanoid habitus with learning difficulties

MFS is not associated with cognitive impairment. If learning difficulties are present, consider XL Fryns syndrome (males), or mosaic trisomy 8, or 15q21 interstitial deletion.

Myotonic dystrophy

This AD condition occasionally presents in the cardiac genetics clinic as query MFS. See 'Myotonic dystrophy (DM1)' in Chapter 3, 'Common consultations', p. 496.

Early-onset, rapidly progressive MFS

Infants with severe phenotypic manifestations of MFS are usually long and floppy due to ligamentous laxity. These children frequently develop significant scoliosis, arachnodactyly, contractures, and rapidly progressing valvular and/or aortic disease. MFS in patients with early severe features usually results from 'de novo' mutations that reside in the central region of FBN1 (exons 24–32). Importantly, classic or mild MFS is also commonly caused by DNMs. So-called 'infantile' or 'neonatal' MFS is not a discrete diagnostic category, but rather an extreme of a phenotypic continuum. Counselling and management should be based upon direct and ongoing observation of the patient in question.

Shprintzen-Goldberg syndrome

Rare AD disorder presenting in infancy with overlapping features of Marfan syndrome and Crouzon syndrome. Caused by heterozygous mutation in SKI.

Genetic counselling

Inheritance and recurrence risk

AD condition with 50% risk to offspring. The rate of sporadic cases, due to de novo FBN1 mutation, approaches 30%. When both parents with normal findings on full clinical assessment (including echo and slit-lamp) have a child with MFS, the recurrence risk is low. Both somatic and germline mosaicism have been described.

Variability and penetrance

The phenotype can be very variable. Ectopia lentis can be discordant between affected related individuals. Some families show fairly consistent severe cardiovascular involvement, but others do not. Penetrance is age-dependent and is crucial in determining 'at-risk' family members.

Prenatal diagnosis and predictive testing

Known pathological FBN1 mutation identified in a first-degree relative allows prenatal genetic testing via CVS in early pregnancy, or amniocentesis at mid pregnancy. In addition, predictive testing is possible and may be offered to facilitate appropriate surveillance and targeted, effective therapeutic recommendations.

Other family members

Parents of an individual with MFS should be offered comprehensive evaluation with clinical assessment, echo, and slit-lamp examination. If parents are not available, or results are unknown, offer evaluation to siblings. All children of an affected individual are at 50% risk and should be offered periodic review. A pathological FBN1 mutation in the proband facilitates assessment of other family members.

Natural history and management

- Progressive dilatation of the aortic root. Beta-blockade has been associated with slowing of progression of aortic root dilatation by decreasing the stress on the aortic wall in some studies. Recent work in animal models suggests that angiotensin receptor blockers (ARBs), such as losartan, may provide greater protection through both reduction in haemodynamic stress and antagonism of TGF-β signalling (Habashi et al. 2006). While a number of studies have suggested a beneficial effect of ARBs in people with MFS, this remains an area of active research. A few very small and/or brief analyses have suggested that either calcium channel blockers or ACE inhibitors may afford some protection; determination of the safety and/or efficacy of these agents in MFS requires further study.

- Scoliosis is usually non-progressive upon the cessation of somatic growth. If a fixed (i.e. non-postural) spinal deformity is noted in a child or adolescent, refer for orthopedic assessment. Bracing and/or surgical stabilization may be required when severe and progressive scoliosis is documented.

- Pneumothorax. Pleurodesis is recommended for recurrent pneumothorax. Avoidance of positive pressure ventilation (e.g. scuba diving) may help mitigate this risk.

- Retinal detachment. Patients with high myopia and increased axial globe length are at increased risk. Contact sports and rapid acceleration/deceleration should be avoided. Retinal detachment is a described, but relatively rare, complication of surgery for ectopia lentis.

- Glaucoma occurs with increased frequency in individuals with ectopia lentis.

Surveillance

- All individuals with MFS should undergo annual echo. Individuals with significant valvular disease or marked aortic root dilatation (>4.5 cm in adults) and rapid aortic expansion (>3 mm/year) should be assessed more frequently. Gravid women should be assessed by echo at each trimester, and more often for a rapidly expanding aorta during pregnancy.

- Initial medical therapy if aortic root diameter >2 SD from mean (consider earlier intervention if child clearly affected and severe cardiovascular phenotype in family). Asthma is a relative contraindication for beta-blockade.

- Patients with an aortic root diameter >5.0 cm are advised to proceed with prophylactic cardiothoracic surgical intervention. Earlier intervention should be considered with rapid aortic root growth (>0.5–1.0 cm/year) or with significant aortic valve dysfunction. Aortic valve-sparing aortic root replacement eliminates the need for anticoagulation and should be considered for patients with preserved or correctable aortic valve function. Mitral valve surgery should be considered in patients with significant mitral valve regurgitation in association with emerging LV dysfunction; mitral valve repair (as opposed to replacement) is often possible.
- Periodic ophthalmic review is appropriate in childhood and early adolescence. Ectopia lentis usually becomes evident early in life and can slowly progress in childhood and early adolescence. Even in the absence of ectopia lentis, adult patients should visit the ophthalmologist annually for assessment and management of visual acuity alterations since glaucoma and early-onset cataracts can develop. It is particularly important to achieve adequate and balanced correction of visual acuity in childhood to avoid amblyopia.
- Growth should be monitored in childhood and adolescence. Interventions to reduce growth potential, such as hormonal treatment and epiphyseal stapling, have fallen out of favour.
- Spine. Annual examination by a primary care physician to assess for scoliosis is advised during childhood and adolescence. Evidence of significant deformity should prompt referral to an orthopaedist.

Lifestyle issues
- Sports. Enquire specifically about leisure pursuits, and assess individually. In general, isometric exercise, e.g. weightlifting, rowing, push-ups, pull-ups, and sit-ups, should be avoided. Contact sports, such as football, basketball, hockey, volleyball, boxing, and wrestling, are contraindicated because of increased risk of retinal detachment and aortic injury from rapid deceleration. Regular recreational aerobic activity, such as walking, swimming, and non-competitive cycling, is not only allowed but is encouraged to promote cardiovascular health.
- The Marfan Association produces a range of booklets for children, teenagers, and adults and also for teachers and can provide help with resources for clothing and shoes.

Emergency situations
- Ocular. Retinal detachment is associated with sudden visual field loss. Although retinal detachment is not life-threatening, unrecognized/untreated detachment can result in blindness. Sudden visual field loss therefore warrants emergency evaluation.
- Pulmonary. Spontaneous pneumothorax results from rupture of pulmonary blebs. Blebs form due to increased air spaces in the lung. Symptoms of spontaneous pneumothorax include chest, neck, or back pain exacerbated by deep breathing, or difficult breathing due to pain. Spontaneous pneumothorax is more common in individuals with connective tissue disorders, presumably from increased signalling in the TGF-β pathway. Symptoms of pneumothorax warrant emergency evaluation.
- Cardiovascular. Aortic dissection is a potentially life-threatening complication of aortic aneurysm. Symptoms of aortic dissection include sudden severe chest pain migrating to the chest, neck, back, abdomen, and/or an extremity. Nausea, vomiting, shortness of breath, and cardiovascular collapse can also accompany aortic dissection. Symptoms of aortic dissection warrant activation of the emergency medical services (call 999) and transport to the nearest hospital with aortic imaging capabilities (CTA, MRA, transoesophageal echo) to confirm or exclude dissection and, if present, to provide appropriate treatment.

Pregnancy
Pregnancy should be carefully planned in women with MFS. Physiologic changes necessary to support maternal and fetal circulation during pregnancy include increases in intravascular volume and cardiac output, which increase maternal cardiovascular demands and increase cardiovascular risk.

If cardiovascular involvement is minor and aortic root diameter is <40 mm, pregnancy is usually tolerated well, with favourable maternal and fetal outcomes and no evidence of aggravation of aortic root dilatation with time (Meijboom et al. 2005).

If there is evidence of cardiovascular compromise, e.g. moderate or more severe aortic regurgitation or aortic root diameter >40 mm, and/or a family history of early dissection, the risk of dissection in pregnancy is increased. The risk of complications is highest as pregnancy approaches term and the risk persists several weeks post-partum.

Echocardiograms establish a baseline for comparison of cardiovascular parameters during and after pregnancy. In addition to echo, baseline MRA or CTA may be advised to assess the distal thoracic and abdominal aorta prior to conception. Although it is impossible to predict which patients will develop aortic dilation during pregnancy, an aortic root dimension exceeding 4 cm at the onset of pregnancy is associated with an increased risk of aortic complications during and after pregnancy.

High-risk obstetric care is recommended for all women with MFS. An echo should be repeated at each trimester of pregnancy. Rapid aortic growth suggests aortic instability, warrants close surveillance, and may require aggressive measures to stabilize the mother. Hospitalization, intensive care unit observation, and IV medical therapy may be indicated. A well-constructed delivery plan that includes high-risk maternal/fetal experts (obstetrics, anaesthesiology, neonatology) can optimize outcome. There is controversy regarding the optimal route of delivery for women with MFS, with options including planned Caesarean section versus a controlled vaginal delivery. Finally, echo is recommended following delivery prior to hospital discharge, and again 2–4 weeks post-partum. A history of aortic root growth during pregnancy or an aortic dimension that infers high risk (>4.0 cm) should lead to consideration of prolonged post-partum observation and/or more frequent imaging. Prophylactic aortic root replacement can diminish (but not eliminate) risk for women with MFS who wish to become pregnant.

Reduced weight in the newborn can occur with beta-blocker use during pregnancy. The effect on birthweight is slightly preferable with metoprolol therapy, compared to atenolol (Wright and Dietz 1999). Both ARBs and ACE inhibitors must be stopped during pregnancy due to a risk of fetal loss and birth defects. Rodent studies caution against use of these agents in the immediate post-partum period due to consequences for renal development.

Support groups: Marfan Association UK, http://www.marfan-association.org.uk; The Marfan Foundation (USA), http://www.marfan.org.

Expert adviser: Hal Dietz, Director, Institute of Genetic Medicine, John Hopkins Hospital, Baltimore, USA.

References

Boileau C, Guo DC, Hanna N, et al. TGFB2 mutations cause familial thoracic aortic aneurysms and dissections associated with mild systemic features of Marfan syndrome. Nat Genet 2012; **44**: 916–21.

Dietz HC, McIntosh I, Sakai LY, et al. Four novel FBN1 mutations: significance for mutant transcript level and EGF-like domain calcium binding in the pathogenesis of Marfan syndrome. Genomics 1993; **17**: 468–75.

GeneTests. http://www.genetests.org.

Glesby MJ, Pyeritz RE. Association of mitral valve prolapse and systemic abnormalities of connective tissue: a phenotypic continuum. JAMA 1989; **262**: 523–8.

Gott VL, Greene PS, Alejo DE, et al. Replacement of the aortic root in patients with Marfan's syndrome. N Engl J Med 1999; **340**: 1307–13.

Habashi JP, Judge DP, Holm TM, et al. Losartan, an AT1 antagonist, prevents aortic aneurysm in a mouse model of Marfan syndrome. Science 2006; **312**: 117–21.

Lee B, Godfrey M, Vitale E, et al., Linkage of Marfan syndrome and a phenotypically related disorder to two different fibrillin genes. Nature 1991 **352**: 330–4.

Lindsay ME, Schepers D, Bolar NA, et al. Loss-of-function mutations in TGFB2 cause a syndromic presentation of thoracic aortic aneurysm. Nat Genet 2012; **44**: 922–7.

Loeys BL, Chen J, Neptune ER, et al. A syndrome of altered cardiovascular, craniofacial, neurogognitive and skeletal development caused by mutations in TGFBR1 or TGFBR2. Nat Genet 2005; **37**: 275–81.

Loeys BL, De Backer J, Van Acker P, et al. Comprehensive molecular screening of the FBN1 gene favors locus homogeneity of classical Marfan syndrome. Hum Mutat 2004; **24**: 140–6.

Loeys BL, Dietz HC, Braverman AC, et al. The revised Ghent nosology for the Marfan syndrome. J Med Genet 2010; **47**: 476–86.

Loeys BL, Schwarze U, Holm T, et al. Aneurysm syndromes caused by mutations in the TGF-beta receptor. N Engl J Med 2006; **355**: 788–98.

Meester JA, Vandeweyer G, et al. Loss-of-function mutations in the X-linked biglycan gene cause a severe syndromic form of thoracic aortic aneurysms and dissections. Genet Med 2016 doi: 10.1038/gim.2016.126.

Meijboom LJ, Vos FE, Timmermans J, Boers GH, Zwinderman AH, Mulder BJ. Pregnancy and aortic root growth in Marfan syndrome: a prospective study. Eur Heart J 2005; **26**: 914–20.

Murdoch JL, Walker BA, Halpern BL, Kuzma JW, McKusick VA. Life expectancy and causes of death in Marfan syndrome. N Engl J Med 1972; **1972**: 804–8.

Online Mendelian Inheritance in Man, OMIM (TM). Center for Medical Genetics, Johns Hopkins University and National Center for Biotechnology Information, National Library of Medicine Baltimore MD and Bethesda MD, 2013.

Putnam EA, Zhang H, Ramirez F, Milewicz DM. Fibrillin-2 (FBN2) mutations result in the Marfan-like disorder, congenital contractural arachnodactyly. Nat Genet 1995; **11**: 456–8.

Regalado ES, Guo DC, Villamizar C, et al. Exome sequencing identifies SMAD3 mutations as a cause of familial thoracic aortic aneurysm and dissection with intracranial and other arterial aneurysms. Circulation Res 2011; **109**: 680–6.

Silverman DI, Burton KJ, Gray J, et al. Life expectancy in the Marfan syndrome. Am J Cardiol 1995; **75**: 157–60.

van de Laar IM, Oldenburg RA, Pals G, et al. Mutations in SMAD3 cause a syndromic form of aortic aneurysms and dissections with early-onset osteoarthritis. Nat Genet 2011; **43**: 121–6.

van de Laar IM, van der Linde D, Oei EH, et al. Phenotypic spectrum of the SMAD3-related aneurysms-osteoarthritis syndrome. J Med Genet 2012; **49**: 47–57.

Wright MJ, Dietz HCI. Connective tissue diseases. In: I McMillan, J Oski (eds.). Oski's principles and practice of pediatrics. Lippincott Raven, Philadelphia, 1999.

Mitochondrial DNA diseases

Disorders following mitochondrial inheritance present some of the most challenging situations in genetic counselling and precise advice may not always be possible at the current time. PND for mitochondrial disorders is highly problematical and expert advice should always be sought where this is considered. An accurate diagnosis enables appropriate screening for other systems that may be affected, e.g. conduction defects and diabetes in KSS. Mitochondrial disorders encoded by nuclear DNA, e.g. FRDA, are discussed elsewhere.

Figures from Sweden (Darin *et al.* 2001) have shown an incidence of mitochondrial respiratory chain (MRC) dysfunction in children under 6 years of age of 1/11 000. The same study showed prevalence figures of 1/21 000 in the paediatric population (<16 years). Studies from the UK looking at adults gave a potential prevalence of 1/8000 and combining the figures for children and adults suggests that MRC disease is far from rare and may occur as frequently as 1/8500.

Mitochondrial DNA (mtDNA) is exclusively maternally inherited, with very rare exceptions (Schwartz and Vissing 2002). It is a circular double-stranded molecule of 16 569bp. The genome encodes two ribosomal RNAs, 22 transfer RNAs involved in translation of mRNA into protein, and 13 polypeptide components of the oxidative phosphorylation (OXPHOS) system. Thousands of copies of mtDNA are present in each nucleated somatic cell. Changes in mtDNA sequence can be inherited or somatic. Human mtDNA has a mutation rate 10–20 times that of nuclear DNA, probably due to failure of proofreading by mtDNA polymerase. In normal individuals, all the copies of mtDNA have the same sequence (homoplasmy); in many patients with mitochondrial disease, there is a mixture of normal and mutant sequence within the same cell (heteroplasmy). A variety of mutations occur in mitochondrial disease, including deletions, duplications, and point mutations. *Point mutations are commonly maternally inherited, while deletions and duplications are most often sporadic.* The percentage of mutant DNA may vary between different tissues and also change with time. Blood levels are a very poor reflection of mutant load in A3243G (MELAS) and rearrangements. Preferential accumulation of mutant mtDNAs in affected tissues appears to explain the progressive nature of mitochondrial disorders.

Individual oocytes from a woman at risk of transmitting mitochondrial disease may contain markedly different levels of mutant mtDNA. There is increasing evidence for a 'bottleneck' early in embryological development, so that all mtDNA in an individual is derived from a small number of progenitors (Brown 1997). The degree of heteroplasmy in the progenitors probably governs the subsequent mutant load in the individual.

Some useful nomenclature follows.

- Homoplasmy. All of an individual's mtDNA is identical.
- Heteroplasmy. The existence of more than one mtDNA type in the same individual, e.g. mitochondria containing a mixture of mtDNA carrying the MELAS 3243 point mutation and mtDNA with the wild-type sequence. In mitochondrial disorders, because of the thousands of mitochondria in each cell, the percentage of mutant and wild-type mtDNAs often varies between different cells and especially between different tissues.

- Mitochondrial depletion syndromes. Conditions caused by a reduction in mtDNA copy number. These are recessive diseases with severe tissue-specific decrease in mtDNA copy number, e.g. Alpers, that are caused by impairment of the mtDNA replication system.
- OXPHOS. Oxidative phosphorylation, the core of the energy-producing pathway in the mitochondrion, is a system of five multisubunit complexes located on the inner mitochondrial membrane. Adenosine triphosphate (ATP) is generated by complex V (ATPase). Seventy of the 83 polypeptide components of the system are encoded by nuclear genes, the other 13 by mtDNA. Some tissues, e.g. brain and muscle, are highly dependent on the OXPHOS system for energy.
- COX. Cytochrome oxidase, complex IV of the OXPHOS system.
- SDH. Succinate dehydrogenase, complex II of the OXPHOS system.

Mitochondrial diseases are often late in being diagnosed, either because they present insidiously or because the clinical features (see Box 3.7) are so heterogeneous that the diagnosis is missed. The organs most often affected in mitochondrial disorders are highly energy-demanding tissues such as the CNS, skeletal and cardiac muscle, pancreatic islets, liver, and kidney. Features that should particularly alert suspicion are highlighted in italics in Box 3.7. Several features together increase the likelihood of an underlying mitochondrial disorder. See also Figure 3.22 showing the clinical spectrum of mitochondrial disease.

Clinical approach

History: key points

Three-generation family tree, with specific enquiry about muscle weakness, vision, hearing, and neurological problems. Extend the family tree as far as possible through the maternal line. If there are other potentially affected members in the family, take a careful history, noting the scope of their problems and the age of onset and progress of their symptoms. Mitochondrial disorders often display extraordinary intrafamilial variability.

Examination: key points

- Growth parameters. Height, weight, OFC.
- Examine the eyes, looking for ptosis and nystagmus and testing for external ophthalmoplegia.
- Neurological examination for hypotonia, myoclonus, and ataxia.
- Ophthalmological examination for pigmentary retinopathy, cataract.

Investigations

- DNA for mutation analysis of mitochondrial genome or nuclear-encoded mitochondrial genes. Note that mtDNA rearrangements are not usually found in blood, while the common point mutations frequently are; both types are seen in muscle. With modern sequencing technology, sequencing of the entire mitochondrial genome is increasingly available. From a clinical perspective, thought needs to be given as to the source of DNA to be analysed, as some mitochondrial

CNS
- Developmental delay/regression
- Generalized seizures
- Ataxia
- *Myoclonus*
- Stroke-like episodes
- Encephalopathy

Muscle
- Myopathy—weakness/fatigue/hypotonia

Eyes
- *Ptosis*
- *External ophthalmoplegia*
- Optic atrophy
- Pigmentary retinopathy
- Cataract
- Sudden loss of vision (Leber hereditary optic neuropathy (LHON))

Ears
- *Sensorineural deafness (including aminoglycoside deafness)*

Heart
- CM
- Conduction defects

Pancreas
- *Diabetes mellitus*

Kidney
- Renal tubular dysfunction (Fanconi syndrome) with generalized amino aciduria and glycosuria

Bone marrow
- Sideroblastic anaemia/pancytopenia

Features highlighted in bold should particularly arouse suspicion of a mitochondrial disorder. NB. *Any* of the above features in combination with *lactic acidosis* is highly suggestive of a mitochondrial disorder. Particular combinations, e.g. *diabetes and sensorineural deafness*, are very suggestive of an underlying mitochondrial disorder.

mutations are tissue-specific and may be difficult to detect in blood-derived DNA.
- ECG for conduction disorder.
- Urinalysis for tubular dysfunction (generalized amino aciduria and glycosuria), which may occur in Pearson syndrome, KSS, and MELAS.
- Blood lactate.
- Blood glucose.
- CK is usually normal or only mildly elevated.
- Consider CSF lactate (important in the investigation of possible Leigh disease).
- Consider muscle biopsy with Gomori trichrome staining for 'ragged red fibres' and staining for COX (complex IV) and SDH (complex II). Occasional COX-negative fibres may be found as a normal variant in individuals >40 years of age, but these never exceed 5%. In

order to gain maximum information, the biopsy should be processed and examined in a specialist facility that can undertake light microscopy, EM, immunostaining, storage of muscle for subsequent assay of individual complex activity, and DNA extraction from muscle for mutation analysis. Muscle biopsy is the single most useful test in the diagnosis of mitochondrial disorders, although occasional patients with Leber hereditary optic neuropathy (LHON) and with mitochondrial myopathy due to mtDNA mutations may have normal biopsies.
- Consider MRI if there are symptoms of encephalopathy, e.g. seizures, regression, ataxia, myoclonus, stroke-like episodes.
- Audiometry.
- Serum levels of FGF21 are increasingly used as a biomarker of mitochondrial disease. They are particularly raised in defects of mtDNA maintenance where they can reduce the need for muscle biopsy substantially (Suomalainen *et al.* 2011).

Specific mitochondrial disorders and genetic advice
Most patients with mtDNA mutations present as apparently sporadic cases.

Chronic progressive external ophthalmoplegia (CPEO)
With or without RP or limb weakness and fatigue is usually caused by a single deletion in mtDNA, although ~30% of cases may be due to nuclear genes (following AD or AR inheritance) involved in mtDNA nucleotide metabolism or replication which cause multiple deletions. It typically presents in teenage or young adult life and usually runs a benign course with little involvement of other organs. Most patients with CPEO do not have a family history and presumably develop from ova in which mutations have arisen *de novo*.
- Recurrence risks. Females with a single mtDNA deletion have a very low (<1–5%) chance of transmitting the disease to their offspring. If mtDNA duplications are present, the recurrence risk is higher.

Kearns–Sayre syndrome (KSS)
A subtype of CPEO with a poorer prognosis. Onset is at <20 years and, in addition to CPEO and pigmentary retinopathy, there is often a cardiac conduction defect and ataxia. Unlike CPEO, the condition is usually life-limiting. Patients with KSS usually have a single mtDNA deletion, but duplications may be found in patients with diabetes and deafness. Most patients with KSS and a single mtDNA deletion do not have a family history and presumably develop from ova in which mutations have arisen *de novo*.
- Recurrence risks. Females with a single mtDNA deletion have a very low (<1–5%) chance of transmitting the disease to their offspring. If mtDNA duplications are present, the recurrence risk is higher.

Leber hereditary optic neuropathy (LHON)
Leber hereditary optic neuritis. NB. Leber has several eponymous conditions, e.g. Leber congenital amaurosis (AR), a congenital retinal dystrophy causing blindness, so ensure that the diagnosis really is LHON before giving genetic advice.

The most common mutation in LHON is 11778 (70%); 3460 accounts for 15% and 14484 for a further 5%. LHON causes a fairly rapid and irreversible loss of vision. It is more penetrant in males than females. Forty

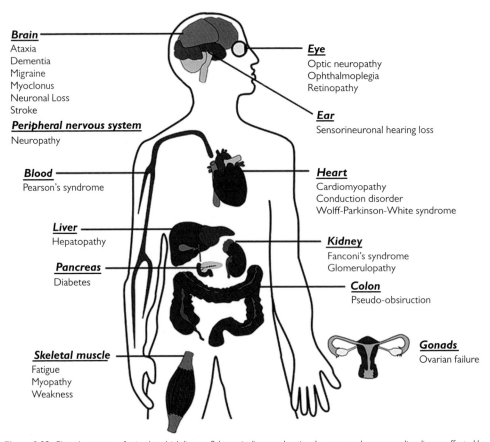

Brain
Ataxia
Dementia
Migraine
Myoclonus
Neuronal Loss
Stroke

Peripheral nervous system
Neuropathy

Blood
Pearson's syndrome

Liver
Hepatopathy

Pancreas
Diabetes

Skeletal muscle
Fatigue
Myopathy
Weakness

Eye
Optic neuropathy
Ophthalmoplegia
Retinopathy

Ear
Sensorineuronal hearing loss

Heart
Cardiomyopathy
Conduction disorder
Wolff-Parkinson-White syndrome

Kidney
Fanconi's syndrome
Glomerulopathy

Colon
Pseudo-obsiruction

Gonads
Ovarian failure

Figure 3.22 Clinical spectrum of mitochondrial disease. Schematic diagram showing the organ and corresponding disease affected by mitochondrial dysfunction.
Reproduced from Chinnery PF, Hudson G., Mitochondrial genetics, *British Medical Bulletin*, volume 106, issue 1, pp. 135–59, 2013. This is an open access article available under the terms of the Creative Commons Attribution 3.0 license (CC BY 3.0) and permits unrestricted reuse, distribution, and reproduction even for commercial purposes, provided the original work is properly attributed.

per cent of patients with G11778A have no family history of the disease. Visual loss is usually irreversible, except with the T14484C mutation where some visual recovery is seen in up to 70% of patients; some visual recovery is also occasionally seen in 3460. The relative risk to women is higher in 3460 families, as the sex ratio is less skewed to males.

Currently there are no effective interventions to prevent visual loss. Advise at-risk family members to avoid known retinal toxins such as smoking and excess alcohol. Age of onset of visual loss is very variable: 5% by age 10 years; 45% by age 20 years; 70% by age 30 years; 80% by age 40 years; 95% by age 50 years; and 100% by age 70 years. The risk diminishes with age. Males who have reached 20 years without problems have halved their lifetime risk; for females, this occurs at 27 years (Harding et al. 1995).

Measuring blood levels is not very helpful in predicting outcome in LHON. The symptom-free maternal relatives may carry identical mutant loads. Some individuals with the G11778A mutation present with an MS-like illness. The G11778 mutation is commonly homoplasmic.

The offspring risks for LHON are summarized in Table 3.29.

Leigh syndrome (subacute necrotizing encephalomyopathy)
See also 'Leigh encephalopathy' in Chapter 3, 'Common consultations', p. 474. Usually presents in infancy with non-specific features such as hypotonia, seizures, and developmental delay. Prevalence ~1/32 000–1/40 000. Spasticity, RP, ataxia, and CPEO may develop later. Blood lactate is often elevated, and CSF lactate is usually significantly elevated. MRI shows bilateral, usually symmetrical, changes in the upper brainstem and thalami. The prognosis for patients presenting in infancy is poor—they usually die within months or a few years. Leigh syndrome is a genetically heterogeneous condition caused by several biochemical defects, including PDH deficiency and OXPHOS defects. A subset of patients carry the mtDNA point mutations T8993G and T8993C (also seen in NARP). Mutations in the nuclear-encoded *Surf1* gene underlie 75% of COX-deficient Leigh syndrome (i.e. 10–20% of all Leigh syndrome) and follow AR inheritance.

Table 3.29 Remaining lifetime risk for LHON at age[*]

	Birth	14 years	26 years	37 years	50 years	61 years
European[†] male	50%	42%	25%	8%	1%	0.07%
European female	No data					
Australian[†] male	20%	17%	10%	3%	0.4%	0.02%
Australian female	4%	3.3%	2%	0.7%	0.1%	0.01%

[*] A mother with 100% mutant has a 99% chance that the child will be the same, so these risks apply to the offspring of these maternal members of the family, i.e. most families stay the same.

[†] The difference between Australian and European risks is thought to be due to environmental factors but could be due to better ascertainment in Australia of all family members.

Reproduced from Traboulsi, *Genetic Diseases of the Eye* (2011) Tab. 'Remaining lifetime risk for LHON at age', p.729. By permission of Oxford University Press, USA.

• Recurrence risks. An empiric risk of 33% was estimated by van Erven *et al.* (1987); this may be an overestimate since the calculation was not corrected for unascertained sibships. See White *et al.* (1999a) for estimate of risk for patients carrying T8993G or T8993C. The recurrence risk for Leigh syndrome due to *Surf1* mutations is 25%.

MELAS (mitochondrial encephalomyopathy–lactic acidosis–strokes)
One of the most common of the mitochondrial disorders (1/10 000) and one of the most *variable*. Ninety per cent of cases are caused by the A3243G point mutation in the tRNA[leu] gene. Despite the acronym, the most common presenting features are diabetes and progressive deafness and some patients do not develop other symptoms. Approximately 10% develop CM. Blood levels in A3243G are a very poor reflection of mutant load and may diminish with age.

• Recurrence risk. Everyone in the A3423G maternal line is at increased risk for diabetes (usual onset in early adult life, initially diet-controlled, but patients usually become insulin-dependent fairly rapidly), deafness (progressive sensorineural), and CM.

• Low load (<30% in muscle, <10% in blood) or asymptomatic or diabetes only: likely lowish offspring risk ~15–25%.

• Moderate load (>50% in muscle) or symptomatic other than diabetes and/or deafness: likely offspring risk >60%.

MERRF (myoclonic epilepsy with ragged red fibres)
In addition to myoclonic epilepsy, the clinical spectrum includes cerebellar ataxia, deafness, and dementia. Caused by mtDNA point mutations, typically A8344G in the tRNA[lys] gene.

• Recurrence risk. In a small analysis of 47 women carrying the A8344G mutation (Chinnery *et al.* 1997), <5% of the offspring were affected when the mutant load in maternal blood was <35%, 15% were affected when the mutant load was 40–59%, 20% when the mutant load was 60–79%, and 80% when the mutant load was 80–100%.

NARP (neurogenic weakness, ataxia, retinitis pigmentosa)
Caused by the T8992G and T8993C mutations (which can also cause a subset of Leigh syndrome).

• Recurrence risks. Risks depend on the base change, T8993G being more severe than T8993A. See White *et al.* (1999a) for further details.

Pearson syndrome
Usually presents in infancy with transfusion-dependent sideroblastic anaemia or pancytopenia often with malabsorption (exocrine pancreatic failure). May develop villous atrophy, diabetes mellitus, renal tubular dysfunction, etc. Caused by mtDNA deletions. Morbidity and mortality are high. If infants survive, their haematology normalizes, the clinical picture then evolves into KSS because the red and white blood cells with higher mutant loads are selected against and gradually lost from the blood, but tissues such as the brain and heart where cells do not turn over rapidly gradually acquire more deletions.

• Recurrence risks. The recurrence risk for pure mtDNA deletions is likely to be very low (<1–5%). If mtDNA duplications are present, the recurrence risk is higher.

Respiratory chain defects where the precise molecular basis is unknown
• Recurrence risks. Genetic counselling of this group is extremely difficult, as they embrace such a wide group of disorders. In the largest study of Leigh disease, recurrence risks were between 1 in 8 and 1 in 4. If, however, a mother carries an mtDNA mutation (which may be unrecognized), then the recurrence risk can be much higher.

Sensorineural deafness
A1555G is the most common mutation but usually only causes hearing impairment in early life if there has been exposure to aminoglycosides (e.g. gentamicin). Hearing loss is progressive. A7445G is the second most common mitochondrial mutation (sometimes associated with palmoplantar keratoderma). 7472insC can cause isolated progressive deafness or deafness with ataxia/dysarthria/myoclonus. Overall, mitochondrial mutations are found in up to 30% of families with members affected by sensorineural deafness in two or more generations related through the maternal line, but only 1% of sporadic early-onset non-syndromic deafness. Age of onset of deafness can be very variable (Estivill *et al.* 1998).

• Recurrence risks. A1555G is homoplasmic in nearly all pedigrees.

Genetic advice
A major problem for genetic counselling is that the correlation between phenotypic severity and the level of mutant mtDNA is poor in many mitochondrial diseases.

Inheritance and recurrence risk
See individual conditions. Offspring of affected males are not at risk.

Variability and penetrance
Mitochondrial disorders often display extraordinary intrafamilial variability, with different family members inheriting different mutant loads.

Prenatal diagnosis
PND for mitochondrially encoded disorders should be undertaken only in conjunction with a centre with specialist expertise in mitochondrial genetics. Each mtDNA mutation needs to be considered separately. The available data from studies of human fetal tissues with mtDNA mutations (White et al. 1999a) suggest that there is little or no tissue variation or selection operating on mtDNA mutations in utero. Current data therefore suggest that mutant load in a prenatal sample (CVS/amniocentesis) does appear to predict the mutant load in most tissues at birth (Thorburn and Dahl 2001). However, the main difficulty lies in accurately predicting the phenotype from the mutant load and, even with expert advice, there may be a high degree of uncertainty.

CVS/amniocentesis may be suitable for women with a low recurrence risk (this approach relies on a woman having a sufficient proportion of oocytes with low mutant loads to have a reasonable chance of a successful outcome). Donor oocyte IVF may be a suitable option for women with moderate to high mutant loads.

Approaches using a donor ovum and either pronuclear transfer or spindle transfer have been developed to enable couples to have a child with both of their nuclear genetic contributions but the mitochondria of the donor ovum.

Predictive testing
This can be offered to maternal relatives; however, as noted in 'Prenatal diagnosis' above, the main difficulty lies in accurately predicting the phenotype from the mutant load. Even with expert advice, there may be a high degree of uncertainty.

Natural history and management
No curative treatment is available. Patients should be under the care of a paediatric neurologist or neurologist and/or metabolic paediatrician/physician.

Surveillance
Check ECG and blood glucose periodically.

Drugs to avoid in mitochondrial disorders
- Sodium valproate inhibits several pathways of intermediate metabolism, so use with caution.
- Barbiturates (used in general anaesthetics). Avoid since they are inhibitors of OXPHOS.
- Gentamicin may cause sensorineural deafness.
- Ciprofloxacin is an mtDNA inhibitor.
- Chloramphenicol is a mitochondrial translation inhibitor.
- Metformin can exacerbate lactic acidosis and has been associated with stepwise deterioration.
- Tetracycline is a mitochondrial translation inhibitor.
- Zidovudine (antiviral agent) causes mitochondrial depletion.

Treatment
There are no specific treatments for disorders due to MRC dysfunction. Early diagnosis and supportive treatment of complications, such as diabetes, CM, epilepsy, and undernutrition, are therefore extremely important. Rare cases of primary coenzyme Q (ubiquinone) deficiency may respond to oral replacement using ubiquinone or idebenone that crosses the blood–brain barrier. Anecdotal reports suggest that patients with complex I deficiency and lipid storage benefit from carnitine treatment and that riboflavin may help some patients with MELAS and A3243G. Other forms of supplementation therapy have been tried without apparent benefit. See European NeuroMuscular Centre (ENMC), http://www.enmc.org.

Support group: The Children's Mitochondrial Disease Network, www.cmdn.org.uk and The Lily Foundation, http://www.thelilyfoundation.org.uk/.

Expert adviser: Joanna Poulton, Professor of Mitochondrial Genetics, University of Oxford, Oxford, UK.

References
Brown GK. Bottlenecks and beyond: mitochondrial DNA segregation in health and disease. J Inherit Metab Dis 1997; **20**: 2–8.

Chinnery PF, Howell N, Lightowlers RN, Turnbull DM. Molecular pathology of MELAS and MERFF: the relationship between mutation load and clinical phenotype. Brain 1997; **120**: 1713–21.

Chinnery PF, Hudson G. Mitochondrial genetics. Br Med Bull 2013; **106**: 135–59.

Darin N, Oldfors A, Moslemi AR, Holme E, Tulinius M. The incidence of mitochondrial encephalomyopathies in childhood: clinical features and morphological, biochemical, and DNA abnormalities. Ann Neurol 2001; **49**: 377–83.

Estivill X, Govea N, Barceló E, et al. Familial progressive sensorineural deafness is mainly due to the mtDNA A1555G mutation and is enhanced by treatment of aminoglycosides. Am J Hum Genet 1998; **62**: 27–35.

Harding A, Sweeney M, Govan GG, Riordan-Eva P. Pedigree analysis in Leber hereditary optic neuropathy in families with a pathogenic mtDNA mutation. Am J Hum Genet 1995; **57**: 77–86.

Leonard JV, Schapiro AHV. Mitochondrial respiratory chain disorders I: mitochondrial DNA defects. Lancet 2000; **355**: 299–304.

Mackey D, Howell N. A variant of Leber hereditary optic neuropathy characterized by recovery of vision and by an unusual mitochondrial genetic etiology. Am J Hum Genet 1992; **51**: 1218–28.

Mackey DA. Mitochondrial diseases. In: El Traboulsi (ed.). Genetic diseases of the eye, p. 729. Oxford University Press, New York, 1998.

Poulton J, Macaulay V, Marchington DR. Transmission, genetic counselling and prenatal diagnosis of mitochondrial DNA disease. In: I Holt (ed.). Genetics of mitochondrial disease, Oxford monographs in medical genetics no. 47, pp. 309–26. Oxford University Press, Oxford, 2003.

Schapira AHV. Mitochondrial diseases (Seminar). Lancet 2012; **374**: 1825–34.

Schwartz M, Vissing J. Paternal inheritance of mitochondrial DNA. N Engl J Med 2002; **347**: 576–80.

Seminars in Medical Genetics. Mitochondrial diseases. Am J Med Genet 2001; **106C** (Issue 1).

Suomalainen A, Elo JM, et al. FGF-21 as a biomarker for muscle-manifesting mitochondrial respiratory chain deficiencies: a diagnostic study. Lancet Neurol 2011; **10**: 806–18.

Thorburn DR, Dahl HH. Mitochondrial disorders: genetics, counseling, prenatal diagnosis and reproductive options. Am J Med Genet C 2001; **106C**: 102–14.

van Erven PM, Cillessen JP, Eekhoff EM, et al. Leigh syndrome, a mitochondrial encephalo(myo)pathy. A review of the literature. Clin Neurol Neurosurg 1987; **89**: 217–30.

White S, Collins V, Wolfe R, et al. Genetic counseling and prenatal diagnosis for the mitochondrial DNA mutations at nucleotide 8993. Am J Hum Genet 1999a; **65**: 474–82.

White SL, Shanske S, Biros I, et al. Two cases of prenatal analysis for the pathogenic T to G substitution at nucleotide 8993 in mitochondrial DNA. Prenat Diagn 1999b; **19**: 1165–68.

Myotonic dystrophy (DM1)

Dystrophia myotonica, Steinert's disease.

Myotonic dystrophy is the most common heritable neuromuscular disorder; in Western Europe, there are two main variants—type 1 (DM1) with a prevalence of 1/8000, and DM2 (see below) which is almost as common as DM1 in Germany, Eastern Europe, and Finland but which becomes progressively less common further West. DM1 is caused by a triplet repeat expansion (CTG) in the non-coding region of the dystrophia myotonica protein kinase (*DMPK*) gene at 19q13.3. The condition is characterized by extreme variability, anticipation, and differential expansion in the maternal and paternal germline.

The normal number of repeats is 4–37 (the most common allele is five triplets (34%); 11, 12, 13, and 14 are also quite common). Alleles of >30 repeats are uncommon (<2%). Affected individuals with DM1 have an increased number of repeats from 50 to many thousands. Less than 100 repeats is usually visible as a clear band, but >100 repeats is usually seen as a smear on Southern analysis due to mitotic instability in triplet repeat number. Pathogenic expansions are liable to expand during both paternal and maternal transmission (but contraction noted in ± 6%). There is potential for much greater expansion if maternally inherited. Women carrying an expansion who are symptomatic or who have clinical signs are at risk of delivering a congenitally affected infant.

Paradoxically, 'protomutations' (50–80 repeats) can be inherited stably through females for several generations but often (70%) result in a large increase into the full disease range of >100 repeats if transmitted by males.

Table 3.30 demonstrates overlaps between the clinical presentation and the repeat size and the current uncertainty of predicting the phenotype on the basis of the molecular results.

Congenital myotonic dystrophy (CMD)

The pregnancy is frequently complicated by polyhydramnios (100% in one series) and talipes, which, combined together, may be the first clue to DM in the family (Zaki et al. 2007). At delivery, severely affected infants are floppy and often have respiratory problems with diaphragmatic hypoplasia and may require ventilatory support. Some severely affected infants may die; the neonatal mortality is 20%. Severe feeding problems may necessitate nasogastric feeding. Infants and young children do not show myotonia at onset of symptoms. Bilateral facial diplegia and a 'tented mouth' and an inability to smile are characteristic features.

Babies who receive ventilatory support through the early weeks/months may subsequently improve and breathe independently and become less floppy. Most will later have significant learning disability requiring specialist educational support and usually ongoing support in adult life, with few living independently. The South Wales survey reported few deaths between the age of 1 and 20 years, but only half survived to the mid 30s and none beyond 40 years (not many studied at this age).

Some individuals with CMD do not have severe neonatal respiratory problems (although usually a history of slow or difficult feeding is elicited) and present later with developmental delay and the characteristic facial appearance. Myotonia usually has its onset in adolescence and other features of classical DM are then gradually superimposed.

Other individuals do not develop clinical features until after 12 months of age. These early and other childhood cases can pose diagnostic difficulty because they frequently present with other features, such as behaviour problems, learning problems, or constipation, without obvious weakness or myotonia until years later.

Clinical approach (to adults)

History: key points

- Three-generation family tree, with specific enquiry for cataracts, diabetes, myotonia, muscle weakness, anaesthetic deaths, etc.
- Neuromuscular:
  - hands 'locking up', e.g. using can opener, turning key in lock, holding steering wheel, peeling potatoes. May be exacerbated by cold weather;
  - weakness, especially hands and ankle (tripping or falls), reduced exercise tolerance.
- Respiratory:
  - chest infections, snoring, morning headaches.
- Cardiac:
  - palpitations, faints, blackout?
- GI:
  - symptoms similar to those of irritable bowel syndrome;
  - choking on food/ difficulty swallowing lumps?
- CNS:
- excessive daytime sleepiness?
- apathy, difficulty initiating actions, motivating;
- fatigue (tire easily);
- sleep with eyes open? Snoring?

Examination: key points

- Facies. Ptosis; a long face with reduced ability to wrinkle the forehead, bury eyelashes, or clench the masseter muscles; male-pattern balding (also seen in affected females). (Absence of external ophthalmoplegia, absence of blepharospasm.)

Table 3.30 Overlap between clinical presentation, CTG repeat size, and phenotype

Number of CTG repeats	Designation	Clinical features
4–37	Normal allele	None
38–49	Premutation	None
50–80	Protomutation	Usually asymptomatic or associated with mild late-onset disease, e.g. cataracts without neuromuscular disease
200–500	Mutation	Usually associated with onset in third and fourth decades
230–1800 (mean 830)	Mutation	Childhood onset, but not usually congenital
>1000	Mutation	May cause congenital myotonic dystrophy

- Sternomastoids. Test muscle power against the hand placed on the side of the chin. Note sternomastoid muscle bulk and power (both often reduced in DM).
- Distal weakness, particularly affecting hand grip, wrist flexion and extension, and ankle dorsiflexion, are characteristic. Proximal weakness does not exclude the diagnosis. (Wasting of the forearm and distal leg muscles is characteristic.)
- Tap the thenar eminence firmly to elicit myotonic contraction.
- Ask the patient to clench the hands into a tight fist, hold, and then quickly release (may elicit grip-myotonia). Alternatively, ask them to grip hold of your index and middle finger and then quickly release (may take many seconds to gradually unfurl the hand).
- DTRs may be normal if mildly affected case, but become difficult to elicit and may be absent in more severely affected individuals.
- Pilomatrixoma. Benign tumour of the hair matrix.
- Ophthalmoscopy—lens dot opacities or stellate cataracts may be easily identified (focus on the iris).

Investigations
- Mutation analysis for $(CTG)_n$ triplet repeat expansion in the *DMPK* gene.
- ECG looking for prolonged PR interval, broad QRS complex, left axis deviation (LAD), and bundle branch block. All indicate early involvement of the cardiac conduction system.
- Blood glucose (diabetes mellitus).
- Ophthalmology referral if suspected cataract. Otherwise recommend regular surveillance by an optometrist/optician. Recent evidence suggests DM1 patients have a greater risk of epiretinal membranes (48%) which are also amenable to surgery (Kersten et al. 2014) if impacting on vision.

Other diagnoses/conditions to consider

Proximal myotonic myopathy (PROMM/DM2)
An AD condition only distinguished from DM after cloning of the myotonin gene. The weakness is predominantly proximal; myotonia is mild, intermittent, and usually subclinical, and muscle pain is a notable feature. PROMM is also known as DM2 and a (CCTG) expansion in the *ZNF9* gene has been found. This mutation should be checked in cases of suspected DM where the expected (CTG) expansion proves negative. Muscle biopsies show preferential type 2 fibre atrophy in contrast to type 1 fibre atrophy seen in DM1 (Vihola et al. 2003).

Congenital non-progressive myotonias
- Thomsen disease (AD) and Becker disease (AR). Characterized by impaired muscle relaxation after forceful contraction (myotonia), which is more pronounced after inactivity and improves with exercise. These diseases are similar, except that transient weakness is seen in Becker disease, but not in Thomsen disease. Mutations in the *CLCN1* chloride channel gene have been found in both types. Blepharospasm is common, especially in the Becker (AR) variant.
- Schwartz–Jampel syndrome. Blepharospasm and skeletal dysplasia. Inheritance is AR with mutation in the perlecan gene (*HSPG2*).

Oculopharyngeal muscular dystrophy (OPMD)
Dysphagia and ptosis are early prominent features, out of proportion to general weakness elsewhere. Ophthalmoplegia may be present. Caused by a GCG triplet expansion in the *PABPN1* gene.

Moebius syndrome
The facial weakness in Moebius syndrome is due to cranial nerve palsy (usually VIth and VIIth), but the facial appearance can be confused with that of DM.

Genetic advice

Inheritance and recurrence risk
Inheritance is AD. The risk of having a child with CMD depends on the sex of the transmitting parent and the clinical features in the parent, and CMD only occurs if the fetus inherits a *DMPK* expansion. See Cobo et al. (1995) for an analysis of CTG repeat sizes in 124 affected mother–child pairs, and more recent data from the same group (Martorell et al. 2007).
- Risk for CMD in offspring of mothers carrying (CTG) expansion.
  - Mothers with minimal disease and a small expansion size (<80 repeats). In such women, the chance of expansion into the CMD range is minimal and the mutation is likely to remain relatively stable.
  - Mothers with neuromuscular involvement and moderate expansion size (200–500 repeats) with no previous children: 10–30% risk of a child with CMD.
  - Mothers with neuromuscular involvement and moderate expansion size (200–500 repeats) with a previous child with CMD: 40–50% risk.
- Risk for CMD in offspring of fathers carrying (CTG) expansion. The risk of transmission of congenital disease from an affected father is very low, with only a few reported cases in the world literature.
- Other offspring risks for males.
  - Males with minimal disease and a small expansion size (<80 repeats). There may be a considerable expansion with offspring at risk for earlier and more severe disease (but not for CMD).
  - Males with neuromuscular involvement and moderate expansion size (200–500 repeats). There is a variable outlook for offspring of an affected male as mutation could contract, stay stable, or expand.

More recent data on 154 DM pregnancies show a huge gender difference in intergenerational size between offspring and transmitting parent—the mean increase when transmitted by the father is 56 CTG repeats (SD 177), compared to 948 CTG repeats (SD 815) when transmitted by the mother (Martorell, et al. 2007), i.e. a difference of 50, compared to just under 1000.

Overall the same.

Variability and penetrance
Affected families exhibit anticipation in their offspring, with a tendency to increasing severity in successive generations. Older generations may be minimally affected, e.g. by cataract alone with no neuromuscular symptoms.

Prenatal diagnosis
Possible by CVS using triplet repeat (CTG) expansion. This will determine whether or not the fetus has inherited the expansion. Predicting prognosis is more difficult. Most (but not all) infants with CMD have expansions of >1000 repeats, though some at this size will have childhood onset. It is usually possible to distinguish whether a fetus is carrying an expansion consistent with minimal or adult-onset disease or an expansion consistent with a risk of CMD. PCR-based assay to determine the size

and presence of normal alleles is quick, but, if only one normal allele is seen, Southern blotting to determine the size of expansion may take 2–3 weeks.

Pre-implantation genetic diagnosis
PGD has now been performed successfully for DM1 for many years, with evidence of good reproductive outcome whether the mother or father is affected. Success does not appear to depend on CTG repeat size in the mother (Verpoest *et al.* 2008, 2010).

Predictive testing
Chance that a sibling/offspring aged 21–40 years with a normal clinical examination carries a (CTG) expansion is 10% (of which only one-half will have significant neuromuscular involvement). When considering predictive testing in a healthy younger person, due consideration needs to be given to potential implications for children, insurance, and financial arrangements.

Other family members
Cascade approach to family screening is appropriate. Males and females are both at risk of idiosyncratic anaesthetic reactions and are especially sensitive to sedatives and opiates; the risk is not high, but deaths of undiagnosed and asymptomatic individuals, especially in the post-operative period, are not rare. Similarly, even mildly affected or asymptomatic women may be at risk of having offspring with CMD. The risk of CMD in offspring of women (21–40 years old) who are entirely clinical normal on examination is low.

Natural history and management
The typical age of onset of symptoms is between 20 and 30 years, though the diagnosis may be delayed when there is no clear family history. The impact of the disease can be obtained from a large study of an affected family in Canada where 20% of affected males and 50% of affected females never worked. Because of its very wide clinical manifestations, the disease does not follow a clear pattern and the rate of progress is difficult to predict. In a large Dutch registry study, the mean age of death in females was 59 years and in males 60 years. The observed survival to the ages of 25, 45, and 65 years was 99%, 88%, and 18%, respectively, compared with an expected survival of 99%, 95%, and 78%, respectively (de Die-Smulders *et al.* 1998). Pneumonia and cardiac arrhythmias are the most frequent primary causes of death (Groh *et al.* 2011).

In young adults, the potential problems to discuss are the following.
- Reproductive issues and fertility. Fertility is reduced in males and females and women have a higher miscarriage rate. They may wish to consider PND or PGD. There are particular obstetric problems:
  - failure to progress in labour;
  - polyhydramnios, 15%;
  - prematurity, <38/40 13%;
  - retained placenta, 10%;
  - PPH, 5%;
  - anaesthetic risks (see 'Potential long-term complications' below).
- Mobility and muscle weakness.
- GI tract; irritable bowel syndrome.
- Consider whether the patient's symptoms could affect driving.

Potential long-term complications
Discuss the benefits of carrying a Medic-alert card and/or jewellery with details of the patient's diagnosis.
- Anaesthetics. There is an increased sensitivity to sedatives and opiates given as premedication. There is an increased risk for adverse reaction to commonly used anaesthetic agents (e.g. suxamethonium), cardiac dysrhythmias, aspiration pneumonia, and prolonged recovery. Consider regional blocks or spinal or epidural anaesthesia. If a general anaesthetic is required, it should be given in a hospital with high dependency unit or intensive care unit facilities for post-operative support and monitoring. Post-operatively, patients with DM are at increased risk for respiratory arrest, dysrhythmias, and chest infections (weak respiratory muscles + sensitivity to opiate analgesia). A preoperative anaesthetic assessment including echo and ECG is advised (Rogers and Clyburn 2004). An anaesthetic leaflet is available from Myotonic Dystrophy Support Group (MDSG; see 'Support groups').
- Diabetes mellitus. Due to insulin resistance.
- Cataract. Posterior subcapsular cataract and/or epiretinal membrane.
- Cardiac involvement. There is clear evidence of an increased risk of conduction disease, but not of ischaemic heart disease. CM is rare in DM1 but has been reported. Ventricular arrhythmias are likely to explain some cases of sudden death. Refer to a cardiologist if the PR interval is >200 ms, QRSd >120 ms, if atrial fibrillation or flutter occur, or the patient is symptomatic (palpitations, syncope). Additional investigations may include Holter monitoring (24-hour tape) or electrophysiological studies. A cardiac pacemaker or ICD may be recommended (Bhakta *et al.* 2011).
- Endocrine disorder with gonadal atrophy and low testosterone in males, premature menopause in females.
- Mildly elevated LFTs are frequently seen in DM1 (and DM2) and do not need investigation, unless they are continuing to rise or are sufficiently elevated to cause clinical concern (Achiron *et al.* 1998; Heatwole *et al.* 2006). Cholelithiasis and/or cholecystitis commonly occur and at unusually young ages in DM1.
- Somnolence. Excessive daytime sleepiness is typical in any type and severity of DM1 and DM2 but may also be a consequence of nocturnal sleep apnoea (Laberge *et al.* 2013). Consider referral for sleep studies.
- Impaired cognitive processing (including dysexecutive functioning) may be apparent in all types of DM1 but may be more pronounced in earlier-onset disease (Axford and Pearson 2013; Sistiaga *et al.* 2013).

Surveillance
Arrange annual follow-up for all affected individuals, usually with a neuromuscular specialist/neurologist or GP. A standardized pattern of assessment is recommended that includes:
- annual ECG with careful assessment of the PR interval and QRS complex; refer if PR >200 ms, QRS >120 ms, atrial fibrillation/flutter, new development of bundle branch block, or symptomatic;
- specific enquiry for symptoms suggestive of diabetes and investigation, if indicated;
- annual FVC;
- consider TFT, LFT, and testosterone.

Recommend careful preoperative assessment if under-going any procedure requiring general anaesthesia or sedation AND careful post-operative monitoring including pre-symptomatic and minimally affected individuals.

Support groups: Myotonic Dystrophy Support Group (MDSG; UK), http://www. myotonicdystrophysupportgroup.org; Myotonic Dystrophy Foundation (MDF; USA), http://www. myotonic.org.

Expert adviser: Mark T. Rogers, Consultant Clinical Geneticist and Honorary Senior Research Fellow, Institute of Medical Genetics, University Hospital of Wales, Cardiff, UK.

References

Achiron A, Barak Y, Magal N, et al. Abnormal liver test results in myotonic dystrophy. J Clin Gastroenterol 1998; **26**: 292–5.

Axford MM, Pearson CE. Illuminating CNS and cognitive issues in myotonic dystrophy: Workshop report. Neuromuscul Disord 2013; **23**: 370–4.

Bennun M, Goldstein B. Continuous propofol anaesthesia for patients with myotonic dystrophy. Br J Anaesth 2000; **85**: 407–9.

Bhakta D, Shen C, Kron J, Epstein AE, Pascuzzi RM, Groh WJ. Pacemaker and implantable cardioverter-defibrillator use in a US myotonic dystrophy type 1 population. J Cardiovasc Electrophysiol 2011; **22**: 1369–75.

Brunner HG, Nillesen W, van Oost BA, et al. Presymptomatic diagnosis of myotonic dystrophy. J Med Genet 1992; **29**: 780–4.

Buxton J, Shelbourne P, Davies J, et al. Detection of an unstable fragment of DNA specific to individuals with myotonic dystrophy. Nature 1992; **355**: 547–8.

Cobo AM, Poza JJ, Martorell L, et al. Contribution of molecular analysis to the estimation of the risk of congenital myotonic dystrophy. J Med Genet 1995; **32**: 105–8.

de Die-Smulders CE, Howeler CJ. Age and causes of death in adult-onset myotonic dystrophy. Brain 1998; **121**: 1557–63.

Gennarelli M, Novelli G, Andreasi Bassi F, et al. Prediction of myotonic dystrophy clinical severity based on the number of intragenic (CTG)n trinucleotide repeats. Am J Med Genet 1996; **65**: 342–7.

Groh WJ, Groh MR, Shen C, et al. Survival and CTG repeat expansion in adults with myotonic dystrophy type 1. Muscle Nerve 2011; **43**: 648–51.

Harley HG, Rundle SA, Reardon W, et al. Unstable DNA sequence in myotonic dystrophy. Lancet 1992; **339**: 1125–8.

Harper PS. Myotonic dystrophy, 3rd edn, Major problems in Neurology series, No. 37. WB Saunders, Philadelphia, 2001.

Harper PS. Myotonic dystrophy—the facts. Oxford University Press, Oxford, 2002.

Heatwole CR, Miller J, Martens B, Moxley RT 3rd. Laboratory abnormalities in ambulatory patients with myotonic dystrophy type 1. Arch Neurol 2006; **63**: 1149–53.

Kersten HM, Roxburgh RH, Child N, et al. Epiretinal membrane: a treatable cause of visual disability in myotonic dystrophy type 1. J Neurol 2014; **261**: 37–44.

Laberge et al. 2013

Martorell L, Cobo AM, Baiget M, Naudó M, Poza JJ, Parra J. Prenatal diagnosis in myotonic dystrophy type 1. Thirteen years of experience: implications for reproductive counselling in DM1 families. Prenat Diagn 2007; **27**: 68–72.

Martorell L, Monckton DG, Sanchez A, Lopez De Munain A, Baiget M. Frequency and stability of the myotonic dystrophy type 1 premutation. Neurology 2001; **56**: 328–35.

Rogers MT, Clyburn PA. Anaesthesia and myotonic dystrophy. In: PS Harper, B van Engelen, B Eymard, DE Wilcox (eds.). Myotonic dystrophy: present management, future therapy. Oxford University Press, Oxford, 2004.

Sistiaga A, Urreta I, Jodar M, et al. Cognitive/personality pattern and triplet expansion size in adult myotonic dystrophy type 1 (DM1): CTG repeats, cognition and personality in DM1. Psychol Med 2010; **40**: 487–95.

Sistiaga et al. 2013

Verpoest W, De Rademaeker M, Sermon K, et al. Real and expected delivery rates of patients with myotonic dystrophy undergoing intracytoplasmic sperm injection and preimplantation genetic diagnosis. Hum Reprod 2008; **23**: 1654–60.

Verpoest W, Seneca S, De Rademaeker M, et al. The reproductive outcome of female patients with myotonic dystrophy type 1 (DM1) undergoing PGD is not affected by the size of the expanded CTG repeat tract. J Assist Reprod Genet 2010; **27**: 327–33.

Vihola A, Bassez G, Meola G, et al. Histopathological differences of myotonic dystrophy type 1 (DM1) and PROMM/DM2. Neurology 2003; **60**: 1854–7.

Zaki M, Boyd PA, Impey L, Roberts A, Chamberlain P. Congenital myotonic dystrophy: prenatal ultrasound findings and pregnancy outcome. Ultrasound Obstet Gynecol 2007; **29**: 284–8.

Zhang J, George AL Jr, Griggs RC, et al. Mutations in the human skeletal muscle chloride channel gene (CLCN1) associated with dominant and recessive myotonia congenita. Neurology 1996; **47**: 993–8.

Neural tube defects

Includes (1) open neural tube defects (NTDs): anencephaly, craniorachischisis, meningomyelocele (open spina bifida cystica), and myelocele (non-cystic open spina bifida); (2) closed NTDs: encephalocele, iniencephaly, meningocele, and spinal dysraphism.

Open NTDs

Result from failure of closure of part or all of the embryonic neural tube during primary neurulation, which occurs during days 18–26 post-fertilization (see Figure 3.23). Approximately 40% of cases are anencephaly, 50% lumbosacral spina bifida (see Figure 3.24), and 10% other open NTDs, including upper spina bifida and craniorachischisis (totally open neural tube). Females are more often anencephalic than males (3:1 ratio), whereas there is no marked sex ratio distortion in open spina bifida.

- NTD prevalence among live births and TOP varies between countries (e.g. most are TOPs in the UK, but all live born in Ireland). Therefore, both types of pregnancy outcome need to be considered in epidemiological comparisons. Frequency of NTDs among miscarriages is also significant but difficult to measure precisely (Creasy and Alberman 1976). Birth prevalence of NTDs was declining in some locations, even before the introduction of periconceptual folate supplementation. Improved maternal nutrition may have contributed, but widespread introduction of PND has led to the largest birth prevalence reductions.
- Combined live birth and TOP rates average one per 1000 pregnancies, but with variation depending on geographical location and ethnicity. Geographical variations include: 0.94 in Europe, 1.3 in Australia, 2.0 in Peru, 4.5 in China (rates per 1000 live births and TOPs, within the last decade) (Abeywardana et al. 2010; Dolk et al. 2010; Ren et al. 2006; Ricks et al. 2012). In the USA, open spina bifida is most prevalent in pregnancies of Hispanic mothers and least prevalent in those of black mothers; White mothers show intermediate frequencies (Agopian et al. 2012).
- Infants of diabetic mothers (Greene 1999) and of epileptic women who take sodium valproate (Yerby

2003) both have an ~10-fold increase in relative risk of NTD. Increased risk of NTDs (3-fold) is also associated with severe pre-pregnancy maternal obesity (Rasmussen et al. 2008).

- Craniorachischisis is the earliest-arising defect when the neural tube fails to initiate closure, leading to a lethal condition in which most of the brain and the whole spine remain open. *Anencephaly* results from subsequent failure of the cranial neural folds to close (day 18 post–fertilization). The forebrain fails to develop and the defect is lethal. Open spina bifida arises when the low spinal neural folds fail to close towards the end of neurulation (days 24–26 post-fertilization) and is generally non-lethal. Neurological function develops in the fetus with spina bifida, even below the level of lesion, but is lost by the time of birth owing to neurodegeneration (Stiefel et al. 2007). Paralysis and lack of sensation are typical sequelae.
- Disorders associated with open spina bifida include hydrocephalus (>90% of cases) and *Chiari II malformation*. The latter is a downward protrusion of the medulla oblongata through the foramen magnum to overlap the spinal cord (can cause lower cranial nerve palsies and central apnoea). It is present in >70% of cases with meningomyelocele and produces increasing symptoms with age. See 'Cerebellar anomalies' in Chapter 2, 'Clinical approach', p. 92.

Closed NTDs

Are heterogeneous conditions in which the early neural tube is abnormal, but not open to the external environment (i.e. there was no failed neural tube closure). Encephalocele occurs in around one per 10 000 established pregnancies. Spinal dysraphism may be much more common, but prevalence figures are not available owing to the highly variable pathology and age of presentation (young child to adult).

- Encephalocele results from herniation of the closed neural tube through bony defects in the skull. Most common is occipital encephalocele, a component of

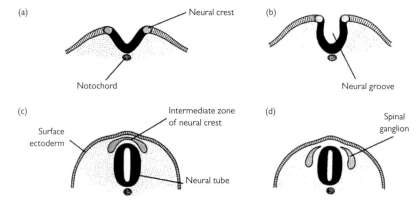

Figure 3.23 Schematic drawing of a number of transverse sections through successively older embryos, showing the formation of the neural folds, neural groove, neutral tube, and neural crest. The cells of the neural crest, initially forming an intermediate zone between the neural tube and surface ectoderm (c), develop into the spinal and cranial sensory ganglia (d).

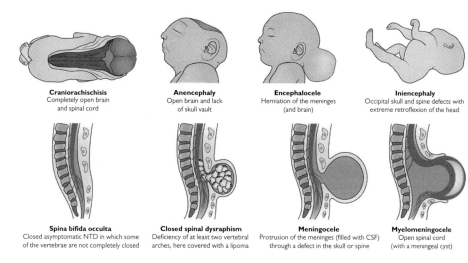

Figure 3.24 Overview of neural tube defects. Schematic representation of several neural tube defects (NTDs). Spina bifida occulta is found in up to 10% of people and usually occurs in the low spinal region. Closed spinal dysraphism has many variants, including lipomyelomeningocele, low-lying conus and thickened filum terminale. CSF, cerebrospinal fluid.
Reprinted by permission from Macmillan Publishers Ltd: *Nature Reviews Disease Primers*, AJ Copp et al., Spina bifida, 1, 15007, copyright 2015, doi:10.1038/nrdp.2015.7.

Meckel syndrome, but also seen non-syndromically. Meninges with/without brain tissue project through an apical defect of the occipital bone, enlarged posterior fontanelle, or high vertebral column defect. Cephaloceles can also be parietal or fronto-ethmoidal, the latter showing high frequencies in oriental populations (Richards 1992). In the spinal region, meningocele probably has a similar pathogenesis, with herniation through a dorsal vertebral defect.

- Iniencephaly is a related severe defect of the cervical spine, including bifid neural arches, with backward flexion of the skull and an extremely short neck. An occipital encephalocele often coexists.
- Spinal dysraphism results from faulty separation of tissue derivatives in the tail bud, the site of secondary neurulation in the caudal-most embryonic region. It often presents as a hairy patch of pigmented or abnormal skin, a subcutaneous mass, a dimple, or a sinus over the lumbosacral spine. Radiology shows failure of fusion of two or more dorsal vertebral arches (usually at L5/S1). Involvement of a single vertebral arch—spina bifida occulta—occurs in 15% of the population (Saluja 1988), is usually asymptomatic, and is detected as a chance radiological finding. It is not thought to confer an increased risk of NTD in offspring.
- A wide range of spinal pathology is included within the 'dysraphism' category, including disorders of the vertebrae (e.g. a midline bony spur), a defective spinal cord (e.g. overdistension of the central canal—hydromyelia), and the presence of ectopic tissues, especially lipoma (as in lipomyelomeningocele). Clinically, tethering of the spinal cord's lower end can be symptomatic, causing lower limb weakness and particularly functional bladder disorders (Lew and Kothbauer 2007). Often associated with anorectal abnormalities, including anal stenosis or atresia.

- Diastematomyelia. A sagittal cleft divides the spinal cord into two halves, each surrounded by its own pia mater. A bony or cartilaginous spur may transfix the cord, fixing it in a low position as the child grows. The cleft is usually in the low thoracic or lumbar region, but cervical clefts have been reported. Often associated with vertebral segmentation defects, open spina bifida, and scoliosis.

Genetics

Syndromic forms occur, particularly encephalocele in Meckel syndrome. NTDs are found as part of several chromosomal disorders (Chen 2007). The majority of open NTDs are sporadic, isolated disorders, occurring at a relatively high frequency and yet rarely present in multi-generational families. This suggests a multifactorial causation, with contribution from environmental (e.g. maternal folate status) and genetic factors. Genetic risk factors have been defined in two main pathways: folate metabolism and planar cell polarity (PCP) signalling. Since these are either rare missense variants or polymorphisms of low relative risk, mutation analysis for NTD-predisposing genes is not routinely used in the clinical setting.

- Folate-related gene polymorphisms have been associated with open NTDs, particularly 5,10-methylene tetrahydrofolate reductase (MTHFR), an essential enzyme of homocysteine remethylation. The C677T and A1298C polymorphisms of MTHFR are associated with ~1.8-fold increased risk of NTDs, a predisposition detected only in non-Hispanic populations (Amorim et al. 2007). Mitochondrial folate metabolic enzymes have also been implicated; the genes encoding enzymes of the glycine cleavage system AMT and GLDC were found to harbour missense variants in NTD cases, but not in unaffected controls (Narisawa et al. 2012).
- The PCP pathway is a non-canonical Wnt signalling cascade required for the initiation of neural tube closure

in mice and other vertebrates. Missense mutations in several genes of the pathway, including *CELSR1* and *VANGL2*, have been detected in NTD cases, but not in unaffected controls (Juriloff and Harris 2012).

Clinical management and prevention

- Post-natal surgical repair of open spina bifida continues to be the mainstay of management for cases that go to term. Insertion of a ventricular shunt to treat associated hydrocephalus is common. Neurological, skeletal, and renal deficits are frequent in post-natal survivors and are treated as appropriate.
- Caesarean section has been advocated, in preference to vaginal delivery, for open spina bifida, as it was claimed to give improved neurological outcome (Luthy et al. 1991), although this has since been questioned (Lewis et al. 2004).
- *In utero* surgical repair is practised in some centres in the USA and was compared with post-natal repair in a randomized controlled clinical trial (Adzick et al. 2011). Fetal surgery led to 50% reduction in shunting for hydrocephalus and significant improvement in spinal neurological function, but a higher rate of premature birth and maternal uterine dehiscence. Long-term outcomes for the child have not been reported.
- PND and TOP have been practised since the 1970s and this is now the most common outcome for open NTDs in the UK and some other countries.
- Primary prevention by folic acid is based on the evidence from a randomized clinical trial in the UK and Hungary that folic acid supplements could prevent 70% of recurrent open NTDs (MRC Vitamin Study Research Group 1991). A subsequent clinical trial showed that a folate-containing multivitamin could also prevent first occurrence of NTDs (Czeizel and Dudás 1992). Most countries now recommend voluntary folic acid supplementation (see below for details of dose level) and some countries have additionally introduced mandatory fortification of staple foods with folic acid. The latter has been associated with variable reductions in NTD prevalence in different geographical regions (Honein et al. 2001; Ricks et al. 2012).

Clinical genetics approach

Most cases involve an isolated NTD, either anencephaly or spina bifida, or both. Care is needed to distinguish between a primary NTD and one that is occurring as a feature of a syndrome, a chromosome anomaly, or a teratogenic exposure. Vertebral anomalies and hydronephrosis are commonly seen as secondary pathology in 'isolated' NTDs.

History: key points

- Three-generation family tree, with enquiry about stillbirths and neonatal deaths.
- Enquiry about diabetes, including gestational, in previous pregnancies.
- Detailed pregnancy history, including enquiry about drug exposure, e.g. anticonvulsants, and pre-conceptual folic acid ingestion.

Examination: key points

- Affected individual. Try to examine the affected individual or obtain a post-mortem report to confirm what type of NTD was present (open or closed?) and whether it was an isolated anomaly. If additional anomalies are found (NB. they occur in >20% of cases), the

possibility of a syndrome or chromosomal anomaly should be revisited. There is an increased incidence of NTDs in association with CHD, diaphragmatic aplasia, and oesophageal atresia.
- Parents or intervening relative. Examine for signs of *spinal dysraphism*, e.g. a hairy patch, pigmented or abnormal skin, a subcutaneous mass, a dimple, or a sinus over the lumbosacral spine associated with failure of fusion of the dorsal vertebral arches (usually at L5/S1), and enquire about bladder control. A spinal cord abnormality may cause asymmetrical lower motor neuron weakness with wasting, diminished reflexes in the lower limb, or spasticity with hyper-reflexia. MRI of the spinal cord indicates if any of these features are present, in which case counsel as if affected by NTD.

Investigations

- If NTD is the only anomaly, karyotyping is not routinely indicated.
- Genomic analysis in presence of features suggestive of a chromosomal or syndromic diagnosis, e.g. genomic array, gene panel, or WES/WGS as available.
- X-ray/MRI if NTD is not adequately defined or if any suspicion of spinal dysraphism in the parent.

Other diagnoses/conditions to consider

Meckel syndrome

Lethal AR syndrome with occipital encephalocele, bilaterally large kidneys with multicystic dysplasia and fibrotic changes of the liver, and PAP. The kidneys are typically filled with thin-walled cysts of various sizes. In Fraser and Lytwyn's study (1981) of 38 secondarily ascertained cases of Meckel syndrome, 100% had cystic dysplasia of the kidney, 63% had an occipital meningocele, 55% had polydactyly, and 18% had no brain malformation. Several genes have now been cloned *MKS1, MKS2 (TMEM216), MKS3 (TMEM67), RPGRIP1L,* and *CEP290,* all of which have a role in ciliary structure and/or function (Logan et al. 2010).

Triploidy

Severe IUGR, syndactyly. See 'Triploidy (69,XXX, 69,XXY, or 69,XYY)' in Chapter 5, 'Chromosomes', p. 694.

Anticonvulsant exposure

Maternal epilepsy and use of sodium valproate, carbamazepine, phenytoin, phenobarbitone, or primidone in the first trimester. Valproate-induced NTDs predominantly affect the lower lumbar and sacral regions. While previously considered as a folate antagonist, valproate is now known to be a potent histone deacetylase inhibitor, and this may be the mechanism of NTD causation (Vassar and Fuchs 1991). Exposure to known folate antagonists (e.g. sulfasalazine, triamterene, or trimethoprim) should also be identified. See 'Fetal anticonvulsant syndrome (FACS)' in Chapter 6, 'Pregnancy and fertility', p. 732.

Genetic advice

Inheritance and recurrence risk

- Anencephaly and spina bifida. See Table 3.31. In non-syndromal NTDs, there is no tendency for the site of the NTD, e.g. anencephaly, high or low spina bifida, to breed true in subsequent affected pregnancies (Drainer et al. 1991).

Table 3.31 Anencephaly and spina bifida: approximate recurrence risks (%) without folate supplementation in relation to population incidence

Relationship of affected individual to 'at-risk' pregnancy	Recurrence risk (%) for population incidence of:		
	0.005	0.002	0.001
One sibling	5	3	2
Two siblings	12	10	10
One second-degree relative	2	1	1
One third-degree relative	1	0.75	0.5
One parent	4	4	4

- Spinal dysraphism. Radiological evidence of two or more absent vertebral arches, with or without symptoms of spinal cord tethering. Currently not clear whether this confers an increased risk of open or closed NTDs. Lipomyelomeningocele has shown no decline in prevalence following the introduction of folic acid fortification (De Wals et al. 2008), suggesting that periconceptual folic acid is likely not protective.

- Spina bifida occulta. Absence of a single vertebral arch as a radiological finding only; in the absence of cutaneous or neurological findings, it is a common variant of normal and not thought to confer an increased risk of NTD to offspring.

Prenatal diagnosis
- USS. Anencephaly is detectable on USS from 11 to 12 weeks' gestation; serial scanning from 16 weeks' gestation is appropriate in high risk pregnancies for detection of spina bifida; large defects may be visible earlier, e.g. from 13 weeks' gestation. Boyd et al. (2000) found the sensitivity of PND by USS in an unselected population to be 98% for anencephaly and 75% for spina bifida. A sensitivity higher than this may be possible when USS is specifically targeted because of increased risk.
- Maternal serum screening for AFP. Serum screening using a cut-off of 2.5 MoM (multiple of the median) at 16 weeks' gestation is a reliable method of screening, with a detection rate for spina bifida of 82% and a false-positive rate of 1.9%. It does not detect closed NTDs (i.e. those covered by intact skin) and is less sensitive in women taking valproate, a known risk factor for NTDs. Hence, AFP screening should be used

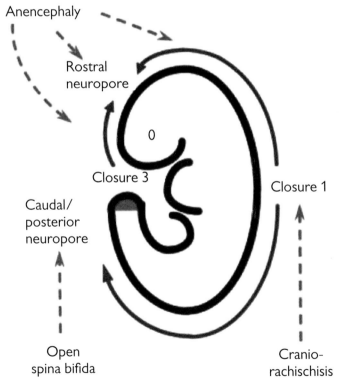

Figure 3.25 Neural tube defects arising from errors in the multisite closure of the neural tube.
Reproduced from AJ Copp et al., Genetics and development of neural tube defects, *Journal of Pathology*, 220, 2, pp. 217–230, Wiley, copyright 2009, Pathological Society of Great Britain and Ireland. Data from Copp AJ, Greene NDE, Murdoch JN. The genetic basis of mammalian neurulation. *Nat Rev Genet* 2003; 4: 784–793; and Greene ND, Copp AJ. Development of the vertebrate central nervous system: formation of the neural tube. *Prenatal Diag* 2009; 29: 303–311.

in conjunction with detailed anomaly USS, especially if monitoring an at-risk pregnancy.

- Amniocentesis. Due to the efficacy of detailed USS in combination with maternal serum screening, amniocentesis is nowadays rarely used for the sole indication of PND of NTD.
- **To prevent first occurrence of NTD**, women who are planning a pregnancy should take 400 µg of folic acid daily from at least 1 month before conception, continuing until the 12th week of pregnancy.
- **To prevent recurrence of NTD**, women who are planning a pregnancy should take 5 mg daily of folic acid from at least 1 month before conception and continuing until the 12th week of pregnancy. High-dose (4 mg) folate prevented ~70% of recurrent NTDs in the MRC randomized clinical trial (MRC Vitamin Study Research Group 1991). No known or suspected adverse effects of folic acid at the proposed 5 mg daily dose have been recorded, and it has no contraindications, though women with epilepsy should have their anticonvulsant treatment reviewed.

Where a recurrence occurs on high-dose folate, reconsider whether there is a syndromal association. It is our practice to continue with high-dose folate supplementation in a subsequent pregnancy, but with little expectation of benefit, and therefore a 10% recurrence risk is appropriate. A clinical trial is currently evaluating whether inositol, a possible adjunct preventive therapy based on animal data, is effective in preventing folate-resistant, recurrent NTDs (Greene et al. 2016).

Other situations where high-dose folate (5 mg/ day) may be appropriate include the following:

- one or other parent has spinal dysraphism with a hairy patch or abnormal skin over a lumbosacral spine with two or more incomplete vertebral arches;
- the mother needs to continue with anticonvulsant therapy during pregnancy or is diabetic or has coeliac disease (or other malabsorption state) or has sickle cell anaemia (BNF 2017);
- affected second-degree relatives, e.g. mother's sib, may be advised to take high-dose folate (5 mg/day) since this should result in an 85% reduction in their absolute risk which is somewhat increased (1–2% versus 0.1–0.5%), compared with the ~36% risk reduction resulting from the standard 400-µg dose.

Long-term outcome

Hunt and Oakeshott (2003) reviewed the outcome of 117 unselected consecutive babies with open spina bifida who had their lesions closed surgically in the immediate neonatal period. Morbidity and mortality were strongly correlated with the level of the sensory deficit, with the best outcome in those with the lowest defects. On review, 35 years later, 54 were still alive of the survivors with a sensory level in infancy below L3, 71% had a CSF shunt, 88% had an IQ of at least 80, 67% were able to walk 50 m, with aids if required, 33% were continent, 58% were living independently and able to drive, and 38% were in open employment.

Support group: SHINE (Spina bifida, Hydrocephalus, Information, Networking, Equality), http://www. shinecharity.org.uk, Tel. 01733 555 988.

Expert adviser: Andrew Copp, Professor of Developmental Neurobiology, University College London, Institute of Child Health, London, UK.

References

Abeywardana S, Bower C, Halliday J, Chan A, Sullivan EA. Prevalence of neural tube defects in Australia prior to mandatory fortification of bread-making flour with folic acid. *Aust N Z J Public Health* 2010; **34**: 351–5.

Adzick NS, Thom EA, Spong CY, et al. A randomized trial of prenatal versus postnatal repair of myelomeningocele. *N Engl J Med* 2011; **364**: 993–1004.

Agopian AJ, Canfield MA, Olney RS, et al. Spina bifida subtypes and sub-phenotypes by maternal race/ethnicity in the National Birth Defects Prevention Study. *Am J Med Genet A* 2012; **158A**: 109–15.

Amorim MR, Lima MA, Castilla EE, Orioli IM. Non-Latin European descent could be a requirement for association of NTDs and MTHFR variant 677C >T: a meta-analysis. *Am J Med Genet A* 2007; **143A**: 1726–32.

Boyd PA, Wellesley DG, De Walle HE, et al. Evaluation of the prenatal diagnosis of neural tube defects by fetal ultrasonographic examination in different centres across Europe. *J Med Screen* 2000; **7**: 169–74.

British National Formulary (BNF) 2017.

Chen CP. Chromosomal abnormalities associated with neural tube defects (I): full aneuploidy. *Taiwan J Obstet Gynecol* 2007; **46**: 325–35.

Copp AJ, Greene NDE. Genetics and development of neural tube defects. *J Pathol* 2010; **220**: 217–30.

Copp AJ, Scott Adzick N, et al. Spina bifida. *Nat Rev Dis Primers* 2015; **1**: 1–18.

Creasy MR, Alberman ED. Congenital malformations of the central nervous system in spontaneous abortions. *J Med Genet* 1976; **13**: 9–16.

Czeizel AE, Dudás I. Prevention of the first occurrence of neural-tube defects by periconceptional vitamin supplementation. *N Engl J Med* 1992; **327**: 1832–5.

De Wals P, Van Allen MI, Lowry RB, et al. Impact of folic acid food fortification on the birth prevalence of lipomyelomeningocele in Canada. *Birth Defects Res A Clin Mol Teratol* 2008; **82**: 106–9.

Dolk H, Loane M, Garne E. The prevalence of congenital anomalies in Europe. *Adv Exp Med Biol* 2010; **686**: 349–64.

Drainer E, May HM, Tolmie JL. Do familial neural tube defects breed true? *J Med Genet* 1991; **28**: 605–8.

Fraser FC, Lytwyn A. Spectrum of anomalies in the Meckel syndrome, or: "Maybe there is a malformation syndrome with at least one constant anomaly". *Am J Med Genet* 1981; **9**: 67–73.

Greene MF. Spontaneous abortions and major malformations in women with diabetes mellitus. *Semin Reprod Endocrinol* 1999; **17**: 127–36.

Greene ND, Leung KY, Gay V, et al. Inositol for the prevention of neural tube defects: a pilot randomised controlled trial. *Br J Nutr* 2016; **115**: 974–83.

Honein MA, Paulozzi LJ, Mathews TJ, Erickson JD, Wong LYC. Impact of folic acid fortification of the US food supply on the occurrence of neural tube defects. *JAMA* 2001; **285**: 2981–6.

Hunt GM, Oakeshott P. Outcome in people with open spina bifida at age 35: prospective community based cohort study. *BMJ* 2003; **326**: 1365–6.

Juriloff DM, Harris MJ. A consideration of the evidence that genetic defects in planar cell polarity contribute to the etiology of human neural tube defects. *Birth Defects Res A Clin Mol Teratol* 2012; **94**: 824–40.

Lew SM, Kothbauer KF. Tethered cord syndrome: an updated review. *Pediatr Neurosurg* 2007; **43**: 236–48.

Lewis D, Tolosa JE, Kaufmann M, Goodman M, Farrell C, Berghella V. Elective cesarean delivery and long-term motor function or ambulation status in infants with meningomyelocele. *Obstet Gynecol* 2004; **103**: 469–73.

Logan CV, Abdel-Hamed Z, Johnson CA. Molecular genetics and pathogenic mechanisms for the severe ciliopathies: insights into neurodevelopment and pathogenesis of neural tube defects. *Mol Neurobiol* 2010; **43**: 12–26.

Luthy DA, Wardinsky T, Shurtleff DB, *et al*. Cesarean section before the onset of labor and subsequent motor function in infants with meningomyelocele diagnosed antenatally. *N Engl J Med* 1991; **324**: 662–6.

MRC Vitamin Study Research Group. Prevention of neural tube defects: results of the Medical Research Council Vitamin Study. *Lancet* 1991; **338**: 131–7.

Narisawa A, Komatsuzaki S, Kikuchi A, *et al*. Mutations in genes encoding the glycine cleavage system predispose to neural tube defects in mice and humans. *Hum Mol Genet* 2012; **21**: 1496–503.

Rasmussen SA, Chu SY, Kim SY, Schmid CH, Lau J. Maternal obesity and risk of neural tube defects: a meta-analysis. *Am J Obstet Gynecol* 2008; **198**: 611–19.

Ren A, Zhang L, Li Z, Hao L, Tian Y, Li Z. Awareness and use of folic acid, and blood folate concentrations among pregnant women in northern China—an area with a high prevalence of neural tube defects. *Reprod Toxicol* 2006; **22**: 431–6.

Richards CG. Frontoethmoidal meningoencephalocele: a common and severe congenital abnormality in South East Asia. *Arch Dis Child* 1992; **67**: 717–19.

Ricks DJ, Rees CA, Osborn KA, *et al*. Peru's national folic acid fortification program and its effect on neural tube defects in Lima. *Rev Panam Salud Publica* 2012; **32**: 391–8.

Saluja PG. The incidence of spina bifida occulta in a historic and modern London population. *J Anat* 1988; **158**: 91–3.

Stiefel D, Copp AJ, Meuli M. Fetal spina bifida: loss of neural function *in utero*. *J Neurosurg* 2007; **106**: 213–21.

Vassar R, Fuchs E. Transgenic mice provide new insights into the role of TGF-alpha during epidermal development and differentiation. *Genes Dev* 1991; **5**: 714–27.

Yerby MS. Management issues for women with epilepsy: neural tube defects and folic acid supplementation. *Neurology* 2003; **61**: S23–6.

Neurofibromatosis type 1 (NF1)

von Recklinghausen disease, MIM (Mendelian Inheritance in Man (database)) number, 162200.

NF1 is an AD disorder, with a birth incidence of one in 2500 and a prevalence of one in 4000. The cardinal features are CALs, neurofibromata, and Lisch nodules in the iris (see Table 3.32). NF1 shows hugely variable expressivity and many of the features of NF1 show age-dependent penetrance.

NF1 is caused by mutations in the *NF1* gene on 17q11.2 that encodes the protein neurofibromin. The *NF1* gene is large, spanning 350 kb of DNA with an mRNA of 11–13 kb and 60 exons. There are three alternatively spliced exons 9a, 23a, and 48a. The mutational spectrum includes nonsense, frameshift, and splice mutations, missense and/or small in-frame deletions, and deletions of the entire *NF1* gene. About 30% of NF1 patients may carry a splice mutation resulting in the production of one or several shortened transcripts (Messiaen et al. 2000). For new mutations, there is a predominance of paternal mutations, but no paternal age effect. About 70% of germline mutations cause truncation of the neurofibromin protein. One of the main functions of the gene is as a guanosine triphosphate (GTP)ase-activating protein (GAP) regulating 'ras' in the cell cycle.

There is a risk of serious complications arising throughout life and regular surveillance is required to try and detect these at an early time when they are potentially treatable.

Clinical approach

History: key points

- Detailed family history, enquiring specifically for other relatives with CALs, lumps, or bumps on their skin and other tumours.
- Previous medical and surgical history (may reveal complications not previously considered to be due to NF1).
- Developmental progress, including schooling difficulties, which are extremely common. Language, reading, visuospatial, neuromotor, and concentration problems are particularly found in NF1.
- Seizures and other neurological symptoms.
- Pain or rapid growth of any soft tissue lesions (indicating possible malignancy).

Examination: key points

- Growth parameters. Height (13% have a height <2 SD), weight, OFC (24% have an OFC >2 SD).
- Skin:
  - CALs. Examine with Woods light if fair-skinned;
  - axillary, neck, or groin freckling (usually appears at 3–5 years of age);
  - most diffuse disfiguring plexiform neurofibromata are apparent within the first 2 years of life, or at least evident by a patch of skin with increased pigmentation;
  - dermal neurofibromata appear from late childhood onwards. They are raised and red purplish in colour and may increase in number and size at puberty and during pregnancy;
  - xanthogranulomata—small, raised yellow lesions often on the forehead that completely disappear in late childhood;
  - some patients with NF1 show a subtle generalized increase in skin pigmentation in comparison with unaffected family members.
- Facial features. Some coarsening of the features, or NS-like features, may be seen (particularly in those with gene deletions).
- Spine. Scoliosis found in 11% and spinal tumours (arrange neurology/neurosurgery opinion and MRI if there are gait abnormalities, spasticity, increased reflexes). If there are no neurological symptoms/signs, consider orthopaedic referral for management of scoliosis.
- If patient <2 years old, check for tibial bowing (pseudarthrosis of the tibia is found in 2%).
- BP. Renal artery stenosis, especially in those under 20 years; at risk for phaeochromocytoma throughout life.
- Heart. Pulmonary stenosis is seen in 1–2% of cases and is associated with non-truncating mutations (Ben-Sachar et al. 2013).

Table 3.32 Diagnostic criteria for NF1 (National Institutes of Health Consensus Development Conference 1988)

Criteria	NF1 patients with this feature (%)*
The patient should have two or more of the following features:	
(1) Six or more café-au-lait spots: • 1.5 cm or larger in post pubertal individuals • 0.5 cm or larger in prepubertal individuals	86.7%
(2) Two or more neurofibromata of any type or one or more plexiform neurofibromata	59.4% (cutaneous neurofibroma)
	45.5% (subcutaneous neurofibroma)
	15.3% (plexiform neurofibroma)
(3) Freckling in the axilla, neck, or groin	83.8% (axillary)
	42.3% (groin)
(4) Optic glioma (tumour in the optic pathway)	
(5) Two or more Lisch nodules (benign iris hamartomas)	63%
(6) Distinctive bony lesion: dysplasia of the sphenoid bone; dysplasia or thinning of the long bone cortex	
(7) First-degree relative with NF1	71.2%

* Data from north-west England register-based study (McGaughran et al. 1999).

Adapted by permission from BMJ Publishing Group Limited, *Journal of Medical Genetics*, Huson et al., A genetic study of von Recklinghausen neurofibromatosis in south east Wales. Guidelines for genetic counselling, volume 26, issue 11, pp. 712–21, Copyright 1989, BMJ Publishing Group Ltd. Data from Mc Gaughran JM et al., A clinical study of neurofibromatosis 1 in north west England. *Journal of Medical Genetics* volume 36, pp 192–6 1999.

- Check visual acuity (VA) in each eye separately and check visual fields (optic pathway gliomas are seen in preschool years; peak incidence is at 4–6 years).
- Precocious puberty (which, if present, is usually found in association with a chiasmal optic glioma).
- Document existing soft tissue lesions carefully, and enquire whether any recent change has been noted.
- Examine the parents for NF1. Do not rely on the patient's own assessment; whereas most adults with full-blown NF1 are aware of this, segmental NF1 is easily missed.

Investigations
- Ophthalmology referral to examine for Lisch nodules (requires slit-lamp). Most authorities recommend annual ophthalmic surveillance for optic glioma in children <6 years old (King et al. 2003). Lisch nodules are not usually present in preschool children.
- Genomic array. Specific dysmorphic facial features, especially hypertelorism, cardiac anomalies, and learning disability, are signs that should lead to the suspicion of a microdeletion at 17q11.2 found in 5% of patients with NF1 (Pasmant et al. 2010). The common 1.4-Mb deletion (type 1 microdeletion) incorporates the *NF1* gene and is caused by unequal homologous recombination of *NF1* repeats; however, some deletion patients have a 1.2-Mb deletion mediated by recombination between *JJAZ1* and its pseudogene (type 2 microdeletion). Kehrer-Sawatski et al. (2004) found a significant frequency of mosaic type 2 microdeletions in sporadic NF1 patients without dysmorphic features or MR and suggest that deletion-sensitive analysis, e.g. FISH or MLPA, should be undertaken in all subjects with NF1 (in whom a mutation is not identified). Recognition is important because of the increased risk of malignant peripheral nerve sheath tumour (MPNST) (de Raedt et al. 2003).
- Molecular DNA analysis. Mutation analysis of *NF1* is available and may be especially helpful in establishing the diagnosis in a borderline patient within a family with a known mutation or in cases with an atypical presentation. It is also necessary for PND or PGD.
- Brain imaging. Some authorities do not advocate routine imaging because of the high frequency of changes of doubtful clinical significance. The main cause of difficulty is the presence of high signal intensity changes, which are predominantly found in the basal ganglia, thalamus, brainstem, and cerebellum. These are called unidentified bright objects (UBOs) or focal abnormal signal intensities (FASI). Imaging, e.g. MRI, is strongly indicated in the presence of:
  - a rapidly expanding head circumference in a baby to exclude aqueduct stenosis;
  - focal neurological signs (the brain and spinal cord need to be considered);
  - epilepsy;
  - visual problems;
  - precocious puberty or failing growth velocity.

Other diagnoses/conditions to consider

In most affected adult individuals, the diagnosis can be made according to the criteria in Table 3.32 and is not in doubt. In most children, the phenotype cannot be distinguished from Legius syndrome.

Legius syndrome This AD condition is characterized by multiple CALs with or without freckling. Other diagnostic NF1 criteria are systematically absent such as Lisch nodules, neurofibromas, optic pathway gliomas, and the typical bone abnormalities of NF1. Legius syndrome is caused by heterozygous mutations in the *SPRED1* gene (Brems et al. 2007) and it is not associated with a tumour predisposition with the exception maybe of a mildly increased risk for acute leukaemia (Pasmant et al. 2015). Some of the children might have learning disabilities and ADHD. The diagnosis can only be made by mutation analysis of the *SPRED1* gene. It is estimated that 2–4% of individuals with a clinical diagnosis of NF1 have Legius syndrome due to a *SPRED1* mutation (Messiaen et al. 2009; Pasmant et al. 2015).

Atypical skin pigmentary changes and unusual disorders of growth can cause diagnostic problems. See 'Patchy pigmented skin lesions (including café-au-lait spots)' in Chapter 2, 'Clinical approach', p. 278 and also 'Lumps and bumps' in Chapter 2, 'Clinical approach', p. 222.

Segmental NF1
Typical skin changes are only found in a segmental distribution. A post-zygotic mutation is the cause (Maertens et al. 2007).

Watson syndrome
CALs, NS-like facies, and pulmonary stenosis. Also due to mutations in neurofibromin, but these usually cause a mutant protein, rather than the truncated protein of NF1.

Neurofibromatosis type 2 (NF2)
This is less common than NF1 but can cause diagnostic confusion. Approximately 43% have a few CALs (with only 4% having >3 spots and none having >6 in Evans's series). NF1-like cutaneous tumours occur in 27%. There is a high incidence of CNS tumours. Spinal neurofibromata seen in NF1 can appear identical to the spinal Schwannomas seen in NF2, both radiologically and at surgery. They are distinct histologically but may need expert review by a neuropathologist for definitive diagnosis. Deafness is a common feature of NF2 due to vestibular Schwannomas but is rare in NF1. See 'Neurofibromatosis type 2 (NF2)' in Chapter 4, 'Cancer', p. 596.

Proteus syndrome
Thickening of the skin on the soles of the feet, macrodactyly, and pigmented skin lesions that look like a linear sebaceous naevus. The lesions are usually asymmetric and may grow rapidly. A specific mosaic mutation in the *AKT1* gene has been reported in affected tissues of Proteus individuals (Marsh et al. 2011).

Recessive mutations in mismatch repair (MMR) genes
Recessive mutations in the MMR genes *PMS2, MLH1, MSH2,* and *MSH6* can cause a phenotype of CALs, axillary freckling, subtle generalized increase in skin pigmentation, PNETs, NHL, and bowel polyps predisposing to bowel cancer. This NF1-like condition has a highly malignant phenotype and follows AR inheritance (Sheridan et al. 2003; Wimmer et al. 2016).

Genetic advice

Counselling the parents of a newly diagnosed child, who is fit and well, but nevertheless is affected with NF1, is challenging. It is necessary to balance the possibility of complications and disfigurement with the equal possibility of a lifetime with few difficulties. Parent support groups with their specialist staff can be a great help to families at this time.

Inheritance and recurrence risk

- Parent affected. The inheritance is AD, with a 50% risk to offspring. The proportion of new mutations is ~50%, although McGaughran et al. (1999) found a lower rate of 28.8% in their register-based study.
- Parents unaffected. If the parents are unaffected (after careful clinical assessment and eye examination) or the proband is known to have a DNM, the recurrence risk is <1%. (Germline mosaicism has been reported by Lazaro et al. (1994) in a clinically normal father who had two affected children and was found to carry an NF1 mutation in 10% of his sperm.) Note the importance of examining the parents for segmental NF1, as a small, but significant, proportion of parents are gonosomal mosaics (see below).
- Parent with segmental NF1. In individuals with mosaic or localized manifestations of NF1 (segmental NF1), disease features are limited to the affected area, which varies from a narrow strip to one quadrant and occasionally to one-half of the body. Distribution is usually unilateral but can be bilateral, either in a symmetrical or asymmetrical arrangement (Ruggieri and Huson 2001). Risks to offspring are generally lower than for parents with non-mosaic NF1, but the exact risk is not definable, varying from <1% to 50%, depending on the degree of gonadal involvement. Animal studies suggest that the risk is proportional to the percentage of body area involved (Ruggieri and Huson 2001). Overall, a figure of 5% may be reasonable.

Variability and penetrance

NF1 is fully penetrant. The frequencies of the most common complications are given in Table 3.33. Many of the features show age-dependent expression (see Table 3.34). NF1 shows highly variable expressivity and it is unwise to predict the manifestations of the condition based on the presence or absence of complications in other family members.

Prenatal diagnosis

Possible by CVS and mutation analysis if the familial mutation is known. Within current UK practice, it is not often requested.

Table 3.33 Frequency of NF1 complications for counselling purposes

Complication	Frequency in NF1 (%)	Risk in NF1	Overall risk in pregnancy in NF1 parent
Intellectual handicap[*]	33.0	1 in 3	1 in 6
Moderate to severe retardation	3.2		
Mild to moderate learning difficulties	29.8		
Developing in childhood with lifelong morbidity	8.5	1 in 12	1 in 24
Severe plexiform neurofibromata of head and neck	1.2		
Scoliosis requiring surgery	5.2		
Severe pseudoarthrosis	2.1 (1.9)		
Treatable complications that can develop	15.7	1 in 6	1 in 12
Aqueduct stenosis	2.1		
Epilepsy	4.2 (4.3)		
Spinal neurofibromata	2.1 (2.1)		
Visceral neurofibromata	2.1		
Endocrine tumours (e.g. phaeochromocytoma)	3.1		
Renal artery stenosis	2.1		
Glomus tumours of the digits	5		
Gastrointestinal stromal tumours	5		
CNS and malignant tumours	4.4–5.2 (9.4)	1 in 20	1 in 40
Optic gliomas	0.7		
Symptomatic	4.5		
Asymptomatic	0.7–1.5		
Other CNS tumours	1.5		
Rhabdomyosarcoma	1.5[**] (8–13)		
Peripheral nerve malignancy			
Breast cancer		Women with NF1 have a 2- to 3-fold increased lifetime risk over population levels with a 4- to 5-fold risk <50 years	

[*] McGaughran et al. (1999) found that learning difficulties of varying severity occurred in 62%.

[**] The median age at diagnosis for malignant peripheral nerve sheath tumours is 26 years.

Adapted by permission from BMJ Publishing Group Ltd.: *Journal of Medical Genetics*, Huson et al, A genetic study of von Recklinghausen neurofibromatosis in south east Wales II. Guidelines for genetic counselling, vol 26, issue 11, 712–21, copyright 1989; and *Journal of Medical Genetics*, McGaughran et al, A clinical study of neurofibromatosis 1 in north west England, vol 36, issue 3, 192–6, copyright 1999.

Table 3.34 Features and complications of NF1 showing age-dependent expression

Feature	Age
Café-au-lait patches	Infancy through childhood; most have six or more patches by 2 years
Sphenoid wing dysplasia	Infancy <2 years
Pseudoarthrosis	Infancy <2 years
Plexiform neurofibroma	Most disfiguring plexiform neurofibromata are evident by 2 years of age
Lisch nodules	Not usually present at birth, 50% by 5 years, 75% by 15 years, 90% by 25 years
Optic glioma	Usually arise in toddler and early childhood years <6 years
Axillary and groin freckling	Childhood
Dermal neurofibromata	Adolescence through adulthood, especially during puberty and pregnancy
Nerve sheath tumours	Adolescence through adulthood

Predictive testing
Clinical examination of at-risk individuals. The children of affected individuals are seen annually if there are no signs to 2 years and then checked once more at 5 years. Genetic testing is possible if the familial mutation is known.

Other family members
Clinical evaluation should be offered, together with mutation testing if the familial mutation is known.

Natural history and management
Potential long-term complications
In the UK the median life expectancy is 70.4 for males and 74 for females with NF1 (Wilding 2012). This reduction is almost entirely due to malignant soft tissue tumours. Some complications present at different ages and this can be useful for reassurance.

- Optic nerve pathway tumours tend to arise in the toddler or early childhood years. Approximately 15% of individuals with NF1 have thickening of the optic nerve tracts visible on MRI scan (Gutmann 2017). A much smaller proportion of these become symptomatic, but all merit careful surveillance. Clinical progression following presentation occurs in less than one-third of patients. Symptoms include loss of VA, decreased field of vision, proptosis, agitation, and behavioural changes, with signs including optic nerve pallor, sometimes with fullness of the optic disc. Most follow a benign course, even when symptomatic. However, a small number impinge on the optic nerves, causing irreversible blindness and, if involving the optic chiasm, can lead to precocious puberty. Tubular expansion of the optic nerves, often with lengthening and kinking, and extension to include the chiasm are highly characteristic of NF1 optic pathway gliomas (OPG). The period for highest risk for the development of OPG in NF1 is the first 6 years of life.
- Xanthogranuloma and juvenile myelomonocytic leukaemia (JMML). An association has been noted between juvenile xanthogranuloma and JMML and >25

cases are recorded in the literature (Morier et al. 1990). Juvenile xanthogranulomas are frequent in young children with NF1 and if there is an increased risk for JMML, it must be very small and does not require screening for leukaemia (Burgdorf and Zelger 2004).
- MPNST. Median age at diagnosis in NF1 patients is 26 years, compared with 62 years in sporadic tumours (Evans et al. 2002). Lifetime risk for peripheral nerve malignancy is 10–15% (Evans 2002; Uustalo 2016). Some originate in existing superficial plexiform tumours, but most arise in deep-seated plexiform neurofibromas, e.g. brachial plexus or sciatic nerve. Almost all MPNSTs present with pain or rapid growth. Any NF1 patient with these symptoms should have rapid access to specialist advice and imaging (MRI and positron emission tomography (PET) scan). Risk may be increased after radiotherapy, so radiation treatment should only be used in NF1 patients when absolutely necessary.
- Breast cancer. Women with NF1 have a 2- to 3-fold increased lifetime risk over population levels, with a 4- to 5-fold risk <50 years.

Surveillance
Arrange follow-up according to the needs of your patient and their family. Options include the following.
- Routine annual follow-up for children with no ongoing problems with a paediatrician:
  - general symptom enquiry;
  - development, behaviour, and schooling;
  - growth parameters (height, weight, OFC) and BP;
  - skin;
  - spine (check for scoliosis);
  - vision (check VA in each eye and check visual fields).
- Routine annual follow-up for adults with no ongoing problems with a GP and with access to specialist NF care:
  - general symptom enquiry;
  - BP;
  - review of the skin;
  - reinforce genetic advice as appropriate.
- Surveillance by a clinical geneticist for patients with ongoing genetic investigations, e.g. workup for possible prenatal testing or features that require surveillance by a doctor with experience of NF1.
- Specialist NF clinic for patients with ongoing surgical or complex medical management or diagnostic issues.
  NB. In addition, all children with NF1 should have annual ophthalmological examinations during the first 6 years of life (King et al. 2003).

Support groups: The Neuro Foundation (UK), http://www.nfauk.org; Children's Tumor Foundation, Ending NF Through Research (USA), http://www.ctf.org; for other countries, Orphanet, http://www.orpha.net/consor/cgi-bin/SupportGroup.php?lng=EN.

Expert adviser: Eric Legius, Clinical Geneticist, Centre for Human Genetics, University Hospital Leuven, Leuven, Belgium.

References
Ben-Shachar S, Constantini S, Hallevi H, et al. Increased rate of missense/in-frame mutations in individuals with NF1-related

pulmonary stenosis: a novel genotype-phenotype correlation. *Eur J Hum Genet* 2013; **21**: 535–9.

Brems H, Chmara M, Sahbatou M, et al. Germline loss-of-function mutations in *SPRED1* cause a neurofibromatosis 1-like phenotype. *Nat Genet* 2007; **39**: 1120–6.

Burgdorf WH, Zelger B. JXG, NF1, and JMML: alphabet soup or a clinical issue? *Pediatr Dermatol* 2004; **21**: 174–6.

De Raedt T, Brems H, Wolkenstein P, et al. Elevated risk for MPNST in NFI microdeletion patients. *Am J Hum Genet* 2003; **72**: 1288–92.

Evans DG, Baser ME, McGaughran J, Sharif S, Howard E, Moran A. Malignant peripheral nerve sheath tumours in neurofibromatosis 1. *J Med Genet* 2002; **39**: 311–14.

Ferner RE. The neurofibromatoses. *Pract Neurol* 2010; **10**: 82–93.

Friedman JM, Gutmann DH, MacCollin M, Riccardi VM. *Neurofibromatosis: phenotype, natural history, and pathogenesis*, 3rd edn. Johns Hopkins University Press, Baltimore, 1998.

Gutmann DH, Ferner RF, et al. Neurofibromatosis type 1. *Nat Rev Dis Primers* 2017; **3**: 17004.

Huson SM, Compston DAS, Harper PS. A genetic study of von Recklinghausen neurofibromatosis in south east Wales II. Guidelines for genetic counselling. *J Med Genet* 1989; **26**: 712–21.

Kehrer-Sawatski H, Kluwe L, Sandig C, et al. High frequency of mosaicism among patients with neurofibromatosis type 1 (NF1) microdeletions caused by somatic recombination of the *JJAZ1* gene. *Am J Hum Genet* 2004; **75**: 410–23.

Kehrer-Sawatzki H, Vogt J, Mußotter T, Kluwe L, Cooper DN, Mautner VF. Dissecting the clinical phenotype associated with mosaic type-2 NF1 microdeletions. *Neurogenetics* 2012; **13**: 229–36.

King A, Listernick R, Charrow J, Piersall L, Gutmann DH. Optic pathway gliomas in neurofibromatosis type 1: the effect of presenting symptoms on outcome. *Am J Med Genet A* 2003; **122A**: 95–9.

Lazaro C, Ravella A, Gaona A, Volpini V, Estivill X. Neurofibromatosis type 1 due to germ-line mosaicism in a clinically normal father. *N Engl J Med* 1994; **331**: 1403–7.

Maertens O, De Schepper S, Vandesompele J, et al. Molecular dissection of isolated disease features in mosaic neurofibromatosis type 1. *Am J Hum Genet* 2007; **81**: 243–51.

Marsh DJ, Trahair TN, Kirk EP. Mutant *AKT1* in Proteus syndrome. *N Engl J Med* 2011; **365**: 2141–2.

McGaughran JM, Harris DI, Donnai D, et al. A clinical study of neurofibromatosis 1 in north west England. *J Med Genet* 1999; **36**: 197–203.

Messiaen LM, Callens T, Mortier G, et al. Exhaustive mutation analysis of the *NF1* gene allows identification of 95% of mutations and reveals a high frequency of unusual splicing defects. *Hum Mutat* 2000; **15**: 541–55.

Messiaen L, Yao S, Brems H, et al. Clinical and mutational spectrum of neurofibromatosis type 1-like syndrome. *JAMA* 2009; **302**: 2111–18.

Morier P, Mérot Y, Paccaud D, Beck D, Frenk E. Juvenile chronic granulocytic leukemia, juvenile xanthogranulomas, and neurofibromatosis. Case report and review of the literature. *J Am Acad Dermatol* 1990; **22**(5 Pt 2): 962–5.

National Institutes of Health Consensus Development Conference. Neurofibromatosis. Conference statement. *Arch Neurol* 1988; **45**: 575–8.

Pasmant E, Sabbagh A, Spurlock G, et al.; members of the NF France Network. NF1 microdeletions in neurofibromatosis type 1: from genotype to phenotype. *Hum Mutat* 2010; **31**: E1506–18.

Pasmant E, Gilbert-Dussardier B, et al. SPRED1, a RAS MAPK pathway inhibitor that causes Legius syndrome, is a tumour suppressor downregulated in paediatric acute myeloblastic leukaemia. *Oncogene* 2015; **34**: 631–8.

Rasmussen SA, Colman SD, Ho VT, et al. Constitutional and mosaic large NF1 gene deletions in neurofibromatosis type 1. *J Med Genet* 1998; **35**: 468–71.

Rasmussen SA, Yang Q, Friedman JM. Mortality in NF1: an analysis using US death certificates. *Am J Hum Genet* 2001; **68**: 1110–18.

Ruggieri M, Huson SM. The clinical and diagnostic implications of mosaicism in the neurofibromatosis. *Neurology* 2001; **56**: 1433–43.

Seminars in Medical Genetics. Neurofibromatosis 1. *Am J Med Genet* 1999; **89C** (Issue 1).

Sheridan E, De Vos M, Hayward B, et al. Recessive mutations in MMR genes are a cause of an NF-1 like phenotype with a highly malignant phenotype and a high recurrence risk. *J Med Genet* 2003; **40**(suppl): S22.

Szudek J, Birch P. Growth in North American white children with NF1. *J Med Genet* 2000; **37**: 933–5.

Uusitalo, E et al. Distinctive cancer associations in patients with neurofibromatosis type 1. *J Clin Oncol* 2016; **34**: 1978–86.

Wilding A, Ingham SL, Lalloo F, et al. Life expectancy in hereditary cancer predisposing diseases: an observational study. *J Med Genet* 2012; **49**: 264–69.

Wimmer K, Rosenbaum T, Messiaen L. Connections between constitutional mismatch repair deficiency syndrome and neurofibromatosis type 1. *Clin Genet* 2016; doi: 10.1111/cge.12904. [Epub Oct 26]

Noonan syndrome and the Ras/MAPK pathway syndromes: neuro-cardio-facial-cutaneous syndromes

Noonan syndrome (NS), cardiofaciocutaneous (CFC) syndrome, LEOPARD syndrome (LS), and Costello syndrome.

These conditions are members of a family of syndromes, with overlapping features, caused by mutations in genes that code for proteins in the Ras/MAPK pathway (see Table 3.35). The mutations lead to activation of the signalling pathway. There have been a number of studies which have given useful clinical information regarding prognosis and surveillance, which are particularly helpful when counselling the parents of newly diagnosed infants, but there is difficulty in the prediction of developmental delay and the severity of cardiac involvement.

Some of the variants seen as germline activating mutations in this group of disorders are encountered as somatic mutations in cancer.

Noonan syndrome (NS)

A relatively common AD disorder affecting ~1/2500 people. It may also occur 'de novo' as a new mutation, but caution is necessary in ascribing unaffected status to a parent, as the typical facial features in childhood become more subtle with time. A family history is reported in 50% of cases. Many individuals with NS probably remain undiagnosed; it is not uncommon to diagnose several members of a family with the condition once a diagnosis is made in the proband. The *PTPN11*, also known as *SHP2*, gene encoding the non-receptor protein tyrosine phosphatase SHP-2 (see Figure 3.26) was the first gene identified. The vast majority of *PTPN11* mutations are located in five of the 15 exons—all are missense.

Fifty to 80% have a cardiac defect and the most common defect is pulmonary stenosis. ASD, VSD, branch pulmonary artery stenosis, tetralogy of Fallot, and coarctation of the aorta are other common structural defects. HCM may occur in 20% and may present at birth, in infancy, or in childhood.

LEOPARD

A very variable AD condition characterized by Lentigines, Ocular hypertelorism, Pulmonary stenosis, Abnormalities of genitalia, Retardation of growth, and Deafness (sensorineural). The lentigines are small (<5 mm) numerous dark brown spots mainly over the face and trunk, and patients commonly present with a provisional diagnosis of NF1. Deafness is variable, ranging from normal to severe. Biventricular obstructive HCM is associated with exon 13 mutations in *PTPN11* (see Table 3.35).

Cardiofaciocutaneous (CFC) syndrome

Is characterized by congenital heart defects, a Noonan-like facial appearance, short stature, ectodermal and GI abnormalities, and MR. Polyhydramnios, fetal oedema, and chylothorax are features. Severe feeding difficulties with postnatal failure to thrive. The hair is typically sparse and curly, and the skin rough and red with keratosis pilaris. The majority of reported cases are sporadic. Mutations found in *MEK1/2, BRAF, KRAS* (see Table 3.35).

Costello syndrome

These infants will present soon after birth and usually there is a history of high birthweight, polyhydramnios, and sometimes prenatally identified CM. Severe feeding difficulties in infancy and Noonan-like features. Hypoglycaemia is common. They develop papillomas around the nose and mouth, and 20% have HCM and others may have a structural defect and chaotic rhythms. The observation that these children were at increased

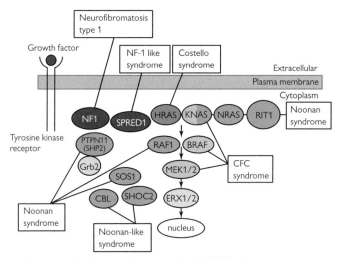

Figure 3.26 Diagram to show genetic disorders caused by genes in the Ras/MAPK pathway.
Reprinted from *American Journal of Human Genetics*, Volume 93, Issue 1, Yoko Aoki, Tetsuya Niihori, Toshihiro Banjo et al., Gain-of-Function Mutations in RIT1 Cause Noonan Syndrome, a RAS/MAPK Pathway Syndrome, pp. 173–180, Copyright 2013, with permission from Elsevier.

Table 3.35 Phenotype associated with some of the Ras/MAPK genes

	LEOPARD syndrome	Noonan syndrome (NS)	Cardiofaciocutaneous (CFC) syndrome	Costello syndrome
PTPN11 Developmental gene and oncogene (juvenile myelomonocytic leukaemia (JMML)) LEOPARD syndrome (LS). Dominant negative effect, i.e. different mode of action than NS mutations	85% mutations in exons 7, 12, or 13. Exon 13 mutations associated with severe biventricular obstructive HCM	Mutations promote active conformation of the protein and hyperactive Ras signalling 50–70% of NS 'Typical' NS phenotype		
RAF1 Missense, gain of function	~10%	NS phenotype HOCM		
SOS1 Missense activating mutation, gain-of-function mutations		NS phenotype Less impairment of growth and development, but ectodermal features of CFC		
SHOC2 Missense and activating S2G mutation		NS with loose anagen hair		
MEK1/2 Missense mutations with some activating action			15% Coagulation defects and lymphoedema not present Relative macrocephaly, pectus deformity, and keratosis pilaris more common than with *BRAF* mutation Most (~90%) have MR	
BRAF Oncogene Mostly missense mutations			70% Severe MR, congenital heart defects, sparse curly hair, optic nerve anomalies, and feeding problems more likely than with *MEK1/2*	
KRAS NS/CFC caused by gain-of-function mutations not found in human cancers (activating mutations in *KRAS* lead to oncogenesis)		Broadest spectrum of clinical features (but only about 5% of NS patients)	Most have CFC phenotypes, significant risk of MR	
HRAS Activating mutations that are also often found somatically mutated in human cancers				Diagnostic for Costello syndrome, usually p.G12 or p.G13 mutation

risk of malignancy helped identify candidate genes. The p.G12 or p.G13 mutation in *HRAS* is diagnostic for Costello syndrome. Most are de novo and there is an increased paternal age association.

Clinical approach

History: key points
- Three-generation family tree, with specific enquiry regarding short stature, congenital heart disease, and learning difficulty.
- Detailed pregnancy history, with specific enquiry for exposure to alcohol and anticonvulsants (phenotypic overlap with some of the dysmorphic features) and

for nuchal thickening/cystic hygroma, pleural effusion, or polyhydramnios. Birthweight usually normal or increased because of oedema.
- Was there failure to thrive or poor feeding in infancy?
- Detailed developmental history (for NS, developmental milestones may be delayed, e.g. sitting at 10/12, walking at 21/12, simple two-word phrases at 31/12; Allanson 2010). LS, often developmentally normal. CFC and Costello syndrome, moderate/severe ID.
- Schooling.
- History of easy bruising or prolonged bleeding after venepuncture, tooth extraction, and surgery.

Examination: key points
- Growth parameters: height (mean height follows 3rd centile until puberty), weight, OFC (usually disproportionately larger than height centile).
- Face. The typical NS face is of a tall forehead, hypertelorism, low-set posteriorly rotated ears with a thickened helix, a short upturned nose, a deeply grooved philtrum with high, wide peaks to the vermilion border of the upper lip, and a small pointed chin. Overall the features may appear coarse, particularly in infancy and childhood.
- Eyes: heavy eyelids or ptosis, epicanthic folds, irides often pale.
- Low posterior hairline and a short neck with redundant skin/webbing.
- Hair.
- Chest: wide-spaced nipples, prominence of the sternum superiorly and depression inferiorly.
- Heart. Structural cardiac defects, particularly pulmonary stenosis and ASD, HCM.
- In males, examine for cryptorchidism (60%).
- Hypotonia and joint hyperextensibility are common in infancy and childhood.
- Skin: lentigines (LEOPARD syndrome). Check carefully for CALs; there is phenotypic overlap with NF1 and it is important not to miss this diagnosis. Dry, eczema, keratosis pilaris.

Investigations
- Genomic array in all sporadic females (phenotypic overlap with 45,X, particularly with NS) and all patients with developmental delay.
- Mutation analysis by gene panel/WES/WGS as appropriate. Give the laboratory plenty of clinical information to ensure correct genes analysed.
- Echo and ECG—if not already done.
- PT, APTT, platelet count—thrombocytopenia, platelet dysfunction, and varied coagulation factor defects (factors V, VIII, XI, and XII, and protein C) may occur alone or in combination in ~50% of patients with NS.
- Eye exam.

Other diagnoses/conditions to consider

Neurofibromatosis (NF1)
The *NF1* and *SPRED1* genes are also part of the Ras/MAPK pathway, so solving the puzzle of why children with NF1/Watson syndrome have similar facial and skin features.

Williams syndrome
Microdeletion on 7q11.23 which encompasses the elastin gene (*ELN*). CHD occurs in 80%; 75% have supravalvular aortic stenosis (SVAS); ~25% have a discrete supravalvular pulmonary stenosis. See 'Congenital heart disease' in Chapter 2, 'Clinical approach', p. 112.

Genetic advice

Inheritance and recurrence risk
NS AD. If one of the parents is affected, a 50% offspring risk is appropriate. If a *PTPN11* mutation is identified and this is not present in either parent, the sibling recurrence risk will be low (small theoretical risk of gonadal mosaicism). Where mutation analysis is not available and the NS appears 'de novo' and both parents have only possible or no signs of NS, an empiric recurrence risk of 5% is appropriate (Sharland et al. 1993).

Parental evaluation should include:
- clinical examination;
- assessment of childhood photographs;
- mutation analysis;
- refer to a cardiologist for clinical evaluation. Echo and ECG.

Variability and penetrance
Features change with age.

Prenatal diagnosis
Monitor for nuchal oedema and polyhydramnios. Pulmonary stenosis is difficult to detect by fetal echo. Lymphatic abnormality with increased nuchal oedema is more common in *PTPN11*. PND possible by CVS or amniocentesis if the familial mutation has been defined.

Natural history and management

Surveillance
- Heart. Specialist cardiological follow-up if a heart defect is identified.
- Growth. Short stature is a very common manifestation of NS and is accompanied by a variable delay in bone age. Bone age is often delayed by ~2 years. If height is <0.4th to 2nd centile, refer to a paediatric growth specialist for further management. Mild delay of puberty is common in both males and females, with a mean age of menarche of 14.5 years. Mean final adult height for males is 162.5 cm (2nd centile) and for females 151 cm (2nd centile). NS found in over half of the females and nearly 40% of males had an adult height below the 3rd percentile. Some centres may consider GH therapy in children with NS.
- Fertility. Normal in females, but may be reduced in males who have had cryptorchidism.
- Hearing. Approximately 30% have chronic serous otitis media in infancy and childhood—increased parental awareness for hearing impairment and low threshold for referral to ENT are appropriate.
- Vision. Over 50% have strabismus and/or a refractive error, so orthoptic referral is appropriate in children at the time of diagnosis.
- Bleeding. Two-thirds of individuals with NS give a history of abnormal bleeding or mild to severe bruising. The coagulopathy is variable and may be subclinical and cause easy bruising or severe surgical haemorrhage.
- Development and education. Early milestones may be delayed (see 'History: key points' above). IQ usually falls in the normal range and most are educated in normal school, but 10–15% require special education. Mild MR is seen in less than one-third (Allanson 2010). Verbal IQ is frequently lower than non-verbal IQ.

Support group: Noonan Syndrome Association, http://www.noonansyndrome.org.uk.

Expert adviser: Michael A. Patton, Emeritus Consultant Clinical Geneticist and Head of the Human Genetics Research Centre, Department of Medical Genetics, St Georges University of London, London, UK.

References
Allanson JE. Noonan syndrome. In: SB Cassidy, JE Allanson (eds.). *Management of genetic syndromes*, 3rd edn, pp. 569–86. John Wiley & Sons, Inc., Hoboken, 2010.

Allanson JE, Hall JG, Van Allen MI. Noonan syndrome: the changing phenotype. *Am J Med Genet* 1985; **21**: 507–14.

Kavamura MI, Pomponi MG, Zollino M, *et al*. *PTPN11* mutations are not responsible for the cardiofaciocutaneous (CFC) syndrome. *Eur J Hum Genet* 2002; **11**: 64–8.

Kelnar CJ. Growth hormone therapy in Noonan syndrome. *Horm Res* 2000; **53**(Suppl 1): 77–81.

Noonan JA, Raaijmakers R, Hall B. Adult height in Noonan syndrome. *Am J Med Genet A* 2003; **123A**: 68–71.

Roberts AE, Araki T, Swanson KD, *et al*. Germline gain-of-function mutations in *SOS1* cause Noonan syndrome. *Nat Genet* 2007; **39**: 70–4.

Schubbert S, Zenker M, Rowe SL, *et al*. Germline *KRAS* mutations cause Noonan syndrome. *Nat Genet* 2006; **38**: 331–6.

Sharland M, Morgan M, Smith G, Burch M, Patton MA. Genetic counselling in Noonan syndrome. *Am J Med Genet* 1993; **45**: 437–40.

Tartaglia M, Mehler EL, Goldberg R, *et al*. Mutations in *PTPN11* encoding the protein tyrosine phosphatase SHP-2 cause Noonan syndrome. *Nat Genet* 2001; **29**: 465–8.

Tartaglia M, Pennacchio LA, Zhao C, *et al*. Gain-of-function *SOS1* mutations cause a distinctive form of Noonan syndrome. *Nat Genet* 2007; **39**: 75–9.

Parkinson's disease

Parkinson's disease is a neurodegenerative disease characterized by tremor, slowness of movement and difficulty initiating movement, rigidity, and poor postural reflexes, affecting 3% of those >75 years of age. This disturbance of motor function is due to the loss of neurons in the substantia nigra and elsewhere, in association with the presence of Lewy bodies (ubiquitinated cytoplasmic protein deposits containing aggregates of α-synuclein) and thread-like proteinaceous inclusions within neurites, also containing α-synuclein (Lewy neurites). It is the second most common neurodegenerative condition after Alzheimer's disease, with a prevalence of 0.5–1% at age 65–69 years and 3% among persons of 75 years and older.

Most cases are sporadic, but there are occasional families with dominant or recessive inheritance. There are few patients with clear Mendelian inheritance, compared with the number of sporadic cases. Typically, Parkinson's disease is a multifactorial neurodegenerative disease caused by an interplay of genetic susceptibility and environmental exposure. Recent research focussed on inherited forms of the disease has delineated a sequence of pathological events whereby deficits in synaptic exocytosis and endocytosis, endosomal trafficking, lysosome-mediated autophagy, and mitochondrial maintenance increase susceptibility to Parkinson's disease (Trinh and Farrer 2013).

Late-onset Parkinson's disease, the most usual form of the disease, does appear to have a familial component. MZ twins with early-onset disease have a very high rate of concordance (much higher than for DZ twins), suggesting a significant genetic component, at least in early-onset disease. Payami et al. (2002) investigated familial aggregation of early- and late-onset Parkinson's disease and found that, compared with controls, the age-specific risk of Parkinson's disease was increased 7.75-fold in the relatives of patients with early-onset disease and nearly 3-fold in the relatives of those with late-onset disease. Kurz et al. (2003), in a Norwegian community-based study, found a 3- to 4-fold increased risk for Parkinson's disease in the families of patients with the disease. Current models favour a rare major Mendelian gene with incomplete and age-dependent penetrance (Maher and Currie 2002).

Nine genetic loci have been reported in the Mendelian forms (PARK1–8 and PARK-10). Rare genetic mutations in the α-synuclein gene (SNCA) result in the aberrant accumulation of this protein, causing toxic gain of function, leading to the development of Parkinson's disease. Singleton et al. (2003) reported a kindred with a triplication of the α-synuclein gene. Additionally over 20 common variants with small effect sizes are now recognized to modulate the risk for PD (Hernadez 2016).

The very rare condition AR juvenile Parkinson's disease may be caused by mutations in parkin (Lucking et al. 2000). Subsequently, heterozygous mutations in parkin have been reported in some apparently sporadic cases of Parkinson's disease, with onset under 60 years (Lucking et al. 2000), and in AD familial Parkinson's disease (Kobayashi et al. 2003). See Table 3.36 for some monogenic causes of Parkinson's disease.

Clinical approach

History: key points
- Three-generation family tree, with careful enquiry about who in the family is/was affected and the age at onset of symptoms, treatment given, and age and cause of death.
- Does the consultand have any symptoms of Parkinson's disease? If so, refer to a neurologist for evaluation.
- Other neurological features in the affected individual or other family members—especially dementia, but also dystonia, ataxia, non-specific tremor, and response to L-dopa (DRD) can present as AD parkinsonism.

Examination: key points
Observe for resting tremor and bradykinesia and other neurological features. If present, refer to a neurologist for evaluation.

Investigations
- Consider storing a DNA sample from an affected member of the family. Mutations in α-synuclein appear to be very rare. Consider next-generation sequencing panel testing/WES/WGS (if available) in familial or early-onset forms of the disease.
- Post-mortem reports are very helpful as the diagnosis is not always accurate in life.

Other diagnoses/conditions to consider

Parkinsonism may be post-encephalitic, drug-induced (antipsychotic agents), or arteriosclerotic and these may all cause confusion with the idiopathic or familial forms of Parkinson's disease. HD in previous generations is not infrequently mistaken for Parkinson's disease.

AD Parkinson's disease
See below.

Tauopathies, e.g. frontotemporal dementia with parkinsonism (including Pick disease)
The second most common presenile dementia after Alzheimer's disease. Mutation in tau gene, AD. See 'Dementia—early onset and familial forms' in Chapter 3, 'Common consultations', p. 386.

Lewy body dementia
One of the three most common causes of dementia in older people (with Alzheimer's disease and vascular dementia). Clinical presentation is typically with fluctuating cognitive impairment, visuospatial dysfunction, marked attentional deficits, psychiatric symptoms (especially complex visual hallucinations), and mild extrapyramidal features (Wilcock 2003).

Fragile X tremor ataxia syndrome (FXTAS)
This is a late-onset disorder characterized by ataxia, dementia, and parkinsonian features that occurs in a substantial proportion of male carriers of a fragile X premutation. See 'Fragile X syndrome (FRAX)' in Chapter 3, 'Common consultations', p. 424.

Gaucher's disease
Carriers for Gaucher's disease due to mutations in GBA (glucocerebrosidase) have a significantly increased risk of developing Parkinson's disease (Beavan and Schapira 2013).

Dopa-responsive dystonia (DRD; Segawa syndrome)
This is a rare condition (prevalence of 0.5–1.0 per million), but important to recognize as it is treatable. Onset is usually in childhood/adolescence and dystonia is the presenting feature. Parkinsonism may also occur. Reflexes may become brisk with extensor plantars. The phenotype in childhood may resemble athetoid cerebral palsy and all children with this condition should have a trial of L-dopa.

Table 3.36 Some monogenic causes of parkinsonism occurring worldwide

| Gene | Inheritance | Disease* | Clinical description | | | | | |
			Dementia	Asymmetry	Resting tremor	Response to L-dopa	Other	Pathology
PARK1 (SNCA)	AD	PD plus DLB* (A53T)	++ (+/no)	+++	+++	+++	Onset typically <45 years	PD plus for DLB A53T
PARK2 (parkin)	Mainly AR, some pseudodominant	PD, dystonia	No	+/no	+/no	+++	Foot dystonia, sleep benefit; insidious course	Nigral cell loss, no Lewy bodies
FTDP17 (tau)	AD	Frontotemporal dementia with parkinsonism	+++	No	No	No	Disinhibition, especially early	Neurofibrillary tangles

* DLB, Lewy body dementia; PD, Parkinson's disease.

Reprinted from *The Lancet Neurology*, vol 2, issue 4, Hardy *et al*, Genes and parkinsonism, pp. 222–8, copyright 2003, with permission from Elsevier.

Inheritance is usually AD with reduced penetrance. The *GCH1* gene codes for an enzyme in the tetrahydrobiopterin pathway. An AR type is due to mutation in the tyrosine hydroxylase gene.

Spinocerebellar ataxia (SCA2 and SCA3)
SCA patients present with gait ataxia that is slowly progressive. See 'Ataxic adult' in Chapter 2, 'Clinical approach', p. 70.

AR juvenile parkinsonism
A rare condition presenting at <40 years with no Lewy bodies or Lewy neuritis at autopsy and caused by LOF mutations in *parkin*, an E3 ubiquitin ligase. Homozygous mutations in *parkin* are found in ~50% of patients with Parkinson's disease in childhood and adolescence, but only ~5% of young adults with the disease.

Benign essential tremor
A common disorder inherited as a late-onset AD condition. May be mistaken for PD.

Genetic advice

Inheritance and recurrence risk
There are a few families with a clearly Mendelian pattern of inheritance (AR or AD) or a defined disease-causing mutation and, in those, counsel as appropriate. For the remainder, advice is based on empiric data.

A 3-fold increase in risk for first-degree relatives of patients with classical Parkinson's disease seems appropriate (Kurtz *et al*. 2003; Payami *et al*. 2002). Given the fairly low prevalence of Parkinson's disease in the population, i.e. 0.5–1% at age 65–69 years and 1–3% among persons of 80 years and older, the absolute risks remain fairly low.

A 7.75-fold increase in risk may be appropriate in first-degree relatives of patients with onset of Parkinson's disease before the age of 50 years (Payami *et al*. 2002).

Variability and penetrance
Penetrance is age-dependent. Factors influencing penetrance are poorly understood.

Prenatal diagnosis
Theoretically possible by CVS for families in which the causative mutation(s) has been identified. However, this is unlikely to be requested, unless there is a family history of exceptionally early-onset disease.

Predictive testing
Theoretically possible if the familial mutation is known and could be offered to at-risk adult members of the family using an approach modelled on the HD predictive testing programme.

Natural history and management
Early treatment of Parkinson's disease involves education for the patient and family, access to support groups, regular exercise, and good nutrition. Dopamine agonists, rather than L-dopa, should be the initial symptomatic therapy (Koller 2002). There is active research into disease-modifying therapies that will provide neurorescue or neuroprotection.

Support group: Parkinson's UK, https://www.parkinsons.org.uk, Tel. 0808 800 0303.

References

Beavan MS, Schapira AH. Glucocerebrosidase mutations and the pathogenesis of Parkinson disease. *Ann Med* 2013; **48**: 511–21.

Hardy J, Cookson MR, Singleton A. Genes and parkinsonism. *Lancet Neurol* 2003; **2**: 221–8.

Hernandez DG, Reed X, Singleton AB. Genetics in Parkinson's Disease: Mendelian versus non-Mendelian inheritance. *J Neurochem* 2016; **139** Suppl: 59–74.

Kobayashi H, Kruger R, Markopoulou K, *et al.* Haploinsufficiency at the alpha-synuclein gene underlies phenotypic severity in familial Parkinson's disease. *Brain* 2003; **126**(pt 1): 32–42.

Koller WC. Treatment of early Parkinson's disease. *Neurology* 2002; **58**(4 suppl. 1): S79–86.

Kurz M, Alves G, Aarsland D, Larsen JP. Familial Parkinson's disease: a community-based study. *Eur J Neurol* 2003; **10**: 159–63.

Lucking CB, Durr A, Bonifati V, *et al.* Association between early-onset Parkinson's disease and mutations in the parkin gene. *N Engl J Med* 2000; **342**: 1560–7.

Maher NE, Currie LJ. Segregation analysis of Parkinson disease revealing evidence for a major causative gene. *Am J Med Genet* 2002; **109**: 191–7.

Nussbaum RL, Ellis CE. Alzheimer's disease and Parkinson's disease. *N Engl J Med* 2003; **348**: 1356–64.

Payami H, Zareparsi S, James D, Nutt J. Familial aggregation of Parkinson disease; a comparative study of early-onset and late-onset disease. *Arch Neurol* 2002; **59**: 848–50.

Polymeropoulos MH, Lavedan C, Leroy E, *et al.* Mutation in the alpha-synuclein gene identified in families with Parkinson's disease. *Science* 1997; **276**: 2045–7.

Samii A, Nutt JG, Ransom BR. Parkinson's disease. *Lancet* 2004; **363**: 1783–93.

Singleton AB, Farrer M, Johnson J, *et al.* Alpha-synuclein locus triplication causes Parkinson's disease. *Science* 2003; **302**: 841.

Trinh J, Farrer M. Advances in the genetics of Parkinson disease. *Nat Rev Neurol* 2013; **9**: 445–54.

Wilcock GK. Dementia with Lewy bodies. *Lancet* 2003; **362**: 1689–90.

Retinitis pigmentosa (RP)

RP is the most common inherited retinal dystrophy, or degeneration, affecting about one in 4000. It is genetically highly heterogeneous following AD, AR, and XLR inheritance, and also being a frequent manifestation of mitochondrial disease. Approximately 15% of UK patients with RP have X-linked retinitis pigmentosa (XLRP), which is a severe form consistently symptomatic in young boys.

In individuals with RP, impaired visual function is associated with the loss of rod and photoreceptors. The disorder is progressive. In RP, there is early loss of rod function, causing reduced sensitivity in the dark and field loss, followed by impaired cone function, causing further field loss; foveal cones are affected late in the disease associated with late deterioration in central vision. Examination of the fundus shows a range of changes, including retinal pigment epithelium disturbance and pigmentary changes in the mid-peripheral retina.

Note that the following are used interchangeably: rod–cone dystrophy = rod–cone degeneration = RP.

To date, >80 genes have been implicated in non-syndromic RP. Many of these can be grouped by function, giving insights into the disease process. These include components of the phototransduction cascade, proteins involved in retinol metabolism and cell–cell interaction, photoreceptor structural proteins, transcription factors, intracellular transport proteins, and splicing factors (Hims et al. 2003).

RP may be isolated or occur as part of systemic disease or syndrome. This section deals only with isolated RP. For RP occurring as part of a systemic disease or syndrome, see 'Retinal receptor dystrophies' in Chapter 2, 'Clinical approach', p. 302.

Clinical approach

The main issues are to: (1) determine that the RP is isolated, rather than part of a syndrome or systemic condition (for the latter, see 'Retinal receptor dystrophies' in Chapter 2, 'Clinical approach', p. 302); (2) confirm that the diagnosis is valid and determine the mode of inheritance; and (3) assess the risk to other family members and to offspring.

History: key points
- Three-generation family tree, or more if there is a suggestion of X-linkage.
- Age of onset and rate of progression.
- Registered as totally or partially sighted?
- Any variability in severity between males and females (suggesting XL inheritance).
- Other medical problems, including obesity, polydactyly, deafness. If there is concomitant congenital sensorineural hearing loss, strongly consider Usher syndrome (~50% are caused by mutations in the *MYO7A* gene).

Examination: key points
- Visual fields and fundal examination, if appropriate.
- Features of coexisting conditions. See 'Retinal receptor dystrophies' in Chapter 2, 'Clinical approach', p. 302.
- Investigations
- ERG and full ophthalmological evaluation of affected individuals. See 'Genetic advice' for advice on carrier testing.

Investigations
- DNA using gene panel/WES/WGS as appropriate. In such a genetically heterogeneous condition, simultaneous interrogation of multiple causative genes is likely to improve the chance of identifying the genetic basis of disease; however, variant interpretation can be challenging.

More extensive investigations are required in sporadically affected individuals and children to exclude syndromes and systemic conditions. See 'Retinal receptor dystrophies' in Chapter 2, 'Clinical approach', p. 302.

Other diagnoses/conditions to consider

Infantile receptor dystrophies
These are inherited disorders of the cones or rods. The most common are the following.

LEBER CONGENITAL AMAUROSIS. Or congenital retinal blindness is one of the most common inherited causes of visual loss in childhood. The rods and cones are lost in the first year or are dead and non-functional at birth. It is generally inherited as an AR trait, but some AD families have been described. Many genes have been identified. It is important to exclude a number of syndromes such as JS, infantile Refsum, Senior–Loken, Lhermitte–Duclos, BBS, and Zellweger syndromes.

ROD MONOCHROMATISM OR ACHROMATOPSIA. Associated with cone dysfunction. The condition is static and the clinical features are poor acuity, nystagmus, early onset of photophobia, and total colour blindness. Mostly AR. Mutations in three genes *CNGA3*, *CNGB3*, and *GNAT2* have been identified.

CONGENITAL STATIONARY NIGHT BLINDNESS. The retina is structurally normal with a normal fundal appearance. Several mechanisms have been described with different genes involved as AD, AR, and XL families have been reported.

CONE–ROD RETINAL DYSTROPHY. Characteristically leads to early impairment of vision. An initial loss of colour vision and VA (due to loss of cone function) is followed by nyctalopia (night blindness) and loss of peripheral visual fields (due to loss of rod function).

Macular degeneration or dystrophy
The rods and cones of the central retina—the macula—are lost to a greater degree than those of the retinal periphery, causing macular dysfunction. In general, a full-field ERG is normal, demonstrating normal rod and cone function.

Genetic advice

Inheritance and recurrence risk
All forms of autosomal inheritance have been found. In ~20%, the inheritance is known to be AR, 20% AD, and 15% XL. In 50% of cases, there is no family history. Many of these individuals may have AR disease, but some will represent de novo AD mutations, AD disease with incomplete penetrance, or XL disease. Absolute generalizations are impossible, but many AR and XL types are often associated with more severe disease with an earlier age of onset.

AFFECTED INDIVIDUALS WITH RP AND KNOWN MODE OF INHERITANCE. Discuss:
- offspring risks;

- possibility of predictive genetic testing in large families and/or those with a known mutation;
- PND only available if known mutation.

XLRP. Two major loci. RP2 (gene *RP2*) at Xp11.23 causes disease in ~15% of XLRP families and RP3 (gene *RPGR*) at Xp21.1 causes disease in ~75% of XLRP families. Some patients with mutations in *RGPR*, which localizes to the photoreceptor-connecting cilia, may have more widespread ciliary dysfunction, e.g. deafness and recurrent sinorespiratory infection (Zito *et al.* 2003) or cone–rod dystrophy.

The great majority of *RPGR* mutations are predicted to result in premature termination of translation. An alternatively spliced exon ORF15 is essential for retinal function. Exon ORF15 is a 'hotspot' for mutation, harbouring 80% of the mutations found within a series of 47 XLRP patients (Vervoort and Wright 2002). Most *RPGR* mutations are unique to single families.

AD RETINITIS PIGMENTOSA (ADRP). ADRP is genetically very heterogeneous. Three genes *RHO* (rhodopsin), *RDS* (peripherin), and *RP1* account for 25–30%, 5–10%, and 5–10% of ADRP cases, respectively (Berson *et al.* 2001).

AR RP is the most genetically heterogeneous of all the types of RP. Generally, there are no common subtypes based on molecular testing.

Variability and penetrance
In general, the earlier the onset, the poorer the prognosis. There is often considerable intrafamilial variability. Some families with ADRP show non-penetrance.

Prenatal diagnosis
Only possible for those with a known mutation.

Predictive testing of apparently unaffected individuals, other family members
- Genetic testing using next-generation sequencing is now possible for those with RP. Testing over 100–150 genes known to cause inherited retinal disease will generally identify pathogenic variants in many patients. Recent pickup rates are around 80% (ADRP), 50% (AR RP), and 90% (XLRP).
- Carrier risk may be determined from the pedigree and female carriers of XLRP can often be detected clinically. Female carriers of XLRP display a broad spectrum of fundus appearance from normal to extensive retinal degeneration; 90% of female carriers have fundus and/or ERG abnormalities.
- In addition to molecular testing, it is possible to arrange for ophthalmological assessment of at-risk individuals. ERG and other investigations can detect the early stages of the disease. Note the age of onset in the family when making an assessment of risk. If the presentation has been in childhood, then a normal examination at age 20 is more reassuring than if the disease is of adult onset.
- See guidelines regarding informed consent.

Natural history and management
Potential long-term complications
Progressive loss of vision.

Surveillance
By an ophthalmologist.

Support groups: RP Fighting Blindness, http://www.rpfightingblindness.org.uk, Tel. 01280 860 363; Foundation Fighting Blindness (USA), http://www.blindness.org.

Expert adviser: Graeme Black, Strategic Director, Manchester Centre for Genomic Medicine, Institute of Human Development, University of Manchester and Central Manchester University Hospitals NHS Foundation Trust, Manchester Academic Health Sciences Centre, St Mary's Hospital, Manchester, UK.

References
Berson EL, Grimsly JL, Adams SM, *et al.* Clinical features and mutations in patients with dominant retinitis-pigmentosa-1 (RP1). *Invest Ophthalmol Vis Sci* 2001; **42**: 2217–24.

Bird AC, Jay B. Diagnosis in inherited retinal disorders. In: AF Wright, B Jay (eds.). *Molecular genetics of inherited eye disorders*, volume 2, pp. 53–88. Harwood Academic Publishers, Chur, Switzerland, 1994.

Cremers FP, van den Hurk JA, den Hollander AI. Molecular genetics of Leber congenital amaurosis. *Hum Mol Genet* 2002; **11**: 1169–76.

Ellingford JM, Barton S, *et al.* Molecular findings from 537 individuals with inherited retinal disease. *J Med Genet* 2016; epub May 11.

Fazzi E, Signorini SG, Scelsa B, Bova SM, Lanzi G. Leber's congenital amaurosis: an update. *Eur J Paediatr Neurol* 2003; **7**: 13–22.

Hims MM, Diager SP, Inglehearn CF. Retinitis pigmentosa: genes, proteins and prospects. *Dev Ophthalmol* 2003; **37**: 109–25.

O'Sullivan J, Mullaney BG, Bhaskar SS, *et al.* A paradigm shift in the delivery of services for diagnosis of inherited retinal disease. *J Med Genet* 2012; **49**: 322–6.

Pacione LR, Szego MJ, Ikeda S, Nishina PM, McInnes RR. Progress toward understanding the genetic and biochemical mechanisms of inherited photoreceptor degenerations. *Annu Rev Neurosci* 2003; **26**: 657–700.

Rivolta C, Sharon D, DeAngelis MM, Dryja TP. Retinitis pigmentosa and allied diseases: numerous diseases, genes and inheritance patterns. *Hum Mol Genet* 2002; **11**: 1219–27.

Vervoort R, Wright AF. Mutations of *RPGR* in X-linked retinitis pigmentosa (RP3). *Hum Mutat* 2002; **19**: 486–500.

Zito I, Downes SM, Patel RJ, *et al.* RPGR mutation associated with retinitis pigmentosa, impaired hearing and sinorespiratory infections. *J Med Genet* 2003; **40**: 609–15.

Rett syndrome

A severe, non-progressive neurodevelopmental disorder that almost exclusively affects females. Prevalence: 1/12 000 female births for classical Rett syndrome. This remains a clinical diagnosis (see Table 3.37), although mutations are found in the *MECP2* gene in ~95% of females with features of classic Rett syndrome. Important groups of females with atypical Rett syndrome—less commonly associated with *MECP2* mutations—include those with a congenital onset, often with early seizures, and those with a mild course and developmental stagnation, rather than a marked regression, often with preserved speech.

Located on Xq28, *MECP2* encodes an abundant DNA-binding protein that may act to maintain the repression of transcription of inactive genes through binding to methylated CpG groups. The range of phenotypes associated with *MECP2* mutations has broadened since the association between such mutations and Rett syndrome was first reported. The phenotypic spectrum now includes females with mild, non-progressive ID, those who previously had a clinical diagnosis of Angelman syndrome (AS) or autism, males with severe neonatal encephalopathy, and males with severe MR and progressive spasticity.

MECP2 mutations in mental retardation

Females

Mutations in *MECP2* are involved in a broad spectrum of phenotypes from classical Rett syndrome to mild intellectual difficulties. The diagnostic yield in those without features of classic Rett syndrome is much lower. Kleefstra et al. (2004) reviewed a cohort of females with unexplained MR and identified two mutations among 63 girls who had been tested for AS and had negative *SNRPN* methylation studies (~7%). One mutation was found in 92 girls who tested negative for *FRAXA* (~1%), and no mutations in girls who had been investigated for PWS and had negative *SNRPN* methylation studies (0%). These results support *MECP2* testing of girls with features suggestive of AS, who have negative *SNRPN* methylation studies. In girls with unexplained MR, additional clinical features should determine whether analysis of *MECP2* is undertaken.

Males

Mutations in *MECP2* have been identified in males with classic Rett syndrome, when somatic mosaicism or Klinefelter's syndrome is usually a feature, and also in a few males with neonatal encephalopathy. It was suggested that mutations in *MECP2* can cause non-specific MR in males and could be responsible for up to 2% of XLMR. Bourdon et al. (2003) undertook a careful review of 354 boys with MR and identified only one potentially pathogenic *MECP2* sequence variation (0.28%), suggesting that the true incidence of *MECP2* mutations in males with non-syndromic MR is likely to be very low. Within the group of males with PPM-X (X-linked psychosis–pyramidal signs–macroorchidism syndrome; also parkinsonian features), however, some may be found with the specific missense mutation A140V. Xq28 duplications encompassing *MECP2* have been reported in males and females. Males present with hypotonia, developmental delay, recurrent infections, and poor speech and may have progressive spasticity.

Table 3.37 Revised diagnostic criteria for Rett syndrome

RTT diagnostic criteria 2010

Consider diagnosis when postnatal deceleration of head growth observed

Required for typical or classic RTT

(1) A period of regression followed by recovery or stabilization[*]

(2) All main criteria and all exclusion criteria

(3) Supportive criteria are not required, although often present in typical RTT

Required for atypical or variant RTT

(1) A period of regression followed by recovery or stabilization[*]

(2) At least two out of the four main criteria

(3) Five out of 11 supportive criteria

Main criteria

(1) Partial or complete loss of acquired purposeful hand skills

(2) Partial or complete loss of acquired spoken language[**]

(3) Gait abnormalities: impaired (dyspraxic) or absence of ability

(4) Stereotypic hand movements such as hand wringing/squeezing, clapping/tapping, mouthing, and washing/rubbing automatisms

Exclusion criteria for typical RTT

(1) Brain injury secondary to trauma (peri- or postnatally), neurometabolic disease, or severe infection that causes neurological problems[***]

(2) Grossly abnormal psychomotor development in first 6 months of life

Supportive criteria for atypical RTT

(1) Breathing disturbances when awake

(2) Bruxism when awake

(3) Impaired sleep pattern

(4) Abnormal muscle tone

(5) Peripheral vasomotor disturbances

(6) Scoliosis/kyphosis

(7) Growth retardation

(8) Small cold hands and feet

(9) Inappropriate laughing/screaming spells

(10) Diminished response to pain

(11) Intense eye communication—'eye pointing'

[*] Because *MECP2* mutations are now identified in some individuals prior to any clear evidence of regression, the diagnosis of 'possible' RTT should be given to those individuals under 3 years old who have not lost any skills but otherwise have clinical features suggestive of RTT. These individuals should be reassessed every 6–12 months for evidence of regression. If regression manifests, the diagnosis should then be changed to definite RTT. However, if the child does not show any evidence of regression by 5 years, the diagnosis of RTT should be diagnosed.

[**] Loss of acquired language is based on best acquired spoken language skill, not strictly on the acquisition of distinct words or higher language skills. Thus, an individual who had learnt to babble but then loses this ability is considered to have a loss of acquired language.

[***] There should be clear evidence (neurological or ophthalmological examination and brain MRI/CT) that the presumed insult directly resulted in neurological dysfunction.

Reproduced with permission from Jeffrey L. Neul et al., Rett syndrome: Revised diagnostic criteria and nomenclature, Annals of Neurology, Volume 68, Issue 6, pp. 944–950, Copyright © 2010 John Wiley and Sons, and American Neurological Association, and the Child Neurology Society.

Clinical approach

The revised diagnostic criteria (2011) include a period of regression as a compulsory criterion for both classic and atypical Rett syndrome.

History: key points
- Perinatal history.
- OFC at birth.
- Developmental milestones (usually normal for first 6–18 months).
- Age at which concerns were first apparent.
- Loss of acquired skills (usually loss of any babble/speech that has been acquired, although sometimes a few words are retained, and loss of hand skills).
- A temporary period of agitation associated with social withdrawal.
- Seizures.
- Impaired sleep/wake cycle.
- Inappropriate laughing/crying spells.

Examination: key points
- Eye contact.
- Observe for stereotypical hand movements (hand wringing, clapping, tapping, mouthing, and flapping).
- Observe for periodic abnormal ventilation (episodes of hyperventilation and breath-holding, valsalva breathing, and hypoventilation) and cyanosis.
- Gait. Usually wide-based dyspraxic/ataxic.
- OFC.
- Examine for altered tone, especially in the lower limbs (tone and DTRs).
- Kyphosis/scoliosis.
- Small/cold hands and feet.

Investigations
- *MECP2* mutation analysis (detection rate ~95% in classic cases).
- Consider genomic array.
- Consider next-generation sequencing panel, which includes *MECP2* and Rett-like disorders, and WES/WGS as appropriate.
- Early epilepsy: consider *CDKL5* and other *EIEE* genes; congenital onset without epilepsy, consider *FOXG1*. See 'Epilepsy in infants and children' in Chapter 3, 'Common consultations', p. 410.

Some diagnoses/conditions to consider

CDKL5

An early infantile epileptic encephalopathy where seizures usually present in the first few months of life though can occur later. Regression associated with seizures can occur; less autonomic features than Rett syndrome and poor eye contact common. Marked hypotonia. May have a normal OFC. Hand stereotypy usually present. There are many other infantile epileptic encephalopathies that may need to be considered in a child presenting with early seizures and developmental delay. See 'Epilepsy in infants and children' in Chapter 3, 'Common consultations', p. 410. Usually *de novo*; one case of gonadal mosaicism reported.

FOXG1

Is often identified on array, showing deletion of 14q12. Sequencing alterations may also be found. First

associated with the congenital variant of Rett in 2008. Usually have severe pre- or postnatal microcephaly, very poor developmental progress from birth, absent speech, tongue thrusting, midline hand stereotypy, and dyskinetic movements. Seizures may occur, but mostly after the first year of life. Do not usually regress. May be dysmorphic with a bulbous nasal tip and full lips. Brain MRI imaging may show partial or complete ACC ± frontal gyral simplification.

MEF2C

Is typically identified by deletion of 5q14.3 on array. Sequencing alterations may be found. Severe developmental delay, hypotonia, absent speech, and hand stereotypy common. May have infantile-onset epilepsy. Have a distinctive appearance with a high broad forehead, thick eyebrows, an anteverted small nose, and a downturned mouth. Various brain abnormalities found.

Pitt Hopkins syndrome

Usually caused by deletions or sequencing alterations in *TCF4*. Present with severe developmental delay, hypotonia, and a distinctive appearance, with a wide mouth, prominent lips, and deep-set eyes, which coarsens with age. In contrast to Rett, they also have long, slim fingers with fetal finger pads and slim feet. Hyperventilation and apnoea tend to occur in mid childhood. The corpus callosum may be hypoplastic.

Angelman syndrome (AS)

Severe MR, rarely with speech, ataxia, dysmorphic facial features, seizures with characteristic EEG, stereotyped hand movements, flapping. Birth OFC normal with deceleration; 30% microcephalic. No regression. See 'Angelman syndrome' in Chapter 3, 'Common consultations', p. 346.

Genetic advice

More than 99% are *de novo*, with mutations usually arising on the paternal chromosome. Familial cases are rare. Mutation screening (sequencing and MLPA) of *MECP2* currently identifies mutations in ~95% of girls with classic Rett syndrome.

Inheritance and recurrence risk

If a mutation is identified, check DNA samples from the parents. If *de novo*, recurrence risk is that of germline mosaicism (i.e. very small but has been described).

Variability and penetrance

Ninety per cent of affected girls have random X-inactivation. Several apparently normal mothers have been shown to have the same *MECP2* mutation as their affected daughters but have extremely skewed X-inactivation. In the few familial cases described, less extreme skewing may cause a milder phenotype.

Prenatal diagnosis

If a mutation is known in the proband, it is possible to offer PND. Since familial cases are so rare, the risk of recurrence needs to be balanced against the risks of invasive testing. However, many parents may wish testing for reassurance in a subsequent pregnancy (perhaps by amniocentesis).

Other family members

If a mutation is identified, check DNA samples from the sisters to exclude the tiny risk that they are gene carriers (arising from parental germline mosaicism) who are normal due to skewed X-inactivation.

Natural history and management

Management

Management is largely symptomatic and supportive, with a focus on nutrition, control of seizures, physiotherapy for the maintenance of mobility (and avoidance, if possible, of scoliosis for which surgery may be required), breathing and communication, increasingly using eye gaze technology. Control of breathing dysrhythmia with non-invasive ventilator support may prove helpful; including overnight, but this has not been established in trials. There is much optimism that rational, perhaps gene-based treatments may be trialled before long although the use of neurotransmitter-modulating treatments has so far not been shown to be effective at improving quality of life.

Potential long-term complications

Cass et al. (2003) undertook a comprehensive assessment of 87 females with Rett syndrome aged from 2 to 44 years. Levels of dependency in individuals with Rett syndrome are high. Almost all have fixed joint deformities and scoliosis in adulthood. Increasingly poor growth is another near-universal feature in older children. Feeding difficulties increased into middle childhood and then reached a plateau. Improvements in mobility into adolescence were followed by a decline in those skills in adulthood. Despite the presence of repetitive hand movements, a range of hand-use skills was seen in individuals of all ages. Cognitive and communication skills were limited, but there was little evidence of deterioration of these abilities with age (Cass et al. 2003). There is an increased mortality rate associated with the diagnosis of Rett syndrome, in part related to the autonomic disturbance of ventilation and heart rhythm and to seizures. This amounts to ~1.2% per annum.

Support groups: Rett UK, http://www.rettuk.org; CDKL5 UK, http://www.curecdkl5.org; International FOXG1 Foundation, http://foxg1.com; Pitt Hopkins Research Foundation, https://pitthopkins.org.

Expert advisers: Angus J. Clarke, Consultant in Clinical Genetics, Institute of Medical Genetics, University Hospital of Wales, Cardiff, UK and Hayley Archer, Department of Medical Genetics, Cardiff University, University Hospital of Wales, Cardiff, UK.

References

Bahi-Buisson N, Nectoux J, Rosas-Vargas H, et al. Key clinical features to identify girls with CDKL5 mutations. Brain 2008; **131**; 2647–61.

Bourdon V, Philippe C, Martin D, Verloès A, Grandemenge A, Jonveaux P. MECP2 Mutations or polymorphisms in mentally retarded boys: diagnostic implications. Mol Diagn 2003; **7**: 3–7.

Cass H, Reilly S, Owen L, et al. Findings from a multidisciplinary clinical case series of females with Rett syndrome. Dev Med Child Neurol 2003; **45**: 325–37.

Clarke A. Rett syndrome. J Med Genet 1996; **33**: 693–9.

Kerr A, Witt Engerstron I (eds.). Rett disorder and the developing brain. Oxford University Press, Oxford, 2001.

Kleefstra T, Yntema HG, Nillesen WM, et al. MECP2 analysis in mentally retarded patients: implications for routine DNA diagnostics. Eur J Hum Genet 2004; **12**: 24–8.

Kortüm F, Das S, Flindt M, et al. The core FOXG1 syndrome phenotype consists of postnatal microcephaly, severe mental retardation, absent language, dyskinesia, and corpus callosum hypogenesis. J Med Genet 2011; **48**: 396–406.

Le Meur N, Holder-Espinasse M, Jaillard S, et al. MEF2C haploinsufficiency caused by either microdeletion of the 5q14.3 region or mutation is responsible for severe mental retardation with stereotypic movements, epilepsy and/or cerebral malformations. J Med Genet 2010; **47**: 22–9.

Neul JL, Kaufmann WE, Glaze DG, et al.; RettSearch Consortium. Rett Syndrome: revised diagnostic criteria and nomenclature. Ann Neurol 2010; **68**: 944–50.

Schollen E, Smeets E, Deflem E, Fryns JP, Matthijs G. Gross rearrangements in the MECP2 gene in three patients with Rett syndrome: implications for routine diagnosis of Rett syndrome. Hum Mutat 2003; **22**: 116–20.

Wan M, Lee SS, Zhang X, et al. Rett syndrome and beyond: recurrent spontaneous and familial MECP2 mutations at CpG hotspots. Am J Hum Genet 1999; **65**: 1520–9.

Sensitivity to anaesthetic agents

There are two main types of inherited sensitivity to anaesthetic agents: suxamethonium sensitivity and malignant hyperthermia (MH)/hyperpyrexia.

Suxamethonium sensitivity

Pseudocholinesterase deficiency, butyrylcholinesterase deficiency.

Suxamethonium (succinylcholine) is a drug used in general anaesthesia to induce to neuromuscular blockade to facilitate tracheal intubation. Suxamethonium is metabolized in the plasma by the non-specific esterase pseudocholinesterase. Normally this happens quickly and the neuromuscular blockade lasts <5 min. Patients who are homozygous or compound heterozygotes for some pseudocholinesterase (BChE) variants produce pseudocholinesterase of abnormal affinity and reduced amount and metabolize the suxamethonium only slowly, resulting in a markedly prolonged neuromuscular blockade and paralysis. Artificial ventilation is used to support the patient until the neuromuscular blockade wears off (usually ~90 min after succinylcholine and ~5 hours after mivacurium). Apnoea after suxamethonium can last for up to 3 days in a highly sensitive individual.

Affected individuals are otherwise entirely asymptomatic (although they may be sensitive to cocaine). The condition follows AR inheritance and therefore siblings are at 1 in 4 risk. The gene encoding pseudocholinesterase is *CHE1* on 3q26.1.

Various low-activity variants are defined on the basis of the levels of cholinesterase and the degree of inhibition by dibucaine, fluoride, and propan-1-ol, e.g. A, F, K, J (see Table 3.38). 'Silent' alleles are also found, due to nonsense mutations/deletions in the *CHE1* gene. Using biochemical assays, the patient's phenotype can be defined. It is often not possible to ascribe a definitive genotype without performing family studies, and therefore usually only the phenotype is reported. Molecular genetic studies may be available in some centres.

The frequency of the atypical variant (A) is 0.017 in Caucasians, giving a homozygous frequency of ~1/3500.

Table 3.38 Classification of pseudocholinesterase variants by biochemical phenotype, genotype, and clinical sensitivity to suxamethonium[*]

Phenotype	Genotype	Sensitivity
U, Usual	U/U, U/S, U/J, U/K, U/A, U/F	Normal
K, Kalow (66% activity) (common)	A/K	Occasionally increased
J, J variant (33% activity)	A/J	Moderately increased
F, Fluoride-resistant (rare, except in Africans)	F/F, F/S, A/F	Moderately increased
A, Atypical (dibucaine-resistant)	A/A, A/S	Markedly increased
S, Silent (no activity)	S/S	Extremely increased

[*] K is in strong linkage disequilibrium with A and is present in most A and J variants, reducing enzyme activity without changing its affinity. The designation AK is often used. Approximately 90% of atypical cholinesterase gene variants are AK and only ~10% are A.

Cholinesterase levels can also be reduced in pregnancy and liver disease and by other drugs. However, any clinical prolongation of effect is small.

Malignant hyperthermia (MH)

MH is a dangerous hypermetabolic state after anaesthesia with suxamethonium and/or volatile halogenated anaesthetic agents such as halothane and methoxyflurane. It affects ~1/20 000 anaesthetized patients and is inherited in an AD manner. MH may also be triggered in susceptible individuals by severe exercise in hot conditions, infections, neuroleptic drugs, and overheating in infants and the overall prevalence is estimated at 1/10 000. The body temperature rises acutely to 40°C or 41°C, with muscle stiffness, tachycardia, sweating, cyanosis, and tachypnoea. Hyperkalaemia, acidosis, and hypercapnia alert the anaesthetist, as well as fever. Dantrolene, which decreases the amount of calcium released from the sarcoplasmic reticulum, is an effective treatment that has reduced case fatality from 70% to 5%.

MH myopathy has a variety of clinical presentations, including heatstroke, gross rhabdomyolysis after a variety of triggers, a chronically raised serum CK, muscle pain, neuroleptic malignant syndrome, and sudden infant death. Muscle histology is usually non-specific and variable.

The inherited abnormalities in MH-susceptible individuals lie in the regulation of myoplasmic calcium. Malignant hyperpyrexia is triggered by a rapid, sustained rise in myoplasmic calcium. Ryanodine, a plant alkaloid that effects calcium release from the sarcoplasmic reticulum (the main store for intracellular calcium), binds to a skeletal muscle calcium release channel—the ryanodine receptor (RYR).

MH is associated with mutations in the *RYR1* or *CACNA1S* gene in 50–70% of affected families; in others, the genetic basis remains unknown. Note, the *RYR1* gene has a large amount of variation, making interpretation problematic in many instances (Gonsalves *et al.* 2013).

- Central-core disease (CCD). All members of a family in which CCD has been diagnosed should be regarded as susceptible to MH. Histochemistry shows striking non-staining lesions extending along type 1 fibres, and there is often type 1 atrophy. CCD is caused by mutation of the RYR (*RYR1*).
- Minicore myopathy. Some patients have mutations in *RYR1*.

Clinical approach

History: key points

- Three-generation family tree, with specific enquiry about anaesthesia.
- Detailed history from the proband regarding experience following anaesthesia.
- For MH, enquire specifically about muscle pains after exercise or episodes of rhabdomyolysis (myoglobinuria).

Investigations

- A 5-ml EDTA sample for molecular genetic analysis, if available (e.g. *CHE1* in suxamethonium sensitivity or *RYR1* in MH).
- For suxamethonium sensitivity, 1–2 ml of serum or heparinized plasma (the sample should not be taken in the immediate post-operative period).

- For MH, measure plasma CK.
- For MH, consider *in vitro* contracture test (increased contractility of skeletal muscle in response to halothane and to caffeine). This provides a specific test to identify susceptibility to MH but requires a muscle biopsy. Molecular genetic analysis is far more accurate, when available.

Genetic advice

Inheritance and recurrence risk

- Suxamethonium sensitivity. AR, with 25% risk to siblings.
- MH. AD, 50% risk to offspring of an affected individual.

Other family members

- Suxamethonium sensitivity. All siblings should be tested biochemically (and molecularly, if available). Parents should also be tested, both to help define the phenotypes and also because the relatively high carrier rate in Caucasians means there is a small chance they too could be affected.
- MH. Consider referral to assess whether parents and offspring. Parents and offspring should be offered *in vitro* muscle testing if an *RYR1* mutation that would enable predictive genetic testing is not identified within a short time.

Natural history and management

Individuals with suxamethonium sensitivity and susceptibility to MH should carry a laminated warning card and consider wearing a Medic-Alert bracelet.

References

Cerf C, Mesguish M, Gabriel I, Amselem S, Duvaldestin P. Screening patients with prolonged neuromuscular blockade after succinylcholine and mivacurium. *Anesth Analg* 2002; **94**: 461–6.

Denborough M. Malignant hyperthermia. *Lancet* 1998; **352**: 1131–6.

Girard T, Urwyler A, Censier K, Mueller CR, Zorzato F, Treves S. Genotype–phenotype comparison of the Swiss malignant hyperthermia population. *Hum Mutat* 2001; **18**: 357–8.

Gonsalves SG, Ng D, Johnston JJ, *et al.* Using exome data to identify malignant hyperthermia susceptibility mutations. *Anaesthesiology* 2013; **119**: 1043–53.

Kalow W, Grant DM. Pharmacogenetics. In: CR Scriver, AL Beaudet, WS Sly, D Valle, B Vogelstein, B Childs (eds.). *The metabolic and molecular bases of inherited diseases*, 8th edn, pp. 225–55. McGraw-Hill Medical, New York, 2001.

Robinson R, Hopkins P, Carsana A, *et al.* Several interacting genes influence the malignant hyperthermia phenotype. *Hum Genet* 2003; **112**: 217–18.

Spinal muscular atrophy (SMA)

SMA is an AR disorder characterized by symmetrical proximal muscle weakness as a consequence of degeneration of the anterior horn cells of the spinal cord. Three classical types are recognized (see below), but these are somewhat arbitrary and there is, in fact, a continuum of clinical severity. Intelligence is unaffected.

- Type I SMA: severe (Werdnig–Hoffmann). Onset of severe muscle weakness and hypotonia in the first few months of life; never able to sit or walk. Fatal respiratory failure usually occurs by age of 2 years and often before 6 months of age. Nearly all present by 6 months and in one-third abnormal fetal movements are reported.
- Type II SMA: intermediate. Onset before 18 months of age (median age 8 months). Ability to sit but not to walk unaided; survival into adult life is usual.
- Type III SMA: mild (Kugelberg–Welander). Onset of proximal muscle weakness after 2 years, ability to walk independently initially; survival into adult life.
- In addition to the three classical types, there is the following.
- Type 0 SMA. A severe form of SMA that is usually fatal in the first months of life. These children present with arthrogryposis multiplex congenita and respiratory compromise. Approximately 50% have homozygous SMN1 deletions; the remainder are not linked to 5q and in a child presenting in early life, the following diagnoses should be considered:
  - spinal muscular atrophy with respiratory distress (SMARD). Some have biallelic mutations in the IGHMBP2 gene on chromosome 11q13 (Grohmann et al. 2003);
  - Brown–Vialetto–Van Laere syndrome. Progressive respiratory insufficiency with hypotonia and bulbar palsy due to biallelic mutations in SLC52A3 (type 1) and SLC52A2 (type 2) (encodes a riboflavin transporter). May respond, in part, to riboflavin (Johnson et al. 2012).

In type I SMA, the absence or dysfunction of SMN1 is reflected in enhanced neuronal death that is already detectable by 12 weeks' gestation. This is associated with a progressive loss of motor neurons towards the neonatal period. The combined birth incidence or early childhood prevalence of all types of SMA is ~1/10 000. All three types are associated with deletions and small intragenic mutations in the survival motor neuron gene SMN1 on 5q13. Wirth (2000) found that 94% of individuals with clinically typical SMA were homozygous for an exon 7 deletion of SMN1, and some of the remaining 6% had one deletion allele and one intragenic mutation. The proportion of disease alleles with SMN1 deletions is highest in type I and lowest in type III. Of individuals with SMA of all three classical types who have identifiable SMN1 mutations, 98% of disease alleles were exon 7 deletions and 2% were small intragenic mutations.

Carrier rate is estimated at 1/50. Most carriers have only one copy of SMN1. However, some unaffected individuals have two copies of SMN1 on one chromosome 5 and no copies on the homologue, complicating carrier detection by dosage analysis. Approximately 7% of unaffected individuals without a family history of SMA have three or four copies of SMN1, suggesting that the 2-copy allele is not uncommon (estimated at 3.3% of SMN1 alleles overall).

SMN2 (SMNc) is highly homologous to its centromeric neighbour SMN1 (SMNt) and is one factor underlying the variable phenotype of SMA. Individuals with type III SMA have, on average, more copies of SMN2 than those with type II or type I disease. However, ~5% of normal individuals lack both copies of SMN2. There are occasional case reports of asymptomatic individuals with homozygous SMN1 deletions—most have an affected sibling and it is likely that the variable severity reflects the variable copy number of SMN2, among other factors, and that mild SMA may develop eventually.

The SMN1/SMN2 gene cluster is prone to gene conversion (a non-reciprocal recombination process that results in an alteration of the sequence of a gene to that of its homologue).

Distal SMA encompasses a heterogeneous group of neuromuscular disorders caused by progressive anterior horn cell degeneration and characterized by progressive motor weakness and muscular atrophy, predominantly in the distal parts of the limbs. Heterozygous mutation in TRPV4 can cause a non-progressive congenital SMA with contractures allelic with HMSN2C (a form of CMT disease).

Clinical approach

History: key points

- Three-generation family tree, with specific enquiry about consanguinity, SMA, and unexplained infant deaths.
- Pregnancy history (reduced fetal movements late in pregnancy?) and delivery.
- Development milestones.
- Subsequent progress. Age of onset of symptoms, loss of mobility, scoliosis, etc.?
- Current level of function.

Examination: key points

- Infant. Assess posture. Infants with type I SMA often lie in a 'frog-leg' posture due to weakness of hip girdle muscles. Assess tone (floppy); look for spontaneous movement. Typically, there is preservation of extraocular movement and small movements of the fingers and toes, but absence of large movements of the limbs. Poor or absent kick with weak or absent withdrawal of the limb in response to pain. Facial muscles are involved, but usually there is some preservation of facial expression. Look carefully for fasciculation. DTRs are usually absent in types 0 and I.
- Child/adult. Careful neurological examination to confirm diagnosis. DTRs may be diminished, rather than absent, in types II and III. May present with delayed motor milestones or proximal muscle weakness (Gower's manoeuvre).

Investigations

- DNA sample for SMN1/SMN2 dosage and mutation analysis (the most common mutation is a deletion of exon 7 in SMN1).
- Next-generation sequencing panel/WES/WGS testing if SMN1/SMN2 analysis normal.
- CK to exclude a muscular dystrophy, unless proven molecular diagnosis of SMA.

Other diagnoses/conditions to consider

See 'Floppy infant' in Chapter 2, 'Clinical approach', p. 154.

Genetic advice

A result showing that an individual with clinically typical SMA is homozygously deleted for SMN1 confirms the diagnosis. Approximately 3.6% of patients with

SMN1-related SMA will be compound heterozygotes for an *SMN1* deletion and an intragenic mutation.

There is some genetic heterogeneity in SMA and Wirth *et al.* (1999) calculated that, in ~1.9% of type I, 1.6% of type II, and 13% of type III patients with typical SMA, including EMG and muscle biopsy results, genes other than *SMN1* are likely to be responsible.

Inheritance and recurrence risk
AR for all, except distal SMA that may be AD, AR, or XL.

NB. A *de novo* deletion occurs in ~1.7% of individuals with SMA. Carrier testing of parents is important as this will have an important effect on recurrence risk and on the counselling and testing of other family members.

Variability and penetrance
Usually the type of SMA will be consistent within a sibship, but with some variability. Within wider families, any type of SMA may occur, i.e. if counselling the uncle of a child who died from type I SMA, the risk that he will have a child with SMA *of any type* will be (1/2 × 1/50 × 1/4 = 1/400), assuming no consanguinity and a negative family history in his partner.

Prenatal diagnosis
Possible by CVS at 11 weeks' gestation if the mutational basis of the SMA in the family is known. Need to genotype both parents prior to CVS. NIPT is under development using a haplotype approach; seek up-to-date advice.

Carrier testing
If an individual at population risk (negative family history) has two copies of *SMN1* on carrier testing, the residual probability that he/she is a carrier is 1/820. If an unaffected sibling of an individual with a homozygous *SMN1* deletion has two copies, the chance that he/she is a carrier reduces from 2/3 to 1/13 (but could be reduced to negligible if it were known that both parents were single-copy carriers).

Other family members
Cascade carrier testing can be offered and is especially important if there is consanguinity.

Natural history and management
Type I SMA
A study of 33 infants with type 1 SMA (De Santis *et al.* 2016) found that none achieved a major developmental milestone e.g. rolling over or sitting independently with conventional therapy, establishing a baseline against which new disease-modifying therapies such as Nusinersen can be assessed. Nusinersen, an anti-sense oligonucleotide specifically designed to alter splicing of SMN2 pre-mRNA to increase the amount of SMN protein has recently been approved by the FDA but continues to be evaluated (Finkel *et al.* 2017). Infants on Nusinersen have been shown to acquire some motor milestones e.g. rolling and sitting independently. Conventionally, infants with a confirmed diagnosis of type I SMA have been offered palliative and terminal care via hospital and community paediatric teams. A recent publication from the USA (Bach *et al.* 2000) challenged this approach showing that long-term ventilation with feeding and physiotherapy support has resulted in prolonged survival (although no improvement in neuromuscular function). Intercurrent chest colds may necessitate periods of hospitalization and intubation. Cognitive development in SMA is normal.

Type II SMA
- Impaired mobility. Patients require specialized physiotherapy and seating input appropriate to the level of disability. Although SMA is said to be a non-progressive disease, many patients do notice a deterioration of mobility with time.
- Feeding difficulty. Patients with type II SMA are at risk of feeding difficulties, e.g. aspiration, which may manifest as recurrent chest infections, and some may require gastrostomy feeding.
- Respiratory insufficiency. Some may experience progressive respiratory failure (a severe scoliosis may exacerbate this) and ultimately may require assisted nocturnal ventilation.
- Scoliosis. Monitoring of scoliosis and appropriate intervention is important in preserving respiratory function in patients with type II SMA, all of whom have pronounced weakness of trunk muscles.
- Cognitive function. In von Gontard *et al.*'s (2002) study, environmentally mediated aspects of intelligence were higher in adolescent patients with SMA than in controls.
- Pregnancy. Successful pregnancy has been reported in women with type II SMA. Pulmonary function may remain stable throughout pregnancy, although it may deteriorate temporarily after delivery.

Type III SMA
The complications listed under type II SMA are much less common in type III.

Support group: Spinal Muscular Atrophy Support UK, http://www.smasupportuk.org.uk.

Expert adviser: Katie Bushby, Act. Res. Chair of Neuromuscular Genetics, Institute of Genetic Medicine, Newcastle University, Newcastle, UK.

References
Bach JR, Niranjan V, Weaver B. Spinal muscular atrophy type 1: a noninvasive respiratory management approach. *Chest* 2000; **117**: 1100–5.

De Sanctis R, Coratti G, *et al.* Developmental milestones in type I spinal muscular atrophy. *Neuromuscul Disord* 2016; **26**(11): 754–9.

Emery AEH. Population frequencies of inherited neuromuscular diseases—a world survey. *Neuromuscul Disord* 1991; **1**: 19–29.

Finkel RS, Chiriboga CA, Vajsar J, *et al.* Treatment of infantile-onset spinal muscular atrophy with nusinersen: a phase 2, open-label, dose-escalation study. *Lancet* 2017; **388**(10063): 3017–26.

Grohmann K, Varon R, Stolz P, *et al.* Infantile spinal muscular atrophy with respiratory distress type 1 (SMARD1). *Ann Neurol* 2003; **54**: 719–24.

Johnson JO, Gibbs JR, Megarbane A, *et al.* Exome sequencing reveals riboflavin transporter mutations as a cause of motor neurone disease. *Brain* 2012; **135**: 2875–82.

Munsat TL, Davies KE. International SMA consortium meeting (26–28 June 1992, Bonn, Germany). *Neuromuscul Disord* 1992; **2**: 423–8.

Ogino S, Leonard DG, Rennert H, Ewens WJ, Wilson RB. Genetic risk assessment in carrier testing for spinal muscular atrophy. *Am J Med Genet* 2002; **110**: 301–7.

Rudnik-Schoneborn S, Breuer C, Zerres K. Stable motor and lung function throughout pregnancy in a patient with infantile spinal muscular atrophy type II. *Neuromuscul Disord* 2002; **12**: 137–40.

von Gontard A, Zerres K, Backes M, *et al.* Intelligence and cognitive function in children and adolescents with spinal muscular atrophy. *Neuromuscul Disord* 2002; **12**: 130–6.

Wirth B. An update on the mutation spectrum of the survival motor neuron gene (*SMN1*) in autosomal recessive spinal muscular atrophy (SMA). *Hum Mutat* 2000; **15**: 228–37.

Wirth B, Herz M, Wetter A, *et al.* Quantitative analysis of survival motor neuron copies: identification of subtle *SMN1* mutations in patients with spinal muscular atrophy, genotype–phenotype correlation, and implications for genetic counselling. *Am J Hum Genet* 1999; **64**: 1340–56.

Stickler syndrome

Hereditary arthro-ophthalmopathy.

Stickler syndrome (OMIM #108300, 604841, 184840) most commonly occurs as an AD inherited connective tissue disorder, with a prevalence estimated at 1:7500 (Carroll et al. 2011). It is most commonly caused by mutations in collagen genes that encode the heterotypic collagen fibrils present in cartilage and vitreous, namely COL2A1, COL11A1, and COL11A2. These genes encode different collagen α-chains that co-assemble into either a type II collagen homotrimer (all three chains being products of the COL2A1 gene) or a type XI collagen heterotrimer that can contain products from all three genes. The COL11A2 gene is not expressed in the eye and mutations in that gene do not result in an eye phenotype. Stickler syndrome types 1 and 2, caused by mutations in COL2A1 and COL11A1, respectively, are the most common cause of inherited retinal detachment and can lead to blindness if untreated, hence the importance of identifying affected individuals (Snead and Yates 1999; Snead et al. 2011). Exon 2 of the COL2A1 gene is alternatively spliced and primarily expressed in the eye, so that exon 2 mutations result in a predominantly 'ocular only' phenotype with minimal systemic manifestations. In these cases, the diagnosis may easily be overlooked without vitreous examination (Snead et al. 2011).

Rare recessive forms of Stickler syndrome exist that are due to mutations in genes encoding type IX collagen (COL9A1 type 4 Stickler syndrome and COL9A2 type 5 Stickler syndrome and COL9A3). In addition, alternative splicing of exon 9 in the COL11A1 gene results in a recessive form of type 2 Stickler syndrome characterized by unusually severe hearing loss.

The major risk in all subgroups is of retinal detachment, particularly through a giant retinal tear, which can occur at any age (Ang et al. 2008, Carroll et al. 2011). The type 1 sub-group have a particularly high risk of retinal detachment and without prophylaxis, 50% will suffer retinal detachment in the second eye within 4 years of the first eye. Prophylaxis reduces the risk of retinal detachment by ~10-fold and is especially important for pre-verbal children who are unlikely to report visual loss (Fincham 2014).

In Stickler et al.'s (2001) survey of 316 patients, 95% had eye problems (retinal detachment in 60%, myopia in 90%, blindness in 4%), 84% had problems with facial structures such as a flat face, a small mandible, or cleft palate, 70% had hearing loss, and 90% had joint problems, primarily laxity and early joint pain from degenerative joint disease. See Box 3.8 for the proposed diagnostic criteria.

The condition exhibits wide inter- and intrafamilial variability. Clefts in Stickler syndrome may be submucous or wide U-shaped, or narrow V-shaped.

Clinical approach

History: key points

- Three-generation family tree, with specific reference to congenital or early-onset myopia, retinal detachment, deafness, joint laxity in youth, premature arthritis in the third to fourth decade, hip and knee problems, and cleft palate.

Examination: key points

- Facial features. Flat midface with a depressed nasal bridge, reduced nasal protrusion, anteverted nares, and micrognathia (most evident in childhood and becoming less distinctive with age).
- Myopia (typically congenital, of high degree, and non-progressive, but 15–20% of patients are not myopic).
- Examine the palate. Submucous cleft often undiagnosed; 25% have a palatal anomaly.
- Joint hypermobility, including hyperextensibility of the knees and elbows (abnormal Beighton score).
- Habitus. Slender extremities, long fingers, and normal height.

Investigations

- Ophthalmological assessment by a vitreoretinal specialist.
- Audiometry very useful to pick up high-tone loss—patients frequently asymptomatic.
- DNA for COL2A1 mutation analysis (congenital 'membranous' anomaly of the vitreous or 'afibrillar' vitreous gel) or COL11A1 ('beaded' vitreous phenotype).
- Consider gene panel, WES/WGS as available. Whole COL2A1 gene analysis for those exhibiting membranous vitreous anomaly. Deep intronic mutations resulting in aberrant splicing are well recognized.

Other diagnoses/conditions to consider

Perthes disease

Perthes disease of the hip can occur in families segregating in an apparently AD fashion with incomplete and variable penetrance. Exclude other familial causes of a dysplastic femoral head such as MED.

Spondyloepiphyseal dysplasia congenita (SEDC)

Patients are very small, with a short trunk and marked lordosis. Myopia, cleft palate, and deafness can occur. Onset is at birth, but severe short stature may not be

---

Box 3.8 Proposed diagnostic criteria for Stickler syndrome

Congenital vitreous anomaly, plus any of:

(1) myopia with onset before 6 years;

(2) rhegmatogenous retinal detachment* or paravascular pigmented lattice degeneration;

(3) joint hypermobility with an abnormal Beighton score ± radiological evidence of joint degeneration/dysplasia;

(4) audiometric confirmation of sensorineural hearing defect;

(5) midline clefting;

(6) first-degree relative with a diagnosis of Stickler syndrome (i.e. meeting the above diagnostic criteria)

* A tear or hole in the retina allows fluid from the vitreous cavity to seep beneath the retina.

Data from Snead MP, Yates JRW. Clinical and molecular genetics of Stickler syndrome. J Med Genet 1999; 5: 353–9.

obvious until 2–3 years of age. In infancy, the vertebral bodies are ovoid or pear-shaped, but later platyspondyly with irregular endplates develops. Odontoid hypoplasia may be a problem. Bone age is markedly delayed and the epiphyses are flattened and fragmented. The capital femoral epiphysis is severely affected. Caused by mutations in *COL2A1*.

Kniest dysplasia
An AD condition with myopia, macrocephaly, platyspondyly, joint enlargement and limitation, lordosis, and atlanto-axial instability. Significant short stature and phalangeal dysplasia are characteristic.

Otospondylomegaepiphyseal dysplasia (OSMED; also known as Weissenbacher–Zweymüller syndrome; STL3)
Eyes are normal. Mutations in *COL11A2*.

Wagner hereditary vitreoretinopathy/erosive retinopathy
Appears predominantly 'ocular' with minimal systemic involvement. An AD eye disorder characterized by early onset cataract, night blindness and pseudo-exotropia (divergent squint). Retinal detachment less common than Stickler. Caused by heterozygous mutations in the *VCAN* gene.

Fibrochondrogenesis
An AR severe skeletal dysplasia due to biallelic mutations in *COL11A1* which is often lethal.

Marshall syndrome
Most 'Marshall syndromes' in the literature, based on facial features, would appear to probably be type 2 Stickler syndrome.

Brittle cornea syndrome
Blue sclerae, progressive high myopia, fragility and rupture of the globe. Due to biallelic variants in ZNF469 and PRDM5. See 'Ehlers-Danlos syndrome (EDS)' in Chapter 3, 'Common consultations', p. 406.

Genetic advice

Inheritance and recurrence risk
AD; 50% risk to offspring of affected individuals.

Variability and penetrance
Wide inter- and intrafamilial variability.

Prenatal diagnosis
Technically feasible in families with a known mutation, but rarely requested.

Predictive testing
Prophylactic retinopexy is appropriate to reduce the risk of retinal detachment. Predictive testing could be used in families with a known mutation to target this more effectively.

Other family members
All first-degree relatives should be examined and offered an expert eye assessment.

Natural history and management

Potential long-term complications
- Eye. Moderate/severe myopia (> −5 D) is common and, in combination with the abnormal vitreous, can result in retinal detachment. The role of retinal

detachment is high and independent of the presence or degree of myopia. Prophylactic retinopexy should be considered in type 1 Stickler syndrome where the risk of retinal detachment and blindness is highest. There is also an increased risk for cataract and glaucoma.
- Ear. Conductive loss due to glue ear is common in young children with Stickler, particularly those with cleft palate. Szymko-Bennett *et al.* (2001) found some sensorineural hearing loss in 60% of adult patients with Stickler. It is milder in type 1 Stickler than in type 2 and generally no more progressive than age-related loss.
- Joint. Joint discomfort from degenerative joint disease is a problem for many Stickler patients in adult life. In one study, 80% of adults had chronic hip pain; 16% had a history of abnormal development of the femoral head in childhood.

Surveillance
Periodic (at least annual) ophthalmological review from infancy.

Support groups: UK patient support group, www.stickler.org.uk; The Vitreoretinal Service at Cambridge University Teaching Hospital, http://www.vitreoretinalservice.org.

Expert adviser: Martin P. Snead, Consultant Vitreoretinal Surgeon, Vitreoretinal Service, Addenbrookes Hospital, Cambridge, UK.

References
Ang A, Poulson AV, Goodburn SF, Richards AJ, Scott JD, Snead MP. Retinal detachment and prophylaxis in type 1 Stickler syndrome. *Ophthalmology* 2008; **115**: 164–8.

Carroll C, Papaioannou D, Rees A, Kaltenthaler E. The clinical effectiveness and safety of prophylactic retinal interventions to reduce the risk of retinal detachment and subsequent vision loss in adults and children with Stickler syndrome: a systematic review. *Health Technol Assess* 2011; **15**: 1–62.

Fincham, GS, Pasea L, *et al.* Prevention of retinal detachment in Stickler syndrome: the Cambridge Prophylactic Cryotherapy protocol. *Ophthalmology*, 2014; **121**: 1588–97.

Richards AJ, McNinch A, Martin H, *et al.* Stickler syndrome and the vitreous phenotype: mutations in COL2A1 and COL11A1. *Hum Mutat* 2010; **31**: E1461–71.

Richards AJ, Fincham G, *et al.* Alternative splicing modifies the effect of mutations in COL11A1 and results in recessive type 2 Stickler syndrome with profound hearing loss. *J Med Genet*, 2013; **50**(11): 765–71.

Richards AJ, Scott JD, Snead MP. Molecular genetics of rhegmatogenous retinal detachment. *Eye* 2002; **16**: 388–92.

Snead MP, McNinch AM, Poulson AV, *et al.* Stickler syndrome: ocular only variants and a key diagnostic role for the ophthalmologist. *Eye* 2011; **25**: 1389–400.

Snead MP, Yates JRW. Clinical and molecular genetics of Stickler syndrome. *J Med Genet* 1999; **5**: 353–9.

Stickler GB, Hughes W, Houchin P. Clinical features of hereditary progressive arthro-ophthalmopathy (Stickler syndrome): a survey. *Genet Med* 2001; **3**: 192–6.

Szymko-Bennett YM, Mastroianni MA, Shotland LI, *et al.* Auditory dysfunction in Stickler syndrome. *Arch Otolaryngol Head Neck Surg* 2001; **127**: 1061–8.

Wilkin DJ, Liberfarb RM, *et al.* Stickler syndrome. In: SB Cassidy, JE Allanson (eds.). *Management of genetic syndromes*, pp. 405–16. Wiley-Liss, New York, 2001.

Thrombophilia

Individuals with thrombophilia have blood that clots more easily than normal. In the normal state, there is a balance between the natural clotting and anticoagulant systems. Both of these systems may be affected by either inherited or acquired (including both intrinsic and environmental) defects. The most common manifestation of thrombophilia is venous thrombosis. The incidence of venous thrombosis is about one per 1000 person-years. In the USA, this leads to 50 000 deaths annually. Venous thromboembolism (VTE) is a multifactorial disorder, with well-characterized examples of gene–gene and gene–environment interactions underlying its pathogenesis. Genetic causes are present in ~25% of unselected venous thrombosis cases and up to 63% of familial cases.

Genetic causes of inherited thrombophilias (hypercoagulabilities) include the following.

- Factor V Leiden (R506Q mutation), causing activated protein C (APC) resistance, was discovered in 1994 and is the most common genetic risk factor for venous thrombosis. Twenty per cent of individuals with an idiopathic first venous thrombosis have this mutation, and 60% of pregnant women with a venous thrombosis have this mutation. Factor V Leiden has also been associated with an increased risk of recurrent pregnancy loss and placental infarction. The factor V Leiden mutation is carried by 4.4% of Europeans and white Americans.
- Prothrombin 20210A mutation (factor II Leiden) is carried by 1–2% of Europeans and white Americans.
- Antithrombin III deficiency.
- Deficiency of protein C. Purified human APC selectively destroys factors Va and VIII:C in human plasma and thus has an important anticoagulant role.
- Deficiency of protein S. Protein S is a vitamin K-dependent plasma protein that inhibits blood clotting by serving as a cofactor for APC. Makris et al. (2000) showed that relatives of a symptomatic individual with protein S deficiency who were also carrying a PROS1 mutation had an ~5-fold relative risk of VTE.

Overall, ~1/3000 individuals has a heritable deficiency of antithrombin III or protein C or protein S.

Acquired or environmental causes include the following.

- Surgical, e.g. post-operative or associated with trauma. Only major surgery is associated with a risk, e.g. abdominal surgery under general anaesthetic or an orthopaedic operation.
- Pregnancy (high factor VIII levels).
- Oestrogens, e.g. oral contraceptive use, HRT.
- Malignancy.
- Immobility, e.g. plaster casts, long-haul flights, stroke with limb weakness.

Patients with post-operative VTE have a very low risk of recurrence and a low incidence of thrombophilic defects (Baglin et al. 2003). Patients with an unprecipitated VTE have a 20% cumulative recurrence rate at 2 years; however, despite 27% of such patients having heritable thrombophilic defects, thrombophilia testing does not allow prediction of a high risk of recurrence (Baglin et al. 2003).

The clinical utility of testing for thrombophilia in patients with VTE is highly contentious. Middeldorp et al. (2001) concluded that the absolute annual incidence of spontaneous VTE in asymptomatic carriers of the factor V Leiden mutation is low and does not justify routine screening of the families of symptomatic patients. Simioni et al. (2002) in a prospective cohort study confirmed that the absolute risk of VTE in heterozygotes for the factor V Leiden mutation is low, with an annual incidence of spontaneous VTE of 0.17% (95% CI, 0.02–0.6) in carriers, compared with 0.1% (95% CI, 0.003–0.56) in non-carriers. However, risk period-related VTE occurred with an incidence of 18% and 5% per risk period in heterozygous carriers and in non-carriers, respectively.

Testing in patients from thrombosis-prone families may be warranted in order to identify individuals who might benefit from thromboprophylaxis during risk periods. If such testing is offered, the clinician needs to have a clear idea before initiating testing in asymptomatic family members that the results will inform clinical management in each individual case. Discuss with colleagues in haematology. See Box 3.9 for the American College of Medical Genetics (ACMG) guidelines on testing for factor V Leiden.

Clinical approach

History: key points

- Three-generation family tree, with specific enquiry regarding:
  - venous thrombosis (note the age of the affected individual and the site of thrombosis). Younger age of onset may indicate homozygosity, particularly for protein S or C deficiency;
  - pulmonary embolus;
  - pregnancy loss and pre-eclampsia;
  - myocardial infarction, particularly in those aged <50 years and women;
  - persistent leg ulcers;
  - childhood stroke.

Ask if there were known additional risk factors at the time of the event such as trauma, pelvic, vascular, or orthopaedic surgery, tumour, immobilization, pregnancy, oestrogen treatment, and other medical conditions.

- Acquired/environmental risk factors affecting the consultand or other affected family members:
  - smoking history;
  - diabetes;
  - lupus.

Examination: key points

Assess for chronic venous hypertension and post-phlebitic syndrome as this is a risk factor for recurrent VTE.

Investigations

- Factor V Leiden or APC resistance is usually performed initially. Patients testing positive for factor V Leiden or APC resistance should be considered for testing for the most common other thrombophilias with overlapping phenotype and for which testing is easy and readily available.
- Prothrombin 20210A variant. The DNA test can be multiplexed with that for factor V Leiden.
- Protein S, protein C, and antithrombin III deficiencies are too genetically heterogeneous for routine molecular genetic testing, but testing by functional coagulation assays may be considered, especially if there is a strong family history of venous thrombosis.

Box 3.9 Testing for factor V Leiden

Testing should be performed in the following circumstances.
* Age <50 years, any venous thrombosis
* Venous thrombosis in unusual sites (such as hepatic, mesenteric, and cerebral veins)
* Recurrent venous thrombosis
* Venous thrombosis and a strong family history of thrombotic disease
* Venous thrombosis in pregnant women or women taking oral contraceptives
* Relatives of individuals with venous thrombosis under age 50 years
* Myocardial infarction in female smokers under age 50 years
  Testing may also be considered in the following situations.
* Venous thrombosis, age >50 years, except when active malignancy is present
* Relatives of individuals known to have factor V Leiden. Knowledge that they have factor V Leiden may influence management of pregnancy and may be a factor in decision-making regarding oral contraceptive use
* Women with recurrent pregnancy loss or unexplained severe pre-eclampsia, placental abruption, intrauterine fetal growth retardation, or stillbirth. Knowledge of factor V Leiden carrier status may influence management of future pregnancies
  Random screening of the general population for factor V Leiden is *not* recommended. Routine testing is *not* recommended for patients with a personal or family history of arterial thrombotic disease. Physicians ordering factor V Leiden testing on a venous thrombosis patient for any of the indications recommended here should also consider the utility of functional, biochemical, and molecular screening for other heritable thrombophilic factors, especially prothrombin 20210A and plasma homocysteine levels.

Reprinted by permission from Macmillian Publishers Ltd: *Genetics in Medicine*, vol 3, issue 2, Grody *et al.*, American College of Medical Genetics Consensus Statement on Factor V Leiden Mutation Testing, copyright 2001.

* Plasma homocysteine levels. Elevation of homocysteine is another potential risk factor in those found to be positive for factor V Leiden.
* Antiphospholipid antibodies can cause APC resistance. Also consider anticardiolipin antibodies and anti-beta 2 glycoprotein antibodies.

Other diagnoses/conditions to consider
Medical conditions
That can cause activation of APC such as lupus.

Homocystinuria
Patients with classic homocystinuria (AR) are at extremely elevated risk of thromboembolism and should probably be tested for other available thrombophilic risk factors. See 'Marfan's syndrome' in Chapter 3, 'Common consultations', p. 484.

Genetic advice
Inheritance and recurrence risk
The genetic thrombophilias are usually inherited as an AD trait. If both parents are carriers for the same disorder, then there is a 1 in 4 risk of a homozygous affected child.

Variability and penetrance
Clinical expression is variable. Although the relative risk of venous thrombosis is increased between 4- and 8-fold for factor V Leiden heterozygotes, the majority of heterozygous individuals never have a thrombotic event. The relative risk depends on gene–gene interaction and gene–environment interaction, so that individuals who carry more than one genetic cause and have additional environmental risks face increasing risks. Homozygotes have an 80-fold risk of venous thrombosis.

Prenatal diagnosis
Not offered for factor V Leiden or prothrombin 20210A.

Predictive testing and testing of other family members
Routine testing of at-risk family members is not recommended for factor V Leiden or prothrombin 20210A, as there is only a mildly increased risk for the individual and testing does not decrease morbidity or mortality (see above). As a general rule, young children should not be tested. Children have special defences against forming blood clots and it is not until they reach puberty that their risk of blood clots due to thrombophilia begins to increase. Teenage daughters of patients with thrombophilia can be considered for testing if the results would influence decisions relating to contraceptive use. For some individuals, there is an indication to test, such as management of a pregnancy or avoidance of hormonal medication (oral contraceptive pill (OCP), HRT), and predictive testing can be offered to adults within families with known mutations after appropriate consent is obtained.

Natural history and management
Potential long-term complications
PREGNANCY. Heterozygosity for factor V Leiden has been linked to 2–3 times the risk of late pregnancy loss and has been associated with a higher risk of pre-eclampsia, abruption, IUGR, and stillbirth, though the risk varies between studies. Individual assessment is required to assess whether the risk of thromboembolism, fetal loss, and pre-eclampsia is greater than the risks related to anticoagulation. Warfarin is a known teratogen with a recognizable embryopathy. Heparin prophylaxis is preferred for those at high risk.

HOMOZYGOTES FOR FACTOR V LEIDEN. Have a higher overall risk of recurrence of VTE than heterozygotes (relative risk, 1.8; 95% CI, 1.0–6.17; Procare Group 2003). Balancing the risk of recurrence against the risk of major bleeding from oral anticoagulation therapy, it appears that factor V Leiden homozygotes with a first VTE are unlikely to benefit from long-term full-dose oral anticoagulant treatment. All these patients should receive short-term prophylaxis during risk situations, particularly during pregnancy (Procare Group 2003). This is also the case for venous thrombosis patients heterozygous for both factor V Leiden and the prothrombin 20210A mutation (co-inheritance occurs in one in 1000 of the population, but in one in 50 of patients with thromboembolism), in whom recurrence risk has been shown to be high.

Surveillance
- Patients on anticoagulants require regular surveillance.
- Advice should be given on ways to modify environmental risks and to report signs or symptoms of thrombosis.
  - Surgical, e.g. post-operative or associated with trauma. Only major surgery is associated with a risk, e.g. abdominal surgery under general anaesthetic or an orthopaedic operation. Heparin injections may be given to reduce thrombosis risk. Minor surgery, such as dental surgery or biopsies under local anaesthetic, are not high-risk situations.
  - Pregnancy (high factor VIII levels).
  - Oestrogens. Consider alternative forms of contraception or progesterone-only preparations if oral contraceptive use is desired. HRT generally confers a 2- to 3-fold increased risk for VTE. Early evidence suggests an interaction of HRT with thrombophilic states such as the factor V Leiden mutation, resulting in a synergistic increase in the risk of VTE (Peverill 2003).
  - Immobility, e.g. long-haul flights (ensure adequate hydration and exercise, and wear venous compression stockings).

Support groups: British Committee for Standards in Haematology (thrombophilia: information for patients and their relatives), http://www.bcshguidelines.com; Thrombosis UK, http://www.thrombosisuk.org.

Expert adviser: Trevor Baglin, formerly Consultant Haematologist, Department of Haematology, Cambridge University Hospitals, Cambridge, UK.

References
Baglin T, Luddington R, Brown K, Baglin C. Incidence of recurrent venous thromboembolism in relation to clinical and thrombophilic risk factors: prospective cohort study. Lancet 2003; 362: 523–6.

British Committee for Standards in Haematology (2003). Guideline on thrombophilia: information for patients and their relatives. http://www.bcshguidelines.com.

Greaves M, Baglin T. Laboratory testing for heritable thrombophilia: impact on clinical management of thrombotic disease annotation. Br J Haematol 2000; 109: 699–703.

Grody WW, Griffin JH, Taylor AK, Korf BR, Heit JA; ACMG Factor V. Leiden Working Group. American College of Medical Genetics consensus statement on factor V Leiden mutation testing. Genet Med 2001; 3: 139–48.

Kujovich JL, Goodnight SH. Factor V Leiden thrombophilia. In: RA Pagon, MP Adam, HH Ardinger, et al. (eds.). GeneReviews®, 2010. http://www.ncbi.nlm.nih.gov/books/NBK1368.

Makris M, Leach M, Beauchamp NJ, et al. Genetic analysis, phenotypic diagnosis, and risk of venous thrombosis in families with inherited deficiencies of protein S. Blood 2000; 95: 1935–41.

Middeldorp S, Meinhardi JR, Koopman MM, et al. A prospective study of asymptomatic carriers of the factor V Leiden mutation to determine the incidence of venous thromboembolism. Ann Intern Med 2001; 135: 322–37.

Peverill RE. Hormone therapy and venous thromboembolism. Best Pract Res Clin Endocrinol Metab 2003; 17: 149–64.

Procare Group. Is recurrent venous thromboembolism more frequent in homozygous patients for the factor V Leiden mutation than in heterozygous patients? Blood Coagul Fibrinolysis 2003; 14: 523–9.

Reich LM, Bower M, Key NS. Role of the geneticist in testing and counseling for inherited thrombophilia. Genet Med 2003; 5: 133–43.

Seligsohn U, Lubetsky A. Medical progress: genetic susceptibility to venous thrombosis. N Engl J Med 2001; 344: 1222–31.

Simioni P, Tormene D, Prandoni P, et al. Incidence of thromboembolism in asymptomatic family members who are carriers of factor V Leiden: a prospective cohort study. Blood 2002; 99: 1938–42.

Zotz RB, Gerhardt A, Scharf RE. Inherited thrombophilia and gestational venous thromboembolism. Best Pract Res Clin Haematol 2003; 16: 243–59.

Tuberous sclerosis (TSC)

TSC is a multisystem disorder characterized by hamartomas (tumour-like lesions) in the brain, skin, and other
organs and often associated with seizures and MR. The
prevalence is ~1/10 000. It can present at any age from
fetal to late adult life and is characterized by highly variable expressivity. The most common presentation is with
infantile spasms or seizures in early childhood, though in
an increasing proportion of cases the first indication of
TSC is the observation of cardiac rhabdomyomas during
routine fetal USS examination (see Table 3.39).

TSC follows AD inheritance, with a high proportion
of cases (60%) caused by new mutations. TSC is caused
by mutations in *TSC1* on 9q (hamartin) or *TSC2* on 16p
(tuberin). Tuberin and hamartin form a tumour suppressor heterodimer that has an important role in the
phosphoinositide 3-kinase (PI3K) signalling pathway and
inhibits the mammalian target of rapamycin (mTOR).
This pathway is a critical regulator of cell growth and
proliferation. The patchy nature of the pathology in TSC
appears to be due to somatic mutation with germline

inactivation of one copy of either *TSC1* or *TSC2* in all
cells (first hit) and subsequent inactivation of the second
copy by somatic mutation (second hit). See Figure 3.27.

Dabora *et al.* (2001) undertook a molecular and
genetic analysis of a cohort of 224 TSC probands.
Sporadic patients with *TSC1* mutations had, on average, milder disease in comparison with patients with
TSC2 mutations, despite being of similar age. They had
a lower frequency of seizures and moderate to severe
MR, fewer subependymal nodules (SENs) and cortical
tubers, less severe kidney involvement, and less severe
facial angiofibroma.

Clinical approach

History: key points

- Three-generation family tree, with careful enquiry for
  TSC, infantile spasms, epilepsy, learning disability, facial
  angiofibromas.
- Specific enquiry for seizures.
- Detailed developmental and behavioural history.

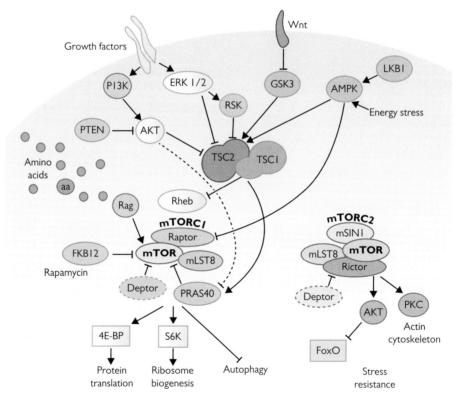

Figure 3.27 The mTOR pathway. A multiprotein complex including mTOR (mTORC1) regulates cell mass through modification of
protein biosynthesis and autophagy. The TSC complex acts as the central controller of mTORC1 activity and is regulated through
various inputs including AMPK.
Reprinted from *Kidney International*, Volume 79, issue 5, Tobias B. Huber, Gerd Walz, E Wolfgang Kuehn, mTOR and rapamycin in
the kidney: signaling and therapeutic implications beyond immunosuppression, pp. 502–511, Copyright 2011, with permission from
Elsevier and the International Society of Nephrology.
* HPFH, hereditary persistence of fetal haemoglobin; MCH, mean corpuscular haemoglobin; MCV, mean corpuscular volume.

Table 3.39 Diagnostic criteria for tuberous sclerosis

Genetic:

- Identification of a pathogenic TSC1 or TSC2 mutation from normal tissue

OR

Clinical:

- definite TSC: either two major features or one major and two minor features;

- possible TSC: either one major feature or two minor features

Major features	Minor features
Hypomelanotic macules (at least 3 of at least 5 mm in diameter)	'Confetti' skin lesions
Angiofibromas (at least three) or fibrous cephalic plaque	Dental enamel pits (>3)
Ungual fibromas (at least two)	Intraoral fibromas (at least two)
Shagreen patch	Retinal achromic patch
Multiple retinal hamartomas	Multiple renal cysts
Cortical dysplasias*	Non-renal hamartomas
Subependymal nodules	
Subependymal giant cell astrocytoma	
Cardiac rhabdomyoma	
Lymphangioleiomyomatosis (LAM)†	
Angiomyolipomas (at least two)†	

* Includes tubers and cerebral white matter radial migration lines.

† A combination of the two major clinical features (LAM and angiomyolipomas) without other features does not meet criteria for a definite diagnosis.

Reprinted from *Pediatric Neurology*, vol 49, issue 4, Northrup and Krueger, Complex Consensus Group. Tuberous Sclerosis Complex Diagnostic Criteria Update: Recommendations of the 2012 International Tuberous Sclerosis Complex Consensus Conference, pp. 243–54, copyright 2013, with permission from Elsevier.

Examination: key points

- Angiofibromas ('adenoma sebaceum') rarely obvious <2 years and may not appear until middle age. Occur in 85% of affected individuals in 'butterfly' distribution over the nose, nasolabial folds, and cheeks, and also the chin. Differentiate from acne by close inspection, showing a lack of involvement of sebaceous glands and the absence of infection. Unlike acne, angiofibromata persist in the same location and do not resolve. May coexist, causing diagnostic uncertainty.
- Hypomelanotic macules ('ash leaf' spots). Occur in 95% of affected individuals by the age of 5 years and are usually the earliest skin feature; may be present from birth or develop in infancy; 0.8% of normal neonates have similar macules, but rarely >3. Typically oval. May need Woods light (360-nm wavelength UV) to visualize them.
- Forehead fibrous plaque. Smooth, raised, flesh-coloured, or yellowish-brown, waxy-looking lesion (a few mm to several cm across), present on the forehead (look under the fringe!). Usually develop in later childhood.
- Shagreen patches. Discoloured, thickened, leathery patches of skin (resembling orange peel), usually over the lumbar region, slightly to one side of the midline. Usually multiple and varying in size (from a few mm

to several cm). Can appear at any age from infancy to puberty and are present in ~50% by early adult life.
- Ungual fibromas. Occur in up to 88% of adults. Look carefully at all fingernails and toenails for pink or red nodules arising in the angle of the nailbed and often causing ridging or guttering of the nail. Usually multiple and more common on the toenails where they may bleed if knocked.
- Dental pits due to enamel hypoplasia. Can occur in normal individuals, so not very specific for TSC. Fibromas similar to the ungual fibromas can occur between teeth.

Investigations

- Refer for ophthalmology assessment. Retinal astrocytic hamartomas are found in 40–50%. They are often multiple and bilateral and can take several forms. The most common are relatively flat, smooth, oval lesions which are semi-transparent and similar in colour to the fundus. Less common are the classic 'mulberry' lesions which are raised, opaque, multinodular, calcified hamartomas, most commonly found in the vicinity of the optic disc. Retinal hamartomas are almost always asymptomatic and only interfere with vision if overlying the macula (rare).
- Cranial imaging. CT will often show SENs along the lateral walls of the lateral ventricles or in the vicinity of the caudate nucleus, particularly if they are calcified. These are the most diagnostic cerebral lesions of TSC and are seen in ~80%. SENs may grow in size and have the propensity to develop into subependymal giant cell astrocytomas (SEGAs). SEGAs typically occur in the head of the caudate nucleus and present with symptoms of hydrocephalus due to obstruction of the foramina of Munro (see 'Natural history and management'). CT may demonstrate cortical tubers (seen in about two-thirds of cases), but these are better visualized by MRI when they are seen in ~95% of cases. FLAIR (fluid attenuated inversion recovery) sequences are the best MRI modality for visualizing cortical tubers. Most patients have 1–10 tubers, but some have more. Tubers may be associated with abnormalities of the underlying white matter such as migrations lines. These radial migration lines are seen in ~20% of MRI scans and are thought to represent hypomyelination and white matter heterotopia. Consider diagnostic specificity, radiation exposure, and availability when assessing whether MRI/CT is preferable. In infants <18 months old, in whom myelination is incomplete, MR imaging may be less good at visualizing tubers and CT may be the preferred investigation if a diagnosis of TSC is suspected on clinical grounds.
- Consider mutation analysis of *TSC1* and *TSC2*. In Dabora et al.'s (2001) series of 224 index cases, mutations were identified in 83% of cases, comprising 138 small *TSC2* mutations, 20 large *TSC2* mutations, and 28 small *TSC1* mutations. The bias in favour of *TSC2* reflects both the larger size of the gene and an intrinsically higher mutation rate.
- Renal USS. Angiomyolipomas (AMLs) are the most common renal manifestation of TSC (see 'Other diagnoses/conditions to consider'). Renal cysts occur in 17–47% of patients with TSC and are often present from early childhood. They are usually multiple and bilateral. In infants, a renal USS is used to identify the

small minority who have a contiguous *TSC2–ADPK1* gene deletion (see 'Other diagnoses/conditions to consider').

- In infants, consider an echo as cardiac rhabdomyomas are common at this age in children with TSC and may be very helpful in making the diagnosis.
- Where possible, perform baseline high-resolution chest CT scan and lung function testing in young adult females. Seek specialist pulmonary opinion for symptomatic LAM. Advise against smoking and use of oestrogen-based contraception. Caution with flying if oxygen-dependent or history of pneumothorax in the last month.

Other diagnoses/conditions to consider
See also 'Patchy hypo- or depigmented skin lesions' in Chapter 2, 'Clinical approach', p. 276.

Contiguous gene deletion involving *TSC2–ADPK1*
A small minority of patients with TSC have a contiguous gene deletion involving *TSC2* and *ADPKD1*, one of the genes encoding ADPKD. Such patients usually present with severe early-onset renal cystic disease, renal enlargement, and radiological appearances of advanced ADPKD, with a poor prognosis for renal function, leading to ESRF in late childhood or early adult life.

Isolated cardiac rhabdomyoma
Cardiac rhabdomyomas identified as an unexpected finding on a routine second- or third-trimester USS (not in the context of PND for TSC) is a well-recognized presentation of TSC and the chance of the baby being affected by TSC in this situation is 39–86%.

Periventricular nodular heterotopia (PVNH) or bilateral periventricular nodular heterotopia (BPNH)
A rare XLD condition causing a localized neuronal migration disorder in females associated with seizures (88% are focal) and prenatal lethality in males. Cranial imaging shows uncalcified periventricular nodules that could be confused with TSC (Jardine *et al.* 1996). PVNH is caused by mutations in filamin A (*FLNA*) that encodes a widely expressed protein that regulates the reorganization of the actin cytoskeleton and hence has an important role in cell migration.

Genetic advice

Inheritance and recurrence risk
AD inheritance, but 60% of cases arise as a result of a new mutation. Germline mutations are less common in *TSC1* than in *TSC2*.

AFFECTED PARENT. If one parent is affected, the risk of inheriting TSC is 50% to each offspring. In view of the variation in disease severity (expressivity), the overall risk of having a child with MR is likely to be 25% or less (since 50% or less of individuals with TSC are mentally retarded).

PARENTS UNAFFECTED. If neither parent is affected with TSC, the risk is 2% due to germline mosaicism (this has been reported for both *TSC1* and *TSC2* and can be either maternal or paternal).

Unless the causative mutation is known, parents of an apparently sporadic case should be evaluated by:
- detailed family tree;
- detailed skin examination, including Woods light exam;
- expert ophthalmological assessment of the fundi;
- consider cranial imaging (CT or MRI);

- consider renal USS.

APPARENTLY UNAFFECTED SIBLINGS. Should be offered a similar evaluation before they plan a family of their own (unless the causative mutation is known, in which case genetic testing should be offered). If both parents of the affected individual have been thoroughly investigated and are unaffected, the need for cranial imaging in the siblings is arguable as the prior risk, with a normal clinical examination, can be estimated to be of the order of <0.2% (2% risk arising from germline mosaicism, with >90% penetrance for skin features, e.g. hypomelanotic macules).

The risk of a *TSC* mutation in the phenotypically normal adult offspring of an affected patient, or the phenotypically normal adult sibling of a sporadic case, is close to that of the general population; hence risk to their offspring is close to population risks. (This assumes the adult offspring/siblings have been determined to be phenotypically normal after clinical examination, including dermatological and ophthalmic assessment, renal USS, or MRI and cranial CT/MRI scans.)

Where a pathogenic mutation is known in the proband gene, testing now replaces detailed clinical evaluation in the assessment of apparently unaffected relatives. Note germline mosaicism risk, so if a DNM is identified (i.e. not present in either parent), genetic testing should still be offered to siblings.

Variability and penetrance
TSC is highly penetrant by adult life; true non-penetrance is rare. TSC is highly variable, hence the need to offer molecular testing to apparently unaffected relatives (or comprehensive clinical and radiographic assessment if the familial mutation is not defined).

Prenatal diagnosis
Possible by CVS where a mutation is known. The risk of a second affected child being born to the phenotypically normal parents of an apparently sporadic case remains significant (1–2%), and PND by gene testing may be offered if a mutation has been identified in the affected child. PGD and NIPT may be options to discuss, depending on the family structure and availability.

Natural history and management
Surveillance and management guidelines were revised by an international expert group in 2012 (Krueger and Northrup 2013).

Affected individuals are at risk of premature death
From epilepsy, cardiac arrhythmias, renal involvement, or complications of giant cell astrocytomas or pulmonary LAM.

Learning disability
Over 50% of individuals with TSC have a normal IQ. Learning disability can be mild to severe but is unusual in individuals who have never had seizures. Children who present with seizures, particularly infantile spasms, in the first 2 years of life are more likely to have learning disability than those who develop seizures later. Onset >5 years is very unlikely to be associated with learning difficulties, unless non-convulsive status epilepticus occurs. Patients with ID have significantly more cortical tubers than those with normal intelligence.

Behavioural problems
Are common. Learning disabilities frequently occur in conjunction with behavioural problems, but not always.

Autism is seen in ~25–61% and more broadly defined pervasive developmental disorders in ~50–86%. Disruptive behavioural disorders characterized by marked hyperactivity and/or attention deficits are common, occurring in 43–59%. Sleep disturbance is very common, especially if a child's epilepsy is poorly controlled.

Seizures

Occur in 80% of individuals with TSC (Joinson *et al.* 2003). The best estimate of the frequency of seizures in familial cases is ~62% (Webb *et al.* 1991)—the frequency of seizures in familial cases is likely to be lower than in sporadic cases for several reasons, including a lower proportion of *TSC2* mutations. A great variety of seizure types can occur, including simple and complex partial (focal) seizures, generalized tonic and tonic–clonic seizures, atonic seizures ('drop attacks'), myoclonic seizures, and infantile spasms. Seizures typically begin in infancy, often in the first few months. The pattern of seizure changes through early childhood. Seizure control can be very difficult and 85% of children who develop seizures still have them by age of 5 years. Most respond, at least to some extent, to anticonvulsants, but a small minority have epilepsy that is refractory to anticonvulsant therapy.

Potential long-term complications

• Giant cell astrocytomas occur in 10–15%. Peak incidence is late childhood through adolescence. Cases present with symptoms of raised intracranial pressure (headaches, vomiting) due to obstruction of the foramina of Munro. Surgery or mTOR inhibitor therapy is indicated for growing or symptomatic lesions.
• Angiomyolipomas of the kidney are common and usually multiple and bilateral, increasing in size and number with age. They are present in 17%, 42%, 65%, and 92% of individuals with TSC by <2 years, 2–5 years, 9–14 years, and 14–18 years, respectively (Jozwiak *et al.* 2000). While often asymptomatic, they can cause renal pain, haematuria, and intrarenal or retroperitoneal haemorrhage and lead to impaired renal function. Embolization is indicated for bleeding lesions and mTOR inhibitor therapy for large non-bleeding lesions.
• Renal cysts occur in 17–47% and are often present from early childhood. They are usually multiple and bilateral. If cysts are numerous, consider the possibility of a contiguous *TSC2–PKD1* gene deletion.
• Symptomatic LAM is uncommon and occurs almost exclusively in adult females. Prognosis can be poor if lung involvement is extensive. It usually presents in adult life but can present earlier. Can cause progressive respiratory impairment and pneumothorax. If symptomatic, refer to a chest physician. mTOR inhibitor therapy appears to slow disease progression.
• Cardiac rhabdomyomas may be identified on USS in fetal life or cause outflow obstruction or arrhythmias in the neonatal period. They usually regress in number and size with age.
• Hepatic hamartomas are present in 25% and are usually of no clinical significance.

Support groups: Tuberous Sclerosis Association (UK), http://www.tuberous-sclerosis.org, Tel. 01527 871 898; Tuberous Sclerosis Alliance (USA), http://www.tsalliance.org, Tel. (toll-free) (800) 225 6872.

Expert adviser: Julian Sampson, Professor and Honorary Consultant in Medical Genetics, Institute of Medical Genetics, Cardiff University Heath Park, Cardiff, UK.

References

Crino PB, Nathanson KL, Henske EP (2006). The tuberous sclerosis complex. *N Engl J Med* 2006; **355**: 1345–56.

Dabora SL, Jozwiak S, Franz DN, *et al.* Mutational analysis in a cohort of 224 tuberous sclerosis patients indicates increased severity of *TSC2*, compared with *TSC1*, disease in multiple organs. *Am J Hum Genet* 2001; **68**: 64–80.

Gamzu R, Achiron R, Hegesh J, *et al.* Evaluating the risk of tuberous sclerosis in cases with prenatal diagnosis of cardiac rhabdomyoma. *Prenat Diagn* 2002; **22**: 1044–7.

Jardine PE, Clarke MA, Super M. Familial bilateral periventricular nodular heterotopia mimics tuberous sclerosis. *Arch Dis Child* 1996; **74**: 244–6.

Joinson C, O'Callaghan FJ, Osborne JP, Martyn C, Harris T, Bolton PF. Learning disability and epilepsy in an epidemiological sample of individuals with tuberous sclerosis complex. *Psychol Med* 2003; **33**: 335–44.

Jozwiak S, Schwartz RA, Janniger CK, Bielicka-Cymerman J. Usefulness of diagnostic criteria of tuberous sclerosis complex in pediatric patients. *J Child Neurol* 2000; **15**: 652–9.

Krueger DA, Northrup H; International Tuberous Sclerosis Complex Consensus Group. Tuberous sclerosis complex surveillance and management: recommendations of the 2012 International Tuberous Sclerosis Complex Consensus Conference. *Pediatr Neurol* 2013; **49**: 255–65.

Kwiatkowski DJ. Genetics of tuberous sclerosis complex. In: DJ Kwiatkowski, VH Whittemore, EA Thiele (eds.). Tuberous sclerosis complex: genes, clinical features and therapeutics, pp. 29–60. Wiley, Wienheim, 2010.

Lewis JC, Thomas HV, Murphy KC, Sampson JR. Genotype and psychological phenotype in tuberous sclerosis. *J Med Genet* 2004; **41**: 203–7.

Northrup H, Krueger DA; International Tuberous Sclerosis Complex Consensus Group. Tuberous sclerosis complex diagnostic criteria update: recommendations of the 2012 International Tuberous Sclerosis Complex Consensus Conference. *Pediatr Neurol* 2013; **49**: 243–54.

Tee AR, Manning BD, Roux PP, Cantley LC, Blenis J. Tuberous sclerosis complex gene products, tuberin and hamartin, control mTOR signaling by acting as a GTPase-activating protein complex toward Rheb. *Curr Biol* 2003; **13**: 1259–68.

Webb DW, Fryer AE, Osborne JP. On the incidence of fits and mental retardation in tuberous sclerosis. *J Med Genet* 1991; **28**: 417–19.

X-linked adrenoleukodystrophy (X-ALD)

ALD, adrenomyeloneuropathy, Schilder disease, sudano-philic leukodystrophy.

X-ALD is an XL metabolic disorder that is associated with accumulations of VLCFAs (see Table 3.40) in the adrenal gland and in the central and peripheral nervous systems. It is caused by mutations in the *ABCD1* gene on Xq28 that encodes a peroxisomal ABC half-transporter (ALDP) of unknown function. The clinical consequences of this are highly variable. ALD is a disease with mixed features of axonal degeneration, leading to myeloneu-ropathy and a severe inflammatory reaction in the cerebral white matter resulting in demyelination. At least six phenotypic variants of X-ALD are recognized (Moser et al. 2000), with childhood cerebral ALD (CCALD) and adrenomyeloneuropathy (AMN) accounting for 80% of cases.

- Childhood cerebral ALD (CCALD). Onset 3–10 years, often presenting with behaviour problems, poor concentration, and decline in school performance. Seizures, spasticity, and dementia occur due to rapidly progressive cerebral demyelination. Once established, the process appears irreversible and most boys die 3–5 years from the onset of symptoms.
- Adolescent cerebral ALD (AdolCALD). As above, but with onset between 10 and 21 years.
- Adult cerebral ALD (ACALD). Rare (1–3%) and usually presenting with predominantly psychiatric symptoms and worsening memory.
- Adrenomyeloneuropathy (AMN). Onset usually in the 20s to 40s. This is the most common phenotype and presents with slowly progressive paraparesis.
- Isolated adrenocortical dysfunction (Addison's disease). Some patients present with isolated adrenocortical dysfunction. Most develop neurological deficits later. Ronghe et al. (2002) identified a man who presented with Addison's at the age of 5 years but was only diagnosed with X-ALD at the age of 34 years when his AMN was recognized.
- Asymptomatic or pre-symptomatic. Mutation carriers with no symptoms.

It is not possible to predict the phenotype by mutation analysis or biochemical assays. There is no apparent genotype–phenotype correlation. Different phenotypes may develop in different family members carrying the same mutation. Some patients have a mixed phenotype, e.g. AMN and Addison's disease. Sometimes the phenotype evolves with time. van Geel et al. (2001) found that, of 68 patients with AMN initially without brain involvement, 13 (19%) later developed cerebral demyelination. Most families have private mutations.

See also Moser et al. (1999) for the largest published experience of plasma VLCFAs. The US Government has recently recommended that X-ALD be added to State newborn screening programmes (Kemper et al. 2017).

Clinical approach

History: key points

- Three-generation family history, with specific enquiry about Addison's disease, gait disturbance, and unexplained deaths in males. Enquire also about other neurological diagnoses in males and females. AMN may be misdiagnosed as multiple sclerosis (MS) or hereditary spastic paraplegia (HSP).
- Detailed developmental history. Are there any recent changes in school performance, personality, and concentration?

Examination: key points

- Examine carefully for spasticity, particularly affecting the lower limbs (abnormal gait, increased tone, increased reflexes, clonus).

Investigations

- Plasma VLCFAs (raised in almost all affected males and in some carrier females).
- DNA for mutation analysis of *ABCD1*.
- Consider testing adrenocortical function in at-risk or affected males by arranging a short Synacthen® test (usually done in early morning with baseline cortisol, followed by administration of Synacthen® and repeat cortisol at 30 min).
- Consider MRI; this is indicated if symptomatic.

Other diagnoses/conditions to consider

Other leukodystrophies

See 'Leukodystrophy/leukoencephalopathy' in Chapter 2, 'Clinical approach', p. 208.

HSP

See 'Hereditary spastic paraplegias (HSP)' in Chapter 3, 'Common consultations', p. 448.

Achalasia–addisonianism–alacrima (AAA) syndrome (Allgrove syndrome)

An AR condition caused by mutations in aladin (*AAAS*) on 12q13, with defective tear production, autonomic dysfunction, and adrenal insufficiency.

Genetic advice

Only 5% of male probands and 1.7% of X-ALD hemizygotes have new mutations (Bezman et al. 2001).

Inheritance and recurrence risk

XLR, with expression in some carrier females (see below).

Variability and penetrance

Female heterozygotes may develop neurological sequelae. In a series of 46 carrier women, Engelen et al.

Table 3.40 Reference ranges for VLCFAs

VLCFA	<1 year	1–10 years	>10 years
C22 (µmol/l)	21–103	33–96	31–98
C24 (µmol/l)	22–87	25–71	24–66
C26 (µmol/l)	0.05–1.97	0.15–0.91	0.15–0.91
C24/C22 ratio	0.00–1.15	0.00–1.01	0.00–0.96
C26/C22 ratio	0.000–0.028	0.000–0.026	0.000–0.022
Phytanate (µmol/l)	0–10	0–15	0–15
Pristanate (µmol/l)	0–1	0–2	0–2

Biochemical Genetics Unit, The Pathology Partnership at Cambridge University Hospitals, UK. Note: results must be interpreted against the reference ranges quoted by the laboratory undertaking the analysis.

(2014) found that X-ALD carriers may develop signs and symptoms of myelopathy (63%) and/or peripheral neuropathy (57%). Especially striking was the occurrence of faecal incontinence (28%). The frequency of symptomatic women increased sharply with age (from 18% in women <40 years to 88% in women >60 years of age). Virtually all (98%) X-ALD carriers had increased VLCFAs in plasma and/or fibroblasts. They did not find an association between the X-inactivation pattern and symptomatic status. Adrenocortical insufficiency is very rare in female heterozygotes and is not routinely tested.

Prenatal diagnosis
Possible by CVS at 11 weeks' gestation by mutation analysis if a familial mutation identified, or by analysis of VLCFAs in cultured chorionic villus cells or amniocytes. PGD may also be available.

Predictive testing
The introduction of BMT raises the issue of predictive testing in at-risk males. Since BMT is a high-risk therapy with a significant morbidity and mortality, it is not usually considered in the complete absence of symptoms/signs. Identification of pre-symptomatic boys permits serial and careful follow-up by neuropsychological profiles and MRI studies at 6- to 12-month intervals, beginning from the age of 3 years with recourse to BMT if initiation of CCALD is identified. BMT should be strongly considered if progressive MRI change is identified, even if neuropsychological function is still intact. BMT is not indicated in boys with normal MRI findings.

Since CCALD does not have its onset before 3 years of age, predictive testing can be considered at any time during the first 2 years of life, with a view to arranging serial MRI and possible workup for BMT from the age of 2.5 years.

VLCFAs are raised even in cord blood in most affected males. However, there are exceptional cases of affected males where plasma levels are within normal limits and abnormalities are only found in fibroblast assays. Mutation analysis is therefore the gold standard for family screening.

• Carrier testing. Fifteen to 20% of female heterozygotes have VLCFA levels within normal limits. Mutation analysis is therefore highly preferable in the evaluation of maternal female relatives. Some labs will accept samples from at-risk female relatives for mutation analysis, even when no sample is available from the proband.

• Extended family. Cascade screening of the extended family provides the opportunity for identifying heterozygous females and pre-symptomatic males.

Natural history and management
A 5- to 10-year follow-up of 12 patients with CCALD (Shapiro et al. 2000) showed the long-term beneficial effect of BMT when the procedure was undertaken at an early stage in the disease. This approach offers hope to families where other males are identified in the pre-symptomatic phase of X-ALD following diagnosis in the proband.

Lorenzo oil (oleic and erucic acids) can lead to improvement in plasma VLCFAs but is of limited value in correcting the accumulation of saturated VLCFAs in the brains of patients with ALD. Aubourg et al. (1993) found no evidence of clinically relevant benefit in a trial of 24 patients, but an international study by Moser et al. (2004) suggested that Lorenzo oil may have a preventative effect.

Surveillance
• Identification of pre-symptomatic boys and serial and careful follow-up by serial (6-monthly) neuropsychological and MRI studies, with recourse to BMT if initiation of CCALD is identified.

• Surveillance for adrenal insufficiency in pre-symptomatic and affected boys.

Support group: ALD Family Support Trust, http://www.aldfst.org.uk.

References
Aubourg P, Adamsbaum C, Lavallard-Rousseau MC, et al. A two-year trial of oleic and erucic acids ('Lorenzo's oil') as treatment for adrenomyeloneuropathy. N Engl J Med 1993; **329**: 745–52.

Bezman L, Moser AB, Raymond GV, et al. Adrenoleukodystrophy: incidence, new mutation rate, and results of extended family screening. Ann Neurol 2001; **49**: 512–17.

Engelen M, Barbier M, Dijkstra IM, et al. X-linked adrenoleukodystrophy in women: a cross-sectional cohort study. Brain 2014; **137**(Pt 3): 693–706.

Kemp S, Pujol A, Waterham HR, et al. ABCD1 mutations and the X-linked adrenoleukodystrophy mutation database: role in diagnosis and clinical correlations. Hum Mutat 2001; **18**: 499–515.

Kemper AR, Brosco T, et al. Newborn screening for X-linked adrenoleukodystrophy: evidence summary and advisory committee recommendation. Genet Med 2017; **19**: 121–6.

Moser H, Dubey P, Fatemi A. Progress in X-linked adrenoleukodystrophy. Curr Opin Neurol 2004; **17**: 263–9.

Moser AB, Kreiter N, Bezman L, et al. Plasma very long chain fatty acids in 3,000 peroxisome disease patients and 29,000 controls. Ann Neurol 1999; **45**: 100–10.

Moser HW, Loes DJ, Melhem ER, et al. X-linked adrenoleukodystrophy: overview and prognosis as a function of age and brain magnetic resonance imaging abnormality. A study involving 372 patients. Neuropediatrics 2000; **31**: 227–39.

Peters C, Charnas LR, Tan Y, et al. Cerebral X-linked adrenoleukodystrophy: the international haematopoietic cell transplantation experience from 1982 to 1999. Blood 2004; **104**: 881–8.

Ronghe MD, Barton J, Jardine PE, et al. The importance of testing for adrenoleucodystrophy in males with idiopathic Addison's disease. Arch Dis Child 2002; **86**: 185–9.

Shapiro E, Krivit W, Lockman L, et al. Long-term effect of bone-marrow transplantation for childhood-onset cerebral X-linked adrenoleukodystrophy. Lancet 2000; **356**: 713–18.

Suzuki Y, Isogai K, Teramoto T, et al. Bone marrow transplantation for the treatment of X-linked adrenoleukodystrophy. J Inherit Metab Dis 2000; **23**: 453–8.

van Geel BM, Bezman L, Loes DJ, Moser HW, Raymond GV. Evolution of phenotypes in adult male patients with X-linked adrenoleukodystrophy. Ann Neurol 2001; **49**: 186–94.

Cancer

Chapter contents

BRCA1 and BRCA2

Dominantly inherited mutations in *BRCA1* and *BRCA2* are the most frequently identified monogenic causes for hereditary breast and breast/ovarian cancers but account for only about 20% of familial breast cancer. The combined contribution of *BRCA1* and *BRCA2* to overall breast cancer is ~2%.

BRCA1 is a large gene with 22 exons, with exon 11 comprising ~60% of the coding sequence. Most mutations are scattered throughout the gene. Eighty-seven per cent of mutations identified are predicted to result in protein truncation or absence of the *BRCA1* protein. The *BRCA1* protein is involved in many important cellular pathways, including DNA repair and regulation of transcription. Several founder mutations are common in specific populations. In the Ashkenazi Jewish population (originating from Central and Eastern Europe, e.g. Poland, Germany, Hungary, Lithuania, Belarus, Ukraine, and Russia), there are two founder mutations in *BRCA1*: c.68_69delAG (BIC: 185delAG) and c.5266dupC (BIC: 5382insC).

BRCA2 is also a large gene, with exons 10 and 11 comprising ~60% of the coding sequence. Mutations are scattered throughout the gene and most are truncating. The *BRCA2* protein is involved in DNA repair, and biallelic mutations in *BRCA2* and rarely *BRCA1* cause Fanconi anaemia (FA). In the Ashkenazi Jewish population (see above), a founder mutation *BRCA2* c.5946delT (BIC: 6174delT) is found in 1–1.5% of Ashkenazi Jews and accounts for ~8% of early-onset breast cancer in that ethnic group. A single mutation—the Icelandic founder mutation c.771_775del5 (BIC: 999del5)—accounts for the majority of Icelandic early-onset familial breast cancer.

Many missense mutations in *BRCA1/2* are of uncertain significance; most will not be pathogenic. Reference to websites may help with interpretation. Multifactorial analysis of data supporting variant classification is important. Since breast cancer is a common disease, there is a stronger possibility than with a rare disease that an observed rare variant may be coincidental, rather than causative.

Somatic testing in tumours has identified a mutational signature suggestive of 'BRCAness' in a higher proportion of tumours than based on germline testing alone. This may be useful for targeted therapies such as PARP inhibition (Davies 2017).

Cancer risks associated with BRCA1

(See Figure 4.1.) Female carriers with a mutation in *BRCA1* have an average risk of breast cancer to age 70 of 65% (range 44–78%), and a 39% (range 18–54%) average risk to age 70 of ovarian cancer (including the Fallopian tubes) (see 'Patterns of cancer' in 'Appendix', p. 846). Where there are multiple affected family members, the risk estimates from the upper end of these ranges are likely to be appropriate due to co-inheritance of possible modifier genes and shared environmental exposure. The relative risk of breast cancer in *BRCA1* carriers, relative to the general population, declines with age from >30-fold below the age of 40 years to 14-fold above the age of 60 years. As a consequence, the incidence of breast cancer diagnosis in *BRCA1* carriers rise to a plateau of ~3–4% per annum in the 40–49 year age group. There is a high risk of contralateral breast cancer in affected carriers; this is highest with age at first diagnosis <40 years and lower with increasing age at first diagnosis. Ovarian

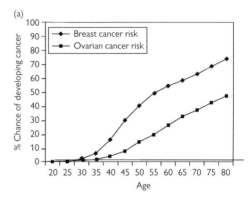

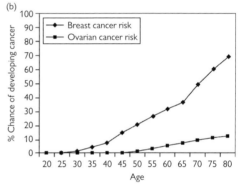

Figure 4.1 (a) *BRCA1*. (b) *BRCA2*.

cancer risks in *BRCA1* carriers are more evenly spread across the age range although increase gradually with increasing age from about 1% per annum at younger ages (40–59 years) and rising to 2% per annum at older ages. For the Ashkenazi founder mutations, the average risk of breast cancer by the age of 70 years is similar for carriers of the *BRCA1* c.68_69delAG and c.5266dupC mutations (64% and 67%, respectively); however, it is much lower for the c.5946delT mutation (43%). The corresponding values for ovarian cancer lifetime risk is 14%, 33%, and 20% in carriers, respectively.

Cancer risks associated with BRCA2

(See Figure 4.1.) Female carriers of a mutation in *BRCA2* have a 45% (CI, 31–56%) risk of breast cancer to age of 70 years and an 11% (CI, 2.4–19%) risk for ovarian cancer (including the Fallopian tubes). Where there are multiple affected family members, the risk estimates from the upper end of these ranges are likely to be appropriate due to co-inheritance of possible modifier genes and shared environmental exposure. The relative risk of breast cancer in *BRCA2* carriers is ~11-fold in all age groups above 40 years and is not significantly higher at younger ages. As a consequence of this, the incidence in *BRCA2* carriers show a pattern parallel to that in the general population, rising steeply up to the age of 50 years and more slowly thereafter. There is a high risk of contralateral breast cancer in affected carriers. Ovarian cancer risks in *BRCA2* carriers are, in contrast, low below the age of 50 years but then increase sharply in the 50–59 year age group. Male mutation carriers are also at increased risk of breast cancer (~6% by 70 years).

BRCA2 mutation carriers are also at increased risk of prostate and pancreatic cancers and possibly also gall bladder/bile duct cancers. The cumulative risk for prostate cancer is 0.1% by the age of 50 years, 1.6% by the age of 60 years, 7.5% by the age of 70 years, and 19.8% by the age of 80 years, and the cumulative risk for all cancers in male mutation carriers is 4% by the age of 50 years, 13% by the age of 60 years, and 32% by the age of 70 years.

Triple-negative breast cancer (TNBC) (oestrogen receptor-, progesterone receptor-, HER2-negative breast cancer)

Accounts for ~12–15% of all breast cancers. In a series of >1800 patients diagnosed with TNBC, but unselected for a family history of breast or ovarian cancer, 8.5% were found to have mutations in *BRCA1*, 2.7% in *BRCA2*, and 1.2% in *PALB2* (Couch et al. 2015).

Clinical approach

History: key points

• Three-generation family tree, with specific enquiry for breast, ovarian, prostate, and other associated cancers.

NB. Benign ovarian tumours, borderline and mucinous malignant tumours, and germ cell tumours are not associated—*BRCA1/2* mutations are mainly associated with serous papillary cystadenocarcinomas. This is important because mucinous and borderline tumours, in particular, are more common at younger ages and the history of ovarian cancer without the pathology can be misleading.

Examination: key points

Usually not necessary for evaluation purposes.

Genetic advice

Counsel a *BRCA1/2* carrier regarding the risks to his/her own health (see Tables 4.1 and 4.2) and arrange appropriate screening and/or risk-reducing surgery

Table 4.1 Table showing risk of cancer by age in *BRCA1/2* carriers

Age (years)	Risk (%) in *BRCA1* carrier of		Risk (%) in *BRCA2* carrier of	
	Breast cancer	Ovarian cancer	Breast cancer	Ovarian cancer
25	0	1	0	0
30	2	1	1	0
35	7	2	4	0
40	16	4	7	0
45	30	8	14	0
50	41	15	20	1
55	50	20	26	3
60	55	27	31	5
65	59	33	36	7
70	64	38	49	9
75	69	43	60	11
80	74	48	69	12

Table 4.2 Cumulative risk of contralateral breast cancer in *BRCA1*, *BRCA2* mutation carriers

	Years since initial breast cancer diagnosis		
	5 years (%)	10 years (%)	20 years (%)
BRCA1 mutation carriers	10.4	25.7	44.4
BRCA2 mutation carriers	6.8	19.5	48.1
Overall	8.6	22.3	45.7

Quoted values are from the adjusted Kaplan–Meier models, which account for delayed entry

Reproduced from *Familial Cancer*, Risk of contralateral breast cancer in BRCA1 and BRCA2 mutation carriers: a 30-year semi-prospective analysis, 14, 4, 2015, pp. 531–538, N.N. Basu et al., © 2017 Springer International Publishing AG. Part of Springer Nature. With permission of Springer.

(Lobb and Meiser 2004). Identify other 'at-risk' members of the family and ensure that the offer of genetic advice, screening, and/or predictive testing is made available to all at-risk relatives from an appropriate age in early adult life.

Penetrance

Please see Table 4.1.

New primary cancer risks

Women who have already had a breast cancer and are found to carry a *BRCA1* or *BRCA2* mutation, will have a higher likelihood of developing a second primary breast cancer and an increased lifetime risk of ovarian cancer. Non-carriers have about a 0.6% risk of developing a new primary breast cancer per annum, *BRCA1* and *BRCA2* carriers with young onset primary cancer have a 2–3% risk per annum. Women should have the opportunity to review their estimated future new primary cancer risks (both ovarian and breast) but this is not necessary as part of their primary cancer treatment. Oncological and genetic risks should be discussed in a multidisciplinary setting; the likelihood of a new primary must be considered in the context of the presenting cancer, its treatment and prognosis. Salpingo-oophorectomy may be appropriate as part of treatment of an oestrogen receptor positive breast cancer. Bilateral mastectomy is not a necessary part of primary cancer treatment and completing all the recommended oncological treatment should take precedence over major reconstructive surgery.

Risk reducing surgery aimed at reducing the risk of future new primary cancers should be considered at an appropriate time depending on age at diagnosis, sub-type of breast cancer, other treatment and likely prognosis.

Predictive testing

When a familial mutation has been defined, predictive testing can be offered to members of the extended family. Since the consequences of the results are profound, this should ideally be done through a clinical genetics service.

Management

Previous studies have reported a breast cancer risk reduction of ~50% after risk-reducing salpingo-oophorectomy in *BRCA1/2* carriers (e.g. Domchek et al. 2010) but may have been subject to several types of bias. Using a study that maximally eliminated bias,

Heemskerk-Gerritsen *et al.* (2015) found no evidence for a protective effect on breast cancer risk. The actual magnitude of risk reduction that might be achieved as a result of a surgically induced premature menopause is still unclear and is either non-existent or much smaller than previously thought.

Since there is no proven method of screening to detect early stages of ovarian cancer, women at high risk may wish to discuss and consider this intervention once their families are complete to address their ovarian cancer risk. The latest NICE guidelines (2013) advise that the health benefits of oestrogen replacement are likely to outweigh any small increase in breast cancer risk due to hormonal exposure. Ideally replacement should consider options for oestrogen-only therapy with topical (intrauterine) delivery of progesterone to protect the endometrium for women who still have a uterus.

Prophylactic mastectomy
Domchek *et al.* (2010), in a prospective multicentre cohort study of 2482 *BRCA1/2* carriers, found no breast cancers in the 247 women with risk-reducing mastectomy, compared with 98 in the 1372 who did not have a risk-reducing mastectomy.

Prophylactic mastectomy is a highly personal decision. Up to 30% of women who undergo the procedure will have surgical complications. The protective effects must be weighed against possible surgical complications and psychological problems and the toxicity of treatment and the chance of dying from a diagnosed breast cancer.

Chemoprevention
Various agents are under trial. A retrospective case analysis showed that treatment of *BRCA1* and *BRCA2* mutation carriers with tamoxifen after surgery for breast cancer reduced the incidence of cancer in the contralateral breast by 50% (Phillips *et al.* 2013).

Physical exercise and avoidance of obesity in adolescence
King *et al.* (2003), in a large study of Ashkenazi Jewish women with inherited mutations in *BRCA1/2*, found that physical exercise and lack of obesity in adolescence were associated with significantly delayed breast cancer onset.

Oral contraceptive pill (OCP)
A case-control study (Narod *et al.* 1998) showed a 60% reduction in frequency of ovarian cancer after 6 years of use, but there are concerns that OCPs could also increase the risk of breast cancer in women with a family history of the disease. Narod *et al.* (2002) have shown that women who are *BRCA1* mutation carriers who have ever used the OCP, or who used the OCP for >5 years, may have an increased risk for early-onset breast cancer (RR 1.2 and 1.33, respectively).

Surveillance strategies
See also 'Cancer surveillance methods' in Chapter 4, 'Cancer', p. 552 especially Table 4.6.
- Mammographic breast screening reduces breast cancer-associated mortality in women in the general population in the age group of 50–65 years.
- Breast USS is used diagnostically to evaluate palpable breast lumps or mammographic abnormalities. Sometimes used for screening very young women (<30 years of age) with a very early-onset family history, but there is no clinical evidence base for using it as a screening tool. It will not detect microcalcification.

- Breast MRI may be more sensitive but less specific than mammography. MRI improves early breast cancer detection in *BRCA* mutation carriers aged <50 years and is recommended for annual surveillance in most guidelines.
- Breast awareness. Women should be advised to be 'breast-aware'; most women with breast cancer find their own lump.
- CA125 (cancer antigen 125) screening and ovarian USS. Of unproven efficacy as a screening method.

Support group: Breast Cancer Now, http://www.breastcancernow.org.

Expert adviser: Diana Eccles, Head of Cancer Sciences, Faculty of Medicine, University Hospital Southampton, Southampton, UK.

References
Antoniou A, Pharoah PD, Narod S, *et al.* Average risks of breast and ovarian cancer associated with mutations in *BRCA1* or *BRCA2* detected in case series unselected for family history: a combined analysis of 22 studies. *Am J Hum Genet* 2003; **72**: 1117–30.

Basu NN, Ingham S, *et al.* Risk of contralateral breast cancer in BRCA1 and BRCA2 mutation carriers: a 30 year semi-prospective analysis. *Fam Cancer* 2015; **14**: 531.

Breast Cancer Information Core (BIC). https://research.nhgri.nih.gov/bic.

Breast Cancer Linkage Consortium. Cancer risks in *BRCA2* mutation carriers. *J Natl Cancer Inst* 1999; **91**: 1310–16.

Couch FJ, Hart SN, Sharma P, *et al.* Inherited mutations in 17 breast cancer susceptibility genes among a large triple-negative breast cancer cohort unselected for family history of breast cancer. *J Clin Oncol* 2015; **33**: 304–11.

Davies H, Glodzik D, *et al.* HRDetect is a predictor of BRCA1 and BRCA2 deficiency based on utational signatures. *Nat Med* 2017; epub Mar13.

Domchek SM, Friebel TM, Singer CF, *et al.* Association of risk-reducing surgery in BRCA1 or BRCA2 mutation carriers with cancer risk and mortality. *JAMA* 2010; **304**: 967–75.

Eisen A, Weber BL. Prophylactic mastectomy for women with BRCA1 and BRCA2 mutations—facts and controversy [editorial]. *N Engl J Med* 2001; **345**: 207–8.

Heemskerk-Gerritsen BA, Seynaeve C, van Asperen CJ, *et al.* Breast cancer risk after salpingo-oophorectomy in healthy BRCA1/2 mutation carriers: revisiting the evidence for risk reduction. *J Natl Cancer Inst* 2015; **107**: pii: djv033.

Kauff ND, Satogopan JM, Robson ME, *et al.* Risk-reducing salpingo-oophorectomy in women with a BRCA1 or BRCA2 mutation. *N Engl J Med* 2002; **346**: 1609–15.

Kennedy RD, Quinn JE, Johnston PG, Harkin DP. BRCA1: mechanisms of inactivation and implications for management of patients [review]. *Lancet* 2002; **360**: 1007–14.

King MC, Marks JH, Mandell JB; New York Breast Cancer Study Group. Breast and ovarian cancer risks due to inherited mutations in BRCA1 and BRCA2. *Science* 2003; **302**: 643–6.

Kriege M, Brekelmans CT, Boetes C, *et al.* Efficacy of MRI and mammography for breast cancer screening in women with a familial or genetic predisposition. *N Engl J Med* 2004; **351**: 427–37.

Leach MO, Boggis CR, Dixon AK, *et al.*; MARIBS study group. Screening with magnetic resonance imaging and mammography of a UK population at high familial risk of breast cancer: a prospective multicentre cohort study (MARIBS). *Lancet* 2005; **365**: 1769–78.

Liberman L. Breast cancer screening with MRI—what are the data for patients at high risk? *N Engl J Med* 2004; **351**: 497–500.

Lobb E, Meiser B. Genetic counseling and prophylactic surgery in women from families with hereditary breast or ovarian cancer [commentary]. *Lancet* 2004; **363**: 1841–2.

Miller AB, To T, Baines CJ, Wall C. Canadian National Breast Screening Study-2: 13-year results of a randomized trial in women aged 50–59 years. *J Natl Cancer Inst* 2000; **92**: 1490–9.

Narod S. What options for treatment of hereditary breast cancer? [editorial]. *Lancet* 2002; **359**: 1451.

Narod SA, Brunet JS, Ghadirian P, et al. Tamoxifen and risk of contralateral breast cancer in *BRCA1* and *BRCA2* mutation carriers: a case-control study. *Lancet* 2000; **356**: 1876–81.

Narod SA, Dube MP, Klijn J, et al. Oral contraceptives and the risk of breast cancer in *BRCA1* and *BRCA2* mutation carriers. *J Natl Cancer Inst* 2002; **94**: 1773–9.

Narod SA, Risch H, Moslehi R, et al. Oral contraceptives and the risk of hereditary ovarian cancer. *N Engl J Med* 1998; **339**: 424–8.

National Institute for Health and Care Excellence. *Familial breast cancer: classification, care and managing breast cancer and related risks in people with a family history of breast cancer.* Clinical guideline CG164, 2013. https://www.nice.org.uk/Guidance/CG164.

Phillips KA, Milne RL, Rookus MA, et al. Tamoxifen and the risk of contralateral breast cancer for *BRCA1* and *BRCA2* mutation carriers. *J Clin Oncol* 2013; **25**: 3091–9.

Rebbeck TR, Lynch HT, Neuhausen SL, et al. Prophylactic oophorectomy in carrieras of *BRCA1* or *BRCA2* mutations. *N Engl J Med* 2002; **346**: 1616–22.

Tabar L, Fagerberg G, Chen HH, et al. Efficacy of breast cancer screening by age. New results from the Swedish Two-County Trial. *Cancer* 1995; **75**: 2507–17.

Teh W, Wilson AR. The role of ultrasound in breast cancer screening. A consensus statement by the European Group for Breast Cancer Screening. *Eur J Cancer* 1998; **34**: 449–50.

Warner E, Plewes DB, Shumak RS, et al. Comparison of breast magnetic resonance imaging, mammography, and ultrasound for surveillance of women at high risk for hereditary breast cancer. *J Clin Oncol* 2001; **19**: 3524–31.

Breast cancer

Breast cancer is the most common form of cancer affecting women. The cumulative incidence of breast cancer in developed countries is 6.3 per 100 women by the age of 70 years, with a lifetime risk of ~10–12%. The western diet is associated both with earlier menarche and with post-menopausal obesity, which, combined with low parity, later first childbirth, and shorter/absent breast-feeding, perhaps largely account for the much higher incidence of breast cancer in the developed world than in many developing countries.

A family history of breast cancer is the strongest known risk factor for breast cancer (other than age)—having an affected first-degree relative approximately doubles a woman's risk. High-risk, highly penetrant Mendelian genes account for only ~20% of the familial relative risk. At a population level, there is a major contribution from weaker genetic susceptibility factors and environmental influences and a modest contribution from moderate-risk genes (see Box. 4.1 for the classification of genes predisposing to breast cancer).

Polygenic breast cancer risk

There are over 100 common genetic variants in non-coding DNA that are associated with small increases in breast cancer risk and evidence that the true number of associated common variants is closer to a thousand, with each individual variant associated with a very small increase in risk. Many familial clusters of breast cancer (or other common cancers) arise on a background of polygenic susceptibility. Mavaddat et al. (2015) modeled the effect on lifetime breast cancer risk of a panel of 77 known susceptibility SNPs. Lifetime risk of breast cancer for women in the lowest and highest quintiles of the polygenic risk score, based on these 77 SNPs, were 5.2% and 16.6%, respectively, for a woman without a family history, and 8.6% and 24.4%, respectively, for a woman with a first-degree family history of breast cancer.

Gene panels for breast cancer

Due to the number of genes and variants potentially predisposing to breast cancer, cancer gene panels are being used more widely. The clinical utility of many of the genes available in these panels is unclear due to rarity and lack of sufficient evidence on which to base reliable lifetime penetrance estimates (Easton et al. 2015). Caution should be exercised when evaluating the clinical actionability of variants in genes with limited aggregate data. Overestimation of risk is likely, due to biases in the selection of cases for research studies.

Factors proven to affect breast cancer risk in the general population

Pregnancy and parity
Breast cancer incidence is transiently increased by pregnancy but is permanently lowered by high parity. The relative risk (RR) of breast cancer decreases by 7% for each birth. Breast cancer incidence is reduced by early first childbirth. Women having their first child at >30 years have double the risk of women having their first child at <20 years.

Breastfeeding
The longer women breastfeed, the more they are protected against breast cancer. The lack of, or short duration of, breastfeeding, typical of women in developed countries, makes a major contribution to the high incidence of breast cancer in these countries. The RR of breast cancer decreases by 4.3% for every 12 months of breastfeeding. This is in addition to a decrease of 7.0% for each birth. This protective effect is more marked in women having an earlier first pregnancy.

Menarche and menopause
Cumulative breast cancer incidence is permanently lowered by late menarche and early menopause.

Obesity
Obesity is associated with an increased risk for post-menopausal breast cancer. Regular physical activity probably reduces the risk of breast cancer, although the quantitative effect is uncertain and the evidence is weak.

Alcohol
Compared with non-drinkers, the RR of breast cancer among women drinking 35–44 g of alcohol/day was 1.32, and for ≥45 g of alcohol/day was 1.46. The RR increased by 7% for each additional 10 g/day (i.e. for each unit or drink of alcohol consumed on a daily basis).

Box 4.1 Classification of genes predisposing to breast cancer

High risk (lifetime risk 40%+)
BRCA1 (see 'BRCA1 and BRCA2' in Chapter 4, 'Cancer', p. 542), BRCA2 (see 'BRCA1 and BRCA2' in Chapter 4, 'Cancer', p. 542), TP53 (see 'Li–Fraumeni syndrome (LFS)' in Chapter 4, 'Cancer', p. 584), PTEN (see 'Cowden syndrome (PTEN hamartoma tumour syndrome (PHTS))' in Chapter 4, 'Cancer', p. 564), CDH1 (see 'Gastric cancer' in Chapter 4, 'Cancer', p. 574), STK11 (see 'Peutz–Jeghers syndrome (PJS)' in Chapter 4, 'Cancer', p. 604), PALB2

Moderate risk (lifetime risk 20–39%+)
CHEK2, ATM (see 'DNA repair disorders' in Chapter 3, 'Common consultations', p. 398), NBN, RAD50, NF1 (see 'Neurofibromatosis type 1 (NF1)' in Chapter 3, 'Common consultations', p. 506), MLH1 (see 'Lynch syndrome (LS)' in Chapter 4, 'Cancer', p. 586), PIK3CA, MRE11, XRCC2
(Three genes originally reported as moderate-risk breast cancer genes have now been discounted—BRIP1, RAD51C, and RAD51D—but they are still considered to be moderate-risk ovarian cancer genes.)

Low-risk predisposition alleles (13–19%)
Over 100 common SNPs have been associated with small increases in risk and act in a multiplicative fashion (see 'Polygenic breast cancer risk' below).

The data suggest that ~4% of breast cancer in developed countries may be attributed to alcohol.

Oral contraceptive pill (OCP)
A meta-analysis suggested that, both for current users and for up to 10 years post-use, there may be a 24% increase (RR, 1.24) in the risk of breast cancer (Collaborative Group on Hormonal Factors in Breast Cancer 2002). Marchbanks et al. (2002) undertook a case-control analysis of 4575 women with breast cancer aged 35–64 years. Overall use of OCPs by women with a family history of breast cancer (affected mother, sister, or daughter) was *not* associated with an increased risk of breast cancer (OR, 0.8). In Marchbanks et al.'s (2002) study, the RR of breast cancer in women aged 35–44 years with a family history of breast cancer and who had ever used OCPs was higher (1.4) than among older women (45–64 years) with a family history, but this difference did not reach significance. Narod et al. (2002) have shown that women who are *BRCA1* mutation carriers who have ever used the OCP or who used the OCP for ≥5 years may have an increased risk of early-onset breast cancer (RR, 1.2 and 1.33, respectively).

Hormone replacement therapy (HRT)
For women in the general population, post-menopausal combined oestrogen and progestin replacement therapy results in an increased risk of breast cancer of 5% per year of use. The risk is substantially higher for combined HRT than for oestrogen replacement therapy alone and does not appear to be influenced by a family history of breast cancer in a first-degree relative (mother, sister, daughter; Ursin et al. 2002). The added risk disappears within ~5 years of cessation of use. In the Million Women Study of breast cancer and HRT (Beral 2003), current users were more likely than never users to develop breast cancer (RR, 1.66), with the risk increasing with the total duration of use. Ten years of HRT use is estimated to result in 19 additional breast cancers per 1000 users of oestrogen–progesterone combinations compared with five additional breast cancers per 1000 users of oestrogen-only preparations. Oestrogen only replacement therapy can lead to endometrial hypertrophy and is only used where a woman has had a hysterectomy or has topical uterine protection (intrauterine device) with progesterone.

Factors suggesting a familial susceptibility gene
* Large number of individuals with breast/ovarian/prostate cancer in the family (on one side of the family).
* Multiple generations affected.
* Young average age at which the breast cancers were diagnosed (>25% of breast cancers diagnosed at <30 years is due to a mutation in a dominant gene; 50% of all breast cancers in the general population are diagnosed after 65 years of age).
* Pattern of different types of cancers occurring within the family.
* Multiple primary cancers in one individual with early age of onset (usually first primary at <50 years).

The combined contribution of *BRCA1* on 17q and *BRCA2* on 13q to overall breast cancer is 2–3%. Close to 10% of women diagnosed with hormone- and HER2 receptor-negative breast cancer before 50 years of age with no known family history will carry a pathogenic *BRCA1* or *BRCA2* variant (Couch et al. 2015). Breast cancer-only families are less likely than breast and ovarian-cancer families to have arisen due to *BRCA1* or *BRCA2* mutations. The probability of a *BRCA1/BRCA2* gene mutation being the main causative factor increases with increasing numbers of affected relatives, younger relatives, and high-grade and receptor-negative breast cancers. Mucinous ovarian cancers are not part of the *BRCA1/2* spectrum of cancers so would not count as affected in assessing the likelihood of detecting a *BRCA1/2* pathogenic variant.

Breast cancer in males
Breast cancer in men is rare, accounting for ~0.8% of diagnoses of all breast cancers. Risk factors include testicular atrophy, benign breast conditions, age, Jewish ancestry, family history, and Klinefelter's syndrome (Giordano et al. 2002). *BRCA2* mutations predispose men to breast cancer and may account for 4–14% of all cases and confers a lifetime risk of ~8%. Most isolated cases of male breast cancer are not due to a *BRCA2* mutation.

Clinical approach
History: key points
* Detailed three-generation family tree, noting in affected relatives their full name and date of birth, the type of cancer, age at diagnosis of cancer, hospital where treated, and, when relevant, age at death. Extend the family tree back as far as possible on the relevant side of the family. Ask questions about the type of treatment relatives have had, as such information may give a clue as to how accurate the reported cancer diagnosis is likely to be.
* Check ancestry. Three founder mutations in *BRCA1/2* in the Ashkenazi Jewish population occur with a combined frequency of 2.5% and may account for >90% of highly penetrant families in that population. There are also founder mutations in many other populations e.g. Iceland and Poland. Founder mutation testing may be appropriate in unaffected individuals in certain circumstances (see 'BRCA1 and BRCA2' in Chapter 4, 'Cancer', p. 542 to the end of the paragraph).

Examination: key points
Examination rarely gives diagnostic information, except where a rare condition, such as Cowden syndrome or Peutz–Jeghers syndrome (PJS), is suspected.

Special investigations
* Confirmation of diagnosis. Reported cases of breast cancer in close relatives are rarely wrong, but it is helpful to know what type of breast cancer, e.g. triple-negative increases the probability of *BRCA1*, low-grade or HER2-amplified both less likely to be *BRCA1*. Reported cases of ovarian cancer, even in close relatives, are often wrong (e.g. cervical, endometrial) or may be of a type (e.g. mucinous or borderline) that can be discounted in evaluating the likely risk of a familial cancer predisposition syndrome. Aim to confirm all diagnoses of ovarian cancer and at least one diagnosis of breast cancer in a family where management decisions hinge on the risk assessment.
* DNA analysis: *BRCA1* and *BRCA2* analysis in a breast or ovarian cancer affected family member (where possible) is indicated based on a >10% probability of finding a pathogenic variant (using BOADICEA analysis a Manchester score of ≥16 to estimate the carrier probability).

Table 4.3 Table showing breast cancer risk categories on which genetic investigation and surveillance decisions are based

	Breast cancer risk category		
	Near population risk	Moderate risk	High risk[1]
Lifetime risk from age 20	<17%	>17% but <30%	30% or greater
Risk between ages 40 and 50	<3%	3–8%	>8%

[1] This group includes known BRCA1, BRCA2, and *TP53* mutations and rare conditions that carry an increased risk of breast cancer such as Peutz–Jeghers syndrome (STK11), Cowden (*PTEN*), and familial diffuse gastric cancer (E-cadherin).

National Institute for Health and Care Excellence (2013) CG 164 Familial breast cancer: Classification and care of people at risk of familial breast cancer and management of breast cancer and related risks in people with a family history of breast cancer. Manchester: NICE. Available from www.nice.org.uk/CG164. Reproduced with permission. Information accurate at time of press. For up-to-date information, please visit www.nice.org.uk.

- Consider DNA storage from a key affected individual if she/he has advanced cancer.
- For Ashkenazi Jewish individuals, one or more relative with breast or ovarian cancer at any age can be offered testing for the Ashkenazi mutations only.
- Women with triple-negative breast cancer <40 years or high-grade serous ovarian cancer without a family history have >10% chance of a *BRCA1/2* mutation, so testing should be offered (Eccles *et al.* 2016).

Genetic advice

Risk assessment

Typically risk is stratified into three classes: near-population risk, moderate risk, and high risk. These classes inform whether genetic investigations are undertaken and what level of surveillance is advised (see Table 4.3 showing breast cancer risk categories on which genetic investigation and surveillance decisions are based).

Where possible, use a carrier probability calculation method with a demonstrated acceptable performance (calibration and discrimination) to determine an individualized risk. The Breast and Ovarian Analysis of Disease Incidence and Carrier Estimation Algorithm (BOADICEA) is freely available software that is used to calculate the risks of breast and ovarian cancers in women based on their family history. It is also used to calculate the probability that they are carriers of cancer-associated mutations in the BRCA1, BRCA2, and other genes (Lee *et al.* 2016) (http://ccge.medschl.cam.ac.uk/boadicea).

Where it is not possible to use BOADICEA or an equivalent program, the Manchester score based on the family history, preferably supplemented with histology, can be used to determine eligibility for *BRCA1/2* testing (see Table 4.4 for the Manchester scoring system and Table 4.5 for adjustments), and the triaging system based on family history outlined in Box 4.2 can be used to determine the class of risk for surveillance.

Penetrance

See discussion in 'BRCA1 and BRCA2' in Chapter 4, 'Cancer', p. 542.

Table 4.4 Manchester scoring system

Cancer and patient age	BRCA1	BRCA2
FBC <30	6	5
FBC 30–39	4	4
FBC 40–49	3	3
FBC 50–59	2	2
FBC >59	1	1
MBC <60	5 (if *BRCA2* tested); for combined, score = 5 without prior testing	8
MBC >59	5 (if *BRCA2* tested); for combined, score = 5 without prior testing	5
Ovarian cancer <60	8	5 (if *BRCA1* tested); for combined, score = 5 without prior testing
Ovarian cancer >59	5	5 (if *BRCA1* tested); for combined, score = 5 without prior testing
Pancreatic cancer	0	1
Prostate cancer <60	0	2
Prostate cancer >59	0	1

Scores are added for each cancer in a direct blood lineage (cancers on the same side of the family). The combined score is determined by adding both the *BRCA1* and *BRCA2* scores without consideration for prior testing, thus MBC scores 5 points for *BRCA1*, and ovarian cancer 5 for *BRCA2*. A combined score of 16 points can be used as a 10% threshold, and 20 points as a 20% threshold in non-founder Western populations. In families with no unaffected family members, a lower threshold could be used. Other tumour types, such as cholangiocarcinoma and ocular melanoma, can contribute to the *BRCA2* score, but the numbers of these tumours is too low to validate a precise score.

FBC, female breast cancer; MBC, male breast cancer.

Reproduced from *Journal of Medical Genetics*, Evans DGR, Eccles DM, et al., A new scoring system for the chances of identifying a *BRCA1/2* mutation outperforms existing models including BRACAPRO, 41(6):474–80, copyright 2004, with permission from BMJ Publishing Group Ltd.

Predictive testing

Possible if there is a known familial mutation. Usually only offered to adults and often deferred until a time at which surveillance may be initiated or intervention such as risk-reducing surgery may be considered.

Management

Breast awareness

A large, well-conducted population-based randomized controlled trial from Shanghai (Thomas *et al.* 2002) shows conclusively that regular breast self-examination does not lead to a reduction in mortality due to breast cancer, compared to no screening at all. Furthermore, women who regularly self-examined had more breast biopsies and diagnoses of benign breast disease than women who did not. 'Breast awareness' should be encouraged instead, so that women understand the importance of seeking prompt advice if they notice any unusual changes in their breasts.

Table 4.5 Calculated adjustments to the Manchester score for predicting *BRCA1* and *BRCA2* mutations according to pathology and receptor status of breast cancer in the index case and the presence of ovarian cancer in the family

Pathology	*BRCA1* adjustment	*BRCA2* adjustment	Notes
Breast			
Her2 +ve	−4*	0	No other alteration to score on basis of pathology needed
Lobular	−2	0	Add or subtract ER status
DCIS only (no invasive cancer)	−1	0	Add or subtract ER status
LCIS only (no invasive cancer)	−4*	0	No other adjustment
Grade 1 IDC	−2	0	Add or subtract ER status
Grade 2 IDC	0	0	Add or subtract ER status
Grade 3 IDC	+2	0	Add or subtract ER status
ER +ve	−1	0	Add or subtract grade
ER −ve	+1	0	Add or subtract grade
Grade 3 triple −ve	+4*	0	No other alteration to score on basis of pathology needed
Ovary			
Epithelial (endometrioid, serous, clear cell, NOS), granulosa cell	0 no change to score	0	No adjustment to ovarian score, i.e. 5 points for cancers >59 years for each gene
Mucinous	No score given for index case or other relative	No score given for index case or other relative	Do not include in scoring at all
Borderline	No score given for index case or other relative	No score given for index case or other relative	Do not include in scoring at all
Germ cell tumours, except granulosa cell	No score given for index case or other relative	No score given for index case or other relative	Do not include in scoring at all

* These adjustments are final, and no further adjustment based on other pathological features is necessary.

DCIS, ductal carcinoma *in situ*; ER, oestrogen receptor; IDC, invasive ductal carcinoma; LCIS, lobular carcinoma *in situ*; NOS, not otherwise specified.

Reproduced from *Journal of Medical Genetics*, Evans DG, Lalloo F, Cramer A, Jones E, Knox F, Amir E, Howell A, Addition of pathology and biomarker information significantly improves the performance of the Manchester scoring system for *BRCA1* and *BRCA2* testing, 46(12):811–7, copyright 2009, with permission from BMJ Publishing Group Ltd.

Box 4.2 Evaluating a family history of breast cancer (use BOADICEA or similar in preference, if accessible)

High risk (>30% lifetime risk, >8% risk between 40 and 50 years of age) criteria
• Clearly dominant pattern of early-onset breast and/or ovarian cancer with an affected first-degree relative
• First-degree relatives where the pattern is consistent with a diagnosis of Li–Fraumeni syndrome

High/moderate risk (25–30% lifetime risk, 5–8% risk between 40 and 50 years of age) criteria
• Clearly dominant pattern of breast and/or ovarian cancer with affected second-degree relatives on the paternal side of the family
• First-degree relative with breast and ovarian cancers with age at diagnosis of first cancer <50 years
• Three relatives diagnosed with breast cancer and/or ovarian cancer, with the breast cancer at average age of 50–60 years (1 in 4 risk) (6–7%)
• Two relatives (one first-degree) with breast cancer diagnosed <40 years

Moderate risk (17–24% lifetime risk, 3–5% risk between 40 and 50 years of age) criteria
• Two relatives diagnosed with breast cancer at any age
• One first-degree relative diagnosed with breast cancer <40 years
• One male relative diagnosed with breast cancer at any age
• One relative with both breast and ovarian cancers (diagnosed at any age)

Slightly increased risk (<1 in 6 lifetime risk) criteria
• One first-degree or a few distant relatives, with no clearly dominant pattern of inheritance and an average age at onset >50 years
• One first-degree relative diagnosed >40 years (assuming negative family history)

Population risk (1 in 11 lifetime risk) criterion
• No family history of breast or ovarian cancer and an average environmental risk profile (1%)

Adapted by permission from BMJ Publishing Group Limited. *Journal of Medical Genetics*, Eccles et al, Guidelines for a genetic risk based approach to advising women with a family history of breast cancer, vol 37, pp. 203–9, copyright 2000.

Women with a family history of breast cancer, with or without a personal history of breast cancer, who have a moderate to high risk of breast cancer on specialist risk estimation and who choose not to have risk-reducing mastectomy may benefit from radiological surveillance of their breasts.
- Ensure digital mammography and breast MRI are performed to national breast screening programme standards. MRI screening was shown to be more cost-effective than mammography for high-risk women with a known *BRCA* or *TP53* mutation or >30% probability of being a mutation carrier.
- Offer annual MRI to women aged 30–49, with or without a personal history of breast cancer, if they have a *BRCA1* or *BRCA2* mutation or have a >30% risk of being a *BRCA* carrier.
- Offer annual mammographic surveillance to women:
  - aged 40–49 years at moderate risk of breast cancer;
  - aged 40–59 years at high risk of breast cancer, but with a ≤30% probability of a *BRCA* or *TP53* mutation;
  - aged 40–59 years with a >30% probability of being a *BRCA* carrier;
  - aged 40–69 years with a known *BRCA1* or *BRCA2* mutation.
- Do not offer mammography to women aged <30 years or to women of any age with a known *TP53* mutation.
- Do not routinely offer USS surveillance to women at moderate or high risk of breast cancer, but consider it when MRI surveillance would normally be offered but is not suitable (e.g. because of claustrophobia) or when results of mammography or MRI are difficult to interpret.

Women at increased genetic risk should be encouraged to adopt healthy lifestyle advice such as weight control, exercise, and minimizing alcohol intake.
*See also Table 4.3, p. 553.

Reproduced from *The BMJ*, D Gareth Evans, John Graham, Susan O'Connell, Stephanie Arnold, Deborah Fitzsimmons, Familial breast cancer: summary of updated NICE guidance, volume 346, copyright 2013, with permission from BMJ Publishing Group Ltd.

Surveillance strategies
Screening should take place in properly conducted studies that are fully audited. NICE guidelines evidence the reasons for MRI in high-risk women. See also 'Cancer surveillance methods' in Chapter 4, 'Cancer', p. 552.

Mammographic surveillance
See Box 4.3.

Reassurance
Reassurance is currently the appropriate management for women where:
- there has been one family member diagnosed with breast cancer at age >40 years;
- there have been two family members diagnosed with breast cancer at age >60 years, *provided that* there has been no bilateral breast cancer, no male breast cancer, and no ovarian cancer.

Standard reassurance (Evans *et al.* 2013) should include written information giving:
- risk information about population level and family history levels of risk;
- breast awareness information;
- lifestyle advice about breast cancer risk, including information about HRT, OCPs, breastfeeding, lifestyle including achieving/maintaining a healthy body weight, restricting alcohol intake and increasing physical activity etc.;
- advice that, if the family history changes, the genetics team should be contacted for an update of the risk assessment.

Support groups: Breast Cancer Now, http://www.breastcancernow.org; The Hereditary Breast Cancer Helpline, http://www.breastcancergenetics. co.uk; Macmillan Cancer Support, https://www.macmillan.org.uk.

Expert advisers: Diana Eccles, Head of Cancer Sciences, Faculty of Medicine, University Hospital Southampton, Southampton, UK and Gareth Evans, Consultant, Manchester Centre for Genomic Medicine, Division of Evolution and Genomic Sciences, St Mary's Hospital, University of Manchester, Manchester, UK.

References
Antoniou A, Pharoah PD, Narod S, et al. Average risks of breast and ovarian cancer associated with mutations in BRCA1 or BRCA2 detected in case series unselected for family history: a combined analysis of 22 studies. Am J Hum Genet 2003; **72**: 1117–30.

Beral V; Million Women Study Collaborators. Breast cancer and hormone-replacement therapy in the Million Women Study. Lancet 2003; **362**: 419–27.

Collaborative Group on Hormonal Factors in Breast Cancer. Breast cancer and breastfeeding: collaborative reanalysis of individual data from 47 epidemiological studies in 30 countries, including 50302 women with breast cancer and 96973 women without the disease. Lancet 2002; **360**: 187–95.

Couch FJ, Hart SN, Sharma P, et al. Inherited mutations in 17 breast cancer susceptibility genes among a large triple-negative breast cancer cohort unselected for family history of breast cancer. J Clin Oncol 2015; **33**: 304–11.

Easton DF, Pharoah PD, Antoniou AC, et al. Gene-panel sequencing and the prediction of breast-cancer risk. N Engl J Med 2015; **372**: 2243–57.

Eccles DM, Balmaôa J, Clune J, et al. Selecting patients with ovarian cancer for germline BRCA mutation testing: findings from guidelines and a systematic literature review. Adv Ther 2016; **33**:129–50.

Evans DG, Eccles DM, Rahman N, et al. A new scoring system for the chances of identifying a BRCA1/2 mutation outperforms existing models including BRACAPRO. J Med Genet 2004; **41**: 474–80.

Evans DG, Graham J, O'Connell S, Arnold S, Fitzsimmons D. Familial breast cancer: summary of updated NICE guidance *BMJ* 2013; **346**: f3829.

Evans DG, Kesavan N, Lim Y, *et al.*; MARIBS Group, Howell A, Duffy S. MRI breast screening in high-risk women: cancer detection and survival analysis. *Breast Cancer Res Treat* 2014; **145**: 663–72.

Evans DG, Lalloo F, Cramer A, *et al* Addition of pathology and biomarker information significantly improves the performance of the Manchester scoring system for *BRCA1* and *BRCA2* testing. *J Med Genet* 2009; **46**: 811–17.

FH01 collaborative teams. Mammographic surveillance in women younger than 50 years who have a family history of breast cancer: tumour characteristics and projected effect on mortality in the prospective, single-arm, FH01 study. *Lancet Oncol* 2010; **11**: 1127–34.

Giordano SH, Buzdar AU, Hortobagyi GN. Breast cancer in men. *Ann Intern Med* 2002: **137**: 678–87.

Hamajima N, Hirose K, Tajima K, *et al.* Alcohol, tobacco and breast cancer—collaborative reanalysis of individual data from 53 epidemiological studies, including 58,515 women with breast cancer and 95,067 women without the disease. *Br J Cancer* 2002; **87**: 1234–45.

Leach MO, Boggis CR, Dixon AK, *et al*; MARIBS study group. Screening with magnetic resonance imaging and mammography of a UK population at high familial risk of breast cancer: a prospective multicentre cohort study (MARIBS). *Lancet* 2005; **365**: 1769–78.

Lee AJ, Cunningham AP, Kuchenbaecker KB, *et al.* BOADICEA breast cancer risk prediction model: updates to cancer incidences, tumour pathology and web interface. *Br J Cancer* 2014; **110**: 535–45.

Marchbanks PA, McDonald JA, Wilson HG, *et al.* Oral contraceptives and the risk of breast cancer. *N Engl J Med* 2002; **346**: 2025–32.

Mavaddat N, Pharoah PD, Michailidou K, *et al.* Prediction of breast cancer risk based on profiling with common genetic variants. *J Natl Cancer Inst* 2015; **107**: pii: djv036.

Narod SA, Dube MP, Klijn J, *et al.* Oral contraceptives and the risk of breast cancer in *BRCA1* and *BRCA2* mutation carriers. *J Natl Cancer Inst* 2002; **94**: 1773–9.

National Institute for Health and Care Excellence. Familial breast cancer: classification, care and managing breast cancer and related risks in people with a family history of breast cancer. Clinical guideline CG164, 2013. https://www.nice.org.uk/Guidance/CG164.

Thomas DB, Gao DL, Ray RM, *et al.* Randomised trial of breast self-examination in Shanghai: final results. *J Natl Cancer Inst* 2002; **94**: 1445–57.

Ursin G, Tseng CC, Paganini-Hill A, *et al.* Does menopausal hormone replacement therapy interact with known factors to increase risk of breast cancer? *J Clin Oncol* 2002; **20**: 699–706.

Cancer surveillance methods

Gastrointestinal (GI) surveillance

Colonoscopy

Bleeding occurs in 30/10 000 colonoscopies; the perforation rate is 10/10 000 colonoscopies, and death results from 1/10 000 colonoscopies. Complications are more likely in the elderly and those with comorbidity or existing disease, e.g. ulcerative colitis, and also include sedative complications (NB. chest disease).

Patients scheduled for a colonoscopy have bowel preparation beforehand, consisting of a low-residue diet for 48 hours and then a liquid diet for 24 hours before the procedure, followed by laxatives, e.g. Picolax®. Most are lightly sedated for the procedure, which, although it is usually uncomfortable to some degree, is only rarely painful. If suspicious lesions are seen, they can be biopsied. Small polyps are usually excision-biopsied; those with a stalk can be snared; larger polyps can often be removed piecemeal if snaring is not possible. Polypectomy is painless but is associated with complications: perforation rate after polypectomy 22/10 000, post-polypectomy bleeding 89/10 000. Mortality after polypectomy is 3.9/10 000, with most fatalities arising in older patients.

Colonoscopy and flexible sigmoidoscopy are both more difficult in women who have had a hysterectomy and this should be discussed. It is a factor to consider in Lynch syndrome (see 'Lynch syndrome (LS)' in Chapter 4, 'Cancer', p. 586) where prophylactic hysterectomy may be considered in women who warrant frequent colonoscopy, because of their endometrial cancer risk.

NB. Colonoscopy will miss ~6% of polyps, usually those <1 cm (Postic et al. 2002).

The background rate of death from colorectal cancer (CRC) at age 50–54 years is 1.8/10 000).

Flexible sigmoidoscopy

Requires less bowel preparation than a colonoscopy (e.g. a sachet of Picolax® on the day before the study or a phosphate mini-enema on the morning of the study). Reaches, at the most, as far as the splenic flexure. Procedure takes ~10 min and is usually performed without sedation. Polypectomy as for colonoscopy, except that if significant lesion/s are found (CRC, polyps larger than 5 mm, three or more adenomas, adenomas 5 mm or smaller with a villous component of >20%, or severe dysplasia), then a colonoscopy will be required to examine the rest of the colon. Flexible sigmoidoscopy may be of considerable utility for population screening but is not recommended as a surveillance method in familial CRC instead of colonoscopy (Atkin et al. 2010). It may be used in screening for polyps in familial adenomatous polyposis (FAP), but this will be as part of a surveillance programme also involving proctoscopy, rigid sigmoidoscopy, and colonoscopy.

Upper GI endoscopy

The complication rate of upper GI endoscopy performed for surveillance is unknown, largely because there is no evidence that it is efficacious, and hence the vast majority of such examinations are performed in symptomatic individuals for diagnosis. The complication rate associated with diagnostic upper GI endoscopy is necessarily high, because of the nature of diseases necessitating such examination, e.g. oesophageal varices, bleeding peptic ulcers, late-presenting cancers. Thus, for example, the death rate in the 30 days following such an examination is about 1/200. There is some evidence to suggest that establishing a baseline in conditions associated with upper GI polyposis is worthwhile, but that continuing upper GI surveillance should be restricted to those with the most severe disease.

Box 4.4 Surveillance for women with no personal history of breast cancer

Offer annual mammographic surveillance to women:
- aged 40–49 years at moderate risk of breast cancer;
- aged 40–59 years at high risk of breast cancer, but with a 30% or lower probability of being a *BRCA* or *TP53* carrier;
- aged 40–59 years who have not had genetic testing but have a >30% probability of being a *BRCA* carrier;
- aged 40–69 years with a known *BRCA1* or *BRCA2* mutation.
    Offer annual MRI surveillance to women:
- aged 30–49 years who have not had genetic testing but have a >30% probability of being a *BRCA1* carrier;
- aged 30–49 years with a known *BRCA1* or *BRCA2* mutation;
- aged 20–49 years who have not had genetic testing but have a >30% probability of being a *TP53* carrier;
- aged 20–49 years with a known *TP53* mutation.
    Surveillance for women with a personal and family history of breast cancer:
- offer annual mammographic surveillance to all women aged 50–69 years with a personal history of breast cancer who:
    - remain at high risk of breast cancer (including those who have a *BRCA1* or *BRCA2* mutation), *and*
    - do not have a *TP53* mutation.
- offer annual MRI surveillance to all women aged 30–49 years with a personal history of breast cancer who remain at high risk of breast cancer, including those who have a *BRCA1* or *BRCA2* mutation.

National Institute for Health and Care Excellence (2013) CG 164 Familial breast cancer: Classification and care of people at risk of familial breast cancer and management of breast cancer and related risks in people with a family history of breast cancer. Manchester: NICE. Available from www.nice.org.uk/CG164. Reproduced with permission. Information accurate at time of press. For up-to-date information, please visit www.nice.org.uk.

Table 4.6 Surveillance strategies for moderate- and high-risk breast cancer National Institute for Health and Care Excellence (2013) *CG164 Familial breast cancer: classification, care and managing breast cancer and related risks in people with a family history of breast cancer.* Available from www.nice.org.uk/CG164. Reproduced with permission. Information accurate at time of press. For up-to-date information, please visit www.nice.org.uk

	Moderate risk	High risk				
Age	Moderate risk of breast cancer[1]	High risk of breast cancer (but with a 30% or lower probability of being a BRCA or TP53 carrier)[2]	Untested but >30% BRCA carrier probability[3]	Known BRCA1 or BRCA2 mutation	Untested but >30% TP53 carrier probability[4]	Known TP53 mutation
20–29	Do not offer mammography	Do not offer mammography	Do not offer mammography	Do not offer mammography	Do not offer mammography	Do not offer mammography
	Do not offer MRI	Do not offer MRI	Do not offer MRI	Do not offer MRI	Annual MRI	Annual MRI
30–39	Do not offer mammography	Consider annual mammography	Annual MRI and consider annual mammography	Annual MRI and consider annual mammography	Do not offer mammography	Do not offer mammography
	Do not offer MRI	Do not offer MRI			Annual MRI	Annual MRI
40–49	Annual mammography	Annual mammography	Annual mammography and annual MRI	Annual mammography and annual MRI	Do not offer mammography	Do not offer mammography
	Do not offer MRI	Do not offer MRI			Annual MRI	Annual MRI
50–59	Consider annual mammography	Annual mammography	Annual mammography	Annual mammography	Mammography as part of the population screening programme	Do not offer mammography
	Do not offer MRI	Do not offer MRI	Do not offer MRI unless dense breast pattern	Do not offer MRI unless dense breast pattern	Do not offer MRI unless dense breast pattern	Consider annual MRI
60–69	Mammography as part of the population screening programme	Mammography as part of the population screening programme	Mammography as part of the population screening programme	Annual mammography	Mammography as part of the population screening programme	Do not offer mammography
	Do not offer MRI	Do not offer MRI	Do not offer MRI unless dense breast pattern	Do not offer MRI unless dense breast pattern	Do not offer MRI unless dense breast pattern	Consider annual MRI
70+	Mammography as part of the population screening programme	Mammography as part of the population screening programme	Mammography as part of the population screening programme	Mammography as part of the population screening programme	Mammography as part of the population screening programme	Do not offer mammography

[1] Lifetime risk of developing breast cancer is at least 17% but <30%.

[2] Lifetime risk of developing breast cancer is at least 30%. High-risk group includes rare conditions that carry an increased risk of breast cancer, such as Peutz–Jeghers syndrome (*STK11*), Cowden syndrome (*PTEN*), and familial diffuse gastric cancer (E-cadherin).

[3] Surveillance recommendations for this group reflect the fact that women who, at first assessment, had a 30% or greater *BRCA* carrier probability and reach 60 years of age without developing breast or ovarian cancer will now have a lower than 30% carrier probability and should no longer be offered MRI surveillance.

[4] Surveillance recommendations for this group reflect the fact that women who, at first assessment, had a 30% or greater *TP53* carrier probability and reach 50 years of age without developing breast cancer or any other *TP53*-related malignancy will now have a lower than 30% carrier probability and should no longer be offered MRI surveillance.

Surveillance strategies for moderate- and high-risk breast cancer National Institute for Health and Care Excellence (2013) *CG164 Familial breast cancer: classification, care and managing breast cancer and related risks in people with a family history of breast cancer.* Available from www.nice.org.uk/CG164. Reproduced with permission. Information accurate at time of press. For up-to-date information, please visit www.nice.org.uk

Upper GI surveillance can be offered to individuals with *CDH1* mutations who are at high risk of developing diffuse gastric centre, but this should only be done in centres with expertise in this condition (Lim *et al.* 2014).

Endometrial surveillance

There is currently no proven efficacious method of surveillance for endometrial cancer in Lynch syndrome (see 'Lynch syndrome (LS)' in Chapter 4, 'Cancer', p. 586).

Various forms of biopsy-based surveillance are possible, e.g. pipelle aspiration, but the evidence base for the use of these is lacking. Progestagen-containing intrauterine devices, e.g. Mirena® coil, may prove to be efficacious, but again studies need to be carried out.

Breast surveillance

Mammographic screening was shown to reduce mortality in women aged 50–64 years from the general population

(Kerlikowske *et al.* 1995). However, it is associated with overdiagnosis and the benefit in breast cancer-related mortality reduction has been brought into question by long-term follow-up studies of the early trials (Miller *et al.* 2014). Current possible methods for surveillance in those at increased familial risk include mammography, USS, and MRI. The efficacy of such techniques in younger women at increased risk is still to be established. However, NICE guidelines for the care of women at risk of familial breast cancer (National Institute for Health and Care Excellence 2013) include recommendations on surveillance (see Box 4.4 and Table 4.6).

Breast MRI
Contrast-enhanced magnetic resonance imaging (CEMRI) provides information about tissue vascularity that is not available from mammography. In many breast cancers, there is neovascularity, and the pattern and time course of enhancement after injection of IV contrast material (e.g. gadolinium) can determine the likelihood of malignancy. MRI can detect otherwise occult breast cancer in high-risk patients and is probably most beneficial in those at highest risk, e.g. carriers of *BRCA* mutations (Kriege *et al.* 2004; Leach *et al.* 2005). Studies that have cumulatively evaluated breast MRI in >1000 high-risk patients found that the technique identified cancer that was not seen on mammography in 4% of cases (Liberman 2004).

Breast self-examination
A large, well-conducted randomized controlled trial from Shanghai (Thomas *et al.* 2002) has shown conclusively that regular breast self-examination does not lead to a reduction in mortality due to breast cancer, compared with no screening at all (Kösters *et al.* 2008). Moreover, self-examination leads to more breast biopsies and diagnoses of benign breast disease. 'Breast awareness' is often encouraged, but the term is open to interpretation and the evidence base for this is absent.

Ovarian surveillance
Routine ovarian cancer screening for the general population is not currently recommended, as there is no research evidence, to date, to support its use.

Potential screening methods for ovarian cancer are either transvaginal ovarian USS or detection of elevated levels of the tumour marker CA125 in the blood. The small proportion of patients diagnosed with stage I ovarian cancer have a good prognosis, in contrast to the majority with advanced disease. The relationship between survival rates and stage thus provides the rationale for such screening. Ovarian surveillance is problematic, even in the high-risk population, as premenopausal women have a variety of both physiological (e.g. menstrual cycle variations) and benign conditions (e.g. endometriosis, ovarian cysts) that can give rise to false-positive abnormalities on USS and CA125. In addition, there is the operative morbidity associated with unnecessary surgery in women with false-positive results, the psychological consequences associated with false-positive results, the false reassurance in women with false-negative results, and the cost implications.

Women from 'high-risk' families with multiple ovarian and/or breast cancers have a 15–45% lifetime risk of ovarian cancer. Understandably, high-risk women are often anxious and seek surveillance. In some countries, there has been widespread introduction of ovarian cancer screening for women over 35 who are from the high-risk population. However, the impact of screening on ovarian cancer in high-risk women has not shown a reduction in mortality (Rosenthal *et al.* 2013). Based on current evidence, surveillance for ovarian cancer is not recommended outside of clinical trials.

Expert adviser: Marc Tischkowitz, Reader and Honorary Consultant Physician in Medical Genetics, Department of Medical Genetics, University of Cambridge and East Anglian Medical Genetics Service, Cambridge, UK.

References
Adams C, Cardwell C, Cook C, Edwards R, Atkin WS, Morton DG. Effect of hysterectomy status on polyp detection rates at screening flexible sigmoidoscopy. *Gastrointest Endosc* 2003; **57**: 848–53.

Atkin WS, Edwards R, Kralj-Hans I, *et al.*; UK Flexible Sigmoidoscopy Trial Investigators. Once-only flexible sigmoidoscopy screening in prevention of colorectal cancer: a multicentre randomised controlled trial. *Lancet* 2010; **375**: 1624–33.

Berek JS. Epithelial ovarian cancers. In: J Berek, N Hacker (eds.). *Practical gynecologic oncology*, 2nd edn, pp. 324–775. Lippincott Williams and Wilkins, Philadelphia, 1994.

Cairns SR, Scholefield JH, Steele RJ, *et al.* British Society of Gastroenterology; Association of Coloproctology for Great Britain and Ireland. Guidelines for colorectal cancer screening and surveillance in moderate and high risk groups (update from 2002). *Gut* 2010; **59**: 666–89.

Kerlikowske K, Grady D, Rubin SM, Sandrock C, Ernster VL. Efficacy of screening mammography: a meta-analysis. *JAMA* 1995; **273**: 149–54.

Kösters JP, Gøtzsche PC. Regular self-examination or clinical examination for early detection of breast cancer. *Cochrane Database Syst Rev* 2008; **3**: CD003373.

Kriege M, Brekelmans CT, Boetes C, *et al.* Efficacy of MRI and mammography for breast cancer screening in women with a familial or genetic predisposition. *N Engl J Med* 2004; **351**: 427–37.

Leach MO, Boggis CR, Dixon AK, *et al.*, MARIBS study group. Screening with magnetic resonance imaging and mammography of a UK population at high familial risk of breast cancer: a prospective multicentre cohort study (MARIBS). *Lancet* 2005; **365**: 1769–78.

Liberman L. Breast cancer screening with MRI: what are the data for patients at high risk? *N Engl J Med* 2004; **351**: 497–500.

Lim YC, di Pietro M, O'Donovan M, *et al.* Prospective cohort study assessing outcomes of patients from families fulfilling criteria for hereditary diffuse gastric cancer undergoing endoscopic surveillance. *Gastrointest Endosc* 2014; **80**: 78–87.

Miller AB, Wall C, Baines CJ, Sun P, To T, Narod SA. Twenty five year follow-up for breast cancer incidence and mortality of the Canadian National Breast Screening Study: randomised screening trial. *BMJ* 2014; **348**: g366.

National Institute for Health and Care Excellence. Familial breast cancer: classification, care and managing breast cancer and related risks in people with a family history of breast cancer. Clinical guideline CG164, 2013. https://www.nice.org.uk/Guidance/CG164.

Postic G, Lewin D, Bickerstaff C, Wallace MB. Colonoscopic miss rates determined by direct comparison of colonoscopy with colon resection specimens. *Am J Gastroenterol* 2002; **97**: 3182–5.

Rosenthal AN, Fraser L, Manchanda R, *et al.* Results of annual screening in phase I of the United Kingdom familial ovarian cancer screening study highlight the need for strict adherence to screening schedule. *J Clin Oncol* 2013; **31**: 49–57.

Thomas DB, Gao DL, Ray RM, *et al.* Randomized trial of breast self-examination in Shanghai: final results. *J Natl Cancer Inst* 2002; **94**: 1445–57.

Colorectal cancer (CRC)

See also 'Familial adenomatous polyposis (FAP) and adenomatous polyposis due to *MUTYH, NTHL1, POLE*, and *POLD1*', p. 568 and 'Lynch syndrome (LS)', p. 586 in Chapter 4, 'Cancer'.

CRC is a common disease. In incidence, it is the third most common cancer in males (after lung and prostate cancers) and the second most common (after breast cancer) in females (Office for National Statistics 1996). Lifetime risks in 1996 in the UK were 1:18 for males and 1:20 for females. Genetic susceptibility accounts for 5% of CRC, but germline mutations in known single genes account for only 1–2% of cases. The shortfall is considered to be due to a combination of more common lower-penetrance genes that are mostly yet to be elucidated. A family history of the disease confers a significantly increased risk to relatives, confirmed in a meta-analysis (Johns and Houlston 2001). The challenge for the geneticist is to try to sort families into: (1) those who are likely to be carrying a germline mutation in a defined gene, conferring a high lifetime risk, and (2) those with a reasonably strong genetic risk who are at moderate risk, and thus to target screening appropriately.

The hallmarks of genetic predisposition to bowel cancer are these.

- Young age at diagnosis. The mean age of diagnosis in sporadic CRC is 60–70 years (in Lynch syndrome (LS), the mean age of diagnosis of CRC is 44 years (although see the section on LS, as this depends on the underlying gene; see http://www.lscarisk.org) and in FAP it is 39 years).
- Multiple tumours. Polyps and/or cancers.
- Family history, both of CRC and tumours at other sites.
- Rare tumours, e.g. small bowel cancers, skin sebaceous tumours, desmoids.

The geneticist's main role is to identify and diagnose those families with a high risk of CRC attributable to, e.g. FAP or LS, and to establish an empiric risk for those at lesser risk to enable appropriate surveillance or reassurance.

The main approach is by integration of information from the family tree, histopathology reports, cancer registry confirmations of diagnosis, and sometimes (e.g. Muir–Torre syndrome and FAP) from features on clinical examination.

CRC is a common disease, but the risk of developing it is markedly skewed towards elderly people; <1% of cases develop the disease <45 years (and <0.1% at <35 years). In addition, most (~70%) sporadic CRC occur in the rectum and sigmoid colon, with about 10% in the caecum and the rest elsewhere in the colon.

Adenomas and polyps

Colorectal adenomas are even more common. Up to one-third of those in their 70s may harbour one or two, but only 1:1000 of the population develop three or more. Large, multiple, dysplastic adenomas and villous (or tubulovillous) histology are all associated with an empiric increased risk of a CRC to the individual. While most (>95%) CRC develop from adenomas, only a minority of adenomas develop into CRC.

Hyperplastic (metaplastic) polyps are similarly common. They are commonly found in association with adenomas, with or without a CRC, but they have a very low chance of causing cancer. So-called serrated adenomas have features of both adenomas and hyperplastic polyps. Patients with a multiplicity of these other sorts of polyp are at an increased empiric risk of CRC. Serrated polyposis syndrome, incorporating metaplastic polyposis, is now a recognized entity (http://www.nzfgcs.co.nz/syndromes/serrated-polyposis-syndrome-%28sps%29).

Ashkenazi Jews

CRC is significantly more common in this population group. This is probably due to a variety and combination of genetic factors. A missense mutation in the *APC* gene (I1307K) is found in 8% of the Ashkenazi Jewish population and is associated with the development of multiple adenomas and metaplastic polyps. Among average-risk Ashkenazi Jews, the adjusted OR was 1.75 (95% CI, 1.26–2.45) (Boursi et al. 2013).

BRAF

BRAF mutations (in particular p.V600E) occur in ~15% of CRC but are rare in LS-related tumours (Jin et al. 2013). Thus, detection of a *BRAF* mutation indicates a probable sporadic cancer.

Consanguinity

In consanguineous families, be aware of the possibility of homozygosity for MMR genes causing constitutional mismatch repair disorder (CMMRD), a rare syndrome including CAL patches along with depigmented lesions, cancer predisposition (especially brain tumours), and GI polyps. See 'Recessive mutations in mismatch repair (MMR) genes' in 'Neurofibromatosis type 1 (NF1)', Chapter 3, 'Common consultations', p. 506.

Hereditary mixed polyposis

This is caused by a 40-kb upstream duplication that leads to increased and ectopic expression of the BMP antagonist *GREM1* (Jaeger et al. 2012). This mutation is more common in individuals of Ashkenazi Jewish heritage.

Mismatch repair (MMR)

Defective MMR occurs in ~15% of all colon cancers and can arise through either of two mechanisms. In <5% of all tumours, it is caused by mutation in MMR genes (e.g. *MLH1, MSH2, MSH6*), i.e. LS, whereas in ~10% of tumours, it is caused by epigenetic silencing of *MLH1* by biallelic methylation (i.e. there is no germline mutation). Defective MMR is rare in rectal cancers, but when it does occur it usually indicates LS.

MUTYH-associated polyposis

This AR condition is characterized by an increased lifetime risk for CRC, some of which may appear to be due to LS as they acquire microsatellite instability (MSI) due to somatic hits in MMR genes. See 'Familial adenomatous polyposis (FAP) and adenomatous polyposis due to *MUTYH, NTHL1, POLE*, and *POLD1*' in Chapter 4, 'Cancer', p. 568.

NTHL1-associated polyposis (NAP)

Biallelic germline truncating mutations in *NTHL1* underlie a novel recessive adenomatous polyposis and CRC predisposition syndrome (Weren et al. 2015). See 'Familial adenomatous polyposis (FAP) and adenomatous polyposis due to *MUTYH, NTHL1, POLE*, and *POLD1'* in Chapter 4, 'Cancer', p. 568.

Small bowel carcinomas

Small bowel carcinomas are very rare in the general population (<0.003%) but occur in predisposition syndromes. Duodenal cancers occur in FAP, though jejunal and ileal cancers are uncommon. Jejunal and ileal carcinomas occur in LS at ~300 times the rate in the general population (duodenal cancers are rare in LS—probably a reflection of the proportion of the small bowel that is the duodenum). So, because of their rarity, small bowel cancers are very significant, but still, less than half are due to LS. So exclude other causes such as coeliac disease and Crohn's disease.

Most of the >13 high-penetrance genes that predispose to CRC primarily predispose to colorectal polyps, and many genes are associated with a specific type of polyp, whether conventional adenomas (*APC, MUTYH, POLE, POLD1, NTHL1*), juvenile polyps (*SMAD4, BMPR1A*), Peutz–Jeghers hamartomas (*LKB1/STK11*), and mixed polyps of serrated and juvenile types (*GREM1*). LS (*MSH2, MLH1, MSH6, PMS2*), by contrast, is associated primarily with cancer risk (Tomlinson 2015).

Clinical approach

History: key points

- Three-generation family tree, with particular emphasis on the history of tumours, benign and malignant, and documentation of age of diagnosis. Try to extend the family tree further on the relevant side if there are individuals with cancer in the grandparental generation.
- Enquire about the health of the consultand. Do they consider themselves in good health? Have they any symptoms, e.g. a change in bowel habit, that are causing them concern? If yes, explore the symptoms further and refer to a gastroenterologist/colorectal surgeon for further evaluation. Be aware that patients presenting to genetics who are especially worried about their family history may actually be symptomatic.
- Obtain histopathology records or cancer registry confirmation. Whenever available, sight of histopathology

records can be critical. A CRC may be found to have occurred in the setting of multiple polyps, or polyps of a particular sort. Be careful not to ascribe too much significance to numbers and types of polyps that are common in the general population. Cases referred with a presumptive diagnosis of FAP usually turn out not to be FAP once the histopathology report is obtained.

- Decide who is affected, i.e. those with CRC, or at least three adenomatous polyps, or one adenomatous polyp, if it occurred at <60 years, or was 1 cm or greater in size, or had tubulovillous/villous or severely dysplastic histology.
- Other relevant Lynch-related tumours, e.g. endometrial (by far the most important), gastric, ovary, ureter/renal pelvis, brain, small bowel, hepatobiliary tract, and skin (sebaceous tumours).

Examination: key points

- Ask about skin lesions in the individual and family; most patients do not regard them as tumours and will not spontaneously report them. Refer to a dermatologist as appropriate—sebaceous adenomas often masquerade as common skin lesions.
- In suspected PJS polyposis, also check for perioral/axillary/inguinal/perianal freckling.
- Ask about, and look for, dental anomalies—extra/missing teeth, dentiginous cysts, osteomas of the jaw (and other sites).
- In suspected FAP, it may be worth looking for congenital hypertrophy of the retinal pigment epithelium (CHRPE). Refer to an ophthalmologist.
- Perhaps the key examination is pathological examination—histopathological reports (medical records, death certificates, cancer registry entries). It can be well worthwhile asking a pathologist with a specialist interest in, e.g. colorectal or skin pathology, to review the histology.

Special investigations

- A combination of IHC (see Table 4.7 on patterns of IHC staining) and MSI, as available, supplemented by

Table 4.7 Underlying causes of microsatellite instability in colorectal and endometrial cancers in genetics clinic patients, by associated pattern of MMR IHC abnormality

	IHC abnormality				Overall
	MLH1 (alone, or in combination with *PMS2*)	*MSH2* (alone, or in combination with *MSH6*)	*MSH6* (alone)	*PMS2* (alone)	
Constitutional *MLH1* mutation	11.8%			2.0%	14%
Constitutional *MLH1* methylation	0.4%				0.4%
Constitutional *MSH2* mutation		14.2%	0.4%		15%
Constitutional *EPCAM* mutation		2.0%			2.0%
Constitutional *MSH6* mutation		0.8%	10.2%		11%
Constitutional *PMS2* mutation				5.9%	5.9%
Acquired *MLH1* methylation	24.0%				24%
Acquired *MLH1* mutation	6.7%				6.7%
Acquired *MSH2* mutation		2.4%			2.4%
Unexplained	10.2%	5.9%	1.6%	1.6%	19%
Total	53%	25%	12%	9%	100%

Reprinted from *Gastroenterology*, Volume 146, Issue 3, Arjen R. Mensenkamp *et al.*, Somatic Mutations in *MLH1* and *MSH2* Are a Frequent Cause of Mismatch-Repair Deficiency in Lynch Syndrome-Like Tumors, pp. 643–646.e8, Copyright 2014, with permission from Elsevier and AGA Institute.

Table 4.8 Age dependency of the probability that a colon cancer with MSI is due to LS

Age (years)	P (MSI)	P (LS)	P (sporadic MSI)	P (MSI tumour is due to LS)*
35	23%	22%	2%	92%
40	16%	14%	2%	90%
45	10%	9%	2%	87%
50	7%	6%	2%	79%
55	6%	4%	2%	60%
60	10%	3%	7%	28%
65	11%	3%	8%	32%
70	14%	3%	11%	23%

* Assuming all LS tumours have MSI.

NB. This applies to colon cancers; MSI is rare in rectal cancers and usually indicates LS.

Reproduced with permission from Frayling, 2016 Frayling I, Berry I, Wallace A, Payne S, Norbury G. *Association for Clinical Genetic Science best practice guidelines for genetic testing and diagnosis of Lynch syndrome.* 2016: http://www.acgs.uk.com/media/998715/ls_bpg_approved.pdf.

Data from: van Lier, M. G., *et al.* Yield of routine molecular analyses in colorectal cancer patients ≤70 years to detect underlying Lynch syndrome. *The Journal of Pathology* 2012; 226: 764–774

BRAF if *MLH1* loss and by *MLH1* hypermethylation, as appropriate (Frayling *et al.* 2016).
- Bear in mind that MSI at a young age is far more predictive of LS than at an older age (see Table 4.8).
- Gene panel and somatic mutation testing is revealing that many cases of MSI tumours with abnormal IHC, but in which no constitutional MMR mutation can be found, are due to somatic mutations in MMR genes caused by constitutional mutations in other genes, e.g. *MUTYH, POLD1/POLE*, etc. (Castillejo *et al.* 2014).
- NB. There is now a strong case for the systematic testing of all, especially younger-onset, cases of CRC in order to find cases of LS (Snowsill *et al.* 2014). NICE guidelines (2017) now recommend MSI or IHC on all colorectal cancers at diagnosis (NICE 2017).
- Consider genomic array—in young-onset cases of CRC (<30 years), CNVs and mutations in genes such as *BUB1* are observed.

Genetic advice
Risk assessment
First, sort out high-risk families.
- Ask the question 'Does or could the family have a defined polyposis?' If so, proceed appropriately for FAP, attenuated (A)FAP, PJS, etc.
- Ask the question 'Does or could this family have LS?' See Boxes 4.5 and 4.6 and see 'Lynch syndrome (LS)' in Chapter 4, 'Cancer', p. 586. If so, proceed appropriately.
- Ask the question 'Could they have some other cancer genetic syndrome, and is the CRC in the family unrelated to it?' (It is also worth considering whether the family history might be due to >1 syndrome, if it is very strong, on both sides, or very early-onset.)

If the family history does not fit with any of the above and it largely or solely consists of CRC, then triage the family into 'high to moderate', 'low to moderate', or 'low' risk, as in familial CRC guidelines (see Table 4.9). Use clinical common sense. Use Table A14 in 'Patterns of cancer', 'Appendix', p. 846 and consider carefully whether there

Box 4.5 Lynch syndrome-associated tumours

- CRC
- Endometrial carcinoma
- Small intestine carcinoma (*MSH2* and *MLH1*)
- Hepatobiliary tract and pancreas cancer (*MSH2* and *MLH1*)
- Gastric cancer (*MSH2* and *MLH1*)
- Ovarian non-serous cancer (*MSH2* and *MLH1*)
- Renal pelvis and ureter carcinoma (*MSH2* and *MSH6*)
- Bladder carcinoma (<60 years) (*MSH2* and *MSH6*)
- Sebaceous gland carcinoma and adenoma (see Muir–Torre syndrome)
- Prostate cancer (*MSH2*)
- Breast cancer (*MLH1*)
- Brain cancer
 For age-related penetrance of LS cancers, see http://www.lscarisk.org.

Reproduced from *Gut*, Pål Møller, Toni Seppälä, Inge Bernstein *et al.*, Cancer incidence and survival in Lynch syndrome patients receiving colonoscopic and gynaecological surveillance: first report from the prospective Lynch syndrome database, 2015, doi:10.1136/gutjnl-2015-309675 with permission from BMJ Publishing Group Ltd.

may be an alternative genetic explanation conferring a significant genetic risk.

Penetrance
St John *et al.* (1993) calculated the OR for developing CRC, and Johns and Houlston (2001) estimated the lifetime risk of dying, given a family history of CRC (see Table 4.10). For FAP, see 'Familial adenomatous polyposis (FAP) and adenomatous polyposis due to *MUTYH, NTHL1, POLE,* and *POLD1*' in Chapter 4, 'Cancer', p. 568 and for LS, see 'Lynch syndrome (LS)' in Chapter 4, 'Cancer', p. 586.

Management
Surveillance
See also 'Cancer surveillance methods' in Chapter 4, 'Cancer', p. 552.

Note that it may not be necessary at the outset to embark on a lifetime regime of colorectal surveillance in those at risk. Consider the possible use of, at least at the outset, one-off colonoscopies to determine if, e.g. polyps are present, perhaps at a young age, in other members of the family. A family at a low/low to moderate level of risk may thus be elevated into a higher-risk group. Not infrequently, relatives may be having somewhat different surveillance regimes when dealt with in other regions—a pragmatic approach may be best. Also bear in mind that, given the pace of advance in imaging techniques and advanced molecular methods of stool analysis, colonoscopy may well become obsolete as the primary method of surveillance in those at increased risk in their lifetime. An upper age when surveillance might cease of 70–75 years is suggested.

Guidelines for CRC screening and surveillance in high- and moderate-risk groups have been published by Cairns *et al.* (2010). For patients with a high-risk and a moderate-risk family history, see Tables A18, A19, and A20 in 'Surveillance for individuals at increased genetic risk of colorectal cancer', 'Appendix', p. 857.

Box 4.6 Different Lynch syndrome clinical criteria

Selection criteria used by Clinical Genetics (Frayling *et al.* 2016)
Note stringency may vary according to whether the selection is for eligibility for MMR testing or cancer surveillance.
   The Amsterdam criteria were developed to identify LS for *research* studies. The Bethesda guidelines were developed to identify patients with CRC who should be tested *clinically* for LS.
1. **Amsterdam (Amsterdam II/revised Amsterdam) criteria** (Vasen HF, Watson P, Mecklin JP, Lynch HT. New clinical criteria for hereditary nonpolyposis colorectal cancer (HNPCC, Lynch syndrome) proposed by the International Collaborative group on HNPCC. *Gastroenterology* 1999; **116**: 1453–6)
• Three or more blood relatives with a Lynch-related cancer (CRC, EC, small intestine, ureter or renal pelvis), and
• Two or more successive generations affected, and
• One relative must be a first-degree relative of the other two, and
• At least one cancer diagnosed <50 years, and
• FAP excluded in colorectal case(s), and
• Tumours pathologically verified.
2. **Revised Bethesda guidelines (2004)** (Umar A, Boland CR, Terdiman JP, *et al.* Revised Bethesda Guidelines for hereditary nonpolyposis colorectal cancer (Lynch syndrome) and microsatellite instability. *J Natl Cancer Inst* 2004; **96**: 261–8)
• At least one CRC <50 years, or
• Synchronous or metachronous CRC or other Lynch-related tumours, any age, or
• MSI CRC <60 years, or
• CRC in one or more first-degree relative with a Lynch-related tumour, one to be diagnosed <50 years, or
• CRC in two or more first or second-degree relatives with Lynch-related tumours, any age.
   These were devised to be more practical than the Amsterdam type criteria. A comparison has found them to be more sensitive but less specific(Syngal S, Fox EA, Eng C, Kolodner RD, Garber JE. Sensitivity and specificity of clinical criteria for hereditary non-polyposis colorectal cancer associated mutations in *MSH2* and *MLH1*. *J Med Genet* 2000; **37**: 641–5).
   Some services will consider testing unaffected individuals where there is an equivalent prior risk of detecting a germline mutation as for familial breast cancer. Examples of such criteria are where there are three or more first- or second-degree relatives with CRC or Lynch-related tumour, all <70 years.

Predictive testing
Feasible, if a condition with a known genetic basis has been diagnosed, e.g. FAP, LS, in which case see relevant sections, e.g. FAP and adenomatous polyposis or LS, PJS, etc.

Education
Educate your patient about the symptoms of CRC, so that he/she is aware of when to seek medical advice and investigation. The most significant symptoms are:
• rectal bleeding;
• a persistent change in bowel habit, usually to looser or more frequent bowel actions;
• abdominal mass;
• unexplained anaemia.

Diet and other environmental or lifestyle influences
As well as a family history, there are numerous other genetic/environmental influences on CRC risk. The magnitude of risk associated with, e.g. a diet rich in red meat or, probably more importantly, poor in fruit and vegetables is about the same as having a single first-degree relative with an adenoma, i.e. twice, and not quite as great as having a single first-degree relative with CRC (2.8 times). How much effect these factors have in those individuals with high-penetrance genes, rather than those with 'moderate' risk, remains to be established, but undoubtedly common genetic variation plays an important part in how an individual interacts with environmental factors. There is no evidence that proprietary dietary supplements make any difference.
   Patients may ask about aspirin prophylaxis. There is good evidence that aspirin (and, to some extent, other NSAIDs) reduces the risk of CRC. The risks of side effects are less in younger individuals but, of course, increase with age. The prophylactic effect of high-dose aspirin in LS has been demonstrated, but current advice regarding its use in LS patients is that this should only be as part of established trials, e.g. CaPP3 (http://www.capp3.org).

Table 4.9 Familial colorectal cancer guidelines on surveillance

Personal or family history of colorectal cancer (CRC)	Refer to Genetics	Tumour studies	Age of initial screen	Bowel screening procedure following normal tumour studies	Bowel screening *if tumour studies are not possible*
>High risk					
Known cancer predisposition syndrome Lynch syndrome, *MYH* polyposis, familial adenomatous polyposis, Peutz–Jeghers, juvenile polyposis, serrated polyposis, *PTEN*-related disorders	Yes	N/A	May start in childhood	Please contact Clinical Genetics for further information	
Fulfils revised Amsterdam criteria: three relatives with CRC or Lynch-related cancer (LRC) (endometrial, ovarian, urinary tract, stomach small bowel, sebaceous tumours, and hepatobiliary tract) • One relative must be a first-degree relative (FDR)* of the other two • Two successive generations affected • One cancer diagnosed <50 years	Yes	Yes	Dependent on family history Consider starting from 35 years	5-yearly colonoscopy until 75 years	Consider mutation analysis and 2-yearly colonoscopy 25–75 years
High/moderate risk					
Three first-degree relatives with CRC/LRC • None <50 years **Two first-degree relatives with CRC** • Average age <60 years	Yes	Yes	50	5-yearly colonoscopy until 75 years	Consider 5-yearly colonoscopy 50–75 years
Low/moderate risk					
One first-degree relative with CRC and one with LRC • Average age <60 years **One first-degree relative with CRC <50 years**	Yes	Yes	55	Colonoscopy at 55 years, then NHS BCSP† if normal	Discuss at cancer meeting
Two first-degree relatives with CRC • Average age >60 years **Both parents with CRC**	No	No	55	N/A	Colonoscopy at 55 years, then NHS BCSP if normal
Near population risk					
All other family history	No	No	60	N/A	NHS BCSP

N/A, not applicable.

* FDR = sibling, parent, or child. Affected relatives must be blood relations through either the maternal or paternal side but can be FDR of each other, not just the consultand.

† NHS BCSP, Bowel Cancer Screening Programme.

If in doubt, please discuss at the cancer meeting.

Courtesy of Dr Ruth Armstrong and Cambridge University Hospitals.

Table 4.10 Odds ratio of dying from CRC

Risk group*	Odds ratio
General population	1.0
Any family history	1.8
One affected FDR (any age)	2.8
One affected FDR <45 years	3.7
Two affected FDRs	5.7

* FDR, first-degree relative.

Data from St John DJB, *et al.* Cancer risk in relatives of patients with common colorectal cancer. *Ann Intern Med* 1993; 118: 785–90.

Update family history

Emphasize the importance of notifying the genetics department of any new diagnoses in the family, as these may significantly change the risk assessment.

Support groups: Lynch Syndrome UK, http://www.lynch-syndrome-uk.org; Macmillan Cancer Support, https://www.macmillan.org.uk; Bowel Cancer UK, www.bowelcancer.org.uk;International Society for Gastrointestinal Hereditary Tumours (InSIGHT), www.insight-group.org.

Expert adviser: Ian M. Frayling, Consultant Genetic Pathologist, Cardiff and Vale University Health Board,

Cardiff University, Institute of Medical Genetics, University Hospital of Wales, Cardiff, UK.

References

Boursi B, Sella T, Liberman E, et al. The APC p.I1307K polymorphism is a significant risk factor for CRC in average risk Ashkenazi Jews. Eur J Cancer 2013; **49**: 3680–5.

Cairns SR, Scholefield JH, Steele RJ, et al.; British Society of Gastroenterology, Association of Coloproctology for Great Britain and Ireland. Guidelines for colorectal cancer screening and surveillance in moderate and high risk groups (update from 2002). Gut 2010; **59**: 666–89.

Castillejo A, Vargas G, Castillejo MI, et al. Prevalence of germline MUTYH mutations among Lynch-like syndrome patients. Eur J Cancer 2014; **50**: 2241–50.

de la Chapelle A. Microsatellite instability [perspective]. N Engl J Med 2003; **349**: 209–10.

Dunlop MG. Guidance of large bowel surveillance for people with two first degree relatives with colorectal cancer or one first degree relative diagnosed with colorectal cancer under 45 years. Gut 2002; **51**(Suppl V): v17–20.

East Anglia Regional Genetics Service. Familial colorectal cancer guidelines, 2013.

Frayling I, Berry I, Wallace A, Payne S, Norbury G. Association for Clinical Genetic Science best practice guidelines for genetic testing and diagnosis of Lynch syndrome, 2016. http://www.acgs.uk.com/media/998715/ls_bpg_approved.pdf.

Giardiello FM, Brensinger JD, Petersen GM. AGA technical review on hereditary colorectal cancer and genetic testing. Gastroenterology 2001; **121**: 198–213.

International Society for Gastrointestinal Hereditary Tumours (InSIGHT). http://www.insight-group.org.

Jaeger E, Leedham S, Lewis A, et al. Hereditary mixed polyposis syndrome is caused by a 40-kb upstream duplication that leads to increased and ectopic expression of the BMP antagonist GREM1. Nat Genet 2012; **44**: 699–703.

Jenkins MA, Baglietto L, Dite GS, et al. After hMSH2 and hMLH1—what next? Analysis of three-generational, population-based, early-onset colorectal cancer families. Int J Cancer 2002; **102**: 166–71.

Jin M, Hampel H, Zhou Z, et al. BRAF V600E mutation analysis simplifies the testing algorithm for Lynch syndrome. Am J Clin Pathol 2013; **140**: 177–83.

Johns LE, Houlston RS. A systematic review and meta-analysis of familial colorectal cancer risk. Am J Gastroenterol 2001; **96**: 2992–3003.

Lindgren G, Liljegren A, Jaramillo E, Rubio C, Lindblom A. Adenoma prevalence and cancer risk in familial non-polyposis colorectal cancer. Gut 2002; **50**: 228–34.

Lynch HT, de la Chapelle A. Hereditary colorectal cancer. N Engl J Med 2003; **348**: 919–32.

Mensenkamp AR, Vogelaar IP, van Zelst-Stams WA, et al. Somatic mutations in MLH1 and MSH2 are a frequent cause of mismatch-repair deficiency in Lynch syndrome-like tumors. Gastroenterology 2014; **146**: 643–6.

Møller P, Seppälä T, Bernstein I, et al. Cancer incidence and survival in Lynch syndrome patients receiving colonoscopic and gynaecological surveillance: first report from the prospective Lynch syndrome database. Gut 2015. pii: gutjnl-2015-309675.

NICE Guidelines: Molecular testing strategies for Lynch syndrome in people with colorectal cancer. www.nice.org.uk/guidance/dg27.

Nusko G, Mansmann U, Kirchner T, Hahn EG. Risk related surveillance following colorectal polypectomy. Gut 2002; **51**: 424–8.

Office for National Statistics (1996). https://www.ons.gov.uk.

Ransohoff DF, Sandler RS. Screening for colorectal cancer. N Engl J Med 2002; **346**: 40–4.

Snowsill T, Huxley N, Hoyle M, et al. A systematic review and economic evaluation of diagnostic strategies for Lynch syndrome. Health Technol Assess 2014; **18**: 1–406.

St John DJ, McDermott FT, Hopper JL, Debney EA, Johnson WR, Hughes ES. Cancer risk in relatives of patients with common colorectal cancer. Ann Intern Med 1993; **118**: 785–90.

Tomlinson I. The Mendelian colorectal cancer syndromes. Ann Clin Biochem 2015; **52**(Pt 6): 690–2.

Vasen HF, Blanco I, Aktan-Collan K, et al.; Mallorca group. Revised guidelines for the clinical management of Lynch syndrome (HNPCC): recommendations by a group of European experts. Gut 2013; **62**: 812–23.

Vasen HF, Möslein G, Alonso A, et al. Guidelines for the clinical management of Lynch syndrome (hereditary non-polyposis cancer). J Med Genet 2007; **44**: 353–62.

Weren RD, Ligtenberg MJ, Kets CM, et al. A germline homozygous mutation in the base-excision repair gene NTHL1 causes adenomatous polyposis and colorectal cancer. Nat Genet 2015; **47**: 668–71.

Wijnen JT, Vasen HF, Khan PM, et al. Clinical findings with implications for genetic testing in families with clustering of colorectal cancer. N Engl J Med 1998; **339**: 511–18.

Winawer SJ, Zauber AG, Gerdes H, et al. Risk of colorectal cancer in the families of patients with adenomatous polyps. National Polyp Study Workgroup. N Engl J Med 1996; **334**: 82–7.

Confirmation of diagnosis of cancer

In cancer genetics, risk assessment usually depends critically on the information reported in the family history. If management decisions, e.g. prophylactic surgery or invasive screening procedures, are going to be based on that information, it is important to confirm its accuracy. In a perfect world, every cancer diagnosis would be confirmed, but, in practice, limited time and resources mean that this is usually impracticable.

Reported cases of breast cancer in close relatives are rarely wrong (inaccurate in 5% in Douglas et al.'s (1999) study), but reported cases of abdominal, and especially gynaecological, cancers often are (inaccurate in 20% in Douglas et al.'s (1999) study). 'Stomach' cancer can mean almost anything abdominal. 'Liver' cancer is usually secondary. 'Womb' cancer includes cervical, as well as endometrial, tumours. Douglas et al. (1999) found that management of 11% of families was changed by information obtained from cancer confirmation.

In practice, it may be reasonable, at least in high-risk families, to confirm:

- all cases of colorectal and GI tract cancer;
- all cases of ovarian cancer;
- at least one diagnosis in a family where prophylactic surgery or screening is being considered;
- at least one diagnosis in a family where mutation screening is instituted on the basis of the family tree (rather than IHC or other histopathological findings in the tumour or clinical features in the proband).

Hierarchy of reliability of confirmation

(1) Pathology report. This is the 'gold standard'.
(2) Cancer Registry report.
(3) Hospital discharge summary.
(4) Death certificate. For relatives who died a long time ago, this may be the only accessible document.

References

Douglas FS, O'Dair LC, Robinson M, Evans DG, Lynch SA. The accuracy of diagnoses as reported in families with cancer: a retrospective study. J Med Genet 1999; 36: 309–12.

Cowden syndrome (PTEN hamartoma tumour syndrome (PHTS))

Introduction
Cowden syndrome (PHTS) is a multiple hamartoma tumour syndrome with a high risk for benign tumours and malignant tumours of the thyroid, breast, endometrium, and kidney. Affected individuals usually have macrocephaly, pathognomonic mucocutaneous skin lesions such as trichilemmomas, and papillomatous papules. Because of the variable, and often subtle, external manifestations of PHTS, many individuals remain undiagnosed; the true prevalence is unknown. The prevalence has been estimated at one in 200 000; likely an underestimate. Up to 85% of individuals who meet the diagnostic criteria for PHTS have a detectable PTEN mutation and fall under the category of PTEN hamartoma tumour syndrome (PHTS). PHTS includes Cowden syndrome and Bannayan–Riley–Ruvalcaba syndrome (BRRS). BRRS is a congenital disorder characterized by macrocephaly, intestinal hamartomatous polyposis, lipomas, and pigmented macules of the glans penis.

Some older papers had reported PTEN mutations in a few patients with Proteus syndrome, a complex, highly variable disorder involving congenital malformations and hamartomatous overgrowth of multiple tissues, as well as connective tissue naevi, epidermal naevi, and hyperostosis, but these individuals are now thought to have PHTS. Proteus syndrome is caused by mosaicism for mutation in AKT1.

Clinical approach
History: key points
- Three-generation family history, with specific attention to benign breast and thyroid disorders, GI polyps, large head size, and learning disabilities. Personal and family history of breast, thyroid, endometrial, and kidney cancers.

Examination: key points
- OFC for macrocephaly, macrocephaly, typically greater than +2SD.
- Careful examination of the oral mucosa for characteristic 'cobblestone' lesions and the skin for pitted keratoses, acral keratoses (verrucous-like lesions), lipomas, and vascular malformations.
- Careful examination of the neck for goitre and nodularity, and the breast for breast lumps.

Clinical diagnosis
A presumptive diagnosis of PHTS is based on clinical signs; by definition, however, the diagnosis of PHTS is made only when a PTEN mutation is identified. Clinical diagnostic criteria for PHTS have been developed to help clinicians identify patients with PHTS. Clinical criteria have been divided into three categories: pathognomonic, major, and minor (see Box 4.7).

Molecular genetic testing
Historically, it was suggested that up to 85% of individuals who meet the diagnostic criteria for CS and 65% of individuals with a clinical diagnosis of BRRS have a detectable PTEN mutation. More recently, it was found that ~25% of individuals who meet the strict diagnostic criteria for CS have a pathogenic PTEN mutation, including large deletions. Approximately 10% of individuals with BRRS who do not have a mutation detected in the PTEN coding sequence have large deletions within, or encompassing, PTEN.

Testing strategy
Given the many protean features of PHTS, the PTEN Cleveland Clinic Risk Calculator was developed as a clinical aid to provide the prior probability of finding a PTEN mutation in children and adults (http://www.lerner.ccf.org/gmi/ccscore).

Optimal PTEN testing for individuals suspected of having PHTS includes:

(1) sequencing of PTEN exons 1–9 and flanking intronic regions. If no mutation is identified, perform:

(2) deletion/duplication analysis. If no mutation is identified, consider:

(3) research testing, especially in those with CS and Cowden-like syndrome:
- PTEN promoter;
- other susceptibility genes for CS: SDHx, PIK3CA, AKT1 mutations, and KLLN epimutations.

Clinical implications
Malignant and non-malignant tumour risk
Individuals with PHTS have a high risk of breast, thyroid, and endometrial cancers. As with other hereditary cancer syndromes, the risk of multifocal and bilateral (in paired organs such as the breasts) cancer is increased. Recent studies suggest higher risks than previously cited, but all include probands ascertained following a cancer diagnosis.

Breast disease
Women with PHTS have as high as a 67% risk for benign breast disease. Prior to gene identification, estimates of lifetime risk to females of developing breast cancer were 25–50%, with an average age of diagnosis of between 38 and 46 years; however, a recent analysis of prospectively accrued and followed probands and family members with a PTEN mutation reveal an 85% lifetime risk for female breast cancer, with 50% penetrance by the age of 50 years.

Thyroid disease
Benign multinodular goitre of the thyroid, as well as adenomatous nodules and follicular adenomas, are common, occurring in up to 75% of individuals with PHTS. The lifetime risk for epithelial thyroid cancer is ~35%. Median age of onset was 37 years and can present as early as 7 years of age. Significantly, follicular thyroid cancer histology is over-represented in adults, compared to the general population in which papillary histology is over-represented and no medullary thyroid carcinoma was observed. Clinicians should be clinically vigilant for other features of PHTS, e.g. macrocephaly, benign tumours in assessing thyroid cancer patients for the possibility of PHTS.

Endometrial disease
Benign uterine fibroids are common among patients with PHTS. Lifetime risk for endometrial cancer is estimated at 28%, with the starting age at risk in the late 30s to early 40s.

Gastrointestinal neoplasias
More than 90% of individuals with a PTEN mutation who underwent at least one upper or lower endoscopy were found to have polyps. Histologic findings varied, ranging from ganglioneuromatous polyps, hamartomatous

Box 4.7 Diagnostic criteria for *PTEN* hamartoma tumour syndrome (PHTS), including Cowden syndrome (CS), Bannayan–Riley–Ruvalcaba syndrome (BRRS), *PTEN*-related Proteus syndrome (PS), and Proteus-like syndrome

A *PTEN* hamartoma tumour syndrome (PHTS) *should be suspected* in individuals with the following clinical features: Cowden syndrome (CS). Based on >3000 prospectively accrued individuals with CS or a Cowden-like syndrome (CSL) from the community, a scoring system (http://www.lerner.ccf.org/gmi/ccscore) that takes into account the phenotype and age at diagnosis has been developed. The scoring system allows input of clinical information on an individual suspected of having CS/CSL and subsequently generates the prior probability of finding a *PTEN* pathogenic variant.

- In adults, a clinical threshold score of ≥10 leads to a recommendation for referral to a genetics professional to consider PHTS.
- In children, macrocephaly and ≥1 of the following leads to the consideration of PHTS:
  - autism or developmental delay;
  - dermatologic features, including lipomas, trichilemmomas, oral papillomas, or penile freckling;
  - vascular features such as AVMs or haemangiomas;
  - GI polyps.

Additionally, consensus diagnostic criteria for CS have been developed (Eng 2001) and are updated each year by the National Comprehensive Cancer Network (National Comprehensive Cancer Network 2015) (see full text; registration required). However, the CS scoring system discussed in this section has been shown to be more accurate than the NCCN diagnostic criteria (Tan *et al.* 2011).

The NCCN consensus clinical diagnostic criteria have been divided into three categories: pathognomonic, major, and minor.

Pathognomonic criteria
- Adult Lhermitte–Duclos disease (LDD), defined as the presence of a cerebellar dysplastic gangliocytoma (Zhou *et al.* 2003).
- Mucocutaneous lesions:
  - trichilemmomas (facial);
  - acral keratoses;
  - papillomatous lesions;
  - mucosal lesions.

Major criteria
- Breast cancer.
- Epithelial thyroid cancer (non-medullary), especially follicular thyroid cancer.
- Macrocephaly (OFC ≥97th percentile).
- Endometrial carcinoma.

Minor criteria
- Other thyroid lesions (e.g. adenoma, multinodular goitre).
- Intellectual disability (IQ ≤75).
- Hamartomatous intestinal polyps.
- Fibrocystic disease of the breast.
- Lipomas.
- Fibromas.
- Genitourinary tumours (especially renal cell carcinoma).
- Genitourinary malformation.
- Uterine fibroids.

An operational diagnosis of CS is made if an individual meets any one of the following criteria:
- pathognomonic mucocutaneous lesions, combined with one of the following:
  - six or more facial papules, of which three or more must be trichilemmoma;
  - cutaneous facial papules and oral mucosal papillomatosis;
  - oral mucosal papillomatosis and acral keratoses;
  - six or more palmoplantar keratoses.
- two or more major criteria;
- one major and three or more minor criteria;
- four or more minor criteria.

In a family in which one individual meets the diagnostic criteria for CS listed above, other relatives are considered to have a diagnosis of CS if they meet *any one* of the following criteria:
- the pathognomonic criteria;
- any one major criterion with or without minor criteria;
- two minor criteria;
- a history of BRRS.

Data from: Eng C. *PTEN Hamartoma Tumor Syndrome* (PHTS) 2001 Nov 29 [Updated 2012 Apr 19]. In: Pagon RA, Bird TD, Dolan CR, *et al.*, editors. *GeneReviews™* [Internet]. Seattle (WA): University of Washington, Seattle; 1993. Available from: http://www.ncbi.nlm.nih.gov/books/NBK1488.

Table 4.11 Table to show cancer risk and screening advice for patients with PTEN hamartoma tumour syndrome (PHTS)

Cancer risk	Risk data	Screening advice
Breast	Cancer—lifetime up to 85%	BRCA-equivalent (annual MRI from age 30, mammography from 40)
	Average age at diagnosis 38–46	
	High incidence of fibrocystic breast disease	
Thyroid	Cancer—lifetime 35% (usually follicular, rarely papillary, never medullary)	As a minimum, screen from 16 by USS and TFT
		Younger as guided by family history or after informed discussion with family
	Median age at diagnosis 37	
	Up to 75% risk of multinodular goitre, adenomatous nodules, and follicular adenomas	Ideally through adult oncology clinic or paediatric endocrinology
Renal	Cancer—lifetime up to 35%	Consider annual urine dip for haematuria from 40
	(mostly papillary)	Consider annual renal USS from 40
	Risk starts late 40s	
Colorectal	Cancer—lifetime up to 9%	Ascertainment colonoscopy at ages 35 and 55
	Risk starts late 30s	Polyp follow-up as required
	More than 50% have polyps, which may be symptomatic	
Skin and vascular system	Melanoma 5%	Baseline dermatological review and appropriate follow-up
	Many non-malignant lesions	
Brain	Lhermitte–Duclos disease—up to 32%	Symptom enquiry
		Brain MRI only if symptomatic
Endometrial	Cancer—lifetime up to 28%	Refer to a specialist gynaecologist at age 35–40 for discussion of screening options and management of non-cancer manifestations
	Risk starts late 30s to early 40s	
	Benign uterine fibroids very common	Consider risk-reducing hysterectomy

UK CGS National Audit 2015.

polyps, and juvenile polyps to adenomatous polyps. Lifetime risk for CRC is estimated at 9%, with the starting age at risk in the late 30s.

Renal cell carcinoma
Lifetime risk for renal cell carcinoma is estimated at 35%, with the starting age at risk in the 40s. The predominant histology is papillary renal cell carcinoma.

Other
Lifetime risk for cutaneous melanoma is estimated at >5%. Brain tumours, as well as vascular malformations affecting any organ, are occasionally seen in individuals with PHTS.

Neurodevelopmental sequelae

Lhermitte–Duclos disease (LDD)
Most, if not all, adult-onset LDD (dysplastic gangliocytoma of the cerebellum, a hamartomatous overgrowth known to be a feature of PHTS) can be attributed to mutations in *PTEN*, even in the absence of other clinical signs of CS/BRRS.

Autism/pervasive developmental disorder and macrocephaly
Germline *PTEN* mutations were identified in individuals with these findings, especially in the presence of other personal or family history consistent with CS/BRRS. The 10–20% prevalence of germline *PTEN* mutations in autism spectrum disorders with macrocephaly has now been confirmed by several independent groups.

Management

Treatment of manifestations
Treatment for the benign and malignant manifestations of PHTS is the same as for their sporadic counterparts.

Cutaneous lesions should be excised only if malignancy is suspected or symptoms (e.g. pain, deformity) are significant.

Surveillance
To detect tumours at the earliest, most treatable stages, the screening recommendations are listed in Table 4.11.

Testing of relatives at risk
PHTS is inherited in an AD manner. The majority of PHTS cases are simplex. Perhaps 10–50% of individuals with PHTS have an affected parent. Each child of an affected individual has a 50% chance of inheriting the mutation and developing PHTS. When a *PTEN* mutation has been identified in a proband, molecular genetic testing of asymptomatic at-risk relatives can identify those who have the family-specific mutation and warrant ongoing surveillance.

Expert adviser: Katherine Lachlan, Consultant Clinical Geneticist, Wessex Clinical Genetics Service, University Hospital Southampton, Princess Anne Hospital, Southampton, UK.

References

Eng C. *PTEN* hamartoma tumor syndrome. In: RA Pagon, TD Bird, CR Dolan, *et al.* (eds.). *GeneReviews®*. University of Washington, Seattle, 2001 (updated 2016). http://www.ncbi.nlm.nih.gov/books/NBK1488.

Mester J, Eng C. Estimate of *de novo* mutation frequency in probands with PTEN hamartoma tumor syndrome. *Genet Med* 2012; **14**: 819–22.

Mester JL, Zhou M, Prescott N, Eng C. Papillary renal cell carcinoma is associated with *PTEN* hamartoma tumor syndrome. *Urology* 2012; **79**: 1187.e1–7.

National Comprehensive Cancer Network (2015). https://www.nccn.org.

Ngeow J, Mester J, Rybicki LA, Ni Y, Milas M, Eng C. Incidence and clinical characteristics of thyroid cancer in prospective series of individuals with Cowden and Cowden-like syndrome characterized by germline PTEN, SDH, or KLLN alterations. J Clin Endocrinol Metab 2011; **96**: E2063–71.

Orloff M, Xin H, Peterson C, et al. Germline PIK3CA and AKT1 mutations in Cowden and Cowden-like Syndromes. Am J Hum Genet 2012; **92**: 76–80.

Pilarski R, Burt R, Kohlman W, Pho L, Shannon KM, Swisher E. Cowden syndrome and the PTEN hamartoma tumor syndrome: systematic review and revised diagnostic criteria. J Natl Cancer Inst 2013; **105**: 1607–16.

Tan MH, Mester JL, Ngeow J, Rybicki LA, Orloff MS, Eng C. Lifetime cancer risks in individuals with germline PTEN mutations. Clin Cancer Res 2012; **18**: 400–7.

Tan MH, Mester J, Peterson C, et al. A clinical scoring system for selection of patients for PTEN mutation testing is proposed on the basis of a prospective study of 3042 probands. Am J Hum Genet 2011; **88**: 42–56.

Zhou XP, Marsh DJ, Morrison CD, et al. Germline inactivation of PTEN and dysregulation of the phosphoinositol-3-kinase/Akt pathway cause human Lhermitte–Duclos disease in adults. Am J Hum Genet 2003; **73**: 1191–8.

Familial adenomatous polyposis (FAP) and adenomatous polyposis due to *MUTYH, NTHL1, POLE,* and *POLD1*

Adenomatous polyposis is genetically heterogeneous. FAP due to mutations in *APC* is AD, whereas *MUTYH*-associated polyposis (MAP) is AR and due to mutations in *MUTYH*. A very rare form of AD polyposis which includes adenomas *inter alia*, and which so far appears restricted to Ashkenazim, is hereditary mixed polyposis syndrome (HMPS).

Colorectal adenomas occur in the general population. Up to 30% of the general population will develop an adenoma or two by the age of 70 years, but only 1:1000 of the population will develop >2 adenomas. Multiplicity of adenomas is empirically associated with a significantly increased risk of CRC.

In terms of numbers of colorectal polyps, the phenotypes of FAP and MAP overlap. Classically, FAP has been defined by >100 adenomatous polyps found in the colorectum at endoscopy (sigmoidoscopy or colonoscopy) or on pathological examination of the colon (after colectomy). Some cases can have thousands of polyps. The term attenuated FAP (AFAP) can be applied to cases and families with <100 adenomas. The colorectal phenotype associated with *APC* mutations can run from a few (zero even, if not yet penetrant) up to thousands of polyps, whereas the phenotype associated with MAP runs from zero to a few hundred polyps. Untreated, the CRC risk in FAP and MAP is very high, but with FAP at a somewhat younger age (98% by age 50 years), compared with MAP (~90% by age 70 years). Hence, the job of the clinical geneticist is to distinguish FAP from MAP, recognizing that 20–30% of cases and families with <100 adenomas remain molecularly undiagnosed.

Familial adenomatous polyposis (FAP)

Complete ascertainment by the Danish FAP Registry has shown the prevalence to be 1:8500, while the incidence appears to be 1.3 new cases per million population per year (but see below).

FAP is due to AD inheritance of germline mutations in the *APC* gene at 5q22.2. Approximately 15–20% of cases arise *de novo*, and about 15% of them are mosaic. Many new cases are undoubtedly due to *de novo APC* mutations, but a significant proportion are due to MAP (*vide infra*).

Multisystem disease: extracolonic features

FAP is associated with a number of extracolonic features (see Table 4.12). Indeed, it is a multisystem disorder. Historically, Gardner described patients with colonic and extracolonic features of FAP, but it is now known that, given close enough examination, all individuals with FAP have extracolonic features. Individuals develop multiple adenomas of both the colorectum and duodenum, with concomitant risk of cancer. Fundic gland polyps develop in the stomach. Desmoid tumours are liable to develop in connective tissue and mesentery, especially in or around the trunk. Characteristic CHRPE develop in the eye. Sebaceous cysts (distinct from the sebaceous adenomas that can develop in MTS due to LS; see 'Lynch syndrome (LS)' in Chapter 4, 'Cancer', p. 586) occur at greater frequency, as do osteomata, dental (dentiginous) cysts, and supernumerary teeth. (NB. Individuals referred as possible FAP because of multiple sebaceous cysts may have

steatocystoma multiplex due to keratin 17 (*KRT17*) mutations.) An increased risk of cancer at several extracolonic sites is also observed, e.g. adrenals, primary brain, thyroid (papillary cancer), primary liver (hepatoblastoma), and hepatobiliary tree.

APC mutations in FAP and AFAP

There are three common FAP-associated *APC* mutations: two recurrent 5-bp deletions—one at codon 1061, the other at codon 1309—and deletion of the whole gene. Together, they account for about 25–30% of mutations; the rest are essentially private point mutations. Less than 1% of cases are due to cytogenetically visible chromosomal mutations involving 5q22, but these are usually associated with a contiguous gene syndrome causing dysmorphic features and learning difficulties, particularly delayed speech.

The hallmark of all FAP-associated *APC* mutations is that they are null, nonsense, or frameshifting; indeed, a priori, any *APC* mutations that appear ostensibly to be missense in nature are most unlikely to be causative of FAP, unless they affect, e.g. message splicing. Deep intronic *APC* mutations revealing pseudoexons have been reported to cause FAP and account, in part, for those families refractory to a molecular diagnosis.

The spectrum of *APC* mutations associated with FAP shows a number of genotype–phenotype correlations. *APC* consists of 2843 codons in 15 exons, exon 15 being exceptionally large. Mutations located between, approximately, codons 160 and 1600 are associated with hundreds of adenomas—classical FAP. Mutations occurring at or near to codon 1300 are associated with thousands of adenomas (and the highest CRC risk). Mutations located 5′ of codon 160 or 3′ of codon 1600 are associated with AFAP. Polyp numbers are related to CRC risk; untreated, those with thousands of polyps develop CRC at a mean age of 28 years, whereas the mean age in those with hundreds of polyps is 44 years, and in those with AFAP is 55 years. Mutations 3′ of codon 1400 are especially associated with desmoid tumours. Indeed, one mutation at codon 1942 (c.5826_5829delCAGA) is associated with *familial infiltrative fibromatosis*, a variant of FAP in which the risk from desmoid tumours is greater than

Table 4.12 Extraintestinal features in FAP

Cancers	Benign lesions
Thyroid (papillary) (2–3%)	Congenital hypertrophy of the retinal pigment epithelium (CHRPE) (70–80%, but see text)
Brain (usually medulloblastoma) (<1%)	Epidermoid cysts (50%)
Hepatoblastoma (~1%)	Osteomas (50–90%)
	Desmoid tumours (10–15%)
	Supernumerary teeth (11–27%)
	Adrenal gland adenomas (7–13%)

that from GI tract cancers. Mutations located 5′ of exon 9 (codons 312–438) are not associated with CHRPE (except for some mutations in exon 6), whereas those located 3′ of exon 9 usually are associated with CHRPE. Mutations located in exon 9 (which is alternately spliced) are not only variably associated with CHRPE, but also with reduced polyp numbers (AFAP). The number of polyps associated with AFAP mutations is highly variable; some individuals may develop no polyps, some >100, and others between one and 100. Only about 10% of those with AFAP have demonstrable *APC* mutations, with about 20% being found to have MAP.

A missense mutation (*APC* p.Ile1307Lys) has been associated with an AFAP-like phenotype in Ashkenazi Jews, while another missense (p.Glu1317Gln) has been variably associated with multiple adenomas in non-Jewish Europeans (as well as being found in 1% of Ashkenazim), but this association may be because it is in linkage disequilibrium with a nonsense mutation at the 5′ end of the gene.

MUTYH-associated polyposis (MAP)

MAP is due to AR inheritance of mutations in *MUTYH*, a DNA repair gene involved in the repair of oxidation damage at 1p34.1. Approximately 25% of cases with >9 adenomas and no evidence of a dominant family history are due to *MUTYH* mutations. There are two common mutations in Northern Europeans (see below). The possible risks, if any, associated with being a *MUTYH* carrier have not been easy to define, but a recent study has concluded: 'The 2-fold increase in CRC risk identified in the present study is comparable with the relative risk of 2.24 seen in individuals from the general population who have at least 1 first-degree relative affected by CRC.31 The present study indicates that screening measures for CRC in the heterozygous relatives of MAP patients need be no more intensive than for this group.' (Jones *et al.* 2009).

However, although individuals found to harbour a common mutation and ascertained through family cancer clinics may have a slightly increased risk of CRC, compared to the general population, the risk in those with one mutation found outside of a clinic appears not to be significantly raised.

Some extracolonic features, such as are observed in FAP due to *APC* mutations, have been reported to occur in a few individuals with MAP, specifically upper GI tumours and CHRPE (see below).

NB. Somatic mutation analysis is revealing that at least a proportion of CRCs in individuals with MAP, but not necessarily many adenomas, can have two somatic mutations in a DNA MMR gene. Thus, they may have MSI and undergo the specific changes on IHC associated with LS but are, in effect, due to MAP. Hence, in individuals who may appear to have LS, but in whom an MMR mutation cannot be found, it is worth checking *MUTYH*.

MUTYH mutations

The current reference sequence in use for *MUTYH* is NM_001128425.1. This is the longest transcript (transcript alpha 5). However, due to alternative splicing of exon 3, nucleotide and amino acid numbering after nucleotide position 157 (amino acid 53) may differ by up to 42 nucleotides (14 amino acids) with the two other reference sequences that have been used historically. Hence, mutations may appear in reports and the literature under one of three different numbering systems, clarified in Table 4.13.

There are two common *MUTYH* point mutations in Northern Europeans—pTyr179Cys and p.Gly396Asp—that together account for ~85% of mutant alleles. The remaining 15% are other point mutations of all classes. In other population groups, p.Glu480X is the prevalent Indian mutation, whereas p.Tyr104X is prevalent in Pakistanis, neither mutation being found in Caucasians. Larger-scale mutations involving whole exons are observed, but they do not appear to be common.

NTHL1-ASSOCIATED POLYPOSIS (NAP). Biallelic germline truncating mutations in *NTHL1* underlie a novel recessive adenomatous polyposis and cancer predisposition syndrome. Weren *et al.* (2012) reported three Dutch families with the same homozygous mutation (NM_002528.c.268C→T,p.Q90*) in the base excision repair gene *NTHL1*. Multiple colorectal adenomas, with or without CRC, were diagnosed in all seven homozygotes, and six received a diagnosis of multiple primary tumours. A subsequent patient, compound heterozygous for *NTHL1* mutations, had <30 multiple colorectal adenomas (that frequently had a villous and focally serrated architecture), together with multiple extracolonic primary tumours (Rivera *et al.* 2015).

POLE- AND POLD1-ASSOCIATED ADENOMATOUS POLYPOSIS. Germline heterozygous variants in *POLE* and *POLD1* encoding the proofreading (exonuclease) domain of DNA polymerases ε and δ cause a high-penetrant multiple adenomatous polyps/CRC syndrome (Palles *et al.* 2013). *POLD1* mutation was also associated with endometrial cancer predisposition. The mutations map to equivalent sites in the proofreading (exonuclease) domain of DNA polymerases ε and δ and are predicted to cause a defect in the correction of mispaired bases inserted during DNA replication.

ADENOMATOUS POLYPOSIS DUE TO MSH3. There is emerging evidence that recessive inheritance of mutations in the mismatch repair proteins MSH3 can cause colorectal adenomatous polyposis (Adam 2016).

HEREDITARY MIXED POLYPOSIS SYNDROME (HMPS). In Ashkenazim, a complex form of adenomatous polyposis which predisposes to CRC is called hereditary mixed polyposis syndrome (HMPS). It is caused by a specific mutation affecting, although not involving, *GREM1* (at 15q13–q22). A 40-kb duplication of the 3′ end of an adjacent gene (*SCG5*) upstream of *GREM1* causes abnormal

Table 4.13 Clarification of mutation numbering systems in *MUTYH*

Original description	Original nucleotide nomenclature	Original protein nomenclature	Interim nucleotide nomenclature	Interim protein nomenclature	Current nucleotide nomenclature	Current protein nomenclature
Y165C	c.494A>G	p.Tyr165Cys	c.527A>G	p.Tyr176Cys	c.536A>G	p.Tyr179Cys
G382D	c.1145A>G	p.Gly382Asp	c.1178G>A	p.Gly393Asp	c.1187G>A	p.Gly396Asp
Y90X	c.270C>G	p.Tyr90X	c.303C>G	p.Tyr101X	c.312C>G	p.Tyr104X
E466X	c.1395G>T	p.Glu466X	c.1429G>T	p.Glu477X	c.1438G>T	p.Glu480X

Courtesy of Sarah Rolleston, Clinical Scientist, All-Wales Medical Genetics Service.

excessive expression of *GREM1* in colorectal mucosal cells. Affected individuals can develop polyps of different types, including conventional adenomas, serrated polyps, Peutz–Jeghers, and juvenile polyps, and they can even, as the name suggests, develop polyps with >1 of these types of histology mixed together.

Brain tumours plus polyposis: Turcot syndrome

Turcot described a syndrome in which colorectal adenomatous polyposis occurred together with a predisposition to primary brain cancers. It has subsequently been shown that Turcot is genetically heterogeneous; some cases are due to *APC* mutations, others not. Quite what proportion, if any, might be due to *MUTYH* mutations remains to be determined, but the association of colorectal polyposis and brain cancers in the first decade of life is now certainly associated with biallelic inheritance of two DNA MMR gene mutations at the same locus, i.e. constitutional mismatch repair deficiency (CMMRD) (see 'Lynch syndrome (LS)' in Chapter 4, 'Cancer', p. 586). Primary brain cancers in FAP, although rare, are more likely to be medulloblastomas, but all types occur.

Clinical approach

It is important to appreciate that a high proportion of FAP patients report being distressed, and there is also evidence that those with *APC* mutations may understand important concepts better when these are explained with pictures, rather than words.

History: key points

- Three-generation family tree, with particular emphasis on history of tumours, benign and malignant, and documentation of histological proof of diagnosis, i.e. >100 adenomas. It is critical to determine the apparent mode of inheritance, i.e. AD or not.
- Ascertain who has had screening or operations for what and when and where.
- Is the family already known to a familial cancer or polyposis registry?
- Ask about possible extracolonic features, e.g. upper GI disease, sebaceous cysts, desmoids/'fibromatosis', osteomata, dental history, ophthalmic history.
- History of learning difficulties?

Examination: key points

- Check for sebaceous cysts, especially scalp and trunk; most patients do not regard them as tumours and will not spontaneously report them.
- Examine the mouth and jaws: teeth, cysts, osteomata.
- Head/neck/trunk/abdominal wall/limb swellings. Desmoids? If so, refer to a surgeon.
- If the patient declares or is found to have an abdominal mass, refer to a gastroenterologist or colorectal surgeon.
- GI tract. Refer to a gastroenterologist or colorectal surgeon (see 'Surveillance and management' below).

Special investigations

- Histopathology. There must be over 100 adenomas in the colorectum to diagnose FAP. If there are fewer than 100 adenomas, then AFAP or 'multiple adenomas' can be diagnosed. Microadenomas in the colorectal mucosa, i.e. adenomas confined to a single crypt ('monocryptal' or 'single-crypt' adenomas), are

a hallmark of FAP/AFAP (but they are found in both *APC*- and *MUTYH*-associated polyposis). Multiple fundic gland polyps in the stomach are characteristic of FAP, but entirely benign.

- Ophthalmology. CHRPE—note that there are various types of these. A single large, pigmented lesion with a pale halo is diagnostic of FAP. Smaller, generally hyperpigmented lesions are not uncommon in the general population but are found at increased frequency in FAP where they are typically multiple/bilateral. The number of lesions tends to be concordant within families and correlates with the site of *APC* mutation. NB. While the presence of significant CHRPE indicates FAP, their absence does not exclude it. See 'Predictive testing' below. If in doubt, refer to an ophthalmologist with expertise in this area, especially in cases of referral from an ophthalmologist who is unfamiliar with the finer points of CHRPE diagnosis in FAP.
- *APC* mutation detection. The laboratory will need to know if AD or possible AR (or *de novo*) inheritance applies. If the family have a particular predilection to desmoids, this may help them in mutation interpretation.
- *MUTYH* mutation detection. The laboratory will wish to know the pattern of inheritance, the ethnic background of the proband/family, if there is a possibility of consanguinity, and polyp numbers. Blood from parents and/or other relatives may be useful, together with details of their phenotype.
- Chromosome analysis or array CGH in cases with learning disability and/or dysmorphic features.
- In Ashkenazim with a phenotype possibly indicating HMPS, consider testing for the 40-kb duplication of the 3′ end of *SCG5* upstream of *GREM1*.

Genetic advice

Risk assessment

- If FAP phenotype and AD inheritance, then a presumptive diagnosis of *APC*-associated FAP can be made, and appropriate counselling given regarding inheritance and possible genetic testing.
- If FAP phenotype, but AD inheritance cannot be demonstrated, i.e. an isolated case or affected sibship, then disease is probably due to *APC* mutation but may be due to *MUTYH*.
- If AFAP phenotype and AD inheritance can be demonstrated, then may be due to *APC* mutation (~10% of cases), but in most cases (90%) the cause is, as yet, elusive (except for rare cases of HMPS).
- If AFAP phenotype (with >9 adenomas) but AD inheritance cannot be demonstrated, i.e. an isolated case or affected sibship, then disease is more likely due to *MUTYH* (~25% of cases) with AR inheritance, but an *APC* mutation cannot be ruled out. However, except in the rare case of HMPS, the cause in the rest remains elusive.

NB. The pattern of inheritance in a particular family may not be obvious until the proband's first-degree relatives have undergone colonoscopy or some other form of diagnostic examination, e.g. for CHRPE.

MUTATIONS. There is usually little difficulty with the interpretation of FAP-related *APC* mutations, as they are almost always (possibly exclusively) null, nonsense, or splice/frameshifting. In apparently *de novo* cases, bear in mind that such individuals may have *MUTYH* mutations.

LINKAGE. In the absence of an *APC* mutation, it is possible to carry out 5q22 linkage studies in families with AD FAP with flanking markers. However, given MAP, all concerned will wish to be absolutely convinced that there is a clear-cut AD family history with histological proof of phenotype, as well as gathering in samples from as many relatives as possible, preferably from >1 generation.

TIMING OF PREDICTIVE TESTING. In FAP, when the *APC* mutation is known, predictive genetic testing for family members should be offered in the early teens, so that colorectal surveillance can be initiated at around the age of 14 years. It has been shown that adolescents adapt well following genetic counselling and testing for FAP. In MAP, genetic testing should be offered such that colorectal surveillance can be started by the early 20s.

CARRIER TESTING IN MAP. This is a common question in the clinic, and it is reasonable to offer testing for common *MUTYH* mutations to spouses of patients with MAP or carriers of MAP. Beware of possible consanguinity.

Penetrance
There is almost complete penetrance, with 50% of FAP patients developing polyps by 15 years and 95% by 35 years. An individual at risk of FAP and found to have a single adenoma on surveillance at a young age must be regarded as a carrier. An adenoma found in an at-risk individual at an older age may be sporadic, but continued surveillance should indicate whether or not this was the case.

Prenatal diagnosis
The possibility of PGD and PND can be discussed with couples. In FAP, more opt for the former than the latter.

Surveillance and management
See also 'Cancer surveillance methods' in Chapter 4, 'Cancer', p. 552.

Surveillance and management of adenomatous polyposis should be based on the patient's phenotype. Surveillance of those at 50% risk of FAP can cease when the carrier risk drops below 1%, i.e. age 40.

Colorectal surveillance
Most individuals with *APC*-associated FAP will start to develop colorectal adenomas in their teens. Thus, surveillance is geared to the detection of these in those at risk, with a view to offering prophylactic surgery at the earliest convenient time. In those with FAP who have not had a prophylactic colectomy, CRC can occur under 20 years of age. This is more likely in those with *APC* mutations at or around codon 1300.

There are subtle differences in the endoscopic methods of polyp surveillance. Most patients will develop polyps detectable on rigid sigmoidoscopy, i.e. in the rectum and sigmoid colon. However, rectal sparing is described, especially in AFAP. Therefore, although rigid sigmoidoscopy is quick and easy to perform, there is a place for flexible sigmoidoscopy (which can also be performed in outpatients and can approach the splenic flexure) and colonoscopy, the latter requiring more extensive preparation and involving day-care admission.

Surveillance strategy will depend on local resources and discussion with the surgical team/endoscopist.

For FAP alternatives are:
• annual sigmoidoscopy from early/mid teenage. Cover for the possibility of rectosigmoid sparing with 5-yearly colonoscopy. Gradually extend the screening interval to 3-yearly, as the patient gets older. Reassure and discharge when the residual risk drops below 1% (i.e. age 40 years in the absence of CHRPE data, but see below);
• annual flexible sigmoidoscopy from 13 to 15 years of age in at-risk family members until 30 years, and then at 3- to 5-yearly intervals until 60 years of age.

NB. This surveillance is *not* appropriate for those at risk of AFAP, because they often exhibit late-onset polyps, rectosigmoid sparing, and wide individual variation in expressivity/penetrance. In such cases, a regime similar to that for LS is more appropriate, i.e. 2-yearly colonoscopy.

Surgical management
Surgical opinion varies, but most plan for prophylactic colectomy in affected individuals between the ages of 16 and 20 years to minimize the risk of malignancy. However, patients with the most severe dense polyposis, e.g. those with mutations at or around codon 1300, may be, given their increased short-term risk of rectal cancer, best managed by restorative proctocolectomy with the formation of an ileoanal pouch. However, for the majority of patients, colectomy and ileorectal anastomosis, with rectal surveillance until mid-life when a proctectomy with ileoanal pouch formation is performed, may be preferred. Undoubtedly, the best results are obtained in specialist centres and it is important for FAP patients to engage with the care of an appropriate surgical team at an early stage.

Upper gastrointestinal tract
There is no established practice as regards the surveillance and management of upper GI polyposis in FAP. Most patients will have gastric fundic polyps, which are entirely benign, but the significant lesions are duodenal adenomas. Now that patients are avoiding CRC by prophylactic colectomy, the overall risk of duodenal cancer is 3–4%, so upper GI disease is increasingly significant. Intensive, e.g. annual, upper GI endoscopy is unpleasant and not without its own risks. There seems to be little point in the surveillance of those with few, less dysplastic adenomas, as they are unlikely to develop duodenal cancer. However, those with more advanced duodenal polyposis (multiple, large, severely dysplastic adenomas) may benefit from some degree of upper GI surveillance, but this remains to be proven. An upper GI endoscopy at around 30 years is reasonable to establish the baseline, with the follow-up interval based on disease severity.

Desmoid tumours
FAP patients are at significantly increased risk of desmoid tumours, and about 10% will develop clinically evident disease. Desmoids are histologically benign but may become clinically malignant, as they encroach on and encase vital organs and structures, particularly in the case of intra-abdominal tumours. They are indolent, difficult to surgically excise completely, and refractory to treatment with chemo- or radiotherapy. Together with upper GI tract disease, they are now one of the leading causes of premature death in FAP.

• Sporadic desmoids are more likely to occur peripherally (limbs), whereas FAP-associated desmoids more commonly arise centrally (head/neck/trunk/abdominal wall/intra-abdominal).

- Families with mutations at or beyond codon 1400 have the highest risk of desmoids, perhaps up to 30–40%. There is no established form of surveillance for occult desmoids, though imaging by CT or MRI may be useful in surgical management.
- A number of FAP families have now been described in which the diagnosis only became apparent when children presented with desmoids.

Non-surgical treatment

Although surgical management of FAP is the mainstay, a number of trials have been or are being carried out into possible chemotherapeutic options. Quoting directly from Vasen et al. (2008):

'Chemoprevention with NSAIDs can be considered in patients following initial prophylactic surgery as an adjunct to endoscopic surveillance, to reduce the rectal polyp burden. The role of selective COX-2 inhibitors in patients with FAP is controversial because of cardiovascular side effects reported for rofecoxib. Therefore, these drugs should only be considered in selected patients without cardiovascular risk factors until more data are available.'

Reproduced from *Gut*, Vansen *et al.*, Guidelines for the clinical management of familial adenomatous polyposis (FAP), 57, 5, pp. 704–13, copyright 2008, with permission from BMJ Publishing Group Ltd.

Support groups: FAP Gene Support Group, http://www.fapgene.com; Macmillan Cancer Support, http://www.macmillan.org.uk/Cancerinformation/Causesriskfactors/Genetics/Cancergenetics/Specificconditions/FAP.aspx.

Expert adviser: Ian M. Frayling, Consultant Genetic Pathologist, Cardiff and Vale University Health Board, Cardiff University, Institute of Medical Genetics, University Hospital of Wales, Cardiff, UK.

References

Adam R, Spier I, et al. Exome sequencing identifies biallelic MSH3 germline mutations as a recessive subtype of colorectal adenomatous polyposis. Am J Hum Genet 2016; **99**: 337–51.

Al-Tassan N, Chmiel NH, Maynard J, et al. Inherited variants of *MYH* associated with somatic G:C→T:A mutations in colorectal tumors. Nat Genet 2002; **30**: 227–32.

Cairns SR, Scholefield JH, Steele RJ, et al. Guidelines for colorectal cancer screening and surveillance in moderate and high risk groups (update from 2002). Gut 2010; **59**: 666–89.

Clark SK, Phillips RK. Desmoids in familial adenomatous polyposis [review]. Br J Surg 1996; **83**: 1494–504.

Douma KF, Aaronson NK, Vasen HF, et al. Psychological distress and use of psychosocial support in familial adenomatous polyposis. Psychooncology 2010; **19**: 289–98.

Frayling IM, Arends MJ. Adenomatous polyposis coli. In: S Maloy, K Hughes (eds.). *Brenner's encyclopedia of genetics*, 2nd edn, volume **1**, pp. 27–9. Academic Press, San Diego, 2013.

Friedl W, Caspari R, Sengteller M, et al. Can APC mutation analysis contribute to therapeutic decisions in familial adenomatous polyposis? Experience from 680 FAP families. Gut 2001; **48**: 515–21.

Jasperson KW, Burt RW. *APC*-associated polyposis conditions. In: RA Pagon, MP Adam, HH Ardinger, et al. (eds.). GeneReviews®, 2014. http://www.ncbi.nlm.nih.gov/books/NBK1345.

Giardiello FM, Brensinger JD, Petersen GM. AGA technical review on hereditary colorectal cancer and genetic testing. Gastroenterology 2001; **121**: 198–213.

Gjone H, Diseth TH, Fausa O, Nøvik TS, Heiberg A. Familial adenomatous polyposis: mental health, psychosocial functioning and reactions to genetic risk in adolescents. Clin Genet 2011; **79**: 35–43.

Healy JC, Reznek RH, Clark SK, Phillips RK, Armstrong P. MR appearances of desmoid tumors in familial adenomatous polyposis. Am J Roentgenol 1997; **169**: 465–72.

Hyer W. Polyposis syndromes: pediatric implications [review]. Gastrointest Endosc Clin N Am 2001; **11**: 659–82, vi–vii.

International Society for Gastrointestinal Hereditary Tumours (InSiGHT). http://www.insight-group.org/guidelines/fap and http://www.insight-group.org/pdf/5-3.pdf [MAP].

Jaeger E, Leedham S, Lewis A, et al. Hereditary mixed polyposis syndrome is caused by a 40-kb upstream duplication that leads to increased and ectopic expression of the BMP antagonist GREM1. Nat Genet 2012; **44**: 699–703.

Jones S, Emmerson P, Maynard J, et al. Biallelic germline mutations in *MYH* predispose to multiple colorectal adenoma and somatic G:C→T: A mutations. Hum Mol Genet 2002; **11**: 2961–7.

Jones N, Vogt S, Nielsen M, et al. Increased colorectal cancer incidence in obligate carriers of heterozygous mutations in MUTYH. Gastroenterology 2009; **137**: 489–94.

Michie S, Bobrow M, Marteau TM. Predictive genetic testing in children and adults: a study of emotional impact. J Med Genet 2001; **38**: 519–26.

Palles C, Cazier JB, Howarth KM, et al. Germline mutations affecting the proofreading domains of *POLE* and *POLD1* predispose to colorectal adenomas and carcinomas. Nat Genet 2013; **45**: 136–44.

Rivera B, Castellsagué E, Bah I, van Kempen LC, Foulkes WD. Biallelic NTHL1 mutations in a woman with multiple primary tumors. N Engl J Med 2015; **373**: 1985–6.

Sampson JR, Dolwani S, Jones S, et al. Autosomal recessive colorectal adenomatous polyposis due to inherited mutations of MYH. Lancet 2003; **362**: 39–41.

Sieber OM, Lamlum H, Crabtree MD, et al. Whole-gene APC deletions cause classical familial adenomatous polyposis, but not attenuated polyposis or 'multiple' colorectal adenomas. Proc Natl Acad Sci U S A 2002; **99**: 2954–8.

Sieber OM, Lipton L, Crabtree M, et al. The multiple colorectal adenoma phenotype, Familial adenomatous polyposis and germline mutations in MYH. N Engl J Med 2003a; **348**: 791–9.

Sieber O, Lipton L, Heinimann K, Tomlinson I. Colorectal tumourigenesis in carriers of the APC I1307K variant: lone gunman or conspiracy? J Pathol 2003b; **199**: 137–9.

Spier I, Horpaopan S, Vogt S, et al. Deep intronic APC mutations explain a substantial proportion of patients with familial or early-onset adenomatous polyposis. Hum Mutat 2012; **33**: 1045–50.

Tomlinson I, Rahman N, Frayling I, et al. Inherited susceptibility to colorectal adenomas and carcinomas: evidence for a new predisposition gene on 15q14–q22. Gastroenterology 1999; **116**: 789–95.

Trimbath JD, Giardiello FM. Review article: genetic testing and counselling for hereditary colorectal cancer. Aliment Pharmacol Ther 2002; **16**: 1843–57.

Vasen HF, Möslein G, Alonso A, et al. Guidelines for the clinical management of familial adenomatous polyposis (FAP). Gut 2008; **57**: 704–13.

Weren RD, Ligtenberg MJ, Kets CM, et al. A germline homozygous mutation in the base-excision repair gene NTHL1 causes adenomatous polyposis and colorectal cancer. Nat Genet 2015; **47**: 668–71.

Gastric cancer

Gastric cancer is the second largest cancer burden worldwide. In the UK, the lifetime risk in the general population is 2.3% for males, and 1.2% for females. Average age at diagnosis in men is 72 years (range 65–80 years), and in women 75 years (range 70–85 years). Survival rates are low (10% at 5 years) due to late presentation and diagnosis. In contrast to the West, Japan has introduced systematic mass screening programmes with oesophago-gastroduodenoscopy (OGD), leading to the increased detection of gastric cancers confined to the mucosa or submucosa. Survival rates for patients with early gastric cancer are >90% at 5 years.

Gastric cancer can be classified histopathologically into two distinct types: intestinal and diffuse (linitis plastica type). The major risk factor for intestinal gastric cancer identified so far is *Helicobacter pylori* infection. However, whether *H. pylori* eradication is an effective cancer prevention measure is not yet proven.

Approximately 10% of cases of gastric cancer involve familial clustering. Cancer predisposition syndromes to consider include:

- LS (HNPCC). Approximately 5% lifetime risk. See 'Lynch syndrome (LS)' in Chapter 4, 'Cancer', p. 586;
- FAP. See 'Familial adenomatous polyposis (FAP) and adenomatous polyposis due to *MUTYH, NTHL1, POLE*, and *POLD1*' in Chapter 4, 'Cancer', p. 568;
- PJS. See 'Peutz–Jeghers syndrome (PJS)' in Chapter 4, 'Cancer', p. 604;
- Hereditary diffuse gastric cancer (HDGC). Approximately 70–80% lifetime risk. See below;
- BRCA2. See 'BRCA1 and BRCA2' in Chapter 4, 'Cancer', p. 542.

Most large familial gastric cancer kindreds show no evidence of LS (HNPCC), and molecular genetic studies show only a low frequency of E-cadherin mutations. Mean age at diagnosis is ~54 years, but there is wide variation. No close association with *H. pylori* has been demonstrated to date.

Hereditary diffuse gastric cancer (HDGC)

HDGC accounts for just 1–3% of gastric adenocarcinomas. Histology is diffuse or 'linitis plastica' type. Hereditary diffuse cancer has a high penetrance (70–80%) and a high mortality rate. It is AD and caused in ~35% of kindreds by inactivating mutations in *CDH1* (E-cadherin). (The overall mutation detection rate in gastric cancer families is ~10%.) It has a strikingly young age of onset, with an average age at diagnosis of 38 years, compared with 60–70 years for sporadic gastric cancer. Following predictive genetic testing, prophylactic total gastrectomy is generally recommended in mutation carriers. For patients without a pathogenic *CDH1* mutation, endoscopic screening can be helpful to identify microscopic foci of signet ring cells indicative of the syndrome. Other patients may opt for endoscopic surveillance to help guide the timing of gastrectomy, though this is not yet proven and the International Consensus guidelines (van der Post 2015) should be followed.

Women with *CDH1* mutations appear to have an increased risk of lobular breast cancer, with a cumulative risk of 39% by age 80 years.

The diagnostic criteria for HDGC are outlined in Figure 4.2.

Oesophageal cancer—tylosis

Tylosis is a rare syndrome presenting with hyperkeratosis of the palms and soles of the feet. AD with variable penetrance.

- Type A tylosis presents in adolescence and is associated with a high risk for oesophageal cancer. Approximately 20% of individuals with type A develop oesophageal cancer (especially in smokers). Onset of malignancy is typically from 50 years. Annual OGD surveillance is recommended.
- Type B tylosis has a neonatal presentation and affected individuals are not at increased risk for oesophageal cancer. Two North American kindreds spanning five and seven generations confirm the benign nature of type B (Maillefer *et al.* 1999). No surveillance is indicated.

Focal palmoplantar keratoderma (tylosis) associated with squamous cell oesophageal cancer (tylosis oesophageal cancer (TOC): type A tylosis) may be caused by heterozygous missense mutation in the *RHBDF2* gene on 17q25 (Blaydon *et al.* 2012).

Clinical approach

History: key points
At least three-generation family tree, with specific enquiry for all forms of cancer, with age at diagnosis. Note the names, dates of birth, and hospital where the diagnosis was made. This information may be helpful in confirming the family history prior to risk assessment.

Examination: key points
Not usually appropriate in an asymptomatic family member, unless there is a family history of oesophageal cancer (examine the palms and soles for hyperkeratosis).

Genetic advice

Risk assessment
Relatives of gastric cancer patients have a 2- to 3-fold increased risk of developing gastric cancer. The risk is elevated for both genders (Imsland *et al.* 2002). The lifetime risk in the general population is 2.3% for males and 1.2% for females.

- The risk with two affected relatives is 1 in 8 to 1 in 10.
- The risk with three affected relatives is 1 in 3.
- The risk in HDGC is AD.

Penetrance
Penetrance in HDGC is high at 70–80% for gastric cancer and ~39% for breast cancer in females.

Predictive testing
Predictive testing is possible if the familial mutation is known. In HDGC, this is used, where possible, to determine which individuals should be offered prophylactic gastrectomy since the procedure has a high morbidity, with some patients having difficulty maintaining adequate nutrition post-surgery, as well as effects on quality of life.

Management

Surveillance strategies
See also 'Cancer surveillance methods' in Chapter 4, 'Cancer', p. 552.

- Consider *H. pylori* screening and eradication.
- Consider regular endoscopy in a specialist centre.
- Consider prophylactic total gastrectomy in HDGC.

Expert adviser: Rebecca Fitzgerald, Professor of Cancer Prevention and Programme Leader, MRC Cancer Unit, Hutchison/MRC Research Centre University

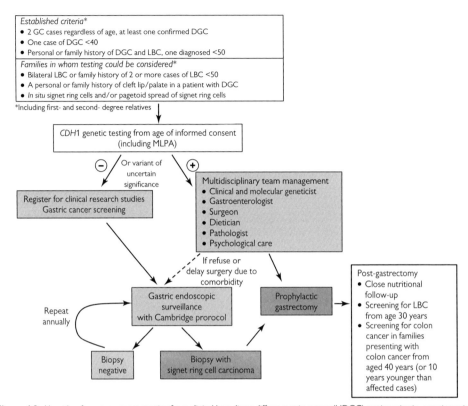

Figure 4.2 Algorithm for management starting from clinical hereditary diffuse gastric cancer (HDGC) testing criteria, genetic testing, role of endoscopy, and gastrectomy. GC, gastric cancer; DGC, diffuse gastric cancer; LBC, lobular breast cancer; MLPA, multiplex ligation probe amplification.
Reproduced from *Journal of Medical Genetics*, Rachel S van der Post *et al.*, Hereditary diffuse gastric cancer: updated clinical guidelines with an emphasis on germline *CDH1* mutation carriers, volume 52, issue 6, pp. 361–374, copyright 2015 with permission from BMJ Publishing Group Ltd.

of Cambridge; Director of Studies in Medicine, and College Lecturer in Medical Sciences, Trinity College, Cambridge, UK.

References

Blaydon DC, Etheridge SL, Risk JM, *et al. RHBDF2* mutations are associated with tylosis, a familial esophageal cancer syndrome. *Am J Hum Genet* 2012; **90**: 340–6.

Blaydon DC, Lind LK, Plagnol V, *et al.* Mutations in AQP5 encoding a water-channel protein, cause autosomal dominant diffuse non-epidermolytic palmo-plantar keratoderma. *Am J Hum Genet* 2013; **93**: 330–5.

Fitzgerald RC, Caldas C. E-cadherin mutations and hereditary gastric cancer: prevention by resection. *Dig Dis* 2002; **20**: 23–31.

Huntsman DG, Carneiro F, Lewis FR, *et al.* Early gastric cancer in young, asymptomatic carriers of germ-line E-cadherin mutations. *N Engl J Med* 2001; **344**: 1904–9.

Imsland AK, Eldon BJ, Arinbjarnarson S, *et al.* Genetic epidemiologic aspects of gastric cancer in Iceland. *J Am Coll Surg* 2002; **195**: 181–6; discussion 186–7.

Maillefer RH, Greydanus MP. To B or not to B: is tylosis B truly benign? Two North American genealogies. *Am J Gastroenterol* 1999; **94**: 829–34.

Risk JM, Evans KE, Jones J, *et al.* Characterization of a 500 kb region on 17q25 and the exclusion of candidate genes as the familial tylosis oesophageal cancer (TOC) locus. *Oncogene* 2002; **21**: 6395–402.

van der Post RS, Vogelaar IP, Carneiro F, *et al.* Hereditary diffuse gastric cancer: updated clinical guidelines with an emphasis on germline *CDH1* mutation carriers. *J Med Genet* 2015; **52**: 361–74.

Weitzel LN, McCahill LE. The power of genetics to target surgical prevention. *N Engl J Med* 2001; **344**: 1942–4.

Gorlin syndrome

Basal cell naevus syndrome, naevoid basal cell carcinoma syndrome.

Gorlin syndrome is an AD condition predominantly caused by mutations in the tumour suppressor gene *PTCH1* on 9q22.3 (~70% of patients), which functions as a receptor for hedgehog. Basal cell carcinomas (BCCs) and other tumours in Gorlin syndrome show loss of heterozygosity (LOH) for *PTCH1* (i.e. the tumours are the consequence of a second hit). The congenital malformations (affecting 5% of patients) are thought to be due to alterations of gene dosage in the dosage-sensitive hedgehog signalling pathway. Gorlin syndrome affects ~1/50 000 individuals.

A small percentage of Gorlin patients have mutations in *SUFU* on 10q24.32 (Smith *et al.* 2014).

The diagnostic criteria for Gorlin syndrome are given in Box 4.8.

Clinical approach

History: key points
- Three-generation family tree, with specific enquiry about skin cancer, jaw cysts, and large head size.
- Past medical history, including any previous surgery.

Examination: key points
- OFC and height to determine whether there is relative macrocephaly.
- Face for mild hypertelorism, frontal bossing, and large jaw.
- Skin for BCCs (may appear in early childhood but usually proliferate from puberty onwards). There may be from few to many 100s of BCCs, but many stay quiescent. More common on the face and sun-exposed areas, but also occur on the trunk. They are raised lesions (1–10 mm in diameter) with a pearly to flesh-coloured to pale brown coloration. Skin tags on the neck that histologically have the appearance of a BCC but do not behave aggressively.
- Palms. Examine for palmar pits, small circular depressions (1–2 mm) in the hard skin of the palms (and sometimes soles), present in 65–80%. Age-dependent.
- Brachydactyly, thumb anomaly.
- Patients who are the first person in their families to be affected may have milder signs because of somatic mosaicism.

Investigations
- DNA (EDTA blood sample) for *PTCH* and *SUFU* mutation sequencing and dosage analysis.
- Genomic array if any features of developmental delay (deletions of *PTCH1* or *SUFU* occur in a proportion of Gorlin patients).
- Chest X-ray to look for bifid, fused, or splayed ribs and hemivertebrae (if diagnosis not secure).
- Skull X-ray (AP and lateral) to look for lamellar falx calcification (present in over 90% of patients by age 20 years) and bridging of the sella turcica.
- Orthopantogram (OPG) in individuals older than 7 years to look for jaw cysts (see 'Management' below).

Genetic advice

Risk assessment
AD; 50% risk to offspring of an affected individual. High new mutation rate; 35–50% of affected individuals have DNMs.

Penetrance
Penetrance is complete, but there is marked intra- and interfamilial variation in expressivity.

Box 4.8 Diagnostic criteria

Diagnosis is based on two major or one major plus two minor criteria.

Major criteria
- More than two BCCs, or one at <20 years, or >10 basal cell naevi
- Odontogenic keratocyst or polyostotic bone cyst
- Three or more palmar/plantar pits
- Bilamellar or early (20 years) calcification of falx cerebri
- A first-degree relative with Gorlin syndrome

Minor criteria
- Congenital skeletal anomaly: bifid, fused, splayed, or missing rib or fused vertebrae
- Macrocephaly (adjusted for height) with bossing
- Congenital malformation: cleft lip/palate (3–8%), pre- or post-axial polydactyly
- Ovarian/cardiac fibroma
- Childhood medulloblastoma
- Lymphomesenteric cysts
- Ocular anomalies (cataract, developmental defects)

Adapted by permission of BMJ Publishing Group, *Journal of Medical Genetics*, D G Evans *et al.*, Complications of the naevoid basal cell carcinoma syndrome: results of a population based study, 30, 6, pp. 460–4, copyright 1993; and adapted with permission from Kimonis *et al.*, Clinical manifestations in 105 persons with nevoid basal cell carcinoma syndrome, *American Journal of Medical Genetics Part A*, vol 69: 299–308, copyright 1997, Wiley.

Predictive testing
Possible if the familial mutation is known or the family is informative for linkage markers.

Prenatal diagnosis
Possible by CVS if the familial mutation is known or the family is informative for linkage markers.

Management
Surveillance strategies
- Skin. BCCs may become locally invasive from puberty onwards. Refer to a dermatologist for annual (or more frequent) monitoring from age 12 years. BCCs are more florid in sun-exposed areas and much less common in those with black skin. Advise liberal use of sunblock, peaked caps, T-shirts, avoidance of midday sun, etc. Avoid treatment by radiation as most (but not all) families respond with multiple new lesions in the treatment field.
- Jaw cysts. Odontogenic keratocysts of both the upper and lower jaws occur from age 7 years. Refer for annual dental screening (OPG) from the age of 8 years. Cysts have an age-dependent penetrance of 80% by 20 years and >90% by 40 years. Make the patient's dentist aware of the diagnosis, or possible diagnosis, of Gorlin syndrome.
- Medulloblastoma affects ~5% and usually presents at ~2.5 years. Smith *et al.* (2014) found a <2% risk in

PTCH1 mutation-positive individuals, with a risk up to 20 times higher in *SUFU* mutation-positive individuals. It is more common in boys than girls (3M:1F). Investigate by MRI (avoid CT, if possible, as ionizing radiation increases the risk for BCCs). *Avoid* radiotherapy, if possible, in treatment as this can result in profuse BCCs in the radiation field.

Support groups: Gorlin Syndrome Group (UK), http://www.gorlingroup.org, Tel. 01772 517 624; Basal Cell Carcinoma Nevus Syndrome Life Support Network, http://www.gorlinsyndrome.org, Tel. (USA) 708 756 3410.

References
Evans DG, Ladusans EJ, Rimmer S, Burnell LD, Thakker N, Farndon PA. Complications of the naevoid basal cell carcinoma syndrome: results of a population based study. *J Med Genet* 1993; **30**: 460–4.

Jones EA, Sajid MI, Shenton A, Evans DG. Basal cell carcinomas in gorlin syndrome: a review of 202 patients. *J Skin Cancer* 2011; **2011**: 217378.

Gorlin RJ. Nevoid basal cell carcinoma syndrome. *Dermatol Clin* 1995; **13**: 113–25.

Kimonis VE, Goldstein AM, Pastakia B, et al. Clinical manifestations in 105 persons with nevoid basal cell carcinoma syndrome [review]. *Am J Med Genet* 1997; **69**: 299–308.

Smith MJ, Beetz C, Williams SG, et al. Germline mutations in SUFU cause Gorlin syndrome-associated childhood medulloblastoma and redefine the risk associated with PTCH1 mutations. *J Clin Oncol* 2014; **32**: 4155–61.

Juvenile polyposis syndrome (JPS)

Juvenile polyps occur sporadically in childhood. They are delicate structures that are prone to haemorrhage, prolapse, and auto-amputation, so they not uncommonly give rise to anaemia. Colonoscopic surveys show that they occur throughout the colorectum, albeit with a slight preponderance of lesions in the rectosigmoid colon. However, there is a group of individuals who develop multiple juvenile polyps, often with a family history of the same or bowel cancer—this is familial juvenile polyposis syndrome (JPS). JPS is an AD condition with variable penetrance, associated with an increased risk of CRC (10–38%) and of gastric and duodenal cancers (15–21%). Adenomatous change can be found within juvenile polyps and this may account for their malignant potential.

The condition is genetically heterogeneous. Constitutional mutations in SMAD4, BMPR1A, and PTEN have all been described in JPS, and the latter is consistent with it overlapping, or being associated, with PHTS, including Cowden/BRRS. Juvenile polyps are also described in Gorlin syndrome due to PTCH mutations. The condition is uncommon, with a prevalence of between 1/100 000 and 1/160 000. Chow and Macrae (2005) have reviewed the condition, including its management.

Diagnostic criteria

In the absence of features suggesting CS/BRRS, JPS is diagnosed when there are:

- >five juvenile polyps in the colon or rectum, or
- juvenile polyps in other parts of the GI tract, or
- any number of juvenile polyps and a positive family history.

Juvenile polyposis of infancy, where the entire GI tract is involved and with protein-losing enteropathy, carries a poor prognosis. Associated features include macrocephaly, clubbing, hypotonia, and absence of a family history. This severe form of early-onset JPS has been associated with a contiguous gene deletion of PTEN and BMPR1A on chromosome 10q23.

Associated clinical features

Clinically, JPS falls into two groups: (1) those individuals with only juvenile polyposis of the GI tract; (2) those with juvenile polyposis of the GI tract plus other features.

Some of the latter group are undoubtedly due to families with PHTS or Gorlin syndrome due to PTCH1 mutations, in which juvenile polyps have occurred. However, cases of JPS due to SMAD4 or BMPR1A mutations have been described, in which dysmorphic/extracolonic features have occurred, suggestive of PHTS. Hereditary haemorrhagic telangiectasia (HHT) occurs in association with JPS (so-called JPS/HHT).

There is wide variation in the phenotype, both inter- and intrafamilial, perhaps not surprising given the genetic heterogeneity. Apart from juvenile polyps in the GI tract, stomach, and colorectum, other clinical features that have been associated with JPS are given in Table 4.14.

Genetics

Mutations in SMAD4 and BMPR1A, components of the TGF-β signal transduction pathway account for most (about 60%) cases:

- SMAD4 on 18q21.1 accounts for about 30% of families. One recurrent 'hotspot' mutation 1372–1375delACAG accounts for about half of SMAD4 cases, i.e. 15–25% of all JPS. Fifteen to 22% of individuals with a SMAD4 mutation develop both HHT and JPS, a condition termed JPS/HHT;
- BMPR1A on 10q23.2 accounts for about 30% of families;
- PTEN on 10q23.31 accounts for a small number of families with features of Cowden syndrome/BRRS;
- PTCH1 on 9q22.32 accounts for a few families with Gorlin syndrome in which juvenile polyps have occurred.

Chromosomal mutations, e.g. del 10q23.2–q23.33 and del 10q22.3–q24.1, have been found in JPS patients, a region encompassing both PTEN and BMPR1A.

Genotype–phenotype

Mutations in SMAD4 are associated with massive gastric polyposis, whereas families with mutations in BMPR1A or undetectable mutations in either gene are not, although such individuals are still liable to low numbers of gastric lesions.

Table 4.14 Clinical features associated with JPS

Feature	Mutations in				
	SMAD4	BMPR1A	PTEN	PTCH1	No mutation identified[*]
Macrocephaly, hypertelorism	Yes	Yes	Yes	Yes	
Mental retardation	Yes		Yes	Yes	Yes
Pulmonary arteriovenous fistulae	Yes				
Ventricular septal defect	Yes	Yes			Yes
Other cardiac defects		Yes			Yes
Thoracic skeletal anomalies	Yes			Yes	
Haemangiomata			Yes	Yes	
Lipomata			Yes	Yes	
Hypospadias					Yes
Genital freckling			Yes	Yes	
Telangiectasia	Yes				

[*] But not necessarily looked for, when reported.

Features of Cowden syndrome/BRRS or Gorlin syndrome in JPS may point to *PTEN* or *PTCH1*, respectively, but are also described in JPS due to *SMAD4* or *BMPR1A* mutations.

Differential diagnosis

The association of JPS with PHTS and Gorlin syndrome has been mentioned above. Although 90% of polyps in children up to 10 years of age are juvenile polyps, other causes of intestinal polyposis in children include:

- Peutz–Jeghers syndrome (PJS), but this has characteristic histology;
- familial adenomatous polyposis (FAP). Rare instances of polyposis before the age of 10 years are described, but the histology is of adenomas;
- Turcot syndrome. This is the co-occurrence of adenomatous polyposis with brain cancer; it may represent cases of either *APC* mutation (so a form of FAP) or CMMRD (see 'Lynch syndrome (LS)' in Chapter 4, 'Cancer', p. 586).

Clinical approach

History: key points
Three-generation family tree, with careful enquiry about possible features of PHTS, Gorlin syndrome, and HHT (see Table 4.14). Take a detailed history of cancer/tumours in other family members (do not forget benign tumours, e.g. haemangiomata, lipomata, etc.).

Examination: key points
- Check for skin, skeletal, neurological, cardiopulmonary, and genitourinary signs (genital freckling?).
- Mouth. Cowden syndrome signs?
- Head circumference.
- Surgical scars, e.g. skin lesions removed and since forgotten about.

Special investigations
- Upper and lower GI endoscopy.
- Radiology/imaging. ICC, skeletal anomalies, or abnormal vertebrae?
- Cranial imaging if cerebellar signs (LDD is a term for dysplastic gangliocytoma of the cerebellum; see 'Cowden syndrome (PTEN hamartoma tumour syndrome (PHTS))' in Chapter 4, 'Cancer', p. 564).
- Specialist review of histopathology. Polyps, skin lesions.
- Genetic testing. Be guided by the clinical features.
  - In cases without features suggestive of PHTS or Gorlin syndrome, carry out germline mutation detection in *SMAD4* first and then *BMPR1A*. If no mutation detected in either gene, review and consider *PTEN* or *PTCH1* testing.
  - In cases with features of PHTS, look in *PTEN*, and then *SMAD4* and *BMPR1A*.
  - In cases with features of Gorlin syndrome, look in *PTCH*, and then *SMAD4, BMPR1A*, and *PTEN*.
- Have a low threshold for requesting a genomic array.

Genetic advice

Risk assessment
AD, with 50% risk of transmission.

Penetrance
Uncertain, and expressivity highly variable and dependent on the underlying cause/gene. Malignant risk is from around 20 years onwards and increases in the fourth

decade of life. Lifetime risk of CRC is up to 68% by age 60 and gastric cancer 15–21%, though these are overall figures and not subdivided by genotype.

Predictive testing
Possible in families with an identified constitutional mutation. Like with FAP, predictive testing should be carried out in teenage, in order to best inform decisions on surveillance and possible prophylactic surgery.

Prenatal diagnosis
Both PGD and PND are possible in families with an identified constitutional mutation.

Management

Surveillance strategies
See also 'Cancer surveillance methods' in Chapter 4, 'Cancer', p. 552.

MANAGEMENT OF PROBANDS AND PROVEN MUTATION CARRIERS. In view of the lifetime risk of death of 1 in 6 in the absence of screening, Cairns et al. (2010) recommend the following surveillance strategy in JPS, in combination with genetic testing of an affected individual:
- 2-yearly colonoscopy and OGD. Extend the interval aged >35 years;
- commence colonoscopy from age 15 years;
- commence OGD from age 25 years;
- consider cardiovascular examination and evaluation for HHT in *SMAD4* mutation carriers.

MANAGEMENT OF AT-RISK FAMILY MEMBERS. In families where a mutation has not been found, it has been recommended to perform upper and lower GI surveillance at least every 10 years from age 15 until 45 years thereafter, following guidelines for CRC screening in the general population. Of course, if any symptoms should develop, the patient should be immediately investigated, as appropriate.

In cases of JPS due to PHTS or *PTCH1*, specific anticancer surveillance directed at sites other than the GI tract should be considered and implemented, as appropriate.

Expert adviser: Karl Heinimann, Consultant Medical Geneticist, Division of Medical Genetics, University Hospital Basel, Basel, Switzerland.

References
Cairns SR, Scholefield JH, Steele RJ, et al. Guidelines for colorectal cancer screening and surveillance in moderate and high risk groups (update from 2002). Gut 2010; **59**: 666–89.

Chow E, Macrae F. A review of juvenile polyposis syndrome. J Gastroenterol Hepatol 2005; **20**: 1634–40.

Dunlop MG. Guidance on gastrointestinal surveillance for hereditary non-polyposis colorectal cancer, familial adenomatous polyposis, juvenile polyposis, and Peutz–Jeghers syndrome. Gut 2002; **51**(Suppl 5): v21–7.

Friedl W, Uhlhaas S, Schulmann K, et al. Juvenile polyposis: massive gastric polyposis is more common in *MADH4* mutation carriers than in *BMPR1A* mutation carriers. Hum Genet 2002; **111**: 108–11.

Gallione CJ, Repette GM. A combined syndrome of juvenile polyposis and hereditary haemorrhagic telangiectasia associated with mutations in *MADH4* (*SMAD4*). Lancet 2004; **363**: 852–9.

Gammon A, Jasperson K, Kohlmann W, Burt RW. Hamartomatous polyposis syndromes. Best Pract Res Clin Gastroenterol 2009; **23**: 219–31.

Haidle JL, Howe JR. Juvenile polyposis syndrome. In: RA Pagon, TD Bird, CR Dolan, et al. (eds.). GeneReviews®, University of

Washington, Seattle, 2003 (updated 2015). http://www.ncbi.nlm.nih.gov/books/NBK1469.

Howe JR, Mitros FA, Summers RW. The risk of gastrointestinal carcinoma in familial juvenile polyposis [review]. *Ann Surg Oncol* 1998; **5**: 751–6.

Howe JR, Ringold JC, Hughes JH, Summers RW. Direct genetic testing for *SMAD4* mutations in patients at risk for juvenile polyposis. *Surgery* 1999; **126**: 162–70.

Howe JR, Shellnut J, Wagner B, et al. Common deletion of *SMAD4* in juvenile polyposis is a mutational hotspot. *Am J Hum Genet* 2002; **70**: 1357–62.

Hyer W. Polyposis syndromes: pediatric implications [review]. *Gastrointest Endosc Clin N Am* 2001; **11**: 659–82, vi–vii.

Iyer NK, Burke CA, Leach BH, Parambil JG. *SMAD4* mutation and the combined syndrome of juvenile polyposis syndrome and hereditary haemorrhagic telangiectasia. *Thorax* 2010; **65**; 745–6.

Jass JR. Juvenile polyposis. In: RKS Phillips, A Spiegelman (eds.). *Familial adenomatous polyposis and other polyposis syndromes*, 1st edn, pp. 203–14. Edward Arnold, London, 1994.

Merg A, Howe JR. Genetic conditions associated with intestinal juvenile polyps [seminar]. *Am J Med Genet C Semin Med Genet* 2004; **129C**: 44–55.

Sayed MG, Ahmed AF, Ringold JR, et al. Germline *SMAD4* or *BMPR1A* mutations and phenotype of juvenile polyposis. *Ann Surg Oncol* 2002; **9**: 901–6.

Syngal S, Brand RE, Church JM, et al. ACG clinical guideline: genetic testing and management of hereditary gastrointestinal cancer syndromes. *Am J Gastroenterol* 2015; **110**: 223–62.

Wirtzfeld DA, Petrelli NJ, Rodriguez-Bigas MA. Hamartomatous polyposis syndromes: molecular genetics, neoplastic risk, and surveillance recommendations [review]. *Ann Surg Oncol* 2001; **8**: 319–27.

Woodford-Richens K, Williamson J, Bevan S, et al. Allelic loss at *SMAD4* in polyps from juvenile polyposis patients and use of FISH to demonstrate clonal origin of the epithelium. *Cancer Res* 2000; **60**: 2477–82.

Zhou XP, Woodford-Richens K, Lehtonen R, et al. Germline mutations in *BMPR1A/ALK3* cause a subset of cases of juvenile polyposis syndrome and of Cowden and Bannayan–Riley–Ruvalcaba syndromes. *Am J Hum Genet* 2001; **69**: 704–11.

Lifestyle factors in cancer: smoking, alcohol, obesity, diet, and exercise

Smoking

Carcinogenic effects of tobacco cause cancer of the lung, pancreas, bladder, and kidney, and (synergistically with alcohol) the larynx, mouth, pharynx (except the naso-pharynx), and oesophagus. Recent evidence suggests that the prevalence of several other types of cancer (stomach, liver, and (probably) cervix) is also increased by smoking.

About 60% of cancers among smokers are due to smoking and tobacco causes one-third of all cancer deaths in developed countries. The rapid increase in the lung cancer incidence rate among continuing smok-ers ceases when they stop smoking—the rate remaining roughly constant for many years in ex-smokers.

Smoking increases the risk of breast cancer in *BRCA2* carriers (Friebel *et al.* 2014).

Alcohol

Alcohol increases the risk of cancers of the oral cavity, pharynx, larynx, oesophagus, liver, and breast.

Obesity

There is now a consensus that cancer is more common in those who are overweight. The evidence on weight is strongest for post-menopausal breast cancer and cancers of the endometrium, gall bladder, and kidney.

A US study (Calle *et al.* 1999) estimated that ~10% of all cancer deaths among American non-smokers (7% in men and 12% in women) are caused by overweight. Bergstrom *et al.* (2001) have estimated that 5% (3% in men and 6% in women) of all incident cancers in the European Union might be prevented if no one had a BMI >25.

Diet

Diet-related factors are thought to account for ~30% of cancers in developed countries (Key 2002). Adequate intakes of fruit and vegetables probably lower the risk for several types of cancer, especially cancers of the GI tract (Key 2002). The significance of other factors, e.g. meat, fibre, and vitamins, is currently unclear.

Exercise

Regular exercise reduces the risk of colon cancer and probably also of breast cancer, although the quantitative effect is uncertain.

General lifestyle advice

Advice to members of the general population is not to smoke and 'to maintain a healthy weight, restrict alco-hol consumption, and select a conventionally balanced diet ensuring an adequate intake of fruit, vegetables, and cereals' (Key 2002). Figure 4.3 illustrates the estimated preventable component for some common cancers. The extent to which such advice can modify the risk of can-cer in individuals who carry, or are at risk of carrying, a mutation in a cancer-predisposing gene is uncertain. However, any reduction in risk, even if very small, may be of benefit.

References

Bergstrom A, Pisani P, Tenet V, Wolk A, Adami HO. Overweight as an avoidable cause of cancer in Europe. *Int J Cancer* 2001; **91**: 421–30.

Calle EE, Thun MJ, Petrelli JM, Rodriguez C, Heath CW Jr. Body-mass index and mortality in a prospective cohort of US adults. *N Engl J Med* 1999; **341**: 1097–105.

Friebel TM, Domcheck SM, Rebbeck TR. Modifiers of cancer risk in *BRCA1* and *BRCA2* mutation carriers: systematic review and meta-analysis. *J Natl Cancer Inst* 2014; **106**: dju091.

Key TJ. Effect of diet on risk of cancer. *Lancet* 2002; **360**: 861–8.

Peto J. Cancer epidemiology in the last century and the next dec-ade. *Nature* 2001; **411**: 390–5.

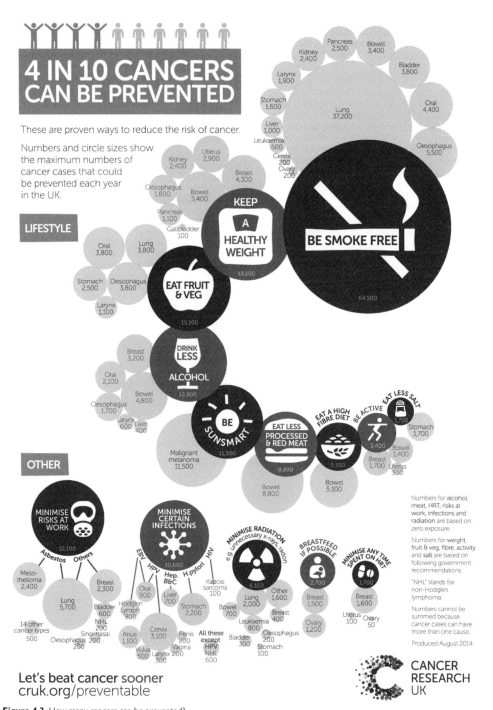

Figure 4.3 How many cancers can be prevented?
Cancer Research UK, http://publications.cancerresearchuk.org/downloads/product/CS_INFOG_PREVENTABLE%20
CANCERS%20POSTER%20IN-DEPTH.pdf, Accessed June 2016.

Li–Fraumeni syndrome (LFS)

LFS is a rare AD disorder of familial and intra-individual clustering of a wide spectrum of neoplasia occurring in children and young adults. Some affected individuals develop multiple primaries. In most families, LFS is caused by germline mutations in *TP53*, a tumour suppressor gene encoding a transcription factor with a crucial role in the regulation of the cell cycle and apoptosis when DNA damage occurs.

TP53 activity is commonly lost by a two-hit process during tumourigenesis in a wide variety of sporadic tumours. In LFS, with a germline *TP53* mutation, LOH leading to inactivation of the wild-type allele by deletion or mutation initiates tumourigenesis.

The diagnostic criteria for classical LFS are as follows.
- Proband with sarcoma diagnosed at <45 years of age, *and*
- At least one first-degree relative with any cancer diagnosed at <45 years of age, *and*
- Another first- or second-degree relative in the lineage with any cancer at <45 years of age or sarcoma at any age.

Although a wide variety of tumours can be seen in LFS kindreds (see Table 4.15), common cancers, such as lung, colon, bladder, prostate, cervix, and ovary, are not found to excess. Breast cancer and sarcomas are numerically the most frequent tumour types, but the greatest increased risk relative to general population rates is for adrenocortical cancer and phyllodes tumour. (Phyllodes tumours are fibroepithelial tumours which range in behaviour from benign (most) to malignant.)

Clinical approach

History: key points
Three-generation family tree, with specific enquiry for cancers, including age at diagnosis, multiple primaries in one individual. Try to obtain full names, dates of birth, and hospital where the diagnosis was made and treatment given, in order to facilitate confirmation.

Examination: key points
Usually not contributory.

Special investigations
DNA for mutation analysis of *TP53*. Mutation detection rate in families fulfilling the classical criteria is ~75%. While there is a need to recognize potential new mutations in families that do not meet LFS criteria, there is a low rate of *TP53* germline mutations in breast/sarcoma families not fulfilling the classical criteria for LFS. Consider mutation analysis for all children with adrenocortical cancer (some without a family history will have a '*de novo*' *TP53* mutation).

Genetic advice

Risk assessment
AD, with 50% risk to offspring of an affected individual.

Penetrance
Cancer risk in *TP53* mutation carriers has been estimated to be 73% in males and nearly 100% in females (the difference being due to breast cancer). However, mutations that are not dominant-negative missense mutations in the core binding domain appear to have lower penetrance (Bougeard et al. 2015).

Predictive testing
Diagnostic testing may be appropriate in an affected child, but predictive testing should be restricted to adults.

Prenatal diagnosis
Possible by CVS if the familial mutation is known.

Management

Surveillance for individuals who are affected by LFS or at high risk is highly problematical. Seek guidance from a unit with expertise in this area. Offer breast screening for females using MRI annually from 20 years. Whole body MRI screening is currently under investigation (Saya 2017).

Expert adviser: Gareth Evans, Consultant, Manchester Centre for Genomic Medicine, Division of Evolution and Genomic Sciences, St Mary's Hospital, University of Manchester, Manchester, UK.

References

Birch JM, Alston RD, McNally RJ, et al. Relative frequency and morphology of cancers in carriers of germline *TP53* mutations. *Oncogene* 2001; **20**: 4621–8.

Bougeard G, Renaux-Petel M, Flaman JM, et al. Revisiting Li-Fraumeni syndrome from *TP53* mutation carriers. *J Clin Oncol* 2015; **33**: 2345–52.

Chompret A. The Li–Fraumeni syndrome. *Biochimie* 2002; **84**: 75–82.

Evans DG, Birch JM, Thorneycroft M, McGown G, Lalloo F, Varley JM. Low rate of *TP53* germline mutations in TP53 mutation breast cancer/ sarcoma families not fulfilling classical criteria for Li–Fraumeni syndrome. *J Med Genet* 2002; **39**: 941–4.

Saya S, Killick F, et al. Baseline results from the UK SIGNIFY study: a whole-body MRI screening study in TP53 mutation carriers and matched controls. *Fam Cancer* 2017; epub Jan 2016.

Villani A, Tabori U, Schiffman J, et al. Biochemical and imaging surveillance in germline *TP53* mutation carriers with Li–Fraumeni syndrome: a prospective observational study. *Lancet Oncol* 2011; **12**: 559–67.

Table 4.15 Tumour types associated with LFS

Strong association	Breast cancer, soft tissue sarcomas (e.g. leiomyosarcoma), osteosarcoma, brain tumours, adrenocortical cancer, Wilms tumour, and phyllodes tumour
Moderate association	Pancreatic cancer, gastric cancer
Weak association	Leukaemias and neuroblastoma

Lynch syndrome (LS)

LS is now the preferred term for what used to be called hereditary non-polyposis colorectal cancer (HNPCC). LS is defined by mutations in DNA MMR genes, whereas HNPCC is now considered more of an overarching term for families without polyposis, but at high risk of CRC, which may or may not harbour constitutional mutations in MMR genes.

LS is due to the AD inheritance of a mutation in one of the components of the DNA MMR system. Constitutional mutations in *MSH2* (2p21) and *MLH1* (3p22.3) were previously considered to be the most common causes of LS, but this is now known to be a function of ascertainment bias, due to the criteria used to justify referral to family cancer clinics. Where systematic testing of colorectal and other LS-associated tumours is carried out, the contributions to LS from all four major MMR genes *MSH2, MLH1, MSH6* (2p16.3: but only 300 kb from *MSH2*), and *PMS2* (7p22.1) appear roughly equal. Recessive inheritance of *MSH3* mutations appears to be a rare cause of adenomatous polyposis and colorectal cancer but if constitutional *PMS1* mutations are a cause of LS, then they are very rare. LS is therefore distinct from the set of AR constitutional DNA repair deficiency diseases that generally manifest with a propensity to multiple tumours and death at an early age. However, where homozygosity or compound heterozygosity of MMR mutations occurs, it causes a classical severe DNA repair disorder (CMMRD). This is characterized by exceptional survival into the second decade of life, the children developing colorectal adenomatous polyposis, primary brain cancers (e.g. PNETs), leukaemia, and CALs. This phenotype is distinct from LS and may well be the cause of at least some cases of Turcot syndrome (see 'Turcot syndrome' below). It is noteworthy that AR inheritance of mutations in *MUTYH*, a DNA repair gene, also predisposes to colorectal adenomatous polyposis (see 'Familial adenomatous polyposis (FAP) and adenomatous polyposis due to *MUTYH, NTHL1, POLE*, and *POLD1*' in Chapter 4, 'Cancer', p. 568).

All classes of mutation are associated with LS. Nonsense, frameshift, splice, and missense point mutations all occur, while an increasing number of whole exon deletions/duplications and rearrangements are being found, especially in *MSH2* where they may account for perhaps a third or more of mutations at that locus. More recently, constitutional methylation of the *MLH1* gene has been described in individuals, and in some families this appears to be transmissible. The 10-Mb paracentric inversion of 2p with a breakpoint involving *MSH2* is now known to be present in the UK, mainland Europe, US, Australia and probes for it are now included in the relevant MLPA kits. Chromosomal or CNV abnormalities are a likely under-ascertained cause of LS.

A small number of families have mutations in *EPCAM*, a gene adjacent to *MSH2*. In these cases, large deletions including the 3′ end of *EPCAM* result in epigenetic silencing of the adjacent *MSH2* gene. The phenotype associated with constitutional mutations of this kind is one largely of CRC, with less of the other tumour types associated with *MSH2* mutations.

Occasional cases of somatic methylation of *MLH1* can cause LS in isolated individuals. This is generally spontaneous and there appears to be little risk to relatives. However, a small percentage of such individuals have rearrangements involving *MLH1* and, for example, *LRRFIP2* (adjacent to *MLH1*), which disrupt *MLH1* and cause methylation. In these cases, the underlying mutation—the rearrangement—is transmissible and is detectable by *MLH1* methylation testing.

LS accounts for 3.3% of all CRCs, and its prevalence is thus at least 1 in 200. Some populations, e.g. Finns, show a founder effect.

Muir–Torre syndrome (MTS)

MTS is the co-occurrence of skin sebaceous tumours, (adenomas, epitheliomas, or carcinomas), with internal malignancy of any kind; sebaceous skin tumours are rare and consistently empirically associated with a high risk of internal cancer. A subset, perhaps the majority, but not all of MTS, is due to LS, as the literature abounds with an association with breast cancer, so LS is not the sole cause of MTS. And, although MTS may be a good indication of LS, it does not unequivocally indicate a diagnosis of LS. Other skin tumours, such as keratoacanthomas, are associated with MTS, but there can often be a fine histological distinction between keratoacanthomas and squamous carcinomas, which may account for the latter also being associated with MTS.

Turcot syndrome

Turcot syndrome is the co-occurrence of colorectal adenomatous polyposis and primary brain cancers. Considered by some to be an AR condition, it is now known that it can be caused by mutations in either *APC* or one of the LS genes; indeed, some cases may be due to AR inheritance of two mutations in the same LS gene (CMMRD; see above).

Pathogenesis

It is important to appreciate that all laboratory tests have finite specificity and sensitivity, and this includes tests that may be performed on tumours to see if they may be due to LS. Hence, while such tests may be good at differentiating sporadic, or at least those which are non-LS, from LS in origin, they should not necessarily be used to deny constitutional mutation testing where other features such as personal or family history suggest LS.

Microsatellite instability

Loss of MMR in a tumour manifests as microsatellite instability (MSI). MSI is defined as the presence of extra alleles at a microsatellite when compared with normal DNA from the same individual. It is due to insertion/deletion mutations at repeats, but it should be borne in mind that, in a cell that has lost MMR, point mutations are occurring all over the genome, somewhat preferentially at repeats. Microsatellites vary in their propensity to show instability, and the frequency with which the same microsatellite is affected in different tumour types also varies. Instability is observed best at mononucleotide repeats, with instability at mononucleotide repeats being somewhat more significant than at dinucleotide repeats. Like any laboratory test, MSI has finite sensitivity and specificity. Current markers used in MSI diagnosis are known to have somewhat reduced sensitivity at detecting MSI in non-CRC, such as endometrial cancers, and in tumours from patients with *MSH6* mutations. Hence, a small, but finite, number of LS-associated tumours may not appear to have MSI (although they may have other indications that they are due to LS such as abnormal MMR protein IHC).

It is important to realize that about 15–20% of sporadic *colon* cancers show MSI, usually due to epigenetic downregulation of *MLH1* by methylation. Thus, unselected colon cancers with MSI have a poor positive predictive value (PPV) for LS, although lack of MSI confers a reasonably good negative predictive value (NPV) of LS. MSI in *rectal* cancers, however, is rare and strongly associated with LS, which can be exploited clinically as it gives an excellent PPV for LS (and NPV when not present). Similarly, MSI is rare in adenomas outside of LS, so giving good values for PPV/NPV. Approximately 15% of sporadic tumours of the types associated with LS also show MSI, e.g. endometrial, ovarian, and gastric tumours. The significance of MSI testing is greatly increased when >1 tumour can be tested from the same individual and/or family.

Immunohistochemistry
It is possible to test tumours for loss or abnormality of MMR protein expression by means of IHC. Abnormality can include patchy expression with loss of nuclear staining, as well as complete loss of expression. Up to 10% of LS tumours that have lost MMR and have MSI do not show any abnormality on IHC. However, when an IHC abnormality is found, it is generally associated with MSI. If it is desired to exclude LS and a tumour shows normal IHC, then it will be necessary to carry out MSI testing.

Current recommendations are that if IHC is performed, then all four MMR proteins should be assessed (*MSH2, MLH1, MSH6,* and *PMS2*). This allows for possible poor tissue fixation, as well as improved detection of concomitant loss of both *MSH2* and *MSH6*, or *MLH1* and *PMS2* in tumours due to constitutional mutations in *MSH2* or *MLH1*, respectively. A small proportion of tumours exhibit unusual patterns of abnormality such as combined loss of *MSH2* and *PMS2*. The major advantage of IHC testing is that it has the power to indicate the gene that is involved, e.g. loss of *MSH2* alone generally indicates a mutation in *MSH2*, and likewise isolated loss of one protein will point to the corresponding gene. Also, loss of both *MSH2* and *MSH6* are seen in tumours due to an underlying *MSH2* mutation, and similarly both *MLH1* and *PMS2* are lost in tumours with an underlying mutation in *MLH1*. As with MSI testing, the value of MMR IHC is considerably enhanced by testing >1 tumour from the same family and/or individual, especially if these are types with a high PPV or are otherwise rare, e.g. rectal cancers, colorectal adenomas, small bowel cancers, sebaceous skin tumours, etc. (as for MSI testing). Consistent IHC abnormality of one MMR protein is excellent evidence for the pathogenicity of a mutation in that gene, which is important, given the number of missense and other difficult-to-interpret mutations that occur in LS.

If a family can be confidently diagnosed clinically as having LS, then the value lies in IHC, indicating which gene is at fault. Whereas, in families that have a lower chance of being due to LS, e.g. high to moderate bowel cancer risk, the greater value lies in excluding LS by not finding MSI. Nevertheless, if an IHC abnormality should be found, then MSI can be implied and the family dealt with accordingly.

NB. Some CRCs due to MAP may exhibit both MSI and abnormal IHC due to somatic MMR gene mutations, and thus appear to be due to LS.

BRAF p.Val600Glu ('V600E')
Somatic mutation in CRCs in the proto-oncogene *BRAF*, predicting substitution of the valine residue at position 600 with glutamate (p.Val600Glu; 'V600E') is highly predictive that the tumour is of sporadic origin and not due to LS. However, sporadic tumours can, and do, occur in individuals with LS, and the absence of *BRAF* p.Val600Glu in a CRC does not exclude LS, although it does perhaps make it somewhat less likely a diagnosis.

BRAF testing is of no use in endometrial cancers.

MLH1 promoter methylation testing
As pointed out, ~15% of sporadic colon cancers exhibit MSI. This is largely due to loss of *MLH1* expression, because both alleles have been inactivated by somatic methylation of the *MLH1* gene promoter. Hence, detection of *MLH1* gene promoter methylation in a tumour is good, although not unequivocal evidence that the tumour is sporadic in origin, for two reasons—occasional sporadic tumours do occur in LS, and constitutional *MLH1* promoter methylation can be found in individuals with LS (and in a few cases, this constitutional *MLH1* methylation is due to a rearrangement and so is transmissible).

Pathology
Multiple adenomas are uncommon in LS, but they do occur. However, if more than, say, half a dozen should be found and there are no other non-colorectal LS-associated tumour types in the family, it would be worth exploring the possibility of attenuated FAP (see 'Familial adenomatous polyposis (FAP) and adenomatous polyposis due to *MUTYH, NTHL1, POLE,* and *POLD1*' in Chapter 4, 'Cancer', p. 568). It is important to note the presence of metachronous or synchronous cancers or adenomas, multiple bowel cancers in particular being a good indicator of LS (see below).

Although LS does not generally predispose to an obvious excess of adenomas, individuals are nonetheless predisposed to CRC. This may be because their adenomas are more likely to progress to carcinomas, and more quickly, than in the general population. There is also reason to suspect that CRCs in LS may also originate along the serrated polyp pathway.

The endometrial cancers in LS are likely to be endometrioid and lower-segment, so beware reports of 'cervical cancer' that may represent endocervical adenocarcinomas. Ovarian cancers in LS are non-serous and thus associated with a lower risk of mortality than ovarian cancers in general. Urothelial cancers in LS are typically transitional cell carcinomas (TCCs). Primary brain cancers are more likely to be astrocytomas/glioblastomas, but all types occur.

NB. Unusual, rare tumours may occur in LS (just as they can in any cancer genetic syndrome).

Tumour spectrum and genotype–phenotype
The major predisposition conferred by LS is to adenocarcinomas of the colon and rectum in both sexes and to endometrial cancer in females. Lifetime risk/penetrance figures vary between genes, studies, and populations, sometimes widely, largely because all previous estimates of cancer risks in LS were based on retrospective, inherently biased studies. Hence, the Prospective Lynch Syndrome Database, based on >25 000 patient years, now provides cancer risks by age, gender, tumour

Table 4.16 Major tumour risk in LS

Site	Risk in LS	Approximate increase over general population	Lifetime UK general population risk[*]
Colorectum	Males: 45% (by 50 years)	~200 times	5.5% (1 in 18)
	70% (by 70 years)		
	80% (lifetime)	16 times	
	Females: 20% (by 50 years)	100 times	5.0% (1 in 20)
	35% (by 70%)		
	40% (lifetime)	8 times	
Endometrium	Females: 10% (by 50 years)	35 times	1.4% (1 in 70)
	40% (by 70 years)		
	50% (lifetime)		

[*] Source: Office for National Statistics. Contains public sector information licensed under the Open Government Licence v3.0. http://www.nationalarchives.gov.uk/doc/open-government-licence/version/3/.

type, and genotype (see http://www.lscarisk.org). Previous estimates of risk are shown in Table 4.16 but should be interpreted in the light of the data from the prospective database. As analysis proceeds, risks of survival after first cancers, risks of subsequent tumours, and survival thereafter will also be presented at http://www.lscarisk.org.

Unlike in the general population, where most bowel cancers occur in the rectum and sigmoid colon, in LS they occur equally throughout the large bowel, thus appearing to have a propensity for 'right-sided' lesions. The young age of onset of cancers in LS is commonly stressed, but it is important to realize that there is bias introduced by familial cancer referral criteria for young onset, and a late-onset tumour cannot be dismissed as sporadic without supporting, e.g. molecular, evidence. As well as colorectal and endometrial cancers, LS also predisposes to a wide variety of tumours at other sites (see http://www.lscarisk.org and Table 4.17). In general, the cancer risks associated with *PMS2* appear to be lower than with the other MMR genes and are later-onset. The cumulative risk (CR) of CRC for male mutation carriers by age 70 years was 19%. The CR among female carriers was 11% for CRC and 12% for EC (ten Broeke *et al.* 2015). A history of LS-associated cancers in the parents (and their kindreds) of individuals identified with CMMRD due to *PMS2* mutations is often singularly lacking.

The risk of developing CRC in *EPCAM* deletion carriers is similar (75% by age 70 years) to the risk in carriers of *MLH1* and *MSH2* mutations, and higher than the risk with *MSH6* mutations. In contrast, the risk of endometrial cancer (12% by age 70 years) is significantly lower in females carrying an *EPCAM* deletion, compared to the risk in *MSH2* or *MSH6* mutation carriers.

Some of the variants (SNPs) identified as modifying CRC risk in the general population have been identified as modifiers in LS.

Recent data, including from the prospective database, show that prostate cancer is a risk associated with *MSH2* mutations and breast cancer is a risk associated with *MLH1* mutations. However, current international guidelines recommend that men with LS should not have prostate surveillance outside of a research study and that women with LS should participate in population breast screening programmes.

Clinical approach

History: key points

- Three-generation family tree, with particular emphasis on history of tumours, benign and malignant. Obtain names and dates of birth of affected relatives, age at diagnosis, and, if possible, details of the hospital where they were treated.
- Ascertain who has had screening or operations for what, when, and where.
- Documentation of histology or cancer registry confirmation:
  - is the family already known to a familial cancer or polyposis registry?

Examination: key points

- Ask about skin lesions in the individual and family; most patients do not regard them as tumours and will not spontaneously report them. Refer to a dermatologist, as appropriate—sebaceous adenomas often masquerade as common skin lesions.
- If the patient declares or is found to have a mass, refer to a surgeon, as appropriate.

Special investigations: key points

- Histopathology. When asking for reports on a known tumour, it is also worth asking if the pathology laboratory has any reports on other, perhaps undeclared, tumours on the same patient, e.g. skin tumours. Ask for a histological review in unusual cases. Note the presence of synchronous cancers or adenomas in bowel cancer reports—each one counts as an independent primary tumour, especially for the purposes of molecular testing, e.g. IHC and MSI. Ask for IHC of MMR proteins and/or MSI testing.
- Tumour testing. Tumour testing should be done by, or in conjunction with, an appropriate molecular or histopathologist. For MSI testing, it is useful to have normal DNA for comparison, ideally from blood, but this is not absolutely essential. Normal DNA may be obtainable from normal tissues.
- Constitutional mutation detection. The laboratory will wish to know about any tumour testing for MSI or IHC that has been carried out in the family. Blood should be taken for DNA testing from at least one affected family member, when possible. It is often useful to

Table 4.17 Cumulative risk (%) of non-colonic and non-endometrial cancers according to the type of MMR gene mutation by age 70 years. See also www.lsrisk.org

Tumour site	Mutation carriers			MLH1			MSH2			MSH6		
	All	M	F	All	M	F	All	M	F	All	M	F
Gastric	0.7–13	6.2/6.7	2.0/2.6	2.1–10.9			0.2–7.8			0–10.4		
Small bowel	0.6–4.2	4.1/12	4.1/3.9	0.4–8			1.1–8			0–3		
Biliary tract	0.6–1.4			1.9-3			0.02–0.4			0		
Pancreas	0.4/3.7			0			0.7			0		
Urinary tract	1.9–4			0.2–2.8	3.7	1.1	2.2–4.1	27.8	11.9	0–0.7		
Upper urinary tract		9.1/9.4	5.4/6.0	1	2.1–4.8	2.4–0.4	15	5.9–20.3	5.8–9.1	2	1.3	0
Bladder		5.5/16.4	3.5/1.9	1	10.8	0	8	12.3	2.6	1	1.3	0
Ovaries			6–13.5			3.4–20			7.5–24			0–1
Brain	1.2–3.7			0.3–1.7			2.5–6.3			0		
Prostate		9.1/30		0				6–18			0–4	
Breast			5.4/14.4			18/17			1.5/11			11

Reproduced from *Gut*, Vasen HFA, *et al.*, Revised guidelines for the clinical management of Lynch syndrome (HNPCC): recommendations by a group of European experts, 62, 6, pp. 812–63, copyright 2013, with permission from BMJ Publishing Group Ltd.

have samples from >1 individual in case segregation studies are needed to determine the pathogenicity or an individual proves to be a phenocopy. If the family is likely to have a mutation (see below), but no point mutation is found, then they may well harbour a large-scale mutation, e.g. whole exon (s) deleted. DNMs have been described, but they are difficult to spot clinically.

- Testing of *MLH1* promoter methylation and *BRAF* p.Val600Glu (see 'Pathogenesis' above) may be helpful where MSI/IHC are abnormal but no germline mutation in an MMR (LS) gene is identified.
- Tumour sequencing to identify somatic mutations is being increasingly used where MSI/IHC are abnormal but no germline mutations are found and *BRAF* or *MLH1* promoter methylation are not helpful.

The interpretation of MMR gene mutations is enabled by, for example, data from tumour testing. The International Society for Gastrointestinal Hereditary Tumours (InSiGHT) has an established database of MMR mutations observed worldwide, and, through a Variant Interpretation Committee, InSiGHT provides classification of mutations via its database at www.insight-group. org/variants/databases. The cancer genetic community is encouraged to submit all occurrences of all MMR variants to the InSiGHT database. In this way, unclassified variants may be classified, and the classification of known variants may be strengthened.

Diagnosis

It is important to note that the Amsterdam criteria (AC) (see Box 4.9) were originally only designed to select families for linkage studies and not to diagnose LS clinically. As such, they had to be necessarily specific, at an acceptable cost to sensitivity. A family with, e.g. only CRC, and that only just fulfils the AC may have odds of a mutation of only 10% or so, whereas a non-AC familial cluster, say, of a woman who has had both endometrial and colorectal cancers and a close relative with a small bowel or ureteric cancer, is highly likely to be due to LS.

LS can be diagnosed either on clinical grounds (e.g. fulfilment of the AC), on clinicopathological grounds, e.g. after tumour testing, or ultimately by a pathogenic constitutional mutation in a DNA MMR gene.

Note that a very young-onset case, e.g. <35 years, is likely to be due to LS, even in the absence of a family history, although mutations in other genes encoding mitotic spindle checkpoint proteins should be considered, such as *BUB1* and *BUB3*, especially in teenage cases. Tumours from such individuals do not exhibit MSI nor generally do those from families with specific *POLD1* and *POLE* mutations, although their family histories may be Lynch-like. It

---

Box 4.9 Amsterdam criteria 2 ('AC2')

All criteria must be satisfied:
- at least three separate relatives* with colorectal cancer (CRC) or LS-related cancer (HRC: see item 2 in the ICG-LS's clinical definition);
- one relative must be a first-degree relative of the other two;
- at least two successive generations affected;
- at least one cancer (CRC or HRC) diagnosed at <50 years of age;
- familial adenomatous polyposis (FAP) excluded in CRC case(s);
- tumours pathologically verified.

* NB. Affected individuals should all be on the same side of the family, e.g. maternal or paternal relatives of the consultand.

Reprinted from *Gastroenterology*, volume 116, issue 6, Hans F.A. Vasen, Patrice Watson, Jukka–Pekka Mecklin, Henry T. Lynch, New clinical criteria for hereditary nonpolyposis colorectal cancer (HNPCC, Lynch syndrome) proposed by the International Collaborative Group on HNPCC, pp. 1453–1456, Copyright 1999, with permission from Elsevier.

is important to bear in mind, however, that tumours may acquire two MMR gene mutations due to an underlying syndrome other than LS, and thus appear to be due to LS when they are due to something else. A rare, characteristic tumour, e.g. small bowel cancer, ureter TCC, skin sebaceous adenoma, is very significant, and synchronous or metachronous bowel cancers are significant. Double primaries, especially colorectal and endometrial, are significant and remember that non-penetrance is common (hence strict adherence to the AC is insensitive).

Given that family histories of cancer are generally poorly taken by non-geneticists, and in any event often not acted upon, allied to the fact that publicity about familial bowel cancer is lacking and so lay individuals have little, if any, idea that their family's history may represent LS, there is a very strong argument for the implementation of systematic testing of relevant tumours to find cases of LS. Some countries, e.g. Denmark and the USA (http://www.lynchscreening.net), have already implemented such programmes and others are considering it, based on positive health economics (http://www.nets.nihr.ac.uk/projects/hta/102801). In the UK, NICE has issued guidance that all colorectal cancers be tested for Lynch syndrome. (NICE 2017). With the distinct possibility of aspirin prophylaxis becoming a reality in LS, systematic screening for LS by tumour testing is becoming an increasing public health consideration.

Genetic advice
LS is an AD disorder, although (often consanguineous) families with CMMRD are now well described. The CMMRD phenotype is quite distinct from LS and may well be the cause of at least some cases of Turcot syndrome (see 'Turcot syndrome' above).

Penetrance in Lynch syndrome is incomplete, sex-limited, and age-dependent—see http://www.lscarisk.org that gives cancer risks by age, gender, tumour type, and genotype, according to the Prospective Lynch Syndrome Database.

Management
Surveillance
See also 'Cancer surveillance methods' in Chapter 4, 'Cancer', p. 552.

COLORECTUM.
- International guidelines recommend colonoscopy every 1–2 years from the age of 25 in those at 100% (i.e. already affected by an HNPCC-related cancer (HRC)) or 50% prior risk of LS.
- Do not forget those who have already developed one (bowel) cancer—they should *not* be discharged from follow-up.
- Liaison with colorectal surgeons is important—an individual with LS who presents with a second or third bowel cancer may wish to consider the option of a more extensive resection as prophylaxis, e.g. panproctocolectomy, rather than hemicolectomy.

ENDOMETRIUM AND OVARIES. Lifetime risk for endometrial cancer (50%) exceeds that for CRC (40%) in women with LS. There is no proven method of effective surveillance for endometrial cancer, so women should be warned of its risk and advised to seek help in case of irregular/post-menopausal bleeding, etc. In some centres, screening may be offered by means of, e.g. pipelle

biopsy, transvaginal ultrasound from age 35–40, and while this is not proven to be of benefit, it may enable detection of premalignant disease and early cancers and so can be offered to mutation carriers. However, any such treatment should be provided as part of a research study. The risk of ovarian cancer in LS appears largely restricted to *MSH2*, and to a lesser component *MLH1*, mutations (www.lsrisk.org). Moreover, the survival of ovarian cancer in LS is better than that associated with the serous ovarian cancers seen with *BRCA1/2*.

Women who have completed childbearing may wish to consider a hysterectomy, though it should be borne in mind that pelvic surgery can make colonoscopy more difficult. Prophylactic hysterectomy with bilateral salpingo-oophorectomy (BSO) does largely prevent the development of endometrial and ovarian cancers and is thus an option to discuss with female mutation carriers who have completed their families. However, there are disbenefits associated with such surgery which needs to be considered. If CRC surgery or prophylaxis is envisaged, the option of combined surgery can be considered.

UROTHELIAL TUMOURS. In view of the lack of evidence for the benefit of surveillance for urinary tract cancer, international guidelines do not recommend surveillance for urinary tract cancer in LS outside the setting of a research project.

STOMACH. There is no regime of gastric surveillance that is of proven benefit.

SKIN. Refer to a dermatologist for management of skin lesions if these are present.

SURVEILLANCE IN GENERAL. LS gene carriers are at increased risk of many tumour types, for most of which it is not possible to offer surveillance of proven efficacy. For most other LS-associated cancer types, there is no proven efficacious surveillance method, but by all means, encourage patients to take part in approved research studies into surveillance. Counsel patients that they should have a low threshold for presentation and their doctors that they should have a low threshold for onward referral. Members of LS families commonly recall stories of delays in diagnosis, especially in individuals who developed cancer at a young age.

ASPIRIN. Regular aspirin significantly reduces the incidence of cancer in LS. The CAPP2 double-blind trial revealed a significant reduction in CRC and other LS-associated cancers among those randomly assigned to aspirin versus those randomly assigned to placebo (Burn et al. 2011). The optimal dose of aspirin in LS will be determined by further randomized studies, e.g. CaPP3 (http://www.capp3.org). International guidelines therefore advise that aspirin should ideally only be prescribed in LS as part of research studies. The option of taking low-dose aspirin should be discussed with gene carriers, including the risks, benefits, and current limitations of available evidence.

Education
Educate your patient about the symptoms of CRC, so that he/she is aware of when to seek medical advice and investigation. The most significant symptoms are:
- rectal bleeding;
- a persistent change in bowel habit, usually to looser or more frequent bowel actions;
- abdominal mass;
- unexplained anaemia.

Future developments

It is important to let those at risk of LS know that current recommendations and surveillance regimes are liable to change or revision as knowledge of the disorder advances. Indeed, they may welcome invitations to take part in clinical trials, e.g. into determining the best dose of aspirin used in prophylaxis (CaPP3).

Support groups: Lynch Syndrome UK, http://www.lynch-syndrome-uk.org, which is part of LS International, http://lynchcancers.com; International Society for Gastrointestinal Hereditary Tumours (InSIGHT), www.insight-group.org.

Expert advisers: Ian M. Frayling, Consultant Genetic Pathologist, Cardiff and Vale University Health Board, Cardiff University, Institute of Medical Genetics, University Hospital of Wales, Cardiff, UK.

References

Arends M, Ibrahim M, Happerfield L, Frayling I, Miller K. Interpretation of immunohistochemical analysis of mismatch repair (MMR) protein expression in tissue sections for investigation of suspected Lynch/hereditary non-polyposis colorectal cancer (HNPCC) syndrome. UK NEQAS ICC & ISH Recommendations, June 2008, issue 1. http://www.research.ed.ac.uk/portal/files/9181795/hnpcc_recommendations_B.pdf.

Burn J, Bishop DT, Mecklin JP, et al. Effect of aspirin or resistant starch on colorectal neoplasia in the Lynch syndrome. N Engl J Med 2008; **359**: 2567–78.

Burn J, Gerdes AM, Macrae F, et al. Long-term effect of aspirin on cancer risk in carriers of hereditary colorectal cancer: an analysis from the CAPP2 randomised controlled trial. Lancet 2011; **378**: 2081–7.

Frayling IM. Microsatellite instability. Gut 1999; **45**: 1–4.

Halford S, Sasieni P, Rowan A, et al. Low-level microsatellite instability occurs in most colorectal cancers and is a nonrandomly distributed quantitative trait. Cancer Res 2002; **62**: 53–7.

Hitchins MP, Ward RL. Constitutional (germline) MLH1 epimutation as an aetiological mechanism for hereditary non-polyposis colorectal cancer. J Med Genet 2009; **46**: 793–802.

International Society for Gastrointestinal Hereditary Tumours (InSiGHT). https://www.insight-group.org.

Jarvinen HJ, Aarnio M, Mustonen H, et al. Controlled 15-year trial on screening for colorectal cancer in families with hereditary nonpolyposis colorectal cancer. Gastroenterology 2000; **118**: 829–34.

Kempers MJ, Kuiper RP, Ockeloen CW, et al. Risk of colorectal and endometrial cancers in EPCAM deletion-positive Lynch syndrome: a cohort study. Lancet Oncol 2011; **12**: 49–55.

Loukola A, Salovaara R, Kristo P, et al. MSI in adenomas as a marker for HNPCC. Am J Pathol 1999; **155**: 1849–53.

Lynch HT, De La Chapelle A. Genetic susceptibility to non-polyposis colorectal cancer. J Med Genet 1999; **36**: 801–18.

Lynch HT, Shaw MW, Magnuson CW, Larsen AL, Krush AJ. Hereditary factors in cancer: study of two large midwestern kindreds. Arch Intern Med 1966; **117**: 206–12.

Lynch HT, Smyrk T, Lynch JF. Molecular genetics and clinical-pathology features of HNPCC (Lynch syndrome): historical journey from pedigree anecdote to molecular genetic confirmation. Oncology 1998; **55**: 103–8.

Mathers JC, Movahedi M, Macrae F, et al. Long-term effect of resistant starch on cancer risk in carriers of hereditary colorectal cancer: an analysis from the CAPP2 randomised controlled trial. Lancet Oncol 2012; **13**: 1242–9.

Metcalf AM, Spurdle AB. Endometrial tumour BRAF mutations and MLH1 promoter methylation as predictors of germline mismatch repair gene mutation status: a literature review. Fam Cancer 2013; **13**: 1–12.

Møller P, Seppälä T, Bernstein I, et al. Cancer incidence and survival in Lynch syndrome patients receiving colonoscopic and gynaecological surveillance: first report from the prospective Lynch syndrome database. Gut 2015; pii: gutjnl-2015-309675.

NHS National Institute for Health Research. HTA–10/28/01: diagnostic strategies for Lynch syndrome, 2014. http://www.nets.nihr.ac.uk/projects/hta/102801.

NICE. Molecular strategies for Lynch syndrome in people with colorectal cancer (DG 27): https://www.nice.org.uk/guidance/dg27

Nilbert M, Planck M, Fernebro E, Borg A, Johnson A. MSI is rare in rectal carcinomas and signifies hereditary cancer. Eur J Cancer 1999; **35**: 942–5.

Offit K, Kauff ND. Reducing the risk of gynecologic cancer in the Lynch syndrome [editorial]. N Engl J Med 2006; **354**: 293–5.

Rothwell PM, Fowkes FG, Belch JF, et al. Effect of daily aspirin on long-term risk of death due to cancer: analysis of individual patient data from randomised trials. Lancet 2011; **377**: 31–41.

Schmeler KM, Lynch HT, Chen LM, et al. Prophylactic surgery to reduce the risk of gynecologic cancers in the Lynch syndrome. N Engl J Med 2006; **354**: 261–9.

ten Broeke SW, Brohet RM, Tops CM, et al. Lynch syndrome caused by germline PMS2 mutations: delineating the cancer risk. J Clin Oncol 2015; **33**: 319–25.

Torre D. Multiple sebaceous tumors. Arch Dermatol 1968; **98**: 549–51.

Trimbath JD, Petersen GM, Erdman SH, Ferre M, Luce MC, Giardiello FM. Café-au-lait spots and early onset colorectal neoplasia: a variant of HNPCC? Fam Cancer 2001; **1**: 101–5.

Vasen HF, Blanco I, Aktan-Collan K, et al.; Mallorca group. Revised guidelines for the clinical management of Lynch syndrome (HNPCC): recommendations by a group of European experts. Gut 2013; **62**: 812–23.

Vasen HF, Möslein G, Alonso A, et al. Guidelines for the clinical management of Lynch syndrome (hereditary non-polyposis cancer). J Med Genet 2007; **44**: 353–62.

Vasen HF, Möslein G, Alonso A, et al. Recommendations to improve identification of hereditary and familial colorectal cancer in Europe. Fam Cancer 2010; **9**: 109–15.

Vasen HF, Sanders EA, Taal BG, et al. The risk of brain tumours in hereditary non-polyposis colorectal cancer (HNPCC). Int J Cancer 1996; **65**: 422–5.

Warthin AS. Heredity with reference to carcinoma, as shown by the study of the cases examined in the pathological laboratory of the University of Michigan, 1895–1913. Arch Intern Med 1913; **12**: 546–55.

Wimmer K, Etzler J. Constitutional mismatch repair-deficiency syndrome: have we so far seen only the tip of an iceberg? Hum Genet 2008; **124**: 105–22.

Win AK, Lindor NM, Jenkins MA. Risk of breast cancer in Lynch syndrome: a systematic review. Breast Cancer Res 2013; **15**: R27.

Multiple endocrine neoplasia (MEN)

Multiple endocrine and other organ neoplasia (MEON)

MEN is defined by the presence of tumours involving two or more endocrine glands in one individual.

The MENs are AD cancer predisposition syndromes, affecting primarily parathyroid, enteropancreatic, endocrine, and pituitary tissues.

Multiple endocrine neoplasia type 1 (*MEN1*)

MEN1 is caused by *inactivating* germline mutations in *MEN1*, a tumour suppressor gene encoding menin, a novel nuclear protein. Menin specifically interacts with FANCD2, a protein encoded by a gene involved in DNA repair (and mutated in some patients with FA) (Jin *et al.* 2003). *MEN1* accounts for ~10% of patients with primary hyperparathyroidism who require surgery. In most patients, hyperparathyroidism is the first manifestation of *MEN1*, but this is not the case in up to 10% of mutation carriers. Unlike sporadic cases of primary hyperparathyroidism, tumours are typically present in one or more parathyroid glands and present at a young age (typically 25–35 years). Disease-specific mortality in *MEN1* is significant, arising largely from the effects of pancreatic islet cell tumours (e.g. gastrinomas and insulinomas) and malignant thymic carcinoid.

Anterior pituitary tumours occur in 30% of *MEN1* patients (most are prolactinomas (60%), somatotrophinomas (GH: 20%), and corticotrophinomas and non-functioning tumours (<15%)). Associated tumours that occur in *MEN1* include adrenal cortical tumours (5%), carcinoid tumours (4–10%), lipomas (1%), facial angiofibromas (88%), and collagenomas (72%).

Familial isolated hyperparathyroidism (FIHP)

An AD condition characterized by uniglandular or multiglandular parathyroid tumours that occur in the absence of other endocrine tumours. Recently, mutations in *MEN1* have been identified in some families, but also consider mutation in the calcium-sensing receptor (CaSR) which causes familial benign hypocalciuric hypercalcaemia.

Screening for *MEN1* should be undertaken in:
- any patient with two or more *MEN1*-associated endocrine tumours;
- any patient <30 years of age with one *MEN1*-associated tumour;
- any first-degree relative of someone with *MEN1*.

Multiple endocrine neoplasia types 2 and 3 (MEN2A, MEN2B now 3)

Mucosal neuroma syndrome or Sipple syndrome.

MEN2 is characterized by the association of medullary thyroid cancer (MTC) and phaeochromocytoma. It is caused by *activating* germline mutations in the *RET* proto-oncogene. MEN2 may be subdivided into three subtypes MEN2A, MEN2B, and familial MTC (FMCT), all with a high risk for MTC arising in the C-cells (calcitonin-producing cells) of the thyroid. MEN2 has now been reclassified as MEN3. The usual age of onset of MTC in MEN2A is in early adult life, in MEN2B in early childhood, and in FMTC in midlife. MEN2 has a prevalence of ~1/30 000. Approximately 60–90% of MEN2 cases are MEN2A, 5% are MEN2B, and 5–35% are FMTC. In MEN2A, signs or symptoms of hyperparathyroidism or phaeochromocytoma rarely present before those of MTC. Kahraman and de Groot (2003) found that in MEN2A, MTC can be present as early as 4 years of age. MTC can occur at an extremely young age in MEN2B and screening is usually commenced at 6 months of age.

The ability of an MTC to oversecrete calcitonin, occasionally together with other hormonally active peptides, e.g. ACTH or calcitonin-gene related peptide (CGRP), leads to unexplained diarrhoea, symptoms of Cushing's syndrome, or facial flushing in many patients with advanced disease. Metastatic spread occurs both locally to regional lymph nodes and to distant sites, e.g. the liver in advanced disease.

Familial medullary thyroid carcinoma (FMTC)

A subtype of MEN2 and caused by mutations in *RET*. An AD condition characterized by MTC, usually diagnosed in middle age, without other features of MEN2.

Table 4.18 Diagnosis of multiple endocrine neoplasia (MEN)

MEN1	MEN2A	MEN2B	Carney
Gene			
MEN1 (menin)	*RET*	*RET*	*PKAR1A*
Locus			
11q13	10q11	10q11	17q22–24
Clinical features			
Parathyroid hyperplasia (95%)	MTC (penetrance 90–95%)	MTC (penetrance 100%)	Lentigines
Pituitary adenomas (30%) (prolactin used for surveillance)	Phaeochromocytomas (50%)	Phaeochromocytomas (50%)	Cardiac myxomas
	Parathyroid hyperplasia (20–30%)	Mucosal neuromas (e.g. lips and tongue)	PPNAD
Pancreatic adenomas (40%): insulinomas gastrinoma (duodenal) VIPoma (rare) glucagonoma (rare)		Marfanoid habitus	Endocrine tumour
		Medullated corneal nerve fibres	
		Multiple diverticulae and megacolon	

MTC, medullary thyroid carcinoma; PPNAD, primary pigmented adrenocortical disease; VIP, vasoactive intestinal peptide.

Screening for MEN2 should be undertaken in:
- any patient with MTC or two or more MEN2-associated endocrine tumours;
- any patient <30 years of age with one MEN2-associated endocrine tumour;
- any patient with mucosal neuromas or somatic features of MEN2B;
- any individual with a first-degree relative with MEN2.

Multiple endocrine neoplasia type 4

Clinically the same features as *MEN1*, but due to LOF mutation in *CDKN1B*. About one-third of *MEN1* patients negative for *MEN1* mutation have MEN4.

Investigate and treat as for *MEN1*.

Table 4.18 summarizes the diagnosis of the different types of MEN.

Other conditions to consider

MEON

MEN can be difficult to distinguish from the following syndromes that may be referred to as MEON (multiple endocrine and other organ neoplasia syndromes).

HYPERPARATHYROIDISM–JAW TUMOUR (HPT-JT) SYNDROME. Caused by mutations in the parafibromin gene (*HRPT2*). An AD disease characterized by the occurrence of parathyroid tumours and fibro-osseous tumours of the jaw bones (mandible and maxilla). Some HPT-JT patients may also develop various cystic and neoplastic renal abnormalities that include Wilms tumours, hamartomas, and polycystic disease. Parathyroid tumours often occur asynchronously in patients with HPT-JT syndrome and, although most of the tumours are benign, the incidence of malignant parathyroid carcinomas is markedly increased in these patients (Shattuck *et al.* 2003).

CARNEY COMPLEX (CNC). CNC is a rare multiple neoplasia syndrome that consists of endocrine (thyroid, pituitary, adrenocortical, and gonadal), non-endocrine (myxomas, particularly atrial myxomas), and neural (schwannomas) tumours. Typically, there are cutaneous pigmented lesions (multiple blue naevi and lentigines). Primary pigmented nodular adrenocortical disease (PPNAD) is the most common endocrine manifestation of CNC. CNC is caused by mutations in *PRKAR1A*, a critical component of the cAMP (cyclic adenosine monophosphate) signalling pathway or another gene (*CNC2*) on 2p16.

VON HIPPEL–LINDAU (VHL) DISEASE. See 'von Hippel–Lindau (VHL) disease' in Chapter 4, 'Cancer', p. 618.

NEUROFIBROMATOSIS TYPE 1 (NF1). See 'Neurofibromatosis type 1 (NF1)' in Chapter 3, 'Common consultations', p. 506.

COWDEN SYNDROME (PHTS). See 'Cowden syndrome (PTEN hamartoma tumour syndrome (PHTS))' in Chapter 4, 'Cancer', p. 564.

MCCUNE–ALBRIGHT SYNDROME. See 'Hemihypertrophy and limb asymmetry' in Chapter 2, 'Clinical approach', p. 164.

Other cancer syndromes and phenocopies

THYROID CANCER. Thyroid cancer accounts for roughly 1% of all new malignant disease. Of these, ~94% are differentiated thyroid cancer (occasionally occurring as a component of Cowden syndrome (*PTEN*) or FAP). Another 5% are MTC, derived from the neuroendocrine C-cells of the thyroid and 1% are anaplastic. Sporadic disease accounts for ~80% of MTC, with presentation usually in the fifth or sixth decade. Twenty per cent of

MTC occurs in the context of an inherited tumour predisposition syndrome, e.g. MEN2A, MEN2B, or FMTC.

SPORADIC PARATHYROID CANCER. Shattuck *et al.* (2003), in an analysis of 15 patients with apparently sporadic parathyroid cancer (no family history and no features of HPT-JT or *MEN1*, etc.), identified three patients with germline mutations in *HRPT2* (the gene mutated in HPT-JT), suggesting that certain patients with apparently sporadic parathyroid carcinoma may have the HPT-JT syndrome or a phenotypic variant.

PHENOCOPIES.
- Individuals in MEN families with one MEN-associated tumour, but no familial mutation;
- Clinical *MEN1* with no *MEN1* mutation, but on further investigation have mutations such as *CDC73* or *CaSR*.

Clinical approach

History: key points

Three-generation family tree, with specific enquiry for the presence of endocrine tumours, age of death, and cause of death.

Examination: key points

In MEN without a known *RET* mutation, examine for physical features of MEN2B, i.e. mucosal neuromas on the lips and tongue, full lips, and Marfanoid habitus.

Special investigations

DNA for mutation analysis of *MEN1* in *MEN1* and of exons 10 and 11 of *RET* in MEN2A, exons 10, 11, 13, and 14 of *RET* in FMTC, and exon 16 of *RET* in MEN2B.

Genetic advice

MEN1

AD, with 50% risk to offspring of an affected individual or mutation carrier. More than 80% of the germline mutations in *MEN1* are inactivating and each kindred has a private mutation. No genotype–phenotype correlation is apparent.

MEN2

AD, with 50% risk to offspring of an affected individual or mutation carrier. For MEN2A, MEN2B, and FMTC, mutations in the tyrosine kinase proto-oncogene *RET* are detectable in 98% of affected family members. Mutations of codon 634 Cys occur in ~85% of MEN2A families. Approximately 95% of individuals with MEN2B have an M918T mutation in exon 16.

Approximately 6% of patients with clinically sporadic MTC carry a germline *RET* mutations, and so genetic testing is offered to all new patients at diagnosis. Initial analysis of the *RET* gene targets exons 10 and 11, the most common sites of mutation. If no mutation is identified, proceed to analyse exons 13–16.

The probability of a *de novo* gene mutation in an index case of MEN2A is 5% and in an index case of MEN2B is 50%.

Penetrance

- In *MEN1*, most are penetrant by 20 years and >90% are penetrant by 30 years, but recent data show that as many as 40% do not present with their first feature of *MEN1* until after age 40 years.
- In MEN2, penetrance is 70% by 70 years.

Predictive testing

- *MEN1*. Genetic testing for *MEN1* in the index cases gives useful information, confirms the clinical diagnosis, and can be used to inform PND/PIGD and predictive testing in other family members. Predictive genetic testing for at-risk family members is of great value in determining which family members are at risk and should be offered annual surveillance.

- MEN2 and familial MTC. *RET* testing has replaced calcitonin in determining which family members are at risk and should be offered prophylactic thyroidectomy.

Prenatal diagnosis
Technically feasible by CVS if the familial mutation is known.

Management

Surveillance strategies

MEN1 AND 4.
- Clinical assessment looking for symptoms and signs of hypercalcaemia, nephrolithiasis, peptic ulcer disease, neuroglycopenia, hypopituitarism, galactorrhoea and amenorrhoea in women, acromegaly, Cushing's disease, visual field loss, subcutaneous lipomas, facial angiofibromas, and collagenomas.
- Annual serum calcium and prolactin from 5 years of age (hypercalcaemia is the first manifestation in 90% of *MEN1* patients). Measurement of GI hormones and specific endocrine function tests should be reserved for individuals who have symptoms and signs of a *MEN1*-associated tumour. See Thakker *et al.* 2012 for further details.

MEN2 AND FMTC. Where the familial mutation is known, predictive genetic testing should be offered at a young age. Prophylactic thyroidectomy is the cornerstone of management for individuals with a *RET* mutation predisposing to MEN2A, MEN2B, or FMTC. See American Thyroid Association Guidelines Task Force (2009) for further details.

In families where the genotype is unknown and for known mutation carriers, screening is recommended in early childhood from age 5 years or earlier in FMTC and MEN2A and from 3–5 years in MEN2B. MTC and C-cell hyperplasia are suspected in the presence of elevated plasma calcitonin concentration.
- 12-monthly clinical assessment looking for symptoms and signs of MTC (lumps in the neck (neck USS), diarrhoea, dysphagia, phaeochromocytoma (hypertension, headaches, palpitations, sweating), hypercalcaemia.
- 12-monthly measurement of serum calcitonin levels.
- 12-monthly 24-hour urine for fractionated metanephrines (phaeochromocytoma).
- 12-monthly measurement of serum calcium and PTH levels.

HPT-JT. Surveillance protocols adapted from Newey *et al.* 2010.
- 6- to 12-monthly serum calcium and PTH (parathyroid tumour).
- 5-yearly panoramic jaw X-ray with neck screening (ossifying jaw fibroma).
- 5-yearly abdominal MRI for renal neoplasia.
- 12-monthly USS for uterine tumour.

Interventions
- *MEN1*. Surgery includes subtotal or total parathyroidectomy, parathyroid cryopreservation, and thymectomy. Proton pump inhibitors or somatostatin analogues

are the main management for oversecretion of most enteropancreatic tumours, except insulin. Surgery on gastrinomas is generally not indicated, and surgery for other enteropancreatic tumours is controversial.
- MEN2 and FMTC. The specific *RET* codon mutation correlates with the age of onset of MTC and the aggressiveness of the tumour and is used to guide management decisions such as whether and when to perform thyroidectomy (Brandi *et al.* 2001). Two strategies are offered to asymptomatic mutation carriers:
  - 6-monthly clinical and biochemical surveillance as above, with recourse to prophylactic thyroidectomy as soon as an abnormal pentagastrin result is obtained (usually around 10–13 years), or
  - total thyroidectomy at 5 years in MEN2A following a predictive test indicating that the child is a mutation carrier (5 years is the earliest age at which metastases have been reported). In MEN2B, metastasis has been reported as young as 2 years and total thyroidectomy at an earlier age is advocated by some.

Support group: Association for Multiple Endocrine Neoplasia Disorders (AMEND), http://www.amend.org.uk.

Expert adviser: Rajesh Thakker May, Professor of Medicine, Radcliffe Department of Medicine, University of Oxford, Oxford Centre for Diabetes, Endocrinology & Metabolism, Churchill Hospital, Oxford, UK.

References

American Thyroid Association Guidelines Task Force, Kloos RT, Eng C, Evans DB, *et al.* Medullary thyroid cancer: management guidelines of the American Thyroid Association. *Thyroid* 2009; **6**: 565–612.

Brandi ML, Gagel RF, Angeli A, *et al.* Guidelines for diagnosis and therapy of MEN type 1 and type 2. *J Clin Endocrinol Metab* 2001; **86**: 5658–71.

Cavaco BM, Barros L, Pannett AA, *et al.* The hyperparathyroidism–jaw tumour syndrome in a Portuguese kindred. *QJM* 2001; **94**: 213–22.

Glascock MJ, Carty SE. Multiple endocrine neoplasia type 1: fresh perspective on clinical features and penetrance. *Surg Oncol* 2002; **11**: 143–50.

Jin S, Mao H, Schnepp RW, *et al.* Menin associates with FANCD2, a protein involved in repair of DNA damage. *Cancer Res* 2003; **63**: 4204–10.

Kahraman T, de Groot JW. Acceptable age for prophylactic surgery in children with multiple endocrine neoplasia type 2a. *Eur J Surg Oncol* 2003; **29**: 331–5.

Newey PJ, Bowl MR, Cranston T, Thakker RV. Cell division cycle protein 73 homolog (*CDC73*) mutations in the hyperparathyroid–jaw tumor syndrome (HPT-JT) and parathyroid tumors. *Hum Mutat* 2010; **31**: 295–307.

Pannett AA, Kennedy AM, Turner JJ, *et al.* Multiple endocrine neoplasia type 1 (*MEN1*) germline mutations in familial isolated primary hyperparathyroidism. *Clin Endocrinol* 2003; **58**: 639–46.

Sandrini F, Stratakis C. Clinical and molecular genetics of Carney complex. *Mol Genet Metab* 2003; **78**: 83–92.

Shattuck TM, Valimaki S, Obara T, *et al.* Somatic and germ-line mutations of the HRPT2 gene in sporadic parathyroid carcinoma. *N Engl J Med* 2003; **349**: 1722–9.

Sherman SI. Thyroid carcinoma. *Lancet* 2003; **361**: 501–11.

Thakker RV. Multiple endocrine neoplasia type 1 (*MEN1*) and type 4 (MEN4). *Mol Cell Endocrinol* 2014; **386**(1–2): 2–15.

Thakker RV, Newey PJ, Walls GV, *et al.* Clinical practice guidelines for multiple endocrine neoplasia type 1 (*MEN1*). *J Clin Endocrinol* 2012; **97**: 2990–3011.

Neurofibromatosis type 2 (NF2)

Central neurofibromatosis, bilateral acoustic neurofibromatosis.

NF2 is an AD disorder caused by inactivating mutations in the tumour suppressor gene merlin (schwannomin) on 22q. Merlin's function as a tumour suppressor has not been elucidated. Schwannomas are benign solitary tumours of the peripheral nerve sheaths. The occurrence of multiple schwannomas usually implies hereditary disease. Vestibular schwannomas (acoustic neuromas), intracranial meningiomas, spinal tumours, peripheral nerve tumours, and presenile lens opacities are common in NF2. The morbidity and mortality of NF2 are largely due to bilateral vestibular schwannomas. These present with hearing loss and tinnitus or vertigo. The diagnostic criteria for NF2 are given in Box 4.10.

In Baser et al.'s (2002a) study of 368 patients, the mean age of first symptoms was 22 years and the mean age of diagnosis was 27 years; 31.5% of patients were diagnosed at <20 years. Life expectancy may be shortened. The risk of mortality increases with decreasing age at diagnosis and is greater in people with intracranial meningiomas, compared with those without meningiomas. The risk of mortality is lower in people with constitutional NF2 missense mutations than in those with other types of mutations (e.g. nonsense or frameshift mutations or large deletions). The clinical features of NF2 are summarized in Table 4.19.

Some patients present young and have an aggressive course; others present in middle life and may have a very slow and indolent course. Two subtypes are recognized.

- Mild (Gardner, type A). Onset >15 years and usually >25 years. Presenting symptoms usually due to bilateral vestibular schwannomas. Skin manifestations minimal and other CNS tumours are rare.
- Severe (Wishardt, type 2B). Onset <30 years and usually <25 years. Meningiomas and spinal tumours occur in large numbers.

Other conditions to consider

The only genetic disorders in which schwannomas occur are: NF2, multiple schwannomatosis, and CNC.

Neurofibromatosis type 1 (NF1)
Important distinguishing features are axillary freckling and Lisch nodules—both are commonly present in NF1 but are very rarely seen in NF2. Spinal neurofibromas seen in NF1 can appear identical to the spinal schwannomas seen in NF2, both radiologically and at surgery. They are distinct histologically but may need expert review by a neuropathologist for definitive diagnosis.

Multiple schwannomas (isolated familial schwannomatosis)
An AD disorder defined as multiple pathologically proven schwannomas without the vestibular tumours diagnostic of NF2. Linkage to 22q, but not to the NF2 locus (MacCollin et al. 2003). Forty per cent of familial cases and 10% of sporadic cases are due to germline SMARCB1 mutation.

Carney complex (CNC)
An AD condition characterized by skin pigmentary anomalies, myxomas (especially atrial), endocrine tumours or overactivity, and schwannomas. See 'Multiple endocrine neoplasia (MEN)' in Chapter 4, 'Cancer', p. 592.

Clinical approach

History: key points
Three-generation family history, with specific enquiry for diagnosis of NF, deafness, and neurosurgery.

Examination: key points
- Careful examination of the skin for NF2 plaques, CALs, cutaneous neurofibromas, and schwannomas.
- Ophthalmological assessment for posterior subcapsular and cortical cataracts and CHRPE or astrocytic hamartomas.

Special investigations
- DNA for mutation analysis of NF2. In apparently sporadic cases, consider starting with mutation analysis of the tumour.
- Cranial and spinal MRI with gadolinium enhancement (if not already performed).
- Audiometry.

Box 4.10 Diagnostic criteria for NF2*

A diagnosis of NF2 is made if one of the following criteria is met:
- bilateral vestibular schwannomas, either proven histologically or seen by MRI with gadolinium enhancement;
- a parent, sibling, or child with NF2 and either: (a) a unilateral vestibular schwannoma *or* (b) two or more of: meningioma, glioma, schwannoma, posterior subcapsular lenticular opacities, and cerebral calcification;
- unilateral vestibular schwannoma and two or more of: meningioma, glioma, schwannoma, posterior subcapsular lenticular opacities, and cerebral calcification;
- multiple meningiomas (two or more) and one or more of: glioma, schwannoma, posterior subcapsular lenticular opacities, and cerebral opacification.

* NB. None of the existing sets of criteria is adequate at initial assessment for diagnosing people with NF2 who present without bilateral vestibular Schwannomas, particularly if there is a negative family history.

Reproduced from *Journal of Medical Genetics*, Evans DGR, Huson SM, et al., A genetic study of type 2 neurofibromatosis: II guidelines for genetic counselling, vol 29, 12, pp. 847–52, copyright 1992, with permission from BMJ Publishing Group Ltd.

Table 4.19 Clinical features of NF2

Clinical feature	Frequency of symptomatic lesions (%)[†]
CNS tumours	
Bilateral vestibular schwannomas	85
Unilateral vestibular schwannoma	6
Meningiomas	45
Spinal tumours (meningiomas, schwannomas)	26
Astrocytomas (usually in brainstem ± upper cervical cord)[+]	4
Ependymomas (usually in brainstem ± upper cervical cord)[+]	2.5
Peripheral nervous system	
Peripheral schwannomas	68
NF2 plaques (slightly raised, roughened skin lesions that may be slightly pigmented; overlying skin is often hairy)	48
Nodular schwannomas	43
NF-like cutaneous neurofibromas	27
Peripheral neuropathy (glove and stocking or mononeuritis)	3
CAL spots	
1–6 spots (only 4% had >3 spots, 0 had >6)	43
Eyes	
Posterior subcapsular cataracts	72.4
Cortical cataracts	41.4
Retinal hamartomas (CHRPEs or astrocytic hamartomas)	8.6

CHRPE, congenital hypertrophy of the retinal pigment epithelium.

[†] NB. A higher frequency of all tumours is found on cranial and spinal MRI; some remain asymptomatic. Lifetime risk of these tumours may also be higher.

[+] It is now recognized that the vast majority of intrinsic brain and spine tumours in NF2 are ependymomas.

Adapted from Evans et al., A clinical study of type 2 neurofibromatosis, *QJM: An International Journal of Medicine*, 1992, 84, 1, pp. 603–18, by permission of the Association of Physicians of Great Britain and Ireland.

Genetic advice

• Familial. AD with 50% risk to offspring. There is strong intrafamilial correlation in the course of the disease, but marked interfamilial variability.
• De novo. About half of all patients are founders with clinically unaffected parents. Kluwe et al. (2003) identified mutations in NF2 in 52% in their cohort of NF2 founders with bilateral vestibular schwannomas and estimated the rate of mosaicism to be 24.8% (58/233). Evans and Wallace (2009) estimated this to be 33%. Almost all individuals with mosaicism have relatively mild disease.

Risk assessment
• AD with 50% risk to offspring of an affected individual.
• De novo. There has only been one report of possible germline mosaicism in NF2. If parental skin and eye examinations and head and spine MRIs are normal,

the recurrence risk is very low, i.e. <1% (Ruggieri et al. 2001). However, transmission risk to offspring of a sporadic case with normal blood DNA analysis is substantially reduced from 50% (Evans and Wallace 2009).

Penetrance
Penetrance is age-dependent and is almost complete by 60 years.

Predictive testing
Possible if the familial mutation is known. If there is no mutation, but there are several affected members and the diagnosis is typical with bilateral vestibular schwannomas, it may be possible to do predictive testing by linkage.

Predictive testing in childhood is warranted since surveillance of 'at-risk' individuals begins in early childhood.

Other family members
If there is no family history, parents <60 years of age should be screened by:
• careful examination of the skin;
• ophthalmological assessment for posterior subcapsular and cortical cataracts and CHRPE or astrocytic hamartomas;
• cranial and spinal MRI with gadolinium enhancement.

Management

Patients with NF2 need care from a team with expertise in skull base surgery, usually comprising a neurosurgeon, an ENT surgeon, an audiologist, etc. NF2 patients who are treated in specialist centres have a significantly lower risk of mortality than those treated in non-specialist centres (Baser et al. 2002a). Vestibular schwannoma growth rates in NF2 are generally higher in younger people but are highly variable, even among multiple NF2 patients of similar ages in the same family. Early microsurgery for small tumours results in optimal preservation of hearing and facial nerve function. Complete removal of a large vestibular schwannoma usually renders the patient completely deaf on the side of the surgery. Brainstem implants may offer hope for some patients. Stereotactic radiotherapy is best reserved for NF2 patients who have particularly aggressive tumours, those who are poor surgical risks, those who refuse surgery, or the elderly. Treatment with bevacizumab has now been shown to have efficacy in treating rapidly growing schwannomas (Plotkin et al. 2009).

Surgery for lesions other than vestibular schwannomas is usually undertaken only when indicated by symptoms.

Surveillance strategies
For mutation carriers and 'at-risk' individuals, i.e. offspring of an affected parent in whom predictive genetic testing is declined or not possible:
• ophthalmological assessment in early childhood;
• annual review for symptomatic lesions until early teens;
• screening for vestibular Schwannomas from early teens;
• full cranial and spinal MRI at 15 years and again at 30 years.

If all imaging studies are normal at 30 years and no other features are present, it is likely that status is unaffected and they may be discharged from surveillance (unless the age of onset of NF2 in the family is late).

Support group: The Neuro Foundation, http://www.nfauk.org.

Expert adviser: Gareth Evans, Consultant, Manchester Centre for Genomic Medicine, Division of Evolution and Genomic Sciences, St Mary's Hospital, University of Manchester, Manchester, UK.

References

Baser ME, Evans DG, Gutmann DH. Neurofibromatosis 2. *Curr Opin Neurol* 2003; **16**: 27–33.

Baser ME, Friedman JM, Wallace AJ, Ramsden RT, Joe H, Evans DG. Evaluation of clinical diagnostic criteria for neurofibromatosis 2. *Neurology* 2002a; **59**: 1759–65.

Baser ME, Friedman JM, Aeschliman D, et al. Predictors of the risk of mortality in neurofibromatosis 2. *Am J Hum Genet* 2002b; **71**: 715–23.

Evans DG, Huson SM, Donnai D, et al. A clinical study of type 2 neurofibromatosis. *QJM* 1992a; **304**: 603–18.

Evans DG, Huson SM, Donnai D, et al. A genetic study of type 2 neurofibromatosis: II guidelines for genetic counselling. *J Med Genet* 1992b; **29**: 847–52.

Evans DG, Wallace A. An update on age related mosaic and offspring risk in neurofibromatosis 2 (NF2). *J Med Genet* 2009; **46**: 792.

Kluwe L, Mautner V, Heinrich B, et al. Molecular study of frequency of mosaicism in neurofibromatosis 2 patients with bilateral vestibular schwannomas. *J Med Genet* 2003; **40**: 109–14.

MacCollin M, Willett C, Heinrich B, et al. Familial schwannomatosis: exclusion of the NF2 locus as the germline event. *Neurology* 2003; **60**: 1968–74.

Ruggieri M, Huson SM. The clinical and diagnostic implications of mosaicism in the neurofibromatoses. *Neurology* 2001; **56**: 1433–43.

Ovarian cancer

The lifetime risk of ovarian cancer in the general population is ~1 in 70 or 1.4%. The majority of women with a family history of ovarian cancer have a single first-degree relative affected with ovarian cancer. If there is no significant cancer history in other members of the family (e.g. breast or bowel), the estimated relative risk of developing ovarian cancer is fairly small at 3.1. In Northern Europe and North America, this equates to a cumulative risk of 4% by age 70 years (Stratton et al. 1999). The relative risk of ovarian cancer in an MZ twin of an affected woman is 6, i.e. twice the sibling risk, indicating that much of the excess familial risk is due to genetic factors, rather than shared environmental factors.

Inherited mutations of BRCA1 in particular, also BRCA2, and to a lesser extent the Lynch syndrome genes MLH1, MSH2, and MSH6 (see 'Lynch syndrome (LS)' in Chapter 4, 'Cancer', p. 586) are known to confer predisposition to ovarian cancer. Together they account for close to half of the excess familial risk of ovarian cancer. Recently mutations in three further genes BRIP1, RAD51C, and RAD51D have been identified in ovarian cancer families.

Mutations in BRCA1 and BRCA2 are thought to be responsible for the majority of families with breast/ovarian and site-specific ovarian cancers (see Box 4.12). Approximately 10–15% of all cases of serous ovarian cancer are attributable to BRCA1/BRCA2 mutations.

Ovarian cancer risks in BRCA1 carriers are low (in absolute terms) below age 40 years; thereafter the incidences are 2% between 40 and 49, 15% from 50 to 59 years, and 22% from 60 to 70. Ovarian cancer risk in BRCA2 carriers are, in contrast, very low below age 50 years (2.6%) but then increase to 5% in the 50–59 year age group and 10% from 60 to 70 years (Chen and Parmigiani 2007).

Very early age at diagnosis may not be a feature of familial ovarian cancer. Stratton et al. (1999) found that, of 202 well-documented families with at least two confirmed cases of epithelial ovarian cancer, only 1.6% were diagnosed at <30 years of age. See Box 4.11 for criteria used to establish high risk of ovarian cancer.

Clinical approach

Where possible, try to obtain confirmation of the diagnosis of ovarian cancer. Ovarian cancer is easily misreported by families (the actual diagnosis may prove to be

---

Box 4.11 Criteria for defining high-risk women where genetic testing for BRCA1/BRCA2 might be indicated

- Ovarian cancer under 50 (high-grade serous papillary)
- Ovarian cancer at any age plus family history of breast cancer under 60
- Two or more cases of ovarian cancer
- A woman with Ashkenazi Jewish ancestry and any family history of breast or ovarian cancer

Data from Eeles et al., Genetic Predisposition to Cancer 2e, Copyright 2004 Taylor & Francis Group Ltd.

Box 4.12 Chance of identifying a BRCA1/2 mutation according to family history

Family history	Chance (%) of identifying mutation in BRCA1/2
At least two cases of ovarian cancer and at least two cases of breast cancer	61
At least three cases of ovarian cancer and >1 case of breast cancer	70
Two cases of ovarian cancer and one case of breast cancer	47
Two cases of ovarian cancer and no cases of breast cancer	20

Reprinted from Best Practice and Research Clinical Obstetrics & Gynaecology, vol 16(4), Pharaoh and Ponder, The Genetics of Ovarian Cancer, pp. 449–68, copyright 2002, with permission from Elsevier.

---

a benign lesion, teratoma, adenocarcinoma of the bowel, uterine cancer, etc.). Krukenberg tumour refers to secondary tumours in the ovaries usually arising from a gastric primary.

History: key points
Three-generation family tree, with particular emphasis on history of cancer (especially ovarian, breast, and bowel) and documentation of age of diagnosis. Try to extend the family tree further on the relevant side if there are individuals with cancer in the grandparental generation.

Examination: key points
Not usually appropriate.

Histopathology is crucial in guiding genetic testing. Around 10–15% of unselected serous ovarian cancers have a BRCA1/BRCA2 mutation, compared to 8% of endometrial cancers. Mucinous and clear cell are over-represented in Lynch syndrome but are not typically seen in BRCA1/BRCA2 (Zhang et al. 2011).

Special investigations
- DNA for BRCA1/2 mutation analysis from an affected member of a family meeting the high-risk criteria. See 'BRCA1 and BRCA2' in Chapter 4, 'Cancer', p. 542.
- IHC or DNA for MMR genes if the family meets Amsterdam criteria (see Box 4.9 in 'Lynch syndrome (LS)', Chapter 4, 'Cancer', p. 586).
- Consider RAD51C/RAD51D testing.

Genetic advice

Risk assessment
This should be done using an established method, e.g. Manchester Score (Evans et al. 2005), BOADICEA (Antoniou et al. 2008).

- Single relative affected <30 years with no other significant family history (e.g. breast cancer or other cancers suggestive of a familial cancer syndrome). Stratton *et al.* (1999) found no *BRCA1/2* mutations among 101 women with ovarian cancer diagnosed at <30 years and no tendency to greater familiality. Overall risks are likely to be similar to those of the sister of an older proband, i.e. 2- to 3-fold increased lifetime risk for ovarian cancer.

- Single relative affected >30 years with no other significant family history (e.g. breast cancer or other cancers suggestive of a familial cancer syndrome). Sister of a woman with 'sporadic' ovarian cancer has a 3-fold increased lifetime risk for ovarian cancer (Stratton *et al.* 1998).
- High-risk women (see criteria for 'high risk' in Box 4.11). High chance of a dominant genetic susceptibility to ovarian and breast cancers.
- It is becoming increasingly common to offer *BRCA1/2* testing to women with serous ovarian cancer regardless of family history (Plaskocinska 2016).

Penetrance
BRCA1 mutation carriers have a 30–50% risk (to age 70 years of ovarian cancer, whereas the risk in *BRCA2* carriers is lower at around 10–20%). The lifetime risk for the Lynch genes and *BRIP1/RAD51C/RAD51D* is around 10%.

Predictive testing
Possible for those families in whom the causative mutation has been defined.

Management

Women with a single affected relative
While the risk of developing ovarian cancer is higher than those of a similar age who are at population risk (RR 3 for first-degree relatives), this increased risk amounts to a cumulative risk of ~4% by age 70 years. In the absence of formal evidence of its efficacy, screening is not currently recommended at this level of risk.

High-risk women and BRCA1/2 carriers
The risk of ovarian cancer among *BRCA1* mutation carriers decreases with parity, tubal ligation, and use of the OCP (hazard ratio = 0.52), and similar patterns are seen in *BRCA2* (Antoniou *et al.* 2009).

PROPHYLACTIC LAPAROSCOPIC SALPINGO-OOPHORECTOMY.
Although the risk of ovarian cancer in carriers of *BRCA1/ BRCA2* mutations is considerably lower than the risk of breast cancer in these carriers, the absence of reliable methods of early detection and the poor prognosis of advanced ovarian cancer make prophylactic salpingo-oophorectomy an option that all female carriers should consider after their families are complete. Kauff *et al.* (2002), in a prospective study of 170 carriers of *BRCA1/ BRCA2* mutations with a mean follow-up of 2 years, found an ovarian cancer hazard ratio of 0.15 after risk-reducing bilateral salpingo-oophorectomy (RRBSO), compared with the surveillance-only group. It was previously thought that RRBSO in premenopausal *BRCA1/BRCA2* mutation carriers led to a significant reduction in breast cancer risk, but recent studies have cast doubt on this (Heemskerk-Gerritsen *et al.* 2015).

Salpingo-oophorectomy must be performed, rather than oophorectomy, as there is increasing evidence that tumours arise in the Fallopian tubes in carriers of *BRCA* mutations. There is a residual risk for primary peritoneal ovarian cancer after oophorectomy.

The risk of developing ovarian cancer at <40 years is low, even in women at high genetic risk. Oophorectomy in premenopausal women precipitates an abrupt menopause. Important side effects include hot flushes, disturbed sleep, vaginal dryness, and increased risk of osteoporosis and heart disease. HRT may be needed in the short term to counteract these side effects.

CHEMOPREVENTION. The oral combined OCP provides a long-term reduction in the risk of ovarian cancer in the general population and in *BRCA1/BRCA22* carriers, but this has to be balanced against the small increased breast cancer risk which reverts to baseline 5 years after stopping.

Surveillance strategies
See also 'Cancer surveillance methods' in Chapter 4, 'Cancer', p. 552.

- Breast surveillance. Due to the high incidence of *BRCA1/2* mutations in high-risk ovarian cancer families (see above), even those in whom an affected family member screens negative for *BRCA1/2* mutations should be managed as if they were at high risk of breast cancer (if serous-type histology is confirmed).
- Serum CA125 estimation and ovarian USS. This is not recommended outside of a clinical trial, as evidence from studies has not shown that screening reduces mortality.
- *BRCA1/2* status and the management of ovarian cancer. There is emerging evidence that *BRCA2* mutation status, in particular, is likely to be an important prognostic and predictive marker in epithelial ovarian cancer. In an analysis of 3879 cases of ovarian cancer (2666 non-carriers, 909 *BRCA1* mutation carriers, and 304 *BRCA2* mutation carriers), adjusted hazard ratios for overall mortality at 5 years were 0.73 for *BRCA1* and 0.49 *BRCA2* mutation carriers, compared with non-carriers (Bolton *et al.* 2012). It also appears that *BRCA1/BRCA2* mutation status provides predictive information regarding the likelihood of response to poly ADP ribose polymerase inhibitors (PARPis). In a study of one such PARPi—olaparib—objective responses were seen in seven of 17 (41%) patients with *BRCA1* or *BRCA2* mutations, compared to 11 of 46 (24%) without mutations (Gelmon *et al.* 2011). If these results are corroborated in further studies, it is likely that *BRCA1/BRCA2* testing will enter mainstream oncological practice and become an integral part of the management of ovarian cancer.

Expert adviser: Marc Tischkowitz, Reader and Honorary Consultant Physician in Medical Genetics, Department of Medical Genetics, University of Cambridge and East Anglian Medical Genetics Service, Cambridge, UK.

References

Antoniou A, Pharoah PD, Narod S, et al. Average risks of breast and ovarian cancer associated with mutations in *BRCA1* or *BRCA2* detected in case series unselected for family history: a combined analysis of 22 studies. *Am J Hum Genet* 2003; **72**: 1117–30.

Antoniou AC, Cunningham AP, Peto J, et al. The BOADICEA model of genetic susceptibility to breast and ovarian cancers: updates and extensions. *Br J Cancer* 2008; **98**: 1457–66.

Antoniou AC, Rookus M, Andrieu N, et al. Reproductive and hormonal factors, and ovarian cancer risk for *BRCA1* and *BRCA2* mutation carriers: results from the International *BRCA1/ 2* Carrier Cohort Study. *Cancer Epidemiol Biomarkers Prev* 2009; **18**: 601–10.

Bolton KL, Chenevix-Trench G, Goh C, et al. Association between BRCA1 and BRCA2 mutations and survival in women with invasive epithelial ovarian cancer. JAMA 2012; **307**: 382–90.

Chen S, Parmigiani G. Meta-analysis of BRCA1 and BRCA2 penetrance. J Clin Oncol 2007; **25**: 1329–33.

Evans DG, Lalloo F, Wallace A, Rahman N. Update on the Manchester Scoring System for BRCA1 and BRCA2 testing. J Med Genet 2005; **42**: e39.

Gelmon KA, Tischkowitz M, Mackay H, et al. Olaparib in patients with recurrent high-grade serous or poorly differentiated ovarian carcinoma or triple-negative breast cancer: a phase 2, multicentre, open-label, non-randomised study. Lancet Oncol 2011; **12**: 852–61.

Heemskerk-Gerritsen BA, Seynaeve C, van Asperen CJ, et al. Breast cancer risk after salpingo-oophorectomy in healthy BRCA1/2 mutation carriers: revisiting the evidence for risk reduction. J Natl Cancer Inst 2015; **107**: pii: djv033.

Kauff ND, Satogopan JM, Robson ME, et al. Risk-reducing salpingo-oophorectomy in women with a BRCA1 or BRCA2 mutation. N Engl J Med 2002; **346**: 1609–15.

NIH Consensus Development Panel on Ovarian Cancer. NIH consensus conference. Ovarian cancer. Screening treatment, and follow-up. JAMA 1995; **273**: 491–7.

Pharaoh PD, Ponder BA. The genetics of ovarian cancer. Best Pract Res Clin Obstet Gynaecol 2002; **16**: 449–68.

Plaskocinska I, Shipman H, et al. New paradigms for BRCA1/BRCA2 testing in women with ovarian cancer: results of Genetic Testing in Epithelial Ovarian Cancer (GTEOC) study.

Stratton JF, Pharaoh PD, Smith SK, Easton D, Ponder BA. A systematic review and meta-analysis of family history and risk of ovarian cancer. Br J Obstet Gynaecol 1998; **105**: 493–9.

Stratton JF, Thompson D, Bobrow L, et al. The genetic epidemiology of early-onset epithelial ovarian cancer: a population-based study. Am J Hum Genet 1999; **65**: 1725–32.

Zhang S, Royer R, Li S, et al. Frequencies of BRCA1 and BRCA2 mutations among 1,342 unselected patients with invasive ovarian cancer. Gynecol Oncol 2011; **121**: 353–7.

Peutz–Jeghers syndrome (PJS)

An AD syndrome consisting of characteristic GI hamartomas, mucocutaneous pigmentation, and predisposition to GI, breast, and other cancers. Patients with PJS are at increased risk of GI intussusception and the development of a variety of malignancies, especially of the GI tract, but also including pancreas, breast, uterine, and gonadal tumours. Prevalence estimates for PJS vary between ~1/8300 and 1/29 000. At least 80-94% of PJS cases have a detectable constitutional mutation in *STK11* (*LKB1*), encoding a serine/threonine kinase on 19p13.3.

Pigmentation

The characteristic freckling of the lips and perioral region develops during childhood but usually fades from the third decade onwards (less so on the buccal mucosa). Although seen in 95% of patients, it is highly variable and not universally present; in some patients, the freckling is florid; in others, it can be extremely subtle. Freckling is also seen around the nostrils, fingers, and toes, and the dorsal and volar aspects of the hands, as well as perianal and perivulval regions. It is not a unique sign and, for example, CNC should be considered in the differential.

Polyps

There is a great variation in phenotype between PJS families. Seventy to 90% of PJS patients have hamartomatous polyps in the small bowel (usually jejunum), 50% have colorectal polyps, and 25% have gastric polyps. The number of polyps per patient is variable, but many fewer than in FAP. PJS polyps tend to be large and pedunculated, and PJS patients commonly present as surgical emergencies in childhood with intussusception, small bowel obstruction, bleeding per rectum, and volvulus. Most polyps do not cause complications but may cause non-specific abdominal pain. Polyps and cancers occur outside of the GI tract, e.g. nose, respiratory tract, uterus, urinary tract, and gall bladder/biliary tree.

Pathology

The histology of PJS polyps is characteristic and diagnostic, consisting of a branched or frond-like pattern in the stroma, termed arborization. Cystic gland dilatation is observed, which may extend into the submucosa and muscularis propria. Juvenile polyps, in contrast, have a lamina propria lacking smooth muscle, but the two types can be confused. Also, small bowel polyps can exhibit 'pseudoinvasion' which can be mistaken for invasive carcinoma. Histological review should therefore be considered.

Molecular pathology

The STK11 serine/threonine kinase is part of the mTOR pathway, and it is therefore not surprising that other hamartomatous polyposis syndromes are caused by constitutional mutations in *PTEN, BMPR1A*, and *SMAD4* and hence the differential diagnosis should include Cowden syndrome, JPS, and CNC. See 'Multiple endocrine neoplasia (MEN)' in Chapter 4, 'Cancer', p. 592. Rare families have been reported linked to loci other than 19p13.3, so genetic heterogeneity is possible, but seemingly rare, and getting rarer as mutation detection improves.

No difference is observed in phenotype between those with missense and truncating *STK11* mutations. In particular, cancer risks do not vary by type and site of mutation.

PJS-associated cancers

A systematic review by Beggs *et al.* (2010) endeavouring to minimize bias and using the data from Giardiello *et al.* (2000) and Hearle *et al.* (2006) provides the best estimates of cancer risks (see Tables 4.20 and 4.21).

CRC risk predominates and a significant rise in risk after the age of 50 is observed. However, female breast and gynaecological cancer risks are also significant. Sex cord tumours (SCTAT) and other, sometimes hormone-secreting, gonadal tumours are also seen, often at a young age.

Diagnostic criteria for PJS

The following is taken from Beggs *et al.* (2010):

'In a single individual, a clinical diagnosis of PJS may be made when any ONE of the following is present:

1. Two or more histologically confirmed PJ polyps.
2. Any number of PJ polyps detected in one individual who has a family history of PJS in close relative(s).
3. Characteristic mucocutaneous pigmentation in an individual who has a family history of PJS in close relative(s).

Table 4.20 Cumulative cancer risk by site and age in Peutz–Jeghers syndrome patients

Type of cancer	Cancer risk by age, % (95% CI)					
	20 years	30 years	40 years	50 years	60 years	70 years
All cancers	2 (0.8–4)	5 (3–8)	17 (13–23)	31 (24–39)	60 (50–71)	85 (68–96)
Gastrointestinal	–	1 (0.4–3)	9 (5–14)	15 (10–22)	33 (23–45)	57 (39–76)
Breast (female)	–	–	8 (4–17)	13 (7–24)	31 (18–50)	45 (27–68)
Gynaecological	–	1 (0.4–6)	3 (0.9–9)	8 (4–19)	18 (9–34)	18 (9–34)
Pancreas	–	–	3 (1–7)	5 (2–10)	7 (3–16)	11 (5–24)
Lung						
Male	–	–	1 (0.1–6)	4 (1–11)	13 (6–28)	17 (8–36)
Female	–	–	1 (0.1–6)	–	–	–

Reproduced from Hearle, N., *et al.* (2006). Frequency and spectrum of cancers in the Peutz-Jeghers syndrome. *Clinical Cancer Research*, 12(10), 3209–3215. With permission from Richard Houlston (reuse of own work).

Table 4.21 Risk ratios, frequencies, and ages of onset of Peutz–Jeghers syndrome cancers by site

Site	Risk ratio (95% CI)	Frequency (%)	Mean age (years)	Age range (years)
Oesophagus	57 (2.5–557)	0.5	67	–
Stomach	213 (96–368)	29	30	10–61
Small bowel	520 (220–1306)	13	42	21–84
Colon	84 (47–137)	39	46	27–71
Pancreas	132 (44–261)	36	41	16–60
Lung	17 (5.4–39)	15	–	–
Testis	4.5 (0.12–25)	9	8.6	3–20
Breast	15.2 (7.6–27)	54	37	9–48
Uterus	16 (1.9–56)	9	–	–
Ovary	27 (7.3–68)	21	28	4–57
Cervix	1.5 (0.31–4.4)	10	34	23–54

Reprinted from *Gastroenterology*, 119(6), Giardiello FM, Brensinger JD, *et al.*, Very high risk of cancer in familial Peutz–Jeghers syndrome, pp. 1447–53, Copyright 2000, with permission from Elsevier and the AGA Institute.

4. Any number of PJ polyps in an individual who also has characteristic mucocutaneous pigmentation.'

Reproduced from *Gut*, Beggs *et al.*, Peutz–Jeghers syndrome: a systematic review and recommendations for management, volume 59, issue 7, pp. 975–86, copyright 2010, with permission from BMJ Publishing Group Ltd.

Aretz *et al.* (2005) correlated the diagnostic criteria for PJS with *STK11* mutation detection rates. Of patients who met the criteria for PJS, >94% had a mutation detected (64% point mutation, 30% deletions).

Differential diagnosis

• JPS (see 'Juvenile polyposis syndrome (JPS)' in Chapter 4, 'Cancer', p. 578) may be confused with PJS, but the histology of the polyps is distinct, although it may necessitate the opinion of a histopathologist specializing in GI pathology. It is well worth asking for histological review.
• HMPS (*CRAC1*; see 'Familial adenomatous polyposis (FAP) and adenomatous polyposis due to *MUTYH*, *NTHL1*, *POLE*, and *POLD1*' in Chapter 4, 'Cancer', p. 568) is not associated with pigmentation and includes adenomas and, so far, has only been described in Ashkenazi Jews.
• LEOPARD syndrome shows abnormal pigmentation, but not the same pattern as in PJS, and is also not associated with polyps.

Clinical approach

History: key points
Three-generation family tree, with careful enquiry about perioral freckling, recurrent abdominal pain, and abdominal surgery. Take a detailed history of cancer in other family members (especially breast, GI, and pancreas).

Examination: key points
• Look carefully for freckling of the lips, buccal mucosa, vulva, anus, fingers, and toes.
• Note skin lentigines.
• Be alert to endocrine signs of sex cord tumours with annular tubules (SCTATs), especially in children, e.g. precocious puberty, oestrogenization, etc.

Special investigations
• Histopathology of polyps/tumours. Consider the opinion of a specialist GI pathologist.
• DNA sample for *STK11* mutation analysis from affected members of the family.

Genetic advice

• PJS is usually due to constitutional mutations in *STK11* (>90%). There is marked inter- and intrafamilial variability of expression in PJS kindreds, unrelated to the mutation type and site within *STK11*.

Risk assessment
AD, 50% risk of inheritance. About 10–20% have apparent new mutations; the remainder are familial.

Penetrance
Almost complete penetrance: 0/17 clinically unaffected at-risk relatives in Ylikorkala *et al.*'s (1999) series showed the disease-associated haplotype. More than 90% have mucocutaneous melanin pigmentation, but this is known to fade after age 20–30 years. Though again, bear in mind the differential diagnoses.

Predictive testing
Possible by direct mutation analysis, if mutation known in the family, or by haplotype analysis if family large enough to establish linkage to 19p13.

Individuals in whom predictive testing has not been possible and in whom screening has shown no polyps and who have no freckling can probably discontinue screening from age 30 years.

Prenatal diagnosis
Technically possible by, for example, CVS if the familial mutation is known.

Management

Beggs *et al.* (2010) comprehensively cover management options. The risks of cancer are significant in both sexes, and recommended surveillance regimes are intensive. The main aim of childhood GI surveillance is to reduce the risk of intussusception, rather than cancer. Current practice is aimed at avoiding the repeated laparotomies of times past for the removal of single, usually small bowel, polyps; if a laparotomy is performed, then the aim should be to remove all polyps, not just the one intussuscepting. Referral to, and management by, a specialized surgical/gastroenterological team experienced in looking after PJS patients is strongly recommended.

Laser and intense pulsed light therapy for mucocutaneous pigmentation has been successfully performed, but their use in routine practice is not currently supported. In cases of psychological morbidity related to pigmentation, referral to a dermatologist and/or a clinical psychologist is advised.

Surveillance strategies

Beggs et al. (2010) have systematically reviewed surveillance options, leading to the following recommendations.

GENERAL.

• Annual FBC and LFTs.

• Annual clinical examination.

GENITAL TRACT.

• Annual examination and testicular examination from birth until 12 years.

• Testicular USS if abnormalities detected at examination.

• Cervical smear with liquid-based cytology (LBC), 3-yearly from age 25 years.

GASTROINTESTINAL.

• Baseline OGD and colonoscopy age 8 years, if:
  • polyps detected, continue 3-yearly until 50 years;
  • no polyps detected, repeat age 18 years, then 3-yearly until 50 years.

• Colonoscopy 1- to 2-yearly after age 50 years.

• Video capsule endoscopy (VCE) of the small bowel every 3 years from age 8 years.

BREAST.

• Monthly self-examination from age 18 years.

• Annual breast MRI from age 25 to 50 years, thereafter annual mammography.

Note that this is not necessarily consistent with other breast surveillance protocols in, for example, *BRCA1/2* cases, and local policies should be decided.

Support group: Bowel Cancer UK, http://www.bowelcanceruk.org.uk; Macmillan Cancer Support, https://www.macmillan.org.uk; International Society of Gastrointestinal Hereditary Tumours (InSIGHT), https://www.insight-group.org.

Expert adviser: Ian M. Frayling, Consultant Genetic Pathologist, Cardiff & Vale University Health Board, Cardiff University, Institute of Medical Genetics, University Hospital of Wales, Cardiff, UK and Richard S. Houlston, Professor, Division of Molecular Pathology, The Institute of Cancer Research, Surrey, UK.

References

Aretz S, Stienen D, Uhlhaas S, et al. (2005). High proportion of large genomic *STK11* deletions in Peutz–Jeghers syndrome. *Hum Mutat* 2005; **26**: 513–19.

Beggs AD, Latchford AR, Vasen HF, et al. Peutz–Jeghers syndrome: a systematic review and recommendations for management. *Gut* 2010; **59**: 975–86.

Giardiello FM, Brensinger JD, Tersmette AC, et al. Very high risk of cancer in familial Peutz–Jeghers syndrome. *Gastroenterology* 2000; **119**: 1447–53.

Hearle N, Schumacher V, Menko FH, et al. (2006). Frequency and spectrum of cancers in the Peutz–Jeghers syndrome. *Clin Cancer Res* 2006; **12**: 3209–15.

Spigelman AD, Murday V, Phillips RK. Cancer and the Peutz–Jeghers syndrome. *Gut* 1989; **30**: 1588–90.

Stratakis CA, Kirschner LS, Carney JA. Clinical and molecular features of the Carney complex: diagnostic criteria and recommendations for patient evaluation [review]. *J Clin Endocrinol Metab* 2001; **86**: 4041–6.

Stratakis CA, Kirschner LS, Taymans SE, et al. Carney complex, Peutz–Jeghers syndrome, Cowden disease, and Bannayan–Zonana syndrome share cutaneous and endocrine manifestations, but not genetic loci. *J Clin Endocrinol Metab* 1998; **83**: 2972–6.

Tomlinson IP, Houlston RS. Peutz–Jeghers syndrome. *J Med Genet* 1997; **34**: 1007–11.

Ylikorkala A, Avizienyte E, Tomlinson IP, et al. Mutations and impaired function of LKB1 in familial and non-familial Peutz–Jeghers syndrome and a sporadic testicular cancer. *Hum Mol Genet* 1999; **8**: 45–51.

Phaeochromocytoma and paraganglioma

The adrenal medulla and ganglia of the sympathetic nervous system are neural crest derivatives. They synthesize and secrete catecholamines (adrenaline, noradrenaline, etc.). Phaeochromocytomas usually arise in the adrenal medulla but can arise outside the adrenal, in the sympathetic chain, where they may be called paragangliomas. Paragangliomas that originate in the sympathetic nervous system are most commonly found in the retroperitoneum but can also occur in the thorax. Paragangliomas that originate in the parasympathetic nervous system can occur adjacent to the aortic arch, neck, and skull base as local 'non-functioning' masses, also called 'glomus tumours' or chemodectomas or head and neck paragangliomas (HNPGLs). Germline mutations in the succinate dehydrogenase subunit genes (most commonly SDHB and SDHD) can cause susceptibility to phaeochromocytomas, paragangliomas and HNPGLs. Classical clinical symptoms of phaeochromocytomas/paragangliomas are paroxysmal headache, sweating, and palpitations, accompanied by hypertension due to the pressor effects of catecholamine release.

Although traditionally ~10% of phaeochromocytomas have been considered to have a genetic origin, the latest studies suggest at least 40% of all cases and 30% of sporadic cases harbour a germline mutation. In addition to a family history, multicentric disease, extra-adrenal location and early age at diagnosis are all risk factors for a germline mutation (Neumann et al. 2002).

The most common genetic causes of phaeochromocytoma are mutations in SDHB, SDHD, VHL, and RET. In addition, there are a number of other, less frequent, non-syndromic causes of inherited phaeochromocytoma/paraganglioma/HNPGL. See Table 4.22 for a summary of genetic conditions predisposing to phaeochromocytoma.

Clinical approach

History: key points

Three-generation family tree, with specific reference to tumour types and features listed in Table 4.22. For SDHD, SDHAF2, and MAX mutations, clinical disease is generally only seen after paternal transmission (i.e. individuals who inherit the mutation from their mother are asymptomatic).

Examination: key points

- Marfanoid body habitus and mucosal neuromas (multiple endocrine dysplasia (MEN2B)).
- Thyroid mass (MEN2).
- Carotid body tumour (familial paraganglioma).
- CALs, axillary freckling, and dermal neurofibromas (NF1).
- Observe the gait, and observe the eyes for nystagmus and past-pointing/dysdiadochokinesia (cerebellar signs in VHL secondary to cerebellar haemangioblastoma).
- Cutaneous leiomyomas.

Special investigations

- DNA for mutation analysis if specific syndrome identified or positive family history, extra-adrenal location, malignancy, or young age at onset. Gene panel tests for multiple genes are available.
- Ophthalmology referral for retinal angiomas (VHL) if no specific syndrome identified.
- Most patients with phaeochromocytoma will have had recent intra-abdominal imaging (usually MRI) as part of their diagnosis which should identify pancreatic cysts and renal cell cancers (VHL).

Table 4.22 Genetic conditions predisposing to phaeochromocytoma

Syndrome*	Gene	Features†	Phaeochromocytoma
MEN2A	RET	MTC, hyperparathyroidism	50
MEN2B	RET	MTC, multiple mucosal neuromas, Marfanoid habitus, hyperparathyroidism	50
Familial paraganglioma	SDHBSDHD‡ SDHA SDHC SDHAF2‡ MAX‡ TMEM127	HNPGLWith SDHB there is a high frequency of malignancy (~30%) and a risk of renal cancer (~15%)	20
VHL	VHL	Cerebellar and CNS haemangioblastoma, renal cell cancer, pancreatic and renal cysts, retinal angiomas	10–20
NF1	NF1	CALs, axillary freckling, dermal neurofibromas	1
HLRCC*	FH	Cutaneous leiomyomas, uterine fibroids, renal cell carcinoma	

* HLRCC, hereditary leiomyomatosis and renal cell carcinoma syndrome (Reed syndrome); MEN, multiple endocrine dysplasia; NF1, neurofibromatosis type 1; VHL, von Hippel–Lindau syndrome.

† CALs, café-au-lait spots; CNS, central nervous system; MTC, medullary thyroid cancer.

‡ Mutations of SDHD, SDHAF2, and MAX show parent of origin effects on penetrance (clinical disease after paternal transmission).

From New England Journal of Medicine, Robert G. Dluhy, Pheochromocytoma—Death of an Axiom, 346, 19, pp. 1486–1488, Copyright © 2008 Massachusetts Medical Society. Reprinted with permission from Massachusetts Medical Society.

Genetic advice

Risk assessment

If a specific syndrome or germline mutation identified, offer screening to all first-degree family members.

Penetrance

See Table 4.22.

Predictive testing

If a specific germline mutation is identified (and you are certain it is disease-causing), offer predictive testing to first-degree relatives in order to target subsequent surveillance.

Management

Surveillance strategies

In genetic conditions predisposing to phaeochromocytoma, screening is usually accomplished by vanillylmandelic acid (VMA) analysis of 24-hour urine samples or plasma metadrenalines (metanephrines) and abdominal imaging (MRI scans). Surveillance for other associated tumours will depend on the genetic cause.

Expert adviser: Eamonn R. Maher, Professor and Honorary Consultant, Department of Medical Genetics, University of Cambridge, Cambridge University Hospitals, Cambridge, UK.

References

Dluhy RG. Phaeochromocytoma—death of an axiom [editorial]. *N Engl J Med* 2002; **346**: 1486–8.

Erlic Z, Rybicki L, Peczkowska M, *et al.* Clinical predictors and algorithm for the genetic diagnosis of phaeochromocytoma patients. *Clin Cancer Res* 2009; **15**: 6389–95.

Jafri M, Maher ER. The genetics of phaeochromocytoma: using clinical features to guide genetic testing. *Eur J Endocrinol* 2012; **166**: 151–8.

Neumann HP, Bausch B, McWhinney SR, *et al.* Germ-line mutations in nonsyndromic phaeochromocytoma. *N Engl J Med* 2002; **346**: 1459–66.

Prostate cancer

Prostate cancer is the most common cancer in men in the UK and is second to lung cancer as a cause of cancer death in males. Like all common cancers, it increases with age and about 60% men are aged >70 years at diagnosis. The lifetime risk is rising and is now 1 in 9 by age 85 years (Cancer Research UK 2014). Earlier diagnosis is associated with better survival; a period analysis has shown that survival has improved over the last 5 years and is now over 80% for men with organ-confined disease. However, a proportion of men are diagnosed when the disease is widespread, and then the 5-year survival after diagnosis is 60%. The problem with prostate cancer screening is that prostate-specific antigen (PSA), a serum marker, can result in a significant proportion of overdiagnosis, although in European studies it has been reported to reduce mortality, but 12–48 men need to be treated with attendant risk of comorbidities of incontinence and impotence to prolong one life.

There are some ethnic differences with black African and Caribbean men at greater risk than Europeans, who have a greater risk than men from Asia.

Some families show clustering of prostate cancer, and in some there is a history of breast cancer in female relatives. The breast cancer gene *BRCA2* (see 'BRCA1 and BRCA2' in Chapter 4, 'Cancer', p. 542) is an important single gene cause of increased risk, though *BRCA2* mutations are only found in about 2% of men who present aged <55 years and 1.2% of men aged 65 years or less at diagnosis. However, men with inherited mutations of *BRCA2* are not only at 5–8.6 times more risk of prostate cancer (the relative risk is even higher at younger ages), but it is also often of a more aggressive type. Male BRCA2 carriers are also at increased risk of breast cancer (~6% by 70 years).

The cumulative risk for prostate cancer in men with *BRCA2* is 10–20% by age 70 and it may only increase the risk at younger ages.

Mutations in the *BRCA1* gene have a smaller effect, increasing a man's risk of prostate cancer by <2-fold in some studies and 4.5-fold in others. There is uncertainty as to whether prostate cancer associated with *BRCA1* mutations is more aggressive and has a worse prognosis, and further studies are needed.

A recent international PSA screening study (the IMPACT study), using a threshold of 3 ng/ml to trigger transrectal ultrasound prostate biopsy, showed that the PPV of biopsy in BRCA2 mutation carriers was 48%, double that in population-based screening studies in men over 55 years, and 66% of the tumours detected were aggressive (intermediate-/high-risk which are groups which are recommended for radical treatment on national guidelines). The novel *HOXB13* G84E variant is associated with a significantly increased risk of hereditary prostate cancer (Ewing *et al.* 2012). The carrier rate of the G84E mutation was increased by a factor of ~20 in 5083 unrelated subjects of European descent who had prostate cancer, with the mutation found in 72 subjects (1.4%), as compared with one in 1401 control subjects (0.1%) ($P = 8.5 \times 10^{-7}$). This mutation was significantly more common in men with early-onset familial prostate cancer (3.1%) than in those with late-onset non-familial prostate cancer (0.6%) ($P = 2.0 \times 10^{-6}$). *HOXB13* is more common in men of Scandinavian descent. Studies

in the UK population have shown that 1.5% of prostate cancer cases have germline G84E mutation in *HOXB13*. It is not associated with aggressive disease features. Recent data have indicated that men in Lynch syndrome families may also have a 2- to 3-fold relative risk of prostate cancer and the IMPACT study is investigating the role of PSA screening in this group. Studies of the BROCA panel of 22 genes in men with 3 or more cases of prostrate cancer in their family history show 7.3% have a predicted loss of function mutation in one of the DNA repair genes in the panel. As yet this is not available as a clinical test.

There are now 112 reported susceptibility loci identified by GWAS (Ahmed, 2015) and these are of low penetrance but the per allele odds ratios are multiplicative and men in the top 1% of the risk distribution have a 5.7 fold relative risk compared with the average of the population; collectively ~30% of the familial risk is due to such variants.

Clinical approach

History
- Three-generation family tree, with specific enquiry for breast, ovarian, prostate, colon, endometrial, and other cancers.

Examination
- Digital rectal examination (DRE).

Investigations
- PSA test. MRI is increasingly used to direct biopsy is indicated if the PSA is raised.
- BRCA1/2 screening if meets Manchester score (see Tables 4.4 and 4.5 in 'Breast cancer', Chapter 4, 'Cancer', p. 546).
- Lynch syndrome screening if meets Lynch syndrome criteria.
- Oncologists are starting to test in trials for germline mutations in DNA repair genes in men with castrate resistant prostate cancer to determine if they can be offered PARP inhibitors.

Genetic advice

If a pathogenic mutation in *BRCA1/2* or Lynch syndrome is identified, this will follow an AD pattern of inheritance with a 50% risk to offspring.

Management

Surveillance
Three screening tests for prostate cancer are available— DRE, imaging with transrectal ultrasound (TRUS) and/or diffusion-weighted (DW)-MRI, and the measurement of PSA levels—but all have problems. There is no UK or US screening programme for prostate cancer in the general white population, but screening by PSA is encouraged in men over 50 years, particularly in African-Americans and those with a family history of at least one first- or second-degree relative with prostate cancer diagnosed at <70 years.

Of the three, the PSA test, a blood test, is the most acceptable, but it fails to be a useful population screening test, mainly because of:
- lack of specificity. Only about a quarter to a third of asymptomatic men with abnormally high PSA levels will

have prostate cancer. Up to two-thirds of men with elevated PSA levels will not have prostate cancer but will suffer the anxiety, discomfort, and risk of follow-up investigations;

• lack of sensitivity. Up to 20% of all men with prostate cancers have normal PSA levels.

Expert adviser: Rosalind Eeles, Professor and Honorary Consultant in Clinical Oncology and Oncogenetics, Division of Genetics & Epidemiology, The Institute of Cancer Research & Royal Marsden NHS Foundation Trust, London, UK.

References

Agaliu I, Karlins E, Kwon EM, et al. Rare germline mutations in the BRCA2 gene are associated with early-onset prostate cancer. Br J Cancer 2007; **97**: 826–31.

Ahmed M, Eeles R. Germline genetic profiling in prostate cancer; latest developments and potential clinical applications. Future Sci OA 2015; **2**: FS087.

Attard G, Parker C, Eeles RA, et al. Prostate cancer. Lancet 2016; **387**: 70–82.

Bancroft EK, Page EC, Castro E, et al. Targeted prostate cancer screening in BRCA1 and BRCA2 mutation carriers: results from the initial round of the IMPACT study. Eur Urol 2014; **66**: 489–99.

Cancer Research UK (2014). http://www.cancerresearchuk.org.

Eeles RA, Goh C, Castro E, et al. The genetic epidemiology of prostate cancer and its clinical implications. Nat Rev Urol 2014; **11**: 18–31.

Eeles RA, Kote-Jarai Z, Olama AA, et al. Identification of seven new prostate cancer susceptibility loci through a genome-wide association study. Nat Genet 2009; **41**: 1116–21.

Ewing CM, Ray AM, Lange EM, et al. Germline mutations in HOXB13 and prostate cancer risk. N Engl J Med 2012; **366**: 141–9.

Renal cancer

Renal cell carcinoma (RCC) is a male-predominant (2:1 ratio) disease with a typical presentation in the sixth and seventh decades of life (median age ~60 years) (Rini et al. 2009). The most common type is clear cell RCC (70–80%). Only about 3% of RCC patients have a positive family history, but studies of rare inherited forms of RCC have provided important insights into the pathogenesis of more common sporadic forms of RCC. Thus, the rare inherited VHL disease (see 'von Hippel–Lindau (VHL) disease' in Chapter 4, 'Cancer', p. 618) is caused by germline mutations in the VHL tumour suppressor gene and most sporadic clear cell RCC harbour somatic VHL mutations (or loss or methylation) that cause biallelic inactivation of the VHL gene (consistent with Knudson's 'two-hit hypothesis'). In addition to VHL disease, there are a number of other syndromic causes of RCC.

Birt–Hogg–Dubé (BHD) syndrome) is a dominantly inherited disorder characterized by the development of facial fibrofolliculomas, pulmonary cysts and pneumothorax, and RCC (20–30% lifetime risk). There may be an increased risk of CRC. BHD is caused by mutations in the FLCN gene and about 5% of patients with features suggestive of inherited RCC (e.g. positive family history or multiple tumours or young age at diagnosis (<35 years)) may harbour a germline FLCN mutation. Germline SDHB mutations, which are most commonly associated with phaeochromocytoma/paraganglioma/HNPGL (see 'Phaeochromocytoma and paraganglioma' in Chapter 4, 'Cancer', p. 608), can predispose to RCC (lifetime risk ~15%) and in some cases present with familial non-syndromic RCC (without evidence of phaeochromocytoma/paraganglioma). Approximately 5% of patients with features suggestive of inherited RCC may harbour a germline SDHB mutation.

Germline mutations in the fumarate hydratase (FH) gene can cause hereditary leiomyomatosis and RCC syndrome (HLRCC). This dominantly inherited disorder is characterized by cutaneous leiomyomas and, in females, multiple uterine leiomyomas (fibroids) at a young age. The lifetime risk of RCC is not well defined, but RCC (typically type 2 papillary or collecting duct RCC) in HLRCC may occur early (youngest reported age 11 years) and typically follows an aggressive course.

Autosomal dominantly inherited activating mutations in the MET proto-oncogene cause hereditary type 1 papillary kidney cancer.

Constitutional chromosome 3 translocations may be associated with dominantly inherited predisposition to clear cell RCC. Individuals with balanced chromosome 3 translocations not ascertained through a personal or family history of RCC are not at significant risk to require surveillance.

Recently germline mutations in BAP1 were reported to predispose to RCC. Though young-onset RCC has occasionally been reported in TSC (see 'Tuberous sclerosis (TSC)' in Chapter 3, 'Common consultations', p. 534), angiomyolipoma is by far the most common renal tumour in this disorder.

Clinical approach

History: key points

• Three-generation family tree, with specific reference to tumour types and features suggestive of a specific syndromic cause (see Table 4.23).

Table 4.23 Types of renal cell carcinoma with their syndromic associations

Histology	Clear cell	Papillary	Variable histopathology
Frequency in sporadic cases	70–80%	10–15% Type 1 and type 2 (more aggressive)	
Hereditary renal cancer syndrome(s)	(a) VHL (tumours tend to be early-onset and multifocal) (b) Constitutional chromosome 3 translocations	(a) Hereditary papillary renal cell carcinoma—type 1 (b) Hereditary leiomyomatosis renal cell carcinoma—type 2	BHD syndrome SDHB mutations BAP1 mutations
Gene	VHL (3p25-26)	(a) C-Met proto-oncogene (7q31-34) (b) Fumarate hydratase (1q42-43)	FLCN (17p11) SDHB BAP1
Renal surveillance strategy for hereditary cancer syndrome	Annual renal MRI or USS in VHL disease from age 16 years Monitor suspicious lesions more frequently and intervene for solid lesions ≥3 cm with nephron-sparing surgery	Annual renal MRI/USS from age ~20 years Annual renal MRI from age ~20 years (or earlier, depending on family history)	Annual renal MRI/USS from age ~20 years Imaging for RCC can be combined with surveillance for phaeochromocytoma/paraganglioma Annual renal MRI/USS from age ~20 years. Surveillance for other manifestations of BAP1-inherited cancer syndrome family history
Syndromic associations	CNS haemangioblastomas, phaeochromocytoma, retinal angiomas, renal, pancreatic, and epididymal cysts, pancreatic endocrine tumours, endolymphatic sac tumours No extrarenal manifestations	(a) No extrarenal manifestations (b) Leiomyomas of skin or uterus, uterine leiomyosarcomas	(a) Cutaneous fibrofolliculomas, lung cysts/pneumothorax, colorectal neoplasia (b) Phaeochromocytoma or paraganglioma or HNPGL (c) Mesothelioma, uveal melanoma, cutaneous melanoma

Examination: key points
- Cutaneous examination for fibrofolliculomas (BHD syndrome) or leiomyomas (HLRCC).

Special investigations
- DNA for mutation analysis if a specific syndrome identified. In non-syndromic cases, analysis of gene panels (e.g. *VHL, MET, FLCN, SDHB, FH, BAP1*) are available. Cytogenetic analysis for constitutional translocation (typically involving chromosome 3).

Genetic advice

Risk assessment
If a specific syndrome or germline mutation identified, offer screening to all first-degree family members.

Penetrance
See above.

Predictive testing
If a specific germline mutation is identified (and you are certain it is disease-causing), offer predictive testing to first-degree relatives in order to target subsequent surveillance.

Management

Surveillance strategies
Individuals at increased risk of RCC are offered annual renal imaging by MRI or USS. In general, small asymptomatic tumours detected on routine surveillance are kept under review and removed when they reach a diameter of 3 cm (e.g. in VHL disease, BHD syndrome). However, in HLRCC, aggressive tumours may not be detected by USS and so annual MRI is indicated (can be considered from age 10 years) and small tumours should be removed and not kept under surveillance.

Expert adviser: Eamonn R. Maher, Professor and Honorary Consultant, Department of Medical Genetics, University of Cambridge, Cambridge University Hospitals, Cambridge, UK.

References

Linehan WM, Pinto PA, Bratslavsky G, *et al*. Hereditary kidney cancer: unique opportunity for disease-based therapy. *Cancer* 2009; **115**: 2252–61.

Maher ER. Genetics of familial renal cancers. *Nephron Exp Nephrol* 2011; **118**: e21–6.

Menko FH, van Steensel MA, Giraud S, *et al*.; European BHD Consortium. Birt–Hogg–Dubé syndrome: diagnosis and management. *Lancet Oncol* 2009; **10**: 1199–206.

Rini BI, Campbell SC, Escudier B. Renal cell carcinoma [seminar]. *Lancet* 2009; **373**: 1119–32.

Woodward ER, Skytte AB, Cruger DG, Maher ER. Population-based survey of cancer risks in chromosome 3 translocation carriers. *Genes Chromosomes Cancer* 2010; **49**: 52–8.

Retinoblastoma

Retinoblastoma (RB) is an embryonic neoplasm of retinal origin caused by mutations in the tumour suppressor gene *RB1* on 13q14. RB affects ~1/20 000 live births and arises predominantly in children <7 years of age (90% of diagnoses are made at <5 years). It can rarely occur antenatally.

The predisposition to RB is inherited as an AD trait. Penetrance can vary. Most mutations are associated with a high (>90%) penetrance, but some mutations have a much lower penetrance. An RB develops according to Knudson's two-hit hypothesis (see Figure 4.4) when both *RB1* alleles are deleted or mutated.

In genetic RB, the first hit is most commonly a mutation (~90–95%) or a deletion (5–10%). The second event is most commonly LOH at syntenic loci over a large segment of 13q (~70%). Less frequently, there is a separate somatic mutation (~30%) or hypomethylation (a few per cent). There is a high new mutation rate in *RB1* and 85% of new germline mutations arise in the paternally derived allele.

The role of the geneticist is to:

(1) provide information to the family, GP, and other clinicians on the aetiology, recurrence risks for different family members, and second tumours;

(2) arrange genetic testing, if appropriate, on the affected child and convey results to the family, GP, and other medical teams;

(3) arrange genetic testing on the wider family, if appropriate, conveying results to the family and GP;

(5) arrange prenatal testing if requested by the family and convey the results to appropriate clinicians.

Terminology

Many of the terms used in the literature overlap and can be confusing.

• Unifocal: one tumour in one eye.
• Unilateral, often used synonymously with unifocal: one eye affected.
• Multifocal: many separate tumours in one eye.
• Bilateral: tumours in both eyes.
• Trilateral: bilateral RB plus a pineoblastoma. Pineoblastomas can, very rarely, develop without obvious tumours in the eyes.
• Genetic or hereditary RB is defined when there is a germline *RB1* mutation affecting all cells in the body and a single somatic hit to the *RB1* gene then initiates tumourigenesis. This will include all trilateral, bilateral, and multifocal RB. It will also include ~10% of unilateral/ unifocal RB.
• Non-genetic/non-hereditary RB occurs when the two hits to the *RB1* gene have occurred only in the tumour and are not present in other cells. This will include the majority of unilateral/unifocal RB.
• Sporadic is used in different contexts, meaning either that there is no family history of RB or being synonymous with non-genetic.

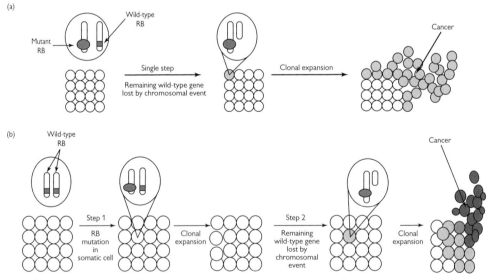

Figure 4.4 Knudson's hypothesis. (a) In individuals with an inherited predisposition to retinoblastoma, every somatic cell contains one intact *Rb* allele and one mutant *Rb* allele. A single somatic mutation is therefore sufficient for loss of *Rb* activity, with subsequent clonal expansion of the double mutant cell and tumour formation. (b) In normal individuals, both copies of *Rb* must be targeted by somatic mutation for *Rb* function to be disrupted. Since the somatic mutation rate is low, the risk of two *Rb* mutations occurring in the same cell is low. This explains the later onset and unifocal nature of retinoblastoma cases that occur in the absence of a family history. Reproduced from David A. Warrell, Timothy M. Cox, and John D. Firth, *Oxford Textbook of Medicine*, Fourth edition, 2003, Figure 1, page 230, with permission from Oxford University Press.

- Mosaicism can be found and can be associated with either unilateral or bilateral RB, depending on the nature of the mutation and the proportion of affected cells.

Second tumours

Survivors of RB who carry a germline mutation in *RB1* are at substantially increased risk for a variety of other tumours. These may include (Errico 2014; Wong 2014):
- osteosarcoma (RR, 200–500: 37% of second primaries), especially if treated with radiotherapy;
- other sarcomas, e.g. soft tissue sarcoma, fibrosarcomas, chondrosarcomas (14% of second primaries);
- malignant melanoma (7%);
- brain tumours (4.5%: excludes pineoblastoma, i.e. trilateral RB, which is not a second primary and occurs in 2.4%).

Widely varying estimates for the probability of a second non-ocular primary in patients with germline *RB1* mutations are found in the literature. Radiotherapy as part of RB treatment further increases the mortality from second tumours. Moll *et al.* (1997) estimate the cumulative incidence of second primary tumours to be 19% at the age of 35 years (RR, 15). The tumours most commonly develop in the second to fourth decades. Overall, the excess risk for a retinoblastoma-related tumour is of the order 6–10%.

Clinical approach

History: key points
- Three-generation (or more extensive) family tree, documenting RB and all other types of tumour.

Examination: key points
- Brief examination of the skin of older patients with hereditary RB, if appropriate.
- Parents of a child with RB should always be examined by an experienced ophthalmologist to look for a spontaneously regressed tumour.

Special investigations
- DNA sample for *RB1* mutation analysis. Mutation identifiable in >95% of families with bilateral or familial RB. For children with unilateral RB, mutation analysis will have a pickup rate of ~8–10% (the majority, but not all, of those with unilateral, but genetic RB).
- When a pathogenic variant is identified in RB1, consideration should be given to targeting deep sequencing of the proband and parental DNA to detect mosaicism, as this will help to inform recurrence risks (Dehainault *et al.* 2016). See 'Timing and origin of new dominant mutations' in Chapter 1, 'Introduction', p. 42.
- Karyotype with FISH for *RB1*. Approximately 3% have an interstitial deletion of 13q14 (many of the children with deletions do have associated dysmorphic features and/or developmental delay, but a significant proportion do not). Such deletions are not detected by conventional molecular genetic techniques and so karyotyping with FISH should be performed on all affected children.
- Linkage exclusion testing can be offered to all families where no mutation has been found in the affected child and siblings are undergoing screening by examination under anaesthesia (EUA) (see 'Predictive testing' below).
- Tumour mutation analysis. This should be preformed routinely on fresh tumour when an embolization is performed. If a mutation is found in tumour, but not in

blood, the mutation cannot have been inherited from a parent and other siblings do not need to be screened or tested. There is a possibility of low-level mosaicism in the affected child and that child's future offspring should be offered mutation analysis.

Genetic advice

Patients with hereditary RB (familial, bilateral, unilateral multifocal, or unilateral, or rarely trilateral or non-penetrant) can transmit the initial *RB1* mutation as an AD trait. Alternatively, the initial *RB1* mutation can arise in retinal cells or their embryonic precursors and not involve the germline. This is the genetic basis for non-hereditary RB (unilateral, unifocal). In 10% of families with hereditary RB, mosaicism for the initial mutation is found either in the proband or in one of the proband's parents. The possibility of mosaicism should always be considered during the genetic counselling of newly identified families with RB.

Empiric risk assessment
- Bilateral RB.
  - Siblings of an affected child (parent unaffected): 5%.
  - Offspring of an affected individual 50% of whom inherit mutation: 45% chance of developing RB (assuming 90% penetrance).
- Unilateral RB.
  - Siblings of an affected child (parents unaffected): 1%.
  - Offspring of an affected individual: 5%. This will include both unilateral and bilateral RB in an affected offspring.

Risk assessment incorporating results of genetic testing

(1) Sporadic bilateral RB or multifocal RB. The assumption is that these are germline *RB1* mutation carriers, with an RR to offspring of 45% (AD inheritance with 90% penetrance). In a few instances, these patients are, in fact, somatic or gonosomal mosaics with a lower offspring risk. In Sippel *et al.*'s (1998) study, all germline mosaics had an initial mutation that was detectable in blood, but there were insufficient data for this to be reliable.

(2) Unilateral simplex RB with *de novo RB1* mutation in blood. Even if the mutation appears *de novo*, i.e. is not detectable in either parent, the possibility of parental germline mosaicism exists and *RB1* testing should be offered to siblings. Offspring risk is 45%.

(3) Unilateral RB with no detectable *RB1* mutation in blood. Estimated risk for developing a tumour in the other eye is 3–5% (because of somatic mosaicism), so regular eye surveillance must be continued. Some risk of germline mosaicism exists, but offspring risk is likely to be small. Look for LOH and *RB1* mutations in tumour tissue. If two intragenic mutations are identified in tumour tissue, but neither is present in blood, a post-zygotic origin has to be assumed and sibs are not at risk.

(4) *RB1* mutation not detectable in a sporadic individual with bilateral or multifocal disease. Consider looking for LOH and *RB1* mutations in tumour tissue. Could be due to an undetectable mutation or mosaicism. NB. There is a significant offspring risk, but this may be <45%. Genetic testing cannot be offered to offspring, so they should undergo screening.

Penetrance and expressivity

For inactivating mutations, penetrance is estimated at 90%. Approximately 30% have a unilateral RB and the rest have bilateral RB. Individuals with partial LOF mutations in *RB1* have a lower penetrance and a higher incidence of unilateral disease. Mosaic individuals have reduced penetrance (60%) and expressivity.

FAMILIES SUGGESTIVE OF REDUCED PENETRANCE. A very rough way of calculating penetrance in a particular family is to calculate the percentage of eyes affected with RB divided by the number of eyes in obligate mutation carriers, e.g. if a grandparent had unilateral RB, a parent was unaffected, and a child had bilateral RB, there are three affected eyes in three people (i.e. six eyes altogether), so the penetrance in that family is 50%. NB. The grandfather may have been a germline mosaic.

Predictive testing

Where a mutation is identified, cascade testing of the family is indicated, starting with parents and siblings and including the extended family as indicated. Parents who do not carry an *RB* mutation present in their affected child should be given a low (not negligible) risk of recurrence, as germline mosaicism can theoretically occur.

Predictive testing of 'at-risk' neonates is appropriate because of the burden of frequent screening by EUA in the early years of life. Those defined as not at risk by mutation analysis or linkage can be excluded from screening.

Linkage analysis can be helpful in families where no mutation has been identified. Linkage exclusion testing can also be helpful for families with either bilateral or unilateral RB when no mutation has been identified. Comparing the RB genotypes in unaffected parents, affected children, and unaffected children gives a 1 in 4 chance of being able to exclude a sibling from screening.

Strategy for assessing risk to siblings and future pregnancies

(1) Screen for *RB1* mutations in the blood of an affected child. If a mutation is identified, parents can be tested to determine whether it is *de novo* or inherited and siblings can be tested.

(2) Linkage exclusion testing: see 'Predictive testing' below.

(3) Genetic analysis of tumour: linkage exclusion testing. If there is LOH, this is presumed to be the result of the 'second hit' and linkage analysis is possible based on the RB genotype, which defines those individuals 'at risk' and enables those not sharing the haplotype to be exempt from/discontinue screening. Offspring will have a low recurrence risk because of the possibility of mosaicism in the affected individual.

(4) Genetic analysis of tumour: mutation analysis. If it is possible to identify the mutations in the tumour tissue and these are not present in the affected child's blood, these define a *de novo* somatic change as the cause of the RB, with no increased risk to siblings who can then be exempt from/discontinue screening.

Prenatal diagnosis

PND by CVS is available in those families in which the *RB1* mutation is known or when a family is informative for linkage.

Management

Treatment

At present, systemic chemotherapy is the first-line treatment, followed by local treatments such as plaques or cryotherapy for accessible tumours or lens-sparing radiotherapy. Radiotherapy is very rarely used, because of the associated risk of second tumours. Proton beam therapy may be used. Enucleation is usually offered or chemotherapy delivered directly to the eye as a first-line treatment for a large unilateral tumour or if the disease is hard to control by other treatments.

Surveillance strategies

- Screening of children at risk of RB (i.e. sibling or child of an affected individual). Any child with an increased risk of RB (including siblings of a child with isolated unilateral RB in whom the risk is only 1%) should be offered EUAs from the age of 2–3 weeks until the age of 3 years. The examinations are offered at decreasing frequency and most children undergo 14 EUAs.
- Surveillance for second non-RB primaries. Increased level of awareness by the patient and GP (with accelerated referral if any concern) and regular skin check for malignant melanoma (can usually be done by patients or their partner, but if there is visual impairment, it could be done by the GP/dermatologist).

Support group: Childhood Eye Cancer Trust, https://chect.org.uk, Tel. 0207 377 5578, Fax. 0207 377 0740, Email: info@chect.org.uk.

Expert adviser: Elisabeth Rosser, Consultant in Clinical Genetics, Department of Clinical Genetics, Great Ormond St Hospital, London, UK.

References

Denainault C, Golmard L, et al. Mosaicism and prenatal diagnosis options: insights from retinoblastoma. *Eur J Hum Genet* 2016; epub Dec 21.

Eng C, Li FP, Abramson DH, et al. Mortality from second tumours among long-term survivors of retinoblastoma. *J Natl Cancer Inst* 1993; **85**: 1121–8.

Errico A. Retinoblastoma–chemotherapy increases the risk of secondary cancer. *Nat Rev Clin Oncol* 2014; **11**: 623.

Lohmann DR, Gerick M, Brandt B, et al. Constitutional *RB1*-gene mutations in patients with isolated unilateral retinoblastoma. *Am J Hum Genet* 1997; **61**: 282–94.

Mohney BG, Robertson DM, Schomberg PJ, Hodge DO. Second nonocular tumors in survivors of heritable retinoblastoma and prior radiation therapy. *Am J Ophthalmol* 1988; **126**: 269–77.

Moll AC, Inhof SM, Bouter LM, Tan KE. Second primary tumors in patients with retinoblastoma. A review of the literature. *Ophthalmic Genet* 1997; **18**: 27–34.

Sippel KC, Fraioli RE, Smith GD, et al. Frequency of somatic and germ-line mosaicism in retinoblastoma: implications for genetic counseling. *Am J Hum Genet* 1998; **62**: 610–19.

Vogel F. Genetics of retinoblastoma. *Hum Genet* 1979; **52**: 1–54.

Warrell DA, Cox TM, Firth JD, Benz EJ Jr (eds.). *Oxford textbook of medicine*, 4th edn. Oxford University Press, Oxford, 2003.

Wong JR, Morton LM, et al. Risk of malignant neoplasms in long-term hereditary retinoblastoma survivors after chemotherapy and radiotherapy. *J Clin Oncol* 2014; **32**: 3284–90.

von Hippel–Lindau (VHL) disease

VHL disease is an AD disorder characterized by a predisposition to a wide variety of tumours, most frequently haemangioblastomas of the cerebellum and spinal cord, retinal angiomas, renal cell carcinoma, phaeochromocytomas, and renal, pancreatic, and epididymal cysts. The gene for VHL on 3p25 encodes a tumour suppressor protein pVHL. pVHL is the recognition component of the E3–ubiquitin ligase complex involved in the degradation of hypoxia-inducible factor-1 (HIF) alpha subunits, a process regulated by oxygen availability and blocked by disease-causing p*VHL* mutations.

The most frequent initial manifestations of VHL are retinal angiomatosis, followed by cerebellar haemangioblastoma, RCC, and phaeochromocytoma (see Table 4.24). The probability of a patient with VHL developing a cerebellar haemangioblastoma, retinal angioma, or RCC by age 60 years is 84%, 70%, and 69%, respectively. The most frequent causes of death are RCC and CNS haemangioblastomas. Haemangioblastomas of the CNS are the most common tumour in VHL, affecting 60–80% of all patients. The average age of presentation for cerebellar haemangioblastomas is 33 years. These tumours are benign but are a major cause of morbidity. Tumours of the endolymphatic sac are rare neuroectodermal neoplasms in the petrous bone originating from inner ear structures, which occur at an increased frequency in VHL. They may present with hearing loss, tinnitus, and vertigo. Pancreatic neuroendocrine tumours may occur in ~10% of patients. Renal, pancreatic, and epididymal cysts are frequent but, apart from providing a clue to the diagnosis, do not cause significant morbidity.

Most germline *VHL* mutations are inactivating (frameshift, nonsense, and deletions of one or more exons). Approximately 30% are missense mutations. There is a strong association between specific missense mutations and susceptibility to phaeochromocytoma.

Clinically, VHL can be subdivided into type 1 (no phaeochromocytoma) and type 2 (phaeochromocytoma present). Most families with a VHL type 2 phenotype also show renal cancer (type 2B), but rare families do not (type 2A). Rare mutations can produce a predisposition to phaeochromocytoma without other manifestations of VHL (type 2C).

Table 4.24 Major complications of VHL and their frequency

Major complications of VHL	Frequency of clinical disease in cross-sectional studies
Retinal angioma	58% (may cause visual loss if not treated, e.g. with laser therapy)
Cerebellar haemangioblastoma	56% (multiple or recurrent in one-third of cases)
Spinal cord haemangioblastoma	14%
Renal cell carcinoma	25% (mean age at diagnosis, 44 years)
Phaeochromocytoma	17% (NB. wide interfamilial differences in frequency)

Clinical approach

History: key points
- Detailed three-generation family tree, with specific enquiry about renal tumours, brain tumours, and visual loss. Extend the family tree of affected individuals as far as possible.
- Detailed past medical history.
- Enquiry about current symptoms.

Examination: key points
- BP.
- If the diagnosis is suspected, careful neurological examination, especially for cerebellar signs.
- Fundoscopy.

Special investigations
If the diagnosis is suspected, arrange:
- DNA sample (EDTA) for *VHL* mutation screening;
- ophthalmology opinion with direct and indirect fundoscopy for retinal angioma;
- brain and abdominal MRI scans;
- 24-hour urine for VMA or blood for plasma metanephrines.

Genetic advice
Approximately 20% are due to new dominant mutations.

Risk assessment
AD, with 50% risk that offspring will inherit the disease-causing mutation. There is considerable variation within families carrying the same mutation.

Penetrance
Penetrance is age-dependent. Mean age at first diagnosis is ~25 years. The proportion of patients who have presented by age 30 years is 65%, by 40 years 85%, by 50 years 95%, and by 60 years 98%.

Predictive testing
Possible if the familial mutation is known. Usually considered prior to the commencement of regular surveillance (e.g. 2–5 years of age).

Prenatal diagnosis
Technically feasible by CVS at 11 weeks' gestation if the familial mutation is known, but not commonly requested.

Management
Surveillance strategies
- Annual BP from age 5 years.
- Annual direct and indirect ophthalmoscopy for detection of retinal angiomas from age 5 years (or when genetic testing performed). More frequent screening may be indicated if angiomas are present.
- Annual renal imaging (MRI or USS) from age 16 years. More frequent renal USS or follow-up MRI imaging may be indicated if there are abnormalities on the renal scan.
- Annual 24-hour urine collection for VMA or plasma metanephrines from 11 years.
- MRI brain scans every 3 years from age 15 years. Patients should be aware that, in many centres, CNS lesions are only removed if symptomatic.

Cerebellar haemangioblastoma

Approximately 30% of all cerebellar haemangioblastomas occur as part of VHL, and full clinical evaluation, combined with mutation screening, should be undertaken in all patients presenting with apparently sporadic cerebellar haemangioblastoma. The younger the patient at diagnosis, the more likely that the patient has VHL. Most haemangioblastomas of the craniospinal axis can be safely and completely excised by surgery. Haemangioblastomas in the CNS often grow at several sites simultaneously; new lesions can arise with time, and the growth pattern of these tumours can be unpredictable. Therefore, resection is deferred until the onset of symptoms to avoid unnecessary surgery (Lonser *et al.* 2003).

Solitary retinal angioma

Solitary retinal angiomas can occur sporadically or be associated with VHL disease. In addition to clinical evaluation, genetic testing should be considered to exclude VHL disease with a high level of certainty. Virtually all patients with multiple retinal angiomas have VHL.

Renal cysts and renal cell carcinoma

Renal cysts may be detected from the second decade; RCC has been detected as early as 16 years. RCC is often, but not invariably, associated with cysts. RCC may be multifocal and bilateral in VHL. Tumours are usually treated with limited partial nephrectomy when they reach 3 cm in diameter. Thereafter, ongoing surveillance is performed, because of the risk of further renal tumours, and this is repeated until a further tumour reaches 3 cm in diameter. This 'nephron-sparing' approach preserves renal function in most patients, but in some cases repeated partial nephrectomies may result in a requirement for renal replacement therapy.

Support group: VHL Alliance, http://www.vhl.org.

Expert adviser: Eamonn R. Maher, Professor and Honorary Consultant, Department of Medical Genetics, University of Cambridge, Cambridge University Hospitals, Cambridge, UK.

References

Decker J, Neuhaus C, Macdonald F, Brauch H, Maher ER. Clinical utility gene card for: von Hippel–Lindau (VHL). *Eur J Hum Genet* 2014; **22**(4). doi: 10.1038/ejhg.2013.180.

Kaelin WG Jr. New cancer targets emerging from studies of the Von Hippel–Lindau tumor suppressor protein. *Ann N Y Acad Sci* 2010; **1210**: 1–7.

Lonser RR, Glenn GM, Walther M, *et al.* von Hippel–Lindau disease. *Lancet* 2003; **361**: 2059–67.

Lonser RR, Kim HJ, Butman JA, Vortmeyer AO, Choo DI, Oldfield EH. Tumors of the endolymphatic sac in von Hippel–Lindau disease. *N Engl J Med* 2004; **350**: 2481–6.

Maher ER, Neumann HP, Richard S. von Hippel–Lindau disease: a clinical and scientific review. *Eur J Hum Genet* 2011; **19**: 617–23.

Maher ER, Yates JR, Harries R, *et al.* Clinical features and natural history of von Hippel–Lindau disease. *QJM* 1990; **283**: 1151–63.

Pugh CW, Ratcliffe PJ. The von Hippel–Lindau tumour suppressor, hypoxia-inducible factor-1 (HIF-1) degradation, and cancer pathogenesis. *Semin Cancer Biol* 2003; **13**: 83–9.

Singh AD, Ahmad NN, Shields CL, Shields JA. Solitary retinal capillary hemangioma. Lack of genetic evidence for von Hippel–Lindau disease. *Ophthalmic Genet* 2002; **23**: 21–7.

Wilms tumour

Nephroblastoma.

Wilms tumour is an embryonal tumour of the kidney, occurring in one in 10 000 children. Most cases present between the ages of 3 and 4 years with an abdominal mass. Ninety per cent present by age 7 years. More than 90% are unilateral. The pathology is complex and typically includes blastemal, stromal, and epithelial elements (triphasic). Stromal-predominant tumours are more common in *WT1* syndromes. Nephrogenic rests (NRs), which are considered to be the precursor cells for Wilms tumour, may be identifiable. A post-mortem study found that these cells are found in about one in 100 neonates against an incidence of Wilms tumour of one in 10 000 children. The position of NRs can differ in Wilms tumour syndromes, e.g. intralobar nephrogenic rests (ILNRs) are common in the *WT1* syndromes and perilobar nephrogenic rests (PLNRs) are common in Wilms tumours found in overgrowth conditions, trisomy 18, and trisomy 13.

Many genes and syndromes have been reported to be associated with Wilms tumour; however, <5% of children with Wilms tumour have a recognizable congenital malformation syndrome. Screening for Wilms tumour in conditions with increased risk has been advocated and is widely practised, although its efficacy is unproven. As the survival of Wilms tumour is so high (90% for localized Wilms tumour and 70% for metastatic disease), an important aim of screening is early detection, so that treatment reduction and consequent decreased treatment-induced morbidity is possible.

Clinical approach

History: key points

- Three-generation family tree.
- Specific enquiry regarding family history of cancer (familial Wilms tumour, LFS, HPT-JT syndrome).
- Pathology report for verification of diagnosis. NB. Stromal-predominant pathology, particularly with rhabdomyoblastic differentiation, is associated with *WT1* syndromes.
- Birth history. Birthweight increased in BWS, SGB syndrome, and Perlman syndrome; decreased in mosaic variegated aneuploidy (MVA), FA, Bloom syndrome, Mulibrey (muscle–liver–brain–eye) nanism (MUL). Neonatal hypoglycaemia (BWS). Feeding difficulties due to tongue enlargement (BWS).
- Renal impairment and glomerulosclerosis (*WT1* syndromes). Mesangial sclerosis (Denys–Drash syndrome (DDS)). Focal segmental sclerosis (Frasier syndrome).
- Genitourinary abnormalities (*WT1* syndromes), FA.
- Developmental delay (WAGR, MVA, Perlman, MUL).
- Dysmorphic features (Perlman, SGB, MVA, FA, Bloom).

Examination: key points

To exclude syndromic associations:

- Height, weight, OFC (increased in BWS, SGB, Perlman; decreased in MVA, FA, Bloom, MUL).
- Eyes. Aniridia (WAGR), cataracts (MVA).
- Hemihypertrophy (BWS, isolated hemihypertrophy (IHH)).
- Macroglossia (BWS).

- Abdominal examination for organ enlargement, umbilical hernia (BWS).
- Genitourinary abnormalities, e.g. cryptorchidism, hypospadias, genital ambiguity.
- Skeletal abnormalities (FA).
- Document any dysmorphic features.
- BP and urinalysis for proteinuria.
- Review imaging and operation notes for evidence of genitourinary malformation.

Special investigations

- Karyotype. XY phenotypic females (DDS), 11p abnormalities (11p13 *WT1*, 11p15 BWS), mosaic aneuploidies (MVA), premature centromere separation (MVA), chromosome breakage (FA, Bloom), trisomies (13, 18), del 2q37.
- FISH or MLPA with 11p13 probes, if aniridia present.
- *WT1* mutation screening (DDS, Frasier: consider in bilateral Wilms tumour cases with genitourinary abnormalities).
- Mutation screening if features of BWS (11p15 MS-MLPA), SGB (*GPC3*) FA-D1 (*BRCA2*), MVA (*BUB1B*), LFS (*TP53*), Bloom (*BLM*), HPT-JT (*HRPT2*), and MUL (*TRIM37*).
- Renal investigations may be indicated.

Syndromic diagnoses to consider

The WT1 syndromes

WAGR (WILMS TUMOUR–ANIRIDIA–GENITOURINARY ANOMALIES–MENTAL RETARDATION). A syndrome due to a microdeletion on 11p13. There is deletion of the Wilms tumour gene WT1, and the adjacent aniridia gene PAX6 on chromosome 11p13. Children have a >50% risk of Wilms tumour. The mean age of diagnosis of Wilms tumour is 29 months. Usually occurs *de novo*, but occasional familial cases reported. Renal failure occurs in ~40% by the age of 20.

DENYS–DRASH SYNDROME (DDS). Classic triad includes Wilms tumour, genitourinary abnormalities that can be severe in males leading to pseudohermaphroditism, and renal impairment that presents with hypertension and proteinuria leading to progressive renal failure. Kidneys show mesangial sclerosis. Caused by constitutional *WT1* mutations, particularly (but not exclusively) missense mutations in the DNA-binding zinc fingers encoded by exons 7–10. The median age at diagnosis of Wilms tumour is 16 months. Usually occurs *de novo*, but non-penetrance in carrier parents has been reported.

FRASIER SYNDROME. Typical features are renal impairment with focal segmental glomerulosclerosis and gonadoblastoma. Wilms tumour less common than in other *WT1*-related disorders. Caused by constitutional *WT1* mutations in intron 9 that alter the ratio of *WT1* splicing isoforms.

NON-SYNDROMIC WILMS TUMOUR. WT1 mutations have been reported in a number of individuals with only one or two of the cardinal features of *WT1*, e.g. with Wilms tumour and undescended testes. *WT1* mutations are identifiable in ~2% of non-syndromic Wilms tumour patients. Bilateral tumours, genitourinary abnormalities, such as undescended testes, and stromal-predominant histology are all associated with an increased risk of *WT1* mutation. There are no current recommendations that any non-syndromic Wilms tumour cases should have *WT1* mutation screening.

FAMILIAL WILMS TUMOUR. Only a very small proportion of Wilms tumour families are due to *WT1* mutations, two out of 39 in a UK series. Genitourinary abnormalities in males are usually present.

NON-SYNDROMIC NEPHROPATHY. Some children with kidney impairment and either mesangial sclerosis or focal segmental glomerulosclerosis, but without the other features of DDS or Frasier syndrome, have been found to carry constitutional *WT1* mutations.

Other syndromes

FAMILIAL WILMS TUMOUR. One to 3% of Wilms tumour cases cluster in families. The majority are AD with reduced and variable penetrance. Genitourinary abnormalities suggest WT1. Loci on 17q21 (FWT1) and 19q13 (FWT2) have been mapped, but genes not yet identified. Some families are unlinked to all known loci, indicating further heterogeneity. Age of onset, bilateral disease, metastatic disease, and/or specific pathology can cluster in some families, but there is extensive intra- and inter-familial variability.

BECKWITH–WIEDEMANN SYNDROME (BWS). Macrosomia, anterior abdominal wall defects, macroglossia, anterior earlobe creases, and posterior helical pits. Caused by dysregulation of imprinted genes on 11p15. Overall risk of Wilms tumour is ~7%, with median age of diagnosis of ~3 years. There is also an increased risk of other embryonal tumours such as hepatoblastoma. The risk of Wilms tumours differs according to the underlying molecular cause and Wilms tumour has not been reported in those with the most common molecular group (KvDMR hypomethylation), who therefore do not need Wilms surveillance. Other groups, including those with no identifiable 11p15 defect, should undergo surveillance. See 'Beckwith–Wiedemann syndrome (BWS)' in Chapter 3, 'Common consultations', p. 358.

SIMPSON–GOLABI–BEHMEL SYNDROME (SGB). XLR disorder due to mutations and deletion in *glypican 3* (Xq26). High birthweight, heavy facies, supernumerary nipples, cryptorchidism, mild/moderate learning disability. See 'Overgrowth' in Chapter 2, 'Clinical approach', p. 272. Risk of Wilms tumour has been estimated at 9%. Rarely, other embryonal tumours have been reported.

ISOLATED HEMIHYPERTROPHY (IHH). Poor clinical definition and true tumour risk uncertain. In Hoyme *et al.*'s (1998) study, tumours developed in 9/168 patients (5.9%), including 3% with Wilms tumour. The risk of Wilms tumour is likely to be >5% in those with high-risk 11p15 defects and Wilms surveillance is recommended in these patients. Wilms surveillance is not currently recommended for those with no identifiable 11p15 defect.

PERLMAN SYNDROME. An AR condition due to mutations in *DIS3L2*, with macrosomia and a high incidence of Wilms tumour (25–50%). Distinctive facial features and high neonatal mortality; learning disability is common.

FANCONI ANAEMIA SUBTYPES D1 AND N (FA-D1 AND FA-N). AR conditions characterized by skeletal abnormalities, short stature, dysmorphic facies, hypersensitivity to DNA cross-linking agents, and haematological malignancies. Eleven subtypes are known. Only subtypes D1 (which is due to biallelic *BRCA2* mutations) and N (due

to biallelic *PALB2* mutations) have an increased risk of Wilms tumour.

MOSAIC VARIEGATED ANEUPLOIDY (MVA). An AR condition due to mutations in *BUB1B*. Characterized by microcephaly, developmental delay, growth retardation, and cataracts. Karyotype shows multiple mosaic monosomies and trisomies, sometimes with premature chromatid separation (PCS). Some cases show only PCS. High incidence of cancer, particularly Wilms tumour.

LI–FRAUMENI SYNDROME (LFS). An AD cancer syndrome due to mutations in *TP53* (17p13), characterized by brain tumours, sarcomas, adrenocortical carcinoma, leukaemia, and young-onset breast cancer. Although at least six *TP53* mutation-positive families have been reported with Wilms tumour, it is not one of the cardinal Li–Fraumeni tumours and the absolute risk of Wilms tumour is low.

TRISOMY 18/TRISOMY 13. Trisomy 18 and trisomy 13 survivors are at increased risk of both Wilms tumour and hepatoblastoma. No increased risk of embryonal tumours in trisomy 21.

CHROMOSOME 2Q37 DELETION. Wilms tumour has been reported in at least three individuals with 2q37 deletion. In all, the centromeric breakpoint was proximal to 2q37.1, rather than the more frequently observed breakpoint of 2q37.3. The overall risk of Wilms tumour has been estimated as <3% in 2q37 deletion. The risk may be primarily in those with deletions extending to 2q37.1.

HYPERPARATHYROIDISM–JAW TUMOUR (HPT-JT) SYNDROME. An AD condition due to mutations in *HRPT2* (1q24), characterized by hyperparathyroidism due to parathyroid tumours, ossifying fibromas of the mandible and maxilla, and renal lesions such as cysts, hamartomas, or Wilms tumour. The risk of Wilms tumour is estimated as <3%.

BLOOM SYNDROME. An AR condition due to mutations in *BLM* (15q26). Characterized by growth retardation, dysmorphic facies, sunlight-sensitive rash, especially on the face, immune deficiency, and malignancies in 20%, including Wilms tumour (<5%). Elevated frequency of chromosomal breaks with increased sister chromatid exchange.

MULIBREY NANISM (MUL). An AR condition, enriched in Finland, caused by mutations in *TRIM37* (17q22). Characterized by prenatal growth failure, constrictive pericarditis, dysmorphic features, and hypoplasia of various endocrine glands causing hormonal deficiency. Less than 3% of MUL patients develop Wilms tumour.

Genetic advice

Recurrence risk

As appropriate for the specific disorder.

For a family with an isolated unilateral Wilms tumour case, the recurrence risk is very low, and screening for siblings is not recommended. Recurrence risk in families with non-syndromic bilateral cases without additional features or family history is also very low, and no screening is recommended in relatives. Offspring risk for individuals with Wilms tumour, particularly bilateral cases, is less clear, as it is only in recent generations that appreciable number of survivors are having children, but currently appears to be <5%. No current recommendations for screening of offspring.

Carrier detection

As for the specific disorder.

Prenatal diagnosis
Only possible in families with a known mutation.

Natural history and further management (preventative measures)

For *WT1* syndromes, long-term monitoring of renal function with annual BP and urinalysis recommended for those without nephropathy, as they may develop renal impairment in adulthood.

Surveillance for Wilms tumour in at-risk individuals
Due to the rarity of Wilms tumour cases occurring in at-risk individuals, it has not been possible to perform randomized studies to evaluate surveillance strategies. In the USA, recommendations based on retrospective studies of BWS and WAGR are for USS screening every 3–4 months until 7–8 years, for individuals deemed to be at increased risk. In the UK, children at >5% risk of Wilms tumour should be offered screening (*WT1* syndromes, familial Wilms tumour, BWS, SGB, Perlman, MVA, FA-D1, FA-N, and patients with IHH who have high-risk 11p15 defects). Screening should be 3- to 4-monthly until 5 years in all conditions, except BWS, SGB, and some familial Wilms tumour pedigrees where it should continue until 7 years.

Support groups: Many of the individual syndromes have their own support group. See Contact a Family, http://www.cafamily.org.uk; Beckwith–Wiedemann Syndrome Support Group (UK), http://bws-support.org.uk.

Expert adviser: Richard Scott, Consultant in Clinical Genetics, Great Ormond Street Hospital NHS Foundation Trust, London, UK.

References

Children's Cancer and Leukaemia Group. http://www.cclg.org.uk.

Hoyme HE, Seaver LH, Jones KL, et al. Isolated hemihyperplasia (hemihypertrophy): report of a prospective multicenter study of the incidence of neoplasia and review. *Am J Med Genet* 1998; **79**: 274–8.

National Wilms Tumor Study. http://www.nwtsg.org.

Pritchard-Jones K. Controversies and advances in the management of Wilms tumour. *Arch Dis Child* 2002; **87**: 241–4.

Scott RH, Stiller CA, Walker L, Rahman N. Syndromes and constitutional chromosomal abnormalities associated with Wilms tumour. *J Med Genet* 2006; **43**: 705–15.

Scott RH, Walker L, Olsen OE, et al. Surveillance for Wilms tumour in at-risk children: pragmatic recommendations for best practice. *Arch Dis Child* 2006; **91**: 995–9.

Chromosomes

Chapter contents

22q11 deletion syndrome

Includes di George syndrome (DGS), Shprintzen or velo-cardiofacial syndrome (VCFS), conotruncal anomaly face syndrome; MIM (Mendelian Inheritance in Man database) no. 188400.

Hemizygous deletion of chromosome 22q11 (del 22q11.2) may cause any combination of the following: cardiac defects; thymic hypoplasia; velopharyngeal insufficiency with cleft palate; parathyroid dysfunction with hypocalcaemia; and a distinctive facial appearance. Microdeletions of 22q11.2 usually encompass ~3 Mb of genomic DNA and are detectable by array CGH or specific FISH analysis. There are several low-copy repeats (LCRs) on chromosome 22 (LCR22). Misalignment between blocks of LCR22s is likely to facilitate the deletion. Most VCFS/DGS patients have a 3-Mb deletion; some have a nested distal deletion breakpoint, resulting in a 1.5-Mb deletion, and a few rare patients have unique deletions, translocations, or point mutations of *TBX1* (Yagi et al. 2003). Overall, ~96% of patients have a defined 1.5–3 Mb deletion including 24–30 genes.

The phenotype (heart outflow tract, velopharyngeal, ear, thymic, and parathyroid abnormalities) arises from a failure to form derivatives of the third and fourth branchial arches during development. Haploinsufficiency of *TBX1* is the major contributor to the phenotype seen with del 22q11 (Yagi et al. 2003). Rare patients with a *TBX1* mutation appear to have a full pharyngeal phenotype, but without the mild learning difficulties often seen in the full del 22q11. The diagnosis should be considered in any child with CHD, cleft palate, or palatal insufficiency. In ~85%, the deletion is *de novo*, with 15% being inherited from a parent.

The diagnosis of del 22q11 may be made antenatally during investigation of a pregnancy in which CHD or a structural renal anomaly (e.g. renal agenesis or multicystic dysplastic kidney) has been identified or when array CGH analysis has been used to investigate other prenatal abnormalities.

Clinical features

There is marked intrafamilial variability in expression. For example, a parent may have a cleft palate and CHD, and a child may have developmental delay, but a normal heart and palate. Common symptoms in childhood include leg pain of unknown cause and constipation.

Growth

Growth retardation is common; 83% have heights/weights <50th centile and 36% are <3rd centile for either height or weight.

Development

Reduced IQ scores, compared with other members of the family, are usual. Severe MR is only found in a small percentage of children with del 22q11. Children with del 22q11 will often require special educational support, especially when these cognitive problems exist in combination with communication difficulties (see 'Communication' below).

Normal development in one-third, mild learning problems in one-third, and moderate learning problems in one-third.

Communication

In excess of 90% have some communication difficulties. These are multifactorial with hypernasality and mild cognitive and language delay, all being important factors contributing to speech delay. Early speech milestones are typically delayed by several months, but use of phrases and sentences may be delayed until 3 years of age or so. Between 3 and 4 years of age, there is often a rapid acceleration in language development.

Behavioural, psychological, and psychiatric problems

These are common, affecting ~93%. Patients often have difficulties in establishing and maintaining friendships. Individuals carrying the 22q11.2 microdeletion are at risk for diverse psychiatric diagnoses across the lifespan, including schizophrenia in a significant minority and anxiety or mood disorders in the majority (Baker and Vortsman 2012). Psychiatric disorders (including bipolar affective disorder and schizophrenia) are described in up to 18% of adults (overall, 6.5% of adults with 22q11 had experienced at least one episode of psychosis). 22q11 deletions account for <2% of individuals with schizophrenia in the general population.

Cardiovascular anomalies

- Fifty to 85% have significant CHD.
- Nearly 20% have tetralogy of Fallot.
- VSD and an interrupted aortic arch are the next most common defects.
- A wide variety of cardiac anomalies have been described, including ASD, truncus arteriosus, right-sided aorta, pulmonary stenosis, aortic valve anomalies, aberrant subclavian arteries, vascular ring, anomalous origin of the carotid artery, TGA, and tricuspid atresia. (Approximately 5% of infants with CHD have del 22q11, depending on the study.)
- Anomalies of the internal carotid arteries and other major neck arteries are frequent.

Otolaryngeal anomalies

- Cleft palate in 9% (± velopharyngeal insufficiency).
- Submucous cleft palate in 5%.
- Velopharyngeal insufficiency in 32%.
- 75% have chronic serous otitis media. Sensorineural hearing loss, often unilateral and mild/moderate, may occur in up to 15%.

Genitourinary anomalies

- Thirty-six per cent have structural renal tract anomalies, including renal agenesis and multicystic dysplastic kidneys, hydronephrosis, and VUR.
- Among male patients, Wu et al. (2002) found a slightly increased incidence of undescended testes (6%) and hypospadias (8%).

Endocrine function

- Thirty to 60% are hypocalcaemic at some time, mostly in the neonatal period, and some have neonatal seizures secondary to hypocalcaemia that cease with calcium supplementation. A few patients have latent or late-onset hypocalcaemia. Taylor et al. (2003) and Greenhalgh et al. (2003) found hypocalcaemia in ~30% and ~42% of children, respectively, outside the neonatal period.

- Shugar *et al.* (2015) conducted a retrospective study of 169 patients (92 males and 77 females) attending a multidisciplinary 22q11 deletion syndrome clinic and found 1.8% had hyperthyroidism and 7.7% had hypothyroidism; 42% of patients with subclinical or prodromal thyroid disease progressed to overt disease.

Immune and haematological status
- Patients with del 22q11 have a variable defect in cell-mediated immunity. Most patients will recover normal or near normal T-cell numbers and function by age 2 years; however, a small group experiences persistent and profound T-cell dysfunction (DGS). There are preliminary data that T-cell number and function may occasionally drop again in adolescence.
- Only 1% have a major abnormality of immune function (Ryan *et al.* 1997).
- Many had a history of recurrent minor infections in the first 2 years of life, which then resolved (Ryan *et al.* 1997).
- Mild thrombocytopenia is common. Idiopathic thrombocytopenic purpura (ITP) is also associated (Levy *et al.* 1997) and idiopathic thrombocytopenia with autoimmune haemolytic anaemia has also been reported. Lawrence *et al.* (2003) found that, even after the exclusion of patients with ITP, the mean platelet count was ~70% of the control population.
- Autoimmune disorders appear to be more common in children with 22q11 deletions than in the general population (Perez and Sullivan 2002). Haemolytic anaemia, T1D, and hypothyroidism/Graves disease have all been reported.

Craniofacial
- Subtle dysmorphic features (see below).
- Approximately 1% have craniosynostosis.

Rare features
- The phenotypic variability observed in a small subset of patients with 22q11DS occurs due to mutations on the non-deleted chromosome which leads to unmasking of AR conditions such as CEDNIK (cerebral dysgenesis (ACC and cortical dysplasia, pachygyria, and PMG), neuropathy, ichthyosis, and keratoderma) caused by mutation in *SNAP29*. Similarly, Kousseff syndrome (sacral myelomeningocele, tetralogy of Fallot, ACC, and microcephaly) and the AR form of Opitz/GBBB syndrome may occur by a similar mechanism. (McDonald-McGinn *et al.* 2013).

Clinical approach

History: key points
- Neonatal problems. Feeding problems (e.g. mild regurgitation through the nose), seizures.
- CHD. Management, e.g. previous surgery.
- Developmental progress, particularly speech.
- History of infections.
- Family history of CHD, cleft palate, psychosis.

Examination: key points
- Growth parameters. Height, weight, OFC.
- Face. Short palpebral fissures with telecanthus, a wide and prominent nasal bridge and root, a small mouth. Ears are round in shape with deficient upper helices.
- Heart. Careful clinical examination.

- Palate. Can the child speak clearly or is his/her speech nasal in quality? Is there a cleft uvula or submucous cleft palate?

Special investigations
Max Appeal, a UK support group, have coordinated a multidisciplinary approach to management at different ages and Table 5.1 is a handy summary to check all surveillance is in place.
- Echocardiogram (unless previously done).
- Renal USS.
- Audiometry. Children with 22q deletion have a high incidence of communication problems. These are multifactorial, but glue ear is a common and treatable cause. Those with sensorineural loss may benefit from hearing aids.
- Plasma calcium. Check at least once during infancy, childhood, adolescence, and pregnancy. It may be a sensible precaution to check plasma calcium on any hospital admission, particularly those for cardiac or palate surgery, or alongside other blood tests whenever these are being performed. Greenhalgh *et al.* (2003) found hypocalcaemia in 42% of school-age children with 22q11.
- Immunology. FBC with platelets and T, B, and NK (natural killer) lymphocyte subsets (if abnormal, discuss management with an immunologist).
- In children older than 4 months, serum immunoglobulins and tetanus, diphtheria, and Hib (*Haemophilus influenzae* type b) antibody titres (if abnormal, discuss management with an immunologist).
- Consider referral to speech therapy and/or to the cleft team for palatal assessment.
- Parental analysis. Using either FISH for 22q11.2, qPCR, or array CGH in both parents.

Pregnancy/neonatal diagnosis
If the diagnosis is made prenatally, fetal echo should be arranged (if not already performed) and plans should be made to anticipate possible problems in the neonatal period arising from:
- CHD (arrange echo in the neonatal period);
- hypocalcaemia—check plasma calcium on day 1;
- feeding problems related to palatal abnormalities, e.g. nasal regurgitation, weak and slow sucking (examine for submucous cleft).

Consider prophylaxis with co-trimoxazole, pending results of immune function (discuss with an immunologist).
In Ryan *et al.*'s (1997) series, 8% of patients died, most within 6 months of birth; all but one death was the result of severe CHD.

Immunizations
No live vaccines should be given (i.e. oral polio, BCG) until immune function has been checked. Then the following should be done.
- MMR (measles, mumps, rubella) vaccine. On a pragmatic basis, offer at 18 months of age to those who have 75% of normal T-cell count and who have responded normally to tetanus and Hib vaccines.
- Use the inactivated polio vaccine, instead of the oral one (since September 2004, the infant immunization schedule (tetanus, diphtheria, polio, Hib, and meningococcus C) in the UK includes no live vaccines, and UK babies with del 22q11 should receive their infant immunizations as usual).

Table 5.1 Recommended assessments

Assessment	At diagnosis	Infancy (0–12 months)	Preschool (1–5 years)	School age (6–11 years)	Adolescence (12–18 years)	Adult (>18 years)
Ionized calcium, PTH[1]	●	●	●	●	●	●
TSH (annual)	●		●	●	●	●
FBC and differential (annual)	●	●	●	●	●	●
Immunologic evaluation[2]	●		●[3]			
Ophthalmology	●		●			
Evaluate palate[4]	●	●	●			
Audiology	●	●	●			●
Cervical spine (>age 4)			●[5]			
Scoliosis exam	●		●		●	
Dental evaluation			●	●	●	●
Renal ultrasound	●					
ECG	●					●
Echocardiogram	●					
Development[6]	●	●	●			
School performance				●	●	
Socialization/functioning	●	●	●	●		●
Psychiatric/emotional/behavioural[7]	●		●	●	●	●
Systems review	●	●	●	●	●	●
Deletion studies of parents	●					
Genetic counselling[8]	●				●	●

[1] In infancy, test calcium levels every 3–6 months, every 5 years through childhood, and every 1–2 years thereafter; thyroid studies annually. Check calcium pre- and post-operatively, and regularly in pregnancy.

[2] In addition to FBC with differential: in the newborn—flow cytometry; and age 9–12 months (prior to live vaccines)—flow cytometry, immunoglobulins, T-cell function.

[3] Evaluate immune function prior to administering live vaccines (see above).

[4] In infancy: visualize the palate and evaluate for feeding problems and nasal regurgitation; in toddlers to adult: evaluate nasal speech quality.

[5] Cervical spine films to detect anomalies: anterior/posterior, lateral, extension, open mouth, and skull base views. Expert opinion is divided about the advisability of routine X-rays. Symptoms of cord compression are an indication for urgent neurological referral.

[6] Motor and speech/language delays are common; rapid referral to early intervention for any delays can help to optimize outcomes.

[7] Vigilance for changes in behaviour, emotional state, and thinking, including hallucinations and delusions; in teens and adults, assessment would include at-risk behaviours (sexual activity, alcohol/drug use, etc.).

[8] See text for details.

Reproduced with kind permission of Max Appeal. Taken from Consensus Document on 22q11 Deletion Syndrome. http://www.maxappeal.org.uk/downloads/Consensus_Document_on_22q11_Deletion_Syndrome.pdf.

- Varicella immunization (as for MMR).
- BCG vaccine should not be given until a risk assessment is carried out that establishes that potential benefit outweighs risk.

Transfusions

Any transfusion products should be CMV-negative and irradiated for children <6 months of age or if there is T-lymphopenia, e.g. CD4 count <500.

Genetic counselling

About 85% of del 22q111.2 arises *de novo*. If either parent is found to carry the 22q deletion, the recurrence risk is 50% for future pregnancies. The affected child will have a 50% risk of transmitting the deletion to his/her offspring in any pregnancy.

If neither parent carries the 22q deletion, the recurrence risk is very small (~1%), but note that there are two reported cases of sibling recurrence presumed due to gonadal mosaicism.

Prenatal diagnosis

Possible by targeted FISH, MLPA, or genomic array after CVS or amniocentesis and potentially by NIPT. Some parents may elect for detailed fetal echo in addition to, or as an alternative to, an invasive procedure (75% of patients with 22q11 will have a cardiac defect, some of which will be detectable by fetal echo).

Support groups: Max Appeal, http://www.maxappeal.org.uk; The 22Crew, http://www.22crew.org; The International 22q11.2 Foundation Inc., http://www.22q.org.

Expert adviser: Judith Goodship, formerly Professor of Medical Genetics, Institute of Human Genetics, Newcastle upon Tyne, UK.

References

Baker K, Vorstman JA. *Is there a core neuropsychiatric phenotype in 22q11.2 deletion syndrome?* Department of Medical Genetics, University of Cambridge, Cambridge, 2012.

Bassett AS, McDonald-McGinn DM, Devriendt K, et al.; International 22q11.2 Deletion Syndrome Consortium. Practical guidelines for managing patients with 22q11.2 deletion syndrome. *J Pediatr* 2011; **159**: 332–9.e1.

Driscoll D, Salvin J, Sellinger B, et al. Prevalence of 22q11 microdeletions in DiGeorge and velocardiofacial syndromes: implications for genetic counselling and prenatal diagnosis. *J Med Genet* 1993; **30**: 813–17.

Dyce O, McDonald-McGinn D, Kirschner RE, Zackai E, Young K, Jacobs IN. Otolaryngologic manifestations of the 22q11.2 deletion syndrome. *Arch Otolaryngol Head Neck Surg* 2002; **128**: 1408–12.

Garabedian M. Hypocalcaemia and chromosome 22q11 microdeletion. *Genet Couns* 1999; **10**: 389–94.

Goodman FR. Congenital abnormalities of body patterning: embryology revisited. *Lancet* 2003; **362**: 651–62.

Greenhalgh KL, Aligianis IA, Bromilow G, et al. 22q11 deletion: a multisystem disorder requiring multidisciplinary input. *Arch Dis Child* 2003; **88**: 523–4.

Hatchwell E, Long F, Wilde J, Crolla J, Temple K. Molecular confirmation of germ line mosaicism for a submicroscopic deletion of chromosome 22q11. *Am J Med Genet* 1998; **78**: 103–6.

Kobrynski LJ, Sullivan KE. Velocardiofacial syndrome, DiGeorge syndrome: the chromosome 22q11.2 deletion syndromes. *Lancet* 2007; **370**: 1443–52.

Lawrence S, McDonald-McGinn DM, Zackai E, Sullivan KE. Thrombocytopenia in patients with chromosome 22q11.2 deletion syndrome. *J Pediatr* 2003; **143**: 277–8.

Levy A, Michel G, Lemerrer M, Philip N. Idiopathic thrombocytopenic purpura in two mothers of children with DiGeorge sequence: a new component manifestation of deletion 22q11? *Am J Med Genet* 1997; **69**: 356–9.

McDermid HE, Morrow BE. Genomic disorders on 22q11. *Am J Hum Genet* 2002; **70**: 1077–88.

McDonald-McGinn DM, Emanuel BS, Zackai EH. 22q11.2 deletion syndrome. In: Pagon RA, Adam MP, Ardinger HH, et al. *Gene Reviews*®. University of Washington, Seattle, 2013. https://www.ncbi.nlm.nih.gov/books/NBK1523.

McDonald-McGinn DM, Fahiminiya S, Revil T, et al. Hemizygous mutations in *SNAP29* unmask recessive conditions and contribute to atypical findings in patients with 22q11DS. *J Med Genet* 2013; **50**: 80–90.

Perez EE, Bokszczanin A, McDonald-McGinn D, Zackai EH, Sullivan KE. Safety of live viral vaccines in patients with chromosome 22q11.2 deletion syndrome (DiGeorge syndrome/velocardiofacial syndrome). *Pediatrics* 2003; **112**: e325.

Perez E, Sullivan KE. Chromosome 22q11.2 deletion syndrome (DiGeorge and velocardiofacial syndromes). *Curr Opin Pediatr* 2002; **14**: 678–83.

Ryan AK, Goodship JA, Wilson DI, et al. Spectrum of clinical features associated with interstitial chromosome 22q11 deletions: a European collaborative study. *J Med Genet* 1997; **34**: 798–804.

Sandrin-Garcia P, Macedo C, Martelli LR, et al. Recurrent 22q11.2 deletion in a sibship suggestive of parental germline mosaicism in velocardiofacial syndrome. *Clin Genet* 2002; **61**: 380–3.

Shugar AL, Shapiro JM, Cytrynbaum C, Hedges S, Weksberg R, Fishman L. An increased prevalence of thyroid disease in children with 22q11.2 deletion syndrome. *Am J Med Genet A* 2015; **167**: 1560–4.

Taylor SC, Morris G, Wilson D, Davies SJ, Gregory JW. Hypoparathyroidism and 22q11 deletion syndrome. *Arch Dis Child* 2003; **88**: 520–2.

Tobias ES, Morrison N, Whiteford ML, Tolmie JL. Towards earlier diagnosis of 22q11 deletion. *Arch Dis Child* 1999; **8**: 513–14.

Wu HY, Rusnack SL, Bellah RD, et al. Genitourinary malformations in chromosome 22q11.2 deletion. *J Urol* 2002; **168**: 2564–5.

Yagi H, Furutani Y, Hamada H, et al. Role of TBX1 in human del 22q11.2 syndrome. *Lancet* 2003; **362**: 1366–73.

47,XXX

Trisomy X syndrome, triple XXX.

47,XXX may be diagnosed incidentally at amniocentesis/CVS. It occasionally comes to light later in life, but usually as an incidental finding. Mosaic karyotypes with combinations of 47,XXX/46,XX/45,X, due to postzygotic non-disjunction, may be found.

The incidence is 1/1000 to 1/1200 female births. There is a significant maternal age effect, with 47,XXX being more common with advanced maternal age, increasing from 1/2500 live births at maternal age of 33 years to 1/450 at 43 years (Hook 1992). It is substantially under-ascertained and the majority of 47,XXX women are unaware of their karyotype.

Clinical features

Physical

A normal female appearance is usual. Tall stature is a consistent finding (>80th percentile). The mean OFC is 10th centile. The frequency of structural urogenital anomalies may be slightly increased.

Puberty

Sexual development and puberty are normal.

Educational

Full-scale IQ averages 10–15 points less than that of siblings. As for 46,XX girls, there is wide variation in ability and attainment, but, of all the sex chromosome trisomies, 47,XXX has shown the highest rate of special educational need. The findings of Bishop et al. (2011) of a cohort of 58 girls, shown in Table 5.2, also confirm a high rate of referral for speech and language therapy (SALT).

Behavioural

There is no increased risk for autism (Bishop et al. 2011), though there is an increased risk for ADHD/hyperactivity, with the highest risk of 50% in a parent report survey by Tartaglia et al. (2012). An American survey of 11 XXX women showed that, during adolescence and young adult life, they were less well-adapted and experienced more stress, work, and relationship problems than their XX siblings. However, overall they were mostly self-sufficient and functioning reasonably well. Sexual orientation is normal.

Fertility

Most 47,XXX women are fertile and have chromosomally normal babies. There may be a slightly increased risk for POF.

Adult life

There may be a modest increase in risk for cardiovascular disease (Swerdlow et al. 2001).

Clinical approach

History: key points (postnatal presentation)

- Developmental milestones, speech and language development, schooling.

Examination: key points (postnatal presentation)

- Height.

Management

- Advise parents that if their daughter shows developmental, behavioural, or educational difficulties, they should have a low threshold for asking for professional help, as early intervention can improve outcome.

Table 5.2 N (%) girls receiving special schooling, registered with special educational needs (SEN), with speech and language therapy (SALT) or a given diagnosis

	Group I		Group II		Siblings	National data**
	XXX	OR	XXX	OR	Sisters	Girls
N	30		28		26	3 992 857
Special schooling	3 (12%)	2.78 (0.3–28.5)	3 (12%)	3.00 (0.3–30.8)	1 (4%)	
SEN	5 (14%)	3.80 (1.5–10.0)	14 (50%)	19.10 (9.1–40.0)	0 (0%)	199 150 (5%)
SALT	7 (24%)	7.61 (0.9–66.7)	17 (61%)	38.64 (4.6–327.7)	1 (4%)	
ASD*	0 (0%)	–	0 (0%)	–	0 (0%)	6680 (0.2%)
Language/literacy problems	0 (0%)	–	2 (7%)	6.00 (1.4–25.3)	0 (0%)	50 520 (1%)
Other*	2 (7%)	–	5 (18%)	–	1 (4%)	
No special needs or diagnosis	16 (55%)	0.39 (0.1–1.3)	5 (18%)	0.07 (0.02–0.3)	20 (77%)	

ORs shown with 95% CI relative to the comparison group shown in bold.

* Diagnoses coded as mutually exclusive.

** Department for Children, Schools and Families (DCSF) Special Educational Needs in England 2008. http://www.dcsf.gov.uk.

ASD, autism spectrum disorder.

Group I consisted of prenatal referrals from regional centres, augmented by ten cases (all prenatally diagnosed) whose parents had joined Unique prior to their first birthday. Group II consisted of those with XXX and XYY karyotypes (either prenatally or postnatally diagnosed) whose parents had joined Unique after their first birthday.

Reproduced from Archives of Disease in Childhood, Bishop DV, Jacobs PA et al, Autism, language and communication in children with sex chromosome trisomies, volume 96, pp. 954–9, 2011 with permission from BMJ Publishing Group Ltd.

- Tartaglia *et al.* (2012) recommends prenatal renal USS in prenatally detected cases.
- There is a small excess of epilepsy/abnormal EEG.
- In general, disclosure of the karyotype on a 'need to know' basis is advised, so that the child is not treated differently or regarded differently by others. Telling a child about their 47,XXX karyotype should be a gradual process extending over many years, with parents being supported in this by health professionals. See Linden *et al.* (2002) for a full discussion of this topic.

Genetic advice

Recurrence risk

Parents of girls with 47,XXX are not routinely karyotyped. The recurrence risk is low (<1%).

Offspring risk

The risk for chromosome anomaly in women with 47,XXX is very low (<1%).

Prenatal diagnosis

PND should be offered to parents and to women with 47,XXX, but there is a fine balance between the very small risk of recurrence and the risk of procedure-associated pregnancy loss. NIPT may be offered as an alternative, where available.

Support group: In the UK via Unique, The Rare Chromosome Disorder Support Group, http://www.rarechromo.org, which produces a detailed information leaflet.

Expert adviser: Nicole Tartaglia, Developmental–Behavioural Paediatrician, Associate Professor of Paediatrics, University of Colorado, School of Medicine, Children's Hospital Colorado, USA.

References

Bishop DV, Jacobs PA, Lachlan K, *et al.* Autism, language and communication in children with sex chromosome trisomies. *Arch Dis Child* 2011; **96**: 954–9.

Christian SM, Koehn D, Pillay R, MacDougall A, Wilson RD. Parental decisions following prenatal diagnosis of sex chromosome anomalies, a trend over time. *Prenat Diagn* 2000; **20**: 37–40.

Harmon RJ, Bender BG, Linden MG, Robinson A. Transition from adolescence to early adulthood: adaptation and psychiatric status of women with 47,XXX. *J Am Acad Child Adolesc Psychiatry* 1998; **37**: 286–91.

Hook EB. Chromosome abnormalities: prevalence, risks and recurrence. In: DLH Brock, CH Rodeck, MA Ferguson-Smith (eds.). *Prenatal diagnosis and screening*, pp. 351–92. Churchill Livingstone, Edinburgh, 1992.

Leggett V, Jacobs P, Nation K, Scerif G, Bishop DV. Neurocognitive outcomes of individuals with a sex chromosome trisomy, XXX, XYY or XXY: a systematic review. *Dev Med Child Neurol* 2010; **52**: 119–29.

Linden MG, Bender BG. Fifty-one prenatally diagnosed children and adolescents with sex chromosome anomalies. *Am J Med Genet* 2002; **110**: 11–18.

Linden MG, Bender BG, Robinson A. Intrauterine diagnosis of sex chromosome aneuploidy. *Obstet Gynecol* 1996; **87**: 468–75.

Linden MG, Bender BG, Robinson A. Genetic counselling for sex chromosome abnormalities. *Am J Med Genet* 2002; **110**: 3–10.

Ratcliffe S. Long term outcome in children of sex chromosome abnormalities. *Arch Dis Child* 1999; **80**: 192–5.

Swerdlow AJ, Hermon C, Jacobs PA, *et al.* Mortality and cancer incidence in persons with numerical sex chromosome abnormalities: a cohort study. *Ann Hum Genet* 2001; **65**(Pt. 2): 177–88.

Tartaglia NR, Avari N, Hutaff-Lee C, Boada R. Attention-deficit hyperactivity disorder symptoms in children and adolescents with sex chromosome aneuploidy: XXY, XXX, XYY, and XXYY. *J Dev Behav Pediatr* 2012; **33**: 309–18.

47,XXY

Klinefelter's syndrome.

Klinefelter's syndrome has a prevalence of 1/600–1/800 male births. There is a significant maternal age effect, with 47,XXY being more common with advanced maternal age, increasing from 1/2500 live births at maternal age of 33 years to 1/300 at 43 years (Hook 1992).

47,XXY is usually either diagnosed prenatally as an unexpected finding at amniocentesis/CVS or in adult life during investigation of male infertility. The majority are probably never diagnosed. Males with Klinefelter's syndrome have a normal lifespan.

Clinical features

Physical

Babies appear normal at birth, although there may be an increased incidence of undescended testes (one-third required orchidopexy in Ratcliffe's (1999) study). Men with 47,XXY tend to be rather tall with a final adult height of 186 cm (compared with 177 cm for 46,XY). There is an increased risk for transient gynaecomastia. If troublesome, surgical reduction can be performed but is rarely necessary (1/19 in Ratcliffe's (1999) study).

Puberty and sexual development

Boys enter puberty normally. By mid puberty, the testes begin to involute, and boys develop hypergonadotrophic hypogonadism with decreased testosterone production. Testes are small in adult life, and men with Klinefelter's syndrome are, with occasional exceptions, infertile. 47,XXY males are no more likely to be homosexual than 46,XY males. Men with 47,XXY have, with the exception of small testes, normal genitalia and normal sexual relations.

Educational

There is a modest decrement in IQ of 10–15 points, when compared with siblings, but IQ varies widely (as for 46,XY) and in Linden and Bender's (2002) study,

the range was 67–133. The majority of 47,XXY (two-thirds) will have more problems with reading and spelling than their 46,XY peers. Nearly half of boys with 47,XXY need speech and language therapy. In Linden and Bender's (2002) study, 70% received additional educational support (usually part-time support in mainstream school); the figure was slightly lower in Bishop et al. (2011) at ~60%, based on a cohort of 19 boys (see Table 5.3).

Behaviour

A higher rate of autism of ~10% (Bishop et al. 2011) and ADHD of 36% (Tartaglia et al. 2012) in 47,XXY has been reported. Gender orientation is normal and there is no evidence for increased aberrant sexual behaviour.

Employment

Ratcliffe (1999) noted that most XXY boys have less skilled jobs than their fathers, but there was no increase in unemployment. Variation is wide and some 47,XXY men will follow professional careers.

Fertility

47,XXY men are generally infertile. Occasionally, men with 47,XXY have a few sperm in their testes, even when none are present in the ejaculate. Testicular sperm extraction and ICSI with IVF offer hope of biological fatherhood to some. New work indicates there may be a critical point in puberty when spermatogenetic function of the testicles could be present. Spermatozoa can be retrieved in a semen sample and in testicular tissue of some adolescent Klinefelter's syndrome patients. Furthermore, the testis may also harbour spermatogonia and incompletely differentiated germ cells. Fertility preservation might best be proposed to adolescent Klinefelter's syndrome patients just after the onset of puberty (Rives et al. 2013), as in early puberty there could be a time when spermatozoa could be detected

Table 5.3 N (%) boys receiving special schooling, registered with special educational needs (SEN), with speech and language therapy (SALT) or a given diagnosis

	Group I		Group I		Group II		Siblings	National data**
	XXY	OR	XYY	OR	XYY	OR	Boys	Boys
N	19		21		37		41	3 992 857
Special schooling	5 (28%)	3.30 (0.8–14.1)	9 (47%)	6.94 (1.8–26.7)	16 (46%)	7.05 (2.1–23.9)	**4 (10%)**	
SEN	6 (32%)	3.60 (1.4–9.4)	10 (48%)	7.10 (3.0–16.6)	29 (78%)	28.0 (12.8–61.5)	4 (10%)	**456 350 (11%)**
SALT	9 (47%)	4.37 (1.3–14.7)	15 (71%)	12.14 (3.5–42.3)	27 (73%)	13.11 (4.4–39.0)	**7 (18%)**	
ASD*	2 (11%)	19.60 (4.5–85.1)	4 (20%)	39.30 (13.8–116.8)	7 (19%)	38.90 (17.1–88.7)	0 (0%)	**23 760 (0.6%)**
Language/literacy problems	1 (5%)	1.80 (0.2–13.1)	1 (5%)	1.60 (0.2–11.8)	0 (0%)	–	2 (5%)	**122 490 (3%)**
Other*	0 (0%)	–	1 (5%)	–	1 (3%)		**1 (3%)**	
No special needs or diagnosis	7 (37%)	0.24 (0.1–0.8)	3 (14%)	0.07 (0.02–0.3)	3 (8%)	0.04 (0.01–0.2)	**27 (68%)**	

ORs shown with 95% CI relative to comparison group (shown in bold).

* Diagnoses coded as mutually exclusive.

** Department for Children, Schools and Families (DCSF) Special Educational Needs in England 2008, http://www.dcsf.gov.uk.

Reproduced from Archives of Disease in Childhood, Bishop DV, Jacobs PA et al, Autism, language and communication in children with sex chromosome trisomies, volume 96, pp. 954–9, 2011 with permission from BMJ Publishing Group Ltd.

in the ejaculate or, if not, at least in the testicular tissue. These could be extracted by testicular sperm extraction, cryopreserved, and used for ICSI therapy later on (Kliesche et al. 2011). Greco et al. (2013) report their experience of 38 azoospermic patients with non-mosaic KS. Spermatozoa were retrieved from 15 patients (~40%) and 26 ICSI cycles were done (16 with cryopreserved sperm). There were 15 pregnancies, leading to the birth of 16 babies. AID and adoption remain important options. Exceptionally, fertility has been reported but is probably the result of a cryptic 47,XXY/46,XY karyotype.

Adult life

There may be a modest increase in risk for diabetes and diseases of the cardiovascular, respiratory, and digestive systems (Swerlow et al. 2001).

Clinical approach

History: key points (postnatal presentation)
- Developmental milestones, speech and language development, schooling.

Examination: key points (postnatal presentation)
- Height.
- Pubertal development (depending on age).

Management

- Advise parents that, if their son shows developmental, behavioural, or educational difficulties, they should have a low threshold for asking for professional help, as early intervention can improve outcome.
- In general, disclosure of the karyotype on a 'need to know' basis is advised, so that the child is not treated differently or regarded differently by others. Telling a child about his 47,XXY karyotype should be a gradual process extending over many years, with parents being supported in this by health professionals. See Linden et al. (2002) for a full discussion of this topic.
- Refer to a paediatric endocrinologist at around 10 years of age for monitoring of growth and measurement of testosterone, FSH, and LH. If studies suggest hypergonadotrophic hypogonadism, testosterone supplementation should be offered. Testosterone supplementation (usually given as IM injections every few weeks or transdermal patches applied daily) improves self-esteem, facial hair growth, and libido. It also has a protective effect in reducing the risk of osteoporosis. There should be consideration of saving sperm at an early age for future use to enable boys with 47,XXY to have children.
- For management of infertility, refer to a reproductive medicine specialist for consideration of AID or assisted conception with IVF and ICSI. Sperm for ICSI may be obtained from ejaculate or testicular biopsy.
- Some of the literature mentions an increased risk of cancer in 47,XXY males. A Danish study of 696 men with Klinefelter's found that the overall cancer incidence is not increased and concluded that no routine cancer screening seems justified (Hasle et al. 1995). Breast cancer is more common in XXY men than in XY men (RR, 20); however, mean age at diagnosis was 72 years and the actual risk (~3%) remains lower than in normal females. There is a very small (<1%) risk of primary mediastinal germ cell tumours that may present with precocious puberty or respiratory symptoms at age 10–30 years.

Genetic advice

Recurrence risk
Parents of boys with XXY are not routinely karyotyped. The recurrence risk is low (<1%).

Offspring risk
There may be an increased risk of aneuploidy (both for sex chromosomes and for +21) and PGD or PND should be discussed. Hennebicq et al. (2001) found a higher frequency of 24,XX and 24,XY sperm than in controls and also a much higher frequency of disomy 21 (6.2% versus 0.4%). Other authors have shown that where focal spermatogenesis is present in non-mosaic Klinefelter's syndrome males, it originates from euploid germ cells and therefore produces normal mature gametes. In support of this finding, at present, the great majority of children born from non-mosaic Klinefelter's syndrome patients are chromosomally normal (Greco et al. 2013).

Prenatal diagnosis
PND should be offered to parents, but there is a fine balance between the very small risk of recurrence and the risk of procedure-associated pregnancy loss. PND is indicated if a patient with Klinefelter's syndrome fathers a pregnancy, because of the increased risk for aneuploidy (see 'Offspring risk' above). NIPT may be offered as an alternative, where available.

Support groups: Klinefelter's Syndrome Association (UK), http://www.ksa-uk.net; Unique (The Rare Chromosome Disorder Support Group), http://www.rarechromo.org, which produces a detailed information leaflet.

Expert adviser: Nicole Tartaglia, Developmental–Behavioural Paediatrician, Associate Professor of Paediatrics, University of Colorado, School of Medicine, Children's Hospital Colorado, USA.

References

Bishop DV, Jacobs PA, Lachlan K, et al. Autism, language and communication in children with sex chromosome trisomies. *Arch Dis Child* 2011; **96**: 954–9.

Greco E, Scarcelli P, Minasi MG, et al. Birth of 16 healthy children after ICSI in cases of nonmosaic Klinefelter syndrome. *Hum Reprod* 2013; **28**: 1155–60.

Hasle H, Mellemgaard A, Nielsen J, Hausen J. Cancer incidence in men with Klinefelter syndrome. *Br J Cancer* 1995; **71**: 416–20.

Hennebicq S, Pelletier R, Bergues U, et al. High risk for trisomy 21 for ICSI conceptus of a Klinefelter patient. *Lancet* 2001; **357**: 2104–5.

Hook EB. Chromosome abnormalities: prevalence, risks and recurrence. In: DLH Brock, CH Rodeck, MA Ferguson-Smith (eds.). *Prenatal diagnosis and screening*, pp. 351–92. Churchill Livingstone, Edinburgh, 1992.

Horowitz M, Wisheart JM, O'Loughlin PD, Morris HA, Need AG, Nordin BE. Osteoporosis and Klinefelter's syndrome. *Clin Endocrinol* 1992; **36**: 113–18.

Hultborn R, Hanson C, Kopf I, et al. Prevalence of Klinefelter's syndrome in male breast cancer patients. *Anticancer Res* 1997; **17**: 4293.

Kliesche S, Zitzmann M, Behre HM. Fertility in patients with Klinefelter syndrome (47,XXY). *Urologe A* 2011; **50**: 26–32.

Linden MG, Bender BG. Fifty-one prenatally diagnosed children and adolescents with sex chromosome anomalies. *Am J Med Genet* 2002; **110**: 11–18.

Linden MG, Bender BG, Robinson A. Intrauterine diagnosis of sex chromosome aneuploidy. *Obstet Gynecol* 1996; **87**: 468–75.

Linden MG, Bender BG, Robinson A. Genetic counselling for sex chromosome abnormalities. *Am J Med Genet* 2002; **110**: 3–10.

Ratcliffe S. Long-term outcome in children of sex chromosome abnormalities. *Arch Dis Child* 1999; **80**: 192–5.

Rives N, Milazzo JP, Perdrix A, *et al.* The feasibility of fertility preservation in adolescents with Klinefelter syndrome. *Hum Reprod* 2013; **28**: 1468–79.

Robinson A, Bender BG, Linden MG. Klinefelter syndrome. In: SB Cassidy, JE Allanson (eds.). *Management of genetic syndromes*, pp. 195–206. Wiley-Liss, New York, 2001.

Swerdlow AJ, Hermon C, Jacobs PA, *et al.* Mortality and cancer incidence in persons with numerical sex chromosome abnormalities: a cohort study. *Ann Hum Genet* 2001; **65**(pt 2): 177–88.

Tartaglia NR, Avari N, Hutaff-Lee C, Boada R. Attention-deficit hyperactivity disorder symptoms in children and adolescents with sex chromosome aneuploidy: XXY, XXX, XYY, and XXYY. *J Dev Behav Pediatr* 2012; **33**: 309–18.

47,XYY

An extra Y chromosome is found in ~1 in 1000 male births. There is no advanced paternal age effect. At least 85% are undiagnosed either pre- or postnatally. Fryns and Kleczkowska (1995) found 75 males with XYY karyotype among nearly 100 000 karyotypes performed in the Leuven cytogenetics laboratory. This is very close to the incidence of XYY in newborn studies and indicates that the frequency of MR/multiple congenital anomaly (MCA) syndromes is not increased in XYY males in general.

Referrals come from two main sources:
- prenatal identification after CVS/amniocentesis for maternal age or suspected fetal abnormality where the 47,XYY karyotype is truly an incidental finding;
- from the investigations of boys with learning and behavioural difficulties where the finding may be of clinical significance (see 'Clinical features' below).

The most common mechanism to produce the extra Y is non-disjunction at meiosis II after a normal chiasmate meiosis I. Post-zygotic mitotic errors and non-disjunction at meiosis II after a nullichiasmate meiosis I are also possible.

Clinical features

Physical
At birth, height, weight, and head circumference show no difference from those of controls. From the age of 2 years, the growth velocity increases until puberty. Boys enter puberty 7–8 cm taller than controls. There are no dysmorphic features.

Puberty
The growth spurt is prolonged with a final height mean of 188 cm (91st to 98th centile). Secondary sexual development is normal, but the onset may be delayed by about 6 months, compared to that of controls.

Educational
There is a small, but significant, lowering of the IQ scores, with the mean 10–15 points lower than that of siblings, but remaining within the normal range. There is an increased incidence of speech/language delay; ~70% have SALT. More than 50% of boys with 47,XYY have special educational needs (Bishop et al. 2011). In Ratcliffe's (1999) study of 19 boys, 54% of the XYY boys had reading difficulties, compared to 18% of controls. Severe MR is rarely found, though only 10% of 47,XYY males in the Bishop et al. (2011) cohort had no special educational needs or diagnosis.

Behaviour
Behavioural problems are more common in males with XYY, especially in those with learning difficulties. In the Bishop et al. (2011) study, around 20% of XYY males had received a diagnosis of autistic spectrum disorders (ASD), which is a 10- to 20-fold increase over even the most liberal prevalence estimate for autism in the general population. Tartaglia et al. (2012) report a 76% risk of ADHD. Medical treatment with psychopharmaceutical stimulants helped in 80%. Forty-seven per cent of the XYY boys in Ratcliffe's (1999) series of 19 boys had been referred to a psychiatrist (control, 9%).

Sexual orientation is normal.

A large Danish study by Stochholm et al. (2012) in a group of 161 men with 47,XYY found the overall risk of conviction (excluding traffic offences) was moderately increased; however, it was similar to controls when adjusting for socio-economic parameters. The mean IQ scores are lower in those with convictions and lowered intelligence appears to be the major risk factor for antisocial and unlawful behaviour.

Employment
Men with XYY were found to move jobs more frequently than controls. The range of jobs described is wide and most XYY males should have normal employment prospects.

Fertility
Most men with XYY are fertile and the majority of sperm in 47,XYY men are chromosomally normal. This may be because XY bivalents and Y univalents are lost during spermatogenesis or by the loss of the additional Y in some primitive sperm cells and a proliferative advantage of XY cells.

Clinical approach (postnatal presentation)

History: key points
- Developmental delay, schooling difficulties, behavioural problems.

Examination: key points (postnatal presentation)
- Height.

Management
- Prenatal detection. Boys detected prenatally have a milder phenotype. This is due to unbiased ascertainment. Advise the parent that, if their son shows developmental, behavioural, or educational difficulties, they should have a low threshold for asking for professional help, as early intervention can improve outcome.
- Postnatal detection. Chromosome testing has often been initiated because of developmental or behavioural difficulties and these boys require careful assessment. If a boy with XYY has dysmorphic features or malformations, they should not be attributed to the 47,XYY karyotype.
- Disclosure of karyotype. See Linden et al. (2002) for a full discussion of this topic. In general, disclosure of the karyotype on a 'need to know' basis is advised, so that the child is not treated differently or regarded differently by others. Telling a child about his 47,XYY karyotype should be a gradual process extending over many years, with parents being supported in this by health professionals.

Genetic advice

Recurrence risk
Fathers of boys with XYY are not routinely karyotyped. The recurrence risk is low (<1%).

Offspring risk
The majority of sperm in 47,XYY men is chromosomally normal and XYY men are not reported to have an increased risk of sons with XYY or XXY.

Prenatal diagnosis
PND should be offered, but there is a fine balance between the very small risk of recurrence and the risk of procedure-associated pregnancy loss. NIPT may be offered as an alternative, where available.

Support group: In the UK via Unique (The Rare Chromosome Disorder Support Group), http://www.rarechromo.org.

Expert adviser: Nicole Tartaglia, Developmental–Behavioural Paediatrician, Associate Professor of Paediatrics, University of Colorado, School of Medicine, Children's Hospital Colorado, USA.

References

Bishop DV, Jacobs PA, Lachlan K, et al. Autism, language and communication in children with sex chromosome trisomies. *Arch Dis Child* 2011; **96**: 954–9.

Fryns JP, Kleczkowska A. XYY syndrome and other Y chromosome polysomies. Mental status and psychosocial functioning. *Genet Couns* 1995; **6**: 197–206.

Gotz MJ, Johnstone EC, Ratcliffe SG. Criminality and antisocial behaviour in unselected men with sex chromosome abnormalities. *Psychol Med* 1999; **29**: 953–62.

Linden MG, Bender BG. Fifty-one prenatally diagnosed children and adolescents with sex chromosome anomalies. *Am J Med Genet* 2002; **110**: 11–18.

Linden MG, Bender BG, Robinson A. Intrauterine diagnosis of sex chromosome aneuploidy. *Obstet Gynecol* 1996; **87**: 468–75.

Linden MG, Bender BG, Robinson A. Genetic counselling for sex chromosome abnormalities. *Am J Med Genet* 2002; **110**: 3–10.

Martin RH, Shi Q, Field LL. Recombination in the pseudoautosomal region in a 47,XYY male. *Hum Genet* 2001; **109**: 143–5.

Ratcliffe S. Long-term outcome in children of sex chromosome abnormalities. *Arch Dis Child* 1999; **80**: 192–5.

Robinson DO, Jacobs PA. The origins of the extra Y chromosome in males with a 47,XYY karyotype. *Hum Mol Genet* 1999; **8**: 2205–9.

Stochholm K, Bojesen A, Jensen AS, Juul S, Gravholt CH. Criminality in men with Klinefelter's syndrome and XYY: a cohort study. *BMJ Open* 2012; **2**: e000650.

Swerdlow AJ, Hermon C, Jacobs PA, et al. Mortality and cancer incidence in persons with numerical sex chromosome abnormalities: a cohort study. *Ann Hum Genet* 2001; **65**(Pt 2): 177–88.

Tartaglia NR, Avari N, Hutaff-Lee C, Boada R. Attention-deficit hyperactivity disorder symptoms in children and adolescents with sex chromosome aneuploidy: XXY, XXX, XYY, and XXYY. *J Dev Behav Pediatr* 2012; **33**: 309–18.

Autosomal reciprocal translocations—background

Chromosome rearrangements are described as balanced or unbalanced. In a balanced rearrangement, the individual has a normal amount of chromosomal material (genes), but a child or adult with an unbalanced rearrangement has additional and/or missing genetic material. Genomic array analysis does not detect balanced translocations. This is an important point for clinicians to note, as a normal array result in a family member at risk for a familial balanced translocation does not indicate whether the translocation has been inherited.

Rearrangements that appear balanced using conventional cytogenetic techniques are described in reports as 'apparently balanced', although imbalance may be detectable using genomic array or exome sequencing technologies. Typical resolution with Giemsa (G)-banding is ~5–10 Mb. When an apparently balanced rearrangement is detected in a phenotypically normal individual, it is assumed to be truly balanced.

In general, a deficiency (monosomy) causes more problems than a similarly sized duplication (trisomy). Chromosome imbalance is usually associated with learning disability with/without congenital anomalies. Dosage-sensitive genes play a critical role in development, and any such genes that are under- or overexpressed will result in phenotypic abnormality. Most published cases (95%) of viable autosomal imbalance fall within a triangle delimited by 4% trisomy and 2% monosomy (see Figure 5.1); chromosomal imbalance falling outside this triangle is likely to result in spontaneous pregnancy loss. Assuming a genome length of ~3,000,000,000 bases (3,000Mb), then 4% equates to ~120Mb and 2% to ~60Mb. N.B. Gene density and dosage sensitivity of genes are not evenly distributed in the genome.

Balanced autosomal reciprocal translocations are common and carried by >0.1% of the population. In simplistic terms, there are four possible outcomes to any pregnancy of a carrier of a balanced autosomal reciprocal translocation. These are a pregnancy with:

- a normal karyotype;
- a balanced autosomal reciprocal translocation (as in the parent);
- an unbalanced product of the translocation resulting in spontaneous pregnancy loss, e.g. miscarriage;
- an unbalanced product of the translocation that is viable resulting in a child with a high likelihood of learning disability with/without congenital anomalies.

One of the important roles of the geneticist is to assess the likelihood of a viable unbalanced outcome. This is likely to be a major factor governing decisions regarding invasive prenatal diagnostic tests (e.g. amniocentesis, CVS).

Chromosomes are not uniform structures and this creates problems in devising methods for predicting the risk of a viable unbalanced outcome. Some regions of the chromosomes are much more gene-rich than others, and none of the computational approaches to this problem are able to account for this. Alternative approaches based on observed outcomes to pregnancies are rather cumbersome and may be subject to ascertainment bias. In practical terms, precision in calculating the likelihood of a viable unbalanced outcome is neither feasible nor necessary. Couples contemplating pregnancy and PND do not make decisions based on values to two decimal places; they need figures that they can evaluate alongside the risks of invasive procedures such as CVS/amniocentesis. Our practice is to define bands of risk: <0.5%; 0.5–1%; 1–5%; 5–10%; and >10%.

Viable imbalance risk

In practice, four different, but complementary, approaches are used to assess the likelihood of a viable unbalanced outcome and determine the risk band.

- Assessment of the family history. Any family ascertained through the birth of a child with an unbalanced product (or TOP with multiple congenital anomalies) is likely to have a high or very high risk (5–10% or >10%).
- Calculation of the haploid autosomal length (HAL) of the imbalance (see 'Haploid autosomal lengths of human chromosomes' in 'Appendix', p. 834). Risks for viability are highest with breakpoints located closest to the telomere, which yield the smallest imbalance.
- Reference to empiric data compiled by Stene and Stengel-Rutowski (1990).
- Literature search using PubMed and resources such as DECIPHER (http://decipher.sanger.ac.uk) to determine whether a viable outcome has been previously reported and, if so, the phenotype.

Different centres use different approaches and most clinicians use a combination to arrive at a risk estimate for a particular family.

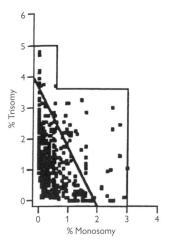

Figure 5.1 Viability of combined duplication/deletion states, according to the amount of imbalance, measured as the percentage of haploid autosomal length (HAL). Most (96%) fall within the triangular area whose hypotenuse lies between 4% duplication/0% deletion and 2% deletion/0% duplication, and a few outliers define an envelope of viable imbalances.
Reproduced from *Human Genetics*, Viability thresholds for partial trisomies and monosomies. A study of 1,159 viable unbalanced reciprocal translocations, volume 93, issue 2, 1994, pp 188–194, Olivier Cohen, With permission of Springer.

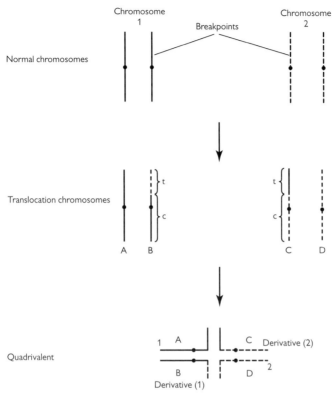

Figure 5.2 This figure shows the generation of a balanced reciprocal translocation between chromosomes 1 and 2, and the formation of a quadrivalent in meiosis. c, centric segment; t, translocated segment.
Reproduced from Ian D Young, *Introduction to Risk Calculation in Genetic Counselling*, Second Edition, 1999, Figure 8.1, page 136, by permission of Oxford University Press, www.oup.com.

Pachytene diagram

This is key to understanding how unbalanced products can arise during meiosis (see Figure 5.2). To construct a pachytene diagram (see Figure 5.3), you need to know the breakpoints and have access to a karyotype ideogram, so that you can identify approximately where, along the length of the chromosomes involved, the breakpoints lie (e.g. Gardner and Sutherland 2011).

The segregation (separation of chromosomes) producing the smallest imbalance is usually found by drawing a line between the homologous segments of the two longest arms of the quadrivalent.

The following are important general principles.

- Alternate segregation produces gametes with normal chromosomes (A + D) or the balanced reciprocal arrangement (B + C) present in the parent.
- Adjacent-1 segregation creates the smallest imbalance when the translocated segments are shorter than the centric segments (A + C and B + D). Overall, it is the most common segregation pattern producing viable imbalance (70%).
- Adjacent-2 segregation creates the smallest imbalance when the translocated segments are longer than the centric segments (A + B and C + D). It is a relatively uncommon segregation pattern to produce viable imbalance (5%).

- 3:1 segregation tends to give rise to the smallest imbalance when one of the non-translocation or derivative chromosomes is very small. (A + B + C) or (B + C + D) give rise to interchange trisomy and (A + B + D) or (A + C + D) give rise to tertiary trisomy—as a mechanism, it accounts for ~25% of viable imbalance. 3:1 segregation is more common in female carriers of a balanced translocation than in male carriers.

Assessing the likelihood of viability

- Risks of viable imbalance are highest with breakpoints located closest to the telomere; the shorter the chromosome segment involved, the more likely it is to be viable.
- Monosomy is much less likely to be viable than trisomy. Monosomy for any whole autosome is not viable; trisomy for whole autosomes is only viable in the case of trisomies 13, 18, and 21.
- Most published cases (96%) of viable autosomal imbalance comprise up to 4% trisomy and up to 2% monosomy, with combinations viable when they fall within a triangle delimited by 4% trisomy/0% monosomy and 2% monosomy/0% trisomy.

Support group: Unique (The Rare Chromosome Disorder Support Group), http://www.rarechromo.org, Tel. 01883 330 766.

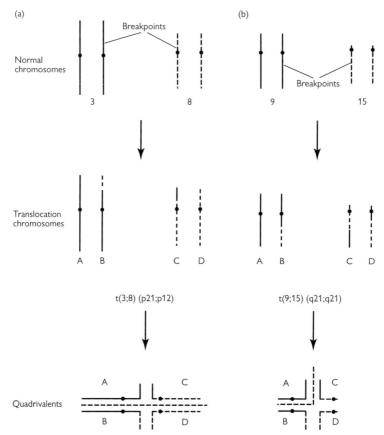

Figure 5.3 Pachytene diagrams drawn to scale for two reciprocal translocations. The bold dashed line indicates the pattern of segregation that will produce the smallest imbalance. In (a), this will be adjacent-1 segregation and in (b) 3:1 segregation resulting in interchange monosomy/trisomy.
Reproduced from Ian D Young, *Introduction to Risk Calculation in Genetic Counselling*, Second Edition, 1999, Figure 8.3, page 139, by permission of Oxford University Press, www.oup.com.

Expert adviser (first edition): Ian D. Young, Consultant Clinical Geneticist, Leicester, England.

References

Cohen O, Cans C, Mermet MA, Demongeot J, Jalbert P. Viability thresholds for partial trisomies and monosomies. A study of 1,159 viable unbalanced reciprocal translocations. *Hum Genet* 1994; **93**: 188–94.

DECIPHER. http://decipher.sanger.ac.uk.

Gardner RJM, Sutherland GR, Shaffer LG. Chromosome anomalies and genetic counseling. *Oxford monographs on medical genetics*, 4th edn. Oxford University Press, New York, 2011.

Jacobs PA. Recurrence risks for chromosome abnormalities. *Birth Defects Orig Art Ser* 1979; **15**(5C): 71–80.

Lindenbaum RH, Bobrow M. Reciprocal translocations in man. 3:1 Meiotic disjunction resulting in 47- or 45-chromosome offspring. *J Med Genet* 1975; **12**: 29–43.

Schinzel A. *Catalogue of unbalanced chromosome aberrations in man*, 2nd edn. de Gruyter, Berlin, 2001.

Stene J, Stengel-Rutowski S. Genetic risks of familial reciprocal and Robertsonian translocation carriers. In: A Daniel (ed.). *The cytogenetics of mammalian autosomal rearrangements*, pp. 3–72. Alan R Liss, New York, 1990.

Young ID. *Introduction to risk calculation in genetic counselling*, 2nd edn. Oxford University Press, Oxford, 1999 [see especially Chapter 8.1, pp. 135–45].

Autosomal reciprocal translocations—familial

See also 'Autosomal reciprocal translocations—background' in Chapter 5, 'Chromosomes', p. 636.

Most rearrangements are unique to a family, but there are a few that appear recurrently, particularly a common translocation (t) between chromosomes 11 and 22. This t(11;22)(q23;q11) is the most frequently occurring non-Robertsonian translocation.

Clinical approach

When an individual is known to either carry or be at risk of carrying, a balanced autosomal reciprocal translocation, an annotated photograph together with an ideogram of the chromosomes involved in the translocation is an invaluable aid to counselling.

History: key points

- Draw a three-generation family tree (or larger if indicated) and enquire about pregnancy loss, stillbirth, neonatal death, and family members with learning disability or congenital anomalies.
- Confirm that the consultand has no health problems or learning disability attributable to the translocation.

Examination: key points

Examine if there are specific indications from the history.

Special investigations

Karyotype your patient if:

- their status is unknown but they are 'at risk' from the family tree and old enough to give their consent and engage with the testing process (see 'Testing for genetic status' in Chapter 1, 'Introduction', p. 38).
- they are a known carrier of a balanced rearrangement where you do not have access to a cytogenetics report defining the breakpoints (especially important if investigation of other family members or PND is planned).

Genetic advice

There is no indication that parents with a structural abnormality are at an increased risk of producing a child with a chromosomal abnormality independent of the parental rearrangement (Jacobs 1979).

Recurrence risk

The main issue is to determine the risk of viable imbalance. A suggested approach (see 'Autosomal reciprocal translocations—background' in Chapter 5, 'Chromosomes', p. 636) is the following.

- (1) Determine breakpoints and construct a pachytene diagram using different coloured pens for the two different chromosomes involved in the translocation.
- (2) Make a rough risk assessment based on knowledge of the family history and length of translocated segments involved. The risk of a viable live birth is highest (>10%) when there is a family history of affected pregnancies continuing to term or when the proposita has been a fetus identified by fetal malformation at an anomaly scan or later in pregnancy.
- (3) Determine whether the product with the smallest imbalance could be viable.
- (4) Determine if a 3:1 segregation (meiotic disjunction) is a likely outcome (more likely when acrocentric chromosomes are involved in the translocation).

Carriers of t(11;22)(q23;q11) are at risk of 3:1 meiotic disjunction, which is found in 5–10% of the offspring of female carriers, resulting in dup(11)(q23-qter) and dup22(pter-q11) (Emanuel syndrome).

- (5) If risk of viable imbalance exists, refine the risk assessment by determining the approximate risk of viable imbalance using a combination of computerized risk assessment based on HAL (see 'Haploid autosomal lengths of human chromosomes' in 'Appendix', p. 834) or Stene and Stengel-Rutowski (1990) tables and a literature search.
- (6) Classify the risk of viable imbalance into one of the risk bands for the purposes of counselling, e.g. <0.5%, 0.5–1%, 1–5%, 5–10%, and >10%.

Prenatal diagnosis

The mainstay of PND is karyotype by amniocentesis/CVS. If the unbalanced product would result in a very subtle anomaly, a genomic array analysis is likely to be far more sensitive than microscopy in detecting an imbalance. If prenatal array analysis is not available, discuss with the lab whether they need to work up FISH probes in order to make a confident PND on preparations from CVS/amniocentesis. If testing is done by genomic array, it will detect unbalanced rearrangements, but not balanced carriers.

For couples with adverse obstetric histories where segregation appears skewed towards unbalanced products, e.g. multiple pregnancy losses due to miscarriage or TOP, IVF with PGD may be an option to consider. See 'Assisted reproductive technology: *in vitro* fertilization (IVF), intracytoplasmic sperm injection (ICSI), and pre-implantation genetic diagnosis (PGD)' in Chapter 6, 'Pregnancy and fertility', p. 706.

Support group: Unique (The Rare Chromosome Disorder Support Group), http://www.rarechromo.org, Tel. 01883 330 766.

Expert adviser (first edition): Ian D. Young, Consultant Clinical Geneticist, Leicester, England

References

Cohen O, Cans C, Mermet MA, Demongeot J, Jalbert P. Viability thresholds for partial trisomies and monosomies. A study of 1,159 viable unbalanced reciprocal translocations. *Hum Genet* 1994; **93**: 188–94.

Gardner RJM, Sutherland GR, Shaffer LG. *Chromosome anomalies and genetic counseling, Oxford monographs on medical genetics*, 4th edn. Oxford University Press, New York, 2011.

Jacobs PA. Recurrence risks for chromosome abnormalities. *Birth Defects Orig Art Ser* 1979; **15**(5C): 71–80.

Lindenbaum RH, Bobrow M. Reciprocal translocations in man. 3:1 Meiotic disjunction resulting in 47- or 45-chromosome offspring. *J Med Genet* 1975; **12**: 29–43.

Ogilvie CM, Braude P, Scriven PN. Successful pregnancy outcomes after preimplantation genetic diagnosis (PGD) for carriers of chromosome translocations. *Hum Fertil (Camb)* 2001; **4**: 168–71.

Stene J, Stengel-Rutowski S. Genetic risks of familial reciprocal and Robertsonian translocation carriers. In: A Daniel (ed.). *The cytogenetics of mammalian autosomal rearrangements*, pp. 3–72. Alan R Liss, New York, 1990.

Young ID. *Introduction to risk calculation in genetic counselling*, 2nd edn. Oxford University Press, Oxford 1999 [see especially Chapter 8.1, pp. 135–45].

Autosomal reciprocal translocations—postnatal

See 'Autosomal reciprocal translocations—background', p. 636 and 'Autosomal reciprocal translocations—familial', p. 640 in Chapter 5, 'Chromosomes'.

Autosomal reciprocal translocations may come to light during the investigation of babies and children with congenital malformations, developmental delay, and/or learning disability, or in the workup of patients with recurrent miscarriage or subfertility. Genomic array is now the first-line investigation of such patients and this investigation does not detect a completely balanced translocation. Array results with a telomeric deletion and/or a telomeric duplication suggest a chromosome rearrangement which may be investigated by FISH and/or conventional karyotype to confirm the result and inform genetic counselling.

The terminology is as follows.

- *De novo*. If the abnormality is not found in either parent, it is described as *de novo* (also consider the possibility of non-paternity).
- Familial. Inherited from a parent.

Normal phenotype

If the child/adult is phenotypically normal, this is likely to be an incidental finding. See 'Autosomal reciprocal translocations—familial' in Chapter 5, 'Chromosomes', p. 640.

Abnormal phenotype

If the child has an abnormal phenotype, continue reading this section.

Clinical approach

History: key points

- Draw a three-generation family tree (or larger, if indicated) and enquire about pregnancy loss, stillbirth, neonatal death, and family members with learning disability or congenital anomalies.
- Document all known malformations in the child and anthropomorphic data.
- Presence of developmental delay.

Examination: key points

- Full clinical examination and documentation of dysmorphic features.

Special investigations

- Arrange for parental chromosome analysis by a method that will detect a balanced translocation to determine whether *de novo* or inherited.
- Clinical photography.
- Consider analysis of genes at the breakpoint(s).

Genetic advice

In the following, it is assumed that the autosomal reciprocal translocation is associated with phenotypic abnormalities.

Apparently balanced rearrangement

This may be an incidental finding if a normal parent carries the same rearrangement.

If it is *de novo*, the chance of the chromosome translocation being the cause is much greater and the following points also need to be considered.

- The translocation is actually unbalanced.
- Unmasking of a recessive allele on the normal homologue.

- There is abnormal gene function as a consequence of the break. Look at the genomic data to see if there is evidence for this and discuss with laboratory scientists.
- Imprinting problems depending on the chromosomes involved. See 'Genomic imprinting' in Chapter 1, 'Introduction', p. 30 for a map of known imprinted genes.

When an abnormality has been detected by light microscopy karyotype, use a genomic array to search for imbalance, and search the literature and databases, such as DECIPHER (http://decipher.sanger.ac.uk), for relevant genes at the breakpoints. If familial, with no phenotype in other family members, consider the possibility of UPD.

Unbalanced rearrangement

This may be found in an infant with multiple malformations or, if the imbalance is smaller, in an older child with milder manifestations. Ascertain if the translocation has been described in the literature/databases and evaluate if the phenotype is compatible. The features, for example of an autosomal deletion (monosomy), may be modified by duplication of the other autosomal segment (trisomy).

Recurrence risk

- *De novo*.
  - Sibling risk. The chance of another affected pregnancy is very small, but offer PND.
  - Offspring risk. See 'Autosomal reciprocal translocations—familial' in Chapter 5, 'Chromosomes', p. 640.
- Familial. If one parent carries a translocation, see 'Autosomal reciprocal translocations—familial' in Chapter 5, 'Chromosomes', p. 640.

Prenatal diagnosis

- *De novo*. Although the chance of another affected pregnancy is low, some families opt for PND for reassurance.
- Familial. If one parent carries a translocation, see 'Autosomal reciprocal translocations—familial' in Chapter 5, 'Chromosomes', p. 640.

Management

If a baby with a *de novo* chromosome abnormality dies, ask permission for a full post-mortem examination and book a follow-up genetic appointment to counsel about the risks of recurrence, and offer family follow-up.

For children with chromosome rearrangements, ensure that:

- the child's medical notes (e.g. GP or family practice notes) are marked with this information;
- the child's parents know that they should request an appointment in the genetics clinic when the child is in his/her mid teens.

Support group: Unique (The Rare Chromosome Disorder Support Group), http://www.rarechromo.org, Tel. 01883 330 766.

Expert adviser (first edition): Ian D. Young, Consultant Clinical Geneticist, Leicester, England

References

DECIPHER. http://decipher.sanger.ac.uk.

Gardner RJM, Sutherland GR, Shaffer LG. *Chromosome anomalies and genetic counseling, Oxford monographs on medical genetics*, 4th edn. Oxford University Press, New York, 2011.

Warburton D. *De novo* balanced chromosome rearrangements and extra marker chromosomes identified at prenatal diagnosis: clinical significance and distribution of breakpoints. *Am J Hum Genet* 1991; **49**: 995–1013.

Autosomal reciprocal translocations—prenatal

See also 'Autosomal reciprocal translocations—background', p. 636 and 'Autosomal reciprocal translocations—familial', p. 640 in Chapter 5, 'Chromosomes'.

Autosomal reciprocal translocations are sometimes identified on karyotyping performed for maternal age indications, increased nuchal translucency, or abnormal USS findings. Determining whether the finding is incidental or, in the case of investigation of abnormal USS findings, causative is crucial.

Balanced translocations are not detected by genomic arrays or NIPT.

Clinical approach

History: key points

- Draw a three-generation family tree (or larger, if indicated) and enquire about pregnancy loss, stillbirth, neonatal death, and family members with learning disability or congenital anomalies.

Examination: key points

- Fetal USS (fetal size and presence of any anomalies).

Special investigations

- Urgent genomic array on fetal DNA (if not already done).
- Arrange for urgent rapid parental chromosome analysis to determine whether inherited or de novo.
- In future, there may be a role for WGS in identifying gene disruption related to a translocation (Talkowski et al. 2012).

Genetic advice

Associated with fetal abnormality

Unbalanced rearrangement. This is likely to be the cause of the fetal abnormality, whether familial or de novo. Define the malformations as well as possible by detailed anomaly scanning. Do a literature/database search for similar karyotypic abnormalities.

APPARENTLY BALANCED REARRANGEMENT. It is imperative to ascertain whether it is de novo and to ensure high-resolution genomic analysis, usually by genomic array. If de novo, then there may be chromosomal loss that is the cause of the abnormalities. Array CGH may add 8.2% to the diagnostic yield, compared with conventional karyotyping, for fetuses with abnormal USS results, and is particularly useful in fetuses with karyotypic balanced translocation or marker chromosomes (Lee et al. 2012). Check the breakpoints for developmental genes and literature reports that may explain the fetal appearance. Counselling will discuss the fact that the chromosome abnormality is likely to be causative, in the absence of another explanation, but there is a chance that it is an incidental finding. If familial, consider if a mechanism such as UPD could be the cause of the abnormalities.

Apparently normal fetus on scan

Usually the indication for pregnancy testing has been an increased risk of Down's syndrome. This is a difficult counselling situation. Parental anxiety is high and there may be no absolute answers.

Unbalanced rearrangement

There is a high risk of disability in a live-born child. Find out about the phenotype associated with the cytogenetic abnormality to aid in counselling the parents and to inform detailed fetal anomaly USS. A further normal USS at ~20 weeks' gestation does not exclude abnormalities presenting later in pregnancy (e.g. polyhydramnios from oesophageal atresia) nor will it help refine the risks of mental handicap or sensory impairment (e.g. hearing, vision). Small size for gestation may be a feature of chromosome imbalance and the presence of 'soft markers' is relevant in this situation.

If there is, or has been, a previous child/pregnancy in the kindred with the same unbalanced product of the translocation, this information can be used to counsel regarding the likely effects of the chromosome imbalance. If familial, arrange follow-up for 'at-risk' members of the family (see 'Autosomal reciprocal translocations—familial' in Chapter 5, 'Chromosomes', p. 640).

Apparently balanced translocation

De novo apparently balanced autosomal reciprocal translocation. The Warburton (1991) study was before the introduction of molecular cytogenetic (array CGH) techniques to assist in the identification of small deletions and duplications. She found one in 2000 pregnancies had a de novo balanced translocation. If truly balanced, then the risk of abnormality is small. The following also need to be considered as all could lead to problems.

- The translocation is actually unbalanced—arrange array CGH.
- Unmasking a recessive allele on the normal homologue.
- There is abnormal gene function as a consequence of the break.
- The potential implications if the breakpoints involve an imprinted region of the genome.

Even though Warburton's (1991) study involved collecting data from many North American laboratories, the amount of information about follow-up is sparse because of the rarity of the occurrence and the lack of information about the effect on neurological development if the pregnancy was terminated.

When the USS was normal, 6.1% of pregnancies had abnormalities at birth or on post-mortem, against the background abnormality rate of ~3%. The 6.1% figure does not include later-onset problems caused by the chromosome imbalance, and the risk of problems, in particular developmental delay, is higher. A 2- to 3-fold risk over the background risk of developmental problems was used (5–10%) when a detailed fetal scan has shown no structural abnormalities and the head size and growth are normal, but parents should understand how the risk figure has been derived. These figures should not be used when CNV has been detected by genomic array; use unbalanced rearrangement data.

FAMILIAL APPARENTLY BALANCED AUTOSOMAL RECIPROCAL TRANSLOCATION. If found in a parent, reassure that the translocation is unlikely to have a phenotypic effect on the fetus. Organize genetic follow-up to discuss the risks of chromosome imbalance in future pregnancies and remember that, at some time in the future, the fetus will be an adult requiring counselling before pregnancy.

Recurrence risk

- De novo. The chance of another affected pregnancy is very small (parental germline mosaicism risk).

- Familial. If one parent carries a translocation, refer to 'Autosomal reciprocal translocations—familial' in Chapter 5, 'Chromosomes', p. 640.

Prenatal diagnosis
- *De novo*. Although the chance of another affected pregnancy is low, some families opt for PND for reassurance.
- Familial. If one parent carries a translocation, refer to 'Autosomal reciprocal translocations—familial' in Chapter 5, 'Chromosomes', p. 640.

Management

If the pregnancy is terminated, arrange for a full post-mortem examination, including clinical photographs, and book a follow-up genetic appointment to counsel about the risks of recurrence and family follow-up. If abnormalities are found, these may confirm the effect of the chromosomal abnormality.

If the pregnancy continues and the fetus is carrying a balanced translocation, ensure that:
- the child is carefully examined at birth;
- the child's medical notes (e.g. GP or family practice notes) are marked with this information;

- the child's parents know that they should request an appointment in the genetics clinic when the child is in his/her mid teens.

Support group: ARC (Antenatal Results and Choices), http://www.arc-uk.org, Tel. 0207 631 0285.

Expert adviser (first edition): Ian D. Young, Consultant Clinical Geneticist, Leicester, England

References

DECIPHER. http://decipher.sanger.ac.uk.

Gardner RJM, Sutherland GR, Shaffer LG. *Chromosome anomalies and genetic counseling, Oxford monographs on medical genetics*, 4th edn. Oxford University Press, New York, 2011.

Lee CN, Lin SY, Lin CH, Shih JC, Lin TH, Su YN. Clinical utility of array comparative genomic hybridisation for prenatal diagnosis: a cohort study of 3171 pregnancies. *BJOG* 2012; **119**: 614–25.

Talkowski ME, Ordulu Z, Pillalamarri V, *et al*. Clinical diagnosis by whole-genome sequencing of a prenatal sample. *N Engl J Med* 2012; **367**: 2226–32.

Warburton D. *De novo* balanced chromosome rearrangements and extra marker chromosomes identified at prenatal diagnosis: clinical significance and distribution of breakpoints. *Am J Hum Genet* 1991; **49**: 995–1013.

Cell division—mitosis, meiosis, and non-disjunction

Mitosis
See Figure 5.4.

Somatic recombination
Pairing of homologous chromosomes, followed by recombination (crossing over), is a central feature of meiosis. In contrast, chromosomes do not generally pair during mitotic cell division, and recombination (homologous or heterologous) is a rare event. Occasional cells do, however, undergo recombination events and this can be an important mechanism in disease. For example, mosaicism for paternal UPD occurring as a result of somatic recombination may underlie some cases of BWS (Kotzot 2001). Somatic recombination can cause LOH, which is often an important step in tumour development.

Meiosis
See Figures 5.5, 5.6, 5.7, and 5.8.

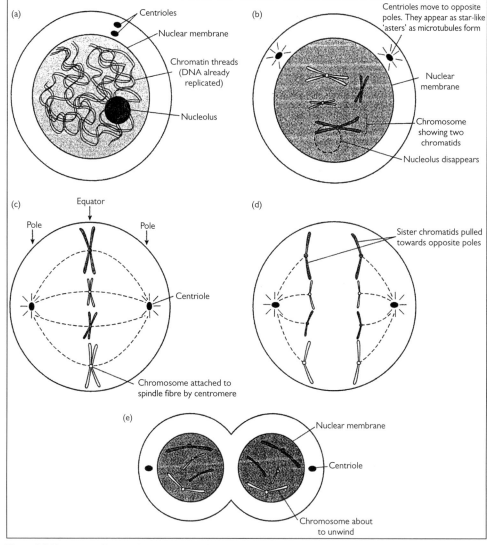

Figure 5.4 The process of mitosis: (a) cell at the end of interphase, (b) prophase, (c) metaphase, (d) anaphase, and (e) telophase. Adapted from *AS level biology*, Bradfield P, et al., Copyright Pearson Education Limited, Longman, London, 2001.

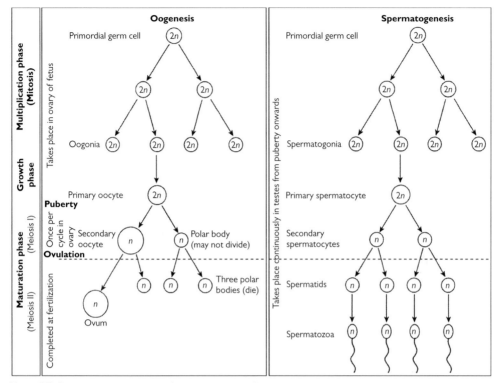

Figure 5.5 Gametogenesis—a comparison between oogenesis and spermatogenesis.
Adapted from AS level biology, Bradfield P., et al., Copyright Pearson Education Limited, Longman, London, 2001.

Female meiosis
Meiosis begins in the fifth month of fetal life in females. When the egg is fertilized, it triggers successive rounds of mitotic cell division. In the fifth month of fetal life, ~33 rounds of mitotic division since fertilization, the fetal ovaries together contain several million oocytes. At this stage, there is a switch from mitosis to meiosis. After progressing through pachytene and into diplotene by the sixth month of fetal life, all of the oocytes are arrested in prophase I.

Table 5.4 A comparison of mitosis and meiosis

Mitosis	Meiosis
Occurs in somatic cells	Occurs in the germline during oogenesis and spermatogenesis
Produces diploid (2n) cells which are genetically identical to each other and to the parent cell	Produces haploid (n) gametes (oocytes and spermatozoa) which are genetically unique because of recombination and independent assortment
Somatic recombination events are rare but can be an important mechanism in disease	Pairing of homologous chromosomes and recombination are key features of meiosis and important in generating genetic diversity
Prophase is short (~30 min)	Prophase is extremely long in female meiosis and lasts from fetal life until puberty and beyond

This phase lasts until puberty and beyond. During a woman's reproductive life, cohorts of oocytes are released from meiotic arrest by progesterone stimulation in each menstrual cycle. The oocytes continue through the first meiotic division but arrest again in metaphase II until fertilization.

At the onset of meiosis in the fifth month of fetal life, the ovaries contain ~8 million oocytes; by the time of birth, this has fallen to 1–2 million as a result of apoptosis. In each monthly cycle, ovulation is accompanied by a wave of apoptosis in oocytes in partially mature follicles.

See Figure 5.5 for a comparison between oogenesis and spermatogenesis.

Male meiosis
In males, mitotic divisions continue to occur in germline stem cell spermatogonia throughout adult life. In a 25-year-old man, about 265 rounds of spermatogonial mitotic division have occurred since fertilization. Gene mutations usually arise as copying errors during replication, and this nearly 9-fold greater number of cell divisions in the male germline before gamete formation is thought to be the basis for the mutation rate being observed to be higher in males than in females.

Meiosis is initiated at puberty when, under hormonal influence, type A spermatogonia switches to type B spermatogonia (germline stem cells). The switch from mitosis to meiosis in type B spermatogonia only occurs in one of the two daughter cells (which becomes a

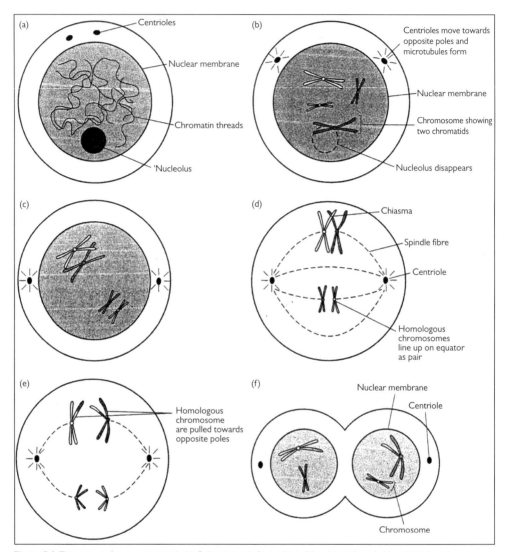

Figure 5.6 The process of meiosis: meiosis 1. (a) Cell at the end of interphase, (b) early prophase 1, (c) mid prophase 1, (d) metaphase 1, (e) anaphase 1, (f) telophase 1.
Adapted from *AS Level Biology*, Bradfield P, et al., Copyright Pearson Education Limited, Longman, London, 2001.

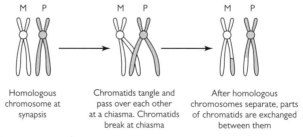

M = maternal chromosome
P = paternal chromosome

Figure 5.7 Diagram to illustrate 'crossing over' (recombination) occurring in late prophase 1, i.e. between (c) and (d) in Figure 5.6.
M, maternal chromosome; P, paternal chromosome.
Adapted from *AS Level Biology*, Bradfield P, et al., Copyright Pearson Education Limited, Longman, London, 2001.

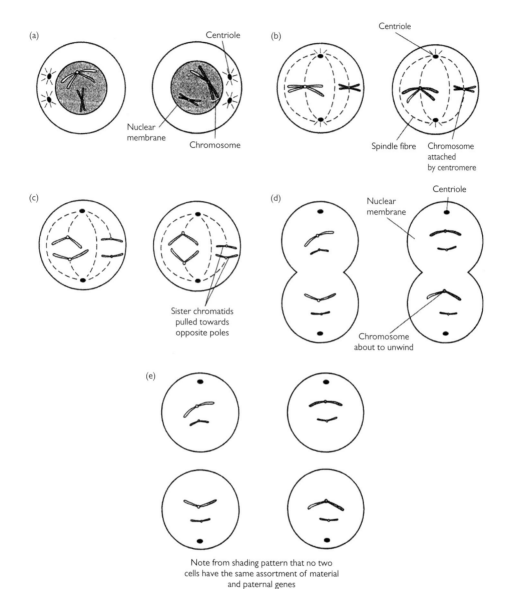

(a)

Centriole

(b)

Centriole

Nuclear
membrane

Chromosome

Spindle fibre   Chromosome
attached
by centromere

(c)

(d)

Centriole

Nuclear
membrane

Sister chromatids
pulled towards
opposite poles

Chromosome
about to unwind

(e)

Note from shading pattern that no two
cells have the same assortment of material
and paternal genes

Figure 5.8 The process of meiosis: meiosis 2. (a) Prophase 2, (b) metaphase 2, (c) anaphase 2, (d) telophase 2, (e) cytokinesis, producing four haploid daughter cells.
Adapted from *AS Level Biology*, Bradfield P, et al., Copyright Pearson Education Limited, Longman, London, 2001.

primary spermatocyte) produced at each type B spermatogonial division (the other stays as a germline stem cell).

Throughout adult life, men produce many tens of millions of spermatogonia, primary spermatocytes, and sperm each day.

Non-disjunction

The failure of homologous chromosomes or sister chromatids to separate appropriately during cell division is called non-disjunction. It results in daughter cells or gametes with an abnormal chromosome number (aneuploidy).

- Meiosis: non-disjunction can arise during meiosis due to: either (1) failure of a pair of homologous chromosomes to separate in meiosis I, or (2) failure of sister chromatids to separate during meiosis II.

• Mitosis: non-disjunction during mitosis arises when sister chromatids fail to separate.

Expert adviser: Andrew Jackson, Professor of Human Genetics, MRC Human Genetics Unit, Institute of Genetics and Molecular Medicine, University of Edinburgh, Edinburgh, UK.

References

Bradfield P, Dodds J, Taylor N. *AS level biology*. Longman, London, 2001.

Gardner RJM, Sutherland GR. *Chromosome abnormalities and genetic counseling, Oxford monographs on medical genetics no. 31*, 3rd edn. Oxford University Press, New York, 2004.

Kotzot D. Complex and segmental uniparental disomy (UPD): review and lessons from rare chromosomal complements. *J Med Genet* 2001; **38**: 497–507.

Chromosomal mosaicism—postnatal

Mosaicism is defined as the presence of two or more cell populations derived from the same conceptus that have subsequently acquired a genetic difference. Mitotic non-disjunction, trisomy rescue, or occurrence of a somatic new mutation can lead to the development of two (or more) genetically distinct cell lines. When post-mitotic non-disjunction involving an autosome occurs, the monosomy cell line is invariably lost and a trisomy lineage exists together with the euploid line, e.g. 47,XY + 8/46,XY. However, with mitotic non-disjunction involving an X chromosome, the monosomy line may persist, e.g. 45,X/46,XX/47,XXX.

Children may be referred after the laboratory has noted mosaicism, but note that screening for mosaicism is not routinely performed, except in girls with Turner syndrome. More commonly, the geneticist is requesting additional investigations because there are clinical signs suggestive of chromosome imbalance or mosaicism.

Mosaicism may be present on genomic array, but the software prediction may not 'call' the abnormality and the clinician needs to make the laboratory aware if you suspect mosaicism. SNP-based arrays are more sensitive for detecting mosaicism frequency than oligoarrays.

Clinical approach

History: key points

- Raised maternal age is a risk factor for trisomy (trisomic rescue can lead to mosaicism).
- Seizures common with some autosomal mosaic karyotypes affecting the brain.

Examination: key points

- Milder phenotype of known chromosomal condition (often mosaic trisomy 21 is detected in this way).
- Asymmetry, particularly noticeable in the limbs.
- Patchy or streaky skin pigmentary changes (hypomelanosis of Ito, diploid/triploid mosaicism).
- Sparse hair in the temporal region (Pallister–Killian syndrome).
- Ear malformation and preauricular tags (mosaic trisomy 22).
- Syndactyly and contractures of the fingers and toes.
- Deep creases on the soles of the feet and hypoplastic patellae (mosaic trisomy 8).
- Extra nipples.

Special investigations

- Genomic array (as discussed above).
- Conventional light microscopy karyotype is usually performed to confirm the array mosaicism result. Ask for an increased number of cells to be analysed. If 30 cells are analysed with no evidence of mosaicism, then this excludes 10% mosaicism with 95% confidence limits.
- If clinical suspicion of mosaicism remains, but array and lymphocyte karyotype normal, consider karyotype and genomic array from another cell lineage, such as fibroblasts, or DNA from a skin biopsy or DNA from a saliva sample. FISH analysis of a buccal smear may be helpful if you suspect a recognized mosaic phenotype.
- Clinical photographs.

Recognizable mosaic phenotypes

Diploid/triploid mosaicism

Arises from partial 'rescue' of a triploid conception with extrusion of the surplus pronucleus at the first cleavage stage and reincorporation at a subsequent cell division so the morula is mosaic (3n/2n). The affected fetus may not survive pregnancy, but some survive to term. Characteristic physical findings are syndactyly, especially of fingers 3/4 and toes 2/3, with bulbous ends of the toes and clinodactyly. There may be body asymmetry and streaky skin hyper- or hypopigmentation. The phenotype usually includes significant ID. Skin chromosome culture may be required to make the diagnosis. Genetic counselling is as for full triploidy. See 'Triploidy (69,XXX, 69,XXY, or 69,XYY)' in Chapter 5, 'Chromosomes', p. 694.

Mosaic tetrasomy 12p (Pallister–Killian syndrome)

As this mosaicism is not detected on routine postnatal lymphocyte testing, clinical recognition of the features is necessary in order that the laboratory can look for evidence of mosaicism in the array and to discuss which other tissues to analyse, e.g. salivary DNA sample. There is variable often severe developmental delay and seizures are common. The prenatal features are listed in 'Chromosomal mosaicism—prenatal' in Chapter 5, 'Chromosomes', p. 654. The facial features are characteristic. The forehead appears large, partly because there is a high hairline and sparse hair over the temples. The mouth is large and the philtrum appears full. Some children have mild coarseness of the facial features.

Mosaic trisomy 8

See 'Mosaic trisomy 8' in Chapter 5, 'Chromosomes', p. 674. The clinical features that suggest the diagnosis are deep longitudinal creases on the soles of the feet, absent or hypoplastic patellae, and contractures of the fingers. There may be no developmental delay or MR of varying degree. An association with haematological and other malignancies has been reported. A fibroblast culture and/ or salivary DNA may be needed to confirm the condition.

Mosaic trisomy 22

The phenotype is variable. Most typical are auricular, cardiac, and renal anomalies, atresia, and radial hypoplasia/aplasia. A Turner-like phenotype is also reported and the degree of MR is difficult to predict. The mosaicism is easier to detect on fibroblasts than in lymphocytes.

Mosaic marker 22

Most cases of CES are de novo, but familial transmission is possible. Urioste et al. (1994) reported a girl, her sister, and her mother who had a supernumerary marker chromosome 22 in mosaic form. Parental karyotypes are important, as some patients with mosaicism for a marker 22 have a normal phenotype (Crolla et al. 1997), and PND should be considered.

Hypomelanosis of Ito

Large areas of the skin may be affected by hypopigmented streaks or whorls distributed along the lines of Blaschko. It may be particularly striking over the trunk. The streaks are mainly present on the limbs and the whorls on the trunk. The lesions are much easier to see under UV light. Swirly hyperpigmentation may also be seen. Seizures and developmental delay are often found. Brain imaging may reveal a migrational abnormality. A mosaic chromosomal aetiology has been found to be the cause in ~60% of reported individuals. The myriad of associated features reflects the extensive variety of aneuploid conditions seen. This pigment pattern can also be seen in otherwise apparently normal individuals. Its cause in them is unknown, but it is presumed to be due to mosaicism for single genes controlling pigment production, particularly for XL conditions (Zweier et al. 2013).

Distinguish from IP. See 'Unusual hair, teeth, nails, and skin' in Chapter 2, 'Clinical approach', p. 330.

Mosaic variegated aneuploidy (MVA)

An AR condition predisposing to mitotic non-disjunction. Affected individuals have growth failure, microcephaly, and ID, often with other congenital malformations, e.g. CHD (Lane et al. 2002) and childhood cancers (e.g. rhabdomyosarcoma, Wilms tumour, leukaemia). Chromosome analysis reveals a heterogeneous mix of aneuploidies, sometimes with a gain or loss of two or three different autosomes in a single cell. Premature centromere separation is a feature in some, but not all, individuals. MVA is caused by biallelic mutations in *BUB1B* which encodes *BUBR1*, a key protein in the mitotic spindle checkpoint (Hanks et al. 2004) and in the centrosomal protein CEP57 (Snape et al. 2011).

Genetic advice

Recurrence risk

The recurrence risk is negligible for mosaicism arising from mitotic non-disjunction or somatic mutation, but a risk arises where it occurs as a result of trisomy rescue, because of the possibility of parental germline mosaicism. It is usually impossible to distinguish between mitotic non-disjunction and trisomy rescue. However, the overall risk to subsequent pregnancies is usually low, except for MVA which is AR with a 25% recurrence risk.

Prenatal diagnosis

Risks of recurrence for mosaicism are usually very low (but see exception below). PND can be offered for reassurance.

PND for MVA is possible (Plaja et al. 2003) and should be offered because of the high recurrence risk (25%).

Support group: Unique (The Rare Chromosome Disorder Support Group), http://www.rarechromo.org, Tel. 01883 330 766.

Expert adviser (first edition): R.J. McKinlay Gardner, Medical Geneticist, Genetic Health Services Victoria and Murdoch Children's Research Institute, Melbourne, Australia.

References

Crolla JA, Howard P, Mitchell C, Long FL, Dennis NR. A molecular and FISH approach to determining karyotype and phenotype correlations in six patients with supernumerary marker (22) chromosomes. Am J Med Genet 1997; **72**: 440–7.

Hanks S, Coleman K, Reid S, et al. Constitutional aneuploidy and cancer predisposition caused by biallelic mutations in *BUB1B*. Nat Genet 2004; **36**: 1159–61.

Lane AH, Aijaz N, Galvin-Parton P, Lanman J, Mangano R, Wilson TA. Mosaic variegated aneuploidy with growth hormone deficiency and congenital heart defects. Am J Med Genet 2002; **110**: 273–7.

Manasse BF, Lekgate N, Pfaffenzeller WM, de Ravel TJ. The Pallister–Killian syndrome is reliably diagnosed by FISH on buccal mucosa. Clin Dysmorphol 2000; **9**: 163–5.

Plaja A, Mediano C, Cano L, et al. Prenatal diagnosis of a rare chromosomal instability syndrome: variegated aneuploidy related to premature centromere division (PCD). Am J Med Genet A 2003; **117A**: 85–6.

Schinzel A. Catalogue of unbalanced chromosome aberrations in man, 2nd edn. de Gruyter, Berlin, 2001.

Snape K, Hanks S, Ruark E, et al. Mutations in *CEP57* cause mosaic variegated aneuploidy syndrome. Nat Genet 2011; **43**: 527–9.

Urioste M, Visedo G, Sanchis A, et al. Dynamic mosaicism involving an unstable supernumerary der(22) chromosome in cat eye syndrome. Am J Med Genet 1994; **49**: 77–82.

Zweier C, Kraus C, Brueton L, et al. A new face of Borjeson–Forssman–Lehmann syndrome? De novo mutations in *PHF6* in seven females with a distinct phenotype. J Med Genet 2013; **50**: 838–47.

Chromosomal mosaicism—prenatal

Mosaicism is defined as the presence of two or more cell populations derived from the same conceptus, but which have subsequently acquired a genetic difference. PND by CVS and amniocentesis relies upon the fact that the fetus, placenta, and membranes are all derived from the fertilized egg and therefore have the same genetic constitution. Occasionally, mitotic non-disjunction, trisomy rescue, or occurrence of a somatic new mutation alters this rule, resulting in two (or more) genetically distinct cell lines. When there is post-zygotic non-disjunction involving an autosome, the monosomy cell line is invariably lost and a trisomy lineage exists together with the euploid line, e.g. 47XY + 8/46XY. When non-disjunction involving an X chromosome occurs, the monosomy line may persist, e.g. 45X/46XX/47XXX.

See Figure 5.9 displaying various types of mosaicism.

Prenatal diagnosis

Mosaicism is diagnosed in 0.3% of amniocenteses and just over 2% of CVS samples (confined placental mosaicism in 1.9% and true fetal mosaicism in 0.19%). Mosaicism is often very difficult to counsel because, although measures can be taken to reduce uncertainty, it is often not possible to provide definitive guidance on outcome. The percentage of abnormal mosaic cells identified at CVS or amniocentesis does not reliably indicate the likelihood of true fetal mosaicism or correlate with phenotypic severity if fetal mosaicism is present.

The introduction of NIPT may also highlight the possibility of mosaicism for aneuploidy and UPD (Bayinder et al. 2015).

Embryonic derivations

- CVS. Direct (short-term culture (STC)) preparations reflect the karyotype of the chorionic cytotrophoblast;

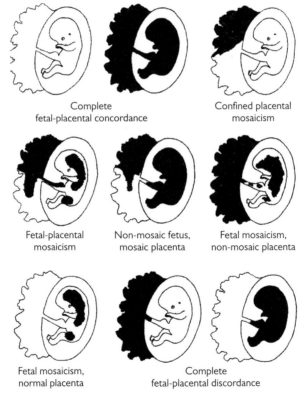

Complete
fetal-placental concordance

Confined placental
mosaicism

Fetal-placental
mosaicism

Non-mosaic fetus,
mosaic placenta

Fetal mosaicism,
non-mosaic placenta

Fetal mosaicism,
normal placenta

Complete
fetal-placental discordance

Figure 5.9 Types of mosaicism of the fetal–placental unit. The fetus is depicted enclosed in its sac to the right, with the chorionic villi comprising the placenta to the left. Grey areas indicate an aneuploid cell line; white areas indicate karyotypic normality. In reality, the distributions of the two cell lines are unlikely to be as clear-cut as is shown here. In the examples showing placental mosaicism, the path taken by the sampling needle will determine whether the abnormality is detected or missed at CVS. The cartoon of the fetus, sac, and placenta is close to the form and about two-thirds the size that actually exists at 10 weeks 0 days (gestational age as measured clinically, dated from the last menstrual period), when the crown–rump length is around 30 mm.

cultured CVS cells (long-term culture (LTC)) reflect the karyotype of the extra-embryonic mesoderm. Cultured chorionic villus cells come from a lineage more closely related to the fetus than direct preparations but are less closely related than amniotic fluid cells.

- Amniocentesis. Cells present in amniotic fluid (amniocytes) are a mixture of cells derived from the amnion, cells shed from the fetal skin, and cells shed from the fetal urinary tract. In order to help in the evaluation of mosaicism, three independent cultures are set up when amniotic fluid cells are cultured. If an *in situ* method is used, independent colonies are assessed.

See Figure 5.10 for cell lineages arising from differentiation in the very early conceptuses.

Definitions

- Pseudomosaicism. The mosaic cell line has arisen during laboratory culture.

- Confined placental mosaicism (CPM). Tissue-specific chromosomal mosaicism affecting the placenta only.
  - Type 1 mosaicism. Placental mosaicism confined to the cytotrophoblast.
  - Type 2 mosaicism. Placental mosaicism confined to the chorionic stroma (extra-embryonic mesoderm).
  - Type 3 mosaicism. Placental mosaicism present in both cell lineages (cytotrophoblast and extra-embryonic mesoderm).
- Classification of *in vitro* mosaicism detected at amniocentesis and CVS.
  - Level I. A single abnormal cell in a flask or colony. Almost always a cultural artefact and routinely not reported. (Worton and Stern (1984) found this in 7.1% of >12 000 amniocentesis samples.)
  - Level II. Two or more cells with the same abnormality in a single flask, or a single abnormal colony in

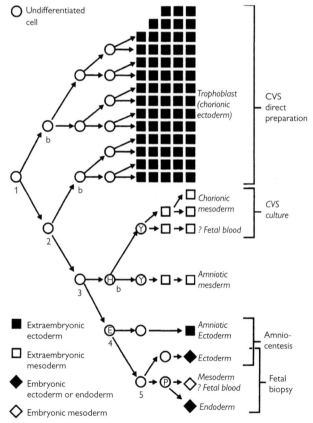

Figure 5.10 Diagram of cell lineages arising from differentiation in the very early conceptus. The fertilized egg (1) produces a trophoblast precursor (1b) and a totipotent stem cell (2), which, in turn, forms another trophoblast precursor (2b) and a stem cell (3) that produces the inner cell mass. The inner cell mass divides into stem cells for the hypoblast (3b) and epiblast (4). The epiblast cell(s) (5) produce the embryonic ectoderm and primitive streak, and the latter is the source of the embryonic mesoderm and endoderm. The cell lineages sampled at various prenatal diagnostic procedures are indicated on the right. E, epiblast; H, hypoblast; P, primitive streak; Y, yolk sac.

Reproduced with permission from Diana W. Bianchi, Louise E. Wilkins-Haug, Allen C. Enders, Elizabeth D. Hayal., Origin of extraembryonic mesoderm in experimental animals: Relevance to chorionic mosaicism in humans, *American Journal of Medical Genetics Part A*, Volume 46, Issue 5, pp. 542–550, Copyright © 1993 John Wiley and Sons.

an *in situ* culture. This is nearly always *pseudomosaicism*. (Worton and Stern (1984) found this in 1.1% of >12 000 amniocentesis samples.) The decision to report this finding is based on an individual case-by-case assessment, largely based on whether the abnormality in question is ever seen in live-borns, e.g. mosaic trisomies 8, 9, 13, 18, and 21.
* Level III. Cells with the same abnormality present in >1 flask; two or more colonies with the same abnormality. (Worton and Stern (1984) found this in 0.3% of >12 000 amniocentesis samples.) This is likely to be a true mosaicism, although not necessarily true fetal mosaicism (see below). In Worton and Stern's (1984) study, 60% of level III mosaicism identified at amniocentesis reflected true fetal mosaicism.

Clinical approach
The finding of a mosaic karyotype on CVS or amniocentesis always requires careful evaluation of the pregnancy as a whole to determine, as far as possible, whether the aberrant cell line is present in the fetus or not and, in the cases of chromosomes 6, 7, 11, 14, 15, 16, and 20, to consider the risk of syndromes associated with imprinting defects due to fetal UPD.

In preparation for the consultation:
* discuss the case with your colleagues both in fetal medicine to determine if there are USS anomalies which is invaluable to the counselling process and in the cytogenetics laboratory to have a clear understanding of the level/type of mosaicism and to plan for further investigations;
* consult a reference book, e.g. Gardner *et al.* (2011);
* undertake a literature search; Kotzot (2008) gives an excellent overview with guidance about testing for UPD and on the variability of UPD phenotypes and concludes that, as a general rule, prenatal UPD testing, following genetic counselling, should be considered if the mosaicism involves chromosomes 6, 7, 11, 14, 15, or 20. See 'Genomic imprinting', Chapter 1, 'Introduction' p. 30.

History: key points
* Brief family tree to include previous pregnancies.
* History of the current pregnancy.
* Raised maternal age is a risk factor for trisomy (trisomic rescue can lead to mosaicism).
* First-trimester screening results.

Examination: key points
Detailed fetal anomaly USS with fetal biometry and specific search for the structural malformations commonly encountered in live births with mosaicism for the chromosome in question.

Mosaic trisomy involving an autosome

MOSAIC TRISOMY 2. Trisomy 2 mosaicism occurs commonly in villus culture, and in most cases the +2 line is present in a small percentage of cells. True trisomy 2 mosaicism is seen in ~1/1000 CVS samples and usually represents CPM; in Sago and Chen's (1997) study, 11/11 had a normal outcome at birth. IUGR may be a feature of some pregnancies with mosaic trisomy 2 identified at CVS (Wolstenholme *et al.* 2001). Fetal trisomy 2 mosaicism identified at amniocentesis is extremely rare; Sago and Chen (1997) report one case with mosaic trisomy 2 and multiple congenital anomalies in 58 000 amniocenteses.

MOSAIC TRISOMY 7. May be identified at CVS but is rarely confirmed at amniocentesis. Most trisomy 7 detected at CVS probably arises by mitotic non-disjunction and is present as CPM. If mosaic trisomy 7 is detected at amniocentesis, the possibility of a meiotic origin with trisomy rescue raises the possibility of UPD leading to a Silver–Russell phenotype with IUGR (Warburton 2002).

MOSAIC TRISOMY 8. No consistent USS anomalies. No IUGR. Variable phenotype. Inconsistencies between CVS, amniocentesis, and fetal blood are reported. See 'Mosaic trisomy 8' in Chapter 5, 'Chromosomes', p. 674.

MOSAIC TRISOMY 9. Cardiac, renal, and brain abnormalities, microphthalmia. Most infants with mosaic trisomy 9 have severe MR.

MOSAIC TRISOMY 13. Holoprosencephaly and midline brain defects, facial clefts, polydactyly. See Wallerstein *et al.* (2000) for further details; see also 'Patau syndrome (trisomy 13)' in Chapter 5, 'Chromosomes', p. 678.

MOSAIC TRISOMY 15. The EUCROMIC study (Hahnemann and Vejerslev 1997) found that the trisomic cell line originates from a meiotic error in about 50% of cases of trisomy 15 CPM, the rest being the result of post-zygotic, mitotic non-disjunction. Amniocentesis is recommended following the finding of a mosaic or non-mosaic trisomy 15 by CVS, in order to check for both UPD (risk for Angelman syndrome (paternal UPD) or PWS (maternal UPD)) and potential true fetal mosaicism.

MOSAIC TRISOMY 16. Usually arises from trisomy rescue. Placental abnormality, IUGR from 16 weeks, structural cardiac defects (particularly VSD). See 'Mosaic trisomy 16' in Chapter 5, 'Chromosomes', p. 676.

MOSAIC TRISOMY 18. IUGR, rocker bottom feet, radial defects, cardiac defects. See Wallerstein *et al.* (2000) for further details; see also 'Edwards' syndrome (trisomy 18)' in Chapter 5, 'Chromosomes', p. 670.

MOSAIC TRISOMY 20. Most cases of apparently full mosaic trisomy 20 are associated with a normal phenotype. FBS is not helpful as the trisomic cells do not appear in blood. Hsu *et al.* (1991) reviewed 103 cases with a PND of trisomy 20 mosaicism through amniocentesis. Approximately 90% were associated with a grossly normal phenotype. James *et al.* (2002) undertook a retrospective review of 14 cases (13 amniocentesis, one CVS) that were ascertained antenatally, all with low levels of mosaicism (8–50%). In 12 cases, the children were physically and developmentally normal, with the longest follow-up being 10 years. Minor anomalies were noted in two and there were no major malformations. This series confirms a much lower incidence of phenotypic abnormalities associated with mosaic trisomy 20, compared to other forms of mosaic aneuploidy. James *et al.* (2002) recommend that, if a detailed anomaly USS is normal, parents be counselled that the risk of abnormality is <10%. Further tests should be performed only on the basis of a clinical indication. Cytogenetic follow-up studies in live-borns should include a culture from urine sediment (Hsu *et al.* 1991).

MOSAIC TRISOMY 21. Search for USS markers of trisomy 21. See Wallerstein *et al.* (2000) for further details; see also 'Down's syndrome (trisomy 21)' in Chapter 5, 'Chromosomes', p. 666.

MOSAIC TRISOMY 22. Cardiac and renal abnormalities, ear malformation, and preauricular tags.

Mosaic sex chromosome abnormality
See 'Sex chromosome mosaicism' in Chapter 5, 'Chromosomes', p. 688.

Mosaicism for a balanced or unbalanced translocation or other structural abnormality
Anomaly, cardiac, and growth scans. See 'Autosomal reciprocal translocations—prenatal' in Chapter 5, 'Chromosomes', p. 644 for details on *de novo* translocations.

Mosaicism for marker chromosome or ring chromosome
See 'Supernumerary marker chromosomes (SMCs)—prenatal', p. 692 and 'Ring chromosomes', p. 682 in Chapter 5, 'Chromosomes'.

Mosaic tetrasomy 12p (Pallister–Killian syndrome)
Diaphragmatic hernia, hydrops, relatively large fetal size. Detectable on amniocentesis and fibroblast culture, but only rarely found in FBS or postnatal blood samples. See 'Coarse facial features' in Chapter 2, 'Clinical approach', p. 106 for further details.

Management
The management of each rearrangement requires specific consideration. Close discussion with the cytogeneticists is recommended to establish if further invasive tests will resolve the question of fetal involvement. In about 50% of cases of level III mosaicism involving an autosome, the findings represent the fetal situation. Possible further investigations:

- amniocentesis if mosaicism was demonstrated in CVS. There is no indication for repeat amniocentesis if the mosaicism was detected at amniocentesis;
- FBS (cordocentesis) may be considered if the mosaicism was identified at amniocentesis or if (as in mosaic trisomy 8) there are instances of mosaicism at CVS not subsequently present in the amniotic fluid but present in fetal blood. However, in most instances, a normal fetal result does not help counselling, as a normal FBS will still not exclude the possibility of low-level fetal mosaicism and puts the pregnancy at increased procedure-based miscarriage risk. In Hsu and Benn's (1999) series reporting mosaic trisomy 16, trisomic cells were never seen in >1% of cultured lymphocytes and so FBS is unlikely to provide helpful information in that situation;
- UPD screen when the mosaicism involves chromosomes with imprinted regions. Parental blood samples may be required.

Important points
- If the mosaicism involves the sex chromosome, there are specific issues relating to the external genitalia, fertility, and gonadal tumour risk. See 'Sex chromosome mosaicism', p. 688 and 'Turner syndrome, 45,X and variants', p. 696 in Chapter 5, 'Chromosomes'.
- For balanced autosomal translocations, true mosaicism is rare and the risk of an abnormal phenotype is low. See 'Autosomal reciprocal translocations—background', p. 636 'Autosomal reciprocal translocations—familial', p. 640 'Autosomal reciprocal translocations—postnatal', p. 642, and 'Autosomal reciprocal translocations—prenatal', p. 644 in Chapter 5, 'Chromosomes' for more detail on *de novo* translocations.

- For unbalanced rearrangements, the risk is higher, and each case needs to be judged on its merits, following a thorough literature search. See 'Autosomal reciprocal translocations—background', p. 636, 'Autosomal reciprocal translocations—familial', p. 640, 'Autosomal reciprocal translocations—postnatal', p. 642, and 'Autosomal reciprocal translocations—prenatal', p. 644 in Chapter 5, 'Chromosomes' for more detail on the likely effect of unbalanced *de novo* translocations.

Genetic advice
Recurrence risk
The recurrence risk is negligible for mosaicism arising from mitotic non-disjunction, but a risk arises where it occurs as a result of trisomy rescue, because of the possibility of parental germline mosaicism. It is usually impossible to distinguish between mitotic non-disjunction and trisomy rescue; however, the overall risk to subsequent pregnancies is usually low.

Prenatal diagnosis
Can be offered in a future pregnancy for reassurance.

Support group: ARC (Antenatal Results and Choices), http://www.arc-uk.org, Tel. 0207 631 0285.

Expert adviser (first edition): R.J. McKinlay Gardner, Medical Geneticist, Genetic Health Services Victoria and Murdoch Children's Research Institute, Melbourne, Australia.

References
Baty BJ, Olsen SB, Magenis RE, Carey JC. Trisomy 20 mosaicism in two unrelated girls with skin hypopigmentation and normal intellectual development. *Am J Med Genet* 2001; **99**: 210–16.

Bayindir B, Dehaspe L, Brison N, et al. Noninvasive prenatal testing using a novel analysis pipeline to screen for all autosomal fetal aneuploidies improves pregnancy management. *Eur J Hum Genet* 2015; **23**: 1286–93.

Bianchi DW, Wilkins-Haug L, Enders AC, Hay ED. Origin of extra-embryonic mesoderm in experimental animals: relevance to chorionic mosaicism in humans. *Am J Med Genet* 1993; **46**: 542–50.

Gardner RJM, Sutherland GR, Shaffer LG. *Chromosome anomalies and genetic counseling*, Oxford monographs on medical genetics, 4th edn. Oxford University Press, New York, 2011.

Hahnemann HM, Vejerslev LO. Accuracy of cytogenetic findings on chorion villus sampling (CVS)—diagnostic consequences of CVS mosaicism and non-mosaic discrepancy in centres contributing to EUCROMIC 1986–1992. *Prenat Diagn* 1997; **17**: 801–20.

Hsu LY, Benn PA. Revised guidelines for the diagnosis of mosaicism in amniocytes. *Prenat Diagn* 1999; **19**: 1081–90.

Hsu LY, Kaffe S, Perlis TE. A revisit of trisomy 20 mosaicism in prenatal diagnosis—an overview of 103 cases. *Prenat Diagn* 1991; **11**: 7–15.

Hsu LY, Yu MT, Neu RL, et al. Rare trisomy mosaicism diagnosed in amniocytes, involving an autosome other than chromosomes 13, 18, 20, and 21: karyotype/phenotype correlations. *Prenat Diagn* 1997; **17**: 201–42.

James PA, Gibson K, McGaughran J. Prenatal diagnosis of mosaic trisomy 20 in New Zealand. *Aust NZ J Obstet Gynaecol* 2002; **42**: 486–9.

Kalousek DK, Vekemans M. Confined placental mosaicism. *J Med Genet* 1996; **33**: 529–33.

Kotzot D. Prenatal testing for uniparental disomy: indications and clinical relevance. *Ultrasound Obstet Gynecol* 2008; **31**:100–5.

Reish O, Wolach B, Amiel A, Kedar I, Dolfin T, Fejgin M. Dilemma of trisomy 20 mosaicism detected prenatally: is it an innocent finding? *Am J Med Genet* 1998; **77**: 72–5.

Robinson WP, McFadden DE, Barrett IJ, et al. Origin of amnion and implications for evaluation of the fetal genotype in cases of mosaicism. *Prenat Diagn* 2002; **22**: 1076–85.

Sago H, Chen E. True trisomy 2 mosaicism in amniocytes and newborn liver associated with multiple system abnormalities. *Am J Med Genet* 1997; **72**: 343–6.

Schinzel A. *Catalogue of unbalanced chromosome aberrations in man*, 2nd edn. de Gruyter, Berlin, 2001.

Schmid M, Stary S, Springer S, Bettelheim D, Husslein P, Streubel B. Prenatal microarray analysis as second-tier diagnostic test: single-center prospective study. *Ultrasound Obstet Gynecol* 2013; **41**: 267–73.

Wallerstein R, Yu MT, Neu RL, et al. Common trisomy mosaicism diagnosed in amniocytes involving chromosomes 13, 18, 20 and 21: karyotype–phenotype correlations. *Prenat Diagn* 2000; **20**: 103–22.

Warburton D. Trisomy 7 mosaicism: prognosis after prenatal diagnosis. *Prenat Diagn* 2002; **22**: 1239–40.

Wolstenholme J, White I, Sturgiss S, Carter J, Plant N, Goodship JA. Maternal uniparental heterodisomy for chromosome 2: detection through 'atypical' maternal AFP/hCG levels, with an update on a previous case. *Prenat Diagn* 2001; **21**: 813–17.

Worton RG, Stern R. A Canadian collaborative study of mosaicism in amniotic fluid cell cultures. *Prenat Diagn* 1984; **4**(Spec No): 131–44.

Deletions and duplications (including microdeletions and microduplications)

Chromosomal deletions and duplications are a major cause of human malformation and ID. Those caused by submicroscopic alterations were not readily detectable when a Giemsa-banded karotype (with a resolution of ~5–10 Mb) was the standard method for chromosome analysis.

The chromosomal phenotype

Many of the children with known microdeletion syndromes, e.g. Williams syndrome, VCFS, share a similar spectrum of abnormalities. Even though differences between patients are enough to distinguish some of these conditions by clinical evaluation, a common pattern of features emerges, including: (1) dysmorphic facial features, (2) unusual growth parameters, (3) developmental delay, and (4) characteristic behaviour that are suggestive of a chromosomal disorder. This has been termed the 'chromosomal phenotype'. However, as more microdeletion disorders are shown to be due to dosage alteration of a single gene contained within the deletion (e.g. KANSL1 in 17q21.31 microdeletion syndrome), the boundary between syndromic forms of ID and chromosomal disorders has become so blurred, such that the term is now less used. Instead, the pattern of features seen in the 'chromosomal phenotype' should be seen as an indication to investigate for a genetic cause (e.g. genomic array/panel/WES/WGS as appropriate).

Molecular karyotyping using arrays

Array-based methods for analysis of genomic copy number across the whole genome may use the level of comparative or absolute hybridization to non-polymorphic probes with/or without assessment of allelic imbalance at individuals SNPs. Compared with G-banded karyotyping, these technologies substantially increases the diagnostic yield and is now the recommended first-line genomic investigation in children with unexplained developmental delay/ID, autism spectrum disorders (ASD), or MCA (Miller et al. 2010) (see Figure 5.13). In comparative hybridization (see Figure 5.11), differentially labelled patient and reference DNA are co-hybridized to an array consisting of thousands of genomic oligonucleotide probes, whereas in absolute hybridization only the patient DNA is required; SNP arrays genotype a large number of polymorphic variants genome-wide to provide data from which regions of altered dosage can be inferred. Some arrays in current use combine absolute hybridization level and SNP approaches.

- 1-Mb array. Three thousand clones are selected to provide coverage of the human genome at ~1-Mb intervals.
- Tiling array. More than 32 000 clones provide complete coverage of the human genome.
- Targeted array. Clones selected to target specific regions of the genome, e.g. custom arrays to detect only known subtelomeric and known microdeletion syndromes.
- SNP array. Oligonucleotides, rather than clones, are used to give coverage of the genome at intervals, e.g. 10-k SNP array which can, like genomic clone arrays, be used to identify regions of copy number change in the genome. Data from SNP arrays can also be analysed to detect UPD/isodisomy and is more sensitive than aCGH at detecting mosaicism (though it will not be a good indicator of the percentage of mosaicism).

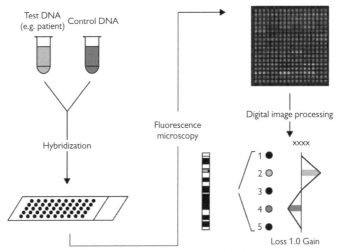

Figure 5.11 Schematic overview of the microarray-based comparative genomic hybridization technique. Test and control DNA are labelled with a green and red fluorochrome, respectively. Both DNAs are hybridized to cloned DNA fragments that have been spotted in triplicate on a glass slide (the array). Images of the fluorescent signals are captured and analysed. Red spots indicate loss of test DNA. Green spots indicate gain of test DNA, and yellow spots indicate the presence of equal amounts of test and control DNA. For a precise evaluation, test to control fluorescence signal ratios are measured for each single clone. These results can be translated in a high-resolution overview of chromosomal changes throughout the whole genome.

Polymorphisms/copy number variants (CNVs)

Large-scale copy number variations (deletions/duplications/amplifications) varying in size from 100 kb to 2 Mb are widely distributed throughout the genome, and a high proportion of them encompass known genes (Iafrate et al. 2004; Sebat et al. 2004). This high level of polymorphism may present challenges in interpreting the result of high-resolution genome-wide techniques and parental studies may be required to aid interpretation of the results. Note that clinical evaluation of the parent is needed to help decide whether a CNV is causative/pathogenic. It is apparent that many of the recurrent CNVs (see below) are variable in expression and may not be fully penetrant.

Subtelomeric rearrangements and deletion syndromes

Telomeric repeat sequences (TTAGGG) cap the termini of every human chromosome (see Figure 5.12). All ends of human chromosomes must have a telomeric cap to be stable. Proximal to these repeat sequences are chromosome-specific repeat sequences, which, in turn, are distal to gene-rich regions. Since the density of genes in the subtelomeric regions is high, small unbalanced rearrangements, e.g. deletions, may lead to a severe phenotype. If a telomere is lost in a terminal deletion, at least three mechanisms exist to maintain the chromosome end: stabilization of a terminal deletion through a process of telomere regeneration ('telomere healing'); retention of the original telomere, producing an interstitial deletion; and formation of a derivative chromosome by obtaining a different telomeric sequence through cytogenetic rearrangement ('telomere capture'; Ballif et al. 2004).

Terminal and subtelomeric deletions may be isolated abnormalities or may have arisen as a consequence of a reciprocal translocation and be associated with a duplication of the reciprocal chromosome.

Clinical features of the recognizable subtelomeric deletions

del (1p36)

Monosomy 1p36 is the most common terminal deletion syndrome (Heilstedt et al. 2003). There is developmental delay and seizures are commonly present. Hypotonia is a common problem in infancy, as well as feeding difficulties and oropharyngeal dyscoordination. Facially, there are deep-set eyes, straight eyebrows, and delayed closure of the fontanelles, and some have orofacial clefts. CHD may be a feature and Ebstein's anomaly and other tricuspid valve defects have been particularly associated with this deletion (Slavotinek et al. 1999).

del (4p) (Wolf–Hirschhorn syndrome)

Characterized by low birthweight and postnatal failure to thrive, microcephaly, developmental delay, and hypotonia. There is a characteristic facial appearance with sagging everted lower eyelids, a 'Greek helmet' profile, a short nose, and a very short philtrum. Patients may have iris colobomata. Seizures are common. Some have a visible deletion with varying breakpoints on 4p; others have a cryptic deletion, requiring FISH to make the diagnosis. From Shannon et al.'s (2001) study, a minimum birth incidence of one in 95 896 was calculated. They found that the crude infant mortality rate was 17% (23/132) and, in the first 2 years of life, the mortality rate was 21% (28/132). Cases with large de novo deletions (proximal to, and including, p15.2) were more likely to have died than those with smaller deletions.

del (5p) (cri du chat syndrome)

This ranges from large visible deletions to smaller deletions of p15 to pter. The characteristic feature is the cat-like cry. Mainardi et al. (2001) investigated the genotype–phenotype correlation in 62 patients with terminal deletions. They found more severe clinical manifestations and developmental delay/MR in individuals with large

Sequence organization of human telomeres

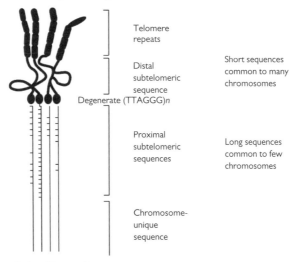

Telomere repeats

Distal subtelomeric sequence
Degenerate (TTAGGG)n

Short sequences common to many chromosomes

Proximal subtelomeric sequences

Long sequences common to few chromosomes

Chromosome-unique sequence

Figure 5.12 Sequence organization of human telomeres.
Courtesy of Sam Knight.

deletions. Their analysis of seven patients with interstitial deletions and one with a small terminal deletion confirmed the existence of two critical regions—one for the typical dysmorphic features and MR in p15.2 and the other for the cat-like cry in p15.3.

del (6p)

Several cases with microscopically visible terminal 6p deletions have been described, and a distinct clinical phenotype has emerged, including developmental delay and severe language impairment, congenital heart malformations, ocular abnormalities, hearing loss, and a characteristic facial appearance (Anderlid et al. 2003). Macrostomia and long, downslanting palpebral fissures may help define the phenotype. The forkhead transcription factor gene FOXC1, involved in a spectrum of anterior eye chamber disorders (Rieger anomaly, congenital glaucoma, and posterior embryotoxin), lies in the distal 6p25 region.

del (7q)

Sacral agenesis and anorectal malformations are associated with deletion of HLXB9 at 7q36 (Currarino syndrome). Deletions may also take out sonic hedgehog SHH and lead to holoprosencephaly. MR is also a feature.

del (9p)

This is a well-known and relatively common telomeric deletion, characterized by trigonocephaly, upward-slanting palpebral fissures, a long philtrum, MR, synophrys, coarse features, and epilepsy. Deletions of 9p24.3 have been associated with 46,XY gonadal dysgenesis and male–female sex reversal (Calvari et al. 2000).

del (9q)

This is a clinically recognizable syndrome characterized by microcephaly, MR, hypotonia, and seizures. Facial features include a dish-shaped midfacial profile, arched eyebrows, synophrys, hypertelorism, a short nose, anteverted nostrils, a cap mouth, a protruding tongue, and micrognathia. Other frequent anomalies are cardiac abnormalities, cryptorchidism, and hypospadias (Iwakoshi et al. 2004). Considerable phenotypic overlap with Down's syndrome in neonates and infants; this phenotype is Kleefstra syndrome and is caused by deletion or heterozygous mutation in EHMT1 located within the region of the chromosome 9q34.3 deletion syndrome.

del (11q)

Distal 11q deletions are known as Jacobsen syndrome. Thrombocytopenia/pancytopenia and cardiac defects are the cardinal features. Mild/moderate MR.

del (15q)

No reports of submicroscopic deletions. Larger visible deletions may lack IGFR1 and have features similar to those of Russell–Silver syndrome (Nagai et al. 2002).

del (16p) (ATR-16 syndrome)

Haemoglobin H disease and MR.

del (17p) (Miller–Dieker syndrome (MDS))

The clinical features of MDS are lissencephaly, microcephaly, and severe MR and the critical region is 17p13.3, which contains the PAFAH1B1 or LIS1 gene. Smaller telomeric deletions of 600 kb or less have been reported in normal individuals (Martin et al. 2002).

del (18p)

Microscopic deletions are associated with a 10% risk of holoprosencephaly.

del (18q)

(de Grouchy syndrome)   Poor growth, narrow ear canal and deafness, proximal thumbs, seizures, and MR.

del (22q13.3)

All individuals reported having severe expressive language delay, behavioural disturbance (hyperactivity, aggressive outbursts), and hypotonia. The facial dysmorphic features are subtle and variable. Overgrowth has been reported. Wilson et al.'s (2003) comparison of clinical features to deletion size showed few correlations. Some measures of developmental assessment did correlate to deletion size; however, all patients showed some degree of MR and severe delay or absence of expressive speech, regardless of deletion size.

del (Xp)

The clinical phenotype of the Xpter deletion in males is well described and depends on which genes are deleted (includes SHOX, CDPX, KAL, and XLI).

dup (Xq)

Distal duplications involving the Xq28 segment cause severe developmental delay in males with hypotonia, recurrent respiratory and other infections, abnormal genitalia, pseudo-obstruction, and premature closure of the fontanelles/metopic suture. The critical region includes the genes MECP2 and FLNA (Sanlaville et al. 2009).

Recurrent microdeletion and microduplication syndromes

Deletion and duplication are expected to occur as reciprocal events caused by low copy repeat (LCR)-mediated non-homologous recombination. Some of the microdeletion syndromes have a recognizable clinical phenotype and were described prior to routine use of microarray, e.g. Williams syndrome due to deletion at 7q11.23. Fewer of the duplications were clinically delineated as often duplication leads to a more benign phenotype than deletion, since trisomy is usually better tolerated than monosomy.

An example of a clinically delineated microduplication syndrome is duplication of 17p11.2 causing HMSN type 1A (CMT1A).

Until the advent of microarrays, inherited copy number variation in the absence of the same phenotype in the parent was considered benign, whereas de novo status supported pathogenicity. While this is broadly the situation for microdeletion syndromes, such as del7q11.23, with a clear phenotype, there are now several common recurring microdeletions and duplications showing incomplete penetrance and variable expressivity that are found at higher frequency in children with neurodisabilities but which may be inherited from an apparently normal parent. These CNVs have become known as predisposing or susceptibility loci for neurodevelopmental disorders.

Predisposing or neurosusceptibility loci

Many of these recurrent microduplications and deletions are factors in the pathogenesis of developmental traits such as autism spectrum disorders (see 'Autism and autism spectrum disorders' in Chapter 3, 'Common consultations', p. 350 for more discussion of the counselling complexities), schizophrenia, and epilepsy, but there are other genetic and environmental factors influencing the penetrance. In order to try and address the counselling of these families, Rosenfeld et al. (2013) have estimated

Table 5.5 Estimated frequency and penetrance of common recurrent deletions and duplications identified by genomic array analysis

Region (gene within region)	Copy number	Coordinates (hg18)	Frequency, postnatal aCGH cases	Frequency, controls	P value (Fisher exact one-tailed test)	Frequency of de novo occurrence in cases	Penetrance estimate, % (95% CI)
Proximal 1q21.1 (RBM8A)	Duplication	chr1: 144.0–144.5 Mb	85/48 637 (0.17%)	10/22,246 (0.04%)	<<0.0001	0/13 (0%)	17.3 (10.8–27.4)
Distal 1q21.1 (GJA5)	Deletion	chr1: 145.0–146.35 Mb	97/33 226 (0.29%)	6/22 246 (0.03%)	<<0.0001	7/39 (17.9%)	36.9 (23.0–55.0)
Distal 1q21.1 (GJA5)	Duplication	chr1: 145.0–146.35 Mb	68/33 226 (0.20%)	6/22,246 (0.03%)	<<0.0001	5/30 (16.7%)	29.1 (16.9–46.8)
15q11.2 (NIPA1)	Deletion	chr15: 20.3–20.8 Mb	203/25 113 (0.81%)	84/22 246 (0.38%)	<<0.0001	0/27 (0%)	10.4 (8.45–12.7)
16p13.11 (MYH11)	Deletion	chr16: 14.9–16.4 Mb	50/33 226 (0.15%)	12/22 246 (0.05%)	<0.0005	5/23 (21.7%)	13.1 (7.91–21.3)
16p12.1 (CDR2)	Deletion	chr16: 21.85–22.4 Mb	62/33 226 (0.19%)	16/22 246 (0.07%)	<0.0002	1/28 (3.6%)	12.3 (7.91–18.8)
Distal 16p11.2 (SH2B1)	Deletion	chr16: 28.65–29.0 Mb	46/33 226 (0.14%)	1/22 246 (0.005%)	<<0.0001	7/21 (33.3%)	62.4 (26.8–94.4)
Distal 16p11.2 (SH2B1)	Duplication	chr16: 28.65–29.0 Mb	35/33 226 (0.11%)	10/22 246 (0.04%)	<0.01	1/8 (12.5%)	11.2 (6.26–19.8)
Proximal 16p11.2 (TBX6)	Deletion	chr16: 29.5–30.15 Mb	146/33 226 (0.44%)	6/22 246 (0.03%)	<<0.0001	33/47 (70.2)*	46.8 (31.5–64.2)
Proximal 16p11.2 (TBX6)	Duplication	chr16: 29.5–30.15 Mb	93/33 226 (0.28%)	9/22 246 (0.04%)	<<0.0001	7/30 (23.3%)	27.2 (17.4–40.7)
17q12 (HNF1B)	Deletion	chr17: 31.8–33.3 Mb	29/33 226 (0.09%)	2/22 246 (0.01%)	<0.0001	5/9 (55.6%)	34.4 (13.7–70.0)
17q12 (HNF1B)	Duplication	chr17: 31.8–33.3 Mb	37/33 226 (0.11%)	5/22 246 (0.02%)	<0.0001	2/9 (22.2%)	21.1 (10.6–39.5)
22q11.21 (TBX1)	Duplication	chr22: 17.2–19.9 Mb	136/48 637 (0.28%)	12/22 246 (0.05%)	<<0.0001	12/47 (25.5%)	21.9 (14.7–31.8)

aCGH, microarray-based comparative genomic hybridization; CI, confidence interval; CNV, copy number variation; <<, much less than.

* Deletions of the proximal 16p11.2 region showed a maternal transmission bias (14/68 mothers identified to be carriers versus 0/38 fathers; two-tailed $P = 0.0018$, Fisher exact test); no parental transmission bias was detected for any other CNV.

Reprinted by permission from Macmillian Publishers Ltd: *Genetics in Medicine*, Rosenfeld and Coe et al., Estimates of penetrance for recurrent pathogenic copy-number variations, 15:478–481, copyright 2013.

a penetrance figure for the most common loci (see Table 5.5). At present, while these figures are a useful aid to counselling, there is no clear consensus about family cascade testing or prenatal testing because of the uncertainties of predicting outcome. For this reason, some laboratories and clinical teams reporting results from prenatal microarrays for diagnostic use (e.g. in a pregnancy for increased nuchal and fetal malformation) do not routinely report syndromes showing substantial levels of incomplete penetrance because the outcome is uncertain and they are unlikely to be the cause of the USS features.

Clinical approach

History: key points
- Draw a three-generation family tree (or larger, if indicated) and enquire about pregnancy loss, stillbirth, neonatal death, and family members with learning disability or congenital anomalies.
- Document all known malformations in the child and anthropomorphic data.
- Presence of developmental delay/MR.

Examination: key points
- Full clinical examination and documentation of dysmorphic features. See 'Dysmorphology examination checklist' in 'Appendix', p. 829.

Special investigations
- Note the importance of undertaking parental studies to determine whether submicroscopic chromosomal anomalies are inherited or de novo (many CNVs are non-pathogenic polymorphisms).
- Note the particular importance of parental studies for subtelomeric rearrangements, because of the possibility of a balanced cryptic translocation in one parent that may have implications for future pregnancies and for the extended family (see 'Autosomal reciprocal translocations—familial' in Chapter 5, 'Chromosomes', p. 640). NB. A genomic array may give a normal result in a parent with a balanced rearrangement, so alternative methods, such as karyotype/FISH/WGS, should be used.

Genetic advice

Recurrence risk
- De novo apparently isolated microdeletion or microduplication. This is very low (~1%), and the recurrence risk is due to mosaicism (either germline mosaicism or low-level gonosomal mosaicism) in one parent.
- Apparently identical microdeletion/microduplication in parent. If an individual carrying the deletion/duplication reproduces, the risk in each pregnancy for a child carrying the deletion/duplication is ~50%. If

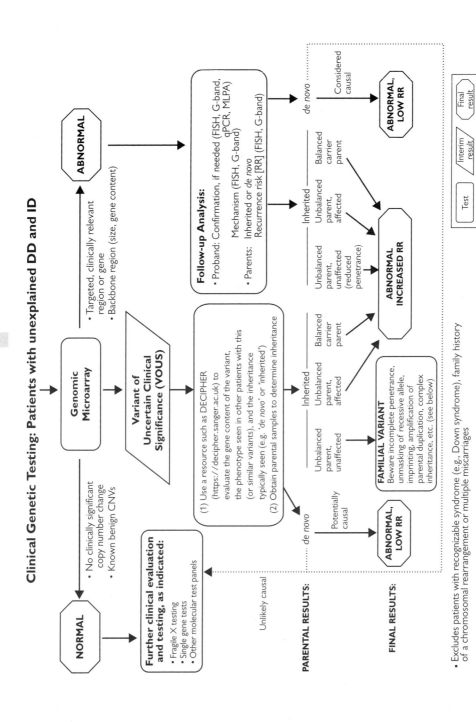

Figure 5.13 Adapted from clinical genetic testing: patients with unexplained developmental delay and intellectual disability.
Reprinted from *The American Journal of Human Genetics*, vol 86(5), Miller DT, Adam MP, *et al.*, Consensus statement: chromosomal microarray is a first-tier clinical diagnostic test for individuals with developmental disabilities or congenital anomalies, pp. 749–64, copyright 2010 with permission from American Society of Human Genetics.

the parent does not have any phenotypic abnormalities, consider the possibility of a polymorphism. If there is a discrepant phenotype between the parent and child, consider:

- a microdeletion unmasking a recessive phenotype, e.g. the CEDNIK (cerebral dysgenesis, neuropathy, ichthyosis and keratoderma) syndrome can be caused by 22q11.21 deletion on one allele and LOF mutation in SNAP29 on the other;
- an imprinted gene;
- incomplete penetrance;
- complex inheritance, as described in 'Predisposing and neurosusceptibility loci' above, for the predisposing or neurosusceptibility loci;
- further amplification of a duplication, e.g. a duplication in a parent expanding to become a triplication in the child or ab extension of a deletion;
- other possibilities.

Prenatal diagnosis

- *De novo* apparently isolated microdeletion or microduplication. PND is possible by CVS/amniocentesis. May be offered/requested for reassurance. Ensure that the phenotype matches with other case reports or with the phenotype of genes known to be deleted/duplicated in the rearrangement, i.e. that the rearrangement is truly pathogenic.
- Parent with an apparently identical microdeletion/microduplication. PND is possible by CVS/amniocentesis. It is offered to those families in which the deletion/duplication is the cause of abnormality. As this may involve the counselling of individuals with learning difficulties, take care to ensure that there is plenty of time for the consultation and appropriate consent for any intervention. Use caution when the abnormality is of variable penetrance (see above). If there is no apparent phenotype, the microdeletion/duplication may be a polymorphism for which PND would not be indicated.

Support group: Unique (The Rare Chromosome Disorder Support Group), http://www.rarechromo.org, Tel. 01883 330 766.

Expert adviser: David FitzPatrick, Paediatric Geneticist, Royal Hospital for Sick Children, Edinburgh, UK.

References

Anderlid BM, Schoumans J, Hallqvist A, et al. Cryptic subtelomeric 6p deletion in a girl with congenital malformations and severe language impairment. *Eur J Hum Genet* 2003; **11**: 89–92.

Ballif BC, Wakui K, Gajecka M, Shaffer LG. Translocation breakpoint mapping and sequence analysis in three monosomy 1p36 subjects with der(1)t(1;1)(p36;q44) suggest mechanisms for telomere capture in stabilizing de novo terminal rearrangements. *Hum Genet* 2004; **114**: 198–206.

Calvari V, Bertini V, De Grandi A, et al. A new submicroscopic deletion that refines the 9p region for sex reversal. *Genomics* 2000; **65**: 203–12.

Carter NP. As normal as normal can be? [comment]. *Nat Genet* 2004; **36**: 931–2.

Ensenauer RE, Adeyinka A, Flynn HC, et al. Microduplication 22q11.2, an emerging syndrome: clinical, cytogenetic, and molecular analysis of thirteen patients. *Am J Hum Genet* 2003; **73**: 1027–40.

Flint J, Knight S. The use of telomere probes to investigate submicroscopic rearrangements associated with mental retardation. *Curr Opin Genet Dev* 2003; **13**: 310–16.

Flint J, Wilkie AO, Buckle VJ, et al. The detection of subtelomeric chromosomal rearrangements in idiopathic mental retardation. *Nat Genet* 1995; **9**: 132–40.

Green EK, Priestley MD, Waters J, Maliszewska C, Latif F, Maher ER. Detailed mapping of a congenital heart disease gene in chromosome 3p25. *J Med Genet* 2000; **37**: 581–7.

Heilstedt HA, Ballif BC, Howard LA, et al. Physical map of 1p36, placement of breakpoints in monosomy 1p36, and clinical characterization of the syndrome. *Am J Hum Genet* 2003; **72**: 1200–12.

Iafrate AJ, Feuk L, Rivera MN, et al. Detection of large-scale variation in the human genome. *Nat Genet* 2004; **36**: 949–51.

Irving M, Hanson H, Turnpenny P, et al. Deletion of the distal long arm of chromosome 10; is there a characteristic phenotype? A report of 15 de novo and familial cases. *Am J Med Genet A* 2003; **123A**: 153–63.

Iwakoshi M, Okamoto N, Harada N, et al. 9q34.3 deletion syndrome in three children. *Am J Med Genet A* 2004; **126A**: 278–83.

Knight SJ, Regan R, Nicod A, et al. Subtle chromosomal rearrangements in children with unexplained mental retardation. *Lancet* 1999; **354**: 1666–81.

Koolen DA, Nillesen WM, Versteeg MH, et al. Screening for subtelomeric rearrangements in 210 patients with unexplained mental retardation using multiple ligation dependent probe amplification (MLPA). *J Med Genet* 2004; **41**: 892–9.

Lorda-Sanchez I, Lopez-Pajares I, Roche MC, et al. Cryptic 6q subtelomeric deletion associated with a paracentric inversion in a mildly retarded child. *Am J Med Genet* 2000; **95**: 336–8.

Mainardi PC, Perfumo C, Cali A, et al. Clinical and molecular characterisation of 80 patients with 5p deletion: genotype–phenotype correlation. *J Med Genet* 2001; **38**: 151–8.

Martin CL, Waggoner DJ, Wong A, et al. 'Molecular rulers' for calibrating phenotypic effects of telomere imbalance. *J Med Genet* 2002; **39**: 734–40.

Miller DT, Adam MP, Aradhya S, et al. Consensus statement: chromosomal microarray is a first-tier clinical diagnostic test for individuals with developmental disabilities or congenital anomalies. *Am J Hum Genet* 2010; **86**: 749–64.

Nagai T, Shimokawa O, Harada N, et al. Postnatal overgrowth by 15q-trisomy and intrauterine growth retardation by 15q-monosomy due to familial translocation t (13; 15): dosage effect of IGF1R? *Am J Med Genet* 2002; **113**: 173–7.

Rauch A, Ruschendorf F, Huang J, et al. Molecular karyotyping using an SNP array for genome wide genotyping. *J Med Genet* 2004; **41**: 916–22.

Rosenfeld JA, Coe BP, Eichler EE, Cuckle H, Shaffer LG. Estimates of penetrance for recurrent pathogenic copy-number variations. *Genet Med* 2013; **15**: 478–81.

Rossi E, Piccini F, Zollino M, et al. Cryptic telomeric rearrangements in subjects with mental retardation associated with dysmorphism and congenital malformations. *J Med Genet* 2001; **38**: 417–20.

Sanlaville D, Schluth-Bolard C, Turleau C. Distal Xq duplication and functional Xq disomy. *Orphanet J Rare Dis* 2009; **4**: 4.

Sebat J, Lakshmi S, Troge J, et al. Large-scale copy number polymorphisms in the human genome. *Science* 2004; **305**: 525–8.

Shannon NL, Maltby EL, Rigby AS, Quarrell OW. An epidemiological study of Wolf–Hirschhorn syndrome: life expectancy and cause of mortality. *J Med Genet* 2001; **38**: 674–9.

Slavotinek A, Shaffer LG, Shapira SK. Monosomy 1p36. *J Med Genet* 1999; **36**: 657–63.

Trask BJ. Human cytogenetics: 46 chromosomes, 46 years and counting. *Nat Rev Genet* 2002; **3**: 769–78.

Vissers LE, de Vries BB, Osoegawa K, et al. Array-based comparative genomic hybridization for the genomewide detection of submicroscopic chromosomal abnormalities. *Am J Hum Genet* 2003; **73**: 1261–70.

Wilson HL, Wong AC, Shaw SR, et al. Molecular characterisation of the 22q13 deletion syndrome supports the role of haploinsufficiency of SHANK3/PROSAP2 in the major neurological symptoms. *J Med Genet* 2003; **40**: 575–84.

Wilson LC, Leverton K, Oude Luttikhuis ME, et al. Brachydactyly and mental retardation: an Albright hereditary dystrophy-like syndrome localised to 2q37. *Am J Hum Genet* 1995; **56**: 400–7.

Yu W, Ballif BC, Kashork CD, et al. Development of a comparative genomic hybridization microarray and demonstration of its utility with 25 well-characterized 1p36 deletions. *Hum Mol Genet* 2003; **12**: 2145–52.

Down's syndrome (trisomy 21)

The chromosomal basis for Down's syndrome can be summarized as follows.

- 95% result from non-disjunction giving rise to trisomy 21;
- 2% result from Robertsonian translocation (especially 14;21), of which 50% are familial;
- 2% result from mosaicism, e.g. post-zygotic non-disjunction (most common) or post-zygotic loss of a chromosome 21 from a trisomic zygote (trisomy rescue);
- 1% result from a variety of chromosome rearrangements; trisomy for 21q22 confers much of the phenotype.

Rapid interphase FISH or qPCR analysis is possible for confirmation of diagnosis where there is high clinical suspicion of Down's syndrome. These are liable to error in detecting mosaicism and some rearrangements causing partial trisomies. Conventional karyotyping is therefore essential to determine the genetic basis for Down's syndrome, i.e. whether there is trisomy 21, a Robertsonian translocation, mosaicism, or an unbalanced chromosome rearrangement involving 21.

The incidence of trisomy 21 conceptions increases strikingly with maternal age (see 'Maternal age' in Chapter 6, 'Pregnancy and fertility', p. 754). There is a high incidence of spontaneous fetal loss during pregnancy. Between ~11 weeks' gestation and term, 43% of affected pregnancies are spontaneously lost, and between ~16 weeks' gestation and term, ~23% are lost (Hook 1992).

The observed live birth prevalence in England is about 54% less than expected, due to screening and subsequent termination, and has remained reasonably constant since 1989 at 1.0 per 1000 births (Wu and Morris 2013).

Clinical features

The neonate with Down's syndrome typically shows marked hypotonia, small ears, upslanting palpebral fissures, a flat facial profile, brachycephaly, etc. See 'Examination: key points' below.

Development

Milestones are delayed, with average age for sitting independently of 6–30 months, walking of 1–4 years, first words of 1–3 years, and toilet training of 2–7 years. Mean IQ in children and young adults with Down's syndrome is 45–48, but there is a wide range of ability. There is some correlation with parental IQ. An educationally based preschool teaching service, such as Portage, is often of benefit.

Education

The trend is towards integration of children with Down's syndrome into mainstream education with additional support, but some will benefit from education in a special school environment, particularly at secondary level.

Adult life

Most people with Down's syndrome will attain a degree of independence, managing their own day-to-day self-care skills and being able to communicate with those around them. Some may be able to live and work independently, although the majority will require some level of supervision on a daily basis.

Life expectancy

The average life expectancy for babies with Down's syndrome born in 2011 was 51 years and the median life expectancy was 58 years (Wu and Morris 2013). CHD is a major factor in increased mortality in infancy and childhood. Survival has increased markedly over a 10- to 20-year view, but nonetheless there remain significant differences in life expectancy, especially in those with CHD (Zhu et al. 2013). Survival figures for patients with Down's syndrome but without CHD (and with Down's syndrome with CHD) are: to age 1 year 90.7% (76.3%), to 5 years 87.2% (61.8%), to 10 years 84.9% (57.1%), and to 30 years 79.2% (49.9%).

Cardiac defects

Forty to 50% have heart problems at birth, half of which are serious and require surgery. The three most common diagnoses in live born infants with Down's syndrome in a Swedish cohort study (1992–2012) were AVSD (42%), VSD (22%), and ASD (16%) (Bergstrom 2016). AVSD, an endocardial cushion defect, is 1000 times more common in children with Down's syndrome than in the general population. Other forms of complex heart disease can occur, including overriding aorta and tetralogy of Fallot.

Other congenital malformations

Overall, the incidence of all congenital anomalies is increased >2-fold in children with Down's syndrome. Many congenital malformations occur more frequently in children with Down's syndrome, particularly duodenal atresia or stenosis and Hirschsprung's syndrome.

Other medical problems

Vision, hearing, sleep-disordered breathing, recurrent infections, coeliac disease, and diabetes. Hypothyroidism occurs in 20–40% and requires specific surveillance. The incidence of leukaemia is about 20-fold higher than in the general population and includes both acute lymphocytic leukaemia (ALL), which occurs in ~2%, and acute non-lymphocytic leukaemia (some of which are acute megakaryoblastic leukaemia).

Seizures

Infantile spasms (IS) or West syndrome (WS) is the most frequent epilepsy syndrome in children with Down's syndrome and occurs in a small minority of children with Down's syndrome (Arya et al. 2011).

Dementia

Adults with Down's syndrome are at very high risk of developing early onset Alzheimer's disease. It is uncommon before the age of 40 years. (Lautarescu 2017). Neuropathological changes appear identical to those seen in Alzheimer's disease.

Clinical approach

History: key points

- Family tree. If the karyotype is already known to be +21, only a brief family tree is required.
- Age of the mother at the time of the birth of her Down's syndrome child.
- Pregnancy history.

Examination: key points
Where appropriate, use clinical photographs to supplement the examination.
- Facial features with upslanting palpebral fissures, a flat facial profile, epicanthic folds, a short nose with a depressed nasal bridge.
- Brachycephaly and patent posterior fontanelle.
- Dermatoglyphics. Single palmar creases and a sandal gap between the hallux and the second toe. Usually, in normal individuals, there are whorl patterns over the hallux and the base of the first metatarsal. In Down's syndrome, the hallucal whorl is often replaced by a loop and the metatarsal whorl by an open pattern with gently curved lines over the ball of the foot.
- Hypotonia, e.g. marked head lag as a newborn. Hypotonia contributes to delayed motor milestones in infancy.
- Heart. Careful clinical assessment due to a high incidence of CHD (40–50%).
- Growth parameters. Height, weight, OFC. Plot on Down's syndrome-specific charts (see http://www.dsmig.org.uk/information-resources/growth-charts).

Special investigations
- Karyotype of the fetus/baby. Parental karyotypes not indicated if straightforward trisomy 21 or mosaic trisomy 21. Parental karyotypes are essential if a translocation or other rearrangement is identified.
- If a clinical diagnosis of Down's syndrome seems likely, yet blood karyotype is normal, consider mosaicism screen using genomic array or conventional cytogenetics and another cell line such as skin biopsy for fibroblast karyotype or buccal smear to investigate the possibility of trisomy 21 mosaicism.
- Echo, if Down's syndrome is diagnosed.

Genetic advice
Recurrence risk
Risk of recurrence of +21 is affected by maternal age and parental germline mosaicism; 10/842 (1.2%) in the Japanese series (Uehara et al. 1999) and 6/1211 (0.5%) in the Dutch series (Sachs et al. 1990) conceived another +21 pregnancy (combined risk 16/2053 is 0.8%). Data from Hook (1992) are stratified by age, but the resulting numbers are very small, and hence the CIs quite wide: at maternal age <30 years, 3/211 (1.4%); 30–34 years, 1/145 (0.7%); 35–39 years, 0/165 (0%); >39 years, 1/112 (0.9%), and total 5/633 (0.8%). Overall, advising a *'slightly <1% recurrence risk' (0.8%) for women <39 years with an age-related risk thereafter* seems reasonable.
- Some women who have had a trisomy 21 conception may have a small increased risk for other aneuploidies (Warburton et al. 2004).
- If the proband has trisomy 21, there is no increased risk to second- and third-degree relatives (Berr and Borghi 1990).
- After two trisomy 21 pregnancies, a 10%+ risk may be appropriate. Strongly consider the possibility of parental germline or gonosomal mosaicism. Examine the parents for features of Down's syndrome and do parental karyotypes with mosaicism screen. In the Dutch study (Sachs et al. 1990), 2/6 couples with recurrent trisomy 21 had evidence of mosaicism. If mosaicism is confined to the gonads, this will not be detected—hence 10%+ risk.

- *De novo* Robertsonian translocation—the risk is low, but recurrence has been reported (Sachs et al. 1990). If parental karyotypes are normal, the risk is certainly <2% (Steinberg et al. 1984).
- If the father carries a Robertsonian translocation involving 21, e.g. rob(14q21q), risk <1%.
- If the mother carries a Robertsonian translocation involving 21, e.g. rob(14q21q), risk 10–15%.
- If the parent carries rob(21q21q) translocation, the risk approaches 100% (unless trisomic rescue occurs).
- If a woman with +21 becomes pregnant, the risk of +21 in the offspring is ~50% (fertility in men with +21 is exceptionally rare).

Family history of Down's syndrome
- Single affected relative. If a sibling, aunt, or uncle has Down's syndrome, try to obtain the karyotype of the affected individual. If +21, there are no added risks to your patient arising from this. If the karyotype is not obtainable and the mother was <40 years old at the time of the affected child's birth, it may be reasonable to offer your patient a karyotype to exclude the very small possibility of a Robertsonian translocation involving 21.
- More than one affected relative on the same side of the family raises the possibility of a Robertsonian translocation involving 21 (e.g. rob14;21). A karyotype of your patient is essential, unless the family has already been carefully investigated.

Prenatal diagnosis
- Possible by CVS or amniocentesis.

Prenatal screening tests
- Nuchal fold thickness at 10–13 weeks' gestation with maternal serum beta-hCG and pregnancy-associated plasma protein A (PAPP-A). NIPT may be available. (Detailed USS alone has a poor detection rate, unless CHD is present.)

Management
At diagnosis, referral should be made to a paediatrician who is able to give the family information about the diagnosis, the likely prognosis, and associated medical problems. This may be a paediatrician based in hospital, a child development centre, or a community paediatrician. There should be regular paediatric review throughout childhood to consider the child's health and development, diagnose and treat associated medical problems, and refer on for therapy or specialist opinions. There should be a schedule of regular health checks for commonly associated problem, e.g. hearing , vision, growth, thyroid function (see schedule of suggested health checks from the Personal Child Health Record insert for babies born with Down's syndrome; guidelines for medical surveillance from the UK & Ireland Down Syndrome Medical Interest Group (http://www.dsmig.org.uk/publications/pchrhealth-chk.html); or health supervision guidelines for children with Down's syndrome from the American Academy of Pediatrics (https://pediatrics.aappublications.org/content/107/2/442).
Regular health checks should continue into adult life.

Support groups: Down's Syndrome Association, http://www.downs-syndrome.org.uk; UK & Ireland

Down Syndrome Medical Interest Group, http://www.dsmig.org.uk; MDS UK (Mosaic Down Syndrome UK), http://www.mosaicdownsyndrome.org; National Down Syndrome Society (USA), http://www.ndss.org.

Expert adviser: Elizabeth Marder, Consultant Paediatrician, Community Child Health, Nottingham Children's Hospital, Nottingham University Hospitals NHS Trust, Nottingham, UK.

References

Arya R, Kabra M, Gulati S. Epilepsy in children with Down syndrome. *Epileptic Disord* 2011; **13**: 1–7.

Bergstrom S, Carr H, et al. Trends in congenital heart defects in infants with Down syndrome. *Pediatrics* 2016; **138**: epub Jun 1.

Berr C, Borghi E. Risk of Down syndrome in relatives of trisomy 21 children. A case-control study. *Ann Genet* 1990; **33**: 137–40.

Bray I, Wright DE, Davies C, Hook EB. Joint estimation of Down syndrome risk and ascertainment rates: a meta-analysis of nine published data sets. *Prenat Diagn* 1998; **18**: 9–20.

Hook EB. Chromosome abnormalities: prevalence, risks and recurrence. In: DLH Brock, CH Rodeck, MA Ferguson-Smith (eds.). *Prenatal diagnosis and screening*, pp. 351–92. Churchill Livingstone, Edinburgh, 1992.

Hunter ASGW. Down syndrome. In: SB Cassidy, JE Allanson (eds.). *Management of genetic syndromes*, pp. 103–29. Wiley-Liss, New York, 2001.

Irving C, Basu A, Richmond S, Burn J, Wren C. Twenty-year trends in prevalence and survival of Down syndrome. *Eur J Hum Genet* 2008; **16**: 1336–40.

Lautarescu BA, Holland AJ, Zaman SH. The early presentation of dementia in people with Down syndrome: a systematic review of longitudinal studies. *Neuropschol Rev* 2017; **27**: 31–45.

Newton R, Puri S, Marder E (eds). *Down syndrome-current perspectives*. MacKeith Press, London, 2015.

Pangalos CG, Talbot CC Jr, Lewis JG, et al. DNA polymorphism analysis in families with recurrence of free trisomy 21. *Am J Hum Genet* 1992; **51**: 1015–27.

Roizen NJ, Patterson D. Down's syndrome [seminar]. *Lancet* 2003; **361**: 1281–9.

Sachs ES, Jahoda MG, Los FJ, Pijpers L, Wladimiroff JW. Trisomy 21 mosaicism in gonads with unexpectedly high recurrence risks. *Am J Med Genet Suppl* 1990; **7**: 186–8.

Steinberg C, Zackai EH, Eunpu DL, Mennuti MT, Emanuel BS. Recurrence rate for *de novo* 21q21q translocation Down syndrome: a study of 112 families. *Am J Med Genet* 1984; **17**: 523–30.

Uehara S, Yaegashi N, Maeda T, et al. Risk of recurrence of fetal chromosomal aberrations: analysis of trisomy 21, trisomy 18, trisomy 13, and 45,X in 1076 Japanese mothers. *J Obstet Gynaecol Res* 1999; **25**: 373–9.

Warburton D, Dallaire L, Thangavelu M, Ross L, Levin B, Kline J. Trisomy recurrence: a reconsideration based on North American data. *Am J Hum Genet* 2004; **75**: 376–85.

Wu J, Morris JK. The population prevalence of Down's syndrome in England and Wales in 2011. *Eur J Hum Genet* 2013; **21**: 1016–19.

Yang Q, Rasmussen A, Friedman JM. Mortality associated with Down's syndrome in the USA from 1983 to 1997: a population-based study. *Lancet* 2002; **359**: 1019–25.

Zhu JL, Hasle H, Correa A, et al. Survival among people with Down syndrome: a nationwide population-based study in Denmark. *Genet Med* 2013; **15**: 64–9.

Edwards' syndrome (trisomy 18)

Trisomy 18 is associated with a high rate of spontaneous loss in pregnancy and very poor outcomes in surviving infants. The spontaneous rate of pregnancy loss from the second trimester onwards is 36% (Hook et al. 1989). Trisomy 18 has an incidence of 1/7900 live births (Parker et al. 2003), with a strong female excess. The great majority are due to de novo meiotic non-disjunction. Eighty-five per cent are maternal in origin and there is a strong maternal age effect (as for trisomy 21).

Presentation may be:
- prenatal:
  - increased nuchal translucency and/or other suspicion, e.g. exomphalos at 11–13 weeks' gestation;
  - abnormal first- or second-trimester maternal serum screen profile (see below);
  - unexpected result at amniocentesis for another indication at 16–18 weeks' gestation;
  - abnormal fetal USS (IUGR, choroid plexus cysts, CHD (usually large VSD), renal defects, exomphalos, overlapping fingers, rocker bottom feet at 19–22 weeks' gestation). There are usually multiple anomalies;
  - IUGR often not noted until 32+ weeks' gestation, or polyhydramnios (30–60%), or IUD.
- neonatal. Neonate with growth retardation and dysmorphic features.

Ninety-four per cent of infants with Edwards' syndrome will have trisomy 18; the remainder have trisomy 18 mosaicism or partial 18q trisomy.

Clinical features

The most striking features in the newborn are small for dates, a short sternum, CHD, and abnormalities of the hands and feet.

Growth retardation

Mean birthweight 2240 g (weight, length, and OFC <3rd centile), with postnatal failure to thrive.

Dysmorphic features

Prominent occiput, simple ears, overriding fingers, often with camptodactyly, nail hypoplasia, short hallux, irregular ribs on chest X-ray, and rocker bottom feet (convex bottom to the foot with a projecting 'heel'). Very pale fundi.

Dermatoglyphics

Usually arches on all ten digits of the hands; this is rarely found in any other condition. (The lens on an auroscope (without the earpiece) is useful for visualizing the fingerprints in a neonate.) Now rarely documented.

Congenital anomalies

At least 90% have CHD, usually VSD ± valve dysplasia. The great majority have polyvalvular dysplasia. Both spina bifida and facial clefts occur more commonly than in the general population.

Developmental disability

Developmental quotient (developmental age/chronological age) averages 0.18, i.e. severe to profound developmental delay, but falls further in older children.

Short life expectancy

Median life expectancy is 4 days (range is large from failure to establish respiration at birth through to 2+ years). Cereda and Carey (2012) reported ~50% of babies with trisomy 18 live longer than 1 week and about 5–10% of children beyond the first year. Baty et al. (1994a) reported a child with +18 who was 19 years old. Seventy per cent of deaths are due to cardiopulmonary arrest; central apnoea is a major factor in the neonatal period and infancy. Survival time is increased for those infants treated intensively.

Wilms tumour has been reported in long-term survivors (see 'Management' below).

Clinical approach

History: key points

- Family tree. If the karyotype is known to be +18, only a brief family tree is required.
- Pregnancy history.

Examination: key points

- Growth parameters.
- Dysmorphic features. See 'Clinical features' above: prominent occiput, simple ears, overriding fingers, a short sternum, short hallux, rocker bottom feet.
- Heart.

Special investigations

- Full karyotype on pregnancy/baby (parental chromosomes not indicated if straightforward +18).
- Chest X-ray usually shows irregularity of the ribs.
- Cardiac echo.
- Clinical photographs.

Management

Nasogastric feeding is usually required initially, which may change to gastrostomy feeding in those surviving beyond 6 months. Gastro-oesophageal reflux is very common—consider prophylaxis. Older infants and children with Edwards' syndrome are at increased risk for Wilms tumour and hepatoblastoma. (The kidneys usually show fetal lobulation.) Photophobia is also common in surviving children.

Genetic advice

Recurrence risk

All sources agree that sibling recurrence risks for non-disjunction trisomy 18 are low, but different sources quote slightly differing rates. Sibling recurrence risk is 0.55% (1/200; Baty et al. 1994a). (0/170 recurrences of +18 in the Japanese series (Uehara et al. 1999) confirm the low risk.) De Souza et al. (2009) showed a higher relative risk for recurrence, particularly in women under 35 years. Cereda and Carey (2012) quote a !% figure to use for counselling.

NB. For mothers aged >37 years, the risk for a +21 pregnancy exceeds that for a recurrence of +18.

Prenatal diagnosis

Invasive PND by CVS/amniocentesis should be offered, but, in view of the low recurrence risk, some couples may prefer the option of surveillance of the pregnancy by a combination of:

- first-trimester screening. A first-trimester trisomy 13/18 risk algorithm is available that combines fetal nuchal translucency thickness and maternal serum free beta-hCG and PAPP-A to estimate risk (Spencer and Nicolaides 2002).
- NIPT. If available, offer NIPT using cell-free fetal DNA (cffDNA) from maternal serum;
- second-trimester screening. Maternal serum screen is now less frequently used. Median levels in pregnancies affected by +18 are all reduced (AFP, 0.43 MoM (multiple of the median); unconjugated oestriol (uE3), 0.43 MoM; and hCG, 0.36 MoM);
- detailed fetal anomaly USS at 19–20 weeks' gestation (high incidence of structural cardiac anomalies, choroid plexus cysts, IUGR, exomphalos, NTD, overlapping fingers, rocker bottom feet).

Combining the above, it should be possible to detect in excess of 80% of affected pregnancies.

Support group: SOFT UK (Support Organisation for Trisomy 18/13), http://www.soft.org.uk.

Expert adviser (first edition): John H. Edwards, Emeritus Professor of Genetics, University of Oxford, Oxford, UK.

References

Baty BJ, Blackburn BL, Carey JC. Natural history of trisomy 18 and trisomy 13: growth, physical assessment, medical histories, survival and recurrence risk. *Am J Med Genet* 1994a; **49**: 175–88.

Baty BJ, Blackburn BL, Carey JC. Natural history of trisomy 18 and trisomy 13: psychomotor development. *Am J Med Genet* 1994b; **49**: 189–94.

Carey JC. Trisomy 18 and trisomy 13 syndromes. In: SB Cassidy, JE Allanson (eds.). *Management of genetic syndromes*, pp. 417–36. Wiley-Liss, New York, 2001.

Carey JC. Introductory comments on special section: trisomy 18. *Am J Med Genet A* 2006; **140A**: 935–6.

Cereda A, Carey JC. The trisomy 18 syndrome. *Orphanet J Rare Dis* 2012; **7**: 81.

De Souza E, Halliday J, Chan A, Bower C, Morris JK. Recurrence risks for trisomies 13, 18, and 21. *Am J Med Genet A* 2009; **149A**: 2716–22.

Hogge WA, Fraer L, Melegari T. Maternal serum screening for fetal trisomy 18: benefits of patient-specific risk protocol. *Am J Obstet Gynecol* 2001; **185**: 289–93.

Hook EB, Topol BB, Cross PK. The natural history of cytogenetically abnormal fetuses detected at midtrimester amniocentesis which are not terminated electively: new data and estimates of the excess and relative risk of late fetal death associated with 47, +21 and some other abnormal karyotypes. *Am J Hum Genet* 1989; **45**: 855–61.

Marion RW, Chitayat D, Hutcheon RG, et al. Trisomy 18 score: a rapid, reliable diagnostic test for trisomy 18. *J Pediatr* 1988; **113**(1 Pt 1): 45–8.

Palomaki GE, Haddow JE, Knight GJ, et al. Risk-based prenatal screening for trisomy 18 using alpha-fetoprotein, unconjugated oestriol and human chorionic gonadotrophin. *Prenat Diagn* 1995; **15**: 713–23.

Parker MJ, Budd JL, Draper ES, Young ID. Trisomy 13 and trisomy 18 in a defined population: epidemiological, genetic and prenatal observations. *Prenat Diagn* 2003; **23**: 856–60.

Root S, Carey JC. Survival in trisomy 18. *Am J Med Genet* 1994; **49**: 170–4.

Spencer K, Nicolaides KH. A first trimester trisomy 13/trisomy 18 risk algorithm combining fetal nuchal translucency thickness, maternal serum free β-hCG and PAPP-A. *Prenat Diagn* 2002; **22**: 877–9.

Uehara S, Yaegashi N, Maeda T, et al. Risk of recurrence of fetal chromosomal aberrations: analysis of trisomy 21, trisomy 18, trisomy 13, and 45,X in 1076 Japanese mothers. *J Obstet Gynaecol Res* 1999; **25**: 373–9.

Inversions

Inversion

Arises after two breaks in a chromosome have occurred and the segment rotates 180° before reinserting. Individuals with an inversion have no phenotypic effect, unless there is chromosomal loss or there is interruption to gene function.

- A pericentric inversion contains the centromere.
- Paracentric inversion. The centromere is outside the inverted area; the inversion is confined to the long or short arm of the chromosome in question.

Submicroscopic inversions

Parental submicroscopic genomic inversions have recently been demonstrated to be present in several genomic disorders, e.g. Angelman syndrome (Gimelli *et al.* 2003), Williams syndrome (Bayes *et al.* 2003). Some progenitor parents carry inversions of LCR sequences and these polymorphisms facilitate misalignment and abnormal recombination between flanking segmental duplications, predisposing to deletion.

De novo apparently balanced chromosome inversions associated with an abnormal phenotype

If it is *de novo*, the chance of a chromosome inversion being the cause of the phenotype is possible (Schluth-Bolard *et al.* 2013) and the following possibilities also need to be considered.

- The inversion is actually unbalanced.
- There is abnormal gene function as a consequence of the break.
- The inversion is unmasking a recessive allele on the normal homologue.

High-resolution arrays have revealed an increased complexity to some *de novo* translocations. Some have increased complexity at the site of the inversion with an associated deletion or other rearrangement, and a proportion may have a deletion or rearrangement elsewhere in the genome.

Clinical approach

Ask your colleagues in cytogenetics to produce an annotated photograph together with an ideogram of the chromosome involved in the inversion. This is an invaluable aid to counselling.

History: key points

- Three-generation family tree, unless the inversion is known to be *de novo*.

Examination: key points

- Ascertain that the phenotype of those carrying the inversion is normal.

Investigations

If there is an abnormal phenotype, undertake genomic array analysis and if the array analysis is normal, consider next-generation sequencing.

Genetic advice

Familial autosomal pericentric inversions

Many pericentric inversions are not associated with a significant risk for offspring with chromosomal imbalance. Of normal offspring, half will have the inversion

and half a normal karyotype. Abnormal gametes are only produced if there is a cross-over between the normal and the inverted chromosome leading to a deletion or duplication. All the recombinants have duplication of one of the non-inverted segments and deficiency of the other.

The main issue is to determine the risk of viable imbalance. The risk of a chromosomally abnormal child depends on the size and type of inversion. Each individual inversion carries its own risk. This is highest when potential imbalance is small and has been documented in the literature as viable (see Ishii *et al.* 1997 or Gardner *et al.* 2011). Recombinants of inversion involving 13, 18, and 21 may be viable, so offer prenatal testing. Some general principles apply.

- Large, symmetrical, pericentric inversion. Small distal segments lead to the possibility of a viable recombinant. Larger distal segments would result in a greater degree of imbalance. This may contribute to infertility or miscarriage, but a low risk of a live-born child with imbalance.
- Small inversions are too small to allow a loop to form and the risk of a viable abnormal offspring is low.
- 'Normal variants'. Certain pericentric inversions are considered polymorphic variants. They appear to have no effect on fertility and no excess of abnormal offspring. These inversions may not be routinely reported by the laboratory or may be classified as a polymorphic variant on a report.

Familial autosomal paracentric inversions

Madan (1995) reviewed 184 cases and concluded that most paracentric inversions are harmless and that the risk of heterozygotes having a child with an unbalanced karyotype is low. Most paracentric inversions are found fortuitously. If recombination occurs, the recombinant products would have two centromeres or no centromere at all and the risk of a viable pregnancy in most situations is low. However, in some cases, it is difficult on a G-banded karyotype to distinguish between a paracentric inversion and a paracentric insertion. The distinction is important because the risk of viable imbalance in the latter case is about 15%. FISH or primed *in situ* labelling (PRINS) studies may be helpful.

Recurrence/offspring risk

- Ten to 15% in families where there has been a previous live birth with an unbalanced recombinant karyotype.
- Discuss each case with laboratory colleagues if there is no help from the family history. The highest risk of a viable pregnancy will be in carriers of large, symmetrical, pericentric inversions with breakpoints close to the telomere and the recombinants of inversions involving chromosomes 13, 18, and 21.

Prenatal diagnosis

PND by CVS/amniocentesis is offered when there is a significant risk of birth of a recombinant offspring.

Management

Family testing may generate unnecessary anxiety and pregnancy testing—consult with laboratory colleagues. Cascade screening of families for carriers of an inversion is not generally undertaken when the risk of viable imbalance is <0.5%.

Support group: Unique (The Rare Chromosome Disorder Support Group, http://www.rarechromo.org, Tel. 01883 330 766.

Expert adviser: Bert de Vries, Clinical Geneticist, Department of Human Genetics, University Hospital Nijmegen, Nijmegen, The Netherlands.

References

Bayes M, Magano LF, Rivera N, Flores R, Pérez Jurado LA. Mutational mechanisms of Williams–Beuren syndrome deletions. *Am J Hum Genet* 2003; **73**: 131–51.

Gardner RJM, Sutherland GR, Shaffer LG. *Chromosome abnormalities and genetic counseling, Oxford monographs on medical genetics no. 31*, 4th edn. Oxford University Press, New York, 2011.

Gimelli G, Pujana MA, Patricelli MG, *et al.* Genomic inversions of human chromosome 15q11–q13 in mothers of Angelman syndrome patients with class II (BP2/3) deletions. *Hum Mol Genet* 2003; **12**: 849–58.

Ishii F, Fujita H, Nagai A, *et al.* Case report of rec (7)dup (7q)inv (7) (p22q22) and a review of the recombinants resulting from parental pericentric inversions on any chromosomes. *Am J Med Genet* 1997; **73**: 290–5.

Kaiser P. Pericentric inversions. Problems and significance for clinical genetics. *Hum Genet* 1984; **68**: 1–47.

Madan K. Paracentric inversions: a review. *Hum Genet* 1995; **96**: 503–15.

Madan K, Nieuwint AW. Reproductive risks for paracentric inversion heterozygotes: inversion or insertion? That is the question [review]. *Am J Med Genet* 2002; **107**: 340–3.

Schluth-Bolard C, Labalme A, Cordier MP, *et al.* Breakpoint mapping by next generation sequencing reveals causative gene disruption in patients carrying apparently balanced chromosome rearrangements with intellectual deficiency and/or congenital malformations. *J Med Genet* 2013; **50**: 144–50.

Mosaic trisomy 8

Mosaic trisomy 8 is a well-recognized syndrome (see below), with an incidence of ~1/30 000 live births. The abnormal cell line tends to disappear from lymphocytes with age; a skin biopsy may be needed to make the diagnosis. There is an M:F ratio of 5:1. Life expectancy is usually normal and most infants have normal birthweight.

Clinical features

- MR. IQ 40–75, but occasionally near normal intelligence.
- Dysmorphic facies with a high prominent forehead and scaphocephaly.
- Contractures of fingers and toes (70%).
- Spinal deformity (65%), e.g. scoliosis, hemivertebrae.
- Cardiac anomalies (25%).
- Renal anomalies.
- Deep palmar, and especially plantar, creases/furrows (75%).
- Agenesis/hypoplasia of the corpus callosum.

Identification at prenatal diagnosis (CVS/amniocentesis)

The identification of mosaic trisomy 8 at CVS is problematic. Empirical observations suggest that, in the majority of cases, there is confined placental mosaicism (CPM) with karyotypic discordance between the placenta and fetus and a normal fetal karyotype. However, the incidence of genuine fetal mosaicism is sufficient that further investigation, e.g. amniocentesis and/or FBS, is indicated. Although further investigations may help to reduce uncertainty, it is not possible to completely eliminate the possibility of fetal mosaicism.

The percentage of abnormal mosaic cells identified at CVS or amniocentesis does not indicate the likelihood of true fetal mosaicism or correlate with phenotypic severity if fetal mosaicism is present.

Clinical approach

History: key points

- Brief family tree to include the nuclear family and previous pregnancies.
- Detailed history of pregnancy and events leading to prenatal investigation. If abnormal fetal USS was the indication, then the finding of +8 mosaicism at CVS/amniocentesis strongly indicates true fetal mosaicism. However, it is more usual that +8 mosaicism is found incidentally during karyotyping for maternal age or increased risk based on maternal serum screening.

Examination: key points

- Prenatal. Detailed fetal anomaly USS with fetal biometry and specific search for spinal, cardiac, and renal malformations.
- Postnatal. Detailed examination with measurement of growth parameters and clinical photographs.

Special investigations

- Amniocentesis (if mosaicism was demonstrated in CVS); there is little justification for repeat amniocentesis if the initial investigation was an amniocentesis.
- FBS (cordocentesis) is advocated by van Haelst *et al.* (2001) if there are USS abnormalities, as false-negative +8 mosaicism has been described following amniocentesis.

Genetic advice

Recurrence risk

Full trisomy 8 is not viable but is sometimes seen in spontaneous pregnancy losses; it arises from errors in maternal meiosis. Mosaic trisomy 8 mainly arises from a euploid conceptus by mitotic non-disjunction, i.e. post-zygotic error. Recurrence risk for mosaic trisomy 8 is therefore negligible.

Prenatal diagnosis

Following a diagnosis of mosaic trisomy 8, an amniocentesis can be offered for reassurance in a subsequent pregnancy, but recurrence risks are lower than the procedure-related risks.

Support group: Unique (The Rare Chromosome Disorder Support Group), http://www.rarechromo.org, Tel. 01883 330 766.

Expert adviser (first edition): R.J. McKinlay Gardner, Medical Geneticist, Genetic Health Services Victoria and Murdoch Children's Research Institute, Melbourne, Australia.

References

Association of Clinical Cytogeneticists (ACC) Working Party on Chorionic Villi in Prenatal Diagnosis. Cytogenetic analysis of chorionic villi for prenatal diagnosis: an ACC collaborative study of U.K. data. *Prenat Diagn* 1994; **14**: 363–79.

van Haelst MM, Van Opstal D, Lindhout D, Los FJ. Management of prenatally detected trisomy 8 mosaicism. *Prenat Diagn* 2001; **21**: 1075–8.

Webb AL, Wolstenholme J, Evans J, Macphail S, Goodship J. Prenatal diagnosis of mosaic trisomy 8 with investigations of the extent and origin of trisomic cells. *Prenat Diagn* 1998; **18**: 737–41.

Mosaic trisomy 16

Trisomy 16 is the most commonly observed trisomy in spontaneous abortions. It occurs in ~1.5% of all clinically detected pregnancies and ~7.5% of all miscarriages. In pregnancies with full trisomy 16, only minimal embryonic development occurs. In virtually all cases, a trisomy 16 conceptus arises from errors in maternal meiosis I. Mosaic trisomy 16 arises by trisomy rescue and there is therefore a risk for maternal UPD.

In the UK, the Association for Clinical Cytogenetics (ACC) guidelines for UPD testing with trisomy 16 states: 'In cases where UPD is excluded, there is still a significant risk of adverse fetal outcome (as judged by lower birth weight and/or fetal malformation). This is attributable to the presence of confined placental mosaicism or cryptic trisomy 16 mosaicism in the fetus or both (Yong et al. 2002, 2003) For this reason, it is particularly important that the implications of a negative UPD result are considered and understood before such testing is initiated.' Eggermann et al. (2004) also conclude that UPD 16 studies in pregnancy do not alter management because of the overlapping features of maternal UPD 16 and biparental disomy 16.

Trisomy 16 detected by CVS most often represents CPM, which can be associated with IUGR, but rarely other phenotypic anomalies. Even when trisomy 16 is confined to the placenta, there is a substantial risk for adverse pregnancy outcomes, e.g. IUGR with IUD, stillbirth, or preterm delivery (possibly due to placental malfunction).

Trisomy 16 detected at amniocentesis is often indicative of true fetal mosaicism that can lead to phenotypic anomalies. In Hsu et al.'s (1998) series where confirmatory chromosome analysis was conducted, 5/8 cases of mosaic trisomy 16 identified at amniocentesis represented true fetal mosaicism and 3/8 represented CPM.

Clinical features

Thirty-three cases of mosaic trisomy, of which 16 were identified at amniocentesis, were reviewed by Hsu et al. (1998). Of 21 continuing pregnancies, 16 (77%) had abnormal outcomes, including neonatal death or liveborns with some combination of IUGR, premature delivery (high risk: 5/5 continuing pregnancies in Hsu et al.'s (1998) personal series were delivered at 29–36 weeks' gestation), CHD, and minor anomalies. The remaining five pregnancies produced infants with an apparently normal phenotype at birth. Ten of 12 (83%) terminated fetuses had an abnormal phenotype. In 20 of the reported cases, the placenta or other extra-embryonic tissues were available for study and 19 (95%) had cells with trisomy 16.

Clinical approach

History: key points
- Brief family tree to include the nuclear family and previous pregnancies.

- Detailed history of pregnancy and events leading to prenatal investigation. Some mosaic +16 pregnancies present with abnormal maternal serum markers (increased AFP or hCG).

Examination: key points
- Prenatal. Detailed fetal anomaly USS with fetal biometry and specific search for structural malformations, e.g. CHD.
- Postnatal. Detailed examination with measurement of growth parameters and clinical photographs.

Special investigations
- Amniocentesis (if mosaicism was demonstrated in CVS). There is little justification for repeat amniocentesis if the initial investigation was an amniocentesis.
- FBS (cordocentesis). In Hsu et al.'s (1998) series, +16 cells were never seen in >1% of cultured lymphocytes and so FBS is unlikely to provide helpful information (see also the table in Hsu et al. (1998) where +16 cells were never identified in fetal blood samples, even in cases with adverse outcomes, e.g. stillbirth or neonatal death).

Genetic advice

Recurrence risk
- Low risk for subsequent pregnancies.

Prenatal diagnosis
- Can be offered for reassurance.

Support group: ARC (Antenatal Results and Choices), http://www.arc-uk.org, Tel. 0207 631 0285.

Expert adviser (first edition): R.J. McKinlay Gardner, Medical Geneticist, Genetic Health Services Victoria and Murdoch Children's Research Institute, Melbourne, Australia.

References

Association for Clinical Cytogenetics. *Prenatal diagnosis best practice guidelines (2009)*, 2009. http://www.acgs.uk.com/media/765666/acc_prenatal_bp_dec2009_1.00.pdf.

Eggermann T, Curtis M, Zerres K, Hughes HE. Maternal uniparental disomy 16 and genetic counseling: new case and survey of published cases. *Genet Couns* 2004; **15**: 183–90.

Hsu W-T, Schepin DA, Mao R, et al. Mosaic trisomy 16 ascertained through amniocentesis: evaluation of 11 new cases. *Am J Med Genet* 1998; **80**: 473–80.

Yong PJ, Barrett IJ, Kalousek DK, Robinson WP. Clinical aspects, prenatal diagnosis, and pathogenesis of trisomy 16 mosaicism. *J Med Genet* 2003; **40**: 175–82.

Yong PJ, Marion SA, Barrett IJ, Kalousek DK, Robinson WP. Evidence for imprinting on chromosome 16: the effect of uniparental disomy on the outcome of mosaic trisomy 16 pregnancies. *Am J Med Genet* 2002; **112**: 123–32.

Patau syndrome (trisomy 13)

Patau syndrome is associated with a high rate of spontaneous loss in pregnancy and very poor outcomes in surviving infants. The spontaneous rate of pregnancy loss from the second trimester onwards is 64% (Hook et al. 1989). Patau syndrome (trisomy 13) has an incidence of 71/9500 live births (Parker et al. 2003). Ninety per cent of cases of Patau syndrome have a trisomy 13 karyotype, while 5–10% are caused by a translocation, usually an unbalanced Robertsonian 13;14. A small proportion is mosaic trisomy 13. The risk of trisomy 13 increases with advanced maternal age, but, even at a maternal age of 40 years, the absolute risk for a live birth with trisomy 13 remains very low at 1/2000. Approximately 90% of trisomy 13 conceptions are due to non-disjunction in maternal meiosis I. The majority of trisomy 13 conceptions result in spontaneous abortion.

The median survival of affected infants in a study by Ramussen et al. (2003) was 7–10 days, with 5–10% surviving to >12 months. Hsu et al. (2007) reported a median survival of 95 days and considered that those infants without holoprosencephaly and exomphalos were less likely to miscarry or be detected prenatally, and survive the longest. Central apnoea may be an important factor in the short life expectancy. Cardiopulmonary arrest is the most common cause of death. Children surviving longer than average are more likely to be mosaic.

Clinical features

- Growth retardation.
- Holoprosencephaly (60–70%).
- Microphthalmia/anophthalmia (60–70%).
- Cutis aplasia (scalp defects).
- Cleft lip/palate (60–70%).
- Cardiac malformations (80%), e.g. ASD or VSD.
- PAP (60–70%) and/or limb reduction defects (occasional).
- Omphalocele.
- Kidney malformations.
- Severe/profound MR.

Clinical approach

History: key points

- Family tree. If the karyotype is known to be trisomy 13, only a brief family tree is required.
- Maternal age.
- Pregnancy history.

Examination: key points

- Growth parameters.
- Dysmorphic features. See 'Clinical features' above: cleft lip/palate, microphthalmos, PAP. Supplement examination with clinical photographs, where possible.

Special investigations

- Full karyotype on pregnancy/baby (parental chromosomes not indicated if straightforward trisomy 13).
- Echo.
- Cranial USS.

Management

Gastro-oesophageal reflux and feeding difficulties are almost invariable in trisomy 13. Aspiration during feeding or from reflux may cause cardiorespiratory arrest.

Genetic advice

Recurrence risk

Recurrence risk is low at ~0.5%. De Souza et al. (2009) showed a higher relative risk for recurrence, particularly in women under 35 years. In one Japanese series (Uehara et al. 1999), 0/46 women with a previous trisomy 13 fetus had a recurrence. NB. For some women, the maternal age-associated risk for trisomy 21 may be higher than the recurrence risk for trisomy 13.

ROBERTSONIAN TRANSLOCATION (13Q;14Q). Carriers of a rob(13;14) translocation have a small (1% or less) risk in each pregnancy of a live-born offspring with trisomy 13. All conceptions that are trisomy 14 will miscarry in early pregnancy. There is an additional small, <0.5% risk of UPD14. See 'Robertsonian translocations' in Chapter 5, 'Chromosomes', p. 684 for additional details and explanations.

DE NOVO ROBERTSONIAN TRANSLOCATION. It is rare for a de novo structural abnormality to recur in a future pregnancy. If parental karyotypes are normal, the risk is likely to be low (<2%) (based on Steinberg et al.'s (1984) figures for de novo 21q21q Down's syndrome).

Prenatal diagnosis

- Possible by CVS at 11 weeks' gestation or amniocentesis at 16 weeks' gestation. Because of the high incidence of structural malformations in trisomy 13, there is a high detection rate (~90%) on fetal anomaly USS. Given the low risks of occurrence or recurrence, some women may elect for detailed fetal anomaly USS, in preference to invasive PND, with recourse to invasive testing if any abnormality is suspected on scan. For a woman with a 1% risk of trisomy 13, the risk following a normal fetal anomaly USS will drop significantly to <0.5% (perhaps as low as 0.2%, based on a 1% prior risk and an 80% detection rate on USS). Spencer and Nicolaides (2002) have devised a first-trimester trisomy 13/18 risk algorithm, combining fetal nuchal translucency thickness and maternal serum free beta-hCG and PAPP-A, that will, for a 0.3% false-positive rate, allow 95% of these chromosomal defects to be identified at 11–14 weeks' gestation.
- NIPT, if available, offer NIPT using cell-free DNA (cff DNA) from maternal serum.

Support group: SOFT UK (Support Organisation for Trisomy 18/13), http://www.soft.org.uk.

Expert adviser (first edition): Ian D. Young, Consultant Clinical Geneticist, Leicester, England.

References

Baty BJ, Blackburn BL, Carey JC. Natural history of trisomy 18 and trisomy 13: I. Growth, physical assessment, medical histories, survival, and recurrence risk. *Am J Med Genet* 1994; **49**: 175–88.

Brewer CM, Holloway SH, Stone DH, Carothers AD, FitzPatrick DR. Survival in trisomy 13 and trisomy 18 cases ascertained from population based registers. *J Med Genet* 2002; **39**: e54.

De Souza E, Halliday J, Chan A, Bower C, Morris JK. Recurrence risks for trisomies 13, 18, and 21. *Am J Med Genet A* 2009; **149A**: 2716–22.

Hook EB, Topol BB, Cross PK. The natural history of cytogenetically abnormal fetuses detected at midtrimester amniocentesis which are not terminated electively: new data and estimates of the excess and relative risk of late fetal death associated with 47, +21 and some other abnormal karyotypes. *Am J Hum Genet* 1989; **45**: 855–61.

Hsu HF, Hou JW. Variable expressivity in Patau syndrome is not all related to trisomy 13 mosaicism. *Am J Med Genet A* 2007; **143A**: 1739–48.

Parker MJ, Budd JL, Draper ES, Young ID. Trisomy 13 and trisomy 18 in a defined population: epidemiological, genetic and prenatal observations. *Prenat Diagn* 2003; **23**: 856–60.

Rasmussen SA, Wong LY, Yang Q, May KM, Friedman JM. Population-based analyses of mortality in trisomy 13 and trisomy 18. *Pediatrics* 2003; **111**: 777–84.

Spencer K, Nicolaides KH. A first trimester trisomy 13/trisomy 18 risk algorithm combining fetal nuchal translucency thickness, maternal serum free β-hCG and PAPP-A. *Prenat Diagn* 2002; **22**: 877–9.

Steinberg C, Zackai EH, Eunpu DL, Mennuti MT, Emanuel BS. Recurrence rate for *de novo* 21q21q translocation Down syndrome: a study of 112 families. *Am J Med Genet* 1984; **17**: 523–30.

Uehara S, Yaegashi N, Maeda T, *et al.* Risk of recurrence of fetal chromosomal aberrations: analysis of trisomy 21, trisomy 18, trisomy 13, and 45,X in 1076 Japanese mothers. *J Obstet Gynaecol Res* 1999; **25**: 373–9.

Prenatal diagnosis of sex chromosome aneuploidy

PND of sex chromosome aneuploidy is almost always incidental, e.g. occurring as an unexpected finding in a karyotype performed to investigate a risk of Down's syndrome. Surveys of consecutive live births show that sex chromosome aneuploidy occurs in 1/400 live births, but, outside of formal studies, sex chromosome aneuploidies are rarely ascertained at birth or in infancy. The frequency at PND is even greater, estimated to be 1/250–1/300 (Ferguson-Smith and Yates 1984).

Sex chromosomes and NIPT

Depending upon the technology used, maternal sex chromosome aneuploidy should be considered when NIPT results suggest fetal sex chromosome aneuploidies (McNamara et al. 2014; Wang et al. 2014). Parents are usually distraught after the news of an abnormal prenatal result. Offering information about the implications of the test result for the pregnancy is entangled in the parental sense of loss for their hope for a 'normal' baby. Experienced and sensitive counselling is needed to try to help parents suffering from the recoil from 'bad news' to assimilate new information about conditions with which most are totally unfamiliar and to make considered and informed decisions about their pregnancy.

Clinical approach

- Take a brief history of the pregnancy and the indications for amniocentesis/CVS that led to the PND. If appropriate, emphasize that the information obtained was not that for which the test was performed, e.g. increased risk of Down's syndrome.
- Briefly discuss what chromosomes are and explain the unexpected findings in this pregnancy.
- Give an account of the particular sex chromosome aneuploidy identified (see '47,XXX', p. 628, '47,XXY', p. 630, '47,XYY', p. 634, and 'Sex chromosome mosaicism', p. 688 in Chapter 5, 'Chromosomes') and what the couple might expect if they continue with the pregnancy, e.g. baby looks entirely normal (with the exception of 45,X if there is a large cystic hygroma) and most would expect to attend mainstream school. Outline management plans (e.g. referral of a 47,XXY boy to a paediatric endocrinologist).
- Engage the couple in discussing their hopes and fears for the pregnancy; enquire about information they have received from other sources (other health professionals, the Internet, libraries), and assess and comment on its validity.
- For 47,XXY, 47,XYY, and 47,XXX, emphasize how infrequently these conditions are diagnosed, compared to the known frequency in the general population. This underdiagnosis reflects how infrequently individuals with sex chromosome aneuploidy come to specialist medical attention.
- Explore the choices open to the couple with regard to their pregnancy (e.g. continuing with or terminating

the pregnancy) and help them to discuss their options and facilitate their decision-making. Discourage a hasty decision, as the couple may need time to adjust to their new situation and assimilate the information provided.

'Patients suffer a loss when they receive a prenatal diagnosis about their fetus. The loss is often not of the fetus that comes to carry the diagnosis but of the fetus the parents hoped they carried. This grief is profound yet does not preclude a woman's ability to welcome an affected fetus into the world.'

Genetic advice

Recurrence risks for 45,X, 47,XXX, 47,XXY, and 47,XYY are all very low and probably not discernibly increased over maternal age-specific rates. PND in future pregnancies should be offered, but the indication for PND is rather weak and there is a fine balance between the very small recurrence risks and the risk of procedure-associated pregnancy loss.

Disclosure of karyotype

See Linden et al. (2002) for a full discussion of this topic. In general, disclosure of the karyotype on a 'need to know' basis is advised, so that the child is not treated differently or regarded differently by others.

Expert adviser: Angela Barnicoat, Consultant Clinical Geneticist, Department of Clinical Genetics, Great Ormond Street Hospital NHS Foundation Trust, London, UK.

References

Biesecker B. Prenatal diagnoses of sex chromosome conditions [editorial]. *BMJ* 2001; **322**: 441.

Ferguson-Smith MA, Yates JR. Maternal age specific rates for chromosome aberrations and factors influencing them: report of a collaborative European study on 52 965 amniocenteses. *Prenat Diagn* 1984; **4**(Spring; 4 Spec. No.): 5–44.

Linden MG, Bender BG. Fifty-one prenatally diagnosed children and adolescents with sex chromosome anomalies. *Am J Med Genet* 2002; **110**: 11–18.

Linden MG, Bender BG, Robinson A. Intrauterine diagnosis of sex chromosome aneuploidy. *Obstet Gynecol* 1996; **87**: 468–75.

Linden MG, Bender BG, Robinson A. Genetic counselling for sex chromosome abnormalities. *Am J Med Genet* 2002; **110**: 3–10.

Ratcliffe S. Long-term outcome in children of sex chromosome abnormalities. *Arch Dis Child* 1999; **80**: 192–5.

McNamara CJ, Limone LA, Westover T, Miller RC. Maternal source of false-positive fetal sex chromosome aneuploidy in noninvasive prenatal testing. *Obstet Gynecol* 2015; **125**: 390–2.

Wang Y, Chen Y, Tian F, et al. Maternal mosaicism is a significant contributor to discordant sex chromosomal aneuploidies associated with noninvasive prenatal testing. *Clin Chem* 2014; **60**: 251–9.

Ring chromosomes

A ring chromosome describes the shape of the chromosome as seen by light microscopy. This section refers to individuals with a 46,r(A) karyotype where the ring comprises a near full-length or full-length autosome. For information on supernumerary ring chromosomes (which are usually very small), refer to 'Supernumerary marker chromosomes (SMCs)—postnatal', p. 690 and 'Supernumerary marker chromosomes (SMCs)—prenatal', p. 692 in Chapter 5, 'Chromosomes'.

Rings are created when breaks occur in the short and long arms of a chromosome, with rejoining of the centric segment at the broken ends or by end-to-end fusion of the telomeres. There is monosomy for any deleted segments.

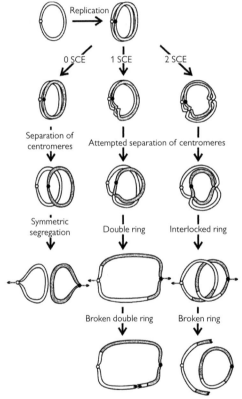

Figure 5.14 Dynamic mosaicism. The single chromatid ring chromosome replicates during interphase. Sister chromatid exchanges (SCEs) may or may not take place. At meiosis, if there are no SCEs (left), segregation is symmetric (dotted arrows represent spindles drawing homologues to opposite poles). If there is one SCE, a double-sized ring is generated (middle). With each centromere being tugged to opposite poles at anaphase (dotted arrows), the chromosome may break. If there are two SCEs in the same direction of rotation (right), the two rings become interlocked. Breakage or other mechanical compromise is the consequence. A second SCE in the opposite direction of rotation would restore the situation.
Reproduced with permission from Gardner RM, Sutherland GR, *Chromosome abnormalities and genetic counselling*, Oxford Monographs on Medical Genetics no. 31, Oxford University Press, New York, USA Copyright © 2004. By permission of Oxford University Press. www.oup.com.

The ring may be disrupted by mitotic cell division. The larger the ring, the greater the likelihood of disruption (see 'Clinical features' below). If the ring is lost, the resulting aneuploidy is likely to be lethal to that cell lineage. Mosaicism for the ring is a frequent finding. Dynamic mosaicism (see Figure 5.14) is sometimes observed where the size of the ring chromosome varies between different cells and different tissues.

Ring chromosomes are rare and most are sporadic. The ascertainment may be:

• during the investigation of a child with developmental delay, dysmorphism, and/or impaired growth—the most common presentation;
• fetal abnormality;
• an incidental finding at amniocentesis/CVS.

With arrays as the first-line investigation in many children, the clue to a ring chromosome is the loss of DNA from the telomeric ends of both arms of the same chromosome. Conventional karyotype will confirm the ring structure.

Clinical features

For all autosomal rings, including those rings that appear to have no loss of chromosomal material, there is a phenotype caused by disturbance to the growth rate. This is believed to be due to mitotic instability from abnormal segregation and sister chromatid exchange (SCE) in somatic cells. If SCE occurs, this prevents symmetrical segregation of the daughter chromosomes, predisposing to breakage of the interlocked or double ring. This is the likely mechanism underlying dynamic changes in the size of the ring chromosome and the tendency for ring chromosome to be 'lost' during cell division. This impairment of cell division may underlie the 'ring chromosome phenotype'. The 'ring chromosome phenotype' is a general phenomenon superimposed to a greater or lesser extent on the phenotype arising from any chromosome imbalance present in the specific chromosome involved in the ring.

'Ring chromosome phenotype'

• Growth failure/short stature.
• Microcephaly.
• MR (variable, but usually moderate to severe).
• Dysmorphic facial features.

Ring X

A ring/marker X chromosome can arise from both maternal and paternal meiotic errors. Large ring X chromosomes generally produce a variant Turner syndrome phenotype and often there is mosaicism for 45,X or 46,XX. Small ring X chromosomes with absence of the *XIST* gene leading to functional X disomy can produce a more severe phenotype with MR, which can be severe (Kubota *et al.* 2002).

Clinical approach

Ask your colleagues in cytogenetics to produce an annotated photograph showing the ring chromosome. This is an invaluable aid to counselling.

History: key points

• Three-generation family tree (unless the ring chromosome is known to be *de novo*), with specific enquiry regarding parental health, development, and education.

- Document the developmental history and medical problems of affected individuals.

Examination: key points
- Prenatal. Detailed fetal anomaly USS.
- Postnatal.
  - Anthropomorphic data: height, weight, and OFC (children with ring chromosomes are usually symmetrically small, except for mosaics with a normal cell line (i.e. those with rings of post-zygotic origin) who may be asymmetric due to different percentages of the abnormal cell line on either side).
  - Document and describe dysmorphic features, preferably supplementing this with clinical photographs.
  - Asymmetry or skin pigmentary abnormalities may be indicators of mosaicism.

Special investigations
- Screen 30 cells to investigate mosaicism.
- Genomic array to identify the chromosome of origin and establish the extent of genomic loss.
- Obtain parental blood samples (Li heparin and EDTA) for karyotyping and genomic array. Request 30 cell screen to investigate for parental mosaicism
- Consider FISH (*XIST*) in girls with r(X). Structural abnormality of the X may disrupt X-inactivation, causing functional X disomy.

Management
Search the OMIM gene map at http://www.ncbi.nlm.nih.gov/htbin-post/Omim/getmap to determine whether there are any disease genes of specific relevance within the deleted regions. Tumour suppressor genes and other important dominant disease genes may need specific surveillance.

Genetic advice
Ninety-nine per cent of rings are sporadic, but there are some familial reports. In a few instances, the ring chromosome has had a minimal or no phenotypic effect.

For the majority of individuals with ring chromosomes, there is associated MR. In 90% of the familial cases, the mother has been the transmitting parent. Ring chromosomes appear to be associated with subfertility in males.

Transmission from mosaic carriers (usually the mother) to offspring may occur, and the phenotype will be difficult to predict, but consider that it may be more severe than in the parent, since the child will inherit a non-mosaic 46,(r). Ring mosaicism in combination with a normal cell line has also been observed in the offspring of parents with mosaicism for a ring and is difficult to explain. This phenomenon may be due to ring opening (Speevak *et al.* 2003).

Recurrence risk
- *De novo* ring. After excluding mosaicism in both parents, the risk is likely to be low (<1%), but data are scant. This is presumably caused by germline association in a few instances.
- Familial (usually maternal). Offspring/recurrence risk is ~40%.

Prenatal diagnosis
- *De novo* ring. PND may be offered by CVS/amniocentesis for reassurance.
- Familial (usually maternal). As this may involve the counselling of individuals with learning difficulties, take care to ensure that there is plenty of time for the consultation and appropriate consent for any intervention.

Support group: Unique (The Rare Chromosome Disorder Support Group), http://www.rarechromo.org, Tel. 01883 330 766.

Expert adviser (first edition): A. Schinzel, Professor, Institute of Medical Genetics, University of Zurich, Schwerzenbach, Switzerland.

References
Daniel A, Malsfiiej P. A series of supernumerary small ring marker autosomes identified by FISH with chromosome probe arrays and literature review excluding chromosome 15. *Am J Med Genet A* 2003; **117A**: 212–22.

Gardner RJM, Sutherland GR, Shaffer LG. *Chromosome abnormalities and genetic counseling, Oxford monographs on medical genetics no. 31*, 4th edn. Oxford University Press, New York, 2011.

Ishmael HA, Cataldi D, Begleiter ML, Pasztor LM, Dasouki MJ, Butler MG. Five new subjects with ring chromosome 22. *Clin Genet* 2003; **63**: 410–14.

Kubota T, Wakui K, Nakamura T, *et al.* The proportion of cells with functional X disomy is associated with the severity of mental retardation in mosaic ring X Turner syndrome females. *Cytogenet Genome Res* 2002; **99**(1–4): 276–84.

Shashi V, White J, Pettenati M, Root S, Bell W. Ring chromosome 17: phenotype variation by deletion size. *Clin Genet* 2003; **64**: 361–5.

Speevak MD, Smart C, Unwin L, Bell M, Farrell SA. Molecular characterization of an inherited ring (19) demonstrating ring opening. *Am J Med Genet A* 2003; **121A**: 141–5.

Robertsonian translocations

These are named after WRB Robertson who described fusion of acrocentric chromosomes in insects. The human acrocentric chromosomes that may be involved in a Robertsonian translocation are 13, 14, 15, 21, and 22. The fused chromosome contains the long arms of the two component chromosomes but lacks some or all of the short arms. The short arms contain the nucleolar organizing regions (NORs), but as there are other copies of these genes, their loss does not have a phenotypic effect. Robertsonian translocations can be classified into two groups, depending on their frequency of occurrence: common (rob(13q14q) and rob(14q21q)) and rare (all remaining possible non-homologous combinations). The common rob(13q14q) and rob(14q21q) are dicentric structures. 'De novo' Robertsonian translocations most commonly arise during oogenesis (Bandyopadhyay et al. 2002).

The balanced carrier has 45 chromosomes. The karyotype of a Robertsonian translocation between chromosomes 14 and 21 in a female is correctly written as 45,XX,rob(14;21)(q10;q10), but often shortened to 45,XX,rob(14q21q).

Non-homologous (heterologous) translocation

Fusion of two different chromosomes, e.g. rob(13q14q).

Homologous translocation

Fusion between homologues, e.g. rob (13q13q). The two arms may derive either from fusion in the zygote of the maternal and paternal chromosomes (in which case the recurrence risk is minimal) or from formation of an isochromosome (Robinson et al. 1994). Isochromosomes, e.g. 45,i(21q) arise when maternal non-disjunction leads to the formation of a nullisomic gamete which results in a monosomic zygote which is 'rescued' by reduplication of the paternal homologue and vice versa.

Frequency

Approximately one in 1000 individuals are carriers of a Robertsonian translocation and the most common is rob(13q14q) with a prevalence of ~1/1300.

Meiosis

Alternate segregation produces normal and balanced gametes, and adjacent segregation produces disomic and nullisomic gametes. Monosomic conceptions either miscarry or do not even progress to a confirmed pregnancy. The main risk for an abnormal phenotype in the child of a balanced carrier is trisomy of 21 or 13 and UPD of 14 or 15.

Miscarriage

Pregnancies of balanced carriers may miscarry. Trisomy 14 and 15 will invariably fail, and most trisomy 22, many trisomy 13, and some trisomy 21 pregnancies will also miscarry. When one partner has a Robertsonian translocation, some couples suffer recurrent miscarriage. For carriers of der(13;14), Engels et al. (2008) reported a miscarriage rate of 28% in females and 20% in the partners of male carriers.

Subfertility

The literature has suggested that males have an increased risk of subfertility. Egozcue et al. (2003), using FISH to analyse decondensed sperm heads, showed, whereas 46,XY males have a mean incidence of disomic sperm (for any chromosome) of ~6.7%, men who are carriers of a Robertsonian translocation produce from 3.4% to 36% of abnormal spermatozoa. Male carriers of der(13;14) have been reported to have a 5- to 10-fold over-representation among infertile couples with oligospermia. Engels et al. (2008) found a male infertility rate of 11% which they concluded was similar to recent population data.

Munne et al. (2000) analysed oocytes harvested from female carriers of rob(13q14q) and rob(14q21q) who were undergoing PGD and found that rob(13q14q) generated 33% of unbalanced, 51% of normal, and 16% of balanced oocytes (n = 69), and rob(14q21q) produced 42% of unbalanced, 37% of normal, and 21% of balanced oocytes (n = 86). Females do not have an increased risk for infertility but do have a higher miscarriage rate, presumably of aneuploid pregnancies.

Familial Down's syndrome

Robertsonian translocations involving 21 are a cause of familial Down's syndrome. See 'Down's syndrome (trisomy 21)' in Chapter 5, 'Chromosomes', p. 666.

Trisomy rescue

This is the 'correction' by mitotic loss of the free homologue in an unbalanced conception. After this has occurred, the fetus may have only maternal or paternal genes for that particular chromosome (UPD), but the karyotype is balanced. This is of importance in chromosomes that are imprinted (see 'Genomic imprinting' in Chapter 1, 'Introduction', p. 30) and there are recognizable syndromes associated with UPD.

Imprinting and UPD

Abnormal phenotypes in children with apparently balanced translocations may be due to genomic imprinting and UPD. Berend et al. (2000) identified 174 prenatally detected acrocentric rearrangements (Robertsonian translocations and isochromosomes). Only 1/168 (0.6%) non-homologous Robertsonian translocations showed UPD (in this instance, UPD 13), but 4/6 (66%) of homologous acrocentric rearrangements showed UPD.

In a later study, Berend et al. (2002) assessed 50 individuals with a balanced isochromosome or Robertsonian translocation who had phenotypic abnormalities. Forty-eight of these had a non-homologous Robertsonian translocation and two of these individuals had UPD. The two with homologous rearrangements both had UPD. Silverstein et al. (2002) reviewed 315 cases (including the above series) analysed for UPD after PND of balanced Robertsonian translocation; of these, two had UPD, giving a risk estimate of 0.65%.

Consider UPD testing for any rearrangement involving 14 or 15, but note that the phenotype with UPD14(mat) is less severe than for UPD14(pat) and UPD15.

Clinical features

- UPD14(pat). Wang Kagami syndrome. Polyhydramnios, postnatal growth retardation, feeding difficulties, a small thorax with 'coat-hanger' ribs, severe developmental delay, a hirsute forehead, small palpebral fissures, and joint contractures. Antenatal appearance may be similar to Jeune syndrome. The mechanism can be either UPD or deletion of the imprinted genes at 14q32.2.

- UPD14(mat). Temple syndrome. Pre- and postnatal growth retardation (similar to SRS). Small hands and feet, hypotonia, macrocephaly, delayed closure of the anterior fontanelle, a flat nasal bridge with a short nose, precocious puberty in some, and normal intelligence or mild delay.
- UPD15(mat). PWS.
- UPD15(pat). Angelman syndrome. See 'Angelman syndrome' in Chapter 3, 'Common consultations', p. 346.

Clinical approach

History: key points
- Draw a three-generation family tree (or larger, if indicated) and enquire about pregnancy loss, stillbirth, neonatal death, and family members with learning disability or congenital anomalies.
- Family history of infertility.
- Family history of Down's syndrome (if translocation involves 21).

Examination: key points
- Document any dysmorphic features.
- Specifically consider if there are features of a UPD syndrome if the translocation involves 14 or 15.

Special investigations
- Karyotype your patient if they are 'at risk' from the family tree or the karyotype is unknown.
- Karyotype parents of children with a Robertsonian translocation.
- Consider UPD testing in children with a balanced karyotype but who have malformations and/or developmental delay consistent with a UPD phenotype. Requires an EDTA sample from the parents and the child.

Genetic advice

If a 'de novo' non-homologous Robertsonian translocation is identified prenatally, the risk of phenotypic abnormality is very low and arises from the small risk of UPD14 or 15 which has been estimated at 0.65% (Silverstein et al. 2002).

If a 'de novo' homologous Robertsonian translocation has arisen in the zygote by fusion of the maternal and paternal homologues, UPD is not a concern and the recurrence risk will be minimal. However, if the translocation is an isochromosome (see above), the risk for UPD is 100%. If the translocation involves chromosomes 14, the resultant phenotype will be UPD14(mat) or UPD14(pat); if it involves chromosome 15, the resultant phenotypes will be Angelman syndrome (paternal UPD) or PWS (maternal UPD). Since chromosomes 13, 21, and 22 do not appear to contain imprinted elements, a phenotypic effect would only arise in the unlikely event that the parent was a carrier for a recessive condition with a locus on the chromosomes in question which was unmasked by the UPD. Altogether, at least 50% of all Robertsonian translocations between homologues show UPD.

Table 5.6 Risks of having a child with aneuploidy or UPD when one parent carries a heterologous Robertsonian translocation

Balanced translocation	Risk of trisomy 13 or 21		Risk of UPD 14 or 15
	Maternal rob	Paternal rob	
rob (13q14q)	<1% (Engels)	<1%	<0.5%*
rob (13q15q)	1%	<1%	<0.5%*
rob (13q21q)	10–15%	<1%	–
rob (13q22q)	1%	<1%	–
rob (14q15q)	–	–	0.5% (mat), <0.5%* (pat)
rob (14q21q)	10–15%	1%	<0.5%*
rob (14q22q)	–	–	<0.5%*
rob (15q21q)	10–15%	<1%	<0.5%*
rob (15q22q)	–	–	<0.5%*
rob (21q22q)	10–15%	<1%	–

* Silverstein showed that the incidence of UPD was 0.65% among fetuses carrying a balanced Robertsonian translocation; since some fetuses will have a normal karyotype, the overall risk for UPD is <0.5%.

Reproduced from *Chromosome Abnormalities and Genetic Counseling* by Gardner and Sutherland (2004) Tab. 'Risks of having a child with anueploidy or UPD when one patient carries an heterologous Robersonian translocation'. By permission of Oxford University Press, USA. www.oup.com.

Recurrence

'DE NOVO' ROBERTSONIAN TRANSLOCATION. The risk is low, but recurrence has been reported (Sachs et al. 1990). If parental karyotypes are normal, the risk is certainly <2% (Steinberg et al. 1984). For homologous Robertsonian translocations, consider using polymorphic markers to study the parental origin of the homologues since this will determine the recurrence risk (see above).

FAMILIAL ROBERTSONIAN TRANSLOCATION. When one parent carries a homologous Robertsonian translocation, e.g. rob(13q13q) or rob(21q21q), their reproductive future is bleak since virtually all conceptions will be either monosomic or trisomic for the chromosome in question. Conceptions trisomic for 14, 15, and most 22 will spontaneously abort, as will the majority of trisomy 13 and some trisomy 21 pregnancies. Donor gametes (AID, donor oocytes) or adoption may enable such a couple to become parents.

Table 5.6 shows the risks when one parent carries a heterologous Robertsonian translocation.

Prenatal diagnosis

ROB(14q21q). As maternal transmission has a 10–15% risk of Down's syndrome, invasive cytogenetic methods of PND should be discussed. The risk for paternal transmission is lower, but still at a level where PND is offered. Nuchal and anomaly scanning and biochemical screening may be preferred by families with recurrent miscarriage or subfertility, but, given the high prior risk, a significant residual risk of Down's syndrome will remain, even if these screening tests are normal. See 'Down's syndrome (trisomy 21)' in Chapter 5, 'Chromosomes', p. 666.

ROB(13q14q). A recent study by Engels et al. (2008) has given useful counselling data. There were no live births with translocation trisomy 13 in 222 pregnancies to carrier parents (123 females, 71 males, 28 unknown parental origin). Translocation trisomy 13 was detected in 13 out of 42 amniocenteses performed and there were five stillbirths at >28 weeks. Unlike trisomy 21, trisomy 13 has more structural anomalies that may be detected on USS by 20 weeks when an USS has a 90% chance of detecting features of trisomy 13. In view of the low risk, and especially where there is a history of miscarriage or subfertility, amniocentesis may be preferable to CVS for a definitive cytogenetic diagnosis. See 'Patau syndrome (trisomy 13)' in Chapter 5, 'Chromosomes', p. 678).

TRANSLOCATION INVOLVING 14 OR 15 AND UPD SCREENING. If a balanced translocation involving chromosome 14 or 15 is identified prenatally, there is a risk (0.65%) of UPD in the fetus. It is unlikely that the fetus with UPD 14 or 15 will have abnormalities that can be accurately assessed by USS, and specific testing using DNA from amniocytes and parental blood is needed to exclude UPD (Silverstein et al. (2002).

Management

- Recurrent miscarriage. If there is no other medical cause for miscarriage, reassurance that most couples will achieve a normal pregnancy eventually may be helpful to the couple. Consider confirmation of a chromosome abnormality in the products of conception.
- Infertility. When translocation couples need assisted conception for subfertility, PGD is a valuable screen for imbalance, even when the risk of a viable chromosome abnormality is low.
- PGD. Consider referral for PGD for a couple with a non-homologous Robertsonian translocation after three or more spontaneous abortions, or if a male with a non-homologous Robertsonian translocation suffers from infertility associated with oligospermia (Bint et al. 2011; Scriven et al. 2001). In practice, PGD is most likely to be considered by women with a translocation involving 21, as the live birth risk for trisomy is low for the other translocations. It will not help carriers for (rob21q21q) and it may not detect UPD.

Family screening

- Offer chromosome analysis to adult members of the family who are 'at risk'.
- If the translocation has been identified through PND or in a child, ensure that the child's medical records contain a recommendation for genetic counselling as a teenager and that parents are fully informed.

Support groups: Unique (The Rare Chromosome Disorder Support Group), http://www.rarechromo.org, Tel. 01883 330 766; Down's Syndrome Association, http://www.downs-syndrome.org.uk; SOFT UK (Support Organisation for Trisomy 13/18), http://www.soft.org.uk.

Expert adviser (first edition): A. Schinzel, Professor, Institute of Medical Genetics, University of Zurich, Schwerzenbach, Switzerland.

References

Bandyopadhyay R, Heller A, Knox-DuBois C, et al. Parental origin and timing of de novo Robertsonian translocation formation. Am J Hum Genet 2002; **71**: 1456–62.

Berend SA, Bejjani BA, McCaskill C, Shaffer LG. Identification of uniparental disomy in phenotypically abnormal carriers of isochromosomes or Robertsonian translocations. Am J Med Genet 2002; **111**: 362–5.

Berend SA, Horowitz J, McCaskill C, Shaffer LG. Identification of uniparental disomy following prenatal detection of Robertsonian translocations and isochromosomes. Am J Hum Genet 2000; **66**: 1787–93.

Bint SM, Ogilvie CM, Flinter FA, Khalaf Y, Scriven PN. Meiotic segregation of Robertsonian translocations ascertained in cleavage-stage embryos—implications for preimplantation genetic diagnosis. Hum Reprod 2011; **26**: 1575–84.

Boué A, Gallano P. A collaborative study of the segregation of inherited chromosome structural rearrangements in 1356 prenatal diagnoses. Prenat Diagn 1984; **4**: 45–67.

Daniel A, Hook EB, Wulf G. Risks of unbalanced progeny at amniocentesis to carriers of chromosomal rearrangements: data from United States and Canadian laboratories. Am J Med Genet 1989; **31**: 14–53.

Egozcue J, Blanco J, Anton E, Egozcue S, Sarrate Z, Vidal F. Genetic analysis of sperm and implications of severe male infertility—a review. Placenta 2003; **24** Suppl S: S62–5.

Engels H, Eggermann T, Caliebe A, et al. Genetic counseling in Robertsonian translocations der(13;14): frequencies of reproductive outcomes and infertility in 101 pedigrees. Am J Med Genet A 2008; **146A**: 2611–16.

Gardner RJM, Sutherland GR, Shaffer LG. Chromosome abnormalities and genetic counseling, Oxford monographs on medical genetics no. 31, 4th edn. Oxford University Press, New York, 2011.

Gianaroli L, Magli MC, Ferraretti AP, et al. Possible interchromosomal effect in embryos generated by gametes from translocation carriers. Hum Reprod 2002; **17**: 3201–7.

Kagami M, Sekita Y, Nishimura G, et al. Deletions and epimutations affecting the human 14q32.2 imprinted region in individuals with paternal and maternal upd(14)-like phenotypes. Nat Genet 2008; **40**: 237–42.

Kovaleva NV, Shaffer LG. Under-ascertainment of mosaic carriers of balanced homologous acrocentric translocations and isochromosomes. Am J Med Genet A 2003; **121A**: 180–7.

McGowan KD, Weiser JJ, Horwitz J, et al. The importance of investigating for uniparental disomy in prenatally identified balanced acrocentric rearrangements. Prenat Diagn 2002; **22**: 141–3.

Munne S, Escudero T, Sandalinas M, Sable D, Cohen J. Gamete segregation in female carriers of Robertsonian translocations. Cytogenet Cell Genet 2000; **90**(3–4): 303–8.

Robinson WP, Bernasconi F, Basaran S, et al. A somatic origin of homologous Robertsonian translocations and isochromosomes. Am J Hum Genet 1994; **54**: 290–302.

Sachs ES, Jahoda MG, Los FJ, Pijpers L, Wladimiroff JW. Trisomy 21 mosaicism in gonads with unexpectedly high recurrence risks. Am J Med Genet Suppl 1990; **7**: 186–8.

Sanlaville D, Aubry MC, Dumez Y, et al. Maternal uniparental heterodisomy of chromosome 14: chromosomal mechanism and clinical follow up. J Med Genet 2000; **37**: 525–58.

Scriven PN, Flinter FA, Braude PR, Ogilvie CM. Robertsonian translocations—reproductive risks and indications for preimplantation genetic diagnosis. Hum Reprod 2001; **16**: 2267–73.

Silverstein S, Lerer I, Sagi M, Frumkin A, Ben-Neriah Z, Abeliovich D. Uniparental disomy in fetuses diagnosed with balanced Robertsonian translocations: risk estimate. Prenat Diag 2002; **22**: 649–51.

Steinberg C, Zackai EH, Eunpu DL, Mennuti MT, Emanuel BS. Recurrence rate for de novo 21q21q translocation Down syndrome: a study of 112 families. Am J Med Genet 1984; **17**: 523–30.

Sex chromosome mosaicism

For example, 45,X/46,XY, 45,X/46,XX, 47,XXY/46,XY, 45,X/47,XXX, and 47,XXX/46,XX.

For 45,X/46,XX, 47,XXY/46,XY, and 47,XYY/46,XY, see 'Turner syndrome, 45,X and variants', p. 696, '47,XXY', p. 630 and '47,XYY', p. 634 in Chapter 5, 'Chromosomes'. The normal cell line generally ameliorates the phenotype. Sex chromosome mosaicism usually arises from mitotic non-disjunction arising in the post-zygotic phase.

The sex chromosome mosaicism may be detected:

(1) during the investigation of fetal hydrops;

(2) in babies and children with ambiguous genitalia or gonadal dysgenesis;

(3) as an incidental finding during prenatal and postnatal investigation for another indication.

The laboratory will usually recommend a karyotype if the original investigation was genomic array.

Sex chromosomes and ageing

Both sex chromosomes show an age-dependent loss. Guttenbach et al. (1995) found a significant correlation between X chromosome loss and ageing, with the frequency of X chromosome loss ranging from 1.5% to 2.5% in prepubertal females, rising to ~4.5–5% in women older than 75 years. Interpretation of low-level mosaicism for a 45,X cell line during routine analysis is dependent on the age of the patient and the clinical phenotype. In males, Y hypoploidy is very low in boys <15 years of age (0.05%) but gradually increases in frequency to 1.34% in men aged 76–80 years.

46,XX/46,XY

Apparent mosaicism of XX/XY, detected through prenatal testing, is usually due to maternal cell contamination (Worton et al. 1984). However, it is rarely due to chimerism because of an admixture of cells from a 'vanishing twin' or because fertilization involved >2 genetically dissimilar gametes.

When detected at CVS/amniocentesis, arrange an anomaly USS to confirm normal male genitalia, and counsel for high probability of a normal 46,XY male.

45,X/46,XY

Incidence is 1.7/10 000 amniocenteses. Individuals with a 45X/46XY karyotype can develop a wide spectrum of phenotypes, including Turner syndrome, mixed gonadal dysgenesis, male pseudohermaphroditism, and phenotypically normal men. There is considerable ascertainment bias in the literature, with many cases identified following karyotyping of babies with ambiguous genitalia or severe hypospadias, but prospective studies of antenatally diagnosed cases show that a phenotypically normal male is the most likely outcome (90%).

- Chang et al. (1990) identified 76 cases in whom 'true mosaicism' was identified (identical chromosome anomaly in two or more flasks/colonies of cultured amniotic fluid cells). Seventy-five were phenotypic males, of whom 72 (95%) had normal male genitalia and three had hypospadias (associated with a micropenis and an abnormal scrotum in one). One of the males with normal male genitalia had a cystic hygroma. The only phenotypic female had clitoromegaly. The degree of amniotic fluid mosaicism does not predict the degree of genital/

gonadal abnormality (21/23 cases with >50% of 45,X were normal male phenotype, whereas the phenotypic female had only 11% of 45,X). Three of 11 (27%) abortuses had abnormal gonadal histology (e.g. ovotestis), of which one had a Fallopian tube on one side and the epididymis on the other. If gonads are dysgenetic, there is a risk for gonadoblastoma. In Chang et al.'s (1990) study, follow-up was available on 23 patients aged 0–4 years. Development and stature were normal, except in one where height was <5th centile.

- Telvi et al. (1999) in a series of 27 prenatally diagnosed cases found no correlation between the proportion of the 45,X/46,XY cell lines in the blood or the fibroblasts and the phenotype. Mild MR was present in four of the patients and two patients showed signs of autism. Three males, apparently normal at birth, developed late-onset abnormalities, such as dysgenetic testes, leading to infertility and Turner syndrome features.

- Hsu (1989) reviewed 54 cases with PND of 45,X/46,XY mosaicism. Of 47 cases with information on phenotypic outcome, 42 cases (89.4%) were reported to be associated with a grossly normal male phenotype. Three cases (6.4%) were diagnosed as having mixed gonadal dysgenesis with internal asymmetrical gonads. Two other cases were questionably abnormal.

The approaches to 45X/47XYY and 45X/46XY/47XYY are broadly similar, except that stature is difficult to predict and there may be chance of tall stature due to the XYY line, as well as short stature due to 45X.

Clinical approach

See 'Turner syndrome, 45,X and variants', p. 696, '47,XXY', p. 630, and '47,XYY', p. 634 in Chapter 5, 'Chromosomes'.

History: key points (postnatal presentation)

- Developmental milestones, speech and language development, schooling.

Examination: key points (postnatal presentation)

- Height (short in 45,X; tall with 47,XXY and 47,XYY; but see individual sections).
- External genitalia (45,X/46,XY).
- Pubertal development (depending on age).
- Features of Turner, Klinefelter's, or XYY syndromes.

Management: 45,X/46,XY

Prenatal presentation

Caution must be used in translating information derived from postnatal diagnosis to PND because of ascertainment bias.

- Detailed anomaly USS to identify genitalia, cystic hygroma; cardiac scan. If the scan shows a Turner-like phenotype, this can be used to help inform pregnancy prognosis.
- Some parents may wish to discuss TOP, particularly if there are USS abnormalities. This is a difficult counselling scenario, as outcome is generally favourable where there is no USS abnormality (see above) (Jeon et al. 2012).
- Postnatal confirmation of the genetic result.

- After birth, these children should be referred to a paediatric endocrinologist for clinical follow-up, USS, and endocrine studies to assess growth and the risk of gonadoblastoma. In a phenotypically normal male with descended testes, the risk is low, but if the testes are not palpable, the risk is higher.

Postnatal presentation

The main management issue is usually the risk of gonadoblastoma. Gravholt *et al.* (2000) undertook a population study in Denmark of the occurrence of gonadoblastoma in females with Turner syndrome and Y chromosome material (detected by karyotype or PCR). The occurrence of gonadoblastoma among Y-positive patients with Turner syndrome was 7–10%. In such patients, the tumour is believed to be present from birth (Gravholt *et al.* 2000).

Genetic advice

Sex chromosome mosaicism usually arises from mitotic non-disjunction arising in the post-zygotic phase.

Recurrence risk

After the birth of a child (or the loss of a pregnancy) with sex chromosome mosaicism, the risk of recurrence is very low.

Prenatal diagnosis

Recurrence risk is very low. PND is discretionary.

Support groups: Klinefelter's Syndrome Association, http://www.ksa-uk.net; Turner Syndrome Support Society, http://www.tss.org.uk.

Expert adviser: Angela Barnicoat, Consultant Clinical Geneticist, Department of Clinical Genetics, Great Ormond Street Hospital NHS Foundation Trust, London, UK.

References

Chang HJ, Clark RD, Bachman H. The phenotype of 45,X/46,XY mosaicism: an analysis of 92 prenatally diagnosed cases. *Am J Hum Genet* 1990; **46**: 156–67.

Gravholt CH, Fedder J, Naeraa RW, Müller J. Occurrence of gonadoblastoma in females with Turner syndrome and Y chromosome material: a population study. *J Clin Endocrinol Metab* 2000; **85**: 3199–320.

Guttenbach M, Koschorz B, Bernthaler U, Grimm T, Schmid M. Sex chromosome loss and aging: *in situ* hybridization studies on human interphase nuclei. *Am J Hum Genet* 1995; **57**: 1143–50.

Hsu LY. Prenatal diagnosis of 45,X/46,XY mosaicism—a review and update. *Prenat Diagn* 1989; **9**: 31–48.

Jeon KC, Chen LS, Goodson P. Decision to abort after a prenatal diagnosis of sex chromosome abnormality: a systematic review of the literature. *Genet Med* 2012; **14**: 27–38.

Nance WE. Genetic tests with a sex-linked marker: glucose-6-phosphate dehydrogenase. *Cold Spring Harbor Symp Quant Biol* 1964; **29**: 415–52.

Plenge RM, Tranebjaerg L, Jensen PK, Schwartz C, Willard HF. Evidence that mutations in the X-linked *DDP* gene cause incompletely penetrant and variable skewed X inactivation. *Am J Hum Genet* 1999; **64**: 759–67.

Telvi L, Lebbar A, Del Pino O, Barbet JP, Chaussain JL. 45,X/46,XY mosaicism: report of 27 cases. *Pediatrics* 1999; **104**(2, pt 1): 304–8.

Warburton D, Dallaire L, Thangavelu M, Ross L, Levin B, Kline J. Trisomy rescue: a consideration based on North American data. *Am J Hum Genet* 2004; **75**: 376–85.

Worton RG, Stern R. A Canadian collaborative study of mosaicism in amniotic fluid cell cultures. *Prenat Diagn* 1984; **4** (Spring Spec No): 131–44.

Supernumerary marker chromosomes (SMCs)—postnatal

Background information for this section is in 'Supernumerary marker chromosomes (SMCs)—prenatal' in Chapter 5, 'Chromosomes', p. 692. Supernumerary marker chromosomes (SMCs) are usually found postnatally in a few children investigated for developmental delay. Marker chromosomes may be ascertained through follow-up of a duplication/triplication on a genomic array. The incidence of SMCs in this group is about 3/1000 against the live birth rate of 0.5/1000 (0.05%), demonstrating that *many markers have no phenotypic effect*. In ~30% of carriers of a small marker chromosome (excluding the ~70% of SMCs derived from one of the acrocentric chromosomes), an abnormal phenotype is observed (Starke *et al.* 2003). Some SMCs have a well-described phenotype that can assist counselling. The two most common are idic(15) and idic(22) where 'idic' stands for isodicentric.

idic(15), also written as idic(15)(pter-q13) or psudic(15)(pter-q12::q13-pter)

A bisatellited isodicentric (idic; symmetrical) or pseudodicentric marker (psudic; asymmetrical). The facial features are not diagnostic, but severe developmental delay and seizures are the usual presenting features (see below). Maternal age is increased and most markers are of maternal origin. Rapid confirmation of the origin is by genomic array or FISH using the SNRPN or other probes for PWS/Angelman syndrome (AS) critical region. Individuals with a 15 marker that does not contain the PW/AS critical region almost invariably have a normal phenotype. Recent molecular studies have revealed a hitherto unrecognized degree of structural heterogeneity in SMCs derived from chromosome 15, and clinical evaluations show that the degree of developmental impairment is proportional to the number of additional copies and extent of the duplication, triplication, or quadruplication conferred by the presence of the chromosome 15 SMC (Roberts *et al.* 2003).

idic(22)

Chromosome 22 SMCs without euchromatin have a low risk of causing abnormalities. Larger markers with euchromatin lead to a variable phenotype from apparently no phenotypic effect to CES.

Cat-eye syndrome (CES): idic 22, alternatively written as idic(22)(pter-q11.2)

The phenotype of CES includes the following:
- coloboma of the iris/choroid;
- other structural eye abnormalities;
- preauricular tags and pits;
- •anal anomalies (anterior displacement of the anus, anal atresia, anal fistulae);
- cardiac defects (TAPVD, tetralogy of Fallot);
- structural renal anomalies, including atresia and ectopia;
- variable developmental delay and MR.

The prognosis for survival is good, except in infants with severe cardiac and renal abnormalities. Parental age is increased and most de novo markers are of maternal origin.

Clinical approach

History: key points
- Three-generation family tree (unless the marker is known to be *de novo*), with specific enquiry regarding parental health, development, and education.

Examination: key points
- Careful clinical assessment. See 'Dysmorphic child' in Chapter 2, 'Clinical approach', p. 134.

Special investigations
- Obtain parental blood samples (Li heparin) for karyotyping. Request 30-cell screen to investigate for parental mosaicism.
- Cytogenetically characterize the marker. A genomic array will be the most useful next step. Where this is not available, use the G-banding pattern to determine whether or not a centromere is present and whether or not it is satellited to help in identification of the origin of the marker and selection of suitable FISH probes and paints.
- If the marker contains euchromatin and is derived from an imprinted region of the genome, initiate UPD studies (requires DNA from the proband and parents).
- Cardiac and renal USS in children with idic(22).

Genetic advice

When the SMC has been identified, search the literature prior to counselling for details of the possible phenotypic effect of the marker. For many of the common markers, there are considerable data. If the marker is mosaic, the phenotype may be modified and milder. If a parent of a child with an abnormal phenotype has an SMC, but no phenotypic features, consider whether the marker or another aetiology is causing the phenotype in the child.

Recurrence risk
- For *de novo* SMCs, the recurrence risk is very low.
- For familial SMCs, the risk of transmission is high but is rarely associated with phenotypic abnormality, idic(22) being an exception to this. Because of the wide phenotypic variability in idic(22), it is possible for a parent carrying the marker to have a normal phenotype and yet have a child who is severely affected (Crolla *et al.* 1997). Where the parent carries an SMC in a mosaic form, the child may inherit this in a mosaic or non-mosaic form. Where both parent and child are mosaic, there may be considerable phenotypic variability (see notes on this point in 'Supernumerary marker chromosomes—prenatal' in Chapter 5, 'Chromosomes', p. 692).

Prenatal diagnosis
- Possible by CVS or amniocentesis.

Support group: Unique (The Rare Chromosome Disorder Support Group, http://www.rarechromo.org, Tel. 01883 330 766.

Expert adviser (first edition): John Crolla, Clinical Molecular Cytogeneticist, Wessex Regional Genetics Laboratories, Salisbury, UK.

References

Buckton K, Spowart G, Newton MS, Evans HJ. Forty four probands with additional 'marker' chromosomes. *Hum Genet* 1985; **69**: 353–70.

Crolla JA, Harvey JF, Sitch FL, Dennis NR. Supernumerary marker 15 chromosomes: a clinical, molecular and FISH approach to diagnosis and prognosis. *Hum Genet* 1995; **95**: 161–70.

Crolla JA, Howard P, Mitchell C, Long FL, Dennis NR. A molecular and FISH approach to determining karyotype and phenotype correlations in six patients with supernumerary marker (22) chromosomes. *Am J Med Genet* 1997; **72**: 440–7.

Crolla JA, Long FL, Rivers H, Dennis NR. FISH and molecular study of autosomal supernumerary marker chromosomes excluding those derived from 15. I: results of 26 new cases. *Am J Med Genet* 1998; **75**: 355–66.

Gardner RJM, Sutherland GR, Shaffer LG. *Chromosome abnormalities and genetic counseling, Oxford monographs on medical genetics no. 31*, 4th edn. Oxford University Press, New York, 2011.

Roberts SE, Maggouta F, Thomas NS, Jacobs PA, Crolla JA. Molecular and fluorescence *in situ* hybridization characterization of the breakpoints in 46 large supernumerary marker 15 chromosomes reveals an unexpected level of complexity. *Am J Hum Genet* 2003; **73**: 1061–72.

Starke H, Nietzel A, Weise A, et al. Small supernumerary marker chromosomes (SMCs): genotype–phenotype correlation and classification. *Hum Genet* 2003; **114**: 51–67.

Supernumerary marker chromosomes (SMCs)—prenatal

Supernumerary marker chromosomes occur in ~0.05% of live births (Buckton et al. 1985) and in 0.04% (Warburton 1991) to 0.08% (Blennow et al. 1994; Hook and Cross 1987) of PND populations. In general, if it can be demonstrated that the SMC contains only heterochromatin, it will almost certainly have no phenotypic effect. A number of SMCs may comprise both heterochromatic (predominantly A-satellite DNA) and euchromatic components, resulting in segmental trisomy or tetrasomy, and consequently these may have effects resulting in developmental aberration(s).

Structurally, SMCs fall into five principal groups: (1) satellited or bisatellited; (2) small metacentrics; (3) small supernumerary ring-shaped chromosomes; (4) so-called 'minutes'; and (5) neocentromeric chromosomes. All the SMCs in group 1 are derived from the acrocentric autosomes (13, 14, 15, 21, or 22), but acrocentric SMCs from phenotypic groups 3 and 4 have also been reported.

Some marker chromosomes, e.g. the 22q derived marker found in CES, contain a duplicated euchromatic segment, resulting in segmental tetrasomy (Crolla et al. 1997; McDermid and Morrow 2002). Overall, 60–80% of SMCs are derived from acrocentric chromosomes, principally 13, 14, 15, and 22, particularly 15 and 22.

About 30% of markers are familial. If the parent carrying the marker has a normal phenotype, there is a low risk of abnormality in most circumstances. Transmission from mosaic parents of SMCs derived from 22 and 15 to non-mosaic children has been reported but is extremely rare, though it may increase the risk of abnormality or UPD (for 15). Another possible scenario is a parent carrying a mosaic 'minute' (all heterochromatic) that is transmitted to the child who is a non-mosaic where the risk is still likely to be low, but each case needs to be considered individually.

Marker chromosomes may be ascertained in the evaluation of a pregnancy with abnormal USS or serum screening findings, or incidentally during antenatal karyotyping. A de novo SMC is found in ~1/2500 amniocenteses. Marker chromosomes may also be ascertained through follow-up of a duplication/triplication on a genomic array.

The clinical outcome of some SMCs is difficult to predict, as they can have different phenotypic consequences because of: (1) differences in euchromatic DNA content; (2) different degrees of mosaicism; and/or (3) UPD of the chromosomes homologous to the SMC. Starke et al. (2003) attempted a genotype–phenotype classification for small marker chromosomes, based on subcentromere-specific multicolour FISH and UPD analysis.

Clinical approach

History: key points

- Three-generation family tree (unless the marker is known to be de novo), with specific enquiry regarding parental health, development, and education.

Examination: key points

- Detailed fetal anomaly USS.

Special investigations

- Obtain parental blood samples (Li heparin) for karyotyping. Request 30-cell screen to investigate for parental mosaicism.

- Cytogenetically characterize the marker. If a genomic array has not been done, this may be the most useful next step. If not available, use the G-banding pattern to determine whether or not it is satellited, as this may help in identification of the origin of the marker and selection of suitable FISH probes.
- Seventy per cent of all SMCs are from the acrocentric autosomes, and 60% of these will be de novo. Prenatal FISH studies must therefore focus on identification of the chromosomal and euchromatic content, particularly of bisatellited de novo SMCs.
  - Approximately 50% will be derived from chromosome 15 and, if FISH shows these (1) to be dicentric for the chromosome 15-specific alpha repeat and (2) to contain two copies of the Prader–Willi/Angelman syndrome critical region (PWACR) (a genomic array may also be used to define this), then this will invariably be associated with a very poor outcome, characterized by severe developmental delay, autistic-like features, behavioural problems, and fitting.
  - If the SMC is a dicentric 15 but does not contain PWACR euchromatin, this will be associated with a normal outcome, providing that UPD(15) is excluded for de novo SMC(15)s of this type. Further discrimination of empirical risk factors associated with dicentric acrocentric SMCs can be carried out using FISH in combination with chromosome 22-specific probes, notably p190.22 (D22Z3; Rocchi et al. 1994) and cosmids cloned from the CES critical region (McDermid and Morrow 2002).
  - SMCs derived from chromosomes 14 and 13/21 (these two centromeres cannot be differentiated between using alphoid probes) are largely associated with a benign postnatal outcome (Crolla et al. 1998).
- Risk assessment associated with non-acrocentric SMCs is more problematical and determination of the chromosomal origin (i.e. after excluding an acrocentric autosomal origin) is probably less useful. However, use of centromere-specific libraries of probes will give a chromosomal origin in most cases, and further use of the relevant chromosomal paint will help to determine (if crudely) the presence of significant additional euchromatin. In this context, Crolla (1998) refined the risk of an abnormal phenotype originally quoted by Warburton (1991) from 15% up to 30% in those cases of de novo autosomal (non-acrocentric) SMCs that contain demonstrable additional euchromatin.

Management

- Where a de novo SMC is found at CVS, the possibility of CPM must be seriously considered but is rarely found.
- If the SMC was identified at *follow-up* amniocentesis or FBS in >1 culture or colony, no further invasive prenatal tests are required.

If the SMC contains euchromatin, further investigation of the pregnancy is indicated, using:

- fetal USS for structural anomalies;
- amniocentesis and/or FBS if SMC detected at CVS.

Genetic advice

When the SMC has been identified, search the literature prior to counselling for details of the possible phenotypic effect.

- Warburton (1991) reported that 13% of pregnancies with SMCs were associated with congenital abnormalities and that some abnormalities were more likely to cause developmental problems.
- Crolla (1998) gives a 30% risk in those cases of *de novo* autosomal (non-acrocentric) SMCs that contain demonstrable euchromatin.
- Daniel and Malsfiiej (2003) reviewed 77 cases with supernumerary small ring marker autosomes and reported that 30% of the prenatally ascertained cases had an abnormal phenotype attributable to the ring.

If the chromosomal origin is unknown, the likelihood of abnormality in the fetus will be increased if:

- the SMC is *de novo*;
- the SMC is large;
- the SMC contains euchromatin; e.g. duplication/triplication on genomic array;
- the SMC is a ring;
- fetal anomalies are identified on USS.

SMC associated with fetal abnormality

Define the malformations as well as possible by detailed anomaly scanning. Do a literature search for similar phenotypic abnormalities in similar markers.

Apparently normal fetus on scan

Usually the indication for pregnancy testing has been an increased risk of Down's syndrome. This is a difficult counselling situation. Parental anxiety is high and there may be no absolute answers. Most of the series of prenatally identified SMCs have limited long-term developmental information. It is particularly important to have comprehensive FISH analyses performed on satellited and bisatellited SMCs, as the SMC(15) containing additional copies of the PWACR will not show abnormalities on USS.

- If the pregnancy is terminated, arrange for a full post-mortem examination and book a follow-up genetic appointment to counsel about the risks of recurrence and family follow-up.
- If the pregnancy continues and the fetus is carrying an SMC, ensure that:
  - the baby is examined at birth by a paediatrician and appropriate genetic and paediatric follow-up is arranged to screen for developmental problems;
  - the child's medical notes (e.g. GP or family practice notes) are marked with this information;
  - the child's parents know that they should request an appointment for genetic counselling when the child is in his/her mid teens.

Recurrence risk

- For *de novo* SMCs, the recurrence risk is very low.
- For familial SMCs, the risk of transmission is high (~50%) but is rarely associated with phenotypic abnormality. Where the parent carries an SMC in a mosaic form, the child may inherit this in a mosaic or non-mosaic form; where both parent and child are mosaic, there may be considerable phenotypic variability.

Prenatal diagnosis

- Possible by CVS or amniocentesis.

Support groups: Unique (The Rare Chromosome Disorder Support Group), http://www.rarechromo.org, Tel. 01883 330 766; ARC (Antenatal Results and Choices), http://www.arc-uk.org, Tel. 0207 631 0285.

Expert adviser (first edition): John Crolla, Clinical Molecular Cytogeneticist, Wessex Regional Genetics Laboratories, Salisbury, UK.

References
Blennow E, Bui TH, Kristoffersson U, et al. Swedish survey on extra structurally abnormal chromosomes in 39 105 consecutive prenatal diagnoses: prevalence and characterization by fluorescence in situ hybridization. Prenat Diagn 1994; **14**: 1019–28.

Buckton K, Spowart G, Newton MS, Evans HJ. Forty four probands with additional 'marker' chromosomes. Hum Genet 1985; **69**: 353–70.

Crolla JA. FISH and molecular studies of autosomal supernumerary marker chromosomes excluding those derived from chromosome 15. II. A review of the literature. Am J Med Genet 1998; **75**: 367–81.

Crolla JA, Harvey JF, Sitch FL, Dennis NR. Supernumerary marker 15 chromosomes: a clinical, molecular and FISH approach to diagnosis and prognosis. Hum Genet 1995; **95**: 161–70.

Crolla JA, Howard P, Mitchell C, Long FL, Dennis NR. A molecular and FISH approach to determining karyotype and phenotype correlations in six patients with supernumerary marker (22) chromosomes. Am J Med Genet 1997; **72**: 440–7.

Crolla JA, Long FL, Rivers H, Dennis NR. FISH and molecular study of autosomal supernumerary marker chromosomes excluding those derived from 15. I: results of 26 new cases. Am J Med Genet 1998; **75**: 355–66.

Crolla JA, Youings SA, Ennis S, Jacobs PA. Supernumerary marker chromosome in man: parental origin, mosaicism and maternal age revisited. Eur J Hum Genet 2005; **13**: 154–60.

Daniel A, Malsfiiej P. A series of supernumerary small ring marker autosomes identified by FISH with chromosome probe arrays and literature review excluding chromosome 15. Am J Med Genet A 2003; **117A**: 212–22.

Gardner RJM, Sutherland GR, Shaffer LG. Chromosome abnormalities and genetic counseling, Oxford monographs on medical genetics no. 31, 4th edn. Oxford University Press, New York, 2011.

Hastings RJ, Nisbet DL, Waters K, Spencer T, Chitty LS. Prenatal detection of extra structurally abnormal chromosomes (ESACs): new cases and a review of the literature. Prenat Diagn 1999; **19**: 436–45.

Hook EB, Cross PK. Extra structurally abnormal chromosomes (ESAC) detected at amniocentesis: frequency in approximately 75,000 prenatal cytogenetic diagnoses and associations with maternal and paternal age. Am J Hum Genet 1987; **40**: 83–101.

Li MM, Howard-Peebles PN, Killos LD, Fallon L, Listgarten E, Stanley WS. Characterization and clinical implications of marker chromosomes identified at prenatal diagnosis. Prenat Diagn 2000; **20**: 138–43.

McDermid HE, Morrow BE. Genomic disorders on 22q11 [review]. Am J Hum Genet 2002; **70**: 1077–88.

Rocchi M, Archidiacono N, Antonacci R, et al. Cloning and comparative mapping of recently evolved human chromosome 22-specific alpha satellite DNA. Somat Cell Mol Genet 1994; **20**: 443–8.

Starke H, Nietzel A, Weise A, et al. Small supernumerary marker chromosomes (SMCs): genotype–phenotype correlation and classification. Hum Genet 2003; **114**: 51–67.

Warburton D. De novo balanced chromosome rearrangements and extra marker chromosomes identified at prenatal diagnosis: clinical significance and distribution of breakpoints. Am J Hum Genet 1991; **49**: 995–1013.

Triploidy (69,XXX, 69XXY, or 69,XYY)

Triploidy is usually identified after pregnancy loss. Triploidy is one of the most frequent chromosome aberrations in first-trimester spontaneous abortions (see Table 6.14 in 'Miscarriage and recurrent miscarriage', Chapter 6, 'Pregnancy and fertility', p. 760). Approximately 7.5% of all spontaneous abortions have a triploid karyotype. In contrast to aneuploidies due to non-disjunction, increased maternal age is not a risk factor and the mechanism of triploidy remains poorly understood (Brancati et al. 2003). The great majority of triploid conceptions are lost in the first trimester, but a few survive into the second trimester; survival into the third trimester is rare and invariably leads to intrauterine or neonatal death. Fetuses with diploid/triploid mosaicism may be more likely to survive longer in pregnancy.

- Digynic (either 69,XXX or 69,XXY), which consists of two maternal sets and one paternal set of chromosomes; arises due to incorporation of the second polar body into the fertilized oocyte.
- Diandric (either 69,XXX, 69,XXY, or 69,XYY), which consists of two paternal sets and one maternal set of chromosomes; arises due to fertilization of an oocyte by two sperms simultaneously.

Triploid pregnancies were reported in 1–2% of all pregnancies in the classic study by Jacobs et al. (1982). However, a recent registry study from Denmark reported 183 triploid pregnancies out of a population of 1.5 million clinically confirmed pregnancies. The majority are associated with molar disease) In the Danish study, there were 29 cases with a living fetus at USS prior to termination. Soft tissue syndactyly and asymmetric growth retardation were common, but the phenotypes were very variable overall, with some near normal fetuses (Joergensen et al. 2014).

Gestational trophoblastic disease

Gestational trophoblastic diseases constitute a spectrum of disorders which includes complete and partial hydatidiform mole (PM), placental-site trophoblastic tumour, and choriocarcinoma. These entities vary in their propensity for local invasion and metastatic spread. Although persistent gestational trophoblastic tumours (GTTs) develop most commonly after a molar pregnancy, they may follow any gestation.

The cause of GTTs remains unknown. If there is a common genetic origin for all GTTs, then it is likely that a combination of an abnormality in the paternal genes associated with deletion of a maternal suppressor gene could explain the patterns seen clinically.

Hydatidiform moles are classified as either complete or partial on the basis of karyotype, gross morphology, and histopathology.

Partial hydatidiform mole (PM)

Usually contains identifiable embryonic or fetal tissues, and the chorionic villi vary in size, with focal swelling, cavitation, and trophoblastic hyperplasia. Ninety to 93% of PMs have a triploid karyotype which is paternally derived (diandric).

Complete hydatidiform mole (CM)

Most complete moles (90%) have a 46,XX karyotype, and the chromosomes are entirely of paternal origin.

Persistent gestational trophoblastic disease and choriocarcinoma

Locally invasive or metastatic gestational trophoblastic neoplasia may develop after either a complete or partial mole. The time interval between the antecedent pregnancy and clinical presentation of choriocarcinoma ranges from a few weeks to years. In the UK, persistent gestational trophoblastic disease occurs after 15% of CMs and 0.5–1% of PMs. The incidence is 1/40 000–1/50 000 in patients following a full-term pregnancy. Whereas the tumour resulting from a CM or PM is usually an invasive mole (which grows more slowly and metastasizes less rapidly than the highly malignant choriocarcinoma), choriocarcinoma can arise in up to 3% of CMs and ~0.1% of PMs. All women with a CM or PM should be placed on hCG follow-up (see http://www.hmole-chorio.org.uk for further details). Treatment is by initial evacuation, followed by chemotherapy which, in the UK, is tailored according to a scoring system introduced by the International Federation of Gynecology and Obstetrics. The outcome is excellent, with cure in >98% of cases registered in the UK.

The recurrence risk for moles is about 1% after one mole and 15–18% after two moles. There are well-reported cases in the literature of familial mole. This is a very rare entity and is characterized by the occurrence of complete moles which have both maternal and paternal chromosomes. The disorder is recessively inherited in the mothers who have the molar pregnancies. Mutations in *NLRP7* and *KHDC3L* have been reported in affected women.

Diploid/triploid mosaicism

Daniel et al. (2003) studied 3n/2n mosaics and two different mechanisms of origin were identified: (1) delayed digyny, by incorporation of a pronucleus from a second polar body into one embryonic blastomere; and (2) delayed dispermy, similarly by incorporation of a second sperm pronucleus into one embryonic blastomere. (In 3n/2n mosaicism, an origin from a diploid gamete is excluded, since all such conceptuses would be simple triploids.) In Daniel et al. (2003)'s study, one fetus with apparent 3n/2n mosaicism was a chimera (formed by the fusion of two zygotes), and in another instance the 3n line was confined to the placenta (CPM). The affected fetus with 3n/2n mosaicism may not survive pregnancy or may survive to term. Characteristic findings are syndactyly, especially of fingers 3/4 and toes 2/3, with bulbous ends of the toes and clinodactyly. There may be body asymmetry and streaky skin hyper- or hypopigmentation. Skin chromosomes may be required to make the diagnosis. Genetic counselling is as for full triploidy.

Clinical features

Digynic
- More likely than diandric to survive to the second trimester.
- Severe IUGR.
- Disproportionately large head. May have holoprosencephaly.
- Abnormally small placenta, oligohydramnios, and abnormal placental Doppler indices.

Diandric
- Accounts for >90% of cases of PMs (focal trophoblastic hyperplasia with villous hydrops, together with identifiable fetal tissue).
- Symmetrical IUGR with structural anomalies (82%), e.g. NTD.
- High maternal serum hCG (80%).
- Big placenta, oligohydramnios, abnormal placental Doppler indices, increased risk of pre-eclampsia.

Clinical approach

History: key points
- Pregnancy history. Events leading to diagnosis of triploidy, e.g. abnormal USS, abnormal maternal serum screening analytes.

Examination: key points
- Not usually relevant.

Special investigations
- Chromosome analysis of the parents is not indicated.
- In familial recurrent hydatidiform moles, especially where the mother's parents are consanguineous, consider the possibility that the mother has a biallelic mutation of *NLRP7* (19q13) or *KDHC3L* (6q13) resulting in recurrent molar pregnancies (Fallahian *et al.* 2013).

Genetic advice

Recurrence risk
The recurrence risk for diandric triploidy with a partial mole is ~1% (Berkowitz *et al.* 2000). Recurrence of triploidy of maternal origin (digynic triploidy) has been described only in a few families (Brancati *et al.* 2003). Overall, recurrence risks are generally very low and probably not much increased over background rates, given that triploidy is found in ~7.5% of all spontaneous abortions and a significant number of cleavage-stage embryos (Munne *et al.* 2002). See above for recurrent hydatidiform mole.

Prenatal diagnosis
PND in future pregnancies is discretionary and not specifically indicated, given that most triploid conceptions will spontaneously fail.

Management
All women with a partial mole should be registered for ongoing hCG monitoring following the pregnancy because of the small risk (0.5%) of malignant transformation. See http://www.hmole-chorio.org.uk for further details.

Support group: Unique (The Rare Chromosome Disorder Support Group), http://www.rarechromo.org, Tel. 01883 330 766.

Expert adviser: Eamonn Sheridan, Professor of Clinical Genetics, University of Leeds, Leeds, UK.

References

Berkowitz RS, Tuncer ZS, Bernstein MR, Goldstein DP. Management of gestational trophoblastic diseases: subsequent pregnancy experience. *Semin Oncol* 2000; **27**: 678–85.

Brancati F, Mingarelli R, Dallapiccola B. Recurrent triploidy of maternal origin. *Eur J Hum Genet* 2003; **11**: 972–4.

Daniel A, Wu Z, Darmanian A, Collins F, Jackson J. Three different origins for apparent triploid/diploid mosaics. *Prenat Diagn* 2003; **23**: 529–34.

Fallahian M, Sebire NJ, Savage PM, Seckl MJ, Fisher RA. Mutations in *NLRP7* and *KHDC3L* confer a complete hydatidiform mole phenotype on digynic triploid conceptions. *Hum Mutat* 2013; **34**: 301–8.

Fox H. Gestational trophoblastic disease. Neoplasia or pregnancy failure? [editorial]. *BMJ* 1997; **314**: 1363.

Genest DR. Partial hydatidiform mole: clinicopathological features, differential diagnosis, ploidy and molecular studies, and gold standards for diagnosis. *Int J Gynecol Pathol* 2001; **20**: 315–22.

Helwani MN, Seoud M, Zahed L, Zaatari G, Khalil A, Slim R. A familial case of recurrent hydatidiform molar pregnancies with biparental genomic contribution. *Hum Genet* 1999; **105**: 112–15.

Jacobs PA, Szulman AE, Funkhouser J, Matsuura JS, Wilson CC. Human triploidy: relationship between paternal origin of the additional haploid complement and development of partial hydatidiform mole. *Ann Hum Genet* 1982; **46**: 223–31.

Jacobs PA, Wilson CM, Sprenkle JA, Rosenshein NB, Migeon BR. Mechanisms of origin of complete hydatidiform mole. *Nature* 1980; **286**: 714–16.

Jauniaux E. Partial moles: from postnatal to prenatal diagnosis. *Placenta* 1999; **20**: 379–88.

Joergensen MW, Niemann I, Rasmussen AA, *et al.* Triploid pregnancies: genetic and clinical features of 158 cases. *Am J Obstet Gynecol* 2014; **211**: 370.e1–19.

Judson H, Hayward BE, Sheridan E, Bonthron DT. A global disorder of imprinting in the human female germline. *Nature* 2002; **416**: 539–42.

Munne S, Sandalinas M, Escudero T, Márquez C, Cohen J. Chromosome mosaicism in cleavage-stage human embryos: evidence of a maternal age effect. *Reprod Biomed Online* 2002; **4**: 223–32.

Seckl MJ, Sebire NJ, Berkowitz RS. Gestational trophoblastic disease. *Lancet* 2010; **376**: 717–29.

Turner syndrome, 45,X, and variants

Turner described the features of this syndrome in 1938, and in 1959 it was found that girls with Turner syndrome (TS) had an absent X chromosome (45,X karyotype). TS affects one in 2500 live female births. The majority (up to 99%) of TS conceptions are lost as spontaneous abortions. The rate of intrauterine lethality between 12 and 40 weeks' gestation is ~65%.

In some females with TS, there may be a normal X chromosome and a structurally rearranged X chromosome. In addition, mosaicism is frequently present, particularly when multiple tissues are tested.

The karyotypes in Birkebaek et al.'s (2002) study of 410 adult females with TS were as follows: 49% had 45,X; 23% had mosaicism with a structural abnormality of the second X; 19% had 45,X/46,XX mosaicism; and 9% had 46,XX and a structural abnormality of the second X (see 'Sex chromosome mosaicism' in Chapter 5, 'Chromosomes', p. 688).

Mosaicism 45,X/46,XY presents the additional problem of the risk of gonadoblastoma and, when detected prenatally, of the phenotypic sex of the child.

Eighty per cent of the X chromosomes in 45,X are of maternal origin. The majority of TS karyotypes are thought to be the result of paternal meiotic errors that generate abnormal sex chromosomes, and the 45,X line is the result of mitotic loss of the abnormal chromosome. Isochromosome Xq and ring/marker X arise from both maternal and paternal meiotic errors. A significant inverse relationship with maternal age is found for 45,X, perhaps reflecting the higher miscarriage rate with advancing maternal age for aneuploidy, as well as euploid conceptions.

Structural abnormalities of the X chromosome found in TS include deletions, duplications, inversions, isodicentric chromosomes, translocations, and rings. Preferential inactivation of the abnormal X is the mechanism that ensures the relatively mild phenotype of TS.

Ring X

Can produce a more severe phenotype, associated with MR, when there is absence of the XIST gene leading to functional X disomy. In mosaic ring X TS females, with a 45,X/46,X,r(X) karyotype, the proportion of cells with functional X disomy may be associated with the severity of MR (Kubota et al. 2002).

Sex chromosomes and ageing

Guttenbach et al. (1995) found a significant correlation between X chromosome loss and ageing, with the frequency of X chromosome loss ranging from 1.5% to 2.5% in prepubertal females, rising to ~4.5–5% in women older than 75 years. The interpretation of low-level mosaicism for a 45,X cell line during routine analysis is dependent on the age of the patient and the clinical phenotype.

Clinical features

There is considerable phenotypic variation in TS. In some girls, there may be few features, other than short stature, to suggest the diagnosis. The phenotype can be sufficiently subtle that a karyotype is routinely included in the evaluation of girls with short stature because otherwise this diagnosis may be missed. The presence of mosaicism affects the phenotype, and the risk of features such as coarctation of the aorta is higher in full 45,X. Please note that many of the structural chromosomal abnormalities

do have specific features; consult with the laboratory and perform a literature search for further information.

Physical features

- Short stature and gonadal dysgenesis are the two features found in the majority of females with TS. The untreated mean adult height is 147 cm, but this is increased following GH therapy in childhood. Physical features, such as a short, broad webbed neck, ptosis, and a low hairline, are secondary to fetal oedema/hydrops. Motor milestones may be slightly delayed.
- Cardiovascular malformations are found in 15–50%, particularly coarctation of the aorta and bicuspid aortic valve, but including ASD and VSD.
- Oedema of the hands and feet is a common finding in the newborn with TS.
- Renal anomalies, including horseshoe kidney, other structural abnormalities, and agenesis, are found in about one-third.

Puberty and sexual development

Poor growth, with no pubertal growth spurt, and absent or minimal breast development is usual. Some women have a few periods but then develop premature menopause and this is more likely in the presence of a 46,XX cell line.

Education

Intelligence is usually normal, but mean IQ is generally 10–15 points lower than that of siblings. Mild speech and language delay is common. Individuals with TS have relative difficulty on measures of spatial/perceptual skills, visual–motor integration, visual memory, and attention (Ross et al. 2000). Most girls with TS attend mainstream schools.

Behaviour

Social adjustment problems are common and some girls/women with TS may have physical features that make them different from their peers. Girls with TS may also have subtle perceptual difficulties, e.g. difficulties with facial affect recognition. In comparison with a control group, McCauley et al. (2001) found that TS girls had significantly more problems in terms of social relationships and school progress. They had fewer friends and spent less time with their friends than the control group. Social difficulties appear to be an area of vulnerability for TS girls. Skuse et al. (1997) found that TS women with a paternally derived X were significantly better adjusted, with superior verbal and higher-order executive function skills that mediate social interactions, than those with a maternally derived X. This observation suggests that there is a genetic locus for social cognition that is imprinted and is not expressed from the maternally derived X chromosome.

Employment

Most women with TS lead independent adult lives, and a recent US study of 240 TS women found that high levels of education and employment were achieved, independent of parental origin of the X chromosome (Gould et al. 2013).

Fertility

The majority of women with TS are infertile. Thirty-one women of the 410 in the Danish survey by Birkebaek et al. (2002) achieved at least one spontaneous pregnancy. However, only women with 45,X/46,XX mosaicism or 46,XX and structural abnormality of the second X gave birth to live children after spontaneous pregnancies. IVF with donor oocytes has resulted in successful pregnancy for some women with TS. In a US survey, Karnis et al. (2003) ascertained 146 TS patients treated, resulting in 101 pregnancies, and drew attention to the ~2% risk for death from rupture or dissection of the aorta in pregnancy. This was supported by similar findings in France, leading to clinical practice recommendations (Cabanes et al. 2010). It is imperative that patients are screened by echo, assessed by a cardiologist, and advised of the potential risks before attempting to become pregnant.

Pregnancy may occur in patients with structural anomalies of the X chromosomes, in which the Xq13–q26 region, containing the genes that are thought to control ovarian function, is spared, or in patients with a mosaic karyotype containing a 46,XX cell line that preserves ovarian function.

Cancer

Breast cancer is very uncommon in women with TS (in contrast, women in the general population have a lifetime risk of ~10%).

Clinical approach

History: key points

- Developmental milestones. The rare presence of significant delay or MR alerts to the possibility of a ring X, X-autosome translocation, or other structural abnormality of the X that alters X-inactivation or causes functional disomy.
- Deafness.

Examination: key points

- Height/length. Plot on TS-specific centile charts.
- Neck short, broad, webbed; low posterior hairline.
- Hands and feet. Puffiness/oedema. Short metacarpals and metatarsals, especially fourth. Small nails.
- Chest. Widely spaced nipples; chest described as shield-shaped. Breast development.
- Cardiovascular system. Delayed femoral pulses, heart murmurs, raised BP.
- Skin. Pigmented naevi.
- Secondary sexual development and external genitalia (if appropriate).

Special investigations

- Genomic array with karyotype with 30-cell count to investigate possible mosaicism.
- Consider FISH (*XIST*) in girls with r(X).
- Echo.
- Renal USS.
- Audiogram.
- Clinical photographs.

Management

Hall et al. noted in 1982 that one-third of TS was diagnosed in the neonatal period, one-third in childhood, and one-third in adolescence. Now many fetuses are found to have TS after oedema or hydrops is seen on nuchal translucency scans performed at 12 weeks' gestation. The postnatal management strategy described below is for the typical TS individual and may require modification to reflect karyotypes other than 45,X.

Antenatal

When TS has been detected due to the presence of fetal oedema/hydrops, there is a high chance that the

pregnancy will be lost naturally. For those women in whom the pregnancy is ongoing, scan for cardiac and renal anomalies. When detected incidentally, with no associated hydrops, the survival may be longer and the phenotype milder. For mosaic karyotypes, the prognosis depends on the proportion of abnormal cells and on the cell line involved. Discuss with the cytogenetic laboratory and use reference literature information.

Neonate

Document physical features. Renal scans and cardiovascular assessment are indicated. Give the parents information about future surveillance.

Childhood

All girls known to have TS should be under the care of a paediatric endocrinologist. Short stature, due to a combination of the loss of growth genes on the X (*SHOX*) and an absent pubertal growth spurt, can be partially corrected by GH in childhood, but the overall gain in height is comparatively small (~5 cm) (Ross et al. 2011) Recurrent otitis media is common, affecting approximately two-thirds of girls (Gungor et al. 2000), and a sensorineural dip in hearing that progresses over time has been observed as early as 6 years of age (Hultcrantz 2003). Careful surveillance for deafness is important to facilitate language acquisition and schooling.

Adolescence

Begin oestrogen replacement therapy, starting at the usual age of puberty. Continue to monitor BP. Deafness and autoimmune disease may present in this age group. Schooling and emotional difficulties may require management.

Adult

In addition to primary ovarian failure, adults with TS are also susceptible to a range of disorders, including osteoporosis, hypothyroidism, hypertension, hyperlipidaemia, and renal and GI disease. The problems of adult life are these.

- Primary ovarian failure. Continue sex hormone replacement. Ovum donation provides an option for some women with TS to become pregnant (see 'Clinical features' above). The prevalence of osteoporosis and bone fractures is not increased significantly in women with TS who are treated with standard oestrogen therapy. Women <150 cm in height are likely to be misdiagnosed with osteoporosis when a real bone density is measured, unless adjustments for body size are made (Bakalov et al. 2003).
- Autoimmune diseases. Hypothyroidism is a common problem; also diabetes mellitus (15%) and inflammatory bowel disease.
- Obesity. Ensure that hypothyroidism has been excluded.
- Deafness. High-frequency sensorineural hearing loss is very common and may be a premature variant of presbycusis. In Gungor et al.'s (2000) study, only one-third had normal audiometry.
- Reduced life expectancy. The life expectancy in TS is reduced due to cardiovascular disease, mainly aortic dissection, which is more common in individuals with pre-existing coarctation and with hypertension. There is also an increase in ischaemic heart disease (Mortensen et al. 2012).
- Bowel. Increased risk of inflammatory bowel disease. GI bleeding due to telangiectasiae.

Surveillance

It is recommended that women stay under the care of an endocrinologist, or a specialist with experience of TS, or preferably a multidisciplinary team (Trolle *et al.* 2012) to coordinate surveillance with the aim of improving life expectancy and reducing morbidity. Suggested screening to include:

- annual assessment of weight and BP. Consider tests of glucose and bone metabolism, LFTs, renal function if symptomatic;
- TFTs—baseline and then as required;
- cardiovascular risk profile;
- bone density scan—baseline as a young adult, then as required;
- hearing test (audiometry).

Genetic advice

The karyotype should include counting 30 cells to establish if there is mosaicism. Parental karyotypes are not requested in the presence of non-mosaic 45,X. Maternal karyotype is indicated when a girl has 46,XX and a structurally abnormal second X. Mosaicism involving 46,XY in the presence of a female phenotype requires consideration of the risk of gonadoblastoma in the residual gonadal tissue (Gravholt *et al.* 2000).

Recurrence risk

After the birth of a child (or the loss of a pregnancy) with 45,X, the risk of recurrence is very low.

Women who carry a structural rearrangement of an X chromosome have a high risk of recurrence and the phenotype may be severe or, more commonly, lethal in pregnancy if the fetus is male.

Offspring risk

Natural fertility is rare. PND should be considered (Tarani *et al.* 1998) because there may be an increased risk for trisomy 21 and 45,X.

Women carrying structural rearrangements are at risk for a similarly affected female or a more severe problem in a male fetus, which may not be viable. PND is possible by either CVS or amniocentesis.

Prenatal diagnosis

Recurrence risk is very low. PND based on this indication should be offered. USS for nuchal translucency at 10–14 weeks and later to examine for any evidence of hydrops may be considered as an alternative (Baena *et al.* 2004). NIPT could be offered, if available.

Support group: Turner Syndrome Support Society, http://www.tss.org.uk.

Expert adviser: Deborah Shears, Consultant in Clinical Genetics, Department of Clinical Genetics, Churchill Hospital, Oxford, UK.

References

Baena N, De Vigan C, Cariati E, *et al.* Turner syndrome; evaluation of prenatal diagnosis in 19 European registries. *Am J Med Genet A* 2004; **129A**: 16–20.

Bakalov VK, Chen ML, Baron J, *et al.* Bone mineral density and fractures in Turner syndrome. *Am J Med* 2003; **115**: 259–64.

Birkebaek NH, Cruger D, Hansen J, Nielsen J, Brunn-Petersen G. Fertility and pregnancy outcome in Danish women with Turner syndrome. *Clin Genet* 2002; **61**: 35–9.

Bondy C, Bakalov VK, Cheng C, Olivieri L, Rosing DR, Arai AE. Bicuspid aortic valve and aortic coarctation are linked to deletion of the X chromosome short arm in Turner syndrome. *J Med Genet* 2013; **50**: 662–5.

Cabanes L, Chalas C, Christin-Maitre S, *et al.* Turner syndrome and pregnancy: clinical practice. Recommendations for the management of patients with Turner syndrome before and during pregnancy. *Eur J Obstet Gynecol Reprod Biol* 2010; **152**: 18–24.

Conway GS, Band M, Doyle J, Davies MC. How do you monitor the patient with Turner's syndrome in adulthood? *Clin Endocrinol (Oxf)* 2010; **73**: 696–9.

Gould HN, Bakalov VK, Tankersley C, Bondy CA. High levels of education and employment among women with Turner syndrome. *J Womens Health (Larchmt)* 2013; **22**: 230–5.

Gravholt CH, Fedder J, Naeraa RW, Müller J. Occurrence of gonadoblastoma in females with Turner syndrome and Y chromosome material: a population study. *J Clin Endocrinol Metab* 2000; **85**: 3199–202.

Güngör N, Böke B, Belgin E, Tunçbilek E. High frequency hearing loss in Ullrich–Turner syndrome. *Eur J Pediatr* 2000; **159**: 740–4.

Guttenbach M, Koschorz B, Bernthaler U, Grimm T, Schmid M. Sex chromosome loss and aging: *in situ* hybridization studies on human interphase nuclei. *Am J Hum Genet* 1995; **57**: 1143–50.

Hall JG, Sybert VP, Williamson RA, Fisher NL, Reed SD. Turner syndrome. *West J Med* 1982; **137**: 32–44.

Hultcrantz M. Ear and hearing problems in Turner's syndrome. *Acta Otolaryngol* 2003; **123**: 253–7.

Karnis MF, Zimon AE, Lalwani SI, Timmreck LS, Klipstein S, Reindollar RH. Risk of death in pregnancy achieved through oocyte donation in patients with Turner syndrome: a national survey. *Fertil Steril* 2003; **80**: 498–501.

Kubota T, Wakui K, Nakamura T, *et al.* The proportion of cells with functional X disomy is associated with the severity of mental retardation in mosaic ring X Turner syndrome females. *Cytogenet Genome Res* 2002; **99**(1–4): 276–84.

Linden MG, Bender BG. Fifty-one prenatally diagnosed children and adolescents with sex chromosome anomalies. *Am J Med Genet* 2002; **110**: 11–18.

Linden MG, Bender BG, Robinson A. Genetic counseling for sex chromosome abnormalities. *Am J Med Genet* 2002; **110**: 3–10.

McCauley E, Feuillan P, Kushner H, Ross JL. Psychosocial development in adolescents with Turner syndrome. *J Dev Behav Pediatr* 2001; **22**: 360–5.

Mortensen KH, Andersen NH, Gravholt CH. Cardiovascular phenotype in Turner syndrome—integrating cardiology, genetics, and endocrinology. *Endocr Rev* 2012; **33**: 677–714.

Ross JL, Quigley CA. Growth hormone plus childhood low-dose estrogen in Turner's syndrome. *N Engl J Med* 2011; **364**: 1230–42.

Ross JL, Roeltgen D, Feuillan P, Kushner H, Cutler GB Jr. Use of estrogen in young girls with Turner syndrome: effects on memory. *Neurology* 2000; **54**: 164–70.

Saenger P. Wikland KA, Conway GS, *et al.* Recommendations for the diagnosis and management of Turner syndrome [review]. *J Clin Endocrinol Metab* 2001; **86**: 3061–9.

Sebire NJ, Snijders RJ, Brown R, Southall T, Nicolaides KH. Detection of sex chromosome abnormalities by nuchal translucency screening at 10–14/40. *Prenat Diagn* 1998; **18**: 581–4.

Skuse DH, James RS, Bishop DV, *et al.* Evidence from Turner's syndrome of an imprinted X-linked locus affecting cognitive function. *Nature* 1997; **387**: 705–8.

Swerdlow AJ, Hermon C, Jacobs PA, *et al.* Mortality and cancer incidence in persons with numerical sex chromosome abnormalities: a cohort study. *Ann Hum Genet* 2001; **65**(Pt 2): 177–88.

Sybert VP, McCauley E. Turner's syndrome. *N Engl J Med* 2004; **351**: 1227–8.

Tarani L, Lampariello S, Raquso G, *et al.* Pregnancy in patients with Turner's syndrome: six new cases and review of literature. *Gynecol Endocrinol* 1998; **12**: 83–7.

Therman E, Susman B. The similarity of phenotypic effects caused by Xp and Xq deletions in the human female: a hypothesis. *Hum Genet* 1990; **90**: 185–6.

Trolle C, Mortensen KH, Hjerrild BE, Cleemann L, Gravholt CH. Clinical care of adult Turner syndrome—new aspects. *Pediatr Endocrinol Rev* 2012; **9**(Suppl 2): 739–49.

Uematsu A, Yorifuji T, Muroi J, *et al.* Parental origin of normal X chromosome in Turner syndrome with various karyotypes: implications for the mechanism leading to generation of a 45,X karyotype. *Am J Med Genet* 2002; **111**: 134–9.

X-autosome translocations

Translocations between an X chromosome and an autosome are different to autosomal translocations, and genetic counselling is more complex, for the following reasons.

X-inactivation

In women, a single X chromosome is functional per diploid adult cell. The other X is described as inactive and this inactivation occurs by the second week following conception. X-inactivation in the embryo is usually a random process. Usually the ratio approximates to 50%. This process is genetically controlled from the X-inactivation centre. The *XIST* gene, in the X-inactivation centre (Xic) at Xq13, is a *cis*-acting gene and only transcribed in the inactive X. The Xist long non-coding RNA (lncRNA) coats the future inactive X chromosome and recruits Polycomb repressive complex 2 (PRC2) to the Xic. Xist then spreads silencing to most of the X chromosome (Simon *et al.* 2013), although some regions escape X-inactivation, notably the pseudoautosomal regions (PARs). Methylation maintains inactivation.

X-inactivation patterns may be assessed by comparing the ratio of the two alleles at a highly polymorphic site, e.g. the CA repeat in the androgen receptor gene, in a non-methylation-sensitive assay with the ratio of the same alleles in a methylation-sensitive assay. The genes at the tip of the short arm of the X in Xp22.3 escape inactivation; this area is known as the pseudoautosomal region (PAR).

Functional disomy

The genes on each X are active—one copy has escaped inactivation. An abnormal phenotype results from overexpression of the affected genes—an important mechanism both in females with apparently balanced X;autosome translocations and in association with X-duplications.

X-inactivation pattern observed in balanced female carriers

Those cells in which the intact X remained active would have functional disomy (see above) for the part of the X that is unable to inactivate because of the translocation. There is selection against this and, in the majority of balanced carriers:
- the 'normal' X that is not involved in the translocation is inactive;
- the two parts of the translocated X are active.

However, in these balanced carriers, phenotypic abnormalities may arise:
- if the chromosomal breakpoint is through a gene;
- if the active X carries an XL mutation;
- if the 'skewing' of X-inactivation varies between different tissues (Hatchwell *et al.* 1996).

In those carriers where the intact X remains active, the genes that are functionally disomic can lead to phenotypic features and developmental delay (e.g. in hypomelanosis of Ito). Also contributing to the phenotype is the possibility of spreading inactivation of genes from the derivative chromosome carrying the Xic into the contiguous region of the autosome.

X chromosome inactivation can spread into an autosome of patients with X;autosome translocations. Sakazume *et al.* (2012) reported a male patient with an X;15 translocation and a PWS phenotype where X chromosome inactivation spread into the paternal chromosome 15 led to the aberrant hypermethylation of *SNRPN* and *OCA2* (with decreased expression) and the PWS-like features and hypopigmentation of the patient.

X-inactivation pattern observed in unbalanced females

The situation is reversed and selective inactivation of the abnormal X (as long as it contains the Xic) gives a milder than expected phenotype. Additionally, spreading of inactivation on to the autosome results in a reduction of trisomy of that section to functional disomy. If there is no Xic in the translocated X, there will be functional partial disomy of the X and autosomal monosomy.

Clinical features

X-linked disease in a female proband. X;autosome translocations that disrupt a disease gene on the X can result in manifestation of the disease in a female, e.g. X;autosome translocations with a breakpoint in Xp21.2 can account for clinical signs of DMD and BMD. Translocations lead to skewed X-inactivation of the normal dystrophin gene at an early stage of development, as there is selection for cells where the normal X is inactive.

Hypomelanosis of Ito

Is characterized by swirly disturbances of skin pigmentation over the trunk and linear or streaky pigmentary disturbance over the limbs. It is known to be associated in many cases with chromosomal mosaicism. While no particular pattern is generally evident for the specific chromosomes involved in such patients, a subgroup of female patients exists in whom the common factor is the presence of a balanced, constitutional X;autosome translocation, with a cytogenetic breakpoint in the pericentromeric region of the X. The phenotype in these cases may result not from the interruption of XL genes, but from the presence of mosaic functional disomy of X sequences above the breakpoint (Hatchwell 1996).

Infertility

- Female infertility. Some female carriers of X;autosome translocations may be infertile. There are critical regions of the X chromosome (Xq13–q22 and Xq22–27) which, if involved with the translocation, may be associated with gonadal dysgenesis (Therman *et al.* 1990). These women are at risk from primary amenorrhoea or POF.
- Male infertility. Males with X;autosome translocations are infertile.

Clinical approach

Ask your colleagues in cytogenetics to produce an annotated photograph together with an ideogram of the chromosomes involved in the translocation. This is an invaluable aid to counselling.

History: key points

- Draw a three-generation family tree (or larger, if indicated, with particular attention to the maternal line)

and enquire about pregnancy loss, stillbirth, neonatal death, and family members with learning disability or congenital anomalies.
- Males with infertility (carriers (?)).
- Ovarian failure.
- Presence of developmental delay.
- Conditions that may be XL.

Examination: key points
- Full clinical examination and documentation of dysmorphic features.
- Neurocutaneous features, especially pigmentary disturbance (hypomelanosis of Ito).

Special investigations
- Genomic array to determine whether there is any loss or gain at the breakpoints.
- Arrange for parental chromosome analysis.

Genetic advice
- *De novo.* X;autosome translocations are usually of paternal origin.
- The mother also has an X;autosome translocation. Discuss with the laboratory the theoretical outcomes of segregation at meiosis. The differences between this type of translocation and an autosomal translocation include the following.
  - A rearrangement with functional disomy of part of the X is likely to have a phenotypic effect and this includes a risk of severe MR.
  - There may be partial Turner, Klinefelter's, or XXX syndromes.
  - The viability of an autosomal imbalance may be improved because of spreading inactivation, such that the abnormality is viable but has a risk of severe phenotypic abnormality.
  - Apparently balanced male hemizygotes have been reported with both normal and abnormal phenotypes, making phenotypic prediction on the basis of the karyotype difficult.

Recurrence risk
- *De novo.* Very low.

- Maternal. Although there is a high risk of imbalance, the difficulty lies in predicting the likely phenotypic effect. Even in mothers and babies with the same chromosome change, the phenotype may be variable.

Prenatal diagnosis
Because of the difficulty in predicting X-inactivation, only 46,XX and 46,XY are accurate predictors of a normal phenotype. USS for evidence of structural abnormality.

Support group: Unique (The Rare Chromosome Disorder Support Group), http://www.rarechromo.org, Tel. 01883 330 766.

References

Gardner RJM, Sutherland GR, Shaffer LG. *Chromosome abnormalities and genetic counseling, Oxford monographs on medical genetics no. 31,* 4th edn. Oxford University Press, New York, 2011.

Hatchwell E. Hypomelanosis of Ito and X; autosome translocations: a unifying hypothesis. *J Med Genet* 1996; **33**: 177–83.

Hatchwell E, Robinson D, Crolla JA, Cockwell AE. X inactivation analysis in a female with hypomelanosis of Ito associated with a balanced X;17 translocation: evidence for functional disomy of Xp. *J Med Genet* 1996; **33**: 216–20.

Powell CM, Taggart RT, Drumheller TC, *et al*. Molecular and cytogenetic studies of an X;autosome translocation in a patient with premature ovarian failure and review of the literature. *Am J Med Genet* 1994; **52**: 19–26.

Sakazume SI, Ohashi H, Sasaki Y, *et al*. Spread of X-chromosome inactivation into chromosome 15 is associated with Prader-Willi syndrome phenotype in a boy with a t(X;15)(p21.1;q11.2) translocation. *Hum Genet* 2012; **131**: 121–30.

Sharp AJ, Spotswood HT, Robinson DO, Turner BM, Jacobs PA. Molecular and cytogenetic analysis of the spreading of X inactivation in X; autosome translocations. *Hum Mol Genet* 2002; **11**: 3145–56.

Simon MD, Pinter SF, Fang R, *et al*. High-resolution Xist binding maps reveal two-step spreading during X-chromosome inactivation. *Nature* 2013; **504**: 465–9.

Therman E, Laxova R, Susman B. The critical region on the human Xq. *Hum Genet* 1990; **85**: 455–61.

Pregnancy and fertility

Chapter contents

Anterior abdominal wall defects

The overall prevalence is 4.3/10 000 births (Overton et al. 2012). The frequent use of antenatal USS and maternal serum AFP has increasingly led to the detection of abdominal wall defects before birth. USS, commonly performed in the first trimester at the dating scan, has taken over from maternal serum AFP measurement as the main method of detection now. The sensitivity of USS detection is ~90% for both gastroschisis and exomphalos. There should be close liaison with neonatal intensive care and paediatric surgery regarding perinatal management. Currently, there is no convincing evidence to support routine LSCS to deliver most abdominal wall defects, unless the defect is very large.

Gastroschisis

Gastroschisis involves herniation of the gut and occasionally the genitourinary tract through an abdominal wall defect to one side (usually the right) of the umbilicus. The defect arises through incomplete closure of the lateral folds of the embryo during the sixth week of gestation. No membrane covers the loops, which float free in the amniotic fluid. Intestinal atresia may occur as a complication of gastroschisis.

Gastroschisis is usually an isolated defect; up to 12–15% of cases have other anomalies (Mastroiacovo et al. 2007). There is no appreciable increase in the incidence of aneuploidy in isolated gastroschisis. Amniocentesis is not indicated if gastroschisis is an isolated finding.

Gastroschisis is strongly associated with young maternal age, mothers under 20 being 12 times more likely to have infants with gastroschisis. In Europe, the total prevalence of gastroschisis has changed from 0.54/10 000 births in 1980–84 to 2.12/10 000 in 2000–2002 (Loane et al. 2007). The increase in risk over time was the same for mothers of all ages. The speed at which the increase has occurred suggests environmental, rather than genetic, risk factors. Over 1 year, in the UK, the overall fetal loss rate of pregnancies with gastroschisis was reported as 1 in 7 (8% TOP, 2% miscarriage, 4% late stillbirth, 5.5% neonatal death) (Overton 2012). Of live births with isolated gastroschisis in the Northern Region study (Rankin et al. 1999), 92.3% were alive at 1 year. The pregnancy should be monitored closely and delivery planned for ~37 weeks' gestation (David et al. 2008). Perinatal management involves normal delivery in a high-risk perinatal centre, with cling film applied over the externalized bowel loops immediately after delivery. Note the association with amyoplasia and intestinal atresia (Reid et al. 1986).

Exomphalos

Exomphalos (omphalocele) is a midline defect with herniation of abdominal contents into the base of the umbilical cord, confined by an amnioperitoneal membrane. In a large exomphalos, the liver, as well as the intestine, may be present in the sac. There is a high incidence of aneuploidy (30%), especially +18 and +13, and the finding of an exomphalos is an indication for karyotyping, e.g. by amniocentesis. Overall, in two-thirds of cases (including those with aneuploidy), there are other structural anomalies, often multiple, especially CHD; in one-third, the exomphalos is an isolated anomaly. Of live births with

isolated exomphalos and a normal karyotype, 95.5% were alive at 1 year and 80% at 11 years (Lakasing et al. 2006).

Exomphalos is a feature of BWS (also characterized by macrosomia, macroglossia, and nephromegaly). If any of these features or a large placenta/polyhydramnios are present, carefully consider this diagnosis. See 'Beckwith–Wiedemann syndrome (BWS)' in Chapter 3, 'Common consultations', p. 358.

Perinatal management involves aiming for a vaginal delivery in a hospital with a neonatal unit, unless the exomphalos is large, in which case delivery should be planned at a high-risk perinatal centre and delivery by Caesarian section may be indicated. There is an increased incidence of respiratory distress syndrome, and blood sugar should be monitored in view of the association with BWS. The baby should be transferred after delivery for treatment in a paediatric surgical centre.

Bladder exstrophy

Bladder exstrophy has an incidence of 1/10 000–1/40 000 births and is more common in males (2.3M:1F). It is caused by incomplete closure of the inferior part of the anterior abdominal wall. The defect starts at 4 weeks' gestation and is caused by failure of migration of mesenchymal cells between the ectoderm of the abdomen and the cloaca. Separation of the pubic bones, a low-set umbilicus, and abnormal genitalia are associated anomalies. Surgical intervention is required to reconstruct the bladder, abdominal wall, and genitalia, with initial surgery usually performed within the first 48 hours after birth.

OEIS (omphalocele and epispadias–exstrophy of the bladder–imperforate anus–spinal anomalies) complex

OEIS is a spectrum of developmental anomalies of increasing severity. OEIS is rare, affecting ~1/200 000. It is probably sporadic with a low recurrence risk, but affected individuals have not reproduced. The majority of males with OEIS have extremely abnormal genitalia.

Body wall complex (body stalk anomaly)

Presence of body wall defects with evisceration of thoracic and/or abdominal organs, often in association with NTD and/or limb deficiency. Scoliosis, abnormalities of the lower extremities, and a short/absent umbilical cord are common features. Maternal serum AFP is usually markedly elevated.

Clinical assessment

History: key points

- Three generation family history including birth weight (Beckwith syndrome).
- Maternal age (young age associated with gastroschisis).
- Maternal diabetes.
- Early pregnancy bleeding and other early pregnancy problems.

Examination: key points

- Detailed fetal anomaly USS to search for other anomalies and assess fetal growth, and in gastroschisis the development of polyhydramnios, a dilated stomach, or dilated bowel, which may be useful prognostic indicators.

Special investigations
- Offer fetal genomic array (e.g. CVS, amniocentesis, or NIPD) in selected cases, e.g. exomphalos.

Genetic advice and management
- Gastroschisis. Isolated gastroschisis has a low sibling recurrence risk of ~1%. For a parent with gastroschisis, the offspring risk is low, with only two reported cases of parent–child occurrence (Schmidt *et al.* 2005).
- Exomphalos. Isolated exomphalos has a low sibling recurrence risk of ~1%.
- Bladder exstrophy is usually a sporadic defect, although occasional familial cases have been reported. Recurrence risk is ~1%. For a parent with bladder exstrophy, the risk to offspring is ~1/70.
- OEIS is probably sporadic with a low recurrence risk, but affected individuals have not reproduced.
- Body wall complex is probably sporadic with a low recurrence risk.

Support group: GEEPS (Gastroschisis Exomphalos Extrophies Parents' Support Network), http://www.geeps.co.uk.

Expert adviser: Anna David, Professor and Consultant in Obstetrics and Maternal Fetal Medicine, Head of Research Department of Maternal Fetal Medicine, Institute for Women's Health, University College London, London, UK.

References
Anteby EY, Yagel S. Route of delivery of fetuses with structural anomalies. *Eur J Obstet Gynecol Reprod Biol* 2003; **106**: 5–9.

Christison-Lagay ER, Kelleher CM, Langer JC. Neonatal abdominal wall defects. *Semin Fetal Nenonatal Med* 2011; **16**: 164–72.

Curry JI, McKinney P, Thornton JG, Stringer MD. The aetiology of gastroschisis. *BJOG* 2000; **107**: 1339–46.

David AL, Tan A, Curry J. Gastroschisis: sonographic diagnosis, associations, management and outcome. *Prenat Diagn* 2008; **28**: 633–44.

Di Tanna GL, Rosano A, Mastroiacovo P. Prevalence of gastroschisis at birth: retrospective study. *BMJ* 2002; **325**: 1389–90.

Heider AL, Strauss RA, Kuller JA. Omphalocele: clinical outcomes in cases with normal karyotypes. *Am J Obstet Gynecol* 2004; **190**: 135–41.

Lakasing L, Cicero S, Davenport M, Patel S, Nicolaides KH. Current outcome of antenatally diagnosed exomphalos: an 11 year review. *J Pediatr Surg* 2006; **41**: 1403–6.

Ledbetter DJ. Congenital abdominal wall defects and reconstruction in pediatric surgery: gastroschisis and omphalocele. *Surg Clin North Am* 2012; **92**: 713–27.

Loane M, Dolk H, Bradbur I. Increasing prevalence of gastroschisis in Europe 1980–2002: a phenomenon restricted to younger mothers? *Paediatr Perinat Epidemiol* 2007; **21**: 363–9.

Mastroiacovo P, Lisi A, Castilla EE, *et al.* Gastroschisis and associated defects: an international study. *Am J Med Genet A* 2007; **143A**: 660–71.

Overton TG, Pierce MR, Gao H, *et al.* Antenatal management and outcomes of gastroschisis in the U.K. *Prenat Diagn* 2012; **32**: 1256–62.

Rankin J, Dillon E, Wright C. Congenital anterior abdominal wall defects in the North of England, 1986–1996: occurrence and outcome. *Prenat Diagn* 1999; **19**: 662–8.

Reid CO, Hall JG, Anderson C, *et al.* Association of amyoplasia with gastroschisis, bowel atresia and defects of the muscular layer of the trunk. *Am J Med Genet* 1986; **24**: 701–10.

Salihu HM, Boos R, Schmidt W, *et al.* Omphalocele and gastroschisis. *J Obstet Gynecol* 2002; **22**: 489–92.

Schmidt AI, Glüer S, Mühlhaus K, Ure BM. Family cases of gastroschisis. *J Pediatr Surg* 2005; **40**: 740–1.

Stone DH, Rimaz S, Gilmour WH. Prevalence of congenital anterior abdominal wall defects in the United Kingdom: comparison of regional registers. *BMJ* 1998; **317**: 1118–19.

Wilcox DT, Chitty LS. Non-visualisation of the fetal bladder: aetiology and management. *Prenat Diagn* 2001; **21**: 977–83.

Assisted reproductive technology: *in vitro* fertilization (IVF), intracytoplasmic sperm injection (ICSI), and pre-implantation genetic diagnosis (PGD)

Assisted reproductive technology (ART) has revolutionized the treatment of infertility. Treatment with ART now accounts for 1–3% of all births in many Western countries. In conjunction with embryo biopsy and analysis of extracted DNA using PCR, aCGH, SNP arrays, or FISH. PGD has been available for an increasing number of genetic disorders since 1990 and can be offered to some patients as an alternative to prenatal diagnosis (PND).

In vitro fertilization (IVF)

Controlled stimulation of the ovaries with exogenous gonadotrophins leads to the recruitment of many follicles (monitored by USS). When the number and size of the developing follicles is deemed appropriate, oocyte maturation is triggered hormonally. Thirty-four to 38 hours later, the oocytes are collected by transvaginal USS-guided aspiration of the follicular fluid. The oocytes are then fertilized *in vitro* with the partner's sperm and any resulting morphologically sound embryos are transferred into the woman's uterus 2–7 days later.

Davies *et al.* (2012) found that 7.2% of infants conceived with IVF had a birth defect diagnosed before the child's fifth birthday, compared with 5.8% in infants conceived without assisted conception treatment in South Australia (adjusted OR, 1.07; 95% CI, 0.90–1.26).

The use of ART increases the risk of having a term singleton with low birthweight (OR, 1.4; 95% CI, 1.1–1.7) (Henningsen *et al.* 2011). In Schieve *et al.*'s (2002) study, infants conceived after ART (IVF, donor oocyte, ICSI) accounted for 0.6% of all infants born to mothers 20 years or older, but 3.5% of low birthweight infants and 4.3% of very low birthweight infants. A possible link has recently been made between *in vitro* conception and certain congenital abnormalities, notably BWS, although the absolute risk appears to be low (BWS; Gosden *et al.* 2003; Maher *et al.* 2003; Odom and Segars 2010). Halliday *et al.* (2004) estimates the risk of BWS after IVF to be one in 4000, but no excess cases were seen in a large Danish Registry study (Lindegaard *et al.* 2005).

Intracytoplasmic sperm injection (ICSI)

ICSI involves the injection of a single sperm directly into the cytoplasm of a mature oocyte. ICSI is favoured for fertility patients where there is male factor infertility, including azoospermia, oligozoospermia, and poor sperm morphology or motility. Additionally, ICSI is used for PCR-based PGD techniques to avoid the risk of extracting extra sperm, buried in the zona pellucida, at embryo biopsy, which would contaminate the assay. Davies *et al.* (2012) found that 9.9% of infants conceived with ICSI had a birth defect before the child's fifth birthday, compared with 5.8% in infants conceived without assisted conception treatment (adjusted OR, 1.57; 95% CI, 1.30–1.90).

Pre-implantation genetic diagnosis (PGD)

PGD has now been available for over two decades and is becoming more widely recognized as a valid clinical service available in many countries. PGD can now be offered for a very wide range of chromosome abnormalities (Mackie Ogilvie *et al.* 2009), originally using FISH analysis but now more commonly array CGH, as well as for almost any single gene disorder, following the development of pre-implantation genetic haplotyping (Renwick *et al.* 2006), direct mutation testing with linked markers, aCGH, and more recently SNP arrays and NGS SNP arrays (Harper and Sengupta 2012).

Most couples requesting PGD do so because they wish to avoid the possibility of terminating a pregnancy following PND. Others may require ART anyway to circumvent a fertility problem that may be caused by a genetic disorder, e.g. CBAVD, as well as the presence of a genetic risk to the offspring.

PGD was first introduced for sexing embryos in the case of XL genetic disorders in 1990 (Handyside *et al.* 1990). In 1992, the first case of a live-born girl after successful PGD for the single gene disorder CF was reported. PGD for single gene disorders moved on a stage further in 1995 with the successful outcome of a pregnancy following PGD for DMD to detect the dystrophin gene deletion. This resulted in a successful non-carrier female pregnancy. Since then, the worldwide development of this service has expanded and the European Society of Human Reproduction and Embryology (ESHRE) published its 13th annual data collection in 2015 from 62 centres internationally (De Rycke *et al.* 2015). The previous 12 data collections were from 57 centres (Harper *et al.* 2010a).

This latest publication reports outcomes of 17 721 cycles of PGD that reached oocyte retrieval (OR). Of these, 6968 oocyte retrievals were reported for chromosome abnormalities, 2814 (1484 sexing only) for XL disease, 7294 for autosomal recessive or dominant monogenic conditions, and 643 for HLA (Human Leucocytic Antigen) typing, This resulted in 12 785 cycles reaching embryo transfer (ET) and a subsequent clinical pregnancy rate of 21% per OR and 29% per ET. A total of 26,737 cycles reached OR for pre-implantation genetic screening (PGS) (performed for couples who do not carry a specific genetic abnormality but who have experienced recurrent IVF failure; the decrease in PGS cases reported in the last data collection is likely to be a consequence of the publication of RCTs that indicated no evidence that PGS improves IVF success rates (Harper et al. 2010b) The data describe the reasons for referral, reproductive histories, and the outcomes of treatment. It is clear that most of the couples requesting PGD have had at least one pregnancy previously that has resulted in a fetus or child with a genetic disorder and that most of these couples do not have any living unaffected children. Cumulative data are reported on 3110 pregnancies, which resulted in 8453 babies born.

Outcome of live-born babies

Evidence suggests that human embryo development *in vitro* is not affected by biopsy at the 8-cell stage (Hardy *et al.* 1990). Most embryo biopsy now takes place at blastocyst stage—day 5–7 of embryo development, with frozen embryo transfer more common. Evidence exists that such strategies do not affect success rate and improve birth weight. (Pelkonen et al. 2010). The need for international collaboration for long-term follow-up of children born as the result of PGD was recognized but is only systematically organized in some provider centres. In general, the outcome following PGD is thought to be the same as that following ICSI without embryo biopsy (Desmyttere et al. 2012).

Worldwide, PGD is now available for a wide range of genetic disorders. Setting up a pre-implantation genetic assay for a specific genetic mutation is time-consuming and labour-intensive, but the availability of PGD for single gene disorders has been revolutionized by the development of pre-implantation genetic haplotyping (PGH), which does not require a mutation-specific assay; instead, informative linked markers either side of the relevant are identified and more recently SNP based platforms, enabling PGD to be offered to any couple carrying a single gene disorder in whom the relevant gene is known and sufficient DNA samples are available to establish the phase (Renwick et al. 2006). Box 6.1 is not designed to give an exhaustive list of conditions for which PGD is available, but it does indicate the conditions for which PGD is commonly requested. A list of all conditions for which PGD is licensed by the Human Fertilisation and Embryology Authority (HFEA) in the UK is available at http://guide.hfea.gov.uk/pgd.

Regulation of PGD

The regulation of PGD worldwide varies from country to country (Geraedts et al. 2001). In many countries where regulations do apply, the bodies responsible for ART will also regulate PGD. The UK Human Fertilisation

---

Box 6.1 Some genetic disorders for which PGD is currently available

Autosomal dominant
- Myotonic dystrophy
- Huntington disease (for known mutation carriers and also exclusion testing for those at 50% risk of having a mutation)
- *BRCA1* and 2

Autosomal recessive
- Cystic fibrosis
- Spinal muscular atrophy
- Beta-thalassaemia
- Sickle-cell disease

X-linked
- Fragile X syndrome
- Alport syndrome
- Duchenne/Becker muscular dystrophy
- Haemophilia
- Hunter syndrome
- Incontinentia pigmenti

Chromosomal disorders[‡]
- Robertsonian translocations
- Reciprocal translocations
- Other chromosomal disorders (inversions, deletions)

[‡] Dependent upon the availability of FISH probes.

Data from the Human Fertilisation and Embryology Authority (HFEA) http://guide.hfea.gov.uk/pgd/.

---

and Embryology Act (HFE Act 1990 and 2008) came into being and, in accordance with the Act, the HFEA was convened in 1990. This regulates all ART, including PGD in the UK.

Success rate

The pregnancy and live birth success rates of PGD are comparable with those for infertile couples undergoing ART. The cumulative ESHRE data suggested an average pregnancy success rate of 29% per embryo transferred (De Rycke 2015), although the success rate varies considerably between different centres. The majority of couples referred for PGD are fertile, so the chance of success, compared with natural conception, must be discussed with couples in detail prior to the start of treatment.

Side effects of treatment

The occurrence of ovarian hyperstimulation syndrome (OHSS) is relatively common but can vary in its clinical severity from mild to severe and life-threatening. In its mildest form, it is likely to occur in 8–23% of cases and, in its severe form, in 0.1–2% of cases. In severe cases, OHSS can incur a hospital admission for a woman undergoing treatment and this is of specific concern for those undertaking PGD who may have a disabled child at home requiring care; however changes to ovarian stimulation protocols have shown reduced risk of OHSS (Youssef et al. 2015).

Misdiagnosis

Twelve cases of misdiagnosis have been reported to ESHRE since data collection started (De Rycke 2015). The technology of single cell analysis is complex and demanding and all couples are made aware of the chance of this happening. There are several possible reasons for misdiagnosis, including mosaicism, although less common in blastocyst biopsy, and allele dropout (ADO), which results in elective amplification of only one of the two parental alleles being studied. ADO could lead to misdiagnosis in a dominant disorder due to loss of the affected allele. Finally, the need to apply large numbers of PCR cycles to obtain an adequate DNA sample from the biopsied single cell creates scope for contamination. Recent evaluation of monogenic strategies concluded that the use of PCR multiplex protocols is the most important criteria for reducing misdiagnosis risk (Dreesen 2014). The risk of misdiagnosis caused by ADO and contamination will be reduced if a sufficient number of informative markers are used.

Special issues

- HLA tissue typing for BMT. One of the most controversial uses of PGD is that of HLA typing to provide a compatible bone marrow-matched child for a sibling with a genetic disorder. The aim of this technology is to analyse the embryos for the genetic disorder concerned and detect an embryo that is both unaffected and an HLA type match for the affected sibling (Verlinsky et al. 2001). This is a highly technically demanding procedure with a limited chance of success, as the chance of each embryo being both unaffected by a recessive condition (3 in 4) and also an HLA match (1 in 4) is only 3/16. In a study of 242 couples undertaking PGD for HLA typing, the chance of successful transplantation was 9.5% (Kahraman 2014). The use of PGD to identify an HLA-matched embryo for a sibling that needs a BMT for a non-genetic reason is even more controversial, as there is no genetic indication for performing an embryo biopsy, but this is required to identify a suitable HLA-matched potential donor.

- Pre-implantation genetic screening (PGS). In July 2001, the HFEA approved in principle the technique of PGS or aneuploidy screening (Ferriman 2001). This technique differs from PGD as it is applied to couples who have had repeated IVF/ICSI failures. It was hoped that by screening the embryos for chromosomal abnormalities, PGS would increase the pregnancy rate among infertile couples of 35 years and over, who were undergoing ART. A more recent meta-analysis shows that PGS does not improve the live birth rate after IVF and, on the contrary, for women of advanced maternal age, PGS significantly lowers the live birth rate, and therefore should not be offered (Mastenbroek et al. 2011). Debate about the value of PGS persists in relation to which patients, if any, should be offered it., Many believe its use should be deferred until the outcome of further large RCTs is known (Sermon et al. 2016).

Expert advisers: Frances Flinter, Consultant Clinical Geneticist, Department of Clinical Genetics, Guy's and St Thomas' NHS Foundation Trust, Guy's Hospital, London, UK and Alison Lashwood, Consultant Genetic Counsellor, Guy's and St Thomas' NHS Foundation Trust, London, UK.

References

Davies M, Moore V, Willson K, et al. Reproductive technologies and the risk of birth defects. N Engl J Med 2012; **366**: 1803–13.

De Rycke M, Belva F, et al. ESHRE PGD Consortium data collection XIII: cycles from January to December 2010 with pregnancy follow-up to October 2011. Hum Reprod 2015; **30**(8): 1763–89.

Desmyttere S, De Rycke M, Liebaers I, et al. Neoonatal follow up of 995 consecutively born children after embryo biopsy for PGD. Hum Reprod 2012; **27**: 288–93.

Dreesen J, Destouni A, et al. Evaluation of PCR-based preimplantation genetic diagnosis applied to monogenic diseases: a collaborative ESHRE PGD consortium study. Eur J Hum Genet 2014; **22**: 1012–8.

Ferriman A. UK approves preimplantation genetic screening technique. BMJ 2001; **323**: 125.

Geraedts JP, Harper J, Braude P, et al. Preimplantation genetic diagnosis (PGD), a collaborative activity of clinical genetic departments and IVF centres. Prenat Diagn 2001; **21**: 1086–92.

Gosden R, Trasler J, Lucifero D, Faddy M. Rare congenital disorders, imprinted genes, and assisted reproductive technology. Lancet 2003; **361**: 1975–7.

Halliday J, Oke K, Breheny S, Algar E, J Amor D. Beckwith–Wiedemann syndrome and IVF: a case-control study. Am J Hum Genet 2004; **75**: 526–8.

Handyside AH, Delhanty J. Preimplantation genetic diagnosis: strategies and surprises. Trends Genet 1997; **13**: 270–5.

Handyside AH, Kontogianni, EH, Hardy K, Winston RM. Pregnancies from biopsied human preimplantation embryos sexed by Y specific DNA amplification. Nature 1990; **344**: 768–70.

Hansen M, Kurinczuk JJ, Bower C, Webb S. The risk of major birth defects after intracytoplasmic sperm injection and in vitro fertilization. N Engl J Med 2002; **346**: 725–30.

Hardy K, Martin K, Leese HJ, Winston RM, Handyside AH. Human preimplantation development in vitro is not adversely affected by biopsy at the 8-cell stage. Hum Reprod 1990; **5**: 708–14.

Harper JC, Coonen E, De Rycke M, et al. ESHRE PGD Consortium data collection X: cycles from January to December 2007 with pregnancy follow-up to October 2008. Hum Reprod 2010; **25**: 2685–707.

Harper JC, Coonen E, Handyside AH, Winston RM, Hopman AH, Delhanty JD. Mosaicism of autosomes in morphologically normal, monospermic preimplantation human embryos. Prenat Diagn 1995; **15**: 41–9.

Harper JC, Sengupta SB. Preimplantation genetic diagnosis: state of the art 2011. Hum Genet 2012; **131**: 175–86.

Henningsen A, Pinborg A, Lidegaard Ø, Vestergaard C, Forman JL, Andersen AN. Perinatal outcome of singleton siblings born after ART and spontaneous conception: Danish national sibling-cohort study. Fertil Steril 2011; **95**: 959–63.

HFEA: Scientific review of the safety and efficacy of methods to avoid mitochondrial disease through assisted conception: 2016 update.

Kahraman S, Beyazyurek C, et al. Successful haematopoietic stem cell transplantation in 44 children from healthy siblings conceived after preimplantation HLA matching. Reprod Biomed Online 2014; **29**: 340–51.

Lidegaard O, Pinborg A, Andersen AN. Imprinting diseases and IVF: Danish National IIVF cohort study. Hum Reprod 2005; **20**: 950–4.

Mackie Ogilvie C, Scriven P. Preimplantation genetic diagnosis for chromosomal rearrangements. In: JC Harper (ed.). Preimplantation genetic diagnosis, 2nd edn, pp 193–202. Cambridge University Press, New York, 2009.

Maher ER, Brueton LA, Bowdin SC, et al. Beckwith–Wiedemann syndrome and assisted reproduction technology (ART). J Med Genet 2003; **40**: 62–4.

Mastenbroek S, Twisk M, van der Veen F, Repping S. Preimplantation genetic screening: a systematic review and meta-analysis of RCTs. Hum Reprod Update 2011; **17**: 454–66.

Odom L, Segars J. Imprinting disorders and assisted conception. Curr Opin Endocrinol Diabetes Obes 2010; **17**: 517–22.

Pelkonen S, Koivunen R, et al. Perinatal outcome of children born after frozen and fresh embryo transfer: the Finnish cohort study 1995-2006. Hum Reprod 2010; **25**: 914–23.

Renwick PJ, Trussler J, Ostad-Saffari E, et al. Proof of principle and first cases using preimplantation genetic haplotyping—a paradigm shift for embryo diagnosis. Reprod Biomed Online 2006; **13**: 110–19.

Schieve LA, Ferre C, Peterson HB, Jeng G, Wilcox LS. Low and very low birth weight in infants conceived with use of assisted reproductive technology. N Engl J Med 2002; **346**: 731–7.

Sermon K, Van Steirteghem A, Liebaers I. Preimplantation diagnosis [review]. Lancet 2004; **363**: 1633–41.

Sermon K, Capalbo A, et al. The why, the how and the when of PGS 2.0: current practices and expert opinions of fertility specialists, molecular biologists, and embryologists. Mol Hum Reprod 2016; **22**: 845–57.

Verlinsky Y, Rechitsky S, Schoolcraft W, Strom C, Kuliev A. Preimplantation diagnosis for Fanconi anemia combined with HLA matching. JAMA 2001; **285**: 3130–3.

Youssef M, Abdelmoty H, et al. GnRH agonist for final oocyte maturation in GnRH antagonist co-treated IVF/ICSI treatment cycles: Systematic review and meta-analysis. J Adv Res 2015; **6**: 341–9.

Bowed limbs

The femur length is measured routinely during the anomaly USS at 18–20 weeks' gestation to compare with other fetal measurements, such as head circumference and abdominal circumference, to assess proportionate growth. Bowing of all the long bones, or an isolated long bone, may be seen at this scan. Alternative terms for bowing include bent or angulated. Bowing is often seen in association with limb shortening.

Clinical assessment

History: key points
- Maternal factors; e.g. IDDM (an association with femoral hypoplasia–unusual facies).
- Raised paternal age.
- Three-generation family history. Note a history of skeletal abnormality, brittle bones/OI, previously affected sibling(s), stillbirth, or neonatal death.
- Consanguinity (AR dysplasias and syndromes).
- Establish an accurate gestational age for the pregnancy (use earliest available USS).

Examination: key points
- Measurements of all long bones and head and abdominal circumference.
- Is there any evidence of asymmetry?
- Are all the bones bowed, or is only one limb or one bone affected?
- If the femora are bowed, check the spine and kidneys.
- *If the features are consistent with a skeletal dysplasia, follow the protocol in 'Short limbs' in Chapter 6, 'Pregnancy and fertility', p. 784, to ensure an accurate assessment of the fetus.*

The particular features to assess in association with bowing are:
- undermineralization of the skull (OI, hypophosphatasia);
- symmetrical bowed femora are most commonly due to campomelic dysplasia or OI types III and IIb;
- short 'crumpled' limbs (OI types IIa and IIc);
- very short limbs and ribs; bowing most obvious in the femora (TD);
- beaded ribs (caused by fractures; OI types IIa and IIc);
- tibia most affected by bowing (campomelic dysplasia (talipes, sex reversal, cardiac defects), OI type IIb, Beemer–Langer syndrome).

A suspected chromosomal disorder or malformation syndrome requires thorough examination of the fetus (see 'Short limbs' in Chapter 6, 'Pregnancy and fertility', p. 784).

Special investigations
- Referral to a specialist centre for scanning may be indicated.
- Consider NIPD/T for TD and/or fetal sexing (for an apparently female fetus on USS, as male fetuses with campomelic dysplasia often show phenotypic sex reversal).
- Molecular analysis. Rapid molecular testing in pregnancy to confirm a skeletal dysplasia is only available for a limited number of conditions. However, a genetic-based diagnosis may be possible in future pregnancies if DNA has been stored from the affected fetus and subsequent testing, e.g. skeletal survey and genetic analysis, reveals a specific genetic diagnosis.

- In fetuses with features of a malformation syndrome, offer fetal genomic array (e.g. CVS, amniocentesis).
- Ensure that DNA is stored for future DNA testing (if the parents consent to this).

Diagnoses to consider

There is considerable overlap with the discussion in 'Short limbs' in Chapter 6, 'Pregnancy and fertility', p. 784.

Thanatophoric dysplasia (TD)
Curved ('telephone receiver') femora found in TD type 1. TD is a sporadic neonatal lethal skeletal dysplasia, caused by *de novo* dominant mutations in *FGFR3* (1/20 000). Consider NIPD for diagnosis. See 'Short limbs' in Chapter 6, 'Pregnancy and fertility', p. 784.

Osteogenesis imperfecta (OI)
Severe forms, e.g. type II, present with short, deformed limbs, often with bowing, angulation, and/or fractures. The fetus may have a narrow chest and some have undermineralization of the skull. Mostly due to dominant mutations in genes encoding type I collagen. Recurrence risk is due to parental germline mosaicism and AR inheritance, and this composite risk was historically estimated at ~7% (Cole and Dalgleish 1995). The more prevalent AD forms of OI are caused by primary defects in type 1 collagen, whereas AR forms are caused by deficiency of proteins which interact with type 1 procollagen for post-translational modification and/or folding (Forlino et al. 2011). See 'Fractures' in Chapter 2, 'Clinical approach', p. 158.

In most populations, recurrence of lethal OI results from parental mosaicism for dominant mutations, but the carrier frequency of recessive forms of OI will impact upon this, such that, in some ethnic groups, the risk of AR OI will exceed that of parental mosaicism. In most populations, the recurrence risk after a single affected pregnancy is 1.3%, but after two affected pregnancies, this rises to 32% (Pyott et al. 2011).

Infantile hypophosphatasia
Usually an AR condition characterized by severe deficiency of chondro-osseous mineralization and caused by mutations in the tissue non-specific alkaline phosphatase gene *TNSALP* on 1p34–36. There is deformity and fracture of the long bones and the skull is undermineralized, assuming a globular shape. Most cases are lethal in the neonatal period. However, there are reports of a good prognosis following the observation of severe long bone bowing in prenatal scans with evidence for AD transmission, particularly maternal. Consult the literature prior to counselling, and consider parental alkaline phosphatase estimation (Wenkert et al. 2011).

Campomelic dysplasia
The tibia shows the most marked bowing and the upper limbs usually appear normal on antenatal imaging. Sex reversal is commonly found, as this dysplasia is caused by haploinsufficiency of the SRY-related gene *SOX9* or by rearrangements and deletions of the 17q24–5 region. Cytogenetic analysis is indicated. The abnormality may not disrupt or delete the *SOX9* gene but may exert a position effect. Parental chromosomes should be performed if the fetus has a chromosome abnormality. Recurrences are due to germline mosaicism for a *SOX9* mutation or chromosome imbalance.

Antley–Bixler syndrome

An AR condition with virilization of females and under-virilization of males due to disordered steroidogenesis. It is caused by biallelic mutation in the *POR* gene encoding cytochrome P450. NIPD with ffDNA may be helpful in establishing the fetal sex. Mothers may become virilized in pregnancy. Maternal urine steroid profiles may contribute to the diagnosis (Reisch et al. 2013). There are phenocopies due to heterozygous mutation of *FGFR2* and also *in utero* exposure to fluconazole (see 'Drugs in pregnancy' in Chapter 6, 'Pregnancy and fertility', p. 718).

FGFR2 bent bone dysplasia syndrome

Heterozygous mutation in *FGFR2*; characteristic findings are bowed bones with midface hypoplasia and an abnormal skull shape due to coronal synostosis. Phenotypic overlap with Antley–Bixler syndrome.

Undiagnosed skeletal dysplasias

Likely to have additional skeletal features, but the precise diagnosis may not be made until after birth. An estimation of whether the condition is likely to be lethal in the neonatal period is needed for counselling purposes and to advise neonatal colleagues. See 'Short limbs' in Chapter 6, 'Pregnancy and fertility', p. 784 for USS predictors of a lethal dysplasia.

Genetic advice and management

Advise, as appropriate, for the specific condition diagnosed.

- Investigation of the fetus and baby with a skeletal dysplasia. A diagnosis is vitally important in order to be able to advise about appropriate management and also recurrence risks. If the pregnancy is terminated or the baby is stillborn, it is possible to get most of the information required, even if a post-mortem examination is refused. See 'Short limbs' in Chapter 6, 'Pregnancy and fertility', p. 784 for a list of important investigations.
- Asymmetrical and/or single bone involvement. This is more likely to be due to a sporadic, vascular,

or environmental factor than a genetic syndrome. Consider the possibility of a somatic mutation.

Support groups: Many of the syndromes have their own support groups. See Contact a Family, http://www.cafamily.org.uk; ARC (Antenatal Results and Choices), http://www.arc-uk.org, Tel. 0207 631 0285.

References

Cole WG, Dalgleish R. Perinatal lethal osteogenesis imperfecta. *J Med Genet* 1995; **32**: 284–9.

Forlino A, Cabral WA, Barnes AM, Marini JC. New perspectives on osteogenesis imperfecta. *Nat Rev Endocrinol* 2011; **7**: 540–57.

Moore CA, Curry CJ, Henthorn PS, et al. Mild autosomal dominant hypophosphatasia: *in utero* presentation in two families. *Am J Genet* 1999; **86**: 410–15.

Parilla BV, Leeth EA, Kambich MP, Chilis P, MacGregor SN. Antenatal detection of skeletal dysplasias. *J Ultrasound Med* 2003; **22**: 255–8.

Pepin M, Atkinson M, Starman BJ, Byers PH. Strategies and outcomes of prenatal diagnosis for osteogenesis imperfecta: a review of biochemical and molecular studies completed in 129 pregnancies. *Prenat Diagn* 1997; **17**: 559–70.

Pyott SM, Pepin MG, Schwarze U, Yang K, Smith G, Byers PH. Recurrence of perinatal lethal osteogenesis imperfect in sibships: parsing the risk between parental mosaicism for dominant mutations and autosomal recessive inheritance. *Genet Med* 2011; **13**: 125–30.

Reisch N, Idkowiak J, Hughes BA, et al. Prenatal diagnosis of congenital adrenal hyperplasia caused by P450 oxidoreductase deficiency. *J Clin End Metab* 2013; **98**: E528–36.

Wenkert D, McAlister WH, Coburn SP, et al. Hypophosphatasia: nonlethal disease despite skeletal presentation *in utero* (17 new cases and literature review). *J Bone Miner Res* 2011; **26**: 2389–98.

Wynne-Davies R, Hall CM, Hurst JA; for the Skeletal Dysplasia Group for Teaching and Research (2004). An approach to the radiological diagnosis of lethal and other skeletal dysplasias presenting at birth. *Occasional Publication* **No. 8c**.

Congenital cystic lung lesions, Currarino syndrome, and sacrococcygeal teratoma

Congenital cystic lung lesions

These are rare and present on USS as a cystic or solid mass in the chest, which needs to be differentiated from a congenital diaphragmatic hernia. Causes of congenital cystic lung lesions include: congenital cystic adenomatoid malformation (CCAM); pulmonary sequestration; congenital lobar emphysema; and bronchogenic cysts. Most cases fare well, but if hydrops is present, the prognosis is worse.

CCAM is diagnosed in ~1/10 000 pregnancies (Kotecha et al. 2012). An increase in growth of the lesions is often noted between 20 and 28 weeks, after which many cases of CCAM improve spontaneously and may disappear from scan view in utero. All cases, however, need postnatal investigation and follow-up with surgery usually reserved for those with symptoms, but the question of malignant transformation potential, although low, has not been completely resolved (Sauvat et al. 2003).

Fetuses with a significant lesion, particularly if associated with mediastinal shift in the third trimester, should be delivered in a unit with facilities for neonatal intensive care and respiratory support, as early surgical treatment may be required. Karyotyping is not indicated, and associated anomalies are rare.

Pulmonary sequestration is a localized area of lung tissue, receiving its own blood supply from an aberrant systemic artery and lacking continuity with the upper respiratory tract. Postnatal surgery is usually offered and successful. Antenatally, it may be distinguished from a CCAM by demonstration of the aberrant blood supply by Doppler, but mixed CCAM/pulmonary sequestration may occur and can confuse.

Currarino syndrome

The combination of partial absence of the sacrum (usually S2–5 only), anorectal anomalies, and a presacral mass constitutes Currarino syndrome. In addition to the triad, urogenital malformations are common and a tethered cord and/or lipoma of the conus should be sought, as early treatment is essential. Severe constipation is the presenting symptom in many cases diagnosed postnatally. The syndrome occurs in the majority of patients as an AD trait associated with mutations (sequence variants and deletions) in the homeobox gene MNX1 (HLXB9) located at 7q36. In Crétolle et al.'s (2008) study, there was poor genotype–phenotype correlation, with nearly one-third of all carriers being clinically asymptomatic. Mutation detection rate was around 50%, but up to 90% in familial cases. Lynch et al. (2000) also provide a good overview.

Sacrococcygeal teratoma

A sacrococcygeal teratoma (SCT) is a germ cell tumour composed of tissues that originate from each of the three layers of the embryonic disc. The incidence is 1/35 000–1/40 000 live births. It is more common in females (1M:4F). SCTs are highly vascular tumours that can grow very rapidly. High-output cardiac failure with hydrops can result and is associated with a poor outlook if present <28/40. There may be associated malformations of the sacrum, vertebrae, and GI or genitourinary tracts. Only a minority of tumours are malignant, but early removal is indicated to reduce this risk.

SCTs are classified as follows.

- Type I. Predominantly external, with only a minimal presacral component (40%).
- Type II. Significant intrapelvic extension (36%).
- Type III. Predominantly internal with abdominal extension.
- Type IV. Completely internal mass.

Reprinted from *Journal of Pediatric Surgery*, volume 9, issue 3, R. Peter Altman, Judson G. Randolph, John R. Lilly, Sacrococcygeal teratoma: American Academy of Pediatrics Surgical Section survey—1973, pp. 389–398, Copyright 1974, with permission from Elsevier.

The pregnancy should be monitored closely for signs of maternal mirror syndrome. The long-term prognosis will depend on the size and type of the lesion, associated malformations, and the gestational age at delivery but is usually excellent following early surgery (Penny 2012).

The great majority of cases are sporadic and the recurrence risk is low.

Of interest, SCTs have been shown to contain human embryonic stem cells (Busch et al. 2009).

Expert adviser: Diana Wellesley, Consultant Clinical Geneticist, Wessex Clinical Genetics Service, Princess Anne Hospital, Southampton, UK.

References

Busch C, Bareiss PM, Sinnberg T, et al. Isolation of three stem cell lines from human sacrococcygeal teratomas. *J Pathol* 2009; **217**: 589–96.

Crétolle C, Pelet A, Sanlaville D, et al. Spectrum of *HLXB9* gene mutations in Currarino syndrome and genotype–phenotype correlation. *Hum Mutat* 2008; **29**: 903–10.

Lynch SA, Wang Y, Strachan T, Burn J, Lindsay S. Autosomal dominant sacral agenesis: Currarino syndrome. *J Med Genet* 2000; **37**: 561–6.

Kotecha S, Barbato A, Bush A, et al. Antenatal and postnatal management of congenital cystic adenomatoid malformation. *Paediatr Respir Rev* 2012; **13**: 162–70.

Penny SM. Sacrococcygeal teratoma: a literature review. *Radiol Technol* 2012; **84**: 11–17.

Sauvat F, Michel JL, Benachi A, Emond S, Revillon Y. Management of asymptomatic neonatal cystic adenomatoid malformations. *J Pediatr Surg* 2003; **38**: 548–52.

Congenital diaphragmatic hernia

The diaphragm develops in early embryonic life and is usually fully formed by 9 weeks' gestation. Congenital diaphragmatic hernia occurs when any of the four components making up the diaphragm (septum transversum, pleuroperitoneal membranes, dorsal mesentery of the oesophagus, and body wall) fails to grow towards each other or to fuse by the eighth week after conception (Wenstrom *et al.* 1991). The most common site for diaphragmatic hernia is the left side, through which the stomach, bowel, spleen, and liver can pass. Poor prognostic features include early diagnosis and the liver in the chest. The main cause of death is pulmonary hypoplasia, due to constrained development of the fetal lungs *in utero*.

Congenital diaphragmatic hernia occurs in ~1/3700 live births (Wenstrom *et al.* 1991).The overall prenatal detection rate by USS is ~60%. They are most commonly detected at the 20 weeks' gestation fetal anomaly scan, but some may present late. In a series of 31 prenatally diagnosed cases from France (Bétrémieux *et al.* 2002), ten fetuses (32%) had associated anomalies, of which four had chromosomal anomalies (trisomy 18, 22q11 deletion) and four had Fryns syndrome. About 30–40% of babies with congenital diaphragmatic hernia have additional major anomalies that most frequently involve the cardiovascular, central nervous, musculoskeletal, and genitourinary systems (Pober 2007).

Congenital diaphragmatic hernia with an abnormal karyotype or other major structural abnormalities, e.g. heart, brain, has a poor outcome. Isolated congenital diaphragmatic hernia, when delivered in a tertiary unit with access to expert neonatal intensive care and paediatric surgical facilities, has a survival rate in excess of 50%. Long-term complications, including feeding difficulties, respiratory problems, and intellectual delay, may occur and parents should be referred to a paediatric surgeon for consultation and discussion of prognosis as soon as possible after PND.

Other causes of a mass in the fetal chest

In the West Midlands Perinatal Institute's (2003) review, 14/121 (12%) PNDs of congenital diaphragmatic hernia made in a fetal medicine centre were false-positive diagnoses. It is important to consider this possibility when counselling parents prenatally. Final diagnoses in the false-positive cases included: CCAM, bronchogenic cyst, hydrothorax, pleural effusions, lung sequestration, duodenal atresia, and gut malrotation. Fetal MRI may be helpful in making the correct diagnosis in difficult cases.

Clinical assessment

History: key points

- Three-generation family tree, with enquiry about consanguinity.

Examination: key points

- Detailed fetal biometry.
- Detailed anomaly USS to detect other structural anomalies.

Special investigations

- Offer fetal genomic array (e.g. CVS, amniocentesis, or NIPT). Karyotyping is indicated, as +18 and +13 are associated with diaphragmatic hernia, and overall about 10% of pregnancies with diaphragmatic

hernia had a chromosomal abnormality in the West Midlands Perinatal Institute's (2003) study. A recent study from Belgium identified genomic imbalance in three of 79 (4%) fetuses with isolated congenital diaphragmatic hernia tested by targeted aGCH (Srisupundit *et al.* 2010). A retrospective study of arrays in infants with CDH identified a likely pathogenic genomic imbalance in 7/28 (25%) (Stark *et al.* 2015).

- Fetal echo. Sixteen per cent have cardiac malformations.

Some diagnoses to consider

Trisomy 18
See 'Edwards' syndrome (trisomy 18)' in Chapter 5, 'Chromosomes', p. 670.

Trisomy 13
See 'Patau syndrome (trisomy 13)' in Chapter 5, 'Chromosomes', p. 678.

Pallister–Killian syndrome (tetrasomy 12p)
Is due to mosaicism for an isochromosome of 12p that is present in skin fibroblasts, but not in blood lymphocytes. Other USS anomalies such as increased nuchal translucency, congenital diaphragmatic hernia, polyhydramnios, rhizomelic limb shortening, and an abnormal facial profile with a prominent philtrum in association with fetal overgrowth are very suggestive of the syndrome, but they are inconstant and may even be absent. Doray *et al.* (2002) propose that, in cases where USS indicators are present, the first investigation should be CVS or placental biopsy and then amniocentesis if the first cytogenetic result is normal. FBS is the least indicated method because of the low frequency of the isochromosome in lymphocytes. In this cytogenetic strategy, FISH and especially interphase FISH on non-cultured cells increase the probability of identifying the isochromosome. See also 'Coarse facial features' in Chapter 2, 'Clinical approach', p. 106.

Cornelia de Lange syndrome (CdLS)
Birth incidence ~1 in 50 000. IUGR often developing in the third trimester), with limb anomalies ranging from short forearms with small hands and tapering fingers to severe limb reduction defects. Upper limb defects are very much more common than lower limb defects. Distinctive craniofacial features (microbrachycephaly, a depressed nasal bridge with anteverted nares, a long smooth philtrum, and micrognathia). The major gene for CdLS is *NIPBL* on 5p13.1. See 'Limb reduction defects' in Chapter 2, 'Clinical approach', p. 212.

Fryns syndrome
A rare AR disorder of multiple congenital abnormalities. The most frequent manifestations of this condition include congenital diaphragmatic hernia, brachytelephalangy and/or nail hypoplasia, polyhydramnios, facial dysmorphism, oro-facial clefting, VSD, CNS anomalies, and genitourinary malformations (Slavotinek 2004). There may be genotypic heterogeneity in Fryns, and McInerney-Leo (2016) recently identified biallelic *PIGN* mutations in two families with a clinical diagnosis of Fryns.

Simpson–Golabi–Behmel (SGB) syndrome
An XLR disorder due to mutations in *GPC3* (Xq26). Overgrowth is of prenatal onset and continues postnatally. Birthweight and birth OFC of affected males are

usually both >97th centile. May have cardiac/GI malformations. See 'Overgrowth' in Chapter 2, 'Clinical approach', p. 272.

Kabuki syndrome
This a common malformation syndrome with diaphragmatic hernia/eventration as a relatively rare presenting feature. Congenital heart disease in ~40%. Diagnosis is not usually made until the characteristic facial appearance at about 12 months. *KMT2D* and *KMD6A* genes. See 'Congenital heart disease' in Chapter 2, 'Clinical approach', p. 112.

Donnai–Barrow syndrome
A rare AR condition characterized by diaphragmatic hernia, exomphalos, absent corpus callosum, hypertelorism, myopia, sensorineural deafness, and increased birthweight (Chassaing et al. 2003), and caused by biallelic mutations in the *LRP2* gene on 2q31 (Kantarci et al. 2007).

Meacham syndrome
A rare disorder characterized by congenital diaphragmatic hernia, cardiac and pulmonary malformations, with sex reversal in karyotypic males (normal female external genitalia or ambiguous genitalia with abnormal male gonads), with some cases caused by heterozygous mutations in *WT1* (Suri et al. 2007).

Lethal multiple pterygium syndrome (LMPS)
An uncommon fetal-onset disorder of unknown aetiology. LMPS results from fetal akinesia commencing in the first or early second trimester. Biallelic germline mutations in the *CHRNG* gene that encodes the γ subunit of the embryonal AChR may cause the lethal form of multiple pterygium syndrome (LMPS). In addition, *CHRNG* mutations and mutations in other components of the embryonal AChR may present with fetal akinesia deformation sequence (FADS) without pterygia (Vogt et al. 2012). See 'Fetal akinesia' in Chapter 6, 'Pregnancy and fertility', p. 724.

Genetic advice and management
For isolated congenital diaphragmatic hernia, the sibling recurrence risk is very low at ~1%.

Repair
The repair is usually through the abdomen, with reduction of herniated contents and excision of any sac preceding the repair. The defect may be closed primarily, or a muscle patch or an inert graft may be needed. Sometimes there is intestinal malrotation requiring a Ladd's procedure to place the intestine in the non-rotated position.

Support groups: CDH UK, http://www.cdhuk.org.uk, Tel. 0800 731 6991; CHERUBS (The Association of Congenital Diaphragmatic Hernia Research, Awareness, and Support), http://www.cherubs-cdh.org.

Expert adviser: Mohnish Suri, Consultant Clinical Geneticist, Nottingham Clinical Genetics Service, Nottinghamshire University Hospitals NHS Trust, Nottingham, UK.

References
Bétrémieux P, Lionnais S, Beuchée A, et al. Perinatal management and outcome of prenatally diagnosed congenital diaphragmatic hernia: a 1995–2000 series in Rennes University Hospital. *Prenat Diagn* 2002; **22**: 988–94.

Chassaing N, Lacombe D, Carles D, Calvas P, Saura R, Bieth E. Donnai–Barrow syndrome: four additional patients. *Am J Med Genet A* 2003; **121A**: 258–62.

Cox PM, Brueton LA, Bjelogrlic P, Pomroy P, Sewry CA. Diversity of neuromuscular pathology in lethal multiple pterygium syndrome. *Pediatr Dev Pathol* 2003; **6**: 59–68.

Doray B, Girard-Lemaire F, Gasser B, et al. Pallister–Killian syndrome: difficulties of prenatal diagnosis. *Prenat Diagn* 2002; **22**: 470–7.

Garne E, Haeusler M, Barisic I, et al. Congenital diaphragmatic hernia: evaluation of prenatal diagnosis in 20 European regions. *Ultrasound Obstet Gynecol* 2002; **19**: 329–33.

Harrison MR, Keller RL, Hawgood SB, et al. A randomized trial of fetal endoscopic tracheal occlusion for severe fetal congenital diaphragmatic hernia. *N Engl J Med* 2003; **349**: 1916–24.

Huddy CL, Boyd PA, Wilkinson AR, Chamberlain P. Congenital diaphragmatic hernia: prenatal diagnosis, outcome and continuing morbidity in survivors. *BJOG* 1999; **106**: 1192–6.

Kantarci S, Al-Gazali L, Hill RS, et al. Mutations in LRP2, which encodes the multiligand receptor megalin, cause Donnai–Barrow and facio-oculo-acoustico-renal syndromes. *Nat Genet* 2007; **39**: 957–9.

Lally KP. Congenital diaphragmatic hernia. *Curr Opin Pediatr* 2002; **14**: 486–90.

Marino T, Wheeler PG, Simpson LL, Craigo SD, Bianchi DW. Fetal diaphragmatic hernia and upper limb anomalies suggest Brachmann–de Lange syndrome. *Prenat Diagn* 2002; **22**: 144–7.

McInerney-Leo AM, Harris JE, Gattas M, et al. Fryns syndrome associated with recessive mutations in PIGN in two separate families. *Hum Mutat* 2016; **37**: 695–702.

Paladini D, Borghese A, Arienzo M, Teodoro A, Martinelli P, Nappi C. Prospective ultrasound diagnosis of Pallister–Killian syndrome in the second trimester of pregnancy: the importance of the fetal facial profile. *Prenat Diagn* 2000; **20**: 996–8.

Pober BR. Overview of epidemiology, genetics, birth defects and chromosome abnormalities associated with CDH. *Am J Med Genet C Semin Med Genet* 2007; **145C**: 158–71.

Slavotinek AM. Fryns syndrome: a review of the phenotype and diagnostic guidelines. *Am J Med Genet A* 2004; **124A**: 427–33.

Srisupundit K, Brady PD, Devriendt K, et al. Targeted array comparative genomic hybridisation (array CGH) identified genomic imbalances associated with isolated congenital diaphragmatic hernia (CDH). *Prenat Diagn* 2010; **30**: 1198–206.

Stark Z, Behrsin J, et al. SNP microarray abnormalities in a cohort of 28 infants with congenital diaphragmatic hernia. *Am J Med Genet* 2015; **167**: 2319–26.

Stege G, Fenton A, Jaffray B. Nihilism in the 1990s: the true mortality of congenital diaphragmatic hernia. *Pediatrics* 2003; **112**(3, pt 1): 532–5.

Suri M, Kelehan P, O'Neill D, et al. WT1 mutations in Meacham syndrome suggest a coelomic mesothelial origin of the cardiac and diaphragmatic malformations. *Am J Med Genet A* 2007; **143A**: 2312–20.

Vogt J, Morgan NV, Rehal P, et al. CHRNG genotype–phenotype correlations in the multiple pterygium syndromes. *J Med Genet* 2012; **49**: 21–6.

Wenstrom KD. Fetal surgery for congenital diaphragmatic hernia [perspective]. *N Engl J Med* 2003; **349**: 1887–8.

Wenstrom KD, Weiner CP, Hanson JW. A five-year statewide experience with congenital diaphragmatic hernia. *Am J Obstet Gynecol* 1991; **165**(4, pt 1): 838–42.

West Midlands Perinatal Institute. West Midlands Congenital Anomaly Register. *Congenital diaphragmatic hernia 1995–2000*. West Midlands Perinatal Institute, Birmingham, 2003.

Williams HJ, Johnson KJ. Imaging of congenital cystic lung lesions. *Paediatr Respir Rev* 2002; **3**: 120–7.

Cytomegalovirus (CMV)

Congenital CMV is diagnosed, investigated, and managed by fetal medicine specialists, paediatricians, and virologists. The geneticist may be involved prior to a definitive diagnosis because the phenotype may overlap with genetic disorders. Therefore, a brief summary of the condition is included in this section. CMV is, by far, the most common serious intrauterine infection, with an incidence of symptomatic disease at birth of 0.1% (Spagno 2001). The severity of infection appears related to gestation at the time of infection—those fetuses acquiring infection in the first trimester have relatively severe consequences, whereas those infected during the third trimester may not suffer severe sequelae.

CMV is a member of the *Herpesviridae* family of viruses. Pregnant women can develop either primary infection, reactivation of the virus, or reinfection during pregnancy. Primary infection is more likely to lead to congenital infection (40%) and disease. Infection does not necessarily equate to sequelae, as the majority of babies born without symptoms will remain healthy—the opposite is true for babies born symptomatic at birth that are at risk of severe complications, mainly deafness and neurodevelopmental delay. In comparison, reactivation or reinfection carry a risk of fetal infection of 1–2% and a <1% risk of sequelae for the baby. In children and adults, most infections are subclinical. The virus is transmitted by close personal contact (saliva, genital tract, breast milk).

CMV is commonly acquired at birth and through the first few months of life, and it is often difficult to distinguish serologically between congenital and postnatally acquired infection.

The *in utero* risk of congenital transmission is not gestation-dependent. The majority of congenitally infected babies do not have any clinical signs and have a good prognosis, though deafness may be late-presenting. Of the 10% with signs, there is a significant mortality and about 20% with typical features die in the perinatal period. Typical features are low birthweight, lethargy, poor feeding, thrombocytopenia, hepatosplenomegaly, ICC, and chorioretinitis (see Table 6.1).

Approximately 60% of survivors with symptomatic neonatal infection have a sensorineural hearing deficit and ~70% have microcephaly, seizures, motor abnormalities, developmental delay, or other cognitive impairment, such that overall 90% of survivors with symptomatic neonatal infection will have a sensory deficit or cognitive impairment.

As CMV is usually subclinical, it is more likely that the condition is considered when scan abnormalities are seen or in babies with features of congenital CMV.

Clinical assessment

History: key points, postnatal
- Birthweight, OFC.
- Lethargy, poor feeding.

Examination: key points, postnatal
- Microcephaly and neurological abnormalities.
- Petechiae.
- Hepatosplenomegaly and jaundice.

Special investigations
- Prenatal.
  - USS: fetal ascites, poor fetal growth, ICC, brain cysts, ventriculomegaly, oligohydramnios.
  - PCR for CMV DNA in amniotic fluid.
  - Maternal CMV serology, CMV IgM, IgG, and IgG avidity.
- Postnatal.
  - Virus isolation from urine used to be the gold standard for diagnosis; however, this has largely been replaced by CMV DNA PCR in urine or saliva in the first 3 weeks of life.
  - Serological testing, e.g. for toxoplasmosis, syphilis, parvovirus, rubella virus, and CMV. Seek expert advice on result interpretation at this age.
  - LFTs, FBC, and platelets (thrombocytopenia).
  - Brain imaging of all symptomatic babies (typical features of congenital CMV infection are ICCs that are predominantly periventricular, periventricular pseudocysts, PMG, and cerebellar hypoplasia).
  - Audiological assessment and follow-up.
  - Ophthalmology referral (chorioretinitis).

Genetic advice and management

Children with proven congenital CMV are not managed by geneticists, but the following points may be useful.
- If there are no clinical signs at birth, the prognosis for normal development is good; ~90% have no sequelae. Hearing loss may develop in 15% of these infants, so refer for formal audiology screen throughout infancy and early childhood up to 6–7 years of age.
- On the other hand, there is a high risk of neurological deficits in babies with typical clinical features of congenital CMV. Microcephaly is the most specific predictor of MR (see Table 6.2).
- Treatment with antivirals (IV ganciclovir for 6 weeks) is offered to babies with symptoms, including CNS involvement at birth. Emerging data suggest that oral antivirals (PO valganciclovir) for longer (6 months) is beneficial for all babies with symptoms not restricted to the CNS.
- Cases of congenital CMV disease have been reported due to reactivation of maternal infection, but, in

Table 6.1 Clinical and laboratory findings in neonates with symptomatic CMV infection

Finding	Percentage of cases
Prematurity (<38 weeks' gestation)	34
IUGR	50
Microcephaly	53
Jaundice	67
Petechiae	76
Purpura	13
Hepatosplenomegaly	60
Thrombocytopenia (platelet count <100 000/mm^3)	77
Haemolytic anaemia	51
Raised ALT (>55 U/l)—mild hepatitis	83

Reproduced from Azam A, Vial Y, et al. Prenatal diagnosis of congenital cytomegalovirus infection. *Obstetrics & Gynecology*, 97(3): 443–8, Copyright 2001 American College of Obstetricians and Gynecologists.

Table 6.2 Neurodevelopmental outcome in symptomatic CMV infection

Symptoms	Outcome
Microcephaly + abnormal CT scan	Mean IQ <50; major motor deficit in 75%
Normal OFC + abnormal CT scan	Mean IQ 70–80; major motor deficit in 37%
Normal OFC + normal CT scan	Mean IQ >90; no major motor deficit

CT, computerized tomography; IQ, intelligence quotient; OFC, occipito-frontal circumference.

Reprinted from *The Journal of Pediatrics*, vol 138(3), Noyola DE, Demmler GJ, et al. Early predictors of neurodevelopmental outcome in symptomatic congenital cytomegalovirus infection. 325–31, copyright 2001 with permission from Elsevier.

general, the risk for significant sequelae is lower in reactivation/reinfection. All infants diagnosed with congenital CMV should be assessed and a decision on whether treatment is required should be made.

- Screening for CMV in pregnancy or at birth is not currently part of routine screening in the UK.
- Consider the AR condition of pseudo-TORCH/micro-cephaly–ICC in babies with signs of congenital infection, but in whom there are no serological features or no virus identified. See 'Intracranial calcification' in Chapter 2, 'Clinical approach' p. 200.
- Refer to the appropriate eye or brain section of Chapter 2, 'Clinical approach', for discussion of other syndromes with some of the features of congenital infections, especially 'Intracranial calcification', p. 200.
- Consider Zika virus. The Zika virus has spread rapidly in the Americas since its first identification in Brazil in early 2015. Rasmussen et al. (2016) conclude that a causal relationship exists between prenatal Zika virus infection and microcephaly and other serious brain anomalies. See https://www.cdc.gov/zika.

Expert adviser: Elani Nastouli, Lead Consultant in Virology, University College Hospital, London, UK.

References

Azam A, Vial Y, Fawer CL, Zufferey J, Hohlfeld P. Prenatal diagnosis of congenital cytomegalovirus infection. *Obstet Gynecol* 2001; **97**: 443–8.

Johnson JM, Anderson BL. Cytomegalovirus: should we screen pregnant women for primary infection? *Am J Perinatol* 2013; **30**: 121–4.

Jones CA, Isaacs D. Predicting the outcome of symptomatic congenital cytomegalovirus infection. *J Paediatr Child Health* 1995; **31**: 70–1.

Kimberlin DW, Jester P, Sanchez PJ, et al. Six months versus six weeks of oral valganciclovir for infants with symptomatic congenital cytomegalovirus (CMV) disease with and without central nervous system (CNS) involvement: Results of a Phase III, randomized, double-blind, placebo-controlled, multinational study, 2013. https://idsa.confex.com/idsa/2013/webprogram/Paper43178.html.

Kimberlin DW, Lin CY, Sánchez PJ, et al. Effect of ganciclovir therapy on hearing in symptomatic congenital cytomegalovirus disease involving the central nervous system: a randomized, controlled trial. *J Pediatr* 2003; **143**: 16–25.

Modlin JF, Grant PE, Makar RS, Roberts DJ, Krishnamoorthy KS. Case records of the Massachusetts General Hospital. Weekly clinicopathological exercises. Case 25–2003: A newborn boy with petechiae and thrombocytopenia. *N Engl J Med* 2003; **349**: 691–700.

Noyola DE, Demmler GJ, Nelson CT, et al. Early predictors of neurodevelopmental outcome in symptomatic congenital cytomegalovirus infection. *J Pediatr* 2001; **138**: 325–31.

Rasmussen SA, Jamieson DJ, Honein MA, Petersen LR. Zika virus and birth defects—reviewing the evidence for causality. *N Engl J Med* 2016; **374**: 1981–7.

Ross SA, Ahmed A, Palmer AL, et al. Detection of congenital cytomegalovirus infection by real-time polymerase chain reaction analysis of saliva or urine specimens. *J Infect Dis* 2014; **210**: 1415–18.

Spagno S. Cytomegaloviruses. In: JS Remington, JO Klein (eds.). *Infectious diseases of the fetus and newborn infant*, 5th edn, pp. 389–424. WB Saunders, Philadelphia, 2001.

Drugs in pregnancy

Sometimes enquiries relate to a drug exposure in an ongoing pregnancy. In this instance, seek advice from the UK Teratology Information Service (UKTIS), a national service which provides information and advice about all aspects of toxicity of drugs and chemicals in pregnancy, at no cost to healthcare professionals in the UK, through a dedicated healthcare professionals enquiry line and written online reviews at https://www.toxbase.org. UKTIS patient information leaflets are also now openly available at 'bumps–best use of medicines in pregnancy' (www.medicinesinpregnancy.org). Equivalent teratology information services are well established around the world. More typically, the geneticist is asked to assess a child with a congenital malformation, dysmorphic features, or developmental delay and to assess whether a known drug exposure during pregnancy is relevant to the child's problems (Rasmussen 2012).

Allopurinol

Allopurinol is rarely used in pregnancy and exposure data are thus very limited. Multiple malformations reminiscent of those observed with mycophenolate embryopathy (below) have been reported in two of the 32 reported cases in the published literature. Given this phenotypic similarity and that allopurinol is a purine analogue, these cases may provide a signal for teratogenicity. Genetic investigation in both cases was, however, limited to microscopic chromosome analysis, and a chance association between exposure and outcome therefore cannot be excluded.

Angiotensin-converting enzyme (ACE) inhibitors

Exposure in the second and third trimesters is associated with ACE-inhibitor fetopathy characterized by renal tubular dysgenesis, prolonged renal failure, anuria and hypotension in the newborn, decreased skull ossification (hypocalvaria), pulmonary hypoplasia, persistent ductus arteriosus, mild to severe IUGR, and fetal or neonatal demise. These effects are attributed to a direct effect of the ACE inhibitors on the fetal renin–angiotensin system (RAS), functional from around 26 weeks' gestation, resulting in fetal hypotension and oligohydramnios with fetal compression (Barr 1994).

It is unclear as to whether ACE inhibitor exposure in the first trimester increases congenital anomaly risk, as studies have yielded conflicting results and suggest that maternal hypertension may itself be linked to an increased risk of certain major malformations in the fetus.

Similar effects have been reported for angiotensin II receptor antagonists (A2RAs).

Anticonvulsants

See 'Fetal anticonvulsant syndrome (FACS)' in Chapter 6, 'Pregnancy and fertility', p. 732.

Carbimazole/methimazole

Exposure during the first trimester (first 7 weeks of pregnancy from last menstrual period reported as the critical 'at-risk' period') confers a variable risk of embryopathy, ranging from 0.8–4.1% in some reports to 11.1% among a cohort of Hong Kong Chinese, suggesting a role for maternofetal genetic factors. Anomalies reported include ectodermal (aplasia cutis, athelia, or hypothelia) (62%), oro-nasal (mainly choanal atresia) (48%), facial dysmorphism (broad forehead, short upslanting palpebral fissure, broad nasal bridge, hypoplastic alae nasi, and thin upper lip) (38%), GI anomaly (mainly patent vitellointestinal duct) (33%), and abdominal wall defect (gastroschisis and omphalocele) (19%). Hypoplastic nipples and developmental delay have also been reported after first trimester exposure to carbimazole (or its active metabolite methimazole) in the treatment of maternal hyperthyroidism. Embryopathy may be more likely at doses in excess of 20 mg/day but has occurred with maternal dose <20 mg/day (Ting et al. 2013; Wilson et al. 1998).

Cocaine

Cocaine causes acute vasoconstriction. Use during pregnancy has been associated with an increased incidence of spontaneous abortion, placental abruption, prematurity, IUGR, sudden infant death syndrome (SIDS), and neurological deficits. Reported malformations include microcephaly and malformations of the skeletal system, limb deficiency, nervous system, GI tract, genitourinary system, and cardiovascular system, although a distinct teratogenic syndrome remains unconfirmed. Exposure in late pregnancy may lead to neonatal withdrawal in the infant (Hoyme et al. 1991).

Fluconazole

Antifungal agent. Although there are only a handful of reports of fetuses with craniosynostosis, orbital hypoplasia, humeroradial synostosis, and femoral bowing (Antley–Bixler syndrome phenocopy) ± cleft palate, cardiovascular malformations, and joint contractures after continuous high-dose (>400 mg/day) exposure in the first trimester, a similar pattern has been observed in animal models. Furthermore, fluconazole inhibits fungal cytochrome P450 sterol CYP51, and mutations in the P450 oxidoreductase (POR) gene and impaired sterol metabolism have been identified in Antley–Bixler syndrome, suggesting a plausible biological mechanism of fluconazole teratogenesis. Single-dose treatments of 150 mg in pregnancy, as typically used in the treatment of thrush, have, however, not been associated with an increased rate of congenital anomalies or a teratogenic embryopathy.

Lithium

Initial reports from the Danish Register of Lithium Babies indicated significantly increased rates of cardiovascular malformations (Schou et al. 1973). A subsequent review of pooled data suggested a more modest risk of Ebstein anomaly of the tricuspid valve (10–20 times greater than in the general population where it occurs in 1/20 000 cases). A prospective controlled study of 148 women found a relative risk of 1.2 for all congenital anomalies and of 3.5 for cardiac anomalies in the babies exposed to lithium (Jacobson et al. 1992). More recent studies have failed to show any increase in risk of cardiac malformations and a recent review of the published literature (Yacobi and Ornoy 2008) highlights the limitations of the earlier data and the number of studies that fail to demonstrate teratogenicity. The authors still recommend a detailed cardiac anomaly scan, as the studies remain underpowered to reach any definitive conclusions.

Lithium has also been reported to affect neonatal thyroid function. A 5-year follow-up of 60 children exposed to lithium in the second and third trimesters found no significant differences in developmental anomalies, compared with non-exposed siblings (Schou 1976). The animal and human data following lithium exposure have been extensively reviewed by Moore (1995)—see Shepard et al. (2002).

Mycophenolate mofetil (MMF)

MMF interferes with purine synthesis and has recently been confirmed as a major teratogen. Increased risk of miscarriage and multiple fetal malformations, similar to those seen in CHARGE syndrome, have been reported following first trimester exposure. Anomalies described include: cleft lip and/or palate, micrognathia and hypertelorism, external auditory canal atresia (EACA) (with and without microtia), tracheo-oesophageal atresia, hydronephrosis, cardiac anomalies, and myelomeningocele Longitudinal developmental data are not yet available.

Oral contraceptive pill (OCP), hormonal pregnancy tests

Meta-analyses and controlled studies (post-1982) do not suggest an increased rate of overall congenital malformations, cardiac malformations, NTDs, or neonatal/infant death. Data regarding risk of limb reduction defects, genital defects, and low birthweight are conflicting. Most of the available data are confounded or limited by the methodology of data collection or analysis.

Retinoids

Retinoids are potent teratogens. The introduction in 1984 of isotretinoin (e.g. Roaccutane®) for oral treatment of severe acne and etretinate for psoriasis led to a spate of birth defects. Etretinate is fat-soluble with an elimination half-life of 120 days or more (and has been taken off the market in the UK because of its teratogenic effects). Acitretin was introduced to replace etretinate since it is excreted from the body rapidly with a half-life of 50–60 hours. However, reverse metabolism of acitretin to etretinate may occur with concurrent exposure to alcohol. The half-life of isotretinoin is 22 hours.

Retinoid embryopathy, associated with systemic exposure, results in some or all of the following abnormalities: CNS defects (hydrocephalus, optic nerve blindness, retinal defects, microphthalmia, posterior fossa defects, and cortical and cerebellar defects); craniofacial defects (microtia or anotia, low-set ears, hypertelorism, depressed nasal bridge, microcephaly, micrognathia, and agenesis or stenosis of external ear canals); cardiovascular defects (TGA, tetralogy of Fallot, VSD, ASD); thymic defects (ectopia and hypoplasia or aplasia); and miscellaneous defects (limb reduction, decreased muscle tone, spontaneous abortion, and behavioural anomalies). Impaired neurodevelopment of varying severity is frequently reported in association with malformation and in up to 60% of exposed children with no obvious structural defects.

Systemic absorption following topical application of retinoids is low and, although data are limited, topical use does not appear to be associated with a teratogenic risk.

Selective serotonin reuptake inhibitors (SSRIs)

There is no confirmed SSRI embryopathy or teratogenic syndrome. There are as many large studies and meta-analyses showing an increased risk of cardiac malformation with use of SSRIs in pregnancy as there are showing no significant association. Debate and disagreement continue as to whether there is an increased risk of specific cardiac anomalies for certain SSRIs, but not others (e.g. paroxetine with RV outflow tract defects, fluoxetine with VSD) (Stephansson et al. 2013).

Statins

Cholesterol is required for SHH signalling. Early case reports and retrospective data collected by the manufacturers which described children with malformations following maternal statin use during fetal organogenesis therefore raised concern. Prospective cohort studies have, however, not provided evidence of an embryopathy or increased risk of adverse outcome but have involved too few women to change current advice to discontinue statins 3 months prior to conception or as soon as pregnancy is recognized (Winterfield et al. 2012). Consideration should be given to the fact that maternal obesity and diabetes are independently associated with an increased risk of fetal anomaly and are likely to be more prevalent among women who are treated with cholesterol-lowering agents.

Warfarin

Warfarin and other coumarin derivatives cross the placenta. Exposure between 6 and 12 weeks' gestation is associated with an embryopathy (chondrodysplasia punctata with nasal hypoplasia and/or stippled epiphyses) in 6–30% of fetuses. CNS malformations and fetoplacental haemorrhage can occur after exposure during any trimester. Exposure near delivery confers a risk of neonatal haemorrhage and neonatal coagulation status should be monitored after birth. The risk of a poor outcome is 80% when the mean daily dose of warfarin is >5 mg, but 3–10% when the mean daily dose is <5 mg (Castellano et al. 2012; Schaefer 2001).

Unfractionated (UFH) and low-molecular-weight heparins (LWMH) do not cross the placenta and are not secreted into breast milk. A change from warfarin to LMWH or UFH is therefore generally advised before 6 weeks of pregnancy, except in situations where the maternal benefit of continued anticoagulation with warfarin is considered to outweigh any potential teratogenic risk (e.g. maternal prosthetic heart valves).

PATIENTS WITH PROSTHETIC HEART VALVES. Pre-pregnancy counselling from a cardiologist and an obstetrician with expertise in fetomaternal medicine and co-management of the pregnancy with a haematologist are advised.

See Table 6.3 (Castellano et al. 2012).

Clinical assessment

History: key points

- What drugs/exposures occurred and at what dose?
- At what gestation was the pregnancy exposed?
- Maternal health (e.g. diabetes, obesity)?
- Family tree to determine whether any malformations noted may have a genetic, rather than a teratogenic, basis.

Examination: key points

Detailed fetal anomaly USS with careful search for structural malformation or other fetal investigations, as appropriate, depending on the nature and timing of exposure.

Table 6.3 Anticoagulation during pregnancy in patients with a prosthetic heart valve

Recommendation	ACC/AHA	ACCP	ESC
Oral anticoagulants	Can be used throughout pregnancy, with substitution by dose-adjusted UFH or LMWH during weeks 6–12 of gestation if preferred by the patient	Can be used throughout pregnancy high-risk patients*, with substitution by LMWH or UFH close to term (time frame not specified, but normally 48 hours before delivery)	If the warfarin dose is ≤5 mg daily, oral anticoagulants throughout pregnancy is the safest regimen (associated with <3% embryopathy)
Heparin derivatives	Monitored UFH or LMWH might be options throughout gestation or during weeks 6–12 of gestation. LMWH dose should be adjusted to give an anti-factor Xa activity	Dose-adjusted and monitored LMWH or UFH throughout pregnancy or during weeks 6–12 of gestation is acceptable. In low-risk patients, LMWH should be given twice daily and the dose adjusted to achieve the manufacturer's peak inhibition of factor Xa 4 hours after subcutaneous injection	LMWH or UFH during weeks 6–12 of gestation should be considered if high-dose warfarin is required to maintain therapeutic anticoagulation. LMWH dose should be adjusted to give an anti-factor Xa activity of 0.8–1.2 units/ml 4–6 hours after administration
Aspirin	Low-dose aspirin in addition to anticoagulation during the second and third trimesters	Low-dose aspirin in addition to anticoagulation in high-risk* patients	Aspirin in addition to anticoagulation is not recommended
Anticoagulation target	INR 3 for all patients with mechanical prosthetic heart valves	INR 2–3 for patients with bileaflet aortic valves without high-risk features*	No INR target recommendation

* First-generation prostheses, mitral valve prostheses, history of thromboembolism, atrial fibrillation, or left ventricular dysfunction.

ACC, American College of Cardiology; ACCP, American College of Chest Physicians; AHA, American Heart Association; ESC, European Society of Cardiology; INR, international normalize ratio; LMWH, low-molecular-weight heparin; UFH, unfractionated heparin.

Reprinted by permission from Macmillian Publishers Ltd: *Nature Reviews Cardiology*, Castellano *et al.* Anticoagulation during pregnancy in patients with a prosthetic heart valve, vol 9(7), 415–424, copyright 2012.

Special investigations

Contact UKTIS for an individual risk assessment and advice and to enable recording of the exposure and outcome by UKTIS for surveillance purposes. UKTIS summaries of the available literature are available at https://www.toxbase.org (free to all NHS healthcare professionals, once registered).

Genetic advice and management

Diagnosis of a teratogenic syndrome is generally on the basis that a genetic or other cause of the anomaly has been excluded. Caution should be exercised where data regarding use of a particular drug in pregnancy are very limited or a teratogenic phenotype has been proposed on the basis of a few case reports where genetic investigation was limited (e.g. allopurinol).

For women who have an infant with a likely teratogenic syndrome, the recurrence risk may be high if they stay on the same medication at the same dose. *Serious consideration must be given to revising her medication in advance of another pregnancy, in conjunction with her physician.*

Nevertheless, while the overall recurrence risk is high, the severity of any effect may be somewhat unpredictable since it is influenced by the pharmacometabolism of the fetoplacental complex which is, in part, genetically determined and may vary between siblings. For example, a woman may stay on the same dose of sodium valproate in three pregnancies but only have one child who is adversely affected.

Information on the longer-term neurodevelopmental effects of many drugs is currently limited, but as the field of neurobehavioural teratology expands, questions regarding an association between *in utero* exposure and conditions such as autism are likely to become more frequent.

Information sources: UK: UK Teratology Information Service, http://www.uktis.org, Tel. 0844 892 0909; Europe: European Network of Teratology Information Services (ENTIS), https://www.entis-org.eu; Canada: Motherisk, http://www.motherisk.org, Tel. (416) 813 6780; USA: OTIS (Organization of Teratology Information Specialists), http://mothertobaby.org, Tel. (866) 626 6847.

Expert adviser: Laura Yates, Consultant in Clinical Genetics (NGS) and Head of Teratology (UKTIS), Institute of Genetic Medicine, Newcastle upon Tyne Hospitals NHS Foundation Trust and Newcastle University, Newcastle upon Tyne, UK.

References

Austin MP, Mitchell PB. Pschotropic medications in pregnant women: treatment dilemmas. *Med J Aust* 1998; **169**: 428–31.

Barr M Jr. Teratogen update: angiotensin-converting enzyme inhibitors. *Teratology* 1994; **50**: 399–409.

Bracken MB. Oral contraception and congenital malformations in offspring: a review and meta-analysis of the prospective studies. *Obstet Gynecol* 1990; **76**: 552–7.

Castellano JM, Narayan RL, Vaishnava P, Fuster V. Anticoagulation during pregnancy in patients with a prosthetic heart valve. *Nat Rev Cardiol* 2012; **9**: 415–24.

Cotrufo M, De Feo M, De Santo LS, *et al.* Risk of warfarin during pregnancy with mechanical valve prostheses. *Obstet Gynecol* 2002; **99**: 35–40.

Holmes LB. Teratogen-induced limb defects. *Am J Med Genet* 2003; **112**: 297–303.

Hoyme HE, Jones KL, Dixon SD, *et al.* Prenatal cocaine exposure and fetal vascular disruption. *Pediatrics* 1990; **85**: 743–7.

Jacobson SJ, Jones K, Johnson K, *et al.* Prospective multicentre study of pregnancy outcome after lithium exposure during first trimester. *Lancet* 1992; **339**: 530–3.

Jilma B, Kamath S, Lip GY. ABC of antithrombotic therapy. Antithrombotic therapy in special circumstances. I—Pregnancy and cancer. *BMJ* 2003; **326**: 37–40.

Koren G, Pastuszak A, Ito S. Drugs in pregnancy [review]. *N Engl J Med* 1998; **338**: 1128–37.

Moore JA. An assessment of lithium using the IEHR evaluative process for assessing human developmental and reproductive toxicity of agents. IEHR Expert Scientific Committee. *Reprod Toxicol* 1995; **9**: 175–210.

Raman-Wilms L, Tseng AL, Wighardt S, Einarson TR, Koren G. Fetal genital effects of first trimester sex hormone exposure: a meta-analysis. *Obstet Gynecol* 1995; **85**: 141–9.

Rasmussen SA. Human teratogens update 2011: can we ensure safety during pregnancy? *Birth Defects Res A* 2012; **94**: 123–8.

Reuvers M. Anticoagulants and antifibrinolytics. In: C Schaefer (ed.). *Drugs during pregnancy and lactation*, pp. 85–92. Elsevier, Amsterdam, 2001.

Schaefer C. Anticoagulants and antifibrinolytics. In: C Schaefer (ed.). *Drugs during pregnancy and lactation*, pp. 312–13. Elsevier, Amsterdam, 2001.

Schou M. What happened to the lithium babies? A follow-up study of children born without malformations. *Acta Psychiatr Scand* 1976; **54**: 193–7.

Schou M, Goldfield MD, Weinstein MR, Villeneuve A. Lithium and pregnancy. I. Report from the Register of Lithium Babies. *Br Med J* 1973; **2**: 135–6.

Shepard TH, Brent RL, Friedman JM, *et al*. Update on new developments in the study of human teratogens. *Teratology* 2002; **65**: 153–61.

Stephansson O, Kieler H, Haglund B, *et al*. Selective serotonin reuptake inhibitors during pregnancy and risk of stillbirth and infant mortality. *JAMA* 2013; **309**: 48–54.

Ting YH, Zhou Y, Lao TT. Carbimazole embryopathy in a Chinese population: case series and literature review. *Birth Defects Res A Clin Mol Teratol* 2013; **97**: 225–9.

Wilson LC, Kerr BA, Wilkinson R, Fossard C, Donnai D. Choanal atresia and hypothelia following methimazole exposure *in utero*: a second report. *Am J Med Genet* 1998; **75**: 220–2.

Winterfield U, Allignol A, Panchaud A, *et al*. Pregnancy outcome following maternal exposure to statins: a multicentre prospective study. *BJOG* 2013; **120**: 463–71.

Yacobi S, Ornoy A. Is lithium a real teratogen? What can we conclude from the prospective versus retrospective studies? A review. *Isr J Psychiatry Relat Sci* 2008; **45**: 95–106.

Female infertility and amenorrhoea: genetic aspects

Infertility is defined by the failure to conceive after 12 months of unprotected intercourse and affects an estimated 14% of the population of reproductive age in the UK (Templeton *et al.* 1990). Despite advances in the diagnosis of causes of subfertility, the inability to conceive remains unexplained in 25–30% of fully investigated couples. The conditions listed here are those that tend to be referred to the genetics clinic for advice; they affect only a small minority of women presenting with infertility.

Primary amenorrhoea

The four most common causes of primary amenorrhoea are gonadal dysgenesis (48.5%), congenital absence of the uterus and vagina (CAUV; 16.2%), gonadotrophin-releasing hormone (GnRH) deficiency (8.3%), and constitutional delay of puberty (6.0%) (Timmreck and Reindollar 2003). For further information on ovarian failure, see 'Premature ovarian failure (POF)' in Chapter 6, 'Pregnancy and fertility', p. 778 and 'Turner syndrome, 45,X and variants' in Chapter 5, 'Chromosomes', p. 696.

Clinical assessment

History: key points
- Three-generation family history.
- Birth history and early development.
- Enquire about breast development, menarche, and menstruation.

Examination: key points
- Detailed assessment is usually undertaken by a gynaecologist/fertility specialist. This includes a general physical exam, assessment of secondary sex characteristics, and pelvic exam.
- Assess whether the neck is short or whether there is any limitation of movement (MURCS (Müllerian duct anomalies–renal aplasia–cervicothoracic somite dysplasia)).

Special investigations
- Usually baseline investigations (e.g. day-3 serum FSH, LH, prolactin, and TFTs; day-21 serum progesterone (as well) and a pelvic USS or MRI) will have been undertaken by the reproductive medicine team. Ovarian and adrenal androgens may also have been measured. In primary amenorrhoea, spot measurements of hormone levels are taken as, without an established menstrual cycle, it is not possible to date the measurements.
- Karyotype (for TS mosaicism or translocation).
- Consider genomic array/WES/WGS if high suspicion of monogenic basis or associated malformation syndrome or strong family history.

Diagnoses to consider

Turner syndrome (TS)
45,X karyotype giving rise to a female phenotype with short stature and streak gonads. See 'Turner syndrome, 45,X and variants' in Chapter 5, 'Chromosomes', p. 696.

Congenital adrenal hyperplasia (CAH)
Non-classical CAH may present with subfertility in adult life. See 'Congenital adrenal hyperplasia (CAH)' in Chapter 3, 'Common consultations', p. 370.

Renal cysts and diabetes syndrome (RCAD, MODY5)
An AD disorder due to mutation in *HNF1B*. Manifestations include genital tract defects occurring in ~20% of women (e.g. bicornuate uterus, vaginal aplasia, rudimentary uterus, etc.); diabetes and gout typically have a later onset. Renal parenchymal defects, such as cystic kidneys or renal agenesis, are common (Edghill *et al.* 2006).

Congenital absence of the uterus and vagina (CAUV)
Also known as Mayer–Rokitansky–Kuster–Hauser syndrome or Müllerian aplasia. Prevalence is 1/4000–1/5000 females. Patients with CAUV are genetically and phenotypically female, with 46,XX karyotype, normal ovaries, breast development, and female patterns of body hair. In most CAUV patients, the uterus, cervix, and upper two-thirds of the vagina are absent; normal Fallopian tubes may be present and caudally attached to two small muscular buds. Most cases are isolated, with only occasional reports of familial occurrence. The aetiology of MRKH syndrome is still largely unknown, probably because of intrinsic heterogeneity (Fontana *et al.* 2016). Elias *et al.* (1984) found only 1/37 female sibs to have a symptomatic uterine anomaly (2.7%), and 0/24 mothers, 0/45 maternal aunts, and 0/50 paternal aunts.

Microdeletions at 16p11.2 and 17q12 were found in 4/38 (10.5%) cases with isolated Müllerian aplasia, and at 16p11.2, 17q12, and 22q11.2 (distal) in 5/25 cases (20%) with syndromic Müllerian aplasia (Nik-Zainal *et al.* 2011). Petrozza *et al.*'s (1997) survey of 17 female infants born through surrogacy to CAUV women did not reveal any CAUV offspring, suggesting it rarely follows AD inheritance.

There is a high incidence of associated anomalies.
- Renal malformations in 30%, e.g. unilateral renal agenesis or ectopia of one or both kidneys. Arrange renal USS.
- Skeletal anomalies, including spinal and limb defects in 11–12%. Arrange cervical spine films.
- Cardiac and hearing defects have also been described but are uncommon.

MURCS (Müllerian duct anomalies–renal aplasia–cervicothoracic somite dysplasia (Klippel–Feil anomaly))
Is thought to be a sporadic disorder and is a subset of CAVV/MRKH (see above).

Complete androgen insensitivity syndrome (CAIS)
Female phenotype with 46,XY karyotype, characterized by primary amenorrhoea due to an absent uterus and absent/sparse pubic and axillary hair. CAIS is due to mutations in the androgen receptor gene. See 'Androgen insensitivity syndrome (AIS)' in Chapter 3, 'Common consultations', p. 344.

Gonadal agenesis/dysgenesis (including 46,XY)
- SRY mutations or deletions of SRY (explains only 15–20% of XY females).
- Approximately 80% of XY females with gonadal dysgenesis are of unknown aetiology. They often have a uterus and streak gonads.

Hypogonadotrophic hypogonadism
The genetic basis for idiopathic hypogonadotrophic hypogonadism is largely unknown. Genes currently

recognized to be involved were reviewed by Silveira et al. (2002) and include *KAL-1* (associated with XL Kallmann syndrome (KS)), GnRH receptor, gonadotrophins, pituitary transcription factors (*HESX1*, *LHX3*, and *PROP-1*), orphan nuclear receptors (*DAX-1*, associated with XL congenital adrenal hypoplasia, and *SF-1*), and three genes also associated with obesity (leptin, leptin receptor, and prohormone convertase 1 (*PC1*)). Treatment comprises induction of puberty and maintenance replacement therapy. Fertility induction treatment is sometimes possible with gametogenesis induced by either exogenous gonadotrophin or pulsatile GnRH therapy. Since pregnancy is dependent on ART and has only recently become available to affected women, there are very few data on offspring risks.

Kallmann syndrome (KS)

Is a genetic condition characterized by the association of hypogonadotrophic hypogonadism and anosmia, with or without other anomalies. It is much less common in females than in males and affects ~1/40 000 females. See 'Male infertility: genetic aspects' in Chapter 6, 'Pregnancy and fertility', p. 750.

Genetic advice and management

* The geneticist's role is to explain the genetic basis of the disorder causing infertility/amenorrhoea. Depending on the specific diagnosis, if ART using the patient's own ova could be used to achieve a pregnancy, then advice about reproductive implications is also appropriate.
* Management of amenorrhoea and infertility is the remit of a specialist in reproductive medicine.
* ART enables pregnancy in some patients. Women with ovarian failure may use a donated ovum to achieve a pregnancy. Women with CAUV may undergo oocyte retrieval and IVF and have their fetus carried by a surrogate mother.

Support groups: Müllerian aplasia, rosagroup@yahoo. co.uk; Infertility Network UK, http://www.infertilitynetworkuk.com, Tel. 01424 732 361.

References

Edghill EL, Bingham C, Ellard S, Hattersley AT. Mutations in hepatocyte nuclear factor-1-beta and their related phenotypes. *J Med Genet* 2006; **43**: 84–90.

Elias S, Simpson JL, Carson SA, Malinak LR, Buttram VC Jr. Genetics studies in incomplete müllerian fusion. *Obstet Gynecol* 1984; **63**: 276–9.

Evers JL. Female subfertility [seminar]. *Lancet* 2002; **360**: 151–9.

Fontana L, Gentikki B, et al. Genetics of Mayer-Rokitansky-Kuster-Hauser (MRKH) syndrome. *Clin Genet* 2016; epub Oct 7.

Kobayashi A, Behringer RR. Developmental genetics of the female reproductive tract in mammals. *Nat Rev Genet* 2003; **4**: 969–80.

Nik-Zainal S, Strick R, Storer M. High incidence of recurrent copy number variants in patients with isolated and syndromic Mullerian aplasia. *J Med Genet* 2011; **48**: 197–204.

Petrozza JC, Gray MR, Davis AJ, Reindollar RH. Congenital absence of the uterus and vagina is not commonly transmitted as a dominant genetic trait: outcomes of surrogate pregnancies. *Fertil Steril* 1997; **67**: 387–9.

Resendes BL, Sohn SH, Stelling JR, et al. Role for anti-Müllerian hormone in congenital absence of the uterus and vagina. *Am J Med Genet* 2001; **98**: 129–36.

Silveira LF, MacColl GS, Bouloux PM. Hypogonadotropic hypogonadism. *Semin Reprod Med* 2002; **20**: 327–38.

Templeton A, Fraser C, Thompson B. The epidemiology of infertility in Aberdeen. *BMJ* 1990; **301**: 148–52.

Timmreck LS, Reindollar RH. Contemporary issues in primary amenorrhea. *Obstet Gynecol Clin North Am* 2003; **30**: 287–302.Fetal akinesia

Fetal akinesia

Fetal akinesia is a lack or severe reduction of spontaneous movement in the fetus. Severe akinesia results in a recognizable deformation sequence manifest on USS with some or all of the following, depending on gestation:

- increased nuchal translucency or hydrops;
- little or no spontaneous movement;
- joint contractures (arthrogryposis), in particular talipes and webbing (pterygia) of the neck, elbows, and knees;
- pulmonary hypoplasia;
- cleft palate and micrognathia;
- IUGR;
- polyhydramnios;
- breech presentation.

In the older literature, this phenotype is referred to as Pena Shokeir syndrome type I.

Clues to the aetiology may be seen on scan or by observation after delivery. Genetic tests are increasingly useful, but a detailed post-mortem is vital in most instances.

Fetal akinesia deformation sequence (FADS) should be differentiated from arthrogryposis secondary to uterine constraint, e.g. bicornuate uterus, oligohydramnios, and skeletal dysplasias.

The primary causes of akinesia are due to defects of the motor pathway (central nervous system and neuromuscular disorders) and there is considerable overlap with the aetiology of arthrogryposis (see 'Arthrogryposis' in Chapter 2, 'Clinical approach', p. 66). These disorders are clinically and genetically heterogeneous. The primary defect may occur at various levels in the motor system, for example:

- **the brain**. Major structural anomalies such as holoprosencephaly may be associated with FADS. Malformations of cortical development, for example perisylvian polymicrogyria with cerebellar hypoplasia due to biallelic mutations in *PI44KA* (Pagnamenta 2015) have been identified in FADS.
- **anterior horn cell and motor neuron**. Lethal arthrogryposis with anterior horn cell disease (LAAHD) is more common in Finland. SMA is not associated with early pregnancy FADS but needs to be considered in the differential diagnosis in surviving babies with later-onset prenatal features;
- **peripheral nervous system**. Axoglial defects resulting in poorly myelinated motor neurones and FADS are caused by autosomal recessive (AR) variants in *CNTAP1*, *ADCY6* and *GPR126* (Laquerriere et al. 2014; Ravenscroft et al. 2013);
- **the neuromuscular junction**. The children of mothers with myasthenia gravis can have arthrogryposis and features of the fetal akinesia sequence, due to the maternal transmission of AChR antibodies to the fetus. Studies of children with a similar phenotype, but without maternal antibodies, led to the discovery of recessive mutations in the embryonal AChR gamma subunit (CHRNG). A continuum of conditions has been shown to be due to mutations in endplate-specific presynaptic, synaptic, and post-synaptic proteins. Complete or severe functional disruption of the fetal AChR causes lethal multiple pterygium syndrome, whereas milder alterations result in fetal hypokinesia

with contractures or a myasthenic syndrome later in life (Michalk et al. 2008). Non-lethal multiple pterygium syndrome is also known as Escobar syndrome;

- **muscle conditions**. AR variants in RYR1 are significant causes of lethal multiple pterygium syndrome (LMPS)/FADS (McKie et al. 2014). Severe nemaline myopathy and forms of muscular dystrophy can also cause FADS.

Clinical assessment

History: key points

- Three-generation family tree, with specific enquiry about previously affected siblings and parental consanguinity.
- Recurrent affected pregnancies with no completely normal babies born between affected siblings may be due to transplacental antibodies in maternal myasthenia gravis. Can occur in asymptomatic mothers.
- Maternal illness such as myotonic dystrophy, myasthenia gravis, congenital infection, and high fever of >39°.
- Early amniocentesis (<14 gestational weeks) and multiple births suggest arthrogryposis due to intrauterine constraint.
- Drugs, e.g. misoprostol, cocaine, may cause intrauterine ischaemia and joint contractures.
- Ethnicity (Finland, *GLE1* mutations).

Examination: key points

- USS features of FADS as already described.
- Fetal/neonatal examination: pattern of joint contractures, pterygia, cleft palate and micrognathia, reduced muscle mass.
- Other associated congenital malformations.
- Maternal features of myasthenia or myotonia.
- Parental joint contractures (AD forms of arthrogryposis).

Special investigations

- Genomic microarray, gene panel, WES or WGS as appropriate/available.
- DNA storage from the fetus and parents.
- Full post-mortem, including neuropathology, muscle histology, and EM (consult with the pathologist to ensure full testing).
- Maternal antibodies to the fetal and adult subunits of AChR and anti-MuSK antibodies.
- Exclude myotonic dystrophy and SMA.
- Consider skin chromosomes for mosaicism (e.g. diploid/triploid mosaic).
- CK, neurophysiology, and muscle biopsy and MRI brain scan may be helpful in surviving infants.

Syndromic diagnoses to consider

Disorders of neuromuscular transmission

For example, lethal multiple pterygium syndrome (LMPS). The features of fetal akinesia may be seen from 12 weeks' gestation and this would indicate a poor prognosis. First reported due to recessive mutations in *CHRNG* (Hoffmann et al. 2006; Morgan et al. 2006). Vogt et al. (2008) analysed 15 cases of LMPS/fetal akinesia without *CHRNG* and found a homozygous

RAPSN frameshift mutation c.1177-1178delAA in a family with three children affected with lethal fetal akinesia sequence. Functional studies were consistent with the hypothesis that, whereas incomplete loss of rapsyn function may cause congenital myasthenia, more severe loss of function can result in a lethal fetal akinesia phenotype. Similarly, the recent observation that biallelic severe LOF mutations in the gene *DOK7* encoding a muscle protein crucial in synaptogenesis can result in a lethal fetal akinesia phenotype, whereas incomplete loss of DOK7 function may cause congenital myasthenia (Vogt et al. 2009). AR mutations in the *CHRND* and *CHRNA1* AChR subunits have also been shown to cause a severe LMPS phenotype (Michalk et al. 2008). Other neuromuscular junction genes are likely to be implicated in this spectrum of conditions.

Congenital myasthenic syndromes (CMS)
CMS are due to genetic mutations in endplate-specific presynaptic, synaptic, and post-synaptic proteins. The first to be identified were *CHRNE* mutations, but subsequent research (Beeson et al. 2008) has studied mutations of proteins involved in clustering the AChR and maintaining the neuromuscular junction structure. Although the CMS are not usually associated with fetal akinesia and joint contractures, an intermediate phenotype comprising prenatal arthrogryposis and neonatal respiratory compromise has been described in association with AR mutations in the AChR subunits *CHRND* and *RAPSN* (Brownlow et al. 2001, Burke et al. 2004).

Anterior horn cell and motor neurone disorders
Lethal congenital contracture syndrome 1 and LAAHD. Nousiainen et al. (2008) have shown that these two conditions are allelic and due to recessive mutations in the *GLE1* gene. The condition was described in Finland and the clinical features are of severe hydrops, micrognathia, and pulmonary hypoplasia. Histopathology shows an anterior horn cell motor neurone loss. The bones are generally thin and the ribs described as being similar to 'fish bones'.

Spinal muscular atrophy (SMA)
See 'Spinal muscular atrophy (SMA)' in Chapter 3, 'Common consultations', p. 526. Does not typically present as fetal akinesia, but there have been reports of infants with homozygous *SMN* mutations and a low *SMN2* copy number with arthrogryposis. AR SMA with respiratory distress (SMARD) is a heterogeneous disorder that may be caused by mutations in the immunoglobulin micro-binding protein gene *IGHMBP2*. Another rare type of SMA—XL infantile SMA (XL-SMA)—presents with hypotonia, areflexia, fractures, arthrogryposis, and infantile death due to respiratory failure and is caused by mutation in *UBE1* (Ramser et al. 2008).

Congenital myopathies
Severe congenital myopathies may present prenatally or at birth with features of fetal akinesia. There may be severe hypotonia with little or no spontaneous movement or respiratory effort at birth. Multiple joint contractures and a DCM may uncommonly be observed. AR variants in *RYR1* were detected in 8% of an LMPS/FADS cohort and thus are a significant cause (McKie et al. 2014). Consideration should be given to potential malignant hyperthermia risks for carrier parents and siblings. Up to half of the severe presentations of nemaline myopathy are due to AR *ACTA1* variants, however AR *NEB* and

KLHL40 variants have also been described in in FADS (Agrawal 2004; Ravenscroft 2013; Wallgren-Petterson et al. 2002). Other severe congenital myopathies with different modes of inheritance may be detected on muscle biopsy studies.

Other causes of fetal akinesia
Metabolic conditions. Glycogen storage disorder type IV and type VII are recognized causes of fetal akinesia.
  Chromosome disorders including trisomy 18, mosaic trisomy 8, and microdeletion syndromes may present with features of fetal akinesia and other congenital malformations.

Syndromes with arthrogryposis
See 'Arthrogryposis' in Chapter 2, 'Clinical approach', p. 66.
• Amyoplasia—1/3 of all those with arthrogryposis. Symmetrical joint contractures with straight elbows, talipes equinovarus, and muscle hypoplasia. Association with gastroschisis and bowel atresias; however, other structural anomalies not usually present; see 'Arthrogryposis' in Chapter 2, 'Clinical approach', p. 66.
• ARC syndrome. See 'Prolonged neonatal jaundice and jaundice in infants below 6 months' in Chapter 2, 'Clinical approach', p. 288.
• Distal arthrogryposis (can be AD). See 'Arthrogryposis' in Chapter 2, 'Clinical approach', p. 66.

Restrictive dermopathy
IUGR, congenital contractures, and tense, easily eroded, and damaged skin, caused by dominant mutations in the *LMNA* gene or AR mutations in the *ZMPSTE24* gene.
• Neu Laxova syndrome (AR variants in *PHGDH* and *PSAT1*) IUGR, microcephaly, and CNS abnormality such as lissencephaly, but the important aetiological clue is the presence of yellow subcutaneous tissue covered by thin, scaly skin and generalized tissue oedema.
• COFS (cerebro-oculo-facial-skeletal syndrome). See 'DNA repair disorders' in Chapter 3, 'Common consultations', p. 398.

Genetic advice and management
• Make every effort to make a precise diagnosis and counsel appropriately.
• If post-mortem declined, limited assessment including muscle biopsy—histology and EM; skeletal X-rays may be helpful.

Inheritance and recurrence risk in the absence of a precise diagnosis
• Recurrence risks are high, with the exception of amyoplasia and some environmental aetiologies such as early amniocentesis. Assume possible AR inheritance, though the empiric risks may be around 15%. Most siblings are similarly affected however intrafamilial variability particularly between more distant relatives may be due to additional variants in other FADS genes, which may modify the severity of the phenotype (Bayram et al. 2016).

Prenatal diagnosis
Definitive PND is possible by CVS if the molecular basis of the fetal akinesia is known. For those where the genetic basis remains undetermined, PND may be possible by serial scanning from 12 weeks' gestation. This

should be reviewed in each pregnancy, as the introduction of genetic disease panels and next-generation sequencing technologies enable a molecular diagnosis to be achieved for more couples. Preimplantation genetic diagnosis (PGD) may be an option for couples if the molecular diagnosis is known.

Support group: The Arthrogryposis Group, http://www.arthrogryposis.co.uk, Tel. 0800 028 4447.

Expert adviser: Julie Vogt, Consultant Geneticist, West Midlands Regional Genetics Service, Birmingham Women's NHS Foundation Trust, Birmingham, UK.

References

Agrawal PB, Strickland CD, Midgett C, et al. Heterogeneity of nemaline myopathy cases with skeletal muscle alpha-actin gene mutations. Ann Neurol 2004; **56**: 86–96.

Bayram Y, Karaca F, et al. Molecular etiology of arthrogryposis in multiple families of mostly Turkish origin. J Clin Invest 2016; **126**: 762–78.

Beeson D, Webster R, Cossins J, et al. Congenital myasthenic syndromes and the formation of the neuromuscular junction. Ann N Y Acad Sci 2008; **1132**: 99–103.

Brownlow S., Webster R., Croxen R., et al. Acetylcholine receptor delta subunit mutations underlie a fast-channel myasthenic syndrome and arthrogryposis multiplex congenita. J Clin Invest 2001; **108**: 125–30.

Burke G, Cossins J, Maxwell S, et al. Distinct phenotypes of congenital acetylcholine receptor deficiency. Neuromuscul Disord 2004; **14**: 356–64.

Hoffmann K, Muller JS, Stricker S, et al. Escobar syndrome is a prenatal myasthenia caused by disruption of the acetylcholine receptor fetal gamma subunit. Am J Hum Genet 2006; **79**: 303–12.

Laquerriere A, Maluenda J, et al. Mutation is CNTNAP1 and ADCY6 are responsible for sever arthrogryposis multiplex congenital with axoglial defects. Hum Mol Genet 2014; **27**: 2279–89.

Michalk A, Stickler S, et al. Acetylcholine receptor pathway mutations explain various fetal akinesia deformation sequence disorders. Am J Med Genet; **2**: 464–76.

Morgan NV, Brueton LA, Cox P, et al. Mutations in the embryonal subunit of the acetylcholine receptor (CHRNG) cause lethal and Escobar variants of multiple pterygium syndrome. Am J Hum Genet 2006; **79**: 390–5.

Michalk A, Stricker S, Becker J, et al. Acetylcholine receptor pathway mutations explain various fetal akinesia deformation sequence disorders. Am J Hum Genet 2008; **2**: 464–76.

Nousiainen HO, Kestilä M, Pakkasjärvi N, et al. Mutations in mRNA export mediator GLE1 result in a fetal motoneuron disease. Nat Genet 2008; **40**: 155–7.

Pagnamenta AT, Howard MF, et al. Germline recessive mutations in PI4KA are associated with perisylvian polymicrogyria, cerebellar hypoplasia and arthrogryposis. Hum Mol Genet 2015; **24**: 3732–41.

Ramser J, Ahearn ME, Lenski C, et al. Rare missense and synonymous variants in UBE1 are associated with X-linked infantile spinal muscular atrophy. Am J Hum Genet 2008; **82**: 188–93.

Ravenscroft G, Miyatake S, et al. Mutations in KLHL40 are a frequent cause of severe autosomal recessive nemaline myopathy. Am J Hum Genet 2013; **93**: 6–18.

Vogt J, Harrison BJ, Spearman H, et al. Mutation analysis of CHRNA1, CHRNB1, CHRND, and RAPSN genes in multiple pterygium syndrome/fetal akinesia patients. Am J Hum Genet 2008; **82**: 222–7.

Vogt J, Morgan NV, Marton T, et al. Germline mutation in DOK7 associated with fetal akinesia deformation sequence. J Med Genet 2009; **46**: 338–40.

Wallgren-Pettersson C, Donner K, Sewry C, et al. Mutations in the nebulin gene can cause severe congenital nemaline myopathy. Neuromuscul Disord 2002; **12**: 674–9.

Fetal alcohol syndrome (FAS)

Sometimes the geneticist is asked to evaluate a child to determine whether his/her learning difficulties or short stature are related to prenatal alcohol exposure. This opinion may be used in court proceedings or care orders and it is important that it is as accurate as possible. It is also crucial to establish this diagnosis because of the potential for preventing recurrence in future pregnancies if the maternal alcohol problems can be treated.

The UK government (Department of Health 2016) recommends that pregnant women should avoid alcohol as a precaution. Although the risk of harm to the baby is low if they have drunk small amounts of alcohol before becoming aware of the pregnancy, there is no 'safe' level of alcohol to drink when you are pregnant.

On other occasions, the history of maternal alcohol exposure is not forthcoming and has to be carefully sought during the evaluation of a child presenting with developmental delay. The incidence of FAS varies, depending on geographical location, but, according to Sampson et al. (1997), the incidence per thousand live births in Seattle (USA) was 2.8 and in Cleveland (USA) 4.6. The combined rate of FAS and alcohol-related neurodevelopmental disorder (ARND) in Seattle was estimated at nearly 1% of all live births. The reduced brain mass and neurobehavioural disturbances associated with human FAS may be related to the recent observation in rats that ethanol can trigger widespread apoptotic neurodegeneration (Ikonomidou et al. 2000).

Quantitative structural MRIs in children with FAS has shown structural abnormalities in several regions of the brain, including the cerebellum, corpus callosum, and basal ganglia. The changes are more frequent and severe in children with dysmorphic facial features (Riley et al. 2004).

- Both high regular intake of alcohol and binge drinking can cause FAS and ARND.

- The critical time period extends throughout pregnancy.
- FAS is associated with high-dose exposure (estimated blood alcohol concentrations to ≥150 mg/dl) delivered at least weekly for at least several weeks in the first trimester, or chronic ingestion of at least 2 g/kg/day of alcohol (1 unit (10 g alcohol) = one glass of table wine = 0.5 pint of beer, lager, or cider = one measure of sherry or vermouth. A standard bottle of spirits = 32 units; a standard bottle of wine = 10 units; a can of extra strong lager = 4 units).
- There is a continuum of risk with population-based studies showing that chronic low-dose exposures to 15 cc of absolute alcohol per day can be associated with reduction in IQ and increased rates of attention and learning problems. These changes are too subtle to detect in an individual but at higher levels of exposure probably merge with ARND.

Box 6.2 gives the clinical features of FAS and Figure 6.1 shows the facial features.

Diagnostic categories

See Stratton et al. 1996.

(1) FAS with confirmed maternal alcohol exposure.
  - Face, CNS neurodevelopmental and growth anomalies.
  - Clear history of alcohol exposure (substantial regular intake or heavy episodic drinking; there may be a history of drunken episodes, withdrawal symptoms, social problems related to drinking, assault, liver problems).

(2) FAS without confirmed maternal alcohol exposure.
  - Face, brain, and growth anomalies.
  - Fostered or adopted child without pregnancy history available.

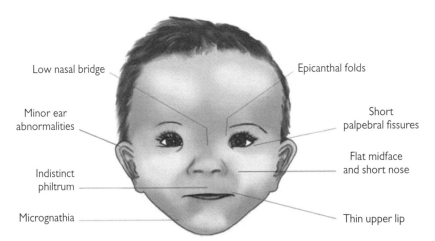

Low nasal bridge

Minor ear abnormalities

Indistinct philtrum

Micrognathia

Epicanthal folds

Short palpebral fissures

Flat midface and short nose

Thin upper lip

Figure 6.1 Facial characteristics that are associated with fetal alcohol exposure.
Reproduced from National Institute on Alcohol Abuse and Alcoholism (NIAAA), Alcohol Alert, 82, US Department of Health and Human Services www.niaaa.nih.gov. All material contained in the Alcohol Alert is in the public domain and may be used or reproduced.

Box 6.2 Clinical features of FAS

Facial features[*]
- Short palpebral fissures
- Flat midface
- Long and flattened philtrum
- Thin vermilion of upper lip

Growth retardation
- Low birthweight for gestational age (<2.5 centile)
- Decelerating weight over time not due to nutrition
- Disproportionately low weight to height relationship

CNS neurodevelopmental anomalies
- Microcephaly or decreased cranial size at birth
- Structural brain anomalies, e.g. partial or complete agenesis of corpus callosum, cerebellar hypoplasia
- Impaired fine motor skills, sensorineural deafness, poor hand–eye coordination, poor tandem gait

Behavioural/cognitive/learning deficits
Complex pattern of behaviour or cognitive abnormalities that are inconsistent with developmental level and cannot be explained by family background or environment alone, such as learning difficulties, deficits in school performance, poor impulse control, problems in social perception, deficits in higher-level receptive and expressive language, poor capacity for abstraction, specific deficits in mathematical skills, or problems in memory, attention, and judgement

[*] Moore *et al.* (2001) have identified six craniofacial measurements that could differentiate individuals with and without prenatal alcohol exposure with 96% accuracy, 98% sensitivity, and 90% specificity.

Data from Elizabeth S. Moore, Richard E. Ward, Paul L. Jamison, Colleen A. Morris, Patricia I. Bader, Bryan D. Hall, The subtle facial signs of prenatal exposure to alcohol: An anthropometric approach, *The Journal of Pediatrics*, 2001, volume 139, issue 2, pp. 215–219.

---

(3) Partial FAS with confirmed maternal alcohol exposure.
  - Clinical features of FAS.
  - Some facial features.
  - Growth retardation or CNS neurodevelopmental abnormalities or behavioural/cognitive/learning deficits.
(4) Alcohol-related birth defects, e.g. CHD, developmental anomalies of the renal tract, etc. This may coexist with category 5.
(5) ARND. CNS neurodevelopmental anomalies or behavioural/cognitive/learning deficits; may coexist with category 4.

Reproduced from Stratton K, Howe C, Battaglia F (Eds.), Institute of Medicine Committee to study fetal alcohol syndrome, *Fetal alcohol syndrome: diagnosis, epidemiology, prevention and treatment*. Reprinted with permission from the National Academies Press, Copyright 1996, National Academy of Sciences.

Clinical assessment

History: key points
- Draw a brief family tree and document parental heights (useful for calculating target parental centile range in the assessment of short stature).
- Obtain a detailed account of maternal alcohol intake throughout pregnancy. If you strongly suspect FAS clinically, you may need to seek information on maternal alcohol intake from several sources, e.g. relatives, obstetric record, or GP.
- Take a careful history of exposures in pregnancy, including medical and recreational drugs.

- Document the birthweight. Are other birth measurements recorded, e.g. OFC?
- Developmental history.

Examination: key points
- Growth parameters. Height, weight, OFC (measure the head size and height of parents for comparison).
- Facial features (see Box 6.2).
- Neurological examination, including developmental assessment.

Special investigations
Whether or not to do further investigations is a matter for individual clinical judgement and will be, in part, dictated by how compelling the evidence for FAS is. It is our usual practice to do the following investigations.
- Genomic array (unless compelling evidence of FAS).
- FRAX, unless microcephalic.
- Consider MRI scan.

Genetic advice and management
Unless the maternal alcohol problem is successfully treated, the recurrence risks in a subsequent pregnancy are high.

Support group: National Organisation for Fetal Alcohol Syndrome UK (NOFAS-UK), http://www.nofas-uk.org.

References
Astley SJ, Clarren SK. A case definition and photographic screening tool for the facial phenotype of fetal alcohol syndrome. *J Pediatr* 1996; **129**: 33–41.

Department of Health. Health risks from alcohol: new guidelines, 2016. https://www.gov.uk/government/consultations/health-risks-from-alcohol-new-guidelines.

Ikonomidou C, Bittigau P, Ishimaru MJ, *et al*. Ethanol-induced apoptotic neurodegeneration and fetal alcohol syndrome. *Science* 2000; **287**: 1056–60.

Jones KL. The effects of alcohol on fetal development. *Birth Defects Res C Embryo Today* 2011; **93**: 3–11.

Mattson SN, Riley EP, Gramling L, Delis DC, Jones KL. Heavy prenatal alcohol exposure with or without physical features of fetal alcohol syndrome leads to IQ deficits. *J Pediatr* 1997; **131**: 718–21.

Moore ES, Ward RE, Jamison PL, Morris CA, Bader PI, Hall BD. The subtle facial signs of prenatal exposure to alcohol: an anthropometric approach. *J Pediatr* 2001; **139**: 215–19.

Riley EP, McGee CL, Sowell ER. Teratogenic effects of alcohol: a decade of brain imaging. *Am J Med Genet C Semin Med Genet* 2004; **127C**: 35–41.

Sampson PD, Streissguth AP, Bookstein FL, *et al*. Incidence of fetal alcohol syndrome and prevalence of alcohol-related neurodevelopmental disorder. *Teratology* 1997; **56**: 317–26.

Stratton K, Howe C, Battaglia F (eds.). *Fetal alcohol syndrome: diagnosis, epidemiology, prevention and treatment, Institute of Medicine Committee to study fetal alcohol syndrome.* National Academy Press, Washington DC, 1996.

Fetal anticonvulsant syndrome (FACS)

Seizure disorders are one of the most common neurological problems affecting women of childbearing age. Approximately 0.5% of pregnant women take anticonvulsant medication to treat epilepsy during pregnancy. Anticonvulsants are also increasingly used to treat other disorders such as migraine and bipolar disorder. Sodium valproate (e.g. Epilim®), phenytoin (e.g. Epanutin®), carbamazepine (e.g. Tegretol®), and phenobarbitone/phenobarbital all have teratogenic potential. Second-generation therapy, such as lamotrigine, vigabatrin, topiramate, and levetiracetam, have been introduced over the past 15+ years, and their teratogenic potential is as yet unclear, though lamotrigine and levetiracetam appear to have a lower teratogenic effect than the first-generation drugs. Collectively antiepileptic drugs are amongst the most common teratogenic drugs prescribed to women of childbearing age (Meador 2016).

For any woman with epilepsy who is contemplating pregnancy, the risks to the fetus of exposure to anticonvulsant therapy must be weighed against the risks of seizure-induced morbidity and mortality, both to the mother and the unborn fetus. Maternal morbidity includes the physical risks of accidents, the social consequences of active epilepsy (e.g. loss of driving licence), and the risk of sudden unexplained death in epilepsy (SUDEP), a documented cause of death in maternal mortality statistics in recent years. Fetal morbidity may be due to the risks of trauma to the baby due to the mother falling, the risks of status epilepticus during pregnancy, and the occurrence of prolonged seizures during labour (1–2% of women with epilepsy will have a convulsion during delivery). One of the major risks for the fetus, however, is the teratogenic effects of some antiepileptic drugs.

Main features of anticonvulsant embryopathy

Overall, there is a fairly solid consensus that treatment with anticonvulsants in pregnancy for whatever reason, i.e. epilepsy or mood disorder, is associated with an *overall 2- to 3-fold increased risk of congenital malformation* (see Table 6.4), compared to the risk in the general population (Dolk and McElhatton 2002; Meador et al. 2008; Wyszynski et al. 2005). The actual risks in a given pregnancy are dependent on the specific drug with individual maternal and fetal metabolism, and genetic susceptibility—factors most likely playing a part. Risks are greater for combination therapy and for higher doses. The lowest risks are with exposure to a drug with lower teratogenic potential used as monotherapy at the lowest dose compatible with adequate seizure control. Growth retardation and microcephaly are uncommon, though the latter may be seen with exposure to some polytherapies. In the meta-analysis carried out by Meador et al. (2008), there was a 7% overall risk of major malformations in women with epilepsy, the risk being 16.8% for polytherapy and 10.7% for valproate (VPA) (see Figure 6.2).

Clinical assessment

History: key points
- Three-generation family tree.
- Detailed enquiry about the precise dose and type of anticonvulsant taken during pregnancy (may need to request the mother's obstetric notes for this information).
- Enquiry about other potential teratogenic exposures during pregnancy, e.g. alcohol, maternal illness.

Box 6.3 Recommendations for the treatment of epilepsy in women of childbearing potential

Whenever possible, treatment should be optimized before pregnancy and the effectiveness assessed before conception, by doing the following.
- Reassess the indication for treatment and consider gradual withdrawal of antiepileptic drugs (AEDs) in women in remission for whom the risk of relapse is low and who are willing to take the risk.
- Select the most appropriate AED for the woman's type of epilepsy and that with the lowest teratogenic potential. VPA* should not be prescribed to female children, female adolescents, and women of childbearing potential or pregnant women, unless other treatments are ineffective or not tolerated.
- Aim for monotherapy with the appropriate AED and try out the lowest effective dosage, in particular for controlling tonic–clonic seizures. Whenever possible, avoid VPA* at doses of 700 mg/day and above (see also bullet point above).
- Measure the plasma concentration of the AED when the dose has been optimized.
- Treatment can be optimized during pregnancy by doing the following.
- Avoid withdrawal or changes of AEDs when pregnancy is already established. Risks generally outweigh possible gains.
- Monitor treatment more closely than normally. Monitor plasma concentrations of lamotrigine in particular and possibly oxcarbazepine and levetiracetam.
- Adjust dose based on seizure control. Consider a dose increase also if there is a pronounced fall in AED plasma concentrations from optimum pre-pregnancy concentrations.
- Offer PND.

* Refer to the guidance and communication materials regarding VPA published by the Medicines and Healthcare products Regulatory Agency (February 2016) and report suspected fetal effects of VPA on a Yellow Card.

Reproduced from *Archives of Disease in Childhood*, Cummings et al., Neurodevelopment of children exposed *in utero* to lamotrigine, sodium valproate and carbamazepine, Vol 96(7): 643–7, copyright 2011, with permission from BMJ Publishing Group Ltd. Data from Medicines and Healthcare products Regulatory Agency (MHRA) Guidance February 2016.

Box 6.4 Box to show the main features of anticonvulsant embryopathy

- *Major malformations.* The major malformations seen most often in anticonvulsant-exposed children are those that also occur commonly in unexposed children: heart defects (ranging from septal defects to complex CHD), hypospadias, talipes, and cleft lip or palate. The risk for NTDs appears to be ~5% with VPA exposure, ~1% with carbamazepine exposure, and not increased for other drugs.
- *Facial features.* These include a short nose with a broad nasal bridge and anteverted nostrils, a thin upper lip; and a wide, featureless philtrum. The facies are more marked with VPA exposure where there may be infraorbital grooves and a small, downturned mouth with an everted lower lip.
- *Musculoskeletal.* Joint laxity, hypoplastic, overlapping toes, and talipes may be seen.
- *Neurodevelopmental problems.* Early studies of neurodevelopment after antiepileptic drug exposure suggested that there was an increased risk for adverse neurodevelopment, but studies were often small and retrospective. In long-term prospective studies, poorer performance after exposure to VPA is a consistent finding (Cummings et al. 2011; Meador et al. 2008; Tomson and Battino 2012). A recent Cochrane systematic review (Bromley et al. 2014) confirmed reduced IQ in the VPA-exposed group with doses above 800 mg daily conferring the most risk. The IQ of children exposed to carbamazepine did not differ from that of unexposed children. Children exposed to antiepileptic drugs have been shown to be at around a 4-fold increased risk for neurodevelopmental disorders, including ADHD and autism (Bromley et al. 2013; Christensen et al. 2013).

- Detailed history of seizures during pregnancy, delivery, and the perinatal period, including birthweight. Were there symptoms of neonatal withdrawal, e.g. jitteriness, seizures, poor feeding?
- Detailed developmental and behavioural history of the child.

Examination: key points

- Height, weight, OFC.
- Eyes. Assess for prominence of the metopic ridge, hypertelorism/telecanthus, epicanthic folds, and infraorbital groove.
- Mouth and nose. Assess shortness of the nose, length of the philtrum, smoothness of the philtrum, thinness of the upper lip, eversion of the lower lip, and cleft lip/palate.
- Hands and feet for joint laxity, nail hypoplasia, stiffness of interphalangeal joints, long overlapping fingers, hypoplastic or overlapping toes, talipes.
- Heart for murmur.
- Hypospadias.
- Examine the back for signs suggesting occult spina bifida.

Special investigations

If there is developmental delay with dysmorphic features, or a family history of learning disability:

- genomic microarray (for other causes of developmental delay, including microdeletion syndromes, predisposing to epilepsy that may have been inherited from the mother, e.g. 15q11.2, 15q13.3, and 16p13.11);
- FRAXA (fragile X syndrome);
- urine amino and organic acids;
- other investigations, as indicated.

Genetic advice and management

Sibling recurrence risk is high if the mother remains on the same drug and dose (estimated at 39–55%; Dean et al. 2002).

If there is a possibility of a subsequent pregnancy (see Box 6.3), refer to a neurologist for assessment as to whether it is appropriate to consider: withdrawal of anticonvulsants (if the mother has not had a seizure for several years); simplification of therapy (monotherapy, rather than polytherapy); or, if the seizures are well controlled, a reduction in dose. Current advice suggests avoiding VPA during pregnancy, if at all possible.

Table 6.4 Rates of major congenital malformations in six different studies.

	Valproate	Carbamazepine	Lamotrigine	Phenobarbital	Phenytoin
International Lamotrigine Pregnancy Registry	–	–	35/1558 (2%)	–	–
Finnish Medical Birth Registry and drug prescription databases	28/263 (11%)	22/805 (3%)	–	–	1/38 (3%)
Swedish Medical Birth Registry	29/619 (5%)	35/1318 (3%)	26/867 (3%)	–	8/119 (7%)
UK Epilepsy and Pregnancy Register	44/715 (6%)	20/900 (2%)	21/647 (3%)	–	3/82 (4%)
North American AED Pregnancy Registry	30/323 (9%)	31/1033 (3%)	31/1562 (2%)	11/199 (6%)	12/416 (3%)
International Registry of Antiepileptic Drugs and Pregnancy (EURAP)	98/1010 (10%)	79/1402 (6%)	37/1280 (3%)	16/217 (7%)	6/103 (6%)

Data are number with major congenital malformations/number exposed to antiepileptic drug monotherapy (%).

AED, antiepileptic drug.

Reprinted from *The Lancet Neurology*, vol 11, Tomson T & Battino D, Teratogenetic effects of antiepileptic drugs, pp. 803–13, copyright 2013 with permission from Elsevier.

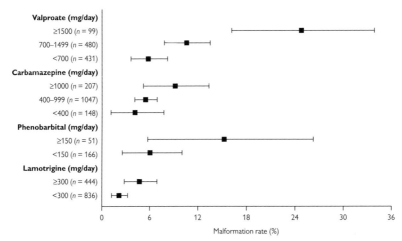

Figure 6.2 Rates of major congenital malformations at 1 year after birth in relation to exposure to antiepileptic drug monotherapy. Note increased risk of fetal malformation with higher maternal dose of anticonvulsant.
Reproduced with permission: EURAP Study Group, Seizure control and treatment in pregnancy: observations from the EURAP epilepsy pregnancy registry. *Neurology*, 66: 354–60, copyright 2006 American Academy of Neurology.

Emphasize to the mother that she should not stop or change her medication without prior discussion with her neurologist. Mothers should take 5 mg folic acid daily pre-conception.

Child with FACS
• Consider referral for vision screening (high incidence of refractive error in FACS and reports of iris and retinal coloboma).
• Consider referral for audiometry (glue ear in 33%).
• Referral for formal developmental assessment if developmental delay.
• Referral to a community paediatrician for ongoing follow-up if significant medical/developmental/behavioural problems.

Future pregnancy
For genetic advice and management for future pregnancy, see above and Figure 6.3.

Features associated with specific anticonvulsant drugs
See Box 6.4.

VALPROATE (VPA). A 10-fold increase in incidence of NTDs. The facial features are characteristic with trigonocephaly, infraorbital grooves, a short nose, a thin upper lip, and a small downturned mouth with an everted lower lip. In Kozma's (2001) survey, the most commonly observed musculoskeletal abnormalities included contractures of small joints and presence of long overlapping fingers (36%), foot deformity (30%), thumb abnormalities (17%), and radial defects (16%). There is a significant risk for cleft palate without cleft lip. The congenital malformations seen after VPA exposure are related to dose in the first trimester, and large daily doses of VPA (>900 mg) have a higher risk of causing malformations and NTDs than smaller doses. In the Australian study by Vajda et al. (2003), the dose of VPA taken was higher in pregnancies with birth defects, compared to those without (mean 2081 mg versus 1149 mg; P <0.0001). High daily doses at the end of pregnancy increase the likelihood of fetal

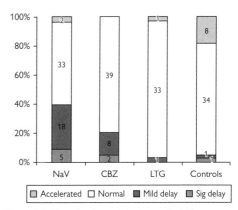

Figure 6.3 Neurodevelopmental outcomes in children exposed to antiepileptic drug monotherapies and in controls. CBZ, carbamazepine; LTG, lamotrigine; NaV, sodium valproate. Reprinted from *The Lancet*, vol 11, issue 9, Tomson T & Battino D, Teratogenetic effects of antiepileptic drugs, pp. 803–13, copyright 2013, with permission from Elsevier.

withdrawal symptoms such as irritability, jitteriness, and neonatal seizures.

In 2005, Wyszynski et al. reported a 10.7% prevalence of major malformations in babies exposed to VPA monotherapy in the first trimester of pregnancy, compared with 2.9% in offspring of women exposed to all other antiepileptic drugs and 1.6% in the normal newborn population. VPA exposure poses the highest risk for developmental effects and autism spectrum disorders.

CARBAMAZEPINE. Some increased risk for NTDs, but less than for VPA. Hypoplastic nails have been specifically noted after carbamazepine therapy. Facial features are less obvious than with VPA. A short nose, full cheeks, and a small mouth and chin have been noted. The philtrum is not shallow as it is with other drug exposures.

LAMOTRIGINE. In 2002, Tennis et al. reported the rate of major malformations was 1.8% among 168 monotherapy-exposed infants. The UK Epilepsy and Pregnancy Registry reported 2.1%, not significantly different from the normal population among 390 monotherapy-exposed infant (Morrow).

LEVETIRACETAM. Though this is a newer drug, studies so far are encouraging with no significant excess of major malformations or neurodevelopmental effects seen after exposure.

Support group: FACS (Fetal Anti Convulsant Syndrome' Association), http://facsa.org.uk.

Expert adviser: Jill Clayton-Smith, Consultant Clinical Geneticist, Manchester Centre For Genomic Medicine, Central Manchester Hospitals NHS Trust, Manchester, UK.

References

Bromley R, Weston J, Adab N, et al. Treatment for epilepsy in pregnancy: neurodevelopmental outcomes in the child. Cochrane Database Syst Rev 2014; **10**: CD010236.

Bromley RL, Mawer GE, Briggs M, et al.; Liverpool and Manchester Neurodevelopment Group. The prevalence of neurodevelopmental disorders in children prenatally exposed to antiepileptic drugs. J Neurol Neurosurg Psychiatry 2013; **84**: 637–43.

Christensen J, Grønborg TK, Sørensen MJ, et al. Prenatal valproate exposure and risk of autism spectrum disorders and childhood autism. JAMA 2013; **309**: 1696–703.

Crawford PM. Managing epilepsy in women of childbearing age. Drug Saf 2009; **32**: 293–307.

Cummings C, Stewart M, Stevenson M, Morrow J, Nelson J. Neurodevelopment of children exposed in utero to lamotrigine, sodium valproate and carbamazepine. Arch Dis Child 2011; **96**: 643–7.

Dean JC, Hailey H, Moore SJ, Lloyd DJ, Turnpenny PD, Little J. Long term health and neurodevelopment in children exposed to antiepileptic drugs before birth. J Med Genet 2002; **39**: 251–9.

Dolk H, McElhatton P. Assessing epidemiological evidence for the teratogenic effects of anticonvulsant medications. J Med Genet 2002; **39**: 243–4.

Glover SJ, Quinn AG, Barter P, et al. Ophthalmic findings in fetal anticonvulsant syndrome(s). Ophthalmology 2002; **109**: 942–7.

Hernandez-Diaz S, Werler MM, Walker AM, Mitchell AA. Folic acid antagonists during pregnancy and the risk of birth defects. N Engl J Med 2000; **343**: 1608–14.

Holmes LB. The teratogenicity of anticonvulsant drugs: a progress report [commentary]. J Med Genet 2002; **39**: 245–7.

Holmes LB, Coull BA, Dorfman J, Rosenberger PB. The correlation of deficits in IQ with midface and digit hypoplasia in children exposed in utero to anticonvulsant drugs. J Pediatr 2005; **146**: 118–22.

Holmes LB, Harvey EA, Coull BA, et al. The teratogenicity of anticonvulsant drugs. N Engl J Med 2001; **344**: 1132–8.

Kozma C. Valproic acid embryopathy: report of two siblings with further expansion of the phenotypic abnormalities and a review of the literature. Am J Med Genet 2001; **98**: 168–75.

Mawhinney E, Craig J, Morrow J, et al. Levetiracetam during pregnancy: results from a UK and Ireland epilepsy and pregnancy register. Neurology 2013; **80**: 400–5.

Meador K, Reynolds MW, Crean S, Fahrbach K, Probst C. Pregnancy outcomes in women with epilepsy: a systematic review and meta-analysis of published pregnancy registries and cohorts. Epilepsy Res 2008; **81**: 1–13.

Meador KJ, Loring DW. Developmental effects of antiepileptic drugs and the need for improved regulation. Neurology 2016; **86**: 297–306.

Shallcross R, Bromley RL, Irwin B, Bonnett LJ, Morrow J, Baker GA; Liverpool Manchester Neurodevelopment Group; UK Epilepsy and Pregnancy Register. Child development following in utero exposure; levetiracetam vs sodium valproate. Neurology 2011; **76**: 383–9.

Tennis P, Eldridge RR; International Lamotrigine Pregnancy Registry Scientific Advisory Committee. Preliminary results on pregnancy outcome in women using lamotrigine. Epilepsia 2002; **43**: 1161–7.

Tomson T, Battino D. Teratogenic effects of antiepileptic drugs. Lancet Neurol 2012; **11**: 803–13.

Vajda FJ, O'Brien TJ, Hitchcock A, Graham J, Lander C. The Australian registry of anti-epileptic drugs in pregnancy: experience after 30 months. J Clin Neurosci 2003; **10**: 543–9.

Wyszynski DF, Nambisan M, Surve T, et al. Increased rate of major malformations in offspring exposed to valproate during pregnancy. Neurology 2005; **64**: 961–5.

Fetomaternal alloimmunization (rhesus D and thrombocytopenia)

Alloimmunization against blood cell alloantigens

Blood cell alloantigen incompatibility between the fetus and mother may occur where the fetus possesses a blood cell alloantigen derived from the father that is not present on the maternal blood cells. Blood cell alloantibodies of the IgG class will cross the placenta and bind their cognate alloantigen. If the expression of the alloantigen is restricted to one type of blood cell, then IgG-mediated blood cell destruction may ensue, resulting in anaemia, thrombocytopenia, or neutropenia, respectively.

Red cell blood groups

- Rhesus D (RhD). About 15% of Caucasian women are RhD-negative. Immunization against RhD is rare because of the introduction of RhD prophylaxis. Severe RhD haemolytic disease of the newborn (HDN) occurs in <100 cases per annum in the UK (620 000 live births).
  - Alloimmunization against red cell alloantigens occurs as a consequence of fetomaternal haemorrhage, which is generally below 4 ml of fetal erythrocytes. The amount of fetomaternal haemorrhage needs to be measured in RhD-negative women within 48 hours after delivery of a RhD-positive baby, so that the amount of RhD prophylaxis can be adjusted in case of bleeds exceeding 4 ml. Abdominal trauma, complications of pregnancy such as vaginal bleeding and abruption, and any invasive procedures carry an increased risk of significant fetomaternal haemorrhage. Such events in RhD-negative women need to be covered with RhD prophylaxis.
  - Prevention of RhD immunization is by injection of anti-D immunoglobulin G (RhD prophylaxis) to all RhD-negative pregnant women at specified times during pregnancy and after delivery in the case of a RhD-positive baby. Once sensitization occurs, RhD prophylaxis is no longer effective.
- Red cell alloantigens other than RhD. HDN because of immunization against red cell blood groups other than RhD is rare but may be severe, i.e. in the case of K(ell) immunization. ABO incompatibility cannot cause severe anaemia in the fetus, but frank haemolysis may occur in the group A or B neonate born to a group O mother.

A routine screening programme to identify women with immunization against red cell alloantigens other than A and B and to identify all RhD-negative women is in place. The aim of this screening programme is to prevent morbidity and mortality due to severe HDN and to provide compatible transfusion support for alloimmunized women. Good antenatal care should prevent the occurrence of hydrops fetalis and cases of severe HDN should be managed in partnership with a fetal medicine team with an interest in HDN and the National Blood Service (NBS). Monitoring of the severity of RhD immunization is by measuring the concentration of anti-D in the maternal serum. In case of a RhD heterozygous partner, fetal RhD genotyping can be performed on maternal plasma from late in the first trimester using ffDNA. See 'Noninvasive prenatal diagnosis/testing (NIPD/T)' in Chapter 6, 'Pregnancy and fertility', p. 764.

Clinical features in the fetus

- The fetus becomes anaemic due to haemolysis caused by maternal IgG anti-D.
- The severity of the anaemia can be determined by periumbilical blood sampling (PUBS).
- Before correction of fetal anaemia became feasible by the transfusion of RhD-negative donor blood, cardiac failure developed as the fetus becomes more anaemic and, in severe cases, progressed to hydrops fetalis.

Management of the at-risk fetus

Since the technical advance of PUBS, survival rates of severe cases have been excellent. Precise data on mortality are lacking but are in the UK thought to be as low as ten per annum. The following investigations are routine:

- prior history of HDN;
- maternal anti-D quantitation in iu/ml;
- RhD phenotyping of the partner;
- in the case of a heterozygous partner, RhD genotyping of the fetus on maternal plasma at booking 20 weeks and if inconclusive 28 weeks (Chitty et al. 2014);
- USS fetal assessment;
- fetal Hb estimation by PUBS and, if required, correction of anaemia by intrauterine, intravascular transfusion;
- amniocentesis has become less popular, as the method of spectrophotometry for bilirubin (Liley index) has its limitations.

Management of the neonate

- RhD antigen and direct antiglobulin test.
- FBC and bilirubin levels.
- Severe HDN may become apparent by the baby rapidly becoming jaundiced, as the immature liver is unable to adequately conjugate the bilirubin and levels of unconjugated bilirubin rise. This is toxic to the brain and, unless treated, may lead to kernicterus. Exchange transfusion is used both to treat the anaemia and to lower the level of bilirubin.

Management of the at-risk neonate

When it is expected that an infant may be severely affected, the paediatricians, haematologist, and NBS should be aware of the likely delivery date, so that preparations for an immediate exchange transfusion at birth (if necessary) have been made. Group O RhD-negative blood from specially selected donors is available from the NBS and must be cross-matched against the serum of the mother. Exchange transfusion because of RhD disease is nowadays rare, as the majority of severe cases will have been transfused in utero.

Neonatal alloimmune thrombocytopenia (NAIT)

NAIT is defined as an isolated thrombocytopenia with a count $<150 \times 10^9/l$ and caused by maternal IgG alloantibodies against platelet-specific alloantigens. So-called human platelet antigen (HPA) antibodies cause severe thrombocytopenia in ~1 per 1200 live births in Caucasians and this is the most frequent cause of severe thrombocytopenia in the otherwise healthy term infant.

In sharp contrast to HDN, NAIT is *frequently observed in a first pregnancy*. No screening for HPA immunization is in place. The presentation is usually through an infant with thrombocytopenic purpura, petechiae, and/or other signs of bleeding. The main clinical concern is the risk of an intracranial haemorrhage during pregnancy, delivery, or in the neonatal period. In Caucasoids, the most commonly encountered HPA antibody is against HPA-1a (formerly P1^{A1}, Zw^a).

The management of the pregnant woman who is known to be alloimmunized against HPA-1a is complex and there are several options. A choice must be based on the history of previous pregnancies (in >90% of cases, the severity of thrombocytopenia will be as or more severe). For high-risk cases, the following approaches are possible.

- HPA genotype the partner and, if heterozygous, determine the HPA genotype of the fetus from a sample of amniotic fluid.
- If the amniotic fluid is positive for the cognate HPA antigen, the following is suggested.
  - Weekly infusion of high-dose IV IgG with or without corticosteroids given to the mother (the preferred approach in North American centres), or
  - Repeated *in utero* transfusions of HPA-compatible platelets from highly selected donors (the preferred treatment approach in some European centres).
  - The least traumatic route of delivery. Generally, a planned Caesarean section is chosen, but there is no good evidence that this reduces the risk of an intracranial bleed in the 'at-risk' neonate.
  - The paediatrician, haematologist, and transfusion service should be informed prior to delivery, so that compatible HPA-matched platelets are available to treat the baby.

The management of a new index case is on basis of the clinical signs of bleeding and the platelet count. In case of overt bleeding or a platelet count <20 × 10^9/l, correction of the count with HPA-1a- and HPA-5b-negative donor platelets is recommended. The results of the serological investigation must not be awaited, as the risk of severe bleeding is assumed to be highest in the first 48 hours after delivery.

Clinical assessment

History: key points
- Previous affected child.
- Fetal loss/miscarriage prior to any blood group testing.

- Pregnancy complications that could cause fetomaternal haemorrhage.

Examination: key points
- Not part of the genetic assessment.

Special investigations
- These are performed by the fetal medicine team and a blood cell genetics/immunology reference centre (see above).

Genetic advice and management

- HDN. A routine preventative screening programme for red blood cell alloimmunization and the risk of HDN is in place. RhD-negative women require antenatal RhD prophylaxis, with a follow-up dose after delivery of an RhD-positive infant. RhD-negative status is generally based on a deletion of the RhD gene and is denoted with the *Rhdd* genotype. The RhD-positive father may be homozygous for D (*DD*), in which case all future children are at risk of RhD immunization, or heterozygous (*Dd*) with a 50% risk.
- NAIT. No screening programme in place. It is important to investigate the HPA antigen status of sisters of childbearing age when the condition has been confirmed in an index case. Families with a severe case history need to be managed in close partnership with a fetal medicine unit and the haematologist and NBS.

Support group: Platelet Disorder Support Association, http://www.pdsa.org.

References

Blanchette VS, Johnson J, Rand M. The management of alloimmune neonatal thrombocytopenia. *Bailliere's Best Pract Res Clin Haematol* 2000; **13**: 365–90.

Bowman J. The management of hemolytic disease in the fetus and newborn. *Semin Perinatol* 1997; **21**: 39–44.

Chitty LS, Finning K, Wade A, *et al*. Diagnostic accuracy of routine antenatal determination of fetal RHD status across gestation: population based cohort study. *BMJ* 2014; **349**: g5243.

Daniels G, Finning K, Martin P, Massey E. Noninvasive prenatal diagnosis of fetal blood group phenotypes: current practice and future prospects. *Prenat Diagn* 2009; **29**: 101–7.

Kaplan C. Immune thrombocytopenia in the foetus and the newborn: diagnosis and therapy. *Transfus Clin Biol* 2001; **8**: 311–14.

Moise KJ Jr. Management of rhesus alloimmunization in pregnancy. *Obstet Gynecol* 2002; **100**: 600–11.

Hyperechogenic bowel

Echogenic bowel, hyperechoic bowel.

Echogenic bowel is a 'soft marker', usually identified as an incidental finding at a routine antenatal USS examination. To be classed as echogenic, the bowel should be of equivalent brightness to the iliac crests. Echogenic fetal bowel is detected in ~0.8% of pregnancies during the second or third trimester (see Table 6.5). In some fetuses, this is a normal variant; however, there is a recognized association with fetal abnormality, in the absence of additional anomalies on scan.

Routine Down's screening, if low risk, has reduced the risk of aneuploidy to nearer 1%.

Intra-amniotic haemorrhage with fetal ingestion of blood pigments can cause echogenic bowel. Other aetiologies include hypoperistalsis (e.g. T21) or decreased fluid content of the meconium (e.g. CF, IUGR).

Simon-Bouy et al. (2003) published a French multicentre study of 682 fetuses with echogenic bowel. Karyotyping, screening for viral infection and CF mutations, were performed in all cases. Pregnancy outcome and postnatal follow-up were known in 91%. Of the 682 cases, of whom 4% had additional anomalies identified on scan, 65.5% had a normal outcome, 3.5% had a significant chromosome anomaly, 3% had CF, and 2.8% had a viral infection—15 with CMV and four with parvovirus; 6.2% were premature; there was IUGR in 4.1%, and an IUD in 1.9%.

The higher risk of an adverse pregnancy outcome was also found in a retrospective Austrian study by Mailath-Pokomy et al. (2012) who looked at 97 cases of isolated fetal echogenic bowel (excluding cases of aneuploidy and major congenital anomaly) and found the incidence of IUGR was 9.9% versus 1.3% in controls and of IUD was 8.9% versus 0.5%.

Clinical approach

History: key points
- Three-generation family tree, with specific enquiry for CF.
- Detailed pregnancy history, noting any pregnancy bleeding, maternal illness/rash, Down's screening, or invasive procedures and results.

Examination: key points
- Fetal biometry.
- Detailed fetal anomaly scan to confirm hyperechogenic bowel and search carefully for other signs of fetal abnormality, placental haemorrhage, etc.
- Doppler measurements—placental and fetal.

Table 6.5 Table to show frequency of some causes of hyperechogenic bowel

Anomaly	Risk
Chromosomal, primarily Down's syndrome (T21)	3–5%, less if low risk T21 screening
Cystic fibrosis (CF)	~3%
Cytomegalovirus (CMV)	~2–3%
Digestive tract anomaly	~3%
Adverse pregnancy outcome, e.g. IUGR, IUD	~7–10%

* IUD, intrauterine death; IUGR, intrauterine growth retardation.

Table 6.6 Bayes theorem

Fetus	CF	Not CF
Echogenic bowel	0.03	0.97
One mutation	$2 \times 0.87 \times 0.13 = 0.2262$	$0.04 \times 0.87 = 0.0348$
Joint probability	$0.03 \times 0.2262 = 0.006786$	$0.97 \times 0.0348 = 0.33756$
Risk of CF in fetus	0.006786/(0.006786 + 0.33756), i.e. 1 in 5.974 or 16.7%	

Special investigations for isolated echogenic bowel
- Offer parental CF carrier testing and maternal serum for investigation of congenital infection.
- Amniocentesis is no longer offered if the Down's screening risk was low.

Genetic advice and management

Note that the population carrier rate for CF varies with ethnicity. Calculations and risks given in Table 6.6 refer to the Caucasian population.

CF MUTATION DETECTED IN BOTH PARENTS. The risk for CF in a fetus with echogenic bowel is very high. Amniocentesis or placental biopsy could be used for diagnostic confirmation if TOP is being considered. Alternatively, if the pregnancy is continuing, confirmation of the neonatal genotype could be made on cord blood at term.

ONE PARENT IS A CF CARRIER. Muller et al. (2002) found an 11% incidence of CF in fetuses with one CF mutation and hyperechogenic bowel. This risk is confirmed using the Hardy–Weinberg principle.
- Full testing for rare CF mutations is not routinely available in a prenatal time frame. There is therefore little value in proving, by amniocentesis, the fetal single CF mutation status, unless confirming the 11% risk would change the outcome of the pregnancy.
- Risks to a fetus with echogenic bowel where one CF mutation has been identified in a fetal sample and one parent is a carrier (where both parents have been screened for common CF mutations) is ~16.7% (see Table 6.6).
- Risks to a fetus with echogenic bowel where no fetal sample is available and one parent is a carrier (where both parents have been screened for common CF mutations) is a complex calculation. Overall risk is ~9.5%
- If negative CF and infection screen and low risk Down's screening, the risk for early-onset IUGR and adverse pregnancy outcome remains. Instigate follow-up growth scans, especially if maternal serum PAPP-A is low or Doppler studies abnormal.

Expert adviser: Diana Wellesley, Consultant Clinical Geneticist, Wessex Clinical Genetics Service, Princess Anne Hospital, Southampton, UK.

References

Al-Kouatly HB, Chasen ST, Streltzoff J, Chervenak FA. The clinical significance of fetal echogenic bowel. *Am J Obstet Gynecol* 2001; **185**: 1035–8.

Bosco AF, Norton ME, Lieberman E. Predicting the risk of cystic fibrosis with echogenic bowel and one cystic fibrosis mutation. *Obstet Gynecol* 1999; **94**: 1020–3.

Mailath-Pokomy M, Klein K, Klebermass-Schrehof K, Hachemian N, Bettelheim D. Are fetuses with isolated echogenic bowel at higher risk for an adverse pregnancy outcome? Experiences from a tertiary referral centre. *Prenat Diagn* 2012; **32**: 1295–9.

Muller F, Simon-Buoy B, Girodon E, *et al.* Predicting the risk of cystic fibrosis with abnormal ultrasound signs of fetal bowel: results of a French collaborative study based on 641 prospective cases. *Am J Med Genet* 2002; **110**: 109–15.

Simon-Bouy B, Satre V, Ferec C, *et al.* Hyperechogenic fetal bowel: a large French collaborative study of 682 cases. *Am J Med Genet A* 2003; **121A**: 209–13.

Hypoplastic left heart

Hypoplastic left heart syndrome (HLHS).

HLHS accounts for 1% of all CHD but is responsible for 25% of deaths from CHD in the first week of life. In addition to the hypoplastic LV, there may be aortic stenosis/atresia, mitral stenosis/atresia, and/or hypoplasia of the aortic arch. At least 21% of fetuses have extracardiac anomalies, including hydrops, hydrocephalus, DWM, etc. (Brackley et al. 2000; Tennstedt et al.1999). In postnatal series, only 10–15% have extracardiac anomalies (Natowicz et al. 1988; Perez-Delboy and Simpson 2003). Siffel et al. (2015) report that the overall survival probability has risen from 0% (1979–84) to 42% (1999–2005). For children who survived the first year long-term survival was ~90%. LV outflow tract malformations, aortic valve stenosis, coarctation of the aorta, and hypoplastic left heart constitute a mechanistically defined subgroup of congenital heart defects that have substantial evidence for a genetic component (with a complex, but most likely oligogenic, pattern of inheritance (McBride et al. 2005), although some individuals have a monogenic cause, e.g. NR2F2.

Clinical assessment

History: key points
- Obtain a three-generation family tree, with specific enquiry regarding CHD.
- History of maternal diabetes.

Examination: key points
- Approximately 5% will have multiple congenital malformations that suggest a specific syndrome diagnosis (Natowicz et al. 1988).
- Detailed fetal USS; 21% have extracardiac anomalies (hydrops, hydrocephalus, DWM, etc.).

Special investigations
- Genomic analysis, e.g. genomic array, gene panel, or WES/WGS as appropriate. Where not available, a karyotype including 22q FISH should be done. Overall, 12% have a chromosomal anomaly (+13, 45,X, +21, +18, del 5, del 11, etc.), but only 6% if the hypoplastic left heart is an isolated finding.
- Consider parental echo since familial clustering of HLHS and bicuspid aortic valve (BAV) may occur (Hinton et al. 2007).

Genetic advice and management

Genetic advice
RECURRENCE RISK FOR FUTURE PREGNANCIES. No figures are available from large prospective series. Brenner et al. (1989) found CHD in 13% of first-degree relatives of hypoplastic left heart patients. Recurrence of hypoplastic left heart occurs in 2–4% in some series (Cox and Wilson, personal communication; Perez-Delboy and Simpson 2003). BAV may occur in asymptomatic parents and first-degree relatives of probands with aortic stenosis, coarctation of the aorta, and HLHS. 0.8% of the general population have BAV, but 7.7% of HLHS relatives had LV outflow

tract malformations or significant CHD in McBride's et al. (2005) study.

In a small study of 38 probands with HLHS by Hinton et al. (2007), the sibling recurrence risk was 8% and for cardiovascular malformation (including BAV) was 22%.

Offer specialist fetal echo in subsequent pregnancies, unless it has been possible to undertake a definitive genetic PND with normal results.

Management
Options open to parents include:
- TOP;
- supportive comfort care for the infant. In the Birmingham series (Brackley et al. 2000), 7/11 died in the first week of life, and a further three within the first 28 days;
- Norwood single ventricle reconstruction. Post-delivery, the baby is duct-dependent (requires prostaglandin E2 infusion if active management is planned, and rapid transfer to a paediatric cardiothoracic centre (in utero transfer may be preferred by some units)). The current literature suggests a 60–80% 5- to 10-year survival expectation (DiBardinino 2015).

Support group: Little Hearts Matter, https://www.lhm.org.uk, 11 Greenfield Crescent, Edgbaston, Birmingham, B15 3AU, Tel. 0121 455 8982, Email: info@lhm.org.

References

Al Turki S, Manickaraj AK, Mercer CL, et al. Rare variants in NR2F2 cause congenital heart defects in humans. Am J Hum Genet 2014; **94**: 574–85.

Brenner JA, Berg KA, Schneider DS, Clark EB, Boughman JA. Cardiac malformations in relatives of infants with hypoplastic left heart syndrome. Am J Dis Child 1989; **143**: 1492–5.

DiBardinino DJ. Long-term progression and survival following Norwood Single Ventricle Reconstruction. Curr Opin Cardiol 2015; **1**: 95–9.

Hinton RB Jr, Martin LJ, Tabangin ME, Mazwi ML, Cripe LH, Benson DW. Hypoplastic left heart syndrome is heritable. J Am Coll Cardiol 2007; **50**: 1590–5.

Lahon H, Schon P, et al. Tetralogy of Fallot, and Hypoplastic Left Heart Syndrome-complex phenotypes meet complex genetic networks. Curr Genomics 2015; **16**: 141–58.

McBride KL, Pignatelli R, Lewin M, et al. Inheritance analysis of congenital left ventricular outflow tract obstruction malformations: segregation, multiplex relative risk, and heritability. Am J Med Genet A 2005; **134A**: 180–6.

Natowicz M, Chatten J, Clancy R, et al. Genetic disorders and major extracardiac anomalies associated with the hypoplastic left heart syndrome. Pediatrics 1988; **82**: 698–706.

Perez-Delboy A, Simpson GG. Ultrasound Med Biol 2003; **29**: S134.

Siffel C, Riehl-Colarusso T, et al. Survival of children with Hypoplastic Heart Syndrome. Paediatrics 2015; **136**; e864.

Tennstedt C, Chaoui R, Korner H, Dietel M. Spectrum of congenital heart defects and extracardiac malformations associated with chromosomal abnormalities: results of a seven year necropsy study. Heart 1999; **82**: 34–9.

Towbin JA, Belmont J. Molecular determinants of left and right outflow tract obstruction. Am J Med Genet 2000; **97**: 297–303.

Imaging in prenatal diagnosis

Ultrasound scanning (USS)

Targeted USS can be very useful in PND or surveillance of conditions characterized by structural anomalies. The role of the geneticist is to assess the genetic risk to the pregnancy and advise the patient and obstetrician on investigations available to manage that risk.

- Detailed fetal anomaly scanning is best interpreted if there is secure dating of the pregnancy. Arrange a dating USS at 8–12 weeks' gestation. At this stage in pregnancy, there is the best correlation between crown–rump length (CRL) and gestation.
- Discuss the limitations of USS. It can detect many major structural anomalies, but not all, e.g. isolated cleft palate without a cleft of the lips and alveolar ridge is very difficult to diagnose; ASD can often be difficult to diagnose; the sonographic signs of some anomalies may present late (hydrocephalus, microcephaly, achondroplasia, some renal anomalies such as AD polycystic disease), or the condition may have a variable presentation. USS does not give information regarding cognition, vision, or hearing (except when there are obvious gross structural CNS defects present).

Dating USS

Is best undertaken at 8–12 weeks' gestation. At this stage in pregnancy, there is a tight correlation between CRL and gestation. It is an important investigation if invasive tests are planned, e.g. CVS or amniocentesis, or if scanning will subsequently be used to monitor fetal growth or limb length.

Nuchal translucency (NT) assessment

Is best undertaken at 11–13^{+6} weeks' gestation. Increased NT can be an indication of a chromosomal anomaly or CHD or a wide variety of other syndromes, the risk of these conditions increasing with the size of the NT. Three millimetres represents the 95th percentile, but many fetuses with a mildly enlarged NT measurement are normal at birth. See 'Oedema—increased nuchal translucency, cystic hygroma, and hydrops' in Chapter 6, 'Pregnancy and fertility', p. 768.

Fetal anomaly scanning

Routine anomaly USS is usually undertaken around 18–22 weeks, at which stage most major structural abnormalities can be identified (Pathak and Lees 2009). If there is a past history of specific structural anomalies or USS is being undertaken for PND, rather than routine obstetric screening, scanning should be arranged in conjunction with a fetal medicine specialist, as the appropriate gestational age at which to scan will vary with the particular condition (see Table 6.7).

Three-dimensional USS

New developments in USS technology enable the image to be presented in three dimensions. This may be particularly valuable when assessing facial features, the fetal brain, and anomalies of the hands and feet where stored volumes can be analysed at the time of the scan or afterwards. Advances in two-dimensional technology have improved imaging considerably.

Fetal echo

Routine obstetric anomaly USS includes a minimum of the four-chamber view of the heart and views of

Table 6.7 Guidelines for timing of fetal ultrasound scanning (USS) for specific congenital malformations

Feature	Time to start USS (weeks gestation)
Anencephaly	11–12
Anterior abdominal wall defects (e.g. gastroschisis/exomphalos)	12
Cleft lip (cleft palate often difficult to visualize)	From 16
Congenital heart disease	11–12 (nuchal scan)
	16 (fetal echo)
	20–22 (review)
Corpus callosum	18+*
Ear anomalies (only detectable if severe)	20
Eyes and orbital spacing	12–14
Facial profile (e.g. severe micrognathia)	14
Fingers and toes (number of digits)	From 12–14
Gender assignment	From 11+†
Ventriculomegaly and hydrocephalus	18 (serial scanning thereafter)
Kidneys and bladder	From 12–14; readily visualized from 16 weeks
Lissencephaly	From 24+‡
Microcephaly	18§
Spina bifida	From 11

* Serial scanning. Absence is usually detectable; hypoplasia is more difficult to determine reliably.

† Sometimes gender cannot be assigned with confidence until 20–22 weeks' gestation.

‡ See 'Lissencephaly, polymicrogyria, and neuronal migration disorders' in Chapter 2, 'Clinical approach', p. 216. Rarely detected prenatally.

§ With serial scanning thereafter. See 'Microcephaly' in Chapter 2, 'Clinical approach', p. 228.

Data from Pathak S, Lees C. Ultrasound structural fetal anomaly screening: an update. *Arch Dis Child Fetal Neonatal Ed.*, 2009, Volume 94, Issue 5.

the outflow tracts are included. If there is suspicion of a CHD, or scanning is being undertaken because of an increased risk of CHD (e.g. family history or increased NT), a more comprehensive study of the fetal heart should be undertaken. Specialist fetal echo includes ventricular outlet views and Doppler assessment of flow across the valves and of the aorta and pulmonary arteries, and visualization of the pulmonary veins.

Fetal sexing

Up to 11–12 weeks' gestation, the external genitalia appear the same in both sexes (although the orientation of the phallus differs, pointing cranially in males and caudally in females), thus allowing gender determination with 90% accuracy at 13–14 weeks. However, this is image quality- and position-dependent; even up to 20 weeks' gestation, it can sometimes be difficult to reliably determine the fetal sex from the appearances of the external genitalia. Analysis of maternal blood for ffDNA enables reliable non-invasive fetal sexing from 8 weeks' gestation (see Table 6.7) and 'Non-invasive prenatal diagnosis/ testing (NIPD/T)', in Chapter 6, p. 764.

Indications for genetic analysis (e.g. genomic array)

There are a few abnormalities that, when seen in isolation in the context of a detailed USS assessment, do not warrant consideration of karyotyping. These include: gastroschisis or unilateral multicystic dysplastic kidney (MCDK) and talipes. The majority of other anomalies will confer an increased risk for a chromosome anomaly, but the need for genetic investigations should be assessed on an individual basis, taking into consideration:

(1) the presence or absence of other USS anomalies;

(2) the level of detail of the USS performed;

(3) other risk factors (maternal age, NT measurement, maternal serum screen result).

Fetal magnetic resonance imaging (MRI)

Fetal MRI requires ultrafast technology to capture images to minimize movement artefact. Currently, fetal MRI is most used for the further delineation of intracranial anomalies, especially neuronal migration defects, and some other complex disorders (Garel 2004) and where the pregnancy is at high risk of CNS malformations (Griffiths *et al.* 2012). Interpretation of images is becoming more standardized; however, there remain limited data on the range of normality at specific gestations. Refer for expert advice. In utero MRI (iuMRI) may improve diagnostic accuracy and confidence for fetal brain anomalies (Griffiths *et al.* 2016).

Support group: ARC (Antenatal Results and Choices), http://www.arc-uk.org, Tel. 0207 631 0285.

Expert adviser: Christoph Lees, Clinical Reader in Obstetrics, Imperial College London, Honorary Consultant in Obstetrics and Head of Fetal Medicine, Imperial College Healthcare NHS Trust, London, UK.

References

Estroff J. Imaging clues in the prenatal diagnosis of syndromes and aneuploidy. *Pediatr Radiol* 2012; **42**(Suppl 1): S5–23.

Garel C. The role of MRS in the evaluation of the fetal brain with an emphasis on biometry, gyration and parenchyma. *Pediatr Radiol* 2004; **34**: 694–9.

Garne E, Loane M, Dolk H, et al. Prenatal diagnosis of severe structural congenital malformations in Europe. *Ultrasound Obstet Gynecol* 2005; **25**: 6–11.

Griffiths PD, Porteous M, Mason G, et al. The use of *in utero* MRI to supplement ultrasound in the foetus at high risk of developmental brain or spine abnormality. *Br J Radiol* 2012; **85**: e1038–45.

Griffiths PD, Bradburn M, et al. Use of MRI in the diagnosis of fetal brain abnormalities in utero (MERIDIAN): a multicentre prospective cohort study. *Lancet* 2016; epub Dec 14.

Pathak S, Lees C. Ultrasound structural fetal anomaly screening: an update. *Arch Dis Child Fetal Neonatal Ed* 2009; **94**: F384–90.

Invasive techniques and genetic tests in prenatal diagnosis

Chorionic villus sampling (CVS) and placental biopsy

See Figure 6.4.

CVS was introduced into clinical practice in the UK during the 1980s. The technique enables sampling of the chorion (developing placenta) during the first trimester of pregnancy. In the second and third trimesters of pregnancy, the same technique is termed placental biopsy. In the first trimester, both transabdominal (TA) and transcervical (TC) approaches may be used to obtain a sample. Most testing is now done by the TA route. The trophoblast and embryo are both derived from the fertilized egg and therefore share the same genetic make-up. This genetic identity is the basis for using CVS as an indirect way of determining the genetic make-up of the fetus. The trophoblast is a highly cellular tissue and ideal for DNA extraction, making this the procedure of choice for many molecular genetic investigations. The mean weight of CVS specimens varies between different centres but, in one study, was 15.2 ± 6.0 mg (Brun et al. 2003). (Larger samples are sometimes needed for biochemical PND requiring enzyme analysis of uncultured CVS material.)

The procedure-associated loss rate is estimated at 1% by most institutions offering CVS testing, though some recent studies (Akolekar et al. 2015) give a lower risk estimate. See Table 6.8 for further information and a comparison with amniocentesis. In early 1990s, two clusters of babies with limb defects following CVS were reported (Burton et al. 1992; Firth et al. 1991), raising the possibility of a causal association between early CVS and transverse limb deficiency (Firth 1997). The risk of limb deficiency extends through the period of limb morphogenesis and slightly beyond, falling from levels 10- to 20-fold above background at ≤9 weeks to levels approaching (or only a few-fold above) background at 11 weeks and beyond (Firth 1997). Stoler et al. (1999), in a review of the literature, found that the frequency of vascular disruption defects, e.g. gastroschisis, intestinal atresias, and club-foot, was significantly increased among CVS-exposed infants, compared with a baseline unexposed population.

Amniocentesis

See Figure 6.5.

Mid-trimester amniocentesis became established during the 1970s as the standard technique for the PND of chromosome abnormalities. With amniocentesis, a 22-gauge spinal needle is directed transabdominally under USS guidance through the wall of the uterus and into a pool of amniotic fluid. Usually ~15 ml of amniotic fluid is withdrawn. The use of USS continuously throughout the procedure, operator experience, and time after gestation are the most important factors determining the risk of post-procedure loss.

The post-procedural loss in Tabor's 11-year national registry study was 1.4% (Tabor et al. 2009), but the more recent findings from Akolekar et al. (2015) (see below) give a lower procedure-related risk of 0.11%. The guidance for risk-related loss given to patients at the same institute as the Akolekar et al. (2015) study is 0.5%.

A retrospective case-control study of 1296 children born following amniocentesis showed no increase in registrable disability (hearing impairment, learning disability, visual problems, and limb anomalies) over a follow-up period of 7–18 years (Baird et al. 1994). See Table 6.8 for further information and a comparison with CVS.

O'Brien et al. (2016) undertook a retrospective analysis of >10 000 amniotic fluid test results. Karyotype failed in 2.3% of tests; failure rate was significantly greater with advancing gestation, reaching 43% at 36–40 weeks. QF-PCR failed in 2.3% of tests and was significantly greater with advancing gestation, reaching 7% at 36–40 weeks. For aCGH, 3.4% failed analysis. In one case, no result was obtainable by any technique.

Early amniocentesis

The Canadian Early and Mid-trimester Amniocentesis Trial (CEMAT) Group (1998) study showed that early amniocentesis (before 13 weeks' gestation) is associated with an increased risk of fetal loss and talipes equinovarus (1.3% versus 0.1%), compared with mid-trimester amniocentesis and should be abandoned.

Comparison of CVS and amniocentesis

The Cochrane review of CVS versus amniocentesis (Alfirevic et al. 2000) concluded that the increase in miscarriages after CVS, compared to amniocentesis, appeared to be procedure-related and that second-trimester amniocentesis appeared to be *safer than CVS*.

More recently, Akolekar et al. (2015) estimated the weighted pooled risks of miscarriage following invasive procedures from analysis of controlled studies including 324 losses in 42 716 women who underwent amniocentesis and 207 losses in 8899 women who underwent CVS. The risk of miscarriage prior to 24 weeks in women who underwent amniocentesis and CVS was 0.81% (95% CI, 0.58–1.08%) and 2.18% (95% CI, 1.61–2.82%), respectively. The background rates of miscarriage in women from the control group that did not undergo any procedures were 0.67% (95% CI, 0.46–0.91%) for amniocentesis and 1.79% (95% CI, 0.61–3.58%) for CVS. The weighted pooled procedure-related risks of miscarriage for CVS and amniocentesis and CVS were 0.11% (95% CI, −0.04 to 0.26%) and 0.22% (95% CI, −0.71 to 1.16%), respectively.

Uncertain results (e.g. mosaicism) are more frequent with CVS than mid-trimester amniocentesis and there are fewer false-positive and false-negative diagnoses. The benefits of earlier diagnosis with CVS must be set against the small additional risk of pregnancy loss and the greater risk of uncertain results. Jauniaux et al. (2000) conclude that mid-trimester amniocentesis remains the safest invasive procedure and that CVS is associated with a higher risk of subsequent pregnancy loss.

Invasive methods may be superseded by non-invasive prenatal testing/diagnosis (NIPT/D) over the coming years. See 'Non-invasive prenatal diagnosis/testing (NIPD/T)' in Chapter 6, 'Pregnancy and fertility', p. 764.

Clinical assessment

For all invasive procedures, the maternal blood group should be known prior to the procedure, and anti-D prophylaxis offered to all Rh-negative women.

- Assess the genetic risk to the pregnancy and offer information about the procedure-related risks to help the patient to assess the risk/benefit for their individual situation.
- Mention the limitations of the technique (normal karyotype does not guarantee a normal baby).

Table 6.8 Comparison of chorionic villus sampling (CVS) and amniocentesis

Feature	CVS	Amniocentesis
Gestation	From 11 weeks' gestation; usually 11–13 weeks' gestation	From 16 weeks' gestation; usually 15–17 weeks' gestation
Post-procedural loss rate (miscarriage risk)	Approximately 1% (Bakker 2016) 0.22% (Akolekar et al. 2015) Risk for counselling and consent purposes ~1%	0.11% (Akolekar et al. 2015) Risk for counselling and consent purposes ~0.5%
Complications	Vaginal spotting/bleeding (1–4%), especially after transcervical (TC) procedures	Amniotic fluid leak causing oligohydramnios
	Intrauterine infection (<0.1%). Amniotic fluid leak after unintentional puncture of amniotic sac (rare)	Increased risk for respiratory problems, e.g. transient tachypnoea of the newborn
Failure to achieve a result	0.21% (Brun et al. 2003)*	This figure is highly correlated with gestation (O'Brien et al. 2016)
		QF-PCR 2.3% (1.9% at 16 weeks to 7.1% at 36 weeks)
		Microarray 3.4% (5.2% at 16 weeks to 0% at 36 weeks). Main cause of failure: lack of DNA
		Karyotype 2.3% (0.3% at 16 weeks to 43.4% at 36 weeks)
Maternal contamination	<1% after microscopic selection of the villi (Brun et al. 2003)	Very low
Mosaicism risk	Confined placental mosaicism in 1.9% and true fetal mosaicism in 0.19% (Wang et al. 1993)	0.3% (with >50% of cases representing true fetal mosaicism)
Timescale for results‡	Interphase trisomy FISH or QF-PCR-based common aneuploidy screen 2–3 days	Interphase trisomy FISH or QF-PCR-based common aneuploidy screen 2–3 days
	Routine microarray 14 days	Routine microarray 14 days
	Routine karyotype around 14 days (cultured cells)	Routine karyotype around 14 days (cultured cells)
	Molecular genetic analysis. CVS is the procedure of choice as DNA can be extracted directly from the trophoblast sample (uncultured), e.g. routine mutation analysis 3- days, mutation analysis requiring Southern blotting, e.g. FRAX, DM1, 10–21 days	Molecular genetic analysis Uncultured 2–3 days (most single gene analysis) Cultured 14 days
	Biochemical diagnosis, e.g. enzyme assay usually within 14–21 days	Biochemical diagnosis, e.g. enzyme assay, usually within 14 days. May be done as part of a screen for hydrops

* Placental biopsy at late gestation, e.g. third trimester, has a higher incidence of culture failure than CVS at 11–13/40. Amniocentesis at late gestation, e.g. third trimester, also has a higher incidence of culture failure than amniocentesis at 15–17/40.

‡ These are intended only as a rough guide. Check with your local laboratory before providing information to patients.

Data from: Akolekar R, Beta J, Picciarelli G, Ogilvie C, D'Antonio F. Procedure-related risk of miscarriage following amniocentesis and chorionic villus sampling: a systematic review and meta-analysis. *Ultrasound Obstet Gynecol.* 2015 Jan;45(1):16-26. doi: 10.1002/uog.14636; Risk of fetal loss associated with invasive testing following combined first-trimester screening for Down syndrome: a national cohort of 147,987 singleton pregnancies, Wulff CB, Gerds TA, Rode L, Ekelund CK, Petersen OB, Tabor A (Danish Fetal Medicine Study Group). *Ultrasound Obstet Gynecol.* 2016 Jan;47(1):38-44. doi: 10.1002/uog.15820. PMID:2658118; and O'Brien AL, Dall'Asta A, Tapon D, Mann K, Ahn JW, Ellis R, Ogilvie C, Lees C, Gestation related karyotype, QF-PCR and CGH-array failure rates in diagnostic amniocentesis. *Prenat Diagn.* 2016 May 18. doi: 10.1002/pd.4843.

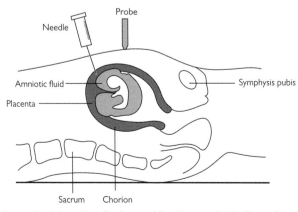

Figure 6.4 Chorionic villus sampling. Adapted from *The Genetics of Renal Disease*, edited by Frances Flinter, Eamon Maher, and Anand Saggar-Malik (2004): By permission of Oxford University Press. www.oup.com.

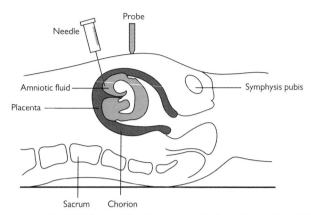

Figure 6.5 Amniocentesis. Adapted from *The Genetics of Renal Disease*, edited by Frances Flinter, Eamon Maher, and Anand Saggar-Malik (2004): By permission of Oxford University Press. www.oup.com.

- Mention the possibility of unexpected results or results that are difficult to interpret if karyotyping is undertaken (e.g. sex chromosome aneuploidy, mosaicism).
- Risks are greater with CVS than amniocentesis.
- Make arrangements for communicating the results.

Special investigations
Important notes.
- PCR-based analyses. For all molecular genetic diagnoses involving PCR, a maternal DNA sample should be available to enable testing for maternal cell contamination.
- Molecular diagnosis of recessive disorders. For all molecular genetic diagnoses for AR disorders, the molecular carrier status of each parent should be defined in advance of PND.
- For XLR disorders. The molecular carrier status of the mother should be defined in advance of PND (but note the risks arising from germline mosaicism).
- Molecular diagnosis of deletions. For all molecular genetic PNDs involving PCR for detection of a large-scale deletion, e.g. SMA, CAH, linkage analysis should be used in conjunction with mutation detection.

Multiple pregnancies

First-trimester USS is necessary to delineate chorionicity; from this, an assessment of the likely zygosity is possible. See 'Twins and twinning' in Chapter 6, 'Pregnancy and fertility', p. 792. Brambati *et al.* (2001) found that determination of the presence or absence of the lambda sign led to a correct assignment of chorionicity in all cases in a series of >200 multiple pregnancies. With this information, it is possible to estimate the likely genetic risks.
- For an MZ pregnancy, the risk that both twins are affected approximates to the risk for a singleton pregnancy.
- For a DZ pregnancy, each twin is assessed independently, as you would do with siblings. Careful consideration needs to be given to the management of the pregnancy if one twin is shown to be affected, whereas the other is normal.

When an invasive procedure is indicated in twins, CVS has, over amniocentesis, the advantage of allowing selective termination to be performed in the first trimester, when the procedure-related risk of pregnancy loss is less than when performed later in pregnancy. It has the disadvantage of leading to ambiguous results in up to 2% of cases (Dommergues 2002). Selective termination in mid trimester carries a 5–10% risk of pregnancy loss or very preterm delivery.

There is debate about the choice of diagnostic procedure. Dommergues (2002) argues that CVS is the choice technique in twin pregnancies at very high risk, while amniocentesis is still indicated in cases at more moderate risk, whereas Brambati *et al.* (2001) state that first-trimester TA CVS is a highly efficient, reliable, and relatively safe approach for genetic diagnosis in twin pregnancies. A literature review by Agarwal and Alfirevic (2012) concluded that there was an excess risk of 1% for both CVS and amniocentesis in twin pregnancies. A precise evaluation of the relative risks of CVS and mid-trimester amniocentesis in twins must await randomized controlled studies.

Support group: ARC (Antenatal Results and Choices), http://www.arc-uk.org, Tel. 0207 631 0285.

Expert adviser: Tessa Homfray, Consultant Medical Genetics, St George's University Hospital, Harris Birthright Unit, Kings College Hospital & Royal Brompton Hospital, London, UK.

References

Agarwal K, Alfirevic Z. Pregnancy loss after chorionic villus sampling and amniocentesis in twin pregnancies: a systematic review. *Ultrasound Obstet Gynecol* 2012; **40**: 128–34.

Akolekar R, Beta J, Picciarelli G, Ogilvie C, D'Antonio F. Procedure-related risk of miscarriage following amniocentesis and chorionic villus sampling: a systematic review and meta-analysis. *Ultrasound Obstet Gynecol* 2015; **45**: 16–26.

Alfirevic Z. Early amniocentesis versus transabdominal chorion villus sampling for prenatal diagnosis. *Cochrane Database Syst Rev* 2000; **2**: CD00077.

Alfirevic Z, Gosden CM, Neilson JP. Chorion villus sampling versus amniocentesis for prenatal diagnosis. *Cochrane Database Syst Rev* 2000; **2**: CD00055.

Bakker M, Birnie E, et al. Total pregnancy loss after chorionic villus sampling and amniocentesis – A cohort study. *Ultrasound Obstet Gynecol* 2016; **34**(1): 19–24.

Baird PA, Yee IM, Sadovnick AD. Population-based study of long-term outcomes after amniocentesis. *Lancet* 1994; **344**: 1134–6.

Brambati B, Tului L, Guercilena S, Alberti E. Outcome of first-trimester chorionic villus sampling for genetic investigation in multiple pregnancy. *Ultrasound Obstet Gynecol* 2001; **17**: 209–16.

Brun JL, Mangione R, Gangbo F, et al. Feasibility, accuracy and safety of chorionic villus sampling: a report of 10 741 cases. *Prenat Diagn* 2003; **23**: 295–301.

Burton BK, Schulz CJ, Burd LI. Limb anomalies associated with chorionic villus sampling. *Obstet Gynecol* 1992; **79**(5, Pt 1): 726–30.

Dommergues M. Prenatal diagnosis for multiple pregnancies. *Curr Opin Obstet Gynecol* 2002; **14**: 169–75.

Firth H. Chorion villus sampling and limb deficiency: cause or coincidence? *Prenat Diagn* 1997; **17**: 1313–30.

Firth HV, Boyd PA, Chamberlain P, et al. Severe limb abnormalities after chorion villus sampling at 56-66 days' gestation. *Lancet* 1991; **337**(8744): 762–3.

Horger EO, Finch H. A single physician's experience with four thousand six hundred genetic amniocenteses. *Am J Obstet Gynecol* 2001; **185**: 279–88.

Jauniaux E, Pahal GS, Rodeck CH. What invasive procedure to use in early pregnancy? *Bailliere's Best Pract Res Clin Obstet Gynaecol* 2000; **14**: 651–62.

O'Brien A, Dall'Asta A, Tapon D, et al. Gestation related karyotype, QF-PCR and CGH-array failure rates in diagnostic amniocentesis. *Prenat Diagn* 2016; **36**: 708–13.

Philip J, Silver RK, Wilson RD, et al. Late first-trimester invasive prenatal diagnosis: results of an international randomized trial. *Obstet Gynecol* 2004; **103**: 1164–73.

Reid R, Sepulveda W, Kyle PM, Davies G. Amniotic fluid culture failure: clinical significance and association with aneuploidy. *Obstet Gynecol* 1996; **87**: 588–92.

Royal College of Obstetricians and Gynaecologists. *Amniocentesis and chorionic villus sampling*. Green-top guideline no. 8, 2010. https://www.rcog.org.uk/globalassets/documents/guidelines/gtg_8.pdf.

Stoler JM, McGuirk CK, Lieberman E, Ryan L, Holmes LB. Malformations reported in chorionic villus sampling exposed children: a review and analytic synthesis of the literature. *Genet Med* 1999; **1**: 315–22.

Tabor A, Alfirevic Z. Update on procedure-related risks for prenatal diagnosis techniques. *Fetal Diagn Ther* 2010; **27**: 1–7.

Tabor A, Philip J, Madsen M, et al. Randomised controlled trial of genetic amniocentesis in 4606 low-risk women. *Lancet* 1986; **1**: 1287–93.

Tabor A, Vestergaard CH, Lidegaard O. Fetal loss rate after chorionic villus sampling and amniocentesis: an 11 year national registry study. *Ultrasound Obstet Gynecol* 2009; **34**: 19–24.

The Canadian Early and Mid-trimester Amniocentesis Trial (CEMAT) Group. Randomised trial to assess safety and fetal outcome of early and midtrimester amniocentesis. *Lancet* 1998; **351**: 242–7.

Wang BB, Rubin CH, Williams J 3rd. Mosaicism in chorionic villus sampling: an analysis of incidence and chromosomes involved in 2612 consecutive cases. *Prenat Diagn* 1993; **13**: 179–90.

Wapner RJ, Evans MI, Davis G, et al. Procedural risks versus theology: chorion villus sampling for Orthodox Jews at less than 8 weeks' gestation. *Am J Obstet Gynecol* 2002; **186**: 1133–6.

Wilson RD. Amniocentesis and chorionic villus sampling. *Curr Opin Obstet Gynecol* 2000; **12**: 81–6.

Low maternal serum oestriol

Maternal serum unconjugated oestriol (uE3) is a component of many antenatal maternal serum screening programmes for Down's syndrome. Occasionally, serum screening reveals very low levels of uE3. In a large Californian programme that studied >100 000 pregnancies, 0.27% had low uE3 levels of ≤0.2 ng/ml, or 0.15 MoM (multiples of the median). IUD occurred in 57% of the 68 women with low uE3 and positive screening results and in 6% of women with low uE3 levels and negative screening results. In viable pregnancies, the most common cause of a low uE3 is XL ichthyosis (XLI). There are a variety of rare disorders that can present with a low maternal serum oestriol (Schoen et al. 2003).

X-linked ichthyosis (steroid sulfatase (STS) deficiency)

STS deficiency or XLI is located at Xp22.3 and affects 1/1300–1/1500 males. Affected males have generalized scaling that usually begins soon after birth. There may be associated corneal opacities that do not affect vision, and there is an increased incidence of cryptorchidism (DiGiovanna and Robinson-Bostom 2003).

In 85–90% of cases, it is caused by a deletion that encompasses the STS gene. In perhaps 5% of cases, the deletion is extensive enough to involve adjacent loci and may sometimes be cytogenetically visible. This can include an adjacent MRX gene, giving rise to learning disability, with autistic spectrum problems and epilepsy in some (Gohlke et al. 2000). Around 10% of patients have point mutations or other intragenic mutations. Valdes-Flores et al. (2001) demonstrated by FISH analysis that most apparently 'sporadic' affected males are due to inherited deletions; 10/12 mothers of apparently sporadic males were carriers in their series. Perinatal risks in pregnancies affected by XLI include:

- failure to initiate labour with prolonged gestation (post-maturity) and a small increased risk of IUD;
- failure to progress in labour.

Clinical approach

(1) Exclude other causes of low uE3.
  - USS to confirm viable pregnancy (and sex of the baby).
  - Check that the mother is not on dexamethasone or a similar medication.
  - If viable female pregnancy, see (5) below.
  - If viable male pregnancy with normal USS, the most likely diagnosis is STS deficiency (XLI). Recalculate the Down's syndrome risk using age, AFP, and hCG and excluding uE3. Offer amniocentesis if high risk. Continue through steps outlined below until a specific diagnosis is reached.
  - Three-generation family tree, with specific enquiry for a family history of XLI. Enquire about the educational attainment of affected males.
  - Obtain maternal blood sample for karyotype, FISH for STS, DNA.

(2) Confirmed family history of XLI with no associated learning or behavioural problems.
  - Reassurance; advice about XLI.

- Advise the obstetrician about perinatal risks (see above).
- Consider implications for other family members.

(3) No family history of XLI; mother has FISH deletion, but no cytogenetically visible deletion.
  - As above.

(4) No family history of XLI and no FISH deletion in mother (uncommon). Probably the mother and baby carry a point mutation or, less likely, the baby has a new mutation that could be a deletion (maybe a large deletion).
  - Offer amniocentesis for karyotype and STS FISH.
  - As above, if diagnosis confirmed.
  - Consider points under (5).

(5) Female pregnancy (rare).
  - Consider AR CAH (very rare and uE3 levels not usually as low as in STS deficiency).
  - Consider AT ACTH deficiency.
  - Consider AR multiple sulfatase deficiency (very rare).
  - Consider SLO syndrome. uE3 levels not usually as low as in STS deficiency. Detailed fetal anomaly USS and amniocentesis for 7-dehydrocholesterol/mutation testing for DHCR7 (Marcos et al. 2009).

(6) Sex reversal (rare).
  - Note that undetectable levels of maternal oestriol may be found in Antley–Bixler syndrome due to mutations in POR (Cragun et al. 2004)—see 'Craniosynostosis' in Chapter 3, 'Common consultations', p. 378. If 46,XY but female genitalia on USS, consider 17-hydroxylase deficiency, lipoid adrenal hypoplasia, and SLO.

Support group: Ichthyosis Support Group, http://www.ichthyosis.org.uk, Tel. 0207 461 9034.

Expert adviser: Anne-Frédérique Minsart, Obstetrician, Department of Obstetrics and Gynaecology, Laboratory of Human Reproduction, Brussels University, Brussels, Belgium.

References

Cragun DL, Trumpy SK, Shackleton CH, et al. Undetectable maternal serum uE3 and postnatal abnormal sterol and steroid metabolism in Antley–Bixler syndrome. Am J Med Genet A 2004; **129A**: 1–7.

DiGiovanna JJ, Robinson-Bostom L. Ichthyosis: etiology, diagnosis, and management. Am J Clin Dermatol 2003; **4**: 81–95.

Gohlke BC, Haug K, Fukami M, et al. Interstitial deletion in Xp22.3 is associated with X linked ichthyosis, mental retardation, and epilepsy. J Med Genet 2000; **37**: 600–2.

Marcos J, Craig WY, Palomaki GE, et al. Maternal urine and serum steroid measurement to identify steroid sulfatase deficiency (STSD) in second trimester pregnancies. Prenat Diagn 2009; **29**: 771–80.

Schoen E, Norem C, O'Keefe J, Krieger R, Walton D, To TT. Maternal serum unconjugated estriol as a predictor for Smith–Lemli–Opitz syndrome and other fetal conditions. Obstet Gynecol 2003; **102**: 167–72.

Valdes-Flores M, Kofman-Alfaro SH, Jimenez Vaca AL, Cuevas-Covarrubias SA. Deletion of exons 1–5 of the STS gene causing X-linked ichthyosis. J Invest Dermatol 2001; **116**: 456–8.

Male infertility: genetic aspects

For a man to be judged normally fertile, the WHO criteria state that he should have a sperm count of 20×10^6/ml and that spermatozoa should show 50% progressive motility and 30% healthy morphology (see Box 6.5). Natural pregnancy is still possible below these cut-off figures, but conception is less likely to occur. A male factor is judged to be the dominant cause of subfertility in 20–26% of couples. Despite advances in the diagnosis of causes of subfertility, the inability to conceive remains unexplained in 25–30% of fully investigated couples. Referrals are usually only made to the genetics clinic when a specific diagnosis with genetic implications has been made.

The following terminology is used in sperm analysis.

- Azoospermia. No sperm seen in the ejaculate.
- Severe oligozoospermia. Sperm count $<10 \times 10^6$/ml.
- Oligozoospermia. Sperm concentration $<20 \times 10^6$/ml.
- Asthenozoospermia. <50% of sperm have normal motility or <25% have any motility.
- Teratozoospermia. <30% of sperm have a normal morphology.

One or more of abnormalities of sperm count, motility, or morphology is found in almost 90% of infertile males. General reviews indicate that 13.7% of non-obstructive azoospermic and 4.6% of oligospermic men have an abnormal karyotype. These mainly consist of an XXY constitution or a Robertsonian or reciprocal translocation (de Braekeleer and Dao 1991). Egozcue *et al.* (2003) have used FISH on decondensed sperm heads to analyse the chromosome constitution of spermatozoa in different populations. In normal males with 46,XY, the mean incidence of disomy in sperm (including all chromosomes) is ~6.7%. Carriers of Robertsonian translocations produce from 3.4% to 36.0% of abnormal sperm, and carriers of reciprocal translocations produce from 47.5% to 81.0% of abnormal spermatozoa.

Box 6.5 Semen analysis (WHO reference values)

The results of semen analysis conducted as part of an initial assessment should be compared with the following WHO reference values:

- semen volume: 1.5 ml or more;
- pH: 7.2 or more;
- sperm concentration: 15 million spermatozoa per ml or more;
- total sperm number: 39 million spermatozoa per ejaculate or more;
- total motility (percentage of progressive motility and non-progressive motility): 40% or more motile or 32% or more with progressive motility;
- vitality: 58% or more live spermatozoa;
- sperm morphology (percentage of normal forms): 4% or more.

Data from Trevor G. Cooper *et al.*, World Health Organization reference values for human semen characteristics, *Human Reproduction Update*, Vol.16, No.3, pp. 231–245, 2010, Advanced Access publication on November 24, 2009 doi:10.1093/humupd/dmp048.

Clinical assessment

History: key points

- Three-generation family tree.
- If CBAVD, detailed enquiry about respiratory symptoms, nasal polyps, chronic sinusitis, pancreatic insufficiency, etc.

Examination: key points

- Usually undertaken by an andrologist/fertility specialist; this includes a general physical examination and an assessment of secondary sex characteristics, testicular size, consistency, and presence/absence of the vas deferens.

Special investigations

- Baseline investigations such as sperm count (semen analysis) will usually have been completed by the reproductive medicine team. These may include hormone tests such as testosterone, FSH, LH, and prolactin and TFTs.
- Karyotype analysis.
- Consider testing for azoospermia factor (AZF) microdeletions
- DNA for mutation analysis of the CF gene (*CFTR*; 70% of males with CBAVD have mutations in both *CFTR* alleles). Consider partner screening if positive (see 'Congenital bilateral absence of the vas deferens (CBAVD)' below).
- If azoospermia with normal karyotype, USS to look for renal agenesis.
- If primary ciliary dyskinesia consider panel/WES/WGS as available.

Diagnoses to consider

Congenital bilateral absence of the vas deferens (CBAVD)
Obstructive azoospermia due to absence of the vas deferens can occur as an AR disorder due to mutations in the CF gene *CFTR*. CBAVD is an almost invariable finding in males with CF. CBAVD can also occur in association with unilateral (or bilateral) renal agenesis; this condition is not associated with mutations in *CFTR*. Advances in reproductive medicine make it possible for some men with CBAVD to father children using percutaneous epididymal sperm aspiration (PESA), ICSI, and IVF techniques.

CBAVD DUE TO CFTR. After careful exclusion of a diagnosis of non-classical CF, AR CBAVD is a more appropriate diagnostic term than 'a variant of CF' in otherwise healthy men. CBAVD males have a much higher incidence of partially functional alleles (e.g. R117H) than men with CF. The other allele may be delta F508. Hence, there is a risk of classical (or non-classical) CF in offspring. In addition, the inefficient 5T splice variant is commonly found in CBAVD males.

- Offer CF mutation analysis to partners of CBAVD males.

CBAVD WITH UNILATERAL RENAL AGENESIS. Abnormal development of the entire mesonephric duct at a very early stage in embryonic development (<9 weeks' gestation) may lead to CBAVD and renal agenesis. This is a less common condition than CBAVD due to *CFTR* (Augarten *et al.* 1994) of males with CBAVD (~20%). In one series of 11 pregnancies achieved, ten had normal

renal anatomy, but one was a male pregnancy with bilateral renal agenesis and CBAVD.
• Offer detailed fetal USS of the renal tract.

Chromosome anomalies
KLINEFELTER'S SYNDROME (47,XXY). The most common chromosomal anomaly causing infertility and hypogonadism. See '47,XXY' in Chapter 5, 'Chromosomes', p. 630.
Y CHROMOSOME ANOMALIES.
• Microdeletions. Approximately 10–15% of men with idiopathic azoospermia or severe oligospermia have AZF deletions. The most frequent microdeletion is AZFc (azoospermia factor c), which removes ~4 Mb from Yq. Homologous recombination between large repeats has been shown to be a mechanism of deletion for AZFa and AZFc, but not for AZFb. However, identical sequences in AZFb and AZFc exist, and this finding could explain deletions found in these regions (Ferlin *et al.* 2003).
  • Natural transmission of AZFc microdeletions from fathers to sons has been reported but is rare, as most men with AZFc deletions require ICSI with IVF to overcome their spermatogenic failure.
  • Patsalis *et al.* (2002) report that there may be a risk of 45X/46XY or 45X karyotype in offspring of males with AZFc microdeletions. Consider offering PGD or PND.
• Isodicentric Y chromosome—idic(Yp). Males with an isodicentric Y chromosome have a male phenotype, because of the presence of the *SRY* gene, but have azoospermia because they have no copies of the *AZF* genes that are required for spermatogenesis (see Figure 6.6).
• 46,XX males. Prevalence is 1/20 000. This condition is usually due to:
  • cryptic translocations involving SRY-bearing Y material and the X chromosomes (FISH for SRY);
  • mosaicism for XX and cell lines involving Y chromosome material;
  • true XX hermaphroditism where both testicular and ovarian tissues persist (findings are variable but may have an ovary on one side and a testis on the other); may be due to mosaicism or chimerism or to mutations in genes in the pathway downstream of SRY.

Monogenic conditions causing meiotic arrest
Meiosis produces haploid gametes from diploid parental cells. This process is unique to the germ cells of the gonads. The synaptonemal complex has a key role in meiosis and consists of several proteins (SYP1, 2, and 3). Miyamoto *et al.* (2003) have identified heterozygous mutations in *SYCP3* in 2/19 men with non-obstructive azoospermia showing maturation arrest.

Hypogonadotrophic hypogonadism
The clinical presentation is often with delayed puberty or lack of masculinization (voice/sexual hair, etc.), rather than infertility. Adolescent and adult males with hypogonadotrophic hypogonadism require testosterone replacement; infertility may be treatable with gonadotrophins or GnRH.
KALLMANN SYNDROME (KS). A genetic condition characterized by the association of hypogonadotrophic hypogonadism and anosmia with or without other anomalies. KS affects about one in 8000 males and one in 40 000 females, with most presentations being of the 'sporadic' type. It can follow AD, AR, or XL inheritance. The gene underlying the XL form of the disease *KAL-1* encodes a glycoprotein anosmin-1 that is involved in the embryonic migration of GnRH-synthesizing neurons and the differentiation of the olfactory bulbs. There is considerable phenotypic variation even within families. Mutations in *FGFR1* or *FGF8* underline an AD form with incomplete penetrance (*KAL2*). Mutations in *PROKR2* and *PROK2* have been found in heterozygous and biallelic states and are likely to be involved in AR KS (*KAL3*) and digenic/oligogenic KS (Dode and Hardelin 2010). Mutations in any of these genes are found in <30% of KS patients.
PRIMARY CILIARY DYSKINESIA (PCD). A genetically heterogeneous recessive disorder of motile cilia, resulting in neonatal respiratory distress, chronic oto-sino-pulmonary disease, and male infertility; organ laterality defects are present in ~50% of individuals. See 'Ciliopathies' in Chapter 3, 'Common consultations', p. 366.

Genetic advice and management
The geneticist's role is to explain the genetic basis of the disorder causing infertility. Depending on the specific diagnosis, if ART could be used to achieve a pregnancy with the patient's own sperm, then advice about reproductive implications is also appropriate. Management of the infertility is the remit of a specialist in reproductive medicine.

Support group: Infertility Network UK, http://www.infertilitynetworkuk.com, Tel. 01424 732 361.

References
Augarten A, Yahav Y, Kerem BS, *et al*. Congenital bilateral absence of vas deferens in the absence of cystic fibrosis. *Lancet* 1994; **344**: 1473–4.

Claustres M, Guittard C, Bozon D, *et al*. Spectrum of CFTR mutations in cystic fibrosis and in congenital absence of the vas deferens in France. *Hum Mutat* 2000; **16**: 143–56.

Cooper TG, Noonan E, von Eckardstein S, *et al*. World Health Organization reference values for human semen characteristics. *Hum Reprod Update* 2010; **16**: 231–45.

De Braekeleer M, Dao TN. Cytogenetic studies in male infertility: a review. *Hum Reprod* 1991; **6**: 245–50.

Dode C, Hardelin JP. Clinical genetics of Kallmann syndrome. *Ann Endocrinol (Paris)* 2010; **71**: 149–57.

Egozcue J, Blanco J, Anton E, Egozcue S, Sarrate Z, Vidal F. Genetic analysis of sperm and implications of severe male infertility—a review. *Placenta* 2003; **24**(Suppl B): S62–5.

Evers JL. Female subfertility [seminar]. *Lancet* 2002; **360**: 151–9.

Ferlin A, Moro E, Rossi A, Dallapiccola B, Foresta C. The human Y chromosome's azoospermia factor b (AZFb) region: sequence,

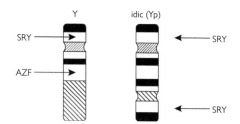

Figure 6.6 (Left) Normal Y chromosome and (right) isodicentric Y chromosome (idic (Yp)). *AZF*, azoospermia factor gene; *SRY*, male-determining gene.

structure, and deletion analysis in infertile men. *J Med Genet* 2003; **40**: 18–24.

Hu Y, Tanriverdi F, MacColl GS, Bouloux PM. Kallmann's syndrome: molecular pathogenesis. *Int J Biochem Cell Biol* 2003; **35**: 1157–62.

McCallum T, Milunsky J, Munarriz R, Carson R, Sadeghi-Nejad H, Oates R. Unilateral renal agenesis associated with congenital bilateral absence of the vas deferens: phenotypic findings and genetic considerations. *Hum Reprod* 2001; **16**: 282–8.

Miyamoto T, Hasuike S, Yogev L, *et al.* Azoospermia in patients heterozygous for a mutation in SYCP3. *Lancet* 2003; **362**: 1714–19.

Oliveira LM, Seminara SB, Beranova M, *et al.* The importance of autosomal genes in Kallmann syndrome: genotype–phenotype correlations and neuroendocrine characteristics. *J Clin Endocrinol Metab* 2001; **86**: 1532–8.

Patsalis PC, Sismani C, Quintana-Murci L, Taleb-Bekkouche F, Krausz C, McElreavey K. Effects of transmission of Y chromosome AZFc deletions. *Lancet* 2002; **360**: 1222–4.

Maternal age

With advanced maternal age, there is an increased risk for the following.

- Subfertility. An increasing incidence of chromosomally abnormal conceptuses with advancing age is a major factor in decline in fertility. Chromosomally abnormal embryos have a lower implantation rate than euploid embryos (Munne 2003).
- Miscarriage. Increased risk due to increased incidence of chromosomally abnormal conceptuses with advanced maternal age and higher miscarriage rate with advancing age for aneuploidy, as well as euploid, conceptions. Risk of early pregnancy loss in a 40-year-old woman is 30–40%.
- Aneuploidy (except 45,X, 47,XYY, triploidy, and de novo rearrangements). Non-disjunction at meiosis I is the main age-dependent factor. Risks increase exponentially with advancing maternal age for +21, +18, +13, and also for 47,XXX and 47,XXY. For the autosomal trisomies, this rise appears to be followed by a levelling off at the extreme upper end of the age range. Marquez et al. (2000) in a study of >1000 cleavage-stage human embryos from patients undergoing IVF found that aneuploidy increased with maternal age, from 3.1% in embryos from 20- to 34-year-old patients to 17% in patients 40 years or older.
  - Eighty per cent of 45,X pregnancies show loss of paternal contribution (may occur post-zygotically). A significant inverse relationship with maternal age is found for live-born 45,X cases, perhaps reflecting the higher miscarriage rate with advancing maternal age for aneuploidy, as well as euploid, conceptions.
- Dizygotic twinning.
- Increased risk of de novo dominant mutation with advancing maternal age, although this is less than with advancing paternal age (see Figure 1.14 in 'Timing and origin of new dominant mutations' in Chapter 1, 'Introduction', p. 42).

Genetic advice and management

- The figures quoted in Table 6.9 are for live births. The risk for Down's syndrome at CVS or amniocentesis is higher, since a proportion of affected pregnancies result in spontaneous fetal loss (miscarriage or IUD). Approximately 43% of affected pregnancies would be lost spontaneously between the time of CVS and term, and ~23% between the time of amniocentesis and term.
- Overall, the risk for any chromosome aneuploidy (e.g. +21, +18, +13, 47,XXX, 47,XXY, which are age-dependent, and 45,X, 47,XYY, triploidy, which are not influenced by maternal age) is approximately double the risk for Down's syndrome.
- For risks arising from combined parental age of a de novo dominant development disorder, see Figure 1.14 in 'Timing and origin of new dominant mutations' in Chapter 1, 'Introduction', p. 42.

References

Ferguson-Smith MA, Yates JR. Maternal age specific rates for chromosome aberrations and factors influencing them: report of a collaborative European study on 52 965 amniocenteses. Prenat Diagn 1984 Spring; 4(Spec no.): 5–44.

Table 6.9 Observed and predicted odds of Down's syndrome live birth by maternal age (after Morris et al. 2002), with suggested counselling odds for use in clinic

Maternal age at child's birth (years)	Counselling odds*	Observed odds	Predicted odds†
17	1:1550	1:1599	1:1504
18	1:1500	1:1789	1:1497
19	1:1450	1:1440	1:1488
20	1:1450	1:1441	1:1476
21	1:1450	1:1409	1:1461
22	1:1450	1:1465	1:1441
23	1:1400	1:1346	1:1415
24	1:1400	1:1396	1:1381
25	1:1350	1:1383	1:1339
26	1:1250	1:1187	1:1285
27	1:1200	1:1235	1:1219
28	1:1150	1:1147	1:1139
29	1:1000	1:1002	1:1045
30	1:950	1:959	1:937
31	1:820	1:837	1:819
32	1:700	1:702	1:695
33	1:570	1:589	1:571
34	1:440	1:430	1:455
35	1:350	1:338	1:352
36	1:260	1:259	1:266
37	1:200	1:201	1:199
38	1:150	1:162	1:148
39	1:110	1:113	1:111
40	1:85	1:84	1:85
41	1:70	1:69	1:67
42	1:55	1:52	1:54
43	1:45	1:37	1:45
44	1:40	1:38	1:39
45	1:35	1:32	1:35
46	1:30	1:31	1:31
47	1:30	1:25	1:29

* Counselling odds are 'rounded' figures for use in the clinic setting.

† Predicted odds are based on the statistical model described by Morris et al. (2002).

Marquez C, Sandalinas M, Bahçe M, Alikani M, Munné S. Chromosome abnormalities in 1255 cleavage-stage human embryos. Reprod Biomed Online 2000; 1: 17–26.

McRae JF, Clayton S, Fitzgerald TW, et al. (2016, under review). Prevalence, phenotype and architecture of developmental disorders caused by de novo mutation. doi: http://dx.doi.org/

10.1101/049056. http://biorxiv.org/content/early/2016/06/16/049056.

Morris JK, Mutton DE, Alberman E. Revised estimates of the maternal age specific live birth prevalence of Down's syndrome. *J Med Screen* 2002; **9**: 2–6.

Munné S. Preimplantation genetic diagnosis and human implantation—a review. *Placenta* 2003; **24**(Suppl B): S70–6.

Maternal diabetes mellitus and diabetic embryopathy

Bell et al. (2012) is the most comprehensive study of this topic, being population-based and including terminations for fetal anomaly at any gestation, late fetal losses, still-births, and malformations diagnosed up to the age of 12 years. Over 400 000 singleton pregnancies were in the study, including 1677 in diabetic women. The incidence of non-chromosomal major congenital malformations among infants of diabetic mothers (IDMs) in this study was 7% (relative risk 4). There was a clear relationship with periconceptual HbA1C; the malformation risk with a periconceptual HbA1c of 10% was 1 in 9, while the risk with a periconceptual HbA1C of 6.1% was 1 in 33. The risk of congenital anomaly increased linearly with increasing HbA1c above 6.3% (45 mmol/mol), by nearly 30% for each 1% (11 mmol/mol) increase. Findings in other large studies and meta-analysis have been similar. There is no significant difference between the incidence of congenital malformations between those with T1D and T2D. Malformation risk is limited to patients who are diabetic at the time of conception and is not found among gestational diabetics.

Table 6.10 lists some features of diabetic embryopathy. Note that even caudal dysplasia sequence, the malformation with the highest relative risk, is as likely to occur in the offspring of a non-diabetic woman as a diabetic woman. In the same spectrum, the relative risk for VATER/VACTERL and sirenomelia are increased, but also more frequent in the offspring of non-diabetic women.

There is nothing in the literature raising concern regarding neurodevelopmental outcome in the offspring of diabetic women.

The mechanism of diabetic embryopathy is not well understood. The diabetic environment appears to simultaneously induce alterations in several interrelated teratological pathways (e.g. disturbances in metabolism of inositol, prostaglandins, and reactive oxygen species). Clinical studies have not established an association between maternal hypoglycaemia and diabetic embryopathy in humans; but animal studies clearly indicate that hypoglycaemia is potentially teratogenic during embryogenesis.

Clinical assessment

History: key points

- Three-generation family tree (to assess whether there is an obvious genetic explanation for any observed malformation).
- Detailed account of the quality of diabetic control periconceptually. What was the HbA1c? Did she experience any hypoglycaemic episodes?

Table 6.10 Relative risk (compared to offspring of non-diabetic women) of having a feature of diabetic embryopathy

Feature	Relative risk
Caudal dysplasia sequence	170
Laterality disturbance	57
Neural tube defects	5
Congenital heart defects	3

Data from Bell et al., Peri-conception hyperglycaemia and nephropathy are associated with risk of congenital anomaly in women with pre-existing diabetes: a population-based cohort study, *Diabetologia*, 2012, volume 55, issue 4, pp 936–947.

- Brief inquiry about other possible teratogenic exposures, e.g. drugs, infection, alcohol.
- If child live-born, detailed perinatal history, birth-weight, and growth parameters.

Examination: key points

- If anomaly identified, examine the parents, e.g. if limb defect in the fetus/child, examine the hands/feet of the parents; if cardiac defect, likewise.

Special investigations

- Maternal serum screening for NTDs (the lab must be informed of maternal diabetes because norms for AFP need to be adjusted).
- Detailed fetal anomaly USS. Wong et al. (2002) found the detection rate for fetal anomalies was lower for diabetic women (30%) than for non-diabetic women (73%), with suboptimal image quality (maternal obesity a major factor (Best et al. 2012)).
- HbA1c (measure of glycaemic control over previous 6–8 weeks). In one series (Wong et al. 2002), periconceptual HbA1c >9% was associated with a high incidence of major anomalies (14.3%).
- Genomic array if multiple anomalies.
- Consider fetal/postnatal echo.

Management of further pregnancies

Diabetic control should be optimized before conception, following NICE guidelines (http://www.nice.org.uk/). All diabetic women need specialist management by an obstetrician with special expertise in fetomaternal medicine.

Expert adviser: Judith Goodship, formerly Professor of Medical Genetics, Institute of Human Genetics, Newcastle upon Tyne, UK.

References

Balsells M, Garcia-Patterson A, Gich I, Corcoy R. Maternal and fetal outcome in women with type 2 versus type 1 diabetes mellitus: a systematic review and metaanalysis. *J Clin Endocrinol Metab* 2009; **94**: 4284–91.

Banhidy F, Acs N, Puhó EH, Czeizel AE. Congenital abnormalities in the offspring of pregnant women with type 1, type 2 and gestational diabetes mellitus: a population-based case-control study. *Congenit Anom (Kyoto)* 2010; **50**:115–21.

Bell R, Glinianaia SV, Tennant PW, Bilous RW, Rankin J. Peri-conception hyperglycaemia and nephropathy are associated with risk of congenital anomaly in women with pre-existing diabetes: a population-based cohort study. *Diabetologia* 2012; **55**: 936–47.

Best KE, Tennant PW, Bell R, Rankin J. Impact of maternal body mass index on the antenatal detection of congenital anomalies. *BJOG* 2012; **119**: 1503–11.

Corrigan N, Brazil DP, McAuliffe F. Fetal cardiac effects of maternal hyperglycemia during pregnancy. *Birth Defects Res A Clin Mol Teratol* 2009; **85**: 523–30.

Eriksson UJ, Borg LA, Cederberg J, et al. Pathogenesis of diabetes-induced congenital malformations. *Ups J Med Sci* 2000; **105**: 53–84.

Garne E, Loane M, Dolk H, et al. Spectrum of congenital anomalies in pregnancies with pregestational diabetes. *Birth Defects Res A Clin Mol Teratol* 2012; **94**: 134–40.

Inkster ME, Fahey TP, Donnan PT, Leese GP, Mires GJ, Murphy DJ. Poor glycated haemoglobin control and adverse pregnancy outcomes in type 1 and type 2 diabetes mellitus: systematic review of observational studies. *BMC Pregnancy Childbirth* 2006; **6**: 30.

Jensen DM, Damm P, Moelsted-Pedersen L, *et al*. Outcomes in type 1 diabetic pregnancies: a nationwide, population-based study. *Diabetes Care* 2004; **27**: 2819–23.

Mills JL, Simpson JL, Driscoll SG, *et al*. Incidence of spontaneous abortion among normal women and insulin-dependent diabetic women whose pregnancies were identified within 21 days of conception. *N Engl J Med* 1988; **319**: 1617–23.

Schwartz R, Teramo KA. Effects of diabetic pregnancy on the fetus and newborn. *Semin Perinatol* 2000; **24**: 120–35.

Wong SF, Chan FY, Cincotta RB, Oats JJ, McIntyre HD. Routine ultrasound screening in diabetic pregnancies. *Ultrasound Obstet Gynecol* 2002; **19**: 171–6.

Maternal phenylketonuria (PKU)

PKU is a treatable AR inherited disorders of metabolism resulting from a deficiency of phenylalanine hydroxylase and characterized by elevation of plasma phenylalanine levels and intellectual disability (ID). It is caused by mutations in the *PAH* gene on 12q24.1. The newborn screening programme for PKU introduced in the 1960s in many countries means that it is now possible to prevent ID in individuals with PKU by strict adherence to a phenylalanine-restricted diet; with optimal dietary control, intelligence can be normal.

The maternal PKU syndrome describes the teratogenicity that occurs secondary to exposure to high levels of maternal phenylalanine *in utero* in children born to mothers with poorly controlled PKU. This is *potentially one of the most teratogenic of all pregnancy complications but can be prevented* by adherence to a low-protein, phenylalanine-restricted diet with reduction of maternal phenylalanine levels, ideally prior to conception and throughout pregnancy.

Teratogenic effects on the offspring are very similar to those of FAS:

- microcephaly: present from birth;
- MR. Reduced cognitive function is a virtually constant feature in offspring of untreated maternal PKU. Also striking hyperactivity and emotional problems;
- CHD, especially tetralogy of Fallot and aortic coarctation;
- IUGR;
- facial dysmorphism:
  - epicanthic folds;
  - maxillary hypoplasia;
  - flattened nasal bridge and upturned nose;
  - long philtrum and thin upper lip;
  - micrognathia.

Clinical assessment

History: key points

- Brief family tree. Enquire specifically for consanguinity.
- Enquire about pre-pregnancy diet and obtain details of the most recent pre-pregnancy maternal blood phenylalanine levels.
- Obtain accurate information about the dating of the pregnancy and dietary control and blood phenylalanine levels during the pregnancy.

Special investigations

- Refer *immediately* for expert dietary advice if the pregnancy is continuing.
- Maternal phenylalanine levels should be monitored 2–3 times weekly in pregnancy. This can be done by blood spot analysis. Aim for stable blood spot phenylalanine of 100–300 µmol/l.
- In women with good metabolic control, obstetric follow-up and USS frequency can be as for a normal pregnancy. In women in whom there are concerns regarding metabolic control, then CHD may be detected on a mid-trimester scan; microcephaly and growth retardation may be identified on third-trimester scans.
- In some women with poor metabolic control, saproterin (a cofactor for the phenylalanine hydroxylase enzyme) may be a useful adjunct to dietary treatment.

Genetic advice and management

- This is an example of a genetic disease (PKU) in the mother that is very harmful (teratogenic) to her unborn infant. The genetic risks are less crucial; the mother is usually a compound heterozygote for mutations in the phenylalanine hydroxylase gene.
- Risk to offspring for PKU if the mother's partner is unrelated and has no family history of PKU is 1/100 (1/50 × 1/2).
- Babies born to mothers with PKU should have standard neonatal screening on day 5 of life (http://newbornbloodspot.screening.nhs.uk).
- Close follow-up and counselling for girls and young women with PKU is essential to maintain awareness of the need for good metabolic control in pregnancy.

Presentation in first trimester

In practice, similar to the general population, many women with PKU have unplanned pregnancies and present already pregnant. A significant relationship between the mean phenylalanine concentration in all trimesters and the occurrence of IUGR, microcephaly, and developmental disability has been shown. The effect appears to be continuous with higher maternal phenylalanine levels being associated with worse outcome (see Tables 6.11 and 6.12). However, data from both the North American Collaborative Study and the UK have suggested that outcome can still be satisfactory when diet is commenced before or up to 8–10 weeks after conception.

Pre-pregnancy counselling

Ideally, women with PKU should receive information about the need for strict dietary control and careful supervision during pregnancy as teenagers. This should include:

- information about teratogenic effects of untreated maternal PKU;
- the need for careful planning of pregnancies with initiation of strict dietary control at least 1 month before conception, aiming for a stable phenylalanine level of 100–300 µmol/l throughout pregnancy;

Table 6.11 Teratogenic effects and frequencies (%) relative to the degree of maternal hyperphenylalanaemia in offspring from untreated maternal phenylketonuria and hyperphenylalanaemia

Abnormality in offspring	Frequency (%) relative to maternal blood phenylalanine level[*]			
	>1200 µmol/l	>1000 µmol/l	>600 µmol/l	200–600 µmol/l
Mental retardation	92	73	22	21
Microcephaly	73	68	35	24
Congenital heart disease	12	15	6	0
Low birthweight	40	52	56	13

[*] To convert from µmol/l to mg/dl, multiply by 0.0165.

Reproduced from Levy H, Ghavami M, Maternal phenylketonuria: a metabolic teratogen, *Teratology*, Vol 53, pp. 176–84, copyright © 1996 Wiley-Liss, Inc and the Teratology Society.

Table 6.12 Maximum accepted blood phenylalanine concentrations and frequency of capillary blood sampling

Age (years)	Blood phenylalanine concentration (μmol/l)	Frequency of capillary blood sampling
0–5	120–360	Weekly
5–10	120–480	Weekly to fortnightly
>10	120–480	Weekly to fortnightly
Adult	120–700	Fortnightly to monthly
Pregnancy	300	Three times weekly

Adapted from the Management of Phenylketonuria (PKU), National Society for Phenylketonuria (UK) Ltd, 2014. Copyright ©: NSPKU (UK) Ltd. All rights reserved.

- the need for specialist dietetic supervision during pregnancy by a centre with an interest in metabolic disease and experienced in the provision of low-protein diets.

Support groups: National Society for Phenylketonuria (NSKPU), http://www.nspku.org; Climb (Children Living with Inherited Metabolic Diseases), http://www.climb.org.uk.

Expert adviser: Elaine Murphy, Consultant in Inherited Metabolic Disease, Charles Dent Metabolic Unit, National Hospital for Neurology and Neurosurgery, London, UK.

References

Koch R, Hanley W, Levy H, et al. The Maternal Phenylketonuria International Study: 1984–2002. *Pediatrics* 2003; **112**: 1523–9.

Lee PJ, Ridout D, Walter JH, Cockburn F. Maternal phenylketonuria: report from the United Kingdom Registry 1978–97. *Arch Dis Child* 2005; **90**: 143–6.

Levy H, Ghavami M. Maternal phenylketonuria: a metabolic teratogen. *Teratology* 1996; **53**: 176–84.

Maillot F, Lilburn M, Baudin J, Morley DW, Lee PJ. Factors influencing outcomes in the offspring of mothers with phenylketonuria during pregnancy: the importance of variation in maternal blood phenylalanine. *Am J Clin Nutr* 2008; **88**: 700–5.

Medical Advisory Panel of the National Society for Phenylketonuria. Management of phenylketonuria. *A consensus document for the diagnosis and management of children, adolescents and adults with phenylketonuria (PKU)*. The National Society for Phenylketonuria (United Kingdom) Ltd., Preston, 2014.

Medical Research Council Working Party on Phenylketonuria. Recommendations on the dietary management of phenylketonuria: report of Medical Research Council Working Party on Phenylketonuria. *Arch Dis Child* 1993; **68**: 426–7.

Phenylalanine hydroxylase locus knowledgebase. http://www.pahdb.mcgill.ca.

Prick BW, Hop WC, Duvekot JJ. Maternal phenylketonuria and hyperphenylalaninemia in pregnancy: pregnancy complications and neonatal sequelae in untreated and treated pregnancies. *Am J Clin Nutr* 2012; **95**: 374–82.

Miscarriage and recurrent miscarriage

Miscarriage is a lay term for spontaneous early pregnancy loss.

- Early pregnancy loss (EPL). Miscarriage or spontaneous abortion at <12 weeks' gestation.
- Spontaneous abortion. Spontaneous pregnancy loss at <24 weeks' gestation.
- Blighted ovum. Empty gestational sac seen on USS with no fetal parts.
- Missed abortion. Fetal parts identified in the gestational sac, but no cardiac activity in pregnancy <24 weeks' gestation.
- Intrauterine fetal death (IUD). Fetal death >24 weeks' gestation, but before onset of labour.
- Recurrent abortion. Three or more consecutive spontaneous abortions.

Twenty-five to 30% of all pregnancies end in EPL. The rate of EPL decreases with gestation. Gestation, maternal age, and previous history are the most important determinants of EPL (see Table 6.13). Risk of miscarriage increases with maternal age; women aged 40 are twice as likely to miscarry as women aged 20, attributable, in part, to increased risk of chromosomally abnormal conceptus with increased maternal age.

At least 50% of miscarriages have a chromosome abnormality. Higher rates of chromosome imbalance (60–70%) have been reported with chromosomal microarray using chorionic villus tissue at the time of diagnosis of EPL (Schaeffer et al. 2004) or from samples that fail to grow in culture (Fritz et al. 2001). The most common findings are shown in Table 6.14.

Dhillon et al. (2014) undertook a meta-analysis comparing conventional G-banded karyotyping with chromosomal microarray and found there was agreement between array and karyotyping in 86.0% of cases (95% CI, 77.0–96.0%). Array detected 13% (95% CI, 8.0–21.0) additional chromosome abnormalities over conventional full karyotyping. In addition, traditional, full karyotyping detected 3% (95% CI, 1.0–10.0%) additional abnormalities over array (e.g. balanced translocations). The incidence of a variant of unknown significance (VUS) being detected was 2% (95% CI, 1.0–10.0%). Overall

molecular cytogenetic techniques offer a higher success rate, shorter reporting times and a more robust analytical pipeline than conventional karyotyping.

Recurrent miscarriage

In Stephenson et al.'s (2002) study of 225 products of conception (POCs) from couples with recurrent miscarriage, 225 (54%) of samples were euploid and 195 (46%) were cytogenetically abnormal (of which 66.5% were trisomic, 19% were polyploid, 9% were 45,X, 4% were unbalanced translocations, and one was 46,X,+21). The distribution of cytogenetic abnormalities in the recurrent miscarriage group was not significantly different from that in controls when stratified for maternal age, although slightly more unbalanced translocations were identified.

De Braekeleer and Dao (1990), in a large study from Quebec of >22 000 couples with two or more spontaneous abortions, found that, in 4.7%, one partner carried a chromosome rearrangement (usually a reciprocal autosomal or Robertsonian translocation) (background rate of 0.5%). Barber et al. (2010) identified 406 balanced rearrangements in 20 432 parents who had experienced recurrent miscarriage (1.9%). These authors questioned the value of karyotyping recurrent miscarriage parents after a review of the number of subsequent prenatally ascertained unbalanced rearrangements in this cohort (n = 4). In 2011, the Royal College of Obstetricians and Gynaecologists (UK) recommended that parental karyotyping be used only following detection of chromosome imbalance in POCs.

Robinson et al. (2001) undertook a study of 54 couples who were ascertained as having two or more documented aneuploid or polyploid spontaneous abortions. He found that the aetiology of trisomy was predominantly a result of meiotic errors related to increased maternal age, regardless of whether the couple has experienced one or multiple aneuploid spontaneous abortions. Furthermore, this was true even when a second spontaneous abortion involves the same abnormality. The overwhelming majority were simply a consequence of the dramatic increase of trisomic conceptions with increased maternal age, and other theoretical possibilities, such as germline mosaicism, factors affecting chromosome structure and segregation, increased sperm aneuploidy in the male partner, or accelerated 'ageing' of the ovaries, did not appear to play a significant role. (However, these data do not exclude some population variability in risk for aneuploidy.)

Clinical assessment

Recurrent miscarriage with normal parental chromosomes is not, in itself, an indication for referral to the genetics clinic. However, if a couple has a significant history of recurrent fetal loss and especially if cytogenetic abnormalities have been identified in POCs, the couple may be referred to the genetics clinic.

History: key points

- Three-generation family tree, noting history of miscarriage, stillbirth, or neonatal death or unexplained handicap/congenital anomaly.

Examination: key points

- Not usually appropriate.

Table 6.13 Incidence of early pregnancy loss (EPL)

	Incidence of EPL (%)
Total loss of conceptions (includes biochemical pregnancies)	50–70
Total clinical miscarriages	25–31
Clinical miscarriages <6 weeks' gestation	18
Clinical miscarriages at 6–9 weeks' gestation	4
Clinical miscarriages at >9 weeks' gestation	3
In primigravidas	6–10
Risk after three miscarriages	25–30
Risk in a 40-year-old woman	30–40

This table was published in *Emery and Rimoin's Principles and Practice of Medical Genetics*, Fourth Edition, David L. Rimoin (ed), Jauniaux E et al., Chapter 63 Early pregnancy loss, Churchill Livingstone, Edinburgh, Copyright Elsevier 2001.

Table 6.14 The most common chromosomal abnormalities leading to miscarriage

Chromosome abnormality	Percentage of	
	Chromosome abnormalities	Spontaneous abortions
Autosomal trisomy[*]	50	25
Triploidy (69,XXX, 69,XXY, 69,XYY)	15	7.5
45,X	10	5
Tetraploidy (92,XXXX or 92,XXYY)	5	2.5
Unbalanced structural chromosome abnormalities[†]	4	2

[*] +16 is the most common, accounting for 30% of trisomies.

[†] 50% de novo; 50% inherited.

Special investigations

- Molecular cytogenetic techniques alone or in combination (e.g. QF-PCR/MLPA) will detect copy number changes (including aneuploidy and unbalanced rearrangements) in POCs. Triploidy will not be detected by comparative genomic hybridization microarray (aCGH) alone. Cytogenetic workup in couples with a history of recurrent miscarriage may be warranted and, if necessary, following POC findings to exclude parental carrier status.
- Other investigations such as antiphospholipid antibodies, lupus anticoagulant and investigations for SLE, protein C, and factor V Leiden are best undertaken in a gynaecological setting.

Genetic advice and management

- If a parental chromosome rearrangement is identified, counsel appropriately. See 'Autosomal reciprocal translocations—familial' in Chapter 5, 'Chromosomes', p. 640.
- If there is no parental chromosome rearrangement, the couples are best managed in a reproductive medicine clinic, rather than a genetics clinic.
- If the karyotype of the abortus is aneuploid, the chance of a successful next pregnancy is higher than if the abortus is euploid (68% subsequent live birth rate versus 41% in Carp et al.'s (2001) series).

- Recurrent pregnancy loss of affected males can occur in some rare XLD disorders such as IP, Goltz syndrome (focal dermal hypoplasia), and OFD syndrome, but it is rarely a presenting feature and together they account for only a very small fraction of recurrent miscarriages.

Support group: The Miscarriage Association, http://www.miscarriageassociation.org.uk.

Expert adviser: Jonathan Waters, Consultant Clinical Scientist, Regional Genetics Service, Great Ormond Street Hospital NHS Trust, London, UK.

References

Barber JC, Cockwell AE, Grant E, Williams S, Dunn R, Ogilvie CM. Is karyotyping couples experiencing recurrent miscarriage worth the cost? *BJOG* 2010; **117**: 885–8.

Carp H, Toder V, Aviram A, Daniely M, Mashiach S, Barkai G. Karyotype of the abortus in recurrent miscarriage. *Fertil Steril* 2001; **75**: 678–82.

De Braekeleer M, Dao TN. Cytogenetic studies in couples experiencing repeated pregnancy losses. *Hum Reprod* 1990; **5**: 519–28.

Dhillon RK, Hillman SC, Morris RK, et al. Additional information from chromosomal microarray analysis (CMA) over conventional karyotyping when diagnosing chromosomal abnormalities in miscarriage: a systematic review and meta-analysis. *BJOG* 2014; **121**: 11–21.

Fritz B, Hallermann C, Olert J, et al. Cytogenetic analyses of culture failures by comparative genome hybridisation (CGH)—re-evaluation of chromosome aberration rates in early spontaneous abortions. *Eur J Hum Genet* 2001; **9**: 539–47.

Jauniaux E, et al. Early pregnancy loss. In: D Rimoin, R Pyeritz, B Korf (eds.). *Emery and Rimoin's principles and practice of medical genetics*, 6th edn, Chapter 34.3. Churchill Livingstone, Edinburgh, 2013.

Robinson WP, McFadden DE, Stephenson MD. The origin of abnormalities in recurrent aneuploidy/polyploidy. *Am J Hum Genet* 2001; **69**: 1245–54.

Royal College of Obstetricians and Gynaecologists. The investigation and treatment of couples with recurrent first-trimester and second-trimester miscarriage. Green-top Guideline No. 17. Royal College of Obstetricians and Gynaecologists, London, 2011.

Schaeffer AJ, Chung J, Heretis K, Wong A, Ledbetter DH, Lese Martin C. Comparative genomic hybridization-array analysis enhances the detection of aneuploidies and submicroscopic imbalances in spontaneous miscarriages. *Am J Hum Genet* 2004; **74**: 1168–74.

Stephenson MD, Awartani KA, Robinson WP. Cytogenetic analysis of miscarriages from couples with recurrent miscarriage: a case-control study. *Hum Reprod* 2002; **17**: 446–51.

Neonatal (newborn) screening (NS)

The UK perspective

As with other screening programmes, the chief aim is to detect conditions that benefit from intervention, management, and surveillance. The UK National Screening Committee (UK NSC) advises the government and currently, in the UK, NS comprises:

- newborn blood spot screening;
- sickle-cell screening;
- newborn hearing assessment;
- newborn physical examination.

In recent years (since January 2015), the range of conditions screened for in newborns via the blood spot has been extended and now comprises:

- phenylketonuria (PKU);
- congenital hypothyroidism (CHT);
- sickle-cell disease (SCD);
- cystic fibrosis (CF);
- medium chain acyl-CoA dehydrogenase (MCAD) deficiency;
- maple syrup urine disease (MSUD);
- isovaleric acidaemia (IVA);
- glutaric aciduria type 1 (GA1);
- homocystinuria (HCU).

These are illustrated in the antenatal and neonatal screening timeline (see Figure A1 in 'Appendix', p. 806).

From the 2005–11 UK data, following the analysis of ~6 million screened newborns, the incidence of conditions for which screening was available is shown in Table 6.15.

Newborn blood spots (formerly known as the Guthrie test, after the American bacteriologist and physician, Robert Guthrie)

This national NS programme was introduced in 1969 for PKU and in 1981 for CHT. These two conditions are the paradigm for meeting the classic screening criteria outlined by Wilson and Jungner in 1968 (Wilson and Jungner 1968), namely affordable, reliable tests for conditions where the initiation of early treatment (within weeks of birth) will prevent the onset of permanent neurological damage. For PKU, the treatment is a low-phenylalanine diet, which can be relaxed from adolescence, and for CHT lifelong replacement of thyroxine. Most cases of CHT result from the congenital absence of the thyroid gland, a disruptive, rather than genetic, condition, which is usually isolated, but sometimes part of a wider syndrome. The newborn test uses dried blood spots on filter paper from a heel-prick and is taken ideally on day 5 (acceptable range days 5–8).

Table 6.15 Incidence of screened conditions

Conditions	Incidence
PKU	1:10 000
CHT	1:3000
MCAD deficiency	1:10 000
CF	1:2500
SCD	1:2400

Data from UK National Screening Committee (UK NSC).

In addition to PKU and CHT, all babies in England are now offered screening for several inborn errors of metabolism, CF, and SCD, all inherited as AR traits. Verbal parental consent is sufficient to undertake NS in the UK.

Medium-chain acyl-CoA dehydrogenase (MCAD) deficiency

MCAD deficiency is an inborn error of fatty acid metabolism and can lead to sudden infant death in some cases. The screening is biochemical, with analysis of the ratio of the medium-chain length acylcarnitines octanoylcarnitine (C8) and decanoylcarnitine (C10).

Maple syrup urine disease (MSUD)

MSUD, also known as branched-chain ketoaciduria, may be caused by mutations in at least three genes, resulting in failure to properly break down three amino acids—leucine, isoleucine, and valine. In addition to poor feeding, lethargy, and irritability, the untreated infant or child may pass urine with a sweet smell, hence the name. Treatment is centred on a special low-protein diet aimed at avoiding the accumulation of these three amino acids.

Isovaleric acidaemia (IVA)

IVA is due to mutations in the gene encoding isovaleryl CoA dehydrogenase (IVD) and this leads to an inability to break down the amino acid leucine. The signs and symptoms are similar to those of MSUD (except for the odour of urine) and treatment centres on a special diet aimed at avoiding the build-up of leucine.

Glutaric aciduria type 1A (GA1)

GA1 is due to homozygous or compound heterozygous mutations of the gene encoding glutaryl CoA dehydrogenase (GCDH) and gives rise to gliosis and neuronal loss in the basal ganglia, secondary to an inability to break down the amino acids lysine, hydroxylysine, and tryptophan. This results in the onset of a movement disorder in infancy, as well as poor feeding, lethargy, vomiting, and breathing difficulties. It is also a cause of subdural and retinal haemorrhage, and therefore should be considered when a non-accidental injury is suspected from these findings. Treatment centres around a special low-protein diet.

Homocystinuria (HCU)

HCU is due to homozygous or compound heterozygous mutations in the gene encoding cystathionine beta-synthase (CBS) and gives rise to increased urinary homocystine and methionine. Untreated, affected individuals slowly develop myopia, ectopia lentis, mild ID, and skeletal anomalies resembling MFS. In some, levels of homocystine can be controlled by vitamin B6 (pyridoxine), but, if unsuccessful, by a special low-protein diet and medication including anticoagulation measures.

Cystic fibrosis (CF)

The first step is the IRT assay, followed by a two-stage mutation analysis of the CFTR gene on all samples with IRT values above the 99.5th centile. This detects affected babies, with two CFTR mutations, and also some carriers (roughly equal in number to those who are affected) who are identified from the mutation analysis but who do not reach the cut-off level for the second IRT analysis or who have a normal sweat test and are thus unaffected with CF. If the newborn proves to be a carrier of CF, both parents are offered carrier testing.

Duchenne muscular dystrophy (DMD
NS for DMD was offered in Wales from 1990 until 2011 and is no longer available; the rationale was to alert the mother/couple (and potentially the wider family) to the risk of recurrence and the option of prevention.

Sickle-cell disease (SCD) screen
This is performed using the blood spot and complements haemoglobinopathy screening already performed in pregnancy and now covers the whole of the UK. As with CF, if the newborn proves to be a carrier of SCD, both parents are offered carrier testing.

Newborn hearing test
Up to 1:500 newborns have congenital hearing impairment, usually isolated and genetic, sometimes part of a wider syndrome. The aim is to detect >40 dB of hearing loss. A combination of the otoacoustic emission test and automated auditory brainstem response is used. The ideal is to offer this within 72 hours of birth, but, in some areas, testing is performed in the community, which inevitably means it will take place slightly later.

Newborn physical examination
For babies born in hospital, the first examination is at 48–72 hours by a paediatrician. For those born at home or in midwife-led units, the examination may be by either the primary care physician or a specially trained midwife. Attention is paid particularly to the examination of the hips for dislocation, auscultation of the heart for murmur, eyes for cataract, and for descended testes in males. The examination is repeated by the primary care physician at 6–8 weeks.

The future
NS is continually under review by the UK NSC, especially as many tests for rare disorders are available and the range of conditions covered in some programmes worldwide is very extensive. Further metabolic disorders are likely to come under consideration in the UK, e.g. galactosaemia, fatty acid oxidation disorders, CAH, and

Hurler's syndrome. Systematic NS for congenital heart disease (CHD) is recommended and is expected to be introduced in due course. Similarly, screening for congenital cataracts and developmental dysplasia of the hips (DDH) was recommended some years ago (2006).

International perspective
NS has been developed for a large number of conditions or inborn errors of metabolism. The USA leads the way with mandated NS in all states. The 'Newborn Screening Saves Lives Act' was signed into law in 2007 with the intention of unifying and expanding the programme nationwide. This is overseen by the Centers for Disease Prevention and Control, and at least 29 conditions are screened for in all states and >50 in some. This includes a wide range of metabolic disorders, as well as SCID. In The Netherlands, NS is voluntary with informed parental consent. Germany screens for 15 conditions, and across the Middle East and North Africa, where rates of consanguinity are high, there is wide variation. In Saudi Arabia, for example, NS covers >10 disorders, but this does not reach the whole population. In general, screening is mandatory or consent is implied.

Expert adviser: Peter Turnpenny, Consultant Clinical Geneticist and Honorary Clinical Professor, University of Exeter, Medical School, Royal Devon & Exeter Healthcare NHS Trust, Exeter, UK.

References
British Inherited Metabolic Diseases Group (BIMDG). http://www.bimdg.org.uk.

Climb (Children Living with Inherited Metabolic Diseases). http://www.climb.org.uk.

National Services Division, NHS Scotland. http://www.nsd.scot.nhs.uk.

Wilson JMG, Jungner G. *Principles and practice of screening for disease. World Health Organization Public Health Papers, No. 34.* World Health Organization, Geneva, 1968. http://apps.who.int/iris/bitstream/10665/37650/17/WHO_PHP_34.pdf.

Public Health England, NHS Screening Programmes. *Newborn blood spot.* https://cpdscreening.phe.org.uk/newbornbloodspot.

Non-invasive prenatal diagnosis/testing (NIPD/T)

Cell-free fetal nucleic acids for non-invasive prenatal diagnosis/testing

Background

Non-invasive prenatal testing (NIPT) is the analysis of genetic material of fetal origin obtained from a sample of maternal blood and used to provide accurate fetal diagnosis without the risk of miscarriage associated with invasive procedures such as CVS or amniocentesis. Recent developments are based on the observation of Lo et al. (1997) that cell-free fetal DNA (cffDNA) and, more recently, cffRNA (Poon et al. 2000) are present in the maternal plasma and serum. ffDNA is mainly derived from placental trophoblasts in the form of apoptotic fragments. Because of its placental origin, cffDNA has been shown to exhibit placental DNA methylation signatures (Lun et al. 2013). cffRNA, on the other hand, appears to have been packaged into microvesicles (Ng et al. 2003).

ffDNA has been detected in maternal plasma as early as the fourth week of gestation and its concentration increases with gestational age. The ratio of maternal to fetal cell-free DNA in maternal plasma is ~60:1; fetal DNA molecules amount to just 10–20% of the total DNA circulating in the maternal plasma.

cffDNA is rapidly cleared from the maternal circulation with an initial rapid phase with a mean half-life of ~1 hour, and a subsequent slower phase with a mean half-life of ~13 hours. The final disappearance of circulating fetal DNA occurs at about 1–2 days post-partum (Yu et al. 2013). Free fetal RNA (ffRNA) has a similar profile half-life in maternal plasma (Chiu et al. 2006). ffDNA levels may be elevated in placental disorders such as pre-eclampsia (PET) and fetal growth restriction.

cffDNA fragments tend to be shorter than maternal fragments, with a dominant peak at ~162 bp and a minor peak at ~340 bp (Fan et al. 2010). This has two important implications: (1) cffDNA concentration can be increased by size fractionation of cell-free DNA in maternal plasma and (2) PND using this approach may not be efficient/reliable for expansions, duplications, or insertions of >200 bp (check with the laboratory).

The analysis of cell-free fetal nucleic acids promises to revolutionize genetic PND/screening. However, like all new tests, large-scale studies will be needed in order to acquire data on false-positive and false-negative rates, to be able to use this technology appropriately in clinical practice.

NIPT for aneuploidy

See Figure 6.7.

Tong et al. (2006) described the detection of fetal trisomy 18 by measuring the ratio between alleles of a gene sequence that exhibited differential DNA methylation between the maternally derived and fetally derived DNA in plasma. Lo et al. (2007b) achieved NIPT for trisomy 21 by determining the ratio between alleles of an SNP in the placentally derived PLAC4 mRNA, which is transcribed from chromosome 21 and isolated from maternal plasma. An alternate method was reported by Dhallan et al. (2007) who used copy number SNP analysis to distinguish fetal DNA from maternal DNA and calculated the ratio of the unique fetal allele signal to the combined maternal and fetal allele signal.

The technology has changed rapidly. Recent developments in this area have been catalysed by approaches that are based on single DNA molecule counting, first described using single-molecule PCR (or so-called digital PCR) (Lo et al. 2007a). Since 2008, it has been demonstrated that next-generation DNA sequencing allows plasma DNA molecule counting to be performed efficiently and robustly (Chiu et al. 2008). Such an approach is designed to detect an increased representation of chromosome 21 DNA molecules in the plasma of women pregnant with trisomy 21 fetuses when compared with euploid pregnancies. A number of large-scale validation studies of such sequencing-based approaches have been published. For all methods evaluated, there is ~1:200 discordance between the NIPT result and fetal result from invasive testing. NIPT to screen for common fetal aneuploidies based on next-generation sequencing, e.g. trisomy 21, has been available commercially since autumn of 2011 and has already been performed in over 500 000 pregnant women in over 15 countries.

NIPT for single gene disorders

This is technically easier where the mutation is not carried by the mother (either paternally inherited or a DNM) (Chiu et al. 2002). It is of particular use in providing molecular confirmation of conditions such as achondroplasia or TD where the scans are suggestive of the diagnosis.

AR disorders are more difficult because of the presence of the maternal mutation but can detect the presence of the mutation on the paternal allele (Lench et al. 2013). PCR, digital PCR, and next-generation sequencing techniques are all under evaluation (Lam et al. 2012; Lun et al. 2008; Tsui et al. 2011).

Clinical approach

Careful USS is mandatory prior to NIPD/T to estimate gestation, multiple pregnancy, and an empty sac of a non-viable pregnancy.

NIPD for fetal sexing

Examples where NIPD should be considered in advance of an invasive procedure include:

- an XL condition for sexing. If female, then further invasive diagnostic testing is not needed;
- CAH where maternal dexamethasone treatment can be stopped in male pregnancies (see 'Genetic advice and management' below);
- conditions with genital ambiguity as a feature, e.g. SLO syndrome.

The usual method to determine the sex of the fetus is the presence of a Y-specific sequence for a male fetus and the absence of Y-specific material in the cffDNA extract in a female fetus.

NIPT for fetal aneuploidy

- May be performed after high-risk first-trimester screening, but increasingly used instead of biochemical/USS screening methods for trisomy 13, 18, and 21.

NIPD for single gene disorders

- De novo conditions.

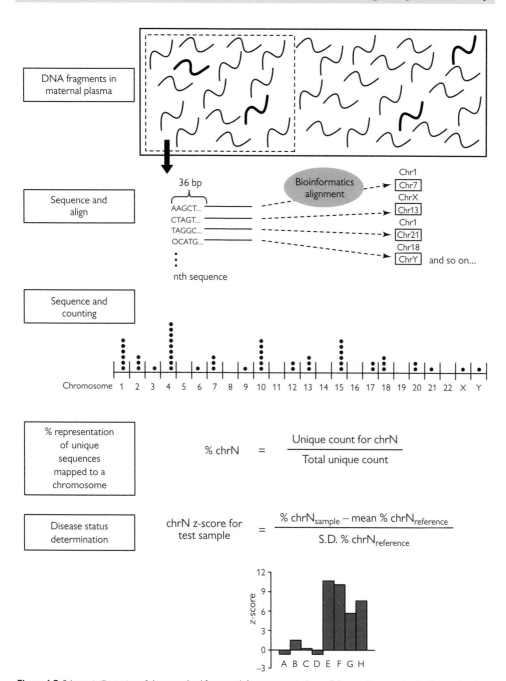

Figure 6.7 Schematic illustration of the procedural framework for using massively parallel genomic sequencing for the non-invasive prenatal detection of fetal chromosomal aneuploidy.
Reproduced from Chiu RWK, Chan KCA *et al.*, Noninvasive prenatal diagnosis of fetal chromosomal aneuploidy by massively parallel genomic sequencing of DNA in maternal plasma, *Proceedings of the National Academy of Sciences*, volume 105, p 20458–63. Copyright (2008) National Academy of Sciences, U.S.A.

- To detect recurrent *de novo* point mutations (e.g. the common achondroplasia mutations in *FGFR3* such as p.Gly380Arg) when short femurs are detected on USS.
- Known mutation: for women at gonadal mosaic risk of recurrence.
- AD conditions: paternally inherited condition with known mutation.
- AR: paternal mutation can guide assessment.

NIPD for rhesus disease

- Fetal RhD disease typing to target immunoprophylaxis.

History: key points

- Establish the genetic diagnosis and whether NIPD for this disorder is appropriate and available.

Examination: key points

- Dating USS—to ensure accurate assessment of gestational age and to determine the number of gestational sacs.

Special investigations

- Maternal blood sample for free fetal nucleic acid analysis. Ensure that arrangements have been made to deliver a sample to the laboratory without delay. Establish with the laboratory whether a second sample will be needed for confirmation of the result.
- Arrange sexing USS from 16/40 to confirm the result from NIPT in pregnancies at risk for an XL disorder.
- Consider repeating free fetal nucleic acid analysis for pregnancies at risk for CAH, since fetal sexing by USS may be unreliable in an affected female fetus.

Points to consider

(1) Failure to detect a specific cffDNA sequence, e.g. a Y-related sequence in a male pregnancy cannot be taken as proof of its absence, since other possibilities include failure of the extraction or amplification steps, or because a proportion of pregnant women have very low fetal DNA fractions.

(2) Failure/inaccuracy due to tiny quantities of DNA (~25 genome equivalents per ml of plasma).

(3) Placental mosaicism. This is present in ~1–2% of CVS samples and has the potential to complicate the analysis and interpretation of free fetal nucleic acids.

(4) Twins. See Qu *et al.* (2013) for determining twin zygosity, and Canick *et al.* (2012) for use of NIPT in the identification of trisomies in multiple pregnancies.

(5) Resolving second gestational sac. In a significant percentage of multiple pregnancies, the second sac resorbs spontaneously during the first trimester.

(6) Although cffDNA can be detected from ~4 weeks' gestation, in practice, fetal testing for aneuploidy using current approaches is more reliable from 10 weeks, by which time there is consistently a greater quantity of ffDNA (Norbury and Norbury 2008).

(7) Maternal chromosomal abnormality or tumour.

Genetic advice and management

High risk for X-linked disorder

In pregnancies at risk for disorders such as DMD, fetal sexing by NIPT obviates the need to proceed to CVS if the pregnancy is identified to be female. Arrange for confirmation of sex either by USS or repeat maternal cffDNA analysis.

High risk for CAH

Fetal sexing by NIPD (as above in 'Clinical approach') may be helpful in the management of pregnancies at risk for CAH. NIPT could potentially provide the diagnosis of CAH non-invasively before the ninth week of gestation (New *et al.* 2014). If a decision is made to initiate dexamethasone therapy (a controversial issue—check current guidelines), therapy would thus be targeted only at mothers carrying an affected female fetus.

Expert adviser: Y. M. Dennis Lo, Li Ka Shing Professor of Medicine and Professor of Chemical Pathology, Department of Chemical Pathology, The Chinese University of Hong Kong, Prince of Wales Hospital, Shatin, New Territories, Hong Kong SAR, China.

References

American College of Obstetricians and Gynecologists Committee on Genetics. Committee Opinion No. **545**: Noninvasive prenatal testing for fetal aneuploidy. *Obstet Gynecol* 2012; **120**: 1532–4.

Canick JA, Kloza EM, Lambert-Messerlian GM, *et al.* DNA sequencing of maternal plasma to identify Down syndrome and other trisomies in multiple gestations. *Prenat Diagn* 2012; **32**: 730–4.

Chitty LS, Bianchi D. Non-invasive prenatal testing: the paradigm is shifting rapidly. *Prenat Diagn* 2013; **33**: 511–13.

Chiu RW, Chan KC, Gao Y, *et al.* Noninvasive prenatal diagnosis of fetal chromosomal aneuploidy by massively parallel genomic sequencing of DNA in maternal plasma. *Proc Natl Acad Sci U S A* 2008; **105**: 20458–63.

Chiu RW, Lau TK, Leung TN, Chow KC, Chui DH, Lo YM. Prenatal exclusion of beta thalassaemia major by examination of maternal plasma. *Lancet* 2002; **360**: 998–1000.

Chiu RW, Lo YM. Noninvasive prenatal diagnosis empowered by high-throughput sequencing. *Prenat Diagn* 2012; **32**: 401–6.

Chiu RW, Lui WB, Cheung MC, *et al.* Time profile of appearance and disappearance of circulating placenta-derived mRNA in maternal plasma. *Clin Chem* 2006; **52**: 513–16.

Dhallan R, Guo X, Emche S, *et al.* A non-invasive test for prenatal diagnosis based on fetal DNA present in maternal blood: a preliminary study. *Lancet* 2007; **369**: 474–81.

Fan HC, Blumenfeld YJ, Chitkara U, Hudgins L, Quake SR. Analysis of the size distributions of fetal and maternal cell-free DNA by paired-end sequencing. *Clin Chem* 2010; **56**: 1279–86.

Hahn S, Chitty LS. Noninvasive prenatal diagnosis: current practice and future perspectives. *Curr Opin Obstet Gynecol* 2008; **20**: 146–51.

Lam KW, Jiang P, Liao GJ, *et al.* Noninvasive prenatal diagnosis of monogenic diseases by targeted massively parallel sequencing of maternal plasma: application to β-thalassemia. *Clin Chem* 2012; **58**: 1467–75.

Lench N, Barrett A, Fielding S, *et al.* The clinical implementation of non-invasive prenatal diagnosis for single-gene disorders: challenges and progress made. *Prenat Diagn* 2013; **33**: 555–62.

Lo YM, Corbetta N, Chamberlain PF, *et al.* Presence of fetal DNA in maternal plasma and serum. *Lancet* 1997; **350**: 485–7.

Lo YM, Lun FM, Chan KC, *et al.* Digital PCR for the molecular detection of fetal chromosomal aneuploidy. *Proc Natl Acad Sci U S A* 2007a; **104**: 13116–21.

Lo YM, Tsui NB, Chiu RW, *et al.* Plasma placental RNA allelic ratio permits noninvasive prenatal chromosomal aneuploidy detection. *Nat Med* 2007b; **13**: 218–23.

Lun FM, Chiu RW, Sun K, *et al.* Noninvasive prenatal methylomic analysis by genomewide bisulfite sequencing of maternal plasma DNA. *Clin Chem* 2013; **59**: 1583–94.

Lun FM, Tsui NB, Chan KC, *et al.* Noninvasive prenatal diagnosis of monogenic diseases by digital size selection and relative mutation dosage on DNA in maternal plasma. *Proc Natl Acad Sci U S A* 2008; **105**: 19920–5.

New MI, Tong YK, Yuen T, *et al.* Noninvasive prenatal diagnosis of congenital adrenal hyperplasia using cell-free fetal DNA in maternal plasma. *J Clin Endocrinol Metab* 2014; **99**: E1022–30.

Ng EK, Tsui NB, Lau K, *et al.* mRNA of placental origin is readily detectable in maternal plasma. *Proc Natl Acad Sci U S A* 2003; **100**: 4748–53.

Norbury G, Norbury CJ. Non-invasive prenatal diagnosis of single gene disorders: how close are we? *Semin Fetal Neonatal Med* 2008; **13**: 76–83.

Poon LL, Leung TN, Lau TK, Lo YM. Presence of fetal RNA in maternal plasma. *Clin Chem* 2000; **46**: 1832–4.

Qu JZ, Leung T, Jiang P, *et al.* Noninvasive prenatal determination of twin zygosity by maternal plasma DNA analysis. *Clin Chem* 2013; **59**: 427–35.

Tong YK, Ding C, Chiu RW, *et al.* Noninvasive prenatal detection of fetal trisomy 18 by epigenetic allelic ratio analysis in maternal plasma: Theoretical and empirical considerations. *Clin Chem* 2006; **52**: 2194–202.

Tsui NB, Kadir RA, Chan KC, *et al.* Noninvasive prenatal diagnosis of hemophilia by microfluidics digital PCR analysis of maternal plasma DNA. *Blood* 2011; **117**: 3684–91.

Yu SC, Lee SW, Jiang P, *et al.* High-resolution profiling of fetal DNA clearance from maternal plasma by massively parallel sequencing. *Clin Chem* 2013; **59**: 1228–37.

Oedema—increased nuchal translucency, cystic hygroma, and hydrops

The reason that chromosomally abnormal fetuses have increased nuchal oedema, cystic hygromas, or hydrops is not well understood. Cystic hygroma per se seems to arise as a result of lymphatic dysplasia and is particularly associated with 45,X (Turner syndrome). Increased nuchal fold thickness/NT may resolve spontaneously (even in a karyotypically abnormal pregnancy). Even when fetal lymphoedema resolves, dysmorphism may result from the tissue distension/displacement that occurred during fetal life, e.g. neck webbing, nuchal skinfolds, hypertelorism and epicanthic folds, low-set ears, wide-spaced nipples.

There is an increased risk of CHD in karyotypically normal pregnancies with increased nuchal fold thickness/cystic hygroma/hydrops. Some structural cardiac anomalies, such as coarctation of the aorta and hypoplastic left heart, may be sequelae of fetal lymphoedema.

Nuchal translucency

Subcutaneous accumulation of fluid at the back of the fetal neck is visualized by USS examination at 10–14 weeks' gestation as increased NT thickness. It is associated with chromosomal abnormalities, a wide range of cardiac defects, and genetic syndromes.

Many pregnancies are now screened for chromosome anomalies (e.g. Down's syndrome) using an algorithm combining nuchal fold thickness measured by USS at 10–14 weeks' gestation with maternal age and maternal serum markers. Using a combination of maternal serum free beta-hCG and PAPP-A and fetal NT thickness, known as the 'combined test', at 12 weeks, the rate of detection of trisomy 21 was 88% for a screen-positive rate of 2% (Kagan et al. 2008).

Cardiac echo is now recommended for all cases with an NT ≥3.5 mm. A review by Mogra et al. (2012) evaluated six recent studies and found that, on average, the prevalence of major cardiac defects in chromosomally normal fetuses with an NT ≥3.5 mm was 6.27% (range 3.1–12.2%). They also looked at eight other studies designed to assess the effectiveness of NT as a screening tool for major cardiac defects. These gave a similar prevalence of 5.88% (2.3–9.7%).

There have been many studies following up pregnancies with a nuchal >3.5 mm and a normal karyotype. Senat et al. (2007) reported that anomalies were found postnatally in 11% of fetuses with negative findings at USS. Bilardo et al (2010) reviewed 451 cases, with the results shown in Table 6.16. Importantly, they also reported that, if the 20-week anomaly scan is entirely normal, the nuchal having completely resolved, then the risk to the fetus returns to the background risk. This key detail was also reported by Souka et al. (2005), but more studies are needed to support this.

Fetal cystic hygroma

Fetal cystic hygroma is an anomaly of the vascular lymphatic system; it can be non-septate or septate, but both are associated with aneuploidy. Graesslin et al.'s (2007) report of 72 cases found that 52.7% had a chromosomal anomaly (37% with trisomy 21). Of the chromosomally normal cases, 18 (52.9%) were live-born, one had Noonan syndrome, another a urinary tract abnormality,

Table 6.16 Outcome of increased nuchal translucency with normal chromosomes

NT (mm)	Fetal death	Structural/ genetic anomalies	Live birth, no defects
95th centile–3.4 mm	2%	6%	92%
3.5–4.4 mm	5%	12%	83%
4.5–5.4 mm	9%	19%	71%
5.5–6.4 mm		42%	58%
≥6.5 mm	50%	30%	20%

Reproduced from Bilardo CM, Timmerman E et al., Increased nuchal translucency in euploid fetuses – what should web e telling the parents?, *Prenatal Diagnosis*, Vol 30(2), pp. 93–102, Copyright 2010 International Society for Prenatal Diagnosis.

and 16 were normal at follow-up of at least 17 months. Thus, 22% overall had no discernable problems. Similarly, Ganapathy et al. (2004) retrospectively analysed 42 cases; 47.6% had aneuploidy (55% with Turner syndrome, 20% with trisomy 21) and 29.4% of the euploid had a major cardiac defect. Regression of the hygroma was noted in 10% of the aneuploid pregnancies and 17.6% of the euploid and so was not useful diagnostically. Boyd et al. (1996) retrospectively analysed 92 cases, of whom 53% had a normal karyotype. High-risk factors were additional anomalies or progression to hydrops or other effusions. For those continued pregnancies with normal chromosomes and no additional risk factors, 89% were normal at follow-up of 1–5 years.

Hydrops

USS definition requires skin oedema >5 mm (over the skull), associated with other serous effusions (ascites, pericardial effusion, hydrothorax) and/or polyhydramnios and/or increased placental thickness (>6 cm in depth). Fetal hydrops is classified as 'immune (fetomaternal alloimmunization)' or 'non-immune'. The latter, accounting for 90% of cases in the Western world, should be considered a non-specific end-stage status of a wide variety of disorders with a high pregnancy loss rate. The most common causes of fetal hydrops are summarized in Table 6.17. Pathophysiological mechanisms are well discussed by Bellini and Hennekam (2012) and include fetal hypomobility, congestive cardiac failure, and obstructed lymphatic flow.

Several metabolic conditions may present *in utero* with hydrops. Pathological examination of the placenta can be particularly helpful in suggesting this. If a fibroblast cell line has been stored, this will allow further biochemical investigations. Frozen amniotic fluid may also be of use in some cases.

Some metabolic disorders with hydrops as a feature include the following.
- Congenital disorders of glycosylation.
- Farber disease (ceraminidase deficiency).
- Galactosialidosis (neuraminidase deficiency with β-galactosidase deficiency).
- Gaucher's disease (β-glucosidase deficiency).
- Glycogen storage disease IV.

Table 6.17 Causes of fetal hydrops

Cause	Number	%
Cardiovascular (structural defects, arrhythmias, tumours, myocardiopathies)	1181	21.7
Chromosomal (45,X and +21, triploidy, and a variety of rare chromosome rearrangements)	727	13.4
Haematological (e.g. haemoglobinopathies, red cell aplasias, dyserythropoiesis)	564	10.4
Fetal infections (e.g. CMV, parvovirus B19)	366	6.7
Thoracic (diaphragmatic hernia, CCAM, short rib skeletal dysplasias, tumours)	327	6.0
Lymphatic dysplasia	310	5.7
Twinning	304	5.6
Syndromic (including inborn errors of metabolism)	297	5.5
Miscellaneous	395	7.2
Unknown	966	17.8

* Total number of cases studied was 5437.

Reproduced from Bellini C, Hennekam RCM et al., Etiology of nonimmune hydrops fetalis: a systematic review, American Journal of Medical Genetics Part A, vol 149A, pp. 844–851, Copyright 2009 Wiley Periodicals, Inc.

- GM1 gangliosidosis (β-galactosidase-1 deficiency).
- I cell disease (mucolipidosis type II).
- MPS I (Hurler), MPS IV, MPS VII (β-glucuronidase deficiency). Can assay glycosaminoglycans (GAGs) in amniotic fluid.
- Multiple sulfatase deficiency (arylsulfatase A and other sulfatases).
- Niemann–Pick A (sphingomyelinase deficiency).
- Niemann–Pick type C disease (cholesterol esterification defect).
- Salla disease and sialic acid storage disease.
- Sialidosis (neuraminidase deficiency).
- Wolman disease (acid esterase).
- (Pearson syndrome (anaemia)—a mitochondrial disorder).

Clinical assessment

History: key points
- Three-generation family tree, with specific reference to previous fetal loss, family history of anaemia, consanguinity.
- Ethnic origin of parents (e.g. α-thalassaemia, G6PD).

Examination: key points
- Detailed fetal anomaly USS at 19–21 weeks' gestation for the presence of structural anomalies and skeletal dysplasias.
- Detailed fetal echo.
- Examine parents for features of Noonan syndrome.

Special investigations
- Fetal karyotype or genomic array, (amniocentesis, CVS, or FBS). Gene panel/WES/WGS including Ras/MAPK panel if available. It may also be possible to arrange biochemical analysis of amniotic fluid and cultured amniocytes, e.g. for lysosomal disorders (some specialist centres offer a 'hydrops screen' for lysosomal storage disorders).
- The obstetrician should consider investigations to exclude fetomaternal alloimmunization (antibody levels), fetal infection (e.g. congenital parvovirus B19), and fetal anaemia.
- If the baby dies, arrange for clinical photography, skeletal radiograph (some skeletal dysplasias may present as hydrops and accurate assessment of fetal limb length is made difficult in the presence of severe oedema), tissue storage (e.g. fibroblast cell line), and DNA storage, and offer post-mortem examination to include the placenta. If there has been fetal akinesia and a muscle abnormality is suspected, a muscle biopsy must be taken as soon as possible after delivery and processed appropriately by pathology staff as an urgent priority.
- For recurrent hydrops without a diagnosis, it is important to set up a fibroblast cell line and freeze amniotic fluid while awaiting the results of the post-mortem and X-rays.
- For severe/lethal hydrops, if the above causes have been excluded, consider whole exome/genome/panel sequencing, especially in consanguineous families.

Genetic advice and management
Make every effort to achieve a diagnosis and counsel as for the specific diagnosis.

Expert adviser: Diana Wellesley, Consultant Clinical Geneticist, Wessex Clinical Genetics Service, Princess Anne Hospital, Southampton, UK.

References
Bellini C, Hennekam RC. Non-immune hydrops fetalis: a short review of etiology and pathophysiology. Am J Med Genet A 2012; **158A**: 597–605.

Bellini C, Hennekam RC, Fulcheri E, et al. Etiology of nonimmune hydrops fetalis: a systematic review. Am J Med Genet A 2009; **149A**: 844–51.

Bilardo CM, Timmerman E, Pajkrt E, van Maarle M. Increased nuchal translucency in euploid fetuses—what should we be telling the parents? Prenat Diagn 2010; **30**: 93–102.

Boyd PA, Anthony MY, Manning N, Rodriguez CL, Wellesley DG, Chamberlain P. Antenatal diagnosis of cystic hygroma or nuchal pad—report of 92 cases with follow-up of survivors. Arch Dis Child Fetal Neonatal Ed 1996; **74**: F38–42.

Ganapathy R, Guven M, Sethna F, Vivekananda U, Thilaganathan B. Natural history and outcome of prenatally diagnosed cystic hygroma. Prenat Diagn 2004; **24**: 965–8.

Graesslin O, Derniaux E, Alanio E, et al. Characteristics and outcome of fetal cystic hygroma diagnosed in the first trimester. Acta Obstet Gynaecol Scand 2007; **86**: 1442–6.

Kagan KO, Wright D, Baker A, Sahota D, Nicolaides KH. Screening for trisomy 21 by maternal age, fetal nuchal translucency thickness, free beta-human chorionic gonadotrophin and pregnancy-associated plasma protein-A. Ultrasound Obstet Gynecol 2008; **31**: 618–24.

Makrydimas G, Souka A, Skentou H, Lolis D, Nicolaides K. Osteogenesis imperfecta and other skeletal dysplasias presenting with increased nuchal translucency in the first trimester. Am J Med Genet 2001; **98**: 117–20.

Mogra R, Alabbad N, Hyett J. Increased nuchal translucency and congenital heart disease. Early Hum Dev 2012; **88**: 261–7.

Nyhan WL, Ozand PT. Atlas of metabolic diseases. Chapman and Hall Medical, London, 1998.

Senat MV, Bussieres L, Couderc S, et al. Long term coutcome of children born after first-trimester measurement of nuchal translucency at the 99th percentile or greater with normal karyotype: a prospective study. Am J Obstet Gynecol 2007; **196**: 531–6.

Souka AP, Von Kaisenberg CS, Hyett JA, Sonek JD, Nicolaides KH. Increased nuchal translucency with normal karyotype. Am J Obstet Gynaecol 2005; **192**: 1005–21.

Spencer K. Aneuploidy screening in the first trimester. Am J Med Genet C 2007; **145C**: 18–32.

Oligohydramnios (including Potter/oligohydramnios sequence)

Up to the 14th week of pregnancy, the amniotic fluid (liquor) is a transudate, predominantly from fetal skin, but some also occurs across the placental membranes. From 14 weeks, the fetal skin keratinizes, so the production of amniotic fluid by transudation is reduced and replaced by fetal urine production. At 16 weeks, the amniotic fluid volume is about 250 ml, increasing to about 800 ml in the third trimester. The volume is kept constant by a balance of fetal swallowing and urine production; thus, conditions that affect either of these processes lead to an abnormal amniotic volume (Beall and Ross 2013). Additionally, if there are fetal malformations (usually associated with the genitourinary tract) or there is amniorrhexis (prelabour, premature, preterm rupture of membranes (PPROM)), then the liquor volume will be significantly reduced. An estimate of the amniotic fluid volume is made by USS measurement of the largest pool of amniotic fluid, the single deepest vertical pool (DVP). This alters with gestational age. The normal range in the third trimester is >3 cm. Below 3 cm indicates too little fluid—oligohydramnios. Complete absence of amniotic fluid is anhydramnios. When the VDP is <1 cm, this may be associated with very high (>95%) perinatal mortality, especially if this occurs between 16 and 24 weeks' gestation.

Oligohydramnios

The prevalence of oligohydramnios in pregnancy is about 5%. The obstetrician will assess for the presence of non-genetic aetiological factors such as uteroplacental insufficiency or PPROM. The overall congenital malformation rate is ~5%, with renal tract malformations the most frequently seen. Bilateral renal agenesis presents with severe oligohydramnios from 14 weeks' gestation (Leung and Suen 2013). Another significant renal anomaly associated with severe oligohydramnios is congenital bladder neck obstruction.

Oligohydramnios, or Potter sequence, is a consequence of the constraint on growth and movement that occurs when the amniotic volume is significantly reduced between 16 and 24 weeks. The main components of the sequence are pulmonary hypoplasia (poor lung development), micrognathia, and postural anomalies such as talipes. The outlook for these babies is very poor but very dependent on the correct diagnosis. Aggressive management of the renal conditions postnatally is possible but associated with high rates of infant mortality. The earlier the development of oligohydramnios, the more severe the effect on lung development, but the cannicular phase of lung development (16–24 weeks) is a critical period. It may be difficult to visualize adequate fetal images on USS when the liquor volume is reduced, and MRI may be increasingly useful.

The role of the geneticist is to identify the single gene conditions with high recurrence risk.

Clinical approach

History: key points

- Three-generation family pedigree, with detailed enquiry about renal tract problems, stillbirths, or neonatal deaths.
- Consanguinity.
- Careful history regarding possible teratogens, in particular ACE inhibitors.

- Bleeding in the first few weeks of gestation or history of early PPROM (early amnio rupture).

Examination: key points

- Renal tract anomalies: cysts, Meckel syndrome (encephalocele, polydactyly, and renal malformation), AR 'infantile' polycystic kidney disease (ARPKD), multicystic dysplastic kidneys (MDK).
- Congenital bladder neck obstruction (urethral atresia or posterior urethral values). Common, but sporadic.
- Microcolon megacystis (hypoperistalsis of bowel/bladder). Mutations of muscarinic AChR M3 (Weber et al. 2011).
- Bright echodense kidneys: Meckel syndrome, ARPKD, *TCF2* mutations.
- Agenesis: Fraser syndrome, BOR syndrome, *RET* mutations, *TCF2* mutations.
- Fetal bladder not seen, with non-functioning kidneys.
- Joint contractures.
- Skull ossification defects: AR renal tubular dysgenesis (RTD), maternal ACE inhibitors.
- Lung morphology: Fraser syndrome, pulmonary hypoplasia.
- Postnatal branchial fistula: BOR syndrome.

Special investigations

- Mother to remain under careful obstetric management.
- Fetal karyotyping is indicated if there is bilateral renal involvement or an additional USS finding. Amniocentesis is not always possible, but consider genomic array analysis in the presence of additional anomalies on scan. CVS/placental biopsy/FBS/NIPD may be useful alternatives. Gene panel/WES/WGS may have an increased diagnostic role in the future.
- Consider fetal MRI if clear USS images cannot be obtained.
- Store DNA from the fetus and parents (fetal trios).
- Parental renal scans prior to genetic advice on recurrence risks may be indicated.

Syndromic diagnoses to consider

Congenital abnormalities of the kidney and urinary tract (CAKUT)

See 'Urinary tract and renal anomalies (congenital anomalies of the kidney and urinary tract—CAKUT)' in Chapter 6, 'Pregnancy and fertility', p. 796 for additional information. Unilateral renal impairment should not lead to significantly reduced liquor volume, as the other kidney can compensate. Bilateral renal agenesis affects 0.12/1000 newborns. Renal agenesis is more common in males (2.45M:1F) and there is a high incidence of associated anomalies. Bilateral MDKs have a complex genetic and syndromic aetiology. Bright hyperechogenic or echodense kidneys may also have a heterogenous genetic aetiology.

Single gene disorders

AUTOSOMAL RECESSIVE POLYCYSTIC KIDNEY DISEASE (ARPKD). Incidence is ~1/20 000 live births. It usually presents in the second or third trimester with large 'bright' kidneys and progressive oligohydramnios.

AUTOSOMAL RECESSIVE RENAL TUBULAR DYSGENESIS (RTD). A severe disorder of renal tubular development, characterized by early-onset and persistent fetal anuria leading to oligohydramnios and the Potter sequence, with additional skull ossification defects. Early death occurs in most cases from anuria, pulmonary hypoplasia, and refractory arterial hypotension. Phenocopy due to maternal ACE inhibitor therapy (Gribouval et al. 2012).

MECKEL (MECKEL–GRUBER) SYNDROME. A lethal AR syndrome with occipital encephalocele, bilaterally enlarged kidneys with multicystic dysplasia, fibrotic changes of the liver, and PAP. The kidneys are typically filled with thin-walled cysts of various sizes. The condition has been subdivided into several types and there is genetic overlap with BBS. It is one of the increasing number of conditions due to abnormalities in ciliary function. The following genes have so far been found to cause Meckel syndrome: MKS1, TMEM67, CEP290, and RPGRIP1L. There is linkage to additional loci in some families, suggesting there are more genes to be found.

BRANCHIO-OTO-RENAL (BOR) SYNDROME. AD due to mutation in EYA1. It is an extremely variable condition and it is important to consider this diagnostic possibility in all babies with renal agenesis. Carefully examine for evidence of branchial fistula(e) and ask about a history of hearing loss. Arrange parental renal scans. See 'Ear anomalies' in Chapter 2, 'Clinical approach', p. 142.

FRASER SYNDROME. An AR disorder with cryptophthalmos, laryngeal stenosis, and syndactyly. Caused by mutation in the FRAS1, GRIP1, or FREM1/2 genes. See 'Ptosis, blepharophimosis, and other eyelid anomalies' in Chapter 2, 'Clinical approach', p. 292. Bilateral hyperechogenic kidneys. There are many other genetic conditions that can also present with this feature; see 'Urinary tract and renal anomalies (congenital anomalies of the kidney and urinary tract—CAKUT)' in Chapter 6, 'Pregnancy and fertility', p. 796.

MÜLLERIAN DUCT ANOMALIES–RENAL APLASIA CERVICOTHORACIC SOMITE DYSPLASIA (MURCS). See 'Female infertility and amenorrhoea: genetic aspects' in Chapter 6, 'Pregnancy and fertility', p. 722.

CHROMOSOMAL DISORDERS. A wide range of chromosomal anomalies have been reported. These may be common autosomal aneuploidies or subtle duplications/rearrangements.

FETAL AKINESIA SYNDROMES. see 'Fetal akinesia' in Chapter 6, 'Pregnancy and fertility', p. 724.

PRELABOUR, PREMATURE RUPTURE OF MEMBRANES (PPROM). This may be associated with trauma (e.g. amniocentesis), polyhydramnios, or preterm delivery. In the majority of cases, there is no clear aetiology. Maternal and fetal infection through the genital tract is a significant risk and may be associated with chorioamnionitis and fetal or (less commonly) maternal death.

Genetic advice and management

Counsel, as appropriate, for the specific condition and refer to other chapters for more information.

Support group: ARC (Antenatal Results and Choices), http://www.arc-uk.org.

Expert advisers: Mark Kilby, Lead for Birmingham Centre for Women's & New Born's Health, University of Birmingham, Birmingham, UK and Fiona L. Mackie, Clinical Research Fellow in Obstetrics and Gynaecology, University of Birmingham, Birmingham Women's Hospital, Birmingham, UK.

References

Beall MH, Ross MG. Manipulation of amniotic fluid volume: homeostasis of fluid volumes. In: MD Kilby, D Oepkes, A Johnson (eds.). *Fetal therapy: scientific basis and critical appraisal of clinical benefits*, pp. 128–36. Cambridge University Press, New York, 2013.

Chhabra S, Dargan R, Bawaskar R. Oligohydramnios: a potential marker for serious obstetric complications. *J Obstet Gynaecol* 2007; **27**: 680–3.

Gribouval O, Morinière V, Pawtowski A, et al. Spectrum of mutations in the renin–angiotensin system genes in autosomal recessive renal tubular dysgenesis. *Hum Mutat* 2012; **33**: 316–26.

TY, Suen SSH. Manipulation of amniotic fluid volume: oligohydramnios and polyhydramnios. In: MD Kilby, D Oepkes, A Johnson (eds.). *Fetal therapy: scientific basis and critical appraisal of clinical benefits*, pp. 137–44. Cambridge University Press, New York, 2013.

Weber S, Thiele H, Mir S, et al. Muscarinic acetylcholine receptor M3 mutation causes urinary bladder disease and a prune-belly-like syndrome. *Am J Hum Genet* 2011; **89**: 668–74.

Paternal age

Maternal age counselling, predominantly for the increased risk of Down's syndrome, has always been an integral part of prenatal screening. Older mothers are more likely to have older partners and often ask if this increases their risk of miscarriage or fetal malformation syndromes. New reproductive techniques have also led to increased interest in paternal age effects.

The association of increased paternal age with single gene conditions, such as achondroplasia and Apert syndrome, has been recognized since 1957 (Penrose 1957). On average, the increase in paternal age in these 'paternal age' disorders is only 3–5 years, so many children are born to young fathers. More recently, the biological basis of this has been elucidated (Choi et al. 2008; Goriely et al. 2005). More than 98% of Apert syndrome is caused by one of two nucleotide substitutions in FGFR2. These authors have demonstrated that, in the case of Apert syndrome, the new mutation is found in foci of increased frequency within most testes; it confers a gain of function that promotes clonal expansion It is this mechanism, rather than the nucleotide being a 'hotspot' for mutation, that leads to the increased Apert risk. A similar mechanism occurs with other FRGR2 mutations associated with Crouzon and Pfeiffer syndrome, FGFR3 (TD, achondroplasia), PTPN11 (Noonan syndrome), HRAS (Costello syndrome), and RET mutations (MEN2A, MEN2B).

Many other genetic conditions, such as NF1 and TBS, show a predominantly paternal origin of mutations without a strong paternal age effect. This most likely reflects the background rate for new mutations in the genome, as recent WGS studies have shown about 80% of new mutations are paternal in origin, with each year of a father's life adding 1–2 mutations on average (Iossifov et al. 2012; Kong et al. 2012). See 'Timing and origin of new dominant mutations' in Chapter1, Introduction, p. 42.

As well as the increase in germ cell mutation, in older men, the sperm quality is reduced by impairment of DNA repair mechanisms and apoptosis. (Rolf and Nieschlag 2001).

Subfertility and miscarriage

Although males may maintain their fertility to old age, as men age, the pregnancy rate is reduced and miscarriage rate increased for both natural conception and after intrauterine insemination (Belloc et al. 2008).

Aneuploidy

There is little evidence for an increase in chromosome abnormality in children born to older fathers. Wyrobek et al. (2006) state that there is no association of increased paternal age with trisomy 21, 18, and 13, Klinefelter's syndrome, Turner syndrome, triple X and XXY, and triploidy. Toriello and Meck (2008) in their ACMG guidance for genetic counselling, while considering that the evidence is weak, nevertheless recommend a discussion about the potential increased risk for Down's syndrome.

Autism, schizophrenia, bipolar disorder, developmental delay

Several large studies have shown an association of increased paternal age in these neurodevelopmental and psychiatric conditions. An increased rate of both de novo small chromosomal abnormalities and de novo paternal origin gene mutation has been described (Iossifov et al. 2012).

De novo dominant mutations

Increased risk of de novo dominant mutation with advancing paternal age, this is greater than with advancing maternal age (see Figure 1.14 in 'Timing and origin of new dominant mutations' in Chapter 1, Introduction, p. 42).

Genetic advice and management

In the absence of a family history, no specific additional paternal age-related testing is recommended (Toriello and Meek 2008). Men with a previous child who has a genetic, chromosomal, or neurodevelopmental problem should receive additional counselling and advice about the risk to another pregnancy.

Recurrence through germline mutation for age-related mutations is low at substantially <1%; please also refer to sections on these conditions for more information.

There is also an increased risk of de novo dominant mutation with advanced paternal age and this is greater than the risk due to advanced maternal age. See Figure 1.15 in 'Timing and origin of new dominant mutations' in Chapter 1, 'Introduction', p. 42 for risk of developmental disorder due to dominant mutation based on combined maternal and paternal age.

Expert adviser: Andrew Wilkie, Nuffield Professor of Pathology, Weatherall Institute of Molecular Medicine, University of Oxford, Oxford, UK.

References

Belloc S, Cohen-Bacrie P. Effect of maternal and paternal age on pregnancy and miscarriage rates after intrauterine insemination. Reprod Biomed Online 2008; **17**: 392–7.

Böhm J, Munk-Schulenburg S, Felscher S, Kohlhase J. SALL1 mutations in sporadic Townes–Brocks syndrome are of predominantly paternal origin without obvious paternal age effect. Am J Med Genet A 2006; **140A**: 1904–8.

Chen XK, Wen SW. Paternal age and adverse birth outcomes: teenager or 40+, who is at risk? Hum Reprod 2008; **23**: 1290–6.

Choi SK, Yoon SR, Calabrese P, Arnheim N. A germ-line-selective advantage rather than an increased mutation rate can explain some unexpectedly common human disease mutations. Proc Natl Acad Sci U S A 2008; **105**: 10143–8.

Goriely A, Hansen RM, Taylor IB, et al. Activating mutations in FGFR3 and HRAS reveal a shared genetic origin for congenital disorders and testicular tumors. Nat Genet 2009; **41**: 1247–52.

Goriely A, McVean GA, van Pelt AM, et al. Gain-of-function amino acid substitutions drive positive selection of FGFR2 mutations in human spermatogonia. Proc Natl Acad Sci U S A 2005; **102**: 6051–6.

Iossifov I, Ronemus M, Levy D, et al. De novo gene disruptions in children on the autistic spectrum. Neuron 2012; **74**: 285–99.

Kong A, Frigge ML, Masson G, et al. Rate of de novo mutations and the importance of father's age to disease risk. Nature 2012; **488**: 471–5.

Penrose LS. Parental age in achondroplasia and mongolism. Am J Hum Genet 1957; **9**: 167–9.

Rolf C, Nieschlag E Reproductive functions, fertility and genetic risks of ageing men. Exp Clin Endocrinol Diabetes 2001; **109**: 68–74.

Saha S, Barnett AG, Foldi C, et al. Advanced paternal age is associated with impaired neurocognitive outcomes during infancy and childhood. PLoS Med 2009; **6**: e40.

Toriello HV, Meck JM. Statement on guidance for genetic counselling in advanced paternal age. ACMG Practice Guidelines. *Genet Med* 2008; **10**: 457–60.

Yang Q, Wen SW, Leader A, Chen XK, Lipson J, Walker M. Paternal age and birth defects: how strong is the association? *Hum Reprod* 2007; **22**: 696–701.

Wyrobek AJ, Eskenazi B, Young S, *et al.* Advancing age has differential effects on DNA damage, chromatin integrity, gene mutations, and aneuploidies in sperm. *Proc Natl Acad Sci U S A* 2006; **103**: 9601–6.

Polyhydramnios

Up to the 14th week of pregnancy, the amniotic fluid (liquor) is a transudate, predominantly from fetal skin, but also some occurs across the placental membranes. From 14 weeks, the fetal skin keratinizes, so the production of amniotic fluid by transudation is less pronounced and replaced by fetal urine production. At 16 weeks, the amniotic fluid volume is ~250 ml, increasing to about 800 ml in the third trimester. The volume is kept constant by a balance of fetal swallowing and urine production; thus, conditions that affect either of these processes lead to an abnormal amniotic volume. Additionally, if there are malformations that disrupt the integrity of the skin, such as anterior abdominal wall defects and NTDs, the amniotic fluid volume is increased by continuing transudation (Beall et al. 2013).

An estimate of the amniotic fluid volume is made by USS measurement of the maximal pool of amniotic fluid, the single deepest vertical pool (DVP). The normal range of DVP change with gestational age but, should not be greater than 8cm. Measurements larger than 8 cm are indicative of too much fluid—polyhydramnios (hydramnios, USA).

Polyhydramnios is found in 1–2% of pregnancies. About 8% have additional fetal anomalies on USS. In up to 60%, the cause is unknown (idiopathic), though these pregnancies carry a 2- to 5-fold increase in perinatal mortality, especially in non-diabetic women (Biggio et al. 1999; Magann et al. 2007).

The maternofetal medicine team will assess for the presence of structural fetal anomalies (predominantly due to upper GI obstruction or brainstem anomalies) or placental anomalies (most commonly chorioangioma). Polyhydramnios may complicate monochorionic multiple pregnancies (with twin-to-twin transfusion syndrome), maternal diabetes (pre-existing or pregnancy-acquired), red cell alloimmunization, and congenital infection (i.e. parvovirus B19) (Leung et al. 2013). The geneticist is asked to assist when there is no obvious obstetric aetiology or, in the presence of fetal multiple malformations, to identify an underlying syndrome or single gene condition.

Clinical approach

History: key points

- Three-generation family pedigree, with detailed enquiry relating to renal tract problems, stillbirths, or neonatal deaths.
- Consanguinity.
- Careful maternal history; diabetes mellitus, features of myotonic dystrophy.
- Presence of other obstetric risk factors such as multiple pregnancy and alloimmunization (i.e. rhesus disease).

Examination: key points

- Detailed level III USS and fetal surveillance to detect the presence of fetal malformations, tumours (i.e. sacrococcygeal teratoma), hydrops, and macrosomia.
- Doppler studies of the middle cerebral artery can screen for fetal anaemia.
- Bowel atresias (upper GI most commonly). Absent or small 'stomach bubble' (tracheo-oesophageal atresia, oesophageal atresia; see 'Oesophageal and intestinal atresia (including tracheo-oesophageal fistula' in Chapter 2, 'Clinical approach', p. 266).

- Double-bubble duodenal atresia (associated with trisomy 21 in 15–20% of prenatal cases).
- Macrosomia (Beckwith syndrome (usually with small omphalocele), maternal glucose intolerance).
- Micrognathia significant enough to cause abnormalities of swallowing (Pierre–Robin and other craniofacial malformations).
- Bilateral talipes (myotonic dystrophy) or fetal akinesia syndrome.
- Severe CNS malformations may indicate a neurological inability to swallow.
- Renal anomalies. Agenesis (VACTERL), bright/cystic (Fryns syndrome, nephroblastomatosis).
- Cardiac defect (VACTERL, CHARGE) involving CM and supraventricular or atrial tachycardia, usually with hydrops fetalis (Costello and CFC syndrome).
- Skeletal dysplasia (mostly lethal dysplasias), congenital diaphragmatic hernia (Fryns, Pallister–Killian (mosaic tetrasomy 12p)).
- Any cause of fetal hydrops. There is overlap between conditions that lead to hydrops and polyhydramnios. See 'Oedema—increased nuchal translucency, cystic hygroma, and hydrops' in Chapter 6, 'Pregnancy and fertility', p. 768.

Special investigations

- Fetal array (e.g. by amniocentesis, CVS, or NIPT in the presence of fetal anomalies).
- DNA storage/and specific testing, if indicated (most helpfully by fetal 'trios'). Gene panel/WES/WGS may have an increased diagnostic role in future.
- Consider maternal testing for myotonic dystrophy (if specific concern).
- Maternal serological testing for CMV, human parvovirus B19, syphilis, and toxoplasmosis, if USS features suggest fetal infection.
- Consider whether biochemistry of the amniotic fluid may be feasible to investigate for Bartter syndrome and congenital diarrhoea (rare).

Syndromic diagnoses to consider

Bowel atresia

- Tracheo-oesophageal fistula/atresia and associated syndromes (see also 'Oesophageal and intestinal atresia (including tracheo-oesophageal fistula' in Chapter 2, 'Clinical approach', p. 266). Particularly look for features of VACTERL and CHARGE, but consider rare single gene aetiology if there is a family history of bowel atresia, e.g. Feingold syndrome, epidermolysis bullosa with pyloric atresia.
- Trisomy 21 with duodenal atresia may present with polyhydramnios.

Neurological conditions

- Myotonic dystrophy (see 'Myotonic dystrophy (DM1)' in Chapter 3, 'Common consultations', p. 496).
- CNS disorders and myopathies.

- FADS. With poor fetal swallowing and impaired fetal movement. See 'Fetal akinesia' in Chapter 6, 'Pregnancy and fertility', p. 724.

Overgrowth syndromes
- BWS (see 'Beckwith–Wiedemann syndrome (BWS)' in Chapter 3, 'Common consultations', p. 358).
- Pallister–Killian syndrome.
- Costello syndrome and CFC syndrome. Increased nuchal measurement, overgrowth, relative macrocephaly. Atrial tachycardia common in Costello syndrome. Germline *HRAS* mutations in patients with Costello syndrome and mutations in *KRAS, BRAF, MEK1*, and *MEK2* and other genes in the RAS pathway in CFC syndrome.

Renal tubular disorders
Prenatal/neonatal Bartter syndrome is a hereditary salt-losing renal tubulopathy due to mutations in genes encoding proteins involved in sodium chloride reabsorption in the ascending limb of Henle. Congenital deafness is seen in patients with *BSND* mutations; transient neonatal hyperkalaemia was present in two-thirds of children with *KCNJ1* mutations. Nephrocalcinosis was constant in *KCNJ1* and *SLC12A1* patients (Brochard *et al.* 2009). These will not be detected *in utero*.

Hemizygous mutations in *MAGED2* cause XL polyhydramnios with prematurity and a severe, but transient, form of antenatal Bartter syndrome (Laghmani *et al.* 2016), with onset of polyhydramnios from 19 to 20 weeks and neonatal polyuria usually ending at 30–33 weeks gestational age (mean gestation at delivery was 28 weeks).

Congenital diarrhoea
Congenital chloride diarrhoea results from biallelic mutation in the *SLC26A3* gene and is characterized by the excretion of large volumes of watery stool containing high levels of chloride, resulting in dehydration, hypokalaemia, and metabolic alkalosis (Hoglund *et al.* 2001). In fetal life, this condition may cause multiple dilated fluid loops of bowel that may be detectable by USS.

Fetal infections
Many fetal infections may cause polyhydramnios. These include acute CMV, toxoplasmosis, and, probably most commonly in Europe, human parvovirus B19. Worldwide, syphilis may be associated with increased liquor, especially if there is associated hydrops.

Genetic advice and management
Counsel, as appropriate, for the specific condition and refer to other chapters for more information.

Support group: ARC (Antenatal Results and Choices), http://www.arc-uk.org.

Expert advisers: Mark Kilby, Lead for Birmingham Centre for Women's & New Born's Health, University of Birmingham, Birmingham, UK and Fiona L. Mackie, Clinical Research Fellow in Obstetrics and Gynaecology, University of Birmingham, Birmingham Women's Hospital, Birmingham, UK.

References
Beall MH, Ross MG. Manipulation of amniotic fluid volume: homeostasis of fluid volumes. In: MD Kilby, D Oepkes, A Johnson (eds.). *Fetal therapy: scientific basis and critical appraisal of clinical benefits*, pp. 128–36. Cambridge University Press, New York, 2013.

Biggio JR, Wenstrom KD, Dubard MB, Cliver SP. Hydramnios prediction of adverse perinatal outcome. *Obstet Gynecol* 1999; **94**: 773–7.

Brochard K, Boyer O, Blanchard A, *et al.* Phenotype–genotype correlation in antenatal and neonatal variants of Bartter syndrome. *Nephrol Dial Transplant* 2009; **24**: 1455–64.

Harman C. Amniotic fluid abnormalities. *Semin Perinatol* 2008; **32**: 288–94.

Hoglund P, Sormaala M, Haila S, *et al.* Identification of seven novel mutations including the first two genomic rearrangements in SLC26A3 mutated in congenital chloride diarrhea. *Hum Mutat* 2001; **18**: 233–42.

Laghmani K, Beck BB, Yang SS, *et al.* Polyhydramnios, transient antenatal Bartter's syndrome and MAGED2 mutations. *N Engl J Med* 2016; **374**: 1853–63.

Leung TY, Suen SSH. Manipulation of amniotic fluid volume: oligohydramnios and polyhydramnios. In: MD Kilby, D Oepkes, A Johnson (eds.). *Fetal therapy: scientific basis and critical appraisal of clinical benefits*, pp. 137–44. Cambridge University Press, New York, 2013.

Lin AE, O'Brien B, Demmer LA, *et al.* Prenatal features of Costello syndrome: ultrasonographic findings and atrial tachycardia. *Prenat Diagn* 2009; **29**: 682–90.

Magann EF, Chauhan SP, Doherty DA, Lutgendorf MA, Magann MI, Morrison JC. A review of idiopathic hydramnios and pregnancy outcomes. *Obstet Gynecol Surv* 2007; **62**: 795–802.

Posterior fossa malformations

Includes Dandy–Walker syndrome, Dandy–Walker variant, Dandy–Walker complex. See 'Cerebellar anomalies' in Chapter 2, 'Clinical approach', p. 92.

Dandy–Walker malformation (DWM) is a developmental anomaly of the posterior fossa. It is characterized by:

- cystic dilatation of the fourth ventricle;
- complete or partial agenesis of the cerebellar vermis;
- enlargement of the posterior fossa, with upward displacement of the tentorium.

DWM is heterogeneous in aetiology. It should be differentiated from Dandy–Walker variant (see below).

Nearly half of fetuses with DWM have a chromosome anomaly. DWM should not be diagnosed prior to 18 weeks' gestation (although it may be suspected earlier). The cerebellar vermis does not finish its development until 17–18 weeks' gestation and, at 15–16 weeks, it is not uncommon to find the cerebellar vermis incompletely formed.

Clinical outcome varies from normal development to severe handicap and perinatal death. Poor fetal or perinatal outcome may be related to extra-CNS malformations, e.g. cardiac defects. Aletebi and Fung (1999) found neurodevelopmental delay in 80% of survivors with follow-up to 4 years of age. Guibaud et al. (2012) report that 4/5 children born with isolated DWM required shunts.

Dandy–Walker variant (DWV)

Cerebellar vermis hypoplasia with some cystic dilation communicating with the fourth ventricle. Very careful assessment is needed to try and ascertain if isolated or part of a syndrome, particularly ciliopathies, wider neurological disorders that may be associated with hydrocephalus or arthrogryposis or SLO syndrome. Isolated DWV generally has a favourable prognosis, but the syndromic conditions may lead to significant disability.

Clinical assessment

History: key points

- Take a detailed three-generation family history and enquire carefully about consanguinity.

Examination: key points

- If identified at 20 weeks' gestation, fetal anomaly USS:
  - look carefully for other CNS malformations, e.g. ventriculomegaly (32%), ACC, holoprosencephaly, lissencephaly, occipital meningocele, or encephalocele;
  - small posterior fossa causes include the many genetic syndromes associated with DWV, rhombencephalosynapsis, pontocerebellar hypoplasias, and cerebellar atrophy (Shekdar 2011);
  - large posterior fossa causes include mainly sporadic developmental disorders such as classic DWM, Blake's pouch cyst, mega cisterna magna, and posterior fossa arachnoid cyst;

- look carefully for extra-CNS malformations, e.g. cardiac defects (40%; chromosomal anomaly or 3C), polydactyly (+13, Joubert), renal anomaly, arthrogryposis, sex reversal.

Special investigations

- Offer genomic analysis/array/karyotype, as available (46% had abnormal karyotype in Ecker et al.'s (2000) series, 6p subtelomeric deletions, Guibaud et al. (2012). Consider gene panel/WES/WGS, as appropriate.
- TORCH screen.
- Consider fetal brain MRI to assess for additional cerebral anomalies and to offer confirmation of the diagnosis by a different scanning modality. Guibaud et al. (2012) highlighted the inaccuracy of magnetic resonance for anatomical analysis of the vermis.

Genetic advice and management

- If a chromosome anomaly is identified, counsel as appropriate.
- If additional findings on USS, this strongly increases the possibility of a syndromic association (e.g. ciliopathy, WWS, SLO). Since many of these conditions follow AR inheritance, there is often a high recurrence risk.
- When the evidence suggests that DWM has not occurred as part of a Mendelian or chromosomal disorder, then the recurrence risk is relatively low, in the order of 1–5% (Murray et al. 1985).

Expert adviser: Charu Deshpande, Consultant Clinical Geneticist, Guy's and St Thomas' NHS Foundation Trust, London, UK.

References

Aletebi FA, Fung KF. Neurodevelopmental outcome after antenatal diagnosis of posterior fossa abnormalities. *J Ultrasound Med* 1999; **18**: 683–9.

Ecker JL, Shipp TD, Bromley B, Benacerraf B. The sonographic diagnosis of Dandy–Walker and Dandy–Walker variant: associated findings and outcomes. *Prenat Diagn* 2000; **20**: 328–32.

Forzano F, Mansour S, Ierullo A, Homfray T, Thilaganathan B. Posterior fossa malformation in fetuses: a report of 56 further cases and a review of the literature. *Prenat Diagn* 2007; **27**: 495–501.

Guibaud L, Larroque A, Ville D, et al. Prenatal diagnosis of 'isolated' Dandy–Walker malformation: imaging findings and prenatal counseling. *Prenat Diagn* 2012; **32**: 185–93.

Kolble N, Wisser J, Kurmanavicius J, et al. Dandy–Walker malformation: prenatal diagnosis and outcome. *Prenat Diagn* 2000; **20**: 318–27.

Murray JC, Johnson JA, Bird TD. Dandy–Walker malformation: etiologic heterogeneity and empiric recurrence risks. *Clin Genet* 1985; **28**: 272–83.

Parisi MA, Dobyns WB. Human malformations of the midbrain and hindbrain: review and proposed classification scheme. *Mol Genet Metab* 2003; **80**: 36–53.

Shekdar K. Posterior fossa malformations. *Semin Ultrasound CT MR* 2011; **32**: 228–41.

Premature ovarian failure (POF)

The median age at menopause in Western populations of women is ~51 years. By convention, menopause that occurs at ages 40–45 years is considered 'early' and occurs in about 5% of women. POF is defined as cessation of menses due to hypergonadotrophic amenorrhoea below the age of 40 years. It occurs in ~1% of women in the general population. Depending upon the age at diagnosis, the probability of a genetic, autoimmune, or idiopathic cause will be more or less likely. At least one-third to one-half of cases remain idiopathic.

Women with POF are usually investigated and managed by a gynaecologist and are only referred to a geneticist if there is a strong family history or if a genetic aetiology seems likely. Normal FSH with elevated oestrogen indicates diminished ovarian reserve. High concentrations of FSH (>20 iu/l) associated with low concentrations of oestradiol are seen in patients with POF.

Among women with idiopathic sporadic POF, ~2% carry a FRAXA premutation. Among women with familial POF, ~14% carry a FRAXA premutation.

Xq26.2–Xq28 appears to contain a critical region for normal ovarian function.

Despite the description of several candidate genes, the cause of POF remains undetermined in the vast majority of cases (Cordts et al. 2011).

DEVELOPMENT OF THE OVARY. After migration of the primordial germ cells into the developing ovary, the population of germ cells increases by mitosis to reach a maximum of 78 million at around 20 weeks' gestation. The population of germ cells declines steadily thereafter by the process of atresia to reach a level of around 1–2 million at birth (Baker 1963).

Clinical assessment

History: key points
- Three-generation family tree, noting age of menopause in relatives and enquiring about family history of learning disability.
- Personal history noting age of menarche and menopause.
- Past medical history. Treatment with cytotoxic agents or radiotherapy for treatment of childhood cancer?

Examination: key points
- Height.
- Examine briefly for physical features of TS, e.g. short, broad, webbed neck and low posterior hairline. Wide carrying angle. Shield-shaped chest. Heart murmur.

Special investigations
- The reproductive medicine team will usually have arranged a hormone analysis and an autoimmune screen.
- Karyotype. In addition, consider mosaicism screen (30 cells) to investigate for TS mosaic.
- FRAXA analysis.

Diagnoses to consider

Turner syndrome (TS)
Typically, in TS, menopause precedes menarche, and there is no evidence of ovarian function, but occasional individuals with TS may menstruate briefly. See 'Turner syndrome, 45,X and variants' in Chapter 5, 'Chromosomes', p. 696.

Mosaic Turner syndrome
Guttenbach et al. (1995) found a significant correlation between X chromosome loss and ageing, with the frequency of X chromosome loss ranging from 1.5% to 2.5% in prepubertal females, rising to ~4.5–5% in women older than 75 years. Thus, interpretation of the significance of low-level 45,X/46,XX mosaicism in a woman with POF can be difficult. Devi et al. (1998) found that, in patients with POF, the percentage of cells with a single X chromosome (mean, 5.50) was significantly greater than in controls of similar age (mean, 2.42), implying that some cases of POF may be attributable to low-level 45,X/46,XX mosaicism.

X-chromosome rearrangements
Some X deletions and translocations are known to be responsible for POF. Xq26.2–Xq28 appears to contain a critical region for normal ovarian function.

Fragile X premutation carrier
Approximately 20% of female premutation carriers will undergo premature menopause (cessation of menses at <40 years), compared to 1% of the general population. The risk appears to be greater for premutations in the 80–100 CGG repeat range. This information may be helpful to carrier women for reproductive planning (e.g. if considering PGD). See 'Fragile X syndrome (FRAX)' in Chapter 3, 'Common consultations', p. 424.

Survivor of radiation- and chemotherapy-treated childhood cancer
Larsen et al. (2003) evaluated ovarian function in 100 survivors of childhood cancer and found that one in every six female survivors had developed POF. Results from survivors with spontaneous menstrual cycles indicated a diminished ovarian reserve, with the expectation that cessation of fertility may occur at an earlier age than normal.

Galactosaemia
The development of POF in females with galactosaemia is more likely if the patient's GALT genotype is Q188R/Q188R and if the mean erythrocyte Gal-1-P is >3.5 mg/dl during therapy.

FSH receptor mutations
Inactivating mutations of the FSH receptor have been described in rare cases of POF. This is a rare AR cause of POF, characterized by high plasma FSH levels associated with very low oestrogen and inhibin B levels. No biological response to high doses of recombinant FSH is detected (Meduri et al. 2003).

Blepharophimosis–ptosis–epicanthus inversus syndrome (BPES)
In this condition, there is a reduced horizontal diameter of the palpebral fissures, droopy eyelids, and a fold of skin that runs from the lower lids inwards and upwards (epicanthus inversus). Mutations in FOXL2, a forkhead transcription factor on 3q, are found in ~67% of patients. Intelligence is mostly normal, except where there is a microdeletion encompassing the gene. In type I BPES, eyelid abnormalities are associated with POF and type II has eyelid defects only. See 'Ptosis, blepharophimosis, and other eyelid anomalies' in Chapter 2, 'Clinical approach', p. 292.

Autoimmune polyendocrinopathy–candidiasis–ectodermal dystrophy (APECED)
A rare AR disorder caused by mutations in the auto-immune regulator (*AIRE*) gene on chromosome 21q22.3. Patients most often suffer from loss of endocrine function in the parathyroid and adrenal glands but may also develop T1D, thyroid disease, or hypogonadism. Hypoparathyroidism is much more common in affected females than in affected males.

Genetic advice and management
Woman with POF should be given HRT at least until the age of 50. HRT is preferable to the contraceptive pill, which will also provide an artificial menstrual cycle but will not allow ovulation to occur. If pregnancy is desired, it can occur while taking HRT, even though the chances of ovulation are extremely unlikely. It is possible to have IVF using donated eggs that have been fertilized by the sperm of the recipient's partner and created embryos can be transferred to the recipient uterus after a special HRT regimen.

Support group: The Daisy Network, https://www.daisynetwork.org.uk.

References
Baker T. A quantitative and cytological study of germ cells in human ovaries. *Proc R Soc London (B)* 1963; **158**: 417–33.

Browne C, Strike P, Jacobs PA. X chromosome loss and ageing. *J Med Genet* 2002; **39**: S30.

Cordts EB, Christofolini DM, Dos Santos AA, Bianco B, Barbosa CP. Genetic aspects of premature ovarian failure: a literature review. *Arch Gynecol Obstet* 2011; **283**: 635–43.

Devi AS, Metzger DA, Luciano AA, Benn PA. 45,X/46,XX mosaicism in patients with idiopathic premature ovarian failure. *Fertil Steril* 1998; **70**: 89–93.

Guerrero NV, Singh RH, Manatunga A, Berry GT, Steiner RD, Elsas LJ 2nd. Risk factors for premature ovarian failure in females with galactosemia. *Pediatrics* 2000; **137**: 833–41.

Guttenbach M, Koschorz B, Bernthaler U, Grimm T, Schmid M. Sex chromosome loss and aging: in situ hybridization studies on human interphase nuclei. *Am J Hum Genet* 1995; **57**: 1143–50.

Laml T, Preyer O, Umek W, Hengstschlager M, Hanzal H. Genetic disorders in premature ovarian failure. *Hum Reprod Update* 2002; **8**: 483–91.

Larsen EC, Muller J, Schmiegelow K, Rechnitzer C, Andersen AN. Reduced ovarian function in long-term survivors of radiation- and chemotherapy-treated childhood cancer. *J Clin Endocrinol Metab* 2003; **88**: 5307–14.

Marozzi A, Manfredini E, Tibiletti MG, *et al.* Molecular definition of Xq common-deleted region in patients affected by premature ovarian failure. *Hum Genet* 2000; **107**: 304–11.

Meduri G, Touraine P, Beau I, *et al.* Delayed puberty and primary amenorrhea associated with a novel mutation of the human follicle-stimulating hormone receptor: clinical, histological, and molecular studies. *J Clin Endocrinol Metab* 2003; **88**: 3491–8.

Meyer G, Badenhoop K. Autoimmune regulator (*AIRE*) gene on chromosome 21: implications for autoimmune polyendo-crinopathy–candidiasis–ectodermal dystrophy (APECED) any more common manifestations of endocrine autoimmunity. *J Endocrinol Invest* 2002; **25**: 804–11.

Santoro N. Mechanisms of premature ovarian failure. *Ann Endocrinol (Paris)* 2003; **64**: 87–92.

Sherman SL. Premature ovarian failure in the fragile X syndrome. *Am J Med Genet* 2000; **97**: 189–94.

Radiation exposure, chemotherapy, and landfill sites

Radiation

Exposure to ionizing radiation during pregnancy may be associated with pregnancy loss, microcephaly, microphthalmia, cataracts, impaired neurodevelopment, and fetal growth restriction. The risk of these adverse outcomes is, however, dependent both on the absorbed dose of radiation (deterministic effects) and the stage of pregnancy during which exposure occurs. Women exposed at any stage of pregnancy to <100 mGy of radiation are not thought to be at an increased risk of the above effects. Case-specific advice may also be sought from teratology information services around the world (http://www.UKTIS.org in the UK).

Radiation-induced heritable diseases or transgenerational effects due to stochastic mutagenesis in maternal or fetal germ cells have not been demonstrated in humans and estimates of genetic risks for protection purposes are based on mouse experiments. The most comprehensive epidemiological study is of the Japanese atomic bomb survivors and their children, which found little evidence for inherited defects attributable to parental radiation. Studies of workers exposed to occupational radiation or of populations exposed to environmental radiation appear too small and exposures too low to convincingly detect inherited genetic damage (Boice et al. 2003). Current risk estimates of germ cell mutation are around one in 200 000 per mGy of exposure.

Diagnostic radiation

Radiation exposure depends on the diagnostic imaging procedure (e.g. estimated fetal absorbed dose for a chest X-ray 0.001 0.01 mGy versus abdominal/chest CT 10–50 mGy). Where serial imaging is being considered, caution must be applied to ensure exposure is within recommended limits (Wall et al. 2009). UK guidelines recommend that pregnant women should not be exposed to doses above 50 mGy to ensure an additional margin of safety below the no observed adverse effect level (NOAEL) of 100 mGy for the deterministic effects described above.

The main consideration is the possible incremental added risk for childhood cancer following fetal exposure.

The estimated background risk of childhood cancer is ~0.2% (one in 500) (Stiller 2007) Observational studies have reported a doubling in the rate of childhood cancer following in utero exposure to diagnostic radiation doses of 25 mGy. Using these data to calculate an absolute childhood cancer risk coefficient, it is therefore suggested that there is an ~1 in 13 000 risk of childhood cancer per mGy of ionizing radiation exposure, independent of the gestational age at which exposure occurs beyond weeks 3–4.

Background radiation in Cambridge, UK is about 2.5 mSv per annum.

Chemotherapy

Two recent studies (Signorello et al. 2012; Stensheim et al. 2013) offer strong evidence that the children of cancer survivors are not at significantly increased risk for congenital anomalies stemming from their parent's exposure to mutagenic cancer treatments. In the study by Signorello et al. (2012) (the Cancer Survivor Study), 4699

offspring were assessed for the incidence of congenital anomalies. One hundred and twenty-nine children had at least one anomaly (prevalence = 2.7%). For children whose mothers were exposed to radiation or alkylating agents versus neither, the prevalence of anomalies was 3.0% versus 3.5% ($P = 0.51$); corresponding figures were 1.9% versus 1.7% ($P = 0.79$) for children of male survivors. In Stensheim et al.'s (2013) case-control study of Norwegian cancer survivors, they compared birth outcomes in 3915 female and male survivors and 144 653 controls from the general population with similar parity. The Norwegian study did find an increased risk for preterm birth among the offspring of female cancer survivors (OR, 1.30 for nullips; OR, 1.89 for primips) and recommended close antenatal follow-up.

Landfill sites

Eighty per cent of the population of the UK live within 2 km of a landfill site.

In Elliott et al.'s (2001) survey of >1 million live births in the UK, the relative risk for women resident within <2 km of a landfill site for all congenital anomalies was 1.01 (adjusted for confounders), i.e. there is a very small excess risk of congenital anomalies. Adjusted risks were 1.05 for NTDs, 1.07 for hypospadias and epispadias, 1.19 for gastroschisis and exomphalos, 1.05 for low birthweight (<2.5 kg), and 1.04 for very low birthweight (<1.5 kg). There was no excess risk for stillbirth. In reality, what this means is: 'this 1% higher rate of birth defects would represent about 100 cases of birth defects each year across England and Wales. This is out of a total of ~12 000 cases of birth defects expected each year in England and Wales' (Troop 2001).

The EUROHAZCON study found a 33% increase in the risk of non-chromosomal anomalies for residents living within 3 km of 21 European hazardous waste landfill sites. A similar effect was found for chromosomal anomalies, with an OR of 1.41 for chromosomal anomalies, in people who lived close to the sites (0–3 km), compared with those who lived further away (3–7 km), after adjustment for confounding by maternal age and socioeconomic status (Dolk et al. 1998). There was a correlation between risk and distance from the site—anomalies included NTDs, cardiac septal defects, anomalies of the great arteries and veins, borderline significance for trachea-oesophageal anomalies, hypospadias, and gastroschisis. However subsequent studies reported smaller increases in risks and confounding from other factors was likely.

Elliott et al. (2009) found a weak spatial association between the risk of certain congenital anomalies and the geographic density of hazardous waste sites, but no excess risk in relation to sites handling non-specialized waste. In a review undertaken in 2011, the UK Health Protection Agency concluded that this study 'did not give grounds for any specific concerns or recommendations relating to the health of pregnant women or those wishing to start a family who live in the vicinity of a landfill site'.

Sources of advice: Information on the fetal effects of these and other exposures in pregnancy is available from teratology information services worldwide. The UK Teratology Information Service (http://www.UKTIS.

org) provides up-to-date information as written reviews on http://www.toxbase.org (free of charge to NHS healthcare professionals) and case-specific risk assessments via a national telephone service, 0844 892 0909.

Expert adviser: Laura Yates, Consultant in Clinical Genetics (NGS) and Head of Teratology (UKTIS), Institute of Genetic Medicine, Newcastle upon Tyne Hospitals NHS Foundation Trust & Newcastle University, Newcastle upon Tyne, UK.

References

www.doh.gov.uk/landfillrep.pdf. Final Landfill Report Dec 2001.

Boice JD Jr, Tawn EJ, Winther JF, et al. Genetic effects of radiotherapy for childhood cancer. *Health Phys* 2003; **85**: 65–80.

Dolk H, Vrijheid M, Armstrong B, et al. Risk of congenital anomalies near hazardous-waste landfill sites in Europe: the EUROHAZCON study. *Lancet* 1998; **352**: 423–7.

Elliott P, Briggs D, Morris S, et al. Risk of adverse birth outcomes in populations living near landfill sites. *BMJ* 2001; **323**: 363–8.

Elliott P, Richardson S, Abellan JJ, et al. Geographic density of landfill sites and risk of congenital anomalies in England. *Occup Environ Med* 2009; **66**: 81–9.

Sharp C, Shrimpton JA, Bury RF. Diagnostic medical exposures: advice on exposure to ionising radiation during pregnancy. *Joint Guidance from National Radiological Protection Board, College of Radiographers, Royal College of Radiologists*. National Radiological Protection Board, Didcot, 1998.

Signorello LB, Mulvihill JJ, Green DM, et al. Congenital anomalies in the children of cancer survivors: a report from the childhood cancer survivor study. *J Clin Oncol* 2012; **30**: 239–45.

Stensheim H, Klungsoyr K, Skjaerven R, Grotmol T, Fosså SD. Birth outcomes among offspring of adult cancer survivors: a population-based study. *Int J Cancer* 2013; **133**: 2696–705.

Stiller C (ed.). *Childhood cancer in Britain: incidence, survival and mortality*. Oxford University Press, Oxford, 2007.

Troop P. Department of Health briefing CEM/CMO/2001/10.

Vrijheid M, Dolk H, Armstrong B, et al. Chromosomal congenital anomalies and residence near hazardous waste landfill sites. *Lancet* 2002; **359**: 320–2.

Wall BF, Meara JR, Muirhead CR, Bury CF, Murray M. Protection of pregnant patients during diagnostic medical exposures to ionising radiation (RCE-9). *Advice from the Health Protection Agency, the Royal College of Radiologists, and the College of Radiographers*. Health Protection Agency, Didcot, 2009.

Rubella

Rubella is a mild viral illness that causes a transient, fine, erythematous macular rash, lymphadenopathy involving post-auricular and suboccipital glands, and, occasionally in adults, arthritis and arthralgia. In unimmunized populations, it is most common among children aged 4–9 years. Clinical diagnosis is unreliable as other viruses can cause a similar picture. The period of infectivity is from about a week before until a week after the onset of the rash. The incubation period is 14–21 days.

Congenital rubella syndrome (CRS)

In contrast to the mild nature of rubella in children, it can cause a devastating embryopathy (see Box 6.6). Maternal rubella infection at 2–10 weeks' gestation results in fetal damage in up to 90% of infants and multiple defects are common; by 16 weeks' gestation, the risk of damage declines to ~10–20%, and fetal damage is rare after this stage in pregnancy.

Some affected infants appear normal at birth, but sensorineural deafness is detected later. Before immunization programmes were introduced, CRS was an important cause of congenital deafness.

Rubella re-infection can occur in individuals with either natural or vaccine-induced antibody. Occasional cases of CRS after re-infection in pregnancy have been reported. Although the risk to the fetus cannot be quantified precisely, it is considered to be low.

Rubella vaccine

- As the vaccine virus is *not* transmitted from vaccinees to susceptible contacts, there is no risk to pregnant women from contact with recently immunized subjects.
- Active surveillance in the USA, UK, and Germany found no cases of CRS following inadvertent immunization shortly before or during pregnancy. There is no evidence that the attenuated vaccine virus is teratogenic. TOP following inadvertent immunization should *not* be recommended (Department of Health 2006). Nevertheless, rubella vaccine should not be given to a woman known to be pregnant and pregnancy should be avoided for 1 month after immunization (Department of Health 2006).

Box 6.6 Features of congenital rubella syndrome

- IUGR
- Microcephaly
- Cataract, pigmentary retinopathy[*], and other eye defects
- Sensorineural deafness[*]
- Cardiac abnormalities, including patent ductus arteriosus (PDA), peripheral pulmonary artery stenosis, and septal defects
- Inflammatory lesions of the brain, liver, lungs, and bone marrow

[*] The only defects that commonly occur in isolation are sensorineural deafness and pigmentary retinopathy.

Epidemiology

Following the introduction of population vaccination programmes, rubella infection and especially CRS have become rare in the UK and most parts of the developed world (see Figure 6.8). Sporadic cases occur in the UK, often associated with travel abroad. Hardelid et al.'s (2009) population-based survey of births occurring in an ethnically diverse English region in 2004 showed that women born in Africa and Asia were 4–5 times more likely to be susceptible to rubella than those born in the UK. If rubella were to re-establish itself in the UK, women who had come to Britain in later childhood or adult life would be at higher risk of acquiring infection in pregnancy than indigenous women.

CRS remains a problem in the developing world where there are an estimated 100 000 CRS births a year, mainly in Africa and South East Asia. In 2012 the World Health Organization published a strategic plan for the global elimination of measles, rubella and congenital rubella (<1 case per 100 000 live births) in at least five of the six WHO Regions by 2020. The WHO Region of the Americas, with no evidence of endemic transmission of rubella or congenital rubella in the previous five consecutive years, confirmed elimination of rubella and congenital rubella in 2015.

Clinical assessment

History: key points, postnatal

- Detailed history regarding timing of exposure to rubella or onset of rash.

Examination: key points, postnatal

- Growth parameters, including OFC.
- Heart.
- Eyes for cataracts, pigmentary retinopathy.

Special investigations: prenatal

- Maternal rubella virus serology. (If the pregnancy may be at risk because of possible contact with a child/adult with rubella, establish the maternal status prior to invasive testing in the fetus.)
- USS: growth retardation, cardiac defects.
- FBS for: (1) PCR for rubella virus RNA in fetal blood and (2) rubella virus-specific IgM. NB. No rubella virus RNA was detectable in amniotic fluid after a maternal rash at 15 weeks' gestation, despite being present in fetal blood (Tang et al. 2003).

Special investigations: postnatal

- Confirmation of congenital infection. Look for rubella virus RNA in serum and urine.
- Serum for rubella virus-specific IgM and IgG.
- Ophthalmology referral (cataract and pigmentary retinopathy).
- Audiometry (sensorineural deafness).
- Echo.
- Consider cranial imaging. ICC can occur (Numazaki and Fujikawa 2003).

Genetic advice and management

In the UK, all children should be immunized with MMR (measles, mumps, and rubella) vaccine at 12–13 months

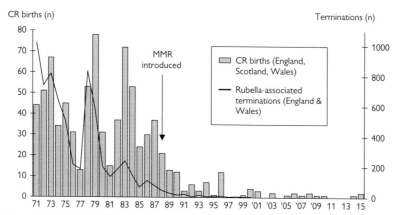

Figure 6.8 Congenital rubella births (NCRSP) 1971–2015 and rubella-associated terminations (ONS) 1971–2000. Terminations data not published since 2000 because of very low numbers.
Reproduced under the Open Government Licence v3.0.

with a second dose in the 4th year of life (Department of Health 2006). This is intended to prevent the circulation of rubella virus by providing high herd immunity, thereby protecting pregnant women from exposure to rubella infection. The vaccine is also available for children, teenagers and adults who did not receive two doses of MMR at earlier ages. Women planning to become pregnant are advised to check their vaccination status with their GP; if there is any indication that they might be susceptible to rubella they should be offered MMR vaccine and advised to avoid conception for one month after receipt of the vaccine. Pregnant women who come into contact with, or have, a rash illness in pregnancy, are advised to seek advice from their GP or midwife immediately, regardless of their vaccination status; they require serological investigation, and should be managed according to the latest guidance issued by Public Health England (PHE 2011).

The antenatal screening programme for rubella susceptibility, which had been in place throughout the UK for over 40 years, ceased in 2016. Pregnant women who have not previously had two doses of MMR should be offered the vaccine post-partum at their 6-week check, to protect any future pregnancy.

Expert adviser: Pat Tookey, Honorary Senior Lecturer, Population Policy and Practice Programme, University College London, Institute of Child Health, London, UK.

References

Department of Health. Immunisation against infectious disease, 3rd edn. The Stationery Office, London, 2006. Updates available at https://www.gov.uk/government/collections/immunisation-against-infectious-disease-the-green-book.

Hardelid P, Cortina-Borja M, Williams D, et al. Rubella seroprevalence in pregnant women in North Thames: estimates based on newborn screening samples. J Med Screen 2009; **16**: 1–6.

Numazaki K, Fujikawa T. Intracranial calcification with congenital rubella syndrome in a mother with serologic immunity. J Child Neurol 2003; **18**: 296–7.

Public Health England. Guidance on viral rash in pregnancy: investigation, diagnosis and management of viral rash illness, or exposure to viral rash illness, in pregnancy, 2011. https://www.gov.uk/government/publications/viral-rash-in-pregnancy.

Tang JW, Aarons E, Hesketh LM, et al. Prenatal diagnosis of congenital rubella infection in the second trimester of pregnancy. Prenat Diagn 2003; **23**: 509–12.

Short limbs

The femur length is measured routinely during the anomaly USS at 18–20 weeks' gestation in order to compare it with other fetal measurements, such as head circumference (HC) and abdominal circumference (AC), to assess proportionate growth.

A short femur may indicate/be a feature of:

- incorrect dates;
- a small normal baby;
- IUGR, which would be very severe to be detected at 20 weeks;
- a chromosomal disorder;
- a skeletal dysplasia;
- a malformation syndrome with IUGR or limb reduction as one of the major features.

The clinical geneticist is asked for an opinion when the fetal medicine specialist suspects a chromosomal disorder, skeletal dysplasia, or malformation syndrome. It is more common for referrals to be made later than 20 weeks after it becomes apparent that the femur length growth is falling away from the centile chart.

See also 'Limb reduction defects', p. 212 and 'Radial ray defects and thumb hypoplasia', p. 296 in Chapter 2, 'Clinical approach'.

Clinical assessment

History: key points

- Maternal factors; age (trisomy), previous IUGR, diseases such as SLE.
- Family history of short stature (do not forget to look at the father!).
- Consanguinity (AR dysplasias and syndromes).
- IDDM (sacral agenesis and an association with femoral hypoplasia, unusual facies).
- Drug exposure. Warfarin may produce a CDP phenotype. Alcohol, phenytoin, and carbamazepine may give limb reduction defects.
- Establish an accurate gestational age for the pregnancy (use the earliest available USS).

Examination: key points

- Maternal and fetal Dopplers to exclude placental insufficiency and review Down's syndrome screening results.
- Measurements of all long bones, HC, thorax, and AC.
- Is there any evidence of asymmetry?
- Are all the bones short, or is only one limb or one bone affected?

If the features are consistent with a skeletal dysplasia, ensure that all the following are scanned and, where possible, measured.

- Long bones:
  - length and degree of shortening;
  - pattern of shortening (proximal, distal, or both);
  - epiphyses for stippling;
  - bowing (camptomelic dysplasia, OI with fractures, hypophosphatasia);
  - bone density/mineralization (OI, achondrogenesis, and hypophosphatasia);
  - fractures (OI, hypophosphatasia).
- Skull:
  - cranial shape (clover-leaf skull in TD);
  - mineralization (reduced in hypophosphatasia, OI IIa/c, and achondrogenesis).
- Vertebral structure:
  - scoliosis;
  - hemivertebrae;
  - (platyspondyly);
  - mineralization.
- Chest:
  - cardiothoracic ratio;
  - rib length and fractures;
  - thoracic:AC ratio.
- Hands and feet:
  - trident hand (TD and achondroplasia), only detectable from 25 weeks' gestation;
  - talipes (diastrophic dysplasia, SEDC, campomelic dysplasia);
  - polydactyly (asphyxiating thoracic dystrophy and short rib polydactyly syndromes, OFD syndrome);
  - absent digits;
  - hitchhiker thumb (diastrophic dysplasia).
- Facial: clefts, profile, frontal bossing (achondroplasia), depressed nasal bridge (CDP), micrognathia (camptomelic dysplasia).
- External genitalia: camptomelic dysplasia, SLO syndrome, and some short rib polydactyly syndromes may have sex reversal (SLO disorder).
- Hydrops.
- Polyhydramnios.

A suspected *chromosomal disorder* or *malformation syndrome* requires thorough examination of the following.

- Limbs for deficiencies such as radial aplasia.
- Intracranial anatomy and NTDs.
- Cardiac anatomy.
- Renal structure.
- Careful examination of the face.
- Fetal size. Many chromosomal disorders and syndromes presenting with short limbs involve low birthweight.
- Placenta, e.g. triploidy.

Special investigations

Referral to a specialist centre for scanning may be indicated.

- Chromosome analysis by CVS/amniocentesis/NIPT, depending on the gestation.
- Molecular analysis. Available for some skeletal dysplasias. Consider NIPD for *FGFR3*-related dysplasia. Note most fetuses with achondroplasia do not have significant shortening at 20 weeks' gestation. Gene panel/WES/WGS has an important role in the diagnosis of skeletal dysplasias and other syndromic disorders.

Genetic advice and management

Chromosomal disorders

- A short femur is one of the USS markers of trisomy 21.
- Fetuses with trisomy 13 or 18 are small but have other distinctive USS features.
- Triploidy. Triploid fetuses are very growth-retarded; the dygynic type is more likely to survive to the second trimester and have relative macrocephaly. See

'Triploidy (69,XXX, 69,XXY, or 69,XYY)' in Chapter 5, 'Chromosomes', p. 694.

- Bilateral radial ray defects are found in trisomy 18 and also in Fanconi syndrome. Routine cytogenetic analysis will not detect chromosomal breaks. See 'Radial ray defects and thumb hypoplasia' in Chapter 2, 'Clinical approach', p. 296 and 'DNA repair disorders' in Chapter 3, 'Common consultations', p. 398.

Syndromes with limb shortening

Most malformation syndromes without a family history will not be diagnosed prenatally. It is impossible to distinguish between a malformation syndrome and a chromosomal disorder by scan and cytogenetic analysis is indicated. A history of IDDM or drug exposure may be significant. If the karyotype is normal, consider the following.

CORNELIA DE LANGE SYNDROME (CDLS). This may present with IUGR and asymmetric radial defects. Birth incidence ~1/50 000. See 'Limb reduction defects' in Chapter 2, 'Clinical approach', p. 212.

RUSSELL–SILVER SYNDROME. This has IUGR, but with a near normal OFC. The head is proportionately large, but usually between the 3rd and 25th centiles. The face is triangular and the mouth downturned. Asymmetry is a key diagnostic feature. About 10% of children have been shown to have maternal UPD of chromosome 7.

SECKEL SYNDROME AND MICROCEPHALIC PRIMORDIAL DWARFISM. These have extreme IUGR and microcephaly (these are very rare syndromes but are included because of their extreme growth retardation). See 'Microcephaly' in Chapter 2, 'Clinical approach', p. 228.

SMITH–LEMLI–OPITZ (SLO) SYNDROME. Has been suspected after the detection of short limbs. Consider maternal urinary steroid profile, as low oestriol may be a clue to this diagnosis. Diagnostic biochemical analysis of sterols is indicated if there are other features of the syndrome. See 'Hypospadias' in Chapter 2, 'Clinical approach', p. 186.

Skeletal dysplasias

There are some dysplasias that can be confidently diagnosed prenatally, either by the USS appearance alone or by USS plus genetic testing, e.g. TD. In some, the diagnosis remains unknown, though attempts should be made to place into a diagnostic group. See 'Skeletal dysplasia charts' in 'Appendix', pp. 853–855. In Parilla *et al.*'s (2003) series of 31 cases of skeletal dysplasia detected antenatally, a final diagnosis was possible in 80%, with eight cases of TD, six of OI, three of achondroplasia, two of Roberts syndrome, and one each of a variety of conditions including EVS syndrome, spondyloepiphyseal dysplasia (SED), metaphyseal dysplasia, etc.

THANATOPHORIC DYSPLASIA (TD). Sporadic neonatal lethal skeletal dysplasia caused by *de novo* dominant mutations in *FGFR3* (1/20 000). The limbs are extremely short, with rolls of redundant skin, and the chest is very narrow causing death from respiratory failure in the immediate neonatal period. The head is relatively large with a prominent forehead and a depressed nasal bridge. In an ongoing pregnancy, confirmation of the diagnosis pre-delivery is indicated in order to plan neonatal management. This is possible by NIPD.

- TD type I. Curved ('telephone receiver') femora and variable (mild) craniosynostosis. Several mutations: Arg248Cys (55%), Tyr373Cys (24%), Ser249Cys (6%), or mutations in the stop codon (10%).

- TD type II. Straight femora and clover-leaf skull (severe craniosynostosis). All have mutation Lys650Glu.

The recurrence risk is low; the possibility of gonadal mosaicism needs to be considered.

ACHONDROPLASIA. See 'Achondroplasia' in Chapter 3, 'Common consultations', p. 334. This is the most common survivable dysplasia and is caused by mutations in the *FGFR3* gene on 4p. Eighty per cent represent new mutations. There are two common mutations G1138A and G1138C, and these mutations lead to increased activity of *FGFR3*. There is a paternal age effect with mutations on the paternally derived chromosome.

The limb lengths are usually on or above the 5th centile until 24 weeks; thus, many do not present until the third trimester. The HC is usually around the 95th centile. Observations of trident hands and frontal bossing are useful. Prenatal confirmation of diagnosis may be possible by NIPD (Chitty *et al.* 2013). Consider plans for delivery in a specialist unit as high risk for cephalopelvic disproportion due to relative macrocephaly in achondroplasia.

OSTEOGENESIS IMPERFECTA (OI). Severe forms, e.g. type II, present with short, deformed limbs, often with bowing, angulation, and/or fractures. There may be a narrow chest and some have undermineralization of the skull. See 'Fractures' in Chapter 2, 'Clinical approach', p. 158 and 'Bowed limbs' in Chapter 6, 'Pregnancy and fertility', p. 710.

INFANTILE HYPOPHOSPHATASIA. An AR condition characterized by severe deficiency of chondro-osseous mineralization caused by mutations in the tissue non-specific alkaline phosphatase gene *TNSALP* on 1p34–36. There is deformity and fracture of the long bones and the skull is undermineralized assuming a globular shape. Blood alkaline phosphatase level is extremely low or undetectable.

DIASTROPHIC DYSPLASIA (DWARFISM). The thumbs are angulated and well described as hitchhiker thumbs. Additional skeletal features are severe bilateral talipes (club-foot), scoliosis, calcification of the costal cartilages, and short stature. The ear pinnae have cysts. Cleft palate may be present. It is an AR skeletal dysplasia caused by mutation in a sulfate transporter gene, now known as *SLC26A2*, but more commonly referred to as *DTDST*. Children with diastrophic dysplasia should be under orthopaedic supervision. Achondrogenesis type IB and atelosteogenesis type II are allelic.

SHORT RIB POLYDACTYLY SYNDROMES. A group of lethal skeletal dysplasias with AR inheritance, characterized by markedly short ribs, short limbs, usually polydactyly, and multiple anomalies of the major organs. At least four types have been recognized, all caused by biallelic mutations in genes encoding components of the primary cilia or cilia regulation (*IFT80, DYNC2H1, WDR60, NEK1*).

- Type 1 (Saldino–Noonan). Narrow thorax with protuberant abdomen and ascites. Urogenital defects and CHD are common.

- Type 2 (Majewski). Midline cleft of the upper lip and relatively normal pelvic and long bones, except for the tibiae, which are oval in shape. Affected infants may also have ambiguous genitalia.

- Type 3 (Verma–Naumoff). Very short ribs and limbs. Some overlap with type 1.

- Beemer–Langer type. Lethal short rib dwarfism. Large head with brain anomalies, e.g. hydrocephalus, etc. Flat face. Short bowed bones. Polydactyly is an inconstant feature.

ACHONDROGENESIS. Achondrogenesis results in still-birth (or neonatal death) and is characterized by severe limb shortening, a relatively large head, a short neck, a short trunk, and a protuberant abdomen. Facial features include a flat nasal bridge and the whole nose is short with anteverted nostrils. Radiologically, ossification of the skull, spine, and pelvis is more deficient in type 1 than in type 2. The long bones are more severely micromelic in type 1 and there are spiky metaphyseal spurs in both, but more so in type 1. It is genetically heterogeneous. Some are due to mutations in *COL2A1* and some have mutations in *SLC26A2*.

UNDIAGNOSED SKELETAL DYSPLASIAS. An estimation of whether the condition is likely to be lethal in the neonatal period is needed for counselling purposes and to advise neonatal colleagues. USS measurements of the fetus, such as the cardiothoracic ratio, and the presence of other malformations are used, but none are particularly accurate. Where possible, plans should be made for a senior paediatrician to be present at the delivery.

Predictors of lethal skeletal dysplasia (after Parilla *et al.* 2003) include:

- early and severe shortening of the long bones;
- femur length:AC ratio <0.16;
- a small chest with short ribs and a high cardiothoracic ratio;
- marked bowing or fractures.

Investigation of the fetus and baby with a skeletal dysplasia
A diagnosis is vitally important in order to be able to advise about appropriate management and also recurrence risks.

- DNA storage. Cord blood, FBS, placental tissue, and skin biopsy can all be used. An increasing number of dysplasias have known mutations.

- Targeted testing of DNA where a specific diagnosis is strongly suspected, e.g. achondroplasia.
- Genomic analysis in presence of features suggestive of a chromosomal or syndromic diagnosis, e.g. genomic array, gene panel, or WES/WGS as appropriate.
- Skin biopsy.
- Radiology: full skeletal survey.
- Clinical photography.
- Clinical measurements.

If the baby dies, it is possible to get most of the information required, even if a post-mortem examination is refused. If a post-mortem is performed, it should include bone histology.

Support group: Many of the syndromes have their own support groups. See Contact a Family, http://www.cafamily.org.uk.

References

Chitty LS, Griffin DR, Meaney C, et al. New aids for the non-invasive diagnosis of achondroplasia, dysmorphic features, chart of fetal size and molecular confirmation using cell-free fetal DNA in maternal plasma. *Ultrasound Obstet Gynecol* 2011; **37**: 283–9.

Chitty LS, Khalil A, Barrett AN, Pajkrt E, Griffin DR, Cole TJ. Safe accurate prenatal diagnosis of thanatophoric dysplasia using ultrasound and free-fetal DNA. *Prenat Diagn* 2013, **33**: 416–23.

Parilla BV, Leeth EA, Kambich MP, Chilis P, MacGregor SN. Antenatal detection of skeletal dysplasias. *J Ultrasound Med* 2003; **22**: 255–8.

Pepin M, Atkinson M, Starman BJ, Byers PH. Strategies and outcomes of prenatal diagnosis for osteogenesis imperfecta: a review of biochemical and molecular studies completed in 129 pregnancies. *Prenat Diagn* 1997; **17**: 559–70.

Talipes (club-foot)

Club-foot usually occurs as an isolated anomaly (77%), but it may reflect an underlying neurological or neuromuscular disorder that postnatally becomes the principal clinical problem. It may also be a feature of a chromosomal disorder (e.g. trisomy 18), syndrome, or NTD. Club-foot may be a consequence of oligohydramnios. Careful assessment is therefore indicated when club-foot is identified antenatally on USS.

Bakalis et al. (2002) undertook a retrospective study of >100 000 pregnancies undergoing routine USS at 18–23 weeks' gestation. The incidence of fetal talipes was 0.1%. Talipes was bilateral in ~60% and unilateral in ~40%. In nearly half of cases, talipes was of complex aetiology, occurring in association with other defects, while in the other half it was idiopathic (isolated). In 19% of cases, an initial diagnosis of idiopathic talipes was changed to complex, because of the subsequent identification of associated features. Adverse outcomes were more frequently associated with bilateral talipes than with unilateral talipes (OR, 3.4).

Several recent genetic studies have identified a key developmental pathway—the PITX1–TBX4 transcriptional pathway—as being important in club-foot aetiology. Both PITX1 and TBX4 are uniquely expressed in the hindlimb (Dobbs and Gurnett 2012).

Talipes may be a presenting feature of a number of malformation syndromes, skeletal dysplasias, and chromosomal disorders chromosomal disorders, such as 22q11 deletion syndrome. See 'Arthrogryposis' in Chapter 2, 'Clinical approach', p. 66 and 'Fetal akinesia' in Chapter 6, 'Pregnancy and fertility', p. 724.

Talipes equinovarus (TEV)

Both the forefoot and the hindfoot are in equinus (plantar-flexed) and varus (rotated towards the midline). Prevalence is 1.6/1000 live births, with a male preponderance (M:F ratio 2:1). The spectrum of disorder ranges from mild positional deformity that corrects easily in the first week or two of life to completely rigid deformity. Many respond to conservative treatment, and fewer require surgery since the introduction of the Ponseti method of serial manipulation, casting, and tenotomy of the Achilles tendon to achieve correction of the club-foot (Laaveg and Ponseti 1980).

Talipes calcaneovalgus

The forefoot is dorsiflexed and everted. Often responds to gentle stretching exercises. The M:F ratio is 0.6:1.

Clinical assessment

History: key points
- Three-generation family tree, with specific enquiry about relatives with club-foot, contractures (distal arthrogryposis), etc.
- History of oligohydramnios (early amniocentesis <14 weeks (Philip et al. 2004), liquor leak, renal abnormality).

Examination: key points
- Detailed fetal anomaly USS.
  - Careful assessment of the whole fetus, with special attention to the brain and spine (exclude NTD and structural brain anomalies) and fetal movement and range of movement of joints (exclude arthrogryposis).

- If additional features are identified, the possibility of a syndrome or chromosomal anomaly is increased.
- Check the amniotic fluid volume.
- Assess if there are features of a skeletal dysplasia.
- Check maternal serum screening results and combine with maternal age in algorithm to determine the risk for trisomy 18 (see 'Edwards' syndrome (trisomy 18)' in Chapter 5, 'Chromosomes', p. 670).
- Assess the mother for myotonic dystrophy.

Special investigations
- Consider karyotype or genomic array (especially if there are other risk factors for aneuploidy, e.g. soft markers on USS, advanced maternal age, abnormal serum screen).
- Consider DNA testing for myotonic dystrophy in the mother if any suggestive features on history/examination.
- For postnatal assessment of severe talipes in conjunction with other problems, e.g. congenital anomalies, consider WES/WGS/panel sequencing as appropriate. See 'Arthrogryposis' in Chapter 2, 'Clinical approach', p. 66.

Genetic advice and management

Prenatally detected club-foot

In an Oxford series (Boyd, personal communication), of 149 cases (1991–2003) identified prenatally, there were six false-positive diagnoses with either no abnormality at birth or positional club-foot only and 110/149 (74%) were isolated anomalies. In a Harvard series (Shipp and Benacerraf 1998) of 68 fetuses, eight (11.8%) were false-positive diagnoses and four (5.9%) had abnormal karyotypes (+21, +18, 47,XXY, 47,XXX). In Malone et al.'s (2000) series of 51 cases of club-foot identified from 27 000 targeted USS, all were confirmed postnatally and no additional malformations were detected. Mean gestation at diagnosis was 21 weeks' gestation. In Carroll et al.'s (2001) series, follow-up was available on only 31/40 live births. Two were false-positive diagnoses, but, of the remainder, 26/29 had a structural defect, for which 21 required surgery, and 3/29 had a positional defect. The largest study is that of Bakalis et al. (2002) (see above). Note the significant proportion of cases thought to be idiopathic at presentation which had additional features when reassessed on subsequent scan or postnatally.

Isolated talipes equinovarus (TEV)

The recurrence risk for sibs in isolated TEV is 3% (risk for sibs of a male patient is 2%; risk for sibs of a female patient is 5%).

Isolated talipes calcaneovalgus

Recurrence risk for sibs is 4.5%.

Support group: STEPS, http://www.steps-charity.org.uk, Tel. 0871 717 0044.

Expert adviser: Tessa Homfray, Consultant Medical Genetics, St George's University Hospital, Harris Birthright Unit, Kings College Hospital & Royal Brompton Hospital, London, UK.

References

Bakalis S, Sairam S, Homfray T, Harrington K, Nicolaides K, Thilaganathan B. Outcome of antenatally diagnosed talipes equinovarus in an unselected obstetric population. *Ultrasound Obstet Gynecol* 2002; **20**: 226–9.

Boyd PA, Chamberlain P, Hicks NR. 6-year experience of prenatal diagnosis in an unselected population in Oxford, UK. *Lancet* 1998; **352**: 1577–81.

Carroll SGM, Lockyer H, Andrews H, *et al*. Outcome of fetal talipes following *in utero* sonographic diagnosis. *Ultrasound Obstet Gynecol* 2001; **18**: 437–40.

Dobbs MB, Gurnett CA. Genetics of clubfoot. *J Pediatr Orthop B* 2012; **21**: 7–9.

Laaveg SJ, Ponseti IV. Long-term results of treatment of congenital club foot. *J Bone Joint Surg Am* 1980; **62**: 23–31.

Malone FD, Marino T, Bianchi DW, Johnston K, D'Alton ME. Isolated clubfoot diagnosed prenatally: is karyotyping indicated? *Obstet Gynecol* 2000; **95**: 437–40.

Philip J, Silver RK, Wilson RD, *et al*. Late first-trimester invasive prenatal diagnosis: results of an international randomized trial. *Obstet Gynecol* 2004; **103**: 1164–73.

Shipp TD, Benacerraf BR. The significance of prenatally identified isolated clubfoot: is amniocentesis indicated? *Am J Obstet Gynecol* 1998; **178**: 600–2.

Wynne-Davies R. Family studies and the cause of congenital club foot, talipes equinovarus, calcaneovalgus and metatarsus varus. *J Bone Joint Surg Br* 1964; **46**: 445–63.

Zwick EB, Kraus T, Maizen C, Steinwender G, Linhart WE. Comparison of Ponseti versus surgical treatment for idiopathic clubfoot: a short-term preliminary report. *Clin Orthop Relat Res* 2009; **467**: 2668–76.

Toxoplasmosis

Congenital toxoplasmosis is diagnosed, investigated, and managed by fetal medicine specialists, paediatricians, and specialists in infectious diseases with laboratory diagnostic support. The geneticist may be involved prior to a definitive diagnosis because the phenotype may overlap with genetic disorders; therefore, a brief summary of the condition is included in this section.

Congenital toxoplasmosis is caused by the parasite *Toxoplasma gondii*. The maternal signs and symptoms of toxoplasmosis include fever, tiredness, and lymphadenopathy, although the infection is often asymptomatic. In the pregnant mother, the infection is caught by eating anything infected or contaminated with the parasite such as:

- raw or undercooked meat;
- food contaminated with cat faeces or with contaminated soil;
- unpasteurized goats milk.

The fetus is infected by transmission of the parasite across the placenta when the mother first acquires the infection during pregnancy. The risk of mother-to-child transmission varies, depending on the point in gestation at which the mother acquires the infection. An analysis, based on all available cohort studies, estimated the risk of transmission as 15% (95% CI, 13–17%) if a mother seroconverted at 13 weeks' gestation, 44% (95% CI, 40, 47) after seroconversion at 26 weeks, and 71% (95% CI, 66, 76) after seroconversion at 36 weeks' gestation. Overall, about one in five babies with congenital infection have clinical signs. The brain and retina are particularly affected and the signs of the disease in neonates and infants include chorioretinitis, hydrocephalus, ICC, and seizures. For infected babies, the risk of clinical signs is highest if the mother acquired the infection in early pregnancy and decreases with gestation of maternal infection.

Antibiotic treatment during pregnancy should be considered, provided treatment can be started shortly after maternal seroconversion. Thiébaut *et al.* (2007) found no clear evidence for an association between early treatment and reduced risk of congenital toxoplasmosis. Gras *et al.* (2005) at the European Multicentre Study on Congenital Toxoplasmosis (EMSCOT) in 2005 concluded that prenatal treatment within 4 weeks of seroconversion reduced the risk of intracranial lesions, compared with no treatment. It is standard clinical practice to use spiramycin to decrease placental transmission, and a combination of pyrimethamine and sulfonamides to treat known fetal infection, but there is no clinical evidence to indicate superior efficacy for either of these treatments. The prognosis for a pregnancy is dependent on the USS features and the degree of damage to the developing CNS (which cannot be reversed by antibiotic treatment), which do not become apparent until 22 weeks' gestation or later.

Children with congenital toxoplasmosis can develop new ocular lesions at any time. By the age of 12 years, about 30% of infected children have one or more retinochoroidal lesions. More than 90% of these children with eye lesions have normal bilateral vision (Snellen 6/12 or better) (Tan *et al.* 2007). Unilateral vision of the eyes affected by lesions is impaired (<6/12) in 19–35% of children. Severe damage to the brain is unusual, affecting only 5% of children with congenital toxoplasmosis.

Typical features include hydrocephalus and calcification of brain tissue, with developmental delay and epilepsy.

Clinical assessment

Screening in pregnancy is not recommended in the UK because of the uncertainty about the effectiveness of treatment and the low incidence of the infection. However, women are advised to avoid sources of infection.

Testing in pregnancy may be warranted for women with symptoms suggestive of *Toxoplasma* infection; the assessment should be under the supervision of a fetal medicine specialist who will decide whether antibiotic treatment (usually spiramycin) in pregnancy is indicated. This will be influenced by the gestation, USS features, and maternal serology (IgM, IgA, and IgG). Making a firm antenatal diagnosis can be problematical due to problems timing the onset of the infection, because IgM titres stay positive for years in some cases. Use of different IgM assays can help and antibody avidity testing may also be useful. Amniocentesis may be offered to assist fetal diagnosis if drugs with serious adverse effects, such as pyrimethamine and sulfadimidine, or TOP are being considered. Diagnosis of toxoplasmosis should be made in conjunction with colleagues in microbiology and a National Reference Laboratory.

History: key points, postnatal

- Birthweight, OFC for microcephaly or to monitor the development of hydrocephalus.
- Lethargy, poor feeding (signs of possible neurological involvement).

Examination: key points, postnatal

- Microcephaly and neurological abnormalities.
- Chorioretinitis.

Special investigations: prenatal

- USS. ICC is the most common USS sign and may occur with or without ventriculomegaly (Gras *et al.* 2005). One or both of these intracranial lesions are found on USS in 10% of newborns with congenital toxoplasmosis. Other fetal anomalies include ICC, hyperechogenic bowel, intrahepatic lesions, and ascites. These abnormalities are rarely detected before 22 weeks' gestation.
- PCR for *T. gondii* DNA in the amniotic fluid.
- Maternal *T. gondii* serology. Go back and check maternal results on booking bloods to try and establish gestation at the onset of infection.
- Consider MRI scan of the fetal brain to establish the extent of cerebral damage.

Special investigations: postnatal

- Confirmation of congenital infection. Check if placental tissue would be of use.
- Brain imaging of all symptomatic babies (toxoplasma is typically associated with enlarged ventricles without cortical malformations).
- Ophthalmology referral (chorioretinitis).

Genetic advice and management

Proven congenital toxoplasmosis is not a genetic condition. Women are advised to consult their obstetrician prior to another pregnancy for repeat serology. Babies with signs of congenital infection, but in whom there are no serological features, may be referred to a geneticist for an opinion. Consider the AR condition of pseudo-TORCH/microcephaly–ICC in babies with signs of congenital infection, but in whom there are no serological features to support the diagnosis.

Refer to the appropriate eye section or brain section of Chapter 2, 'Clinical approach', for discussion of other syndromes with some of the features of congenital infections.

Support group: ARC (Antenatal Results and Choices), http://www.arc-uk.org.

Expert adviser: Ruth Gilbert, Professor of Clinical Epidemiology, UCL GOS Institute of Child Health, London, UK.

References

Gras L, Wallon M, Pollak A, et al.; European Multicentre Study on Congenital Toxoplasmosis. Association between prenatal treatment and clinical manifestations of congenital toxoplasmosis in infancy: a cohort study in 13 European centres. *Acta Paediatr* 2005; **94**: 1721–31.

Martin S. Congenital toxoplasmosis. *Neonatal Netw* 2001; **20**: 23–30.

Members of the European Multicentre Study on Congenital Toxoplasmosis (EMSCOT); Writing committee: Gilbert RE, Cortina-Borja M, Tan HK, et al. http://www.ucl.ac.uk/paediatric-epidemiology/EMSCOT/emscot.html.

Mombro M, Perathoner C, Leone A, et al. Congenital toxoplasmosis: assessment of risk to newborns in confirmed and uncertain maternal infection. *Eur J Pediatr* 2003; **162**: 703–6.

Monatora SG, Liesenfeld O. Toxoplasmosis [seminar]. *Lancet* 2004; **363**: 1965–76.

Thiébaut R, Leproust S, Chêne G, Gilbert R; SYROCOT (Systematic Review on Congenital Toxoplasmosis) study group. Effectiveness of prenatal treatment for congenital toxoplasmosis: a meta-analysis of individual patients' data. *Lancet* 2007; **369**: 115–22.

Tan HK, Schmidt D, Stanford M, et al.; European Multicentre Study on Congenital Toxoplasmosis (EMSCOT). Risk of visual impairment in children with congenital toxoplasmic retinochoroiditis. *Am J Ophthalmol* 2007; **144**: 648–53.

Twins and twinning

Twins occur in one in 80 live births but increased in developed countries with increasing maternal age at conception and increased use of IVF. They have a special place in Greek mythology and ancient legends. Classical twin studies have played a key role in defining the 'heritability' of a trait by studying the concordance in monozygotic (MZ) versus dizygotic (DZ) twins. Many aspects of twin pregnancies, including prematurity and maternal physiology, make them different from singleton pregnancies. The incidence of MZ twins is increased ~4-fold in babies born following IVF.

'Vanishing' twin
Only 29% of women with a twin pregnancy on USS at <10 weeks' gestation will give birth to twins. Hence, there is ~70% loss rate in twin pregnancies.

Congenital anomalies
Congenital anomalies occur in at least 10% of all twin pregnancies. The congenital anomaly rate is probably higher in MZ than in DZ twins, partly due to the increased burden of anomalies arising from vascular disruption and possibly because, in the earliest phase of embryonic development, the cytoplasm of a single egg cell supports the nutritional requirements of two embryos prior to implantation. Both MZ and DZ twins have an increased risk for deformational congenital anomalies, associated with constraint and intrauterine crowding, such as greater moulding of the head, craniosynostosis, dislocated hips, bowing of the legs, and club-feet.

Disruptions in MZ twins, including hemifacial microsomia, limb reduction defects, and amyoplasia and bowel atresia, are probably related to the shared placental circulation unique to MZ twins, with differences in vascular flow leading to vascular compromise.

Dizygotic (DZ) twins ('non-identical twins')
DZ twins share the same genetic similarity as siblings, i.e. they have 50% of their nuclear DNA in common and they have a 25% risk to be concordant for AR disorders. DZ twins have separate placentas and membranes (dichorionic diamniotic; see Figure 6.9(a)), although they might be fused and even have vascular connections. At least 8% of DZ twins show some level of chimerism in blood lymphocytes. This is also occasionally seen in singletons (possibly arising from a 'vanished' twin). The introduction of artificial reproductive technologies (ARTs) has led to an 'epidemic' of DZ twins.

There are now six published cases of DZ twins with a monochorionic placenta. This exceptionally rare phenomenon has been documented using fibroblast DNA and seems to be more common after ART. The bone marrow of one twin may take over both bone marrows.

Factors increasing DZ twinning rate
- Raised gonadotrophin levels. Older, taller, heavier mothers and nulliparas. The peak incidence is at 37 years.
- Fertility drugs, e.g. clomiphene. These promote superovulation with a markedly increased risk for DZ twinning.
- Familial factors. Women with a family history of DZ twinning are more likely to have DZ twins.

- Ethnicity. The rate of DZ twinning varies widely between different populations. It is low in Asian populations with an incidence of 4/1000, intermediate in Europeans and Northern Americans at 10–14/1000, and high in Africans at 26–40/1000.

Types of DZ twinning
- Superfecundation. More than one egg fertilized in the same menstrual cycle.
- Superfetation (rare). Implantation of a second fertilized egg in a uterus containing a pregnancy.
- Polar body twins (rare). Fertilization of the nucleus of the egg and the polar body by two different sperms.

Monozygotic (MZ) twins ('identical twins')
Traditionally, MZ twins are considered to be genetically identical. MZ twinning occurs at the same rate worldwide. In MZ twinning, a single egg is fertilized by a single sperm. MZ twins account for 3–4/1000 births in the UK. Manipulation of the environment around the time of conceptions can induce MZ twinning in animals; the MZ twinning rate is increased 4-fold in IVF pregnancies. Milki *et al.* (2003) reported an MZ twinning rate of 5.6% with blastocyst transfer, compared with 2% following day 3 transfer (cleavage stage). The placentation of MZ twinning is thought to be determined by the time at which twinning occurs following fertilization (see Table 6.18 and Figure 6.10). Twenty-five to 30% of MZ twins have completely separate placentas and membranes; 70–75% share one placenta with monochorionic diamniotic membranes, and 1–2% have one set of membranes and one placenta (monochorionic, monoamniotic; see Figure 6.9(b)). Monochorionic placentas of all types are prone to have vascular connections that can lead to twin–twin transfusion syndrome, twin reverse arterial perfusion sequence (TRAP), and disruptive congenital anomalies (see above).

Types of MZ twin
- Acardiac. ~1/35 000 births. The normal twin supports the acardiac twin, with risk of cardiac failure and hydrops in the normal twin.
- Fetus papyraceus. Frequent if looked for. Co-twin dies in second or third trimester and is delivered at term, often attached to the placenta.
- Concordant MZ twins. The great majority of MZ twins.
- Discordant MZ twins. This arises due to new dominant mutation, chromosomal aneuploidy, copy number variation, differential X-inactivation (Valleix *et al.* 2002), imprinting loss/gain (Weksberg *et al.* 2002), mitotic recombination, and differential mitochondrial load. As a result, everyone, including MZ twins, is genetically unique.
- Mirror image twins. Ten to 15% of MZ twins. Twinning occurs late in development during the establishment of the body axis (just prior to the formation of conjoined twins).

DISCORDANCE. Discordance between MZ twins has been noted for chromosomal anomalies, single gene disorders, skewed X-inactivation, genomic imprinting defects, mitochondrial disturbances, and minisatellites. These factors need to be borne in mind during PND, since MZ twins could be discordant for chromosomal

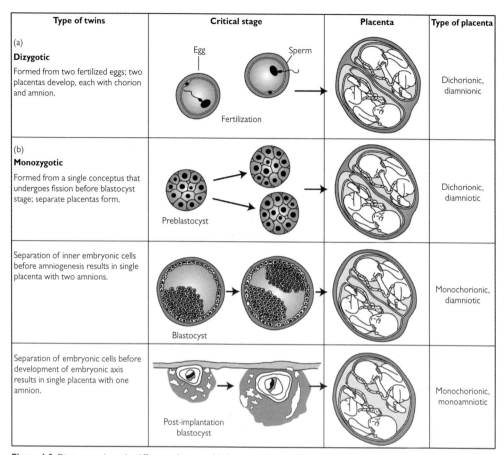

Type of twins	Critical stage	Placenta	Type of placenta
(a) **Dizygotic** Formed from two fertilized eggs; two placentas develop, each with chorion and amnion.	Egg Sperm Fertilization		Dichorionic, diamnionic
(b) **Monozygotic** Formed from a single conceptus that undergoes fission before blastocyst stage; separate placentas form.	Preblastocyst		Dichorionic, diamniotic
Separation of inner embryonic cells before amniogenesis results in single placenta with two amnions.	Blastocyst		Monochorionic, diamniotic
Separation of embryonic cells before development of embryonic axis results in single placenta with one amnion.	Post-implantation blastocyst		Monochorionic, monoamniotic

Figure 6.9 Diagram to show the differences between (a) dizygotic twins and (b) monozygotic twins.

anomalies, chromosomal mosaicism, imprinting defects and new dominant mutations.

VASCULAR SHUNTS. MZ twins are at risk of placental vascular anastomoses that may be arterioarterial, venovenous, or arteriovenous. They predispose to a variety of congenital anomalies due to vascular disruption: microcephaly; porencephaly; hydranencephaly; gastroschisis; intestinal atresia; and transverse limb reduction defects. If the co-twin dies in the second or third trimester, MZ twins are at greatly increased risk of cerebral palsy (perhaps due to embolization or disturbance of the coagulation balance arising from the dying/dead twin).

Clinical assessment

History: key points

- Family tree with history of twinning, and determine ethnicity.
- Pregnancy and delivery. Were there separate placentas? Were there separate amniotic sacs?

Table 6.18 Placentation of MZ twins in relationship to timing of twinning after fertilization

Placentation of MZ twins	Time of twinning after fertilization	% of all MZ pregnancies surviving to term	Comment
Dichorionic diamniotic	Separation by day 3	25	Early separation leads to completely separate placentation
Monochorionic diamniotic	4–8 days	70–75	Single placenta with separate amniotic sacs
Monochorionic monoamniotic	9–12 days	1–2	Risk of tangled cords
Conjoined twins	13–14 days	Rare	75% are female

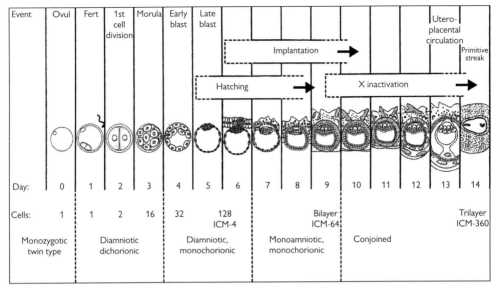

Figure 6.10 Schematic drawing of normal human embryonic development with timing of monozygotic twinning superimposed. Reprinted from *The Lancet*, Vol. 362, Issue 9385, Hall, Twinning, pp. 735–743, Copyright 2003, with permission from Elsevier.

- Subsequent growth and development. How similar are the twins? Can strangers tell them apart?

Examination: key points
- Careful examination of MZ (monochorionic) twins for congenital anomalies.
- Growth parameters.
- Examine as for the issue in question. Are the twins concordant or discordant for the problem?

Special investigations
- DNA for zygosity testing; may need to use a buccal swab or skin fibroblasts if a single placenta. Documentation of zygosity at birth (using cord blood) may be considered for all same-sex dichorionic twins.
- Careful examination of the placenta.

Genetic advice and management
Zygosity testing sufficient for routine clinical practice can usually be accomplished using a relatively small number (e.g. seven or more) of highly polymorphic microsatellite markers. Microsatellite polymorphisms are based on short tandem repeats, usually di-, tri-, or tetranucleotides, that can be typed by PCR and give a discrete allele with a precise repeat number.

Support groups: The Multiple Births Foundation, http://www.multiplebirths.org.uk, Tel. 0208 383 3519;

Tamba (Twins and Multiple Births Association), http://www.tamba.org.uk, Tel. 0870 770 3305.

Expert adviser: Judith Hall, Professor Emerita of Paediatrics and Medical Genetics, UBC & Children's and Women's Health Centre of British Columbia, Department of Medical Genetics, British Columbia's Children's Hospital, Vancouver, Canada.

References

Glingianaia SV, Rankin J, Wright C, et al. A multiple pregnancy register in the north of England. *Twin Res* 2002; **5**: 436–9.

Hall JG. Twinning [review]. *Lancet* 2003; **362**: 735–43.

Milki AA, Jun SH, Hinckley MD, Behr B, Giudice LC, Westphal LM. Incidence of monozygotic twinning with blastocyst transfer compared to cleavage-stage transfer. *Fertil Steril* 2003; **79**: 503–6.

Painter JN, Medland SJ, Montgomery GW, et al. Twins and twinning. In: DL Rimoin, RE Pyeritz, BR Korf (eds.). *Emery and Rimoin's principles and practice of medical genetics*, **volume 1**, 6th edn, pp. 53–8. Churchill Livingstone, New York, 2016.

Valleix S, Vinciguerra C. Skewed X-chromosome inactivation in monochorionic diamniotic twin sisters results in severe and mild haemophilia A. *Blood* 2002; **100**: 3034–6.

Weksberg R, Shuman C, Caluseriu O, et al. Discordant KCNQ1OT1 imprinting in sets of monozygotic twins discordant for Beckwith–Wiedemann syndrome. *Hum Mol Genet* 2002; **11**: 1317–25.

Urinary tract and renal anomalies (congenital anomalies of the kidney and urinary tract—CAKUT)

Congenital anomalies of the kidney and urinary tract anomalies are common, comprising ~15% of all pre-natally detected congenital anomalies. About 25% are associated with other anomalies. Renal tract anomalies are found in ~250–300 syndromes and ~35% of all chromosome anomalies.

The main presentations of renal tract anomalies on fetal USS are:

(1) renal parenchymal defects such as agenesis or hypoplasia;

(2) cystic or 'bright' kidneys;

(3) oligohydramnios: fetal urine production accounts for the majority of amniotic fluid production from 14 weeks' gestation. Any impairment in fetal urine output will manifest as oligohydramnios;

(4) ureteric tract dilatation (hydronephrosis).

Dysplastic kidneys can be of any size, ranging from mas-sive kidneys distended with multiple large cysts of up to 9 cm in diameter that are termed multicystic dysplastic kidneys (MCDK) to normal-sized or small kidneys with or without cysts that are echogenic.

In embryological terms, either multicystic dysplasia or renal agenesis or both may occur if the complex mor-phogenesis of the kidney is disturbed. Dysplastic kidneys identified on antenatal USS may even disappear com-pletely, both before and after birth, suggesting that many patients diagnosed with renal agenesis may originally have had dysplasia.

Patients with kidney parenchymal defects have a higher prevalence of genetic disorders and worse renal and overall survival, compared to patients with isolated hydronephrosis. The presence of extrarenal defects is also predictive of worse renal survival, possibly due to higher genetic load (Quirino et al. 2012; Sanna-Cherchi et al. 2009).

Numerous kindreds have been described with AD and AR inheritance of aplasia, hypoplasia, dysplasia, and other urinary tract abnormalities including vesicoureteral reflux (VUR), duplications, and horseshoe kidneys. The exact familial incidence of renal/urinary tract disease is unknown. However, Roodhooft et al. (1984) looked at index cases with bilateral agenesis/severe dysplasia and reported that 9% of relatives had renal malforma-tions (the most common anomaly being unilateral renal agenesis). Within the same family, individuals can display a spectrum of phenotypes, ranging from mild renal asym-metry to severe MCDK, suggesting these phenotypes share a common pathogenetic origin.

Upper tract defects: kidney parenchymal abnormalities

Renal agenesis

Unilateral renal agenesis occurs in 0.15/1000 newborns, and bilateral renal agenesis affects 0.12/1000 newborns. Renal agenesis is more common in males (2.45M:1F). Bilateral renal agenesis presents with severe oligohydram-nios beyond 14 weeks' gestation and Potter sequence (pulmonary hypoplasia, micrognathia, talipes), and there is a high incidence of associated anomalies. Unilateral renal agenesis may be an incidental finding or discovered during the investigation of a renal tract disorder. There may be hypertrophy of the contralateral kidney. The ipsi-lateral ureter and Fallopian tube may be absent.

SYNDROMES ASSOCIATED WITH RENAL AGENESIS.

- VATER (vertebral defects–anal atresia–tracheo-oesophageal fistula–(o)esophageal atresia–renal anomalies)/VACTERL (vertebral defects–anal atre-sia–cardiac anomalies–tracheo-oesophageal fistula–(o) esophageal atresia–renal anomalies–limb defects). See 'Radial ray defects and thumb hypoplasia' in Chapter 2, 'Clinical approach', p. 296.

- MURCS (Müllerian duct anomalies–renal aplasia–cer-vicothoracic somite dysplasia). See 'Female infertil-ity and amenorrhoea: genetic aspects' in Chapter 6, 'Pregnancy and infertility', p. 722.

- BOR syndrome (branchio-oto-renal). See 'Ear anoma-lies' in Chapter 2, 'Clinical approach', p. 142.

- Fraser syndrome. An AR disorder with cryptophthal-mos and syndactyly. See 'Ptosis, blepharophimosis, and other eyelid anomalies' in Chapter 2, 'Clinical approach', p. 292.

Multicystic dysplastic kidney (MCDK)

MCDK most commonly presents as an incidental find-ing on prenatal USS. Sonographically, an MCDK is large, often very large, and irregularly bright with large cystic areas all but replacing the renal substance. Unilateral MCDK occurs in 1/3000–1/5000 births and liquor volume is usually normal. Bilateral MCDK occurs in 1/10 000 births and there is oligohydramnios.

Lazebnik et al. (1999) reviewed 102 prenatally diag-nosed cases. In unilateral cases, abnormality of the contralateral kidney is common (33%). Associated non-renal anomalies occur frequently with both unilateral (26%) and bilateral (67%) MCDK and increase the risk of a chromosome anomaly when present. Males are more likely than females to be affected (2.4M:1F), but females are twice as likely to have bilateral disease. There is a strong association between dysplasia and obstruction, and the lower urinary tract should always be carefully assessed. Twenty to 50% have a genitourinary anomaly on the contralateral side, e.g. VUR or pelvi-ureteral junc-tion (PUJ) obstruction. Ten per cent have contralateral renal agenesis. Most MCDKs involute, both pre- and postnatally.

- Unilateral MCDK. In Lazebnik et al.'s (1999) study, unilateral MCDK without associated renal or non-renal anomalies was not associated with an abnormal chromosome study and resulted in favourable out-comes. In Aubertin et al.'s (2002) study of 73 cases of apparently isolated MCDK, +21 was found in one fetus and genitourinary defects were subsequently identified in 33% and non-renal abnormalities in 16%. Karyotyping is not generally undertaken in unilateral MCDK.

- Bilateral MCDK. Karyotyping is indicated if there is bilateral renal involvement or an additional USS finding. A wide range of chromosome anomalies are associ-ated with MCDK, including a variety of deletions/duplications that may often not be detectable on a routine antenatal karyotype. If there is an associated cardiac anomaly, offer 22q.11 FISH.

Unilateral MCDK can be familial but is most commonly a sporadic anomaly. Belk et al.'s (2002) study did not find significant renal anomalies in any of the 94 first-degree relatives of unilateral MCDK index cases, so formal screening of relatives is not recommended.

Large 'bright' or hyperechogenic kidneys

The term 'hyperechogenic' or 'bright' kidneys is used to describe renal tissue that is brighter than the liver or spleen. Sonographically, polycystic kidneys are large and uniformly 'bright'. Initial kidney development is unremarkable, but subsequently cysts develop; adjacent functioning renal tissue is compromised and may eventually lead to renal insufficiency. In AR polycystic kidney disease (ARPKD; infantile polycystic kidney disease), the cysts only arise from the collecting ducts. In AD polycystic kidney disease (ADPKD; adult polycystic kidney disease), cysts arise from all areas of the nephron or collecting duct. There are usually numerous small cysts in ARPKD; fewer, larger cysts are more characteristic of ADPKD.

Recent data indicated that a molecular diagnosis is possible in up to 15–20% of patients with renal agenesis, hypoplasia, or dysplasia; 5–10% have a mutation in *PAX2*, *HNF1B*, *DSTYK*, *SALL1*, *SIX1*, or *EYA1* (Thomas et al. 2011; Weber et al. 2006) and another 10% have a major genomic imbalance (Sanna-Cherchi et al. 2012). Conditions to consider in these cases include the following.

RELATIVELY COMMON SYNDROMES FEATURING KIDNEY PARENCHYMAL DEFECTS.

- Renal cysts and diabetes (RCAD) syndrome (also known as MODY5). An AD disorder due to mutation in *HNF1B*. About 80% of patients present at birth with a renal parenchymal defect such as cystic kidneys or renal agenesis. Other manifestations include genital tract defects; diabetes and gout typically have a later onset. Mutations are present in 3–5% of patients with renal hypoplasia/aplasia/dysplasia.
- Renal coloboma syndrome. An AD disorder due to mutation in *PAX2*, characterized by retina colobomas and hearing and renal defects. The renal abnormalities may occur without retinal or hearing defects. Mutations account for 3–5% with renal hypoplasia/aplasia/dysplasia.
- *DSTYK* mutations. This is a recently described AD syndrome. Mutations in the *DSTYK* gene cause a spectrum of urinary tract malformations, including renal agenesis and hypoplasia and ureteric obstruction, and account for 2.3% of urinary tract malformations (Sanna-Cherchi et al. 2013).
- di George/velocardiofacial syndrome (DGS/VCFS). This is caused by deletions on 22q11.2. Most commonly associated with cardiac malformations, neuropsychiatric defects, and immune deficiency. Up to one-third of patients have renal developmental defects. See '22q11 deletion syndrome' in Chapter 5, 'Chromosomes', p. 624.
- Submicroscopic genomic imbalances. A recent microarray study demonstrated that 10.5% of 522 children with renal agenesis, hypoplasia, or dysplasia have a genomic disorder that was not suspected by a standard clinical evaluation. Thirty-five distinct disorders were identified in 55 patients; the most common imbalances were in the RCAD and di George/velocardiofacial

loci. The majority of these disorders were previously associated with neuropsychiatric disorders (Sanna-Cherchi et al. 2012). Half of these pathogenic CNVs were inherited from an apparently unaffected parent. Pathogenic CNVs were also detected in 8% of children with all-cause chronic renal disease, permitting reclassification of diagnosis (Verbitsky el al. 2015). The CNVs may also impact neurocognition and therefore have additional significance (Verbitsky et al. 2017, in press).

- ARPKD. Incidence is ~1/20 000 live births. It usually presents in the second or third trimester with large 'bright' kidneys and progressive oligohydramnios. Prognosis is usually poor. All have hepatic and renal involvement, but the clinical spectrum is very diverse. Both kidneys are symmetrically involved and markedly enlarged. Individual cysts are not detectable on antenatal USS. It is caused by mutations in *PKHD1* ('polyductin') on 6p12, which is among the largest human genes. It has a minimum of 86 exons assembled into a variety of alternatively spliced transcripts (Onuchic et al. 2002). Both truncating and non-conservative missense mutations are described. All patients with two truncating mutations display a severe phenotype with perinatal or neonatal demise, while patients surviving the neonatal period bear at least one missense mutation (certain missense mutations produce a severe phenotype) (Bergmann et al. 2004). There is a subgroup in which the disease phenotype is milder and who may survive into teenage years and early adulthood (Zerres et al. 1993).
- ADPKD. Rarely, ADPKD may present in fetal or neonatal life with large hyperechogenic kidneys; individual cysts may also be detectable. Prognosis is good for fetal life and early childhood, unless there is oligohydramnios, which is extremely uncommon. If ADPKD does develop prenatally in a family, there is an increased likelihood that further affected children will also present early (Zerres et al. 1993). Individuals with ADPKD who develop cysts in fetal life may be at risk for earlier onset of complications, e.g. hypertension and renal impairment. See 'Autosomal dominant polycystic kidney disease (ADPKD)' in Chapter 3, 'Common consultations', p. 354.
- Bardet–Biedl syndrome (BBS). An AR syndrome characterized by polydactyly, obesity, developmental delay, hypogonadism, and rod–cone dystrophy. Prenatally, large echogenic kidneys and polydactyly are the only detectable features. BBS is highly heterogeneous, with mutations in at least 15 different genes identified to date. See 'Ciliopathies' in Chapter 3, Common conditions', p. 358.
- Beckwith–Wiedemann syndrome (BWS). Increased renal echogenicity, hydronephrosis, and cysts may be seen, in addition to large kidneys and generalized overgrowth. Other features detectable antenatally include exomphalos and a large tongue and increased liquor. See 'Beckwith–Wiedemann syndrome (BWS)' in Chapter 3, 'Common consultations', p. 358.

RARE SYNDROMES FEATURING KIDNEY PARENCHYMAL DEFECTS.

- Oral–facial–digital (OFD) syndrome type 1. An XLD ciliopathy characterized by pre- and post-axial polydactyly, complex clefts, and renal cysts. See 'Ciliopathies' in Chapter 3, 'Common consultations', p. 366.

- Meckel–Gruber. An AR disorder with occipital encephalocele, microcephaly, cleft lip and palate, large multicystic kidneys, and PAP. Considerable phenotypic variation is possible, even between sibs. See 'Neural tube defects' in Chapter 3, 'Common consultations', p. 500.
- Trisomy 13. Other congenital malformations are usually present, e.g. holoprosencephaly, PAP, orofacial clefting, and cardiac defects.
- Zellweger. An AR peroxisome disorder with severe hypotonia, seizures, and nystagmus. Antenatally, multiple renal cysts may be seen bilaterally as may cerebral ventriculomegaly. PND is possible by quantification of VLCFAs at CVS.

Lower tract defects: hydronephrosis, reflux, and bladder defects

Hydronephrosis

Hydronephrosis is a relatively common finding on prenatal USS which usually resolves spontaneously. Congenital hydronephrosis can be due to pyelectasis (dilatation of the fetal renal pelvis), ureteropelvic junction obstruction, and ureterovesical obstruction. Mild pyelectasis is a very common finding, seen in 0.5–1% of pregnancies, and is often incidental, with no significant long-term sequelae. Isolated hydronephrosis, in the absence of kidney parenchymal defects or extrarenal anomalies, also has a good prognosis (Quirino et al. 2012; Sanna-Cherchi et al. 2009). Most patients can be managed expectantly with appropriate follow-up postnatal imaging. The presence of bilateral hydronephrosis, renal failure, lower urinary tract obstruction, and bladder or cloacal exstrophy usually requires more intensive medical or surgical intervention.

Congenital urethral obstruction

In males, this is usually due to maldevelopment of the urethra, ranging from complete urethral atresia to posterior urethral valves (PUVs) that form around the membranous/prostatic urethra. In the female bladder, outflow obstruction is rare and may be the result of 'cloacal plate abnormalities' with associated anomalies of the genital tract (e.g. vagina and uterus) and bowel. Cloacal plate anomalies can also occur in males.

According to Thomas et al. (2001), the following are predictors of early-onset renal failure in congenital urethral obstruction:

- dilatation detectable at <24 weeks' gestation;
- moderate/severe upper tract dilatation (renal pelvis anteroposterior diameter ≥10 mm in second trimester);
- thick-walled bladder;
- oligohydramnios;
- USS evidence of renal dysplasia, i.e. echogenic cortex, microcystic renal change.

Vesico-ureteric reflux (VUR)

VUR is common (~1% of all live births) and is usually an asymptomatic and self-limiting disease. Poor prognostic features are high-grade reflux and scarring at birth. Chronic pyelonephritis and reflux nephropathy remain important causes of end-stage renal failure in adult life. Medical management (prophylactic antibiotics) and surgical management are equally effective. In some families, VUR appears to follow an AD pattern of inheritance with highly variable penetrance and expression; in others, there may be a polygenic basis.

Risk factors for VUR are:
- dilatation of the renal pelvis on antenatal USS;
- an affected sibling;
- an affected parent.

MANAGEMENT OF A NEONATE AT RISK FOR VUR. Management is complex and optimal management varies with the sex of the baby and the severity of the antenatal findings. Prophylactic antibiotics from birth are indicated in some infants, and various imaging modalities, e.g. USS, micturating cystourethrogram (MCUG), and functional scans (e.g. dimercaptosuccinic acid (DMSA) scans), are possible. This is a controversial area and neonates should be managed in conjunction with a paediatrician with expertise in this field.

Prune-belly syndrome

Abdominal muscle deficiency, megaureter, megacystis, and undescended testis, affecting 1/30 000. Almost all cases are male. Sibling recurrence risk is low (<1%). Discordant MZ twins have been reported.

Occasionally, the bladder is enlarged due to non-obstructive causes, e.g. neuropathic bladder (consider spinal USS in early infancy) or MMIH syndrome (see 'Visceral myopathy (megacystis–microcolon–intestinal hypoperistalsis (MMIH) syndrome)' below).

The urofacial syndrome (UFS)

An AR disorder of bladder innervation, characterized by severe and early-onset urinary incontinence and incomplete bladder emptying. Patients have dysmorphic bladders, dilatation of the ureter and renal pelvis, and VUR. Affected individuals have a characteristic facial grimace when trying to smile. In addition, one-third have constipation or faecal soiling. UFS is caused by mutations in either the HPSE2 or LRIG2 genes, which are expressed in autonomic nerves of the bladder.

Visceral myopathy (megacystis–microcolon–intestinal hypoperistalsis (MMIH) syndrome)

Familial visceral myopathy may be caused by heterozygous mutation in ACTG2, with incomplete penetrance or biallelic variants in MYH11. Can present in pregnancy with megacystis, oligohydramnios or polyhydramnios, or normal liquor volume. Prognosis is variable but can be poor if extensive gut involvement necessitating surgery and/or total parenteral nutrition (Wangler et al. 2014).

The spectrum of conditions with visceral myopathy also includes chronic intestinal pseudo-obstruction (CIPO) and a multi-system smooth muscle dysfunction syndrome (MSMDS) (Moreno et al. 2016).

Clinical assessment of pregnancy with renal tract anomalies

History: key points

- Three-generation family tree, with detailed enquiry about renal tract problems, other congenital anomalies, neuropsychiatric disease, stillbirths, or neonatal deaths.
- Careful history regarding possible teratogens (alcohol, diabetes, rubella, ACE inhibitors).

Examination: key points

- Detailed fetal anomaly USS, with careful attention to the genitourinary tract and scrutiny for other malformations.

Special investigations

- Offer amniocentesis as indicated in the text.

- Consider parental USS (not indicated for unilateral MCKD or mild pyelectasis).
- If the USS suggests renal parenchymal involvement (e.g. bright kidneys) and the pregnancy fails or is terminated, strong consideration should be given to archiving DNA and obtaining a renal biopsy or full post-mortem assessment.

Genetic advice and management

- Attempt to exclude monogenic, syndromic, and copy number disorder causes insofar as this is possible.
- Genomic analysis is recommended in patients with kidney parenchymal defects (aplasia/agenesis/dysplasia), particularly if they have extrarenal developmental defects, e.g. genomic array, gene panel, or WES/WGS as available. Microarrays should be considered as a first line diagnostic test in children with renal hypoplasia/dysplasia as they have a 10% diagnostic rate.

Recurrence risks

- Renal agenesis. Recurrence risk for sibs is 3–8% for bilateral renal agenesis. There may be some additional risk for unilateral renal agenesis.
- Perinatal lethal MCDK. Empiric recurrence risk for sibs in 3.6%, but only 0.2% for cousins.
- Non-lethal MCDK. Empiric recurrence risk for normal parents of a child with isolated MCDK is small, of the order of 2–3%. If one parent is affected, the recurrence risk is 15–20%.
- Conditions with renal parenchymal cysts. Counsel for specific diagnosis (see text).
- Congenital urethral obstruction. Sibling risks are small.
- VUR. There is a high sibling recurrence risk (20–45%) when siblings are carefully evaluated (e.g. MCUG). There is a high offspring risk for children of affected parents (~15–20%).

Expert adviser: Ali Gharavi, Professor of Medicine and Chief, Division of Nephrology, Columbia University, New York, USA.

References

Aubertin G, Cripps S, Coleman G, et al. Prenatal diagnosis of apparently isolated unilateral multicystic kidney: implications for counselling and management. Prenat Diagn 2002; **22**: 388–94.

Belk RA, Thomas DF, Mueller RF, Godbole P, Markham AF, Weston MJ. A family study and the natural history of prenatally detected unilateral multicystic dysplastic kidney. J Urol 2002; **167**(2 Pt 1): 666–9.

Bergmann C, Senderek J, Küpper F, et al. PKHD1 mutations in autosomal recessive polycystic kidney disease (ARPKD). Hum Mutat 2004; **23**: 453–63.

Chudleigh T. Mild pyelectasis. Prenat Diagn 2001; **21**: 936–41.

Chudleigh PM, Chitty LS, Pembrey M, Campbell S. The association of aneuploidy and mild fetal pyelectasis in an unselected population: the results of a multicenter study. Ultrasound Obstet Gynecol 2001; **17**: 197–202.

De Bruyn R, Gordon I. Postnatal investigation of fetal renal disease. Prenat Diagn 2001; **21**: 984–91.

Lazebnik N, Bellinger MF, Ferguson JE 2nd, Hogge JS, Hogge WA. Insights into the pathogenesis and natural history of fetuses with multicystic dysplastic kidney disease. Prenat Diagn 1999; **19**: 418–23.

Moreno CA, Metze K, Lomazi EA, et al. Visceral myopathy: Clinical and molecular survey of a cohort of seven new patients and state of the art of overlapping phenotypes. Am J Med Genet A 2016; **170**(11): 2965–74.

Onuchic LF, Furu L, Nagasawa Y, et al. PKHD1, the polycystic kidney and hepatic disease 1 gene, encodes a novel large protein containing multiple immunoglobulin-like plexin-transcription-factor domains and parallel beta-helix 1 repeats. Am J Hum Genet 2002; **70**: 1305–17.

Pilu G, Nicolaides KH. Features of chromosomal defects. In: G Pilu, KH Nicolaides. Diagnosis of fetal abnormalities: the 18–23 week scan, pp. 99–104. Parthenon Publishing, Carnforth, 1999.

Quirino IG, Diniz JS, Bouzada MC, et al. Clinical course of 822 children with prenatally detected nephrouropathies. Clin J Am Soc Nephrol 2012; **7**: 444–51.

Roodhooft AM, Birnholz JC, Holmes LB. Familial nature of congenital absence and severe dysgenesis of both kidneys. N Engl J Med 1984; **310**: 1341–5.

Sanna-Cherchi S, Kiryluk K, Burgess KE, et al. Copy-number disorders are a common cause of congenital kidney malformations. Am J Hum Genet 2012; **91**: 987–97.

Sanna-Cherchi S, Ravani P, Corbani V, et al. Renal outcome in patients with congenital anomalies of the kidney and urinary tract. Kidney Int 2009; **76**: 528–33.

Sanna-Cherchi S, Sampogna RV, Papeta N, et al. Mutations in DSTYK and dominant urinary tract malformations. N Engl J Med 2013; **369**: 621–9.

Thomas DF. Prenatal diagnosis: does it alter outcome? Prenat Diagn 2001; **21**: 1004–11.

Thomas R, Sanna-Cherchi S, Warady BA, Furth SL, Kaskel FJ, Gharavi AG. HNF1B and PAX2 mutations are a common cause of renal hypodysplasia in the CKiD cohort. Pediatr Nephrol 2011; **26**: 897–903.

Verbitsky M, Sanna-Cherchi S, et al. Genomic imbalance in pediatric patients with chronic kidney disease. J Clin Invest 2015; **125**: 2171–8.

Verbitsky M, Kogan AJ. Genomic disorders and neurocognitive impairment in pediatric CKD. J Am Soc Nephrol 2017; Mar 27.

Wangler MF, Gonzaga-Jauregui C, Gambin T, et al. Heterozygous de novo or inherited mutations in the smooth muscle (ACTG2) gene underlie megacystis–microcolon–hypoperistalsis syndrome. PLoS Genet 2014; **10**: e1004258.

Weber S, Moriniere V, Knüppel T, et al. Prevalence of mutations in renal developmental genes in children with renal hypodysplasia: results of the ESCAPE study. J Am Soc Nephrol 2006; **17**: 2864–70.

Wellesley D, Howe DT. Fetal renal anomalies and genetic syndromes. Prenat Diagn 2001; **21**: 992–1003.

Winyard P, Chitty L. Dysplastic and polycystic kidneys: diagnosis, associations and management. Prenat Diagn 2001; **21**: 924–35.

Zerres K, Rudnik-Schoneborn S, Deget F. Childhood onset autosomal dominant polycystic kidney disease in sibs: clinical picture and recurrence risk. German Working Group on Paediatric Nephrology. J Med Genet 1993; **30**: 583–8.

Zerres K, Rudnik-Schoneborn S, Deget F, et al. Autosomal recessive polycystic kidney disease in 115 children: clinical presentation, course and influence of gender. Arbeitsgemeinschaft fur Padiatrische, Nephrologie. Acta Paediatr 1996; **85**: 437–45.

Varicella

Varicella (chickenpox) is an acute disease caused by varicella-zoster virus (VZV) that is transmitted by personal contact or droplet spread. It is highly contagious, since the rate of transmission among household contacts is ~90%. Since chickenpox is so common in childhood, over 90% of adults in temperate countries are immune. An effective vaccine is available but is not universally administered in all countries. The incubation period is 2–3 weeks. Chickenpox is usually a mild illness in childhood but can be more serious in adults, especially pregnant women who are at risk of fulminating varicella pneumonia. Herpes zoster (shingles) is the reactivation of VZV, which can occur many years later.

Fetal varicella syndrome

This rare syndrome comprises one or more birth defects, including limb hypoplasia, skin scarring usually involving one or a few dermatomes, and damage to the eyes and CNS. Women who develop chickenpox during the first 20 weeks of pregnancy have a 1–2% risk of having a baby with fetal varicella infection. Most cases follow maternal varicella between 13 and 20 weeks' gestation (Enders et al. 1994). The risk of fetal varicella syndrome is minimal before 8 weeks' gestation and after 24 weeks. Some infants who acquire varicella during the pregnancy and have no birth defects go on to develop shingles later after birth.

In the case of maternal herpes zoster, the risk of fetal varicella is very low (0 in a series of 366 women; Enders et al. 1994).

Neonatal varicella

This is a potentially devastating infection of the neonate, following maternal varicella near the time of delivery. The risk is highest, of the order of 50%, in cases of birth between 4 days before and 2 days after the maternal rash. Neonatal symptoms include skin lesions, ulcerated necrotic or haemorrhagic lesions, as well as life-threatening systemic disease (pneumonia, liver failure, encephalitis, and coagulopathy). The risk is increased in preterm infants.

Management of contact during pregnancy

- If a pregnant woman has no history of chickenpox or zoster and has recently been in direct contact with a case of chickenpox or zoster, immediately test a blood sample for VZV IgG immunity. Pregnant woman with no immunity to VZV should be offered zoster immune globulin (ZIG) without delay in these circumstances.
- The diagnosis of chickenpox is usually clinically evident. In case of doubt and in the absence of a history of contact, the diagnosis can be confirmed by testing the mother's blood to document seroconversion.

Management of the mother

- Maternal varicella can be a serious, and even fatal, condition (risk of pneumonitis and encephalitis).
- Seek advice from an infectious diseases expert and give consideration to the use of aciclovir.

Management of the pregnancy

- In cases of varicella before 24 weeks, perform detailed fetal USS, with particular attention to the limbs, CNS, and eyes. Repeat USS monthly. Consider amniocentesis (after the end of scarring) with VZV PCR of amniotic fluid for fetal diagnosis.
- In cases of varicella near term, start treatment with valacyclovir and attempt to delay delivery. In cases of maternal varicella between −4 days and +2 days of birth, the neonate should be hospitalized and treated with aciclovir.

Expert adviser: Laurent Mandelbrot, Professor, Department of Obstetrics and Gynaecology, Hôpital Louis Mourier, Assistance Publique-Hôpitaux de Paris, Colombes, France.

References

Enders G, Miller E, Craddock-Watson J, et al. Consequences of varicella and herpes zoster in pregnancy: prospective study of 1739 cases. Lancet 1994; **343**: 1547–50.

Mandelbrot L. Fetal varicella—diagnosis, management and outcome. Prenat Diagn 2012; **32**: 511–18.

Royal College of Obstetricians and Gynaecologists. Chickenpox in pregnancy. Green-top guideline No. 13, 2015. https://www.rcog.org.uk/globalassets/documents/guidelines/gtg_13.pdf.

Ventriculomegaly

Ventriculomegaly in a fetus is an increase in the size of the cerebral ventricles, as measured by USS. This finding is associated with an increased risk of other structural brain malformations, fetal chromosomal abnormalities, congenital anomalies and infections, syndromes, perinatal death, and childhood developmental delay (Wax *et al.* 2003). A wide range in the incidence of mild ventriculomegaly is reported in the literature (1.5–20/1000 fetuses).

- Normal. Axial sonograms of the brain through the atrium of the lateral ventricle demonstrate that the normal atrial diameter remains relatively constant from 14 weeks' gestation. The atrium has a mean diameter of 7.6 ± 0.6 mm (SD). Atrial diameters exceeding 10 mm (above 4 SDs) suggest ventriculomegaly, with a low false-positive rate (Cardoza *et al.* 1988).
- Mild ventriculomegaly. The lateral ventricle diameter measures 10–12 mm.
- Moderate ventriculomegaly. The lateral ventricle diameter measures 12.1–15 mm.
- Severe ventriculomegaly. The lateral ventricle diameter measures >15 mm (Gaglioti *et al.* 2009).

Hydrocephalus has a birth incidence of 4–8/10 000 live births and stillbirths. Congenital malformations of the CNS (e.g. spina bifida), infections (congenital infection or meningitis), and haemorrhage can all give rise to hydrocephalus.

It is important to attempt to distinguish between ventriculomegaly caused by conditions where the ventricles appear large due to poor brain growth, infections, and other insults and ventriculomegaly caused by hydrocephalus due to CSF obstruction or poor CSF absorption (see Figure 6.11). All types of ventriculomegaly are associated with other brain malformations, chromosomal anomalies, and syndromes, but severe ventriculomegaly has a higher frequency of hydrocephalus and structural intracranial anomalies.

The prognosis for ventriculomegaly depends on the underlying diagnosis, the gestational age at diagnosis, and whether the condition is progressive. It is important to determine if the ventriculomegaly is isolated or associated with other malformations. Sonographically, isolated mild ventriculomegaly is associated with a significantly better prognosis than non-isolated mild ventriculomegaly (Goldstein *et al.* 1990). Studies have shown that the majority of fetuses with additional abnormalities can be detected with a combination of detailed scans and chromosomal analysis.

Mild ventriculomegaly may resolve with no neurological deficit (Falip *et al.* 2007; Signorelli *et al.* 2004). Alternatively, mild ventriculomegaly may be associated with serious neurological disability in many chromosomal and genetic disorders. Overall, isolated mild ventriculomegaly resolves in about two-thirds before birth, with no apparent neurodevelopmental sequelae (see 'Genetic advice and management' below). Management and counselling for mild ventriculomegaly are challenging and difficult tasks.

Clinical assessment

History: key points

- Detailed three-generation family tree. Extend further on the maternal side, if possible. Enquire specifically for other relatives with hydrocephalus, unexplained stillbirths, spasticity, or mental handicap.
- Consanguinity. AR genetic syndromes.
- Enquire about infections, trauma, and bleeding disorders in the mother.

Examination: key points

The main aim is to determine if the ventriculomegaly is isolated or associated with an intracranial malformation or a non-CNS anomaly. Over 60% of fetuses with dilated cerebral ventricles have another abnormality on scan. In severe ventriculomegaly, about two-thirds of

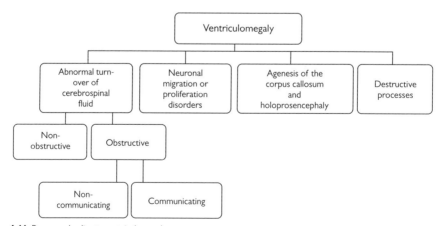

Figure 6.11 Processes leading to ventriculomegaly.
Reproduced from Gaglioti P, Manuela O *et al.*, The significance of fetal ventriculomegaly: etiology, short- and long-term outcomes, *Prenatal Diagnosis*, 2009; 29: 381–388, with permission from Wiley and the International Society for Prenatal Diagnosis.

these are intracranial (particularly ACC) and one-third are extracranial.

- Other intracranial anomalies. Document which ventricles are dilated, if bilateral/unilateral, and if there has been progression. Look at the development of the corpus callosum.
- Detailed fetal anomaly USS, looking for extracranial anomalies. Particularly examine the spine (NTDs).

Special investigations

- Genomic array/karyotype. Should be considered in all patients. In mild ventriculomegaly, the range of abnormal results varies from 3% to 14%, but if increased maternal age risk is excluded, the risk of aneuploidy is about 3.5% (Gaglioti *et al.* 2009). In isolated severe ventriculomegaly, there is a low risk of chromosomal abnormality, but amniocentesis is indicated because identification of an anomaly gives further evidence for poor prognosis.
- CMV and toxoplasmosis screen (10–20% of severe ventriculomegaly). Consider Zika virus in women with possible exposure in pregnancy (Honein *et al.* 2017).
- Screen for neonatal alloimmune thrombocytopenia (NAIT).
- Consider fetal MRI. Mehta *et al.* (2005) reviewed the usefulness of MRI in fetuses with ventriculomegaly. MRI is better than USS at detecting abnormalities of callosal and gyral development, cerebellar hypoplasia, porencephaly, vermian cysts, and subependymal and cortical tubers (features of TSC; see 'Tuberous sclerosis (TSC)' in Chapter 3, 'Common consultations', p. 534). The diagnosis changed in 45/145 cases, with MRI better in later gestation at identifying significant abnormalities.
- Store DNA from the fetus if pregnancy is terminated, in case features of a single gene disorder are found at post-mortem in which case request gene panel/WES/WGS as appropriate.
- Strongly recommend non-invasive post mortem (including brain MRI) or detailed post-mortem, including neuropathology, in terminated fetuses. As neuropathology takes extra time (brain requires fixing), ensure that the parents give the correct consent for this procedure. Despite clear appearances of ventriculomegaly on prenatal USS, these appearances may not be confirmed at post-mortem.

Diagnoses to consider

The following are conditions to consider in fetuses with ventriculomegaly.

Hydrocephalus

'TRUE' ISOLATED HYDROCEPHALUS. This is secondary to a relative or complete block to CSF flow. This is divided into communicating and non-communicating hydrocephalus. XL hydrocephalus with aqueduct stenosis may present in this way. For more details, see 'Hydrocephalus' in Chapter 2, 'Clinical approach', p. 172.

HYDROCEPHALUS WITH AN NTD. See 'Neural tube defects' in Chapter 3, 'Common consultations', p. 500.

Structural brain anomalies that may be associated with, or confused with, ventriculomegaly

HOLOPROSENCEPHALY (HPE). During embryonic life, the forebrain vesicle divides along the dorsal midline to form the cerebral hemispheres. Failure, or partial failure, of this cleavage results in alobar HPE, where the two lateral ventricles are replaced by a single midline ventricle that is often greatly enlarged, to part fusion of the frontal lobes (lobar HPE). Other midline forebrain structures, including the olfactory bulbs and tracts, optic bulbs and tracts, corpus callosum, thalamus, hypothalamus, and pituitary, are frequently also affected.

About 50% of HPE has a chromosomal aetiology. Trisomy 13 is the most common abnormality, but many other anomalies have been described. Particularly exclude loci known to have been associated with HPE. Triploidy may be found in fetuses with HPE. Genomic array is indicated.

The most common single gene associated with HPE is sonic hedgehog *SHH*. See 'Holoprosencephaly (HPE)' in Chapter 2, 'Clinical approach', p. 168.

HYDRANENCEPHALY. Scans show a small rim of cerebral cortex, but the cerebellum and brainstem may be normal. Disruption to the carotid artery supply is one cause. Enquire about early pregnancy bleeding and trauma. May be confused with HPE.

ARACHNOID AND PORENCEPHALIC CYSTS. An arachnoid cyst is a cystic cavity within the arachnoid membrane. Hydrocephalus can occur by obstruction and reduced CSF resorption. The majority of arachnoid cysts are sporadic. See 'Structural intracranial anomalies (agenesis of the corpus callosum, septo-optic dysplasia, and arachnoid cysts)' in Chapter 2, 'Clinical approach', p. 320.

Single gene disorders

X-linked hydrocephalus

The neural cell adhesion molecule L1CAM plays a key role during neurodevelopment. The gene encoding L1CAM maps to Xq28, and males with a mutation in this gene have a phenotype characterized by a combination of corpus callosum hypoplasia, MR, adducted thumbs, spastic paraplegia, and hydrocephalus. There is a high degree of intra- and interfamilial variability. See 'Hydrocephalus' in Chapter 2, 'Clinical approach', p. 172.

Muscle–eye–brain (MEB) disease (Walker–Warburg syndrome (WWS))

AR disorders that share the combination of cerebral neuronal migration defects (type II lissencephaly), ocular abnormalities, and CMD. The features of WWS are hydrocephalus, agyria, retinal dystrophy, and sometimes an encephalocele—thus its alternative name of HARD ± E. Syndromes are due to genes in the *O*-mannosylation pathway (the *POMT1* gene in WWS and *POMGNT1* in MEB).

Pseudo-TORCH

This is an AR condition with ICC, therefore mimicking congenital infection. The OFC is usually microcephalic. See 'Intracranial calcification' in Chapter 2, 'Clinical approach', p. 200.

Chromosomal disorders

Exclude chromosomal disorders in fetuses with additional malformations. Counsel as appropriate.

Genetic advice and management

Isolated ventriculomegaly

There have been a number of prospective studies to try and establish the natural history of fetal ventriculomegaly. Nevertheless, management of mild fetal ventriculomegaly and counselling of parents remain difficult, as the cause of the ventriculomegaly and the absolute risk and degree of possible resulting handicap often cannot be determined with confidence (Wyldes and Watkinson 2004).

Pooling of data by Gaglioti et al. (2009) on the outcome of isolated ventriculomegaly showed a normal outcome in 94% of fetuses with mild ventriculomegaly, in 76% with moderate ventriculomegaly, and in 28% with severe ventriculomegaly. The numbers in the severe ventriculomegaly group is small, probably reflecting the fact that many parents had opted for TOP in this group, but it is this group that typically present for genetic counselling either during pregnancy or after delivery.

Mild ventriculomegaly

Ensure that all investigations have been done to exclude other malformations, chromosome abnormalities, etc. Most have a good prognosis, but there remains the possibility of serious disabling neurological conditions. The condition may resolve and these children have a good prognosis. Progression and persistence of the ventriculomegaly during pregnancy are of concern.

Severe ventriculomegaly

The risk for disability is highest in this group, but postmortem often gives good diagnostic information to inform genetic counselling. After careful consideration of the differential diagnosis and a post-mortem that does not reveal any features suggestive of a genetic or chromosomal disorder, counsel as for isolated hydrocephalus:

- the empiric risk for sibs of an isolated case is ~5%, with all studies showing a higher risk for male sibs of an affected male;
- the risk for male sibs of an isolated male case with aqueduct stenosis is higher (5–10%), unless *L1CAM* has been excluded;
- children of consanguineous parents may have hydrocephalus as part of an AR condition.

If there is incomplete information, the recurrence risk cannot be accurately assessed.

Support groups: Shine (Spina bifida, Hydrocephalus, Information, Networking, Equality), http://www.shinecharity.org.uk, Tel. 01733 555 988; ARC (Antenatal Results and Choices), http://www.arc-uk.org, Tel. 0207 631 0285.

Expert adviser: Charu Deshpande, Consultant Clinical Geneticist, Guy's and St Thomas' NHS Foundation Trust, London, UK.

References

Cardoza JD, Goldstein RB, Filly RA. Exclusion of fetal ventriculomegaly with a single measurement: the width of the lateral ventricular atrium. *Radiology* 1988; **169**: 711–14.

Falip C, Blanc N, Maes E, et al. Postnatal clinical and imaging follow-up of infants with prenatal isolated mild ventriculomegaly: a series of 101 cases. *Pediatr Radiol* 2007; **37**: 981–9.

Futagi Y, Suzuki Y, Toribe Y, Morimoto K. Neurodevelopmental outcome in children with fetal hydrocephalus. *Pediatr Neurol* 2002; **27**: 111–16.

Gaglioti P, Oberto M, Todros T. The significance of fetal ventriculomegaly: etiology, short- and long-term outcomes. *Prenat Diagn* 2009; **29**: 381–8.

Goldstein RB, La Pidus AS, Filly RA, Cardoza J. Mild lateral cerebral ventricular dilatation *in utero*: clinical significance and prognosis. *Radiology* 1990; **176**: 237–42.

Graham E, Duhl A, Ural S, Allen M, Blakemore K, Witter F. The degree of antenatal ventriculomegaly is related to paediatric neurological morbidity. *J Matern Fetal Med* 2001; **10**: 258–63.

Honein MA, Dawson AL, Petersen EE, et al. Birth defects among fetuses and infants of US women with evidence of possible Zika virus infection during pregnancy. *JAMA* 2017; **317**(1): 59–68.

Kelly EN, Allen VM, Seaward G, Windrim R, Ryan G. Mild ventriculomegaly in the fetus, natural history, associated findings and outcome of isolated mild ventriculomegaly: a literature review. *Prenat Diagn* 2001; **21**: 697–700.

Mehta TS, Levine D. Imaging of fetal cerebral ventriculomegaly: a guide to management and outcome. *Semin Fetal Neonatal Med* 2005; **10**: 421–8.

Robson S, Webster S, Smith M, McCormick K, Embleton N. Outcome of mild/moderate fetal cerebral ventriculomegaly. *J Obstet Gynaecol* 2003; **23**(Suppl 1): S22–23.

Signorelli M, Tiberti A, Valseriati D, et al. Width of the fetal lateral ventricular atrium between 10 and 12 mm: a simple variation of the norm? *Ultrasound Obstet Gynecol* 2004; **23**: 14–18.

Wax JR, Bookman L, Cartin A, Pinette MG, Blackstone J. Mild fetal cerebral ventriculomegaly: diagnosis, clinical associations, and outcomes. *Obstet Gynecol Surv* 2003; **58**: 407–14.

Wyldes M, Watkinson M. Isolated mild fetal ventriculomegaly [review]. *Arch Dis Child Fet Neonat Ed* 2004; **89**: F9–13.

Appendix

Appendix contents

Antenatal and neonatal screening timelines

For a timeline of antenatal and newborn screening, see Figure A1.

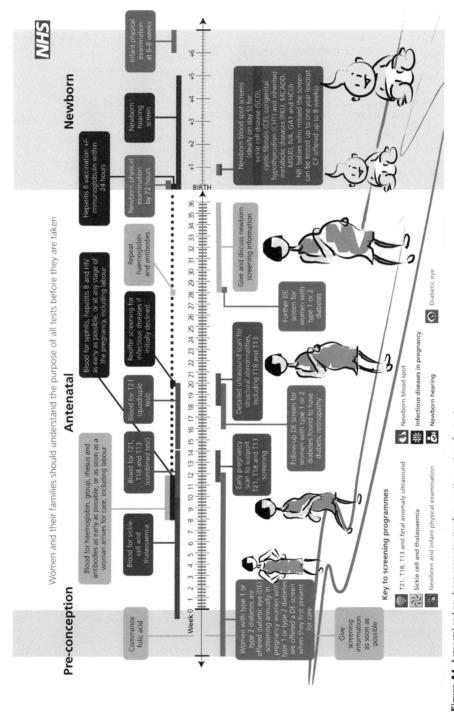

Figure A1 Antenatal and newborn screening timeline—optimum times for testing.
© Crown Copyright 2016. This information was originally developed by Public Health England Screening (https://www.gov.uk/topic/population-screening-programmes) and is used under the Open Government Licence v3.0.

Bayes' theorem

Bayes' theorem as applied to X-linked (XLR) disorders where males do not reproduce (e.g. Duchenne muscular dystrophy (DMD)).

This provides a method of modifying the prior risk by the introduction of conditional factors (such as number of unaffected sons).

Important notes

- v = mutation rate in male gametes and m = mutation rate in female gametes.
- For DMD, $v = m$.
- Prior probability that any female is a carrier of a sex-linked recessive disorder with a genetic fitness of zero = $4m$ (see Young (1999) for formal proof).
- Probability that the daughter of a non-carrier will become a carrier as a result of a new mutation is $2m$ (she has two X chromosomes), whereas probability that the son of a non-carrier will be affected as a result of a new mutation is m (he has one X chromosome).
- Terms of m^2 or m^3 are ignored for the purposes of these calculations as they are so small. Similarly $1 - 4m$ is approximated to 1 because the $4m$ term is so tiny in comparison.

- Mothers with two or more affected children or carrier daughters are assumed to be carriers. (The possibility of gonadal mosaicism is generally not considered in making these calculations.)
- Identify the closest female relative from whom both the consultand and all the affected male relatives are descended—the 'dummy consultand' or I1 in the worked examples.
- Information must never be used twice.

Worked examples

The five worked examples refer to parts (a)–(e), respectively, of Figure A2. In Figure A2, the person for whom the genetic risk is being calculated is marked by an arrow. The roman numerals denote the row/generation (going top to bottom) and the arabic numerals the position (left to right) in that row, so that III2 is the second person in the third generation (bottom row). Circles denote females and squares males. Black squares indicate affected males. The required result for the arrowed proband is given in boldface type.

1. See part (a) of Figure A2. II2 is a carrier as she has an affected brother and son. I1 is a carrier as she has an

Table A1 Relative probability of the dystrophin mutation arising in carriers using Bayes' theorem

		I1 is a carrier (C)		I1 is not a carrier (NC)	
Prior probability		$4m$		$1 - 4m = 1$	
II1	C		NC	C	NC
Prior	1/2		1/2	$2m$	1
Conditional (1 affected son)	1/2		m	1/2	m
Joint probability	m		$(2m^2)$	m	m
Relative probability		m	:		$2m$
Absolute probability		$m/m + 2m$		$2m/m + 2m$	
		1/3		2/3	

The probability that I1 is a carrier is 1/3; therefore, the probability that her daughter is a carrier is 1/6.

Adapted by permission from BMJ Publishing Group Limited. *Journal of Medical Genetics*, Bundey S. Calculation of genetic risks in Duchenne muscular dystrophy by geneticists in the United Kingdom, volume 15, pp. 249–53, Copyright © 1978 BMJ Publishing Group.

Table A2 Relative probability of the dystrophin mutation arising in carriers using Bayes' theorem

		I1 is a carrier (C)		I1 is not a carrier (NC)	
Prior probability		$4m$		$1 - 4m = 1$	
Conditional (4 normal sons)		$1/2 \times 1/2 \times 1/2 \times 1/2$		1	
II1	C		NC	C	NC
Prior	1/2		1/2	$2m$	1
Conditional (1 affected son)	1/2		m	1/2	m
Joint probability	$m/16$		$(m^2/8)$	m	m
Relative probability		$m/16$	:		$2m$
Absolute probability		$m/33m$		$32m/33m$	
		1/33		32/33	

The probability that I1 is a carrier is 1/33; therefore, the probability that her daughter is a carrier is 1/66.

Adapted by permission from BMJ Publishing Group Limited. *Journal of Medical Genetics*, Bundey S. Calculation of genetic risks in Duchenne muscular dystrophy by geneticists in the United Kingdom, volume 15, pp. 249–53, Copyright © 1978 BMJ Publishing Group.

Table A3 Relative probability of the dystrophin mutation arising in carriers using Bayes' theorem

	I1 is a carrier (C)				I1 is not a carrier (NC)
Prior probability	4m				1 − 4m =1
Conditional (3 normal sons)	1/2 × 1/2 × 1/2				1
II1	C		NC	C	NC
Prior	1/2		1/2	2m	1
Conditional (1 affected son)	1/2		m	1/2	m
Joint probability	m/8		(m²/4)	m	m
Relative probability		m/8	:		2m
Absolute probability		m/17m			16m/17m
		1/17			16/17

The probability that I1 is a carrier is 1/17; therefore, the probability that her daughter is a carrier is 1/34.

Adapted by permission from BMJ Publishing Group Limited. *Journal of Medical Genetics*, Bundey S. Calculation of genetic risks in Duchenne muscular dystrophy by geneticists in the United Kingdom, volume 15, pp. 249–53, Copyright © 1978 BMJ Publishing Group.

Table A4 Relative probability of the dystrophin mutation arising in carriers using Bayes' theorem

	II5 is a carrier (NC)		II5 is not a carrier (C)
Prior probability	1/34		33/34
Conditional (1 normal son)	1/2		1
Joint probability	1/68		33/34
Relative probability	1	:	66
Absolute probability	1/67		66/67

The probability that II5 is a carrier is 1/67.

Adapted by permission from BMJ Publishing Group Limited. *Journal of Medical Genetics*, Bundey S. Calculation of genetic risks in Duchenne muscular dystrophy by geneticists in the United Kingdom, volume 15, pp. 249–53, Copyright © 1978 BMJ Publishing Group.

affected son and a carrier daughter (ignoring germline mosaicism). If I1 is a carrier, her daughter has a 1/2 risk of being a carrier, and her grand-daughter has a carrier risk of 1/4.

Table A5 Relative probability of the dystrophin mutation arising in carriers using Bayes' theorem

	I1 is a carrier (C)			I1 is not a carrier (NC)
Prior probability	4m			1 − 4m =1
II1	C	NC	C	NC
Prior	1/2	1/2	2m	1
Conditional (4 normal sons)	(1/2)⁴	1	(1/2)⁴	1
Conditional (1 affected son)	1/2	m	1/2	m
Joint probability	m/16	(2m²)	m/16	m
Relative probability	m	:		17m
Absolute probability	1/18			17/18

The probability that I1 is a carrier is 1/18; therefore, the probability that her daughter is a carrier is 1/36.

Note: m is a small number, so 1 − m = 1, m² = 0.

Adapted by permission from BMJ Publishing Group Limited. *Journal of Medical Genetics*, Bundey S. Calculation of genetic risks in Duchenne muscular dystrophy by geneticists in the United Kingdom, volume 15, pp. 249–53, Copyright © 1978 BMJ Publishing Group.

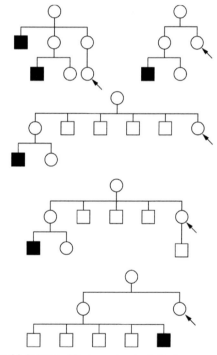

Figure A2 Pedigrees of Duchenne muscular dystrophy requesting the genetic risks run by the female relatives marked by arrow.
Adapted by permission from BMJ Publishing Group Limited. *Journal of Medical Genetics*, Bundey S. Calculation of genetic risks in Duchenne muscular dystrophy by geneticists in the United Kingdom, volume 15, pp. 249–53, Copyright © 1978 BMJ Publishing Group.

2. See part (b) of Figure A2 and Table A1. In this family tree, there is uncertainty as to where the dystrophin mutation has arisen. Is it present in the maternal grandmother, or has it arisen *de novo* in the affected boy (III1) or in his mother (II1)? Bayes' theorem can help to establish the relative probabilities.

3. See part (c) of Figure A2 and Table A2. This family tree is similar to that shown in part (b), except for the addition

of four unaffected boys. This substantially reduces the chance that I1 is a carrier. This 'conditional' information is put into the Bayes' calculation to derive the carrier risk.

4. See part (d) of Figure A2 and Table A3. This family tree is similar to that shown in part (c), but there are fewerunaffected males in generation II and there is additional conditional information since the consultand has a normal son (see Table A4).

5. See part (e) of Figure A2 and Table A5. In this family tree, there is uncertainty as to where the dystrophin mutation has arisen. Has it arisen *de novo* in the affected boy (III5) or in his mother (II1) or in the maternal grandmother (I1)? The affected boy has four normal brothers. This conditional information substantially reduces the chance that his mother (II1) or his maternal grandmother (I1) are carriers for a dystrophin mutations. Bayes' theorem can help to establish the relative probabilities.

References

Bundey S. Calculation of genetic risks in Duchenne muscular dystrophy by geneticists in the United Kingdom. *J Med Genet* 1978; **15**: 249–53.

Young ID. *Introduction to risk calculation in genetic counselling*, 2nd edn. Oxford University Press, Oxford, 1999.

Carrier frequency and carrier testing for autosomal recessive disorders

The Hardy–Weinberg equation

In a large randomly mating population with a disease caused by mutations at a single locus, it is possible to calculate the carrier frequency from a knowledge of the incidence of affected individuals in the population.

If N is the normal allele and n is the disease allele, then NN is the homozygous normal state, nn is the homozygous affected state, and Nn is the carrier state.

The frequency of the three genotypes can be determined from the binomial expression $(p + q)^2$, where p and q are the frequencies of the normal and disease alleles, respectively, and $p + q = 1$:

Frequency of NN = p^2 Normal
Frequency of Nn = $2pq$ Carrier
Frequency of nn = q^2 Affected

The carrier rate can be calculated as:

Carrier rate = $2pq = 2(1-q)q = 2q-2q^2$.

If the disease is rare, e.g. 1/1000 or less, the $2q^2$ term becomes very small and, for the purposes of clinical risk

estimation, can be ignored and so the carrier rate can be approximated to ~$2q$,

Carrier rate ~$2(q^2)^{1/2}$, i.e. $2q$
or $2 \times$ (disease frequency for rare diseases)$^{1/2}$,

e.g. for a rare disease with a frequency of 1/90 000, the carrier rate is $2(1/90\ 000)^{1/2} = 2 \times 1/300 = 1/150$. Table A7 gives a guide to gene and carrier frequencies for different disease frequencies.

The following sources may be helpful in finding disease frequencies from which carrier frequencies can be derived: The Frequency of Inherited Disorders Database (FIDD), https://medicapps.cardiff.ac.uk/fidd; Online Mendelian Inheritance in Man (OMIM), https://www.ncbi.nlm.nih.gov.

Table to show data about carrier frequency and carrier testing for a sample of autosomal recessive disorders

See Table A6.

Table A6 Table to show data about carrier frequency and carrier testing for a sample of autosomal recessive disorders

Disease*	Carrier frequency in general population	Gene	Carrier testing for	
			Relatives at increased risk	Individuals at population risk
Alpha-1 antitrypsin deficiency	1/25 for Z and 1/17 for S alleles in northern European population	SERPINA1	Alpha-1 antitrypsin phenotyping on sample of clotted blood	Alpha-1 antitrypsin phenotyping on sample of clotted blood
Batten disease or juvenile neuronal lipofuscinosis (JNCL)	LB rate 0.46/10 000, i.e. ~1/20 000. Note genetic heterogeneity: LB rate for CLCN3 ~1/30 000, giving a carrier rate for CLCN3 of ~1/85	CLCN1 (21%), CLCN2 (7%), CLCN3 (72%)	Common 1-kb deletion of exons 7 and 8 in CLCN3	Common 1-kb deletion of exons 7 and 8 in CLCN3
Congenital adrenal hyperplasia (CAH)	1/50 for CYP21	CYP21	In classic CAH, ~20–25% have a gene deletion and ~30% have an intron 2 splice-site mutation. The missense mutation V281L is the most common mutation in non-classic CAH	Possible for the common mutations
Congenital deafness: connexin 26 type	1/50 in European, North American, and Mediterranean populations	GJB2	Possible if mutations have been defined in the proband	Possible for common 35delG mutation
Cystic fibrosis (CF)	1/23 in Caucasians (see 'Cystic fibrosis (CF)' in Chapter 3, 'Common consultations', p. 382 for other ethnic groups)	CFTR	Available by direct mutation analysis if mutation in proband is known	Possible using commercial multiplex mutation assay
Friedreich's ataxia	1/85	Frataxin	Analysis for triplet repeat (GAA)$_n$ expansion	Analysis for triplet repeat (GAA)$_n$ expansion
Galactosaemia	1/105	GALT1	Mutation analysis of GALT1	Screen for common Q188R mutation
Gaucher	1/25 in Ashkenazi population	GBA	Analysis of acid beta-glucosidase enzyme. Mutation analysis of GBA	Four common mutations of GBA in the Ashkenazi population
Haemochromatosis	1/10 in northern European populations (see 'Haemochromatosis' in Chapter 3, 'Common consultations', p. 430 for more details)	HFE	Mutation analysis for C282Y and H63D	Mutation analysis for C282Y and H63D

Table A6 Continued

Disease*	Carrier frequency in general population	Gene	Carrier testing for	
			Relatives at increased risk	Individuals at population risk
Hurler	1/60	IDUA	Mutation analysis of IDUA (two common nonsense mutations W402X and Q70X). Enzyme analysis of alpha-L-iduronidase	Two common nonsense mutations W402X and Q70X
Krabbe	Very rare, more common in Druze and Sicilian populations	GALC	Mutation analysis of GALC Enzyme analysis of glycosyl ceramidase	
Metachromatic leukodystrophy	1 in 40 000 LB, 1/100	ARSA	Mutation analysis of ARSA Enzyme analysis of arylsulfatase A gene	
Phenylketonuria (PKU) 1/50		PAH	Mutation analysis of PAH Linkage analysis Enzyme analysis	Mutation analysis of PAH for common mutations
Sanfilippo (MPS III)	1/65 000 LB (all types)	SGSH (type A)	Mutation analysis of SGSH Enzyme analysis of heparan N-sulfatase	
		NAGLU (type B)	Mutation analysis of NAGLU Enzyme analysis of alpha-N-acetylglucosaminidase	
Spinal muscular atrophy (SMA)	1/50	SMN1	Mutation analysis for exon 7 deletion in SMN1	Mutation analysis for exon 7 deletion in SMN1
Tay–Sachs disease	1/30 in Ashkenazi Jewish populations	HEXA	Mutation analysis of HEXA Enzyme analysis of hexosaminidase A gene	Mutation analysis in Jewish population Enzyme analysis in non-Jewish population

* Please refer to the relevant sections of this book for a fuller account.

Table A7 Carrier and gene frequencies for representative values of disease frequency

Disease frequency (q^2)	Gene frequency (q)	Carrier frequency ($2pq$)
1/100	1/10	2/11
1/400	1/20	71/10
1/900	1/30	71/15
1/1000	1/32	71/16
1/1600	1/40	71/20
1/2000	1/45	71/23
1/5000	1/71	71/35
1/10 000	1/100	71/50
1/15 000	1/122	71/60
1/20 000	1/141	71/70
1/25 000	1/158	71/80
1/30 000	1/173	71/85
1/40 000	1/200	71/100
1/50 000	1/224	71/110
1/60 000	1/245	71/125
1/70 000	1/265	71/135
1/80 000	1/283	71/140
1/90 000	1/300	71/150
1/100 000	1/316	71/160
1/150 000	1/387	71/200
1/200 000	1/448	71/225

Carrier and gene frequencies for representative values of disease frequency

See Table A7 for carrier frequencies.

For the top ten most common carrier frequencies by population, see Table A8.

Top ten most common carrier frequencies by population

See Table A8, p. 812.

Reference

Scriver CR, Beaudet AL, Sly WS, Valle D (eds.). *The metabolic and molecular bases of inherited disease*, 8th edn. McGraw-Hill, New York, 2001.

Table A8 Top ten most common carrier frequencies by population

Disease	Counsyl frequency (1 in)	Counsyl 95% CI (1 in)	Literature frequency (1 in)	# Tested	Screening?
All populations (N = 23,453)					
α-1-Antitrypsin deficiency	13.1	12–14	11.5	15,484	×
Cystic fibrosis	27.8	26–30	31.7	23,369	Y
DFNB1	42.6	39–47	42.8	15,799	×
Spinal muscular atrophy	57.1	52–63	54	23,127	1
Familial Mediterranean fever	64.2	57–73	Unknown	15,854	×
Smith–Lemli–Opitz syndrome	68.2	60–78	123	15,825	×
Sickle cell disease/β-thalassemia	69.6	63–78	158	21,360	×
Gaucher disease	76.7	69–87	200	21,473	×
Factor XI deficiency	92.0	80–108	Rare	15,724	×
Achromatopsia	97.5	85–115	123	15,798	×
Northwestern Europe (N = 12,915)					
α-1-Antitrypsin deficiency	10.2	10–11	11.4	8,570	×
Cystic fibrosis	22.9	21–25	28	12,870	Y
DFNB1	46.0	40–54	33.2	8,735	×
Spinal muscular atrophy	49.9	45–57	47	12,730	1
Smith–Lemli–Opitz syndrome	50.3	44–59	123.9	8,750	×
MCAD deficiency	73.5	62–90	61.7	8,749	×
Hereditary fructose intolerance	90.1	75–113	81.1	8,744	×
Achromatopsia	91.0	76–114	123	8,734	×
Hereditary thymine-uraciluria	96.4	80–122	33	8,680	×
Familial Mediterranean fever	99.5	82–126	Unknown	8,756	×
Ashkenazi Jewish (N = 2,410)					
Factor XI deficiency	12.6	11–15	8	1,501	×
Familial Mediterranean fever	13.2	11–16	10.5	1,513	×
Gaucher disease	16.8	14–20	17	2,384	1
DFNB1	21.3	17–28	21	1,509	×
Cystic fibrosis	21.6	18–27	29	2,402	Y
α-1-Antitrypsin deficiency	24.2	19–32	16	1,452	×
Hexosaminidase A deficiency	26.9	22–34	27.4	2,366	Y
SCAD deficiency	29.1	23–40	Unknown	1,511	×
Familial dysautonomia	41.8	33–57	31	2,385	Y
CPT II deficiency	43.2	33–65	Rare/too few patients worldwide	1,512	×
Hispanic (N = 2,302)					
α-1-Antitrypsin deficiency	9.1	8–11	9.2	1,608	×
Cystic fibrosis	52.1	40–74	59	2,294	Y
DFNB1	67.6	48–114	100	1,623	×
Spinal muscular atrophy	81.2	59–130	68	2,274	1
Sickle cell disease/β-thalassemia	83.1	60–138	128	2,077	×
Pompe disease	134.7	85–326	100	1,616	×
CDG-Ia	135.4	86–328	Unknown	1,625	×
Smith–Lemli–Opitz syndrome	135.5	86–328	No reliable data	1,626	×
Familial Mediterranean fever	136.6	86–331	Unknown	1,639	×
Phenylalanine hydroxylase deficiency	162.8	99–462	Unknown	1,628	×

Table A8 Continued

Disease	Counsyl frequency (1 in)	Counsyl 95% CI (1 in)	Literature frequency (1 in)	# Tested	Screening?
African American (N = 1,193)					
Sickle cell disease/β-thalassemia	9.7	8–12	10	1,121	1
α-1-Antitrypsin deficiency	29.2	21–50	37.3	672	×
Cystic fibrosis	74.2	50–149	84	1,188	Y
Pompe disease	112.5	61–800	59.7	675	×
Spinal muscular atrophy	117.8	72–334	72	1,178	1
Galactosemia	169.5	82–∞	94	678	×
Gaucher disease	213.2	109–4,770	34.6	1,066	×
DFNB1	226.0	99–∞	25.3	678	×
Hereditary fructose intolerance	226.0	99–∞	Unknown	678	×
Smith–Lemli–Opitz syndrome	339.0	127–∞	137.8	678	×
South Asia (N = 1,123)					
Achromatopsia	23.5	18–35	123	798	×
Sickle cell disease/β-thalassemia	30.1	23–45	25	1,055	1
Cystic fibrosis	40.1	29–64	118	1,122	Y
Spinal muscular atrophy	73.3	48–153	52	1,099	1
Hereditary thymine-uraciluria	99.8	58–371	33	798	×
DFNB1	99.9	58–372	148	799	×
Citrullinemia type 1	212.0	93–∞	Unknown	636	×
MLC	212.0	93–∞	Unknown	636	×
Biotinidase deficiency	266.3	116–∞	123	799	×
Tyrosinemia type I	266.3	116–∞	173	799	×
Eastern Asia (N = 1,121)					
DFNB1	22.2	17–34	33–200	756	×
Sickle cell disease/β-thalassemia	78.0	50–178	50	1,014	1
Spinal muscular atrophy	85.5	55–195	59	1,111	1
Gaucher disease	96.9	59–275	Unknown	969	×
Achromatopsia	189.0	91–	123	756	×
Cystic fibrosis	223.6	115–5011	242	1118	Y
α-1-Antitrypsin deficiency	249.0	109–	450	747	×
Pendred syndrome	252.0	110–	51	756	×
Pompe disease	366.5	137–	112	733	×
CPT II deficiency	378.0	142–∞	Rare/too few patients worldwide	756	×
Southern Europe (N = 1,063)					
α-1-Antitrypsin deficiency	17.0	13–24	13.1	715	×
Cystic fibrosis	35.3	26–55	28	1,059	Y
DFNB1	37.2	26–67	33.2	745	×
Spinal muscular atrophy	40.3	29–66	47	1,049	1
Sickle cell disease/β-thalassemia	52.4	36–97	50	996	1
Familial Mediterranean fever	74.5	46–211	Unknown	745	×
Phenylalanine hydroxylase deficiency	74.6	46–211	50.5	746	×
Pompe disease	81.9	49–260	100	737	×
Smith–Lemli–Opitz syndrome	82.9	49–263	Unknown	746	×
Hereditary thymine-uraciluria	105.1	59–495	33	736	×

(Continued)

Table A8 Continued

Disease	Counsyl frequency (1 in)	Counsyl 95% CI (1 in)	Literature frequency (1 in)	# Tested	Screening?
Middle East (N = 512)					
Familial Mediterranean fever	24.5	17–49	Variable (1/10–1/20)	392	×
Sickle cell disease/β-thalassemia	5.1	31–165	30 (but variable)	469	×
Hereditary thymine-uraciluria	54.9	31–256	33	384	×
Achromatopsia	55.1	31–257	123	386	×
Cystic fibrosis	63.1	37–234	91	505	Y
Spinal muscular atrophy	72.4	41–340	25	507	1
DFNB1	77.6	40–1627	83	388	×
Inclusion body myopathy 2	96.5	47–∞	15 (Iranian Jews), unknown in others	386	×
Hereditary fructose intolerance	97.0	47–∞	Unknown	388	×
Smith–Lemli–Opitz syndrome	129.3	57–∞	Rare	388	×

Confidence intervals computed as Wilson 95% score interval. Some listed diseases overlap in definition in terms of genetic variants. Specific variants tested for each disease listed here are given in Supplementary Table B. Please refer to Supplementary Table C for citations to previous literature. CDG-Ia, congenital disorder of glycosylation type Ia; CI, confidence intervals; CPT II deficiency, carnitine palmitoyltransferase II deficiency; DFNB1, GJB2-related DFNB 1 nonsyn- dromic hearing loss and deafness; MCAD deficiency, medium chain acyl-CoA dehydrogenase deficiency; MLC, megalencephalic leukoencephalopathy with subcortical cysts; SCAD deficiency, short chain acyl-CoA dehydrogenase deficiency; Y, both ACMG and ACOG recommend offering screening to this population; 1, one of ACMG/ACOG recommend offering screening to this population; ×, neither ACMG/ACOG recommend offering screening to this population.

Reprinted by permission from Macmillan Publishers Ltd: Genetics in Medicine, Lazarin GA et al., An empirical estimate of carrier frequencies for 400+ casual Mendelian variants: results from an ethnically diverse clinical sample of 23,453 individuals, volume 15, issue 3, pp. 178–186, copyright 2013.

Centile charts for boys' height and weight

In the centile charts that follow (see Figures A3 to A10), there is a normal distribution—approximately 68%, 95%, and 99.6% fall within the mean 91, 2, and 3 standard deviations (SD), respectively.

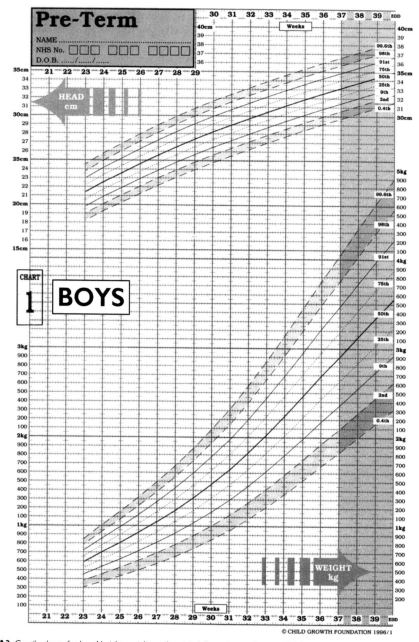

Figure A3 Centile charts for boys' height, weight, and occipital–frontal circumference (OFC) (preterm).
© Child Growth Foundation, reproduced with permission.

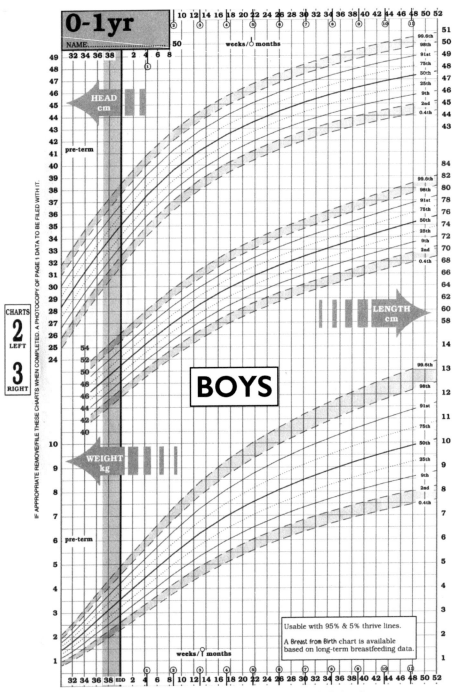

Figure A4 Centile charts for boys' height, weight, and occipital–frontal circumference (OFC) (0–1 year).
© Child Growth Foundation, reproduced with permission.

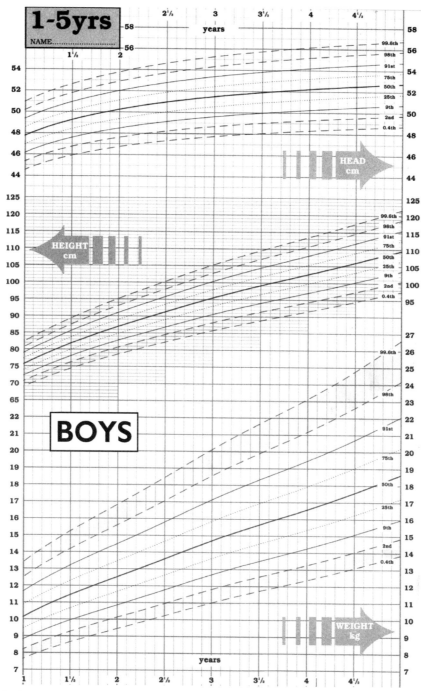

Figure A5 Centile charts for boys' height, weight, and occipital–frontal circumference (OFC) (1–5 years).
© Child Growth Foundation, reproduced with permission.

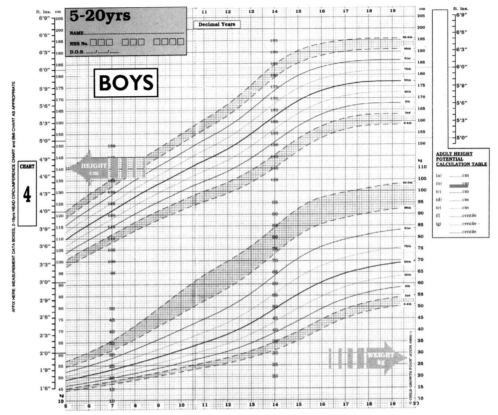

Figure A6 Centile charts for boys' height, weight, and occipital–frontal circumference (OFC) (5–20 years).
© Child Growth Foundation, reproduced with permission.

Centile charts for girls' height and weight

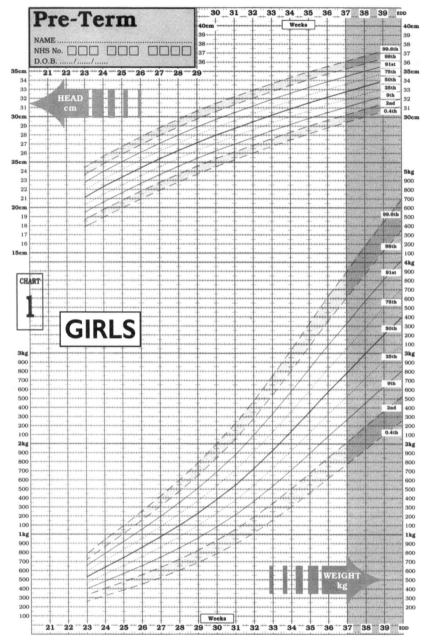

Figure A7 Centile charts for girls' height, weight, and occipital–frontal circumference (OFC) (preterm).
© Child Growth Foundation, reproduced with permission.

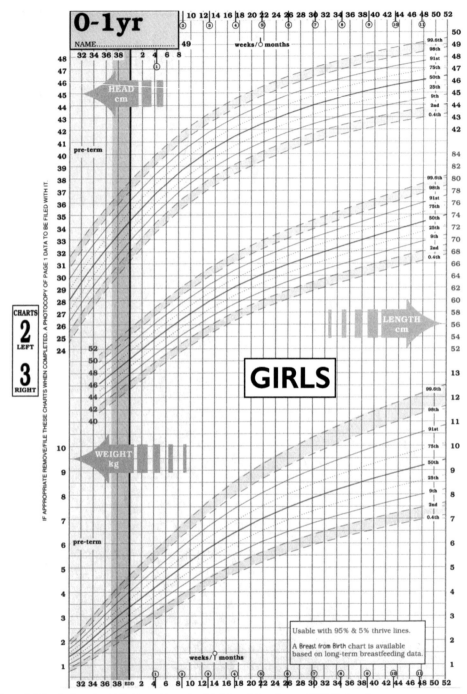

Figure A8 Centile charts for girls' height, weight, and occipital–frontal circumference (OFC) (0–1 year).
© Child Growth Foundation, reproduced with permission.

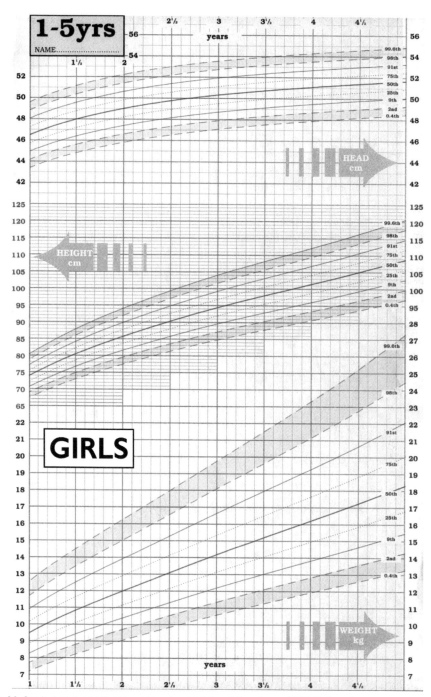

Figure A9 Centile charts for girls' height, weight, and occipital–frontal circumference (OFC) (1–5 years).
© Child Growth Foundation, reproduced with permission.

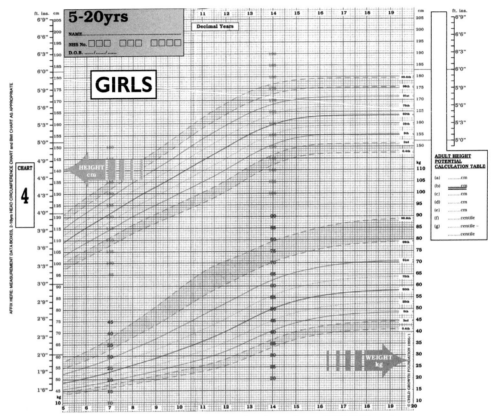

Figure A10 Centile charts for girls' height, weight, and occipital–frontal circumference (OFC) (5–20 years).
© Child Growth Foundation, reproduced with permission.

Centile charts for occipital–frontal circumference (OFC)

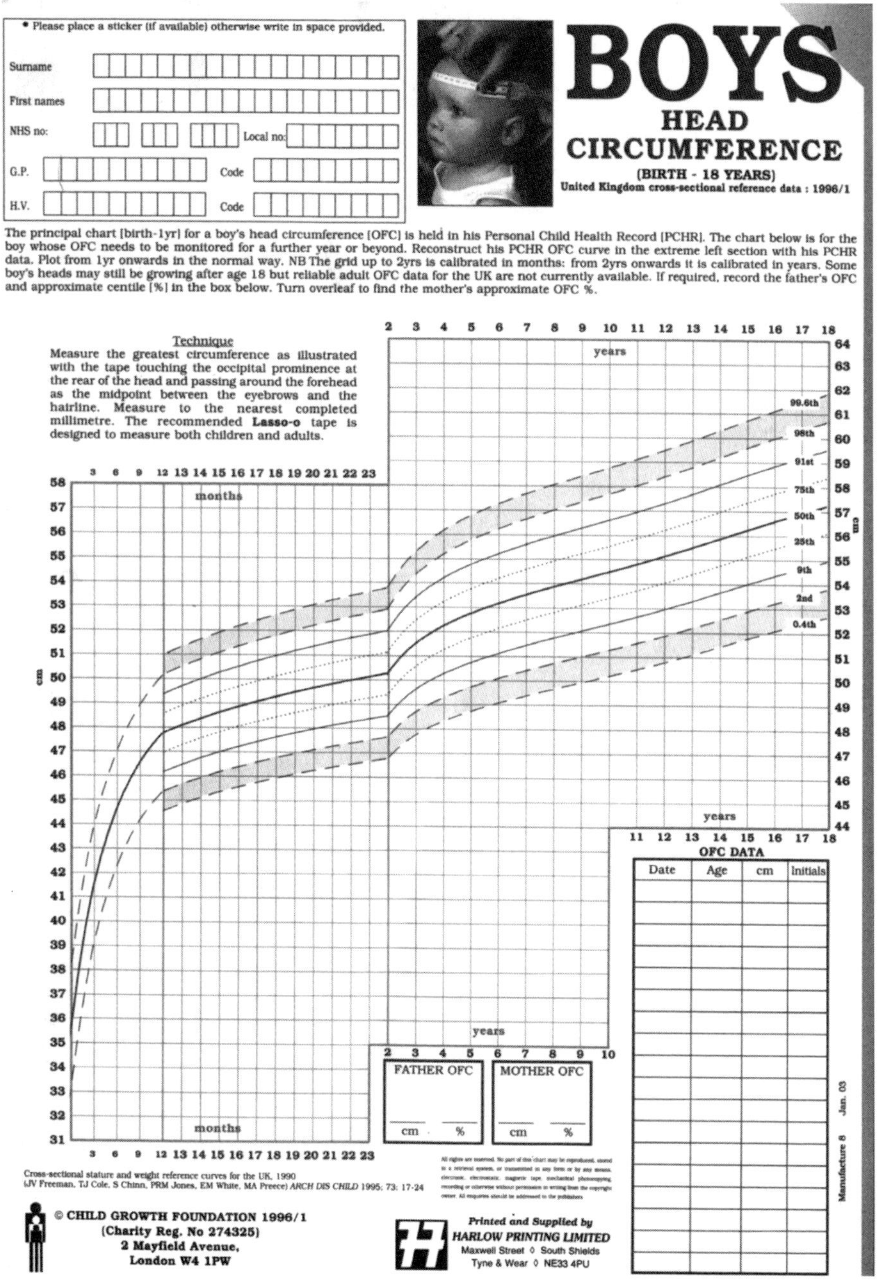

Figure A11 Boys: head circumference chart. Birth–18 years.
© Child Growth Foundation, reproduced with permission.

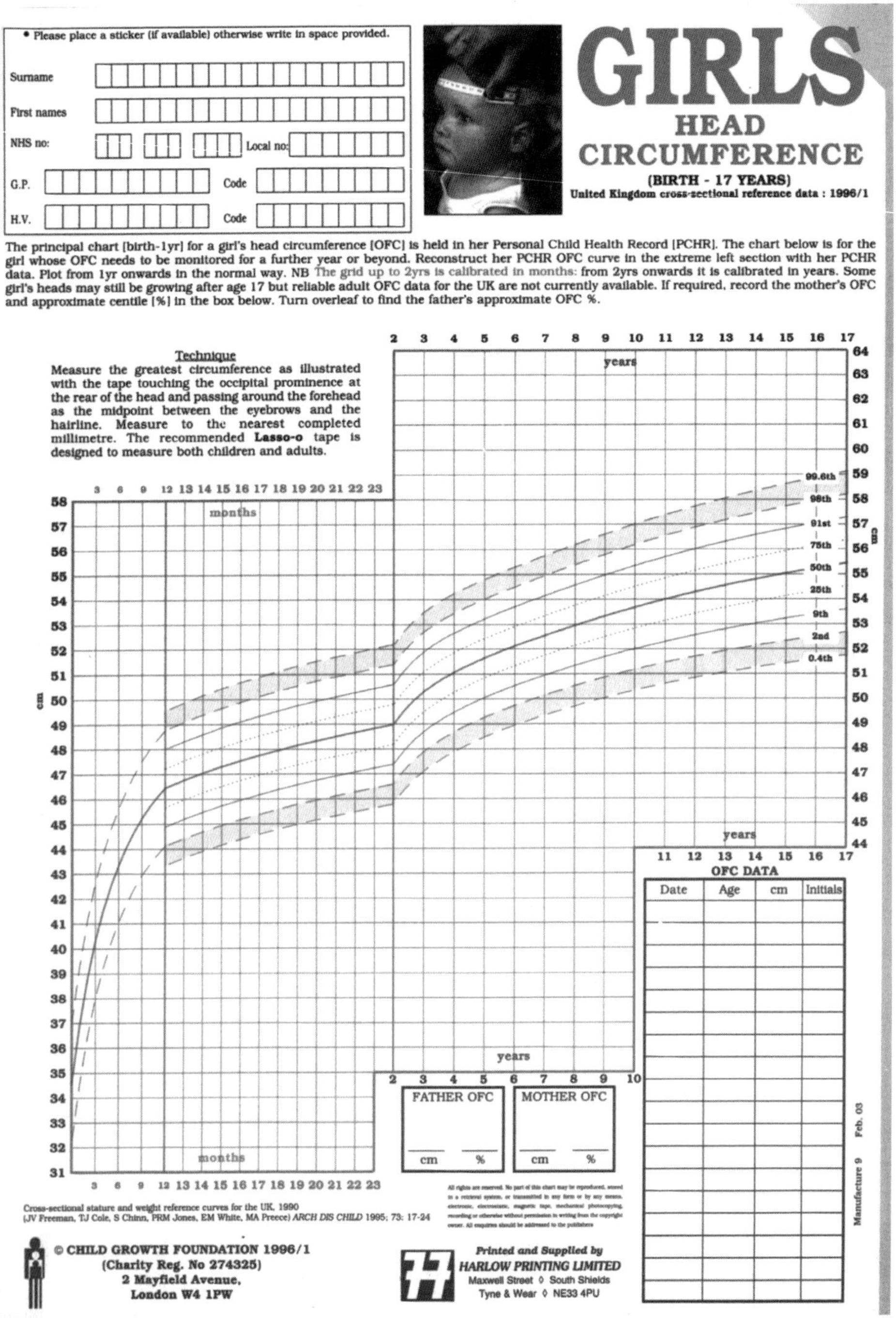

• Please place a sticker (if available) otherwise write in space provided.

Surname

First names

NHS no: Local no:

G.P. Code

H.V. Code

GIRLS
HEAD CIRCUMFERENCE
(BIRTH - 17 YEARS)

United Kingdom cross-sectional reference data : 1996/1

The principal chart [birth-1yr] for a girl's head circumference [OFC] is held in her Personal Child Health Record [PCHR]. The chart below is for the girl whose OFC needs to be monitored for a further year or beyond. Reconstruct her PCHR OFC curve in the extreme left section with her PCHR data. Plot from 1yr onwards in the normal way. NB The grid up to 2yrs is calibrated in months: from 2yrs onwards it is calibrated in years. Some girl's heads may still be growing after age 17 but reliable adult OFC data for the UK are not currently available. If required, record the mother's OFC and approximate centile [%] in the box below. Turn overleaf to find the father's approximate OFC %.

Technique

Measure the greatest circumference as illustrated with the tape touching the occipital prominence at the rear of the head and passing around the forehead as the midpoint between the eyebrows and the hairline. Measure to the nearest completed millimetre. The recommended **Lasso-o** tape is designed to measure both children and adults.

OFC DATA

Date	Age	cm	Initials

FATHER OFC: cm %

MOTHER OFC: cm %

Cross-sectional stature and weight reference curves for the UK, 1990 (JV Freeman, TJ Cole, S Chinn, PRM Jones, EM White, MA Preece) *ARCH DIS CHILD* 1995; 73: 17-24

© CHILD GROWTH FOUNDATION 1996/1
(Charity Reg. No 274325)
2 Mayfield Avenue,
London W4 1PW

Printed and Supplied by
HARLOW PRINTING LIMITED
Maxwell Street ◊ South Shields
Tyne & Wear ◊ NE33 4PU

Manufacture 9 Feb. 03

Figure A12 Girls: head circumference chart. Birth–17 years.
© Child Growth Foundation, reproduced with permission.

CK (creatine kinase) levels in carriers of Duchenne muscular dystrophy (DMD)

Currently, molecular genetic analysis enables detection of deletions and duplications of the dystrophin gene in ~65–70% of boys with DMD. If a dystrophin mutation is detected, this allows robust carrier detection in the families of boys (although the possibility of germline mosaicism in the mother of a sporadic case should always be remembered). In future, the ability to undertake sequencing of the dystrophin gene should enable the great majority of families to have robust carrier detection. Carrier detection by assessment of CK levels (see Table A9) is *fallible and should only be used as a last resort* when molecular methodology has failed to identify a mutation in a boy with biopsy-proven DMD.

NB. Carriers of autosomal recessive (AR) limb–girdle dystrophies may sometimes have a mildly elevated CK so, unless the diagnosis of DMD has been proven by molecular genetic analysis, it is important to ensure that the diagnosis in the proband is well founded and based on muscle biopsy.

Important points

- Women should refrain from intense exercise, e.g. running, aerobics, for 48 hours before the sample is taken.
- CK levels should be expressed in iu/l.
- Take the average of three separate values—each sample taken on a different occasion and the sample should preferably be processed by the laboratory on the day of sampling. The repeat samples need to be taken some time apart, preferably at monthly intervals.
- CK levels are reduced during pregnancy. *Consistently elevated levels would be very suggestive of carrier status in an 'at-risk' female, but results within the normal range in pregnancy are probably uninterpretable.*
- The proportion of carriers of BMD who show elevated levels of CK is lower than for DMD and so the same tables/graphs *cannot* be used for the two conditions.

Reference

Sibert JR, Harper PS, Thompson RJ, Newcombe RG. Carrier detection in Duchenne muscular dystrophy. Evidence from a study of obligatory carriers and mothers of isolated cases. *Arch Dis Child* 1979; **54**: 534–7.

Table A9 Table of likelihood of carrier status for DMD based on serum creatine kinase (CK) level*

Relative risk of being

CK level (iu/l)*	Carrier	Not carrier
0–40	0.12	1
40–49	0.12	1
50–59	0.16	1
60–69	0.27	1
70–79	0.46	1
80–89	0.86	1
90–99	1.67	1
100–109	3.28	1
110–119	6.49	1
120–129	12.79	1
130–139	25.12	1
140–149	49.02	1
150–159	94.34	1
160–169	180.9	1
= 170	Carrier	

*Important note. These data should be *used in conjunction with analysis of the family tree* to provide conditional information in a Bayesian calculation; they are not intended for 'standalone' assessment of carrier status. Laboratory measurements of CK vary and these data were derived in a laboratory where an upper limit of normal (95%) for adult females was 100 iu/l. Consult with your laboratory and do not use these data if the upper limit of normal in your laboratory differs appreciably from this value. (It may be possible to adjust the value by proportion, e.g. if the upper limit of normal in your laboratory is 200 iu/l, then by dividing the CK level by 2, the table could then be used to obtain an approximation of the probability.)

Conversion charts—imperial to metric

See Figure A13. Conversion for height and weight can easily be found by typing the original height/weight into a search engine such as Google.

Tools for calculation of the BMI are also readily available online.

oz	g	lb oz	g	lb oz	g	lb oz	g	lb oz	g	lb oz	g
		1lb 0oz	454g	2lb 0oz	907g	3lb 0oz	1361g	4lb 0oz	1815g	5lb 0oz	2268g
1oz	28.35g	1lb 1oz	482g	2lb 1oz	936g	3lb 1oz	1389g	4lb 1oz	1843g	5lb 1oz	2296g
2oz	57g	1lb 2oz	510g	2lb 2oz	964g	3lb 2oz	1418g	4lb 2oz	1872g	5lb 2oz	2325g
3oz	85g	1lb 3oz	539g	2lb 3oz	992g	3lb 3oz	1446g	4lb 3oz	1900g	5lb 3oz	2353g
4oz	113g	1lb 4oz	567g	2lb 4oz	1021g	3lb 4oz	1474g	4lb 4oz	1928g	5lb 4oz	2381g
5oz	142g	1lb 5oz	595g	2lb 5oz	1049g	3lb 5oz	1503g	4lb 5oz	1956g	5lb 5oz	2410g
6oz	170g	1lb 6oz	624g	2lb 6oz	1077g	3lb 6oz	1531g	4lb 6oz	1985g	5lb 6oz	2438g
7oz	199g	1lb 7oz	652g	2lb 7oz	1106g	3lb 7oz	1559g	4lb 7oz	2013g	5lb 7oz	2467g
8oz	227g	1lb 8oz	680g	2lb 8oz	1134g	3lb 8oz	1588g	4lb 8oz	2041g	5lb 8oz	2495g
9oz	255g	1lb 9oz	709g	2lb 9oz	1162g	3lb 9oz	1616g	4lb 9oz	2070g	5lb 9oz	2523g
10oz	284g	1lb 10oz	737g	2lb 10oz	1191g	3lb 10oz	1644g	4lb 10oz	2098g	5lb 10oz	2552g
11oz	312g	1lb 11oz	766g	2lb 11oz	1219g	3lb 11oz	1673g	4lb 11oz	2126g	5lb 11oz	2580g
12oz	340g	1lb 12oz	794g	2lb 12oz	1247g	3lb 12oz	1701g	4lb 12oz	2155g	5lb 12oz	2608g
13oz	369g	1lb 13oz	822g	2lb 13oz	1276g	3lb 13oz	1730g	4lb 13oz	2183g	5lb 13oz	2637g
14oz	397g	1lb 14oz	850g	2lb 14oz	1304g	3lb 14oz	1758g	4lb 14oz	2211g	5lb 14oz	2665g
15oz	425g	1lb 15oz	879g	2lb 15oz	1333g	3lb 15oz	1786g	4lb 15oz	2240g	5lb 15oz	2693g

lb oz	g	lb oz	g	lb oz	g	lb oz	g	lb oz	g	lb oz	g
6lb 0oz	2722g	7lb 0oz	3175g	8lb 0oz	3629	9lb 0oz	4082g	10lb 0oz	4536g	11lb 0oz	4990g
6lb 1oz	2750g	7lb 1oz	3204g	8lb 1oz	3657g	9lb 1oz	4111g	10lb 1oz	4564g	11lb 1oz	5018g
6lb 2oz	2778g	7lb 2oz	3232g	8lb 2oz	3686g	9lb 2oz	4139g	10lb 2oz	4593g	11lb 2oz	5047g
6lb 3oz	2807g	7lb 3oz	3260g	8lb 3oz	3714g	9lb 3oz	4168g	10lb 3oz	4621g	11lb 3oz	5075g
6lb 4oz	2835g	7lb 4oz	3289g	8lb 4oz	3742g	9lb 4oz	4196g	10lb 4oz	4649g	11lb 4oz	5103g
6lb 5oz	2863g	7lb 5oz	3317g	8lb 5oz	3771g	9lb 5oz	4224g	10lb 5oz	4678g	11lb 5oz	5132g
6lb 6oz	2892g	7lb 6oz	3345g	8lb 6oz	3799g	9lb 6oz	4253g	10lb 6oz	4706g	11lb 6oz	5160g
6lb 7oz	2920g	7lb 7oz	3374g	8lb 7oz	3827g	9lb 7oz	4281g	10lb 7oz	4735g	11lb 7oz	5188g
6lb 8oz	2948g	7lb 8oz	3402g	8lb 8oz	3856g	9lb 8oz	4309g	10lb 8oz	4763g	11lb 8oz	5216g
6lb 9oz	2977g	7lb 9oz	3430g	8lb 9oz	3884g	9lb 9oz	4338g	10lb 9oz	4791g	11lb 9oz	5245g
6lb 10oz	3005g	7lb 10oz	3459g	8lb 10oz	3912g	9lb 10oz	4366g	10lb 10oz	4820g	11lb 10oz	5273g
6lb 11oz	3034g	7lb 11oz	3487g	8lb 11oz	3941g	9lb 11oz	4394g	10lb 11oz	4848g	11lb 11oz	5302g
6lb 12oz	3062g	7lb 12oz	3515g	8lb 12oz	3969g	9lb 12oz	4423g	10lb 12oz	4876g	11lb 12oz	5330g
6lb 13oz	3090g	7lb 13oz	3544g	8lb 13oz	3997g	9lb 13oz	4451g	10lb 13oz	4905g	11lb 13oz	5358g
6lb 14oz	3119g	7lb 14oz	3572g	8lb 14oz	4026g	9lb 14oz	4479g	10lb 14oz	4933g	11lb 14oz	5387g
6lb 15oz	3147g	7lb 15oz	3601g	8lb 15oz	4054g	9lb 15oz	4508	10lb 15oz	4961g	11lb 15oz	5415g

Figure A13 Birthweight—imperial to metric conversion chart.

Denver Developmental Screening Test

For the Denver Developmental Screening Test, see Figure A14.

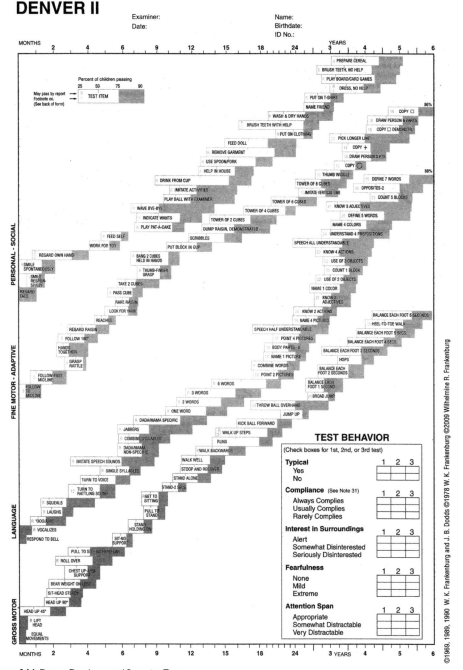

Figure A14 Denver Developmental Screening Test.
© 1969, 1989, 1990 W.K. Frankenburg and J.B. Dodds, © 1978 W.K. Frankenburg, © 2009 Wilhelmine R. Frankenburg. The Denver Developmental Screening Test is available from Hogrefe Ltd., Hogrefe House, Albion Place, Oxford, OX1 1QZ, UK.

DIRECTIONS FOR ADMINISTRATION

1. Try to get child to smile by smiling, talking or waving. Do not touch him/her.
2. Child must stare at hand several seconds.
3. Parent may help guide toothbrush and put toothpaste on brush.
4. Child does not have to be able to tie shoes or button/zip in the back.
5. Move yarn slowly in an arc from one side to the other, about 8" above child's face.
6. Pass if child grasps rattle when it is touched to the backs or tips of fingers.
7. Pass if child tries to see where yarn went. Yarn should be dropped quickly from sight from tester's hand without arm movement.
8. Child must transfer cube from hand to hand without help of body, mouth, or table.
9. Pass if child picks up raisin with any part of thumb and finger.
10. Line can vary only 30 degrees or less from tester's line. |/
11. Make a fist with thumb pointing upward and wiggle only the thumb. Pass if child imitates and does not move any fingers other than the thumb.

12. Pass any enclosed form. Fail continuous round motions.	13. Which line is longer? (Not bigger.) Turn paper upside down and repeat. (pass 3 of 3 or 5 of 6)	14. Pass any lines crossing near midpoint.	15. Have child copy first. If failed, demonstrate.

When giving items 12, 14, and 15, do not name the forms. Do not demonstrate 12 and 14.

16. When scoring, each pair (2 arms, 2 legs, etc.) counts as one part.
17. Place one cube in cup and shake gently near child's ear, but out of sight. Repeat for other ear.
18. Point to picture and have child name it. (No credit is given for sounds only.)
    If less than 4 pictures are named correctly, have child point to picture as each is named by tester.

19. Using doll, tell child: Show me the nose, eyes, ears, mouth, hands, feet, tummy, hair. Pass 6 of 8.
20. Using pictures, ask child: Which one flies?...says meow?...talks?...barks?...gallops? Pass 2 of 5, 4 of 5.
21. Ask child: What do you do when you are cold?...tired?...hungry? Pass 2 of 3, 3 of 3.
22. Ask child: What do you do with a cup? What is a chair used for? What is a pencil used for?
    Action words must be included in answers.
23. Pass if child correctly places and says how many blocks are on paper. (1,5).
24. Tell child: Put block **on** table; **under** table; **in front of** me, **behind** me. Pass 4 of 4.
    (Do not help child by pointing, moving head or eyes.)
25. Ask child: What is a ball?...lake?...desk?...house?...banana?...curtain?...fence?...ceiling? Pass if defined in terms of use, shape, what it is made of, or general category (such as banana is fruit, not just yellow). Pass 5 of 8, 7 of 8.
26. Ask child: If a horse is big, a mouse is ___? If fire is hot, ice is ___? If the sun shines during the day, the moon shines during the ___? Pass 2 of 3.
27. Child may use wall or rail only, not person. May not crawl.
28. Child must throw ball overhand 3 feet to within arm's reach of tester.
29. Child must perform standing broad jump over width of test sheet (8 1/2 inches).
30. Tell child to walk forward, ⟳⟳⟳⟳→ heel within 1 inch of toe. Tester may demonstrate.
    Child must walk 4 consecutive steps.
31. In the second year, half of normal children are non-compliant.

OBSERVATIONS:

Figure A14 Continued

Distribution of muscle weakness in different types of muscular dystrophy

For the distribution of predominant muscle weakness in different types of dystrophy, see Figure A15.

Reference

Emery AE. The muscular dystrophies. *BMJ* 1998; **317**: 991–5.

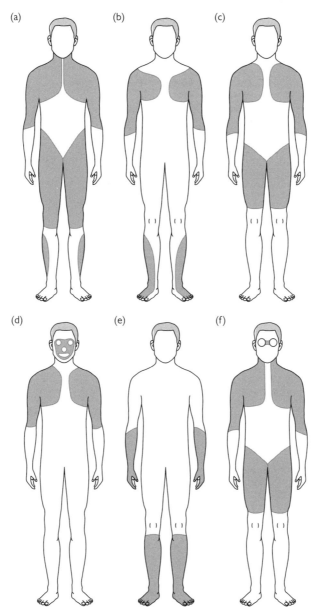

Figure A15 Distribution of predominant muscle weakness in different types of dystrophy: (a) Duchenne-type and Becker-type; (b) Emery–Dreifuss; (c) limb–girdle; (d) facioscapulohumeral; (e) distal; and (f) oculopharyngeal.
Reproduced from *The BMJ*, Alan E H Emery, The muscular dystrophies, volume 317, p. 991, Copyright © 1998, with permission from BMJ Publishing Group Ltd.

Dysmorphology examination checklist

For the dysmorphology examination checklist, see Table A10.

Table A10 Dysmorphology examination checklist*

Growth parameters†	Length/height ...... cm	Weight ...... kg	OFC ...... cm
	Length/height ...... centile†	Weight ...... centile	OFC ...... centile
Stature	Proportionate ☐ Disproportionate ☐ If disproportionate, further measurements:		
	Span ...... cm		Lower segment ...... cm
	Upper segment ...... cm		Sitting height ...... cm
Build	Normal ☐ Describe, e.g. truncal obesity		
Face	Overall impression Normal ☐		
	Dysmorphic features, familial ☐		
	Dysmorphic features, non-familial ☐		
Skin	Normal ☐ Describe birth marks, neurocutaneous stigmata, e.g. café-au-lait spots,		
	Pigmentary anomalies,		
	Cutis laxa, tight skin or unusual texture		
Cranium	Normal ☐ Describe skull shape, e.g. brachycephaly		
	Fontanelle: describe if large/small/additional		
Ears	Normal ☐ Describe size and position		
	Structure, e.g. creases		
	Pits or tags		
Eyes	Normal ☐ Describe whether eyes are deepset or prominent		
	Spacing, e.g. hypertelorism		
	Epicanthic folds		
	Palpebral fissures, e.g. length/angle/everted		
	Eyebrows, e.g. interrupted, arched, straight		
Nose	Normal ☐ Describe, e.g. long/short		
	Nasal bridge, e.g. hypoplastic/prominent		
	Nasal tip, e.g. bulbous		
	Nares, e.g. anteverted		
Philtrum	Normal ☐ Describe, e.g. long/short/smooth		
Mouth	Normal ☐ Describe, e.g. small/large		
	Lips, e.g. thin/full/cleft		
	Tongue, e.g. large/furrowed		
	Palate, e.g. cleft palate		
	Frenulum, e.g. single/missing/multiple		
	Gums, e.g. thickened gums		
	Teeth, e.g. size/shape/eruption		
Chin	Normal ☐ Describe, e.g. small chin (micrognathia), prominent chin (prognathism)		
Hands/feet and limbs	Normal ☐ Describe fingers, e.g. polydactyly, syndactyly, brachydactyly		
	Palmar and plantar creases		
	Nails, e.g. hypoplastic, dysplastic		
Chest	Normal ☐ Describe chest shape, e.g. pectus excavatum/carinatum		
	Nipples, e.g. inverted/supranumerary		
Heart	Normal ☐ Describe, e.g. murmurs		
Abdomen (including genitalia)	Normal ☐ Describe, e.g. organomegaly, hypospadias		
Back	Normal ☐ Describe, e.g. scoliosis		
Nervous system	Normal ☐ Describe gait, e.g. ataxic, high stepping		
	Posture, e.g. frog-legged		
	Tone, e.g. spastic, hypotonic		
	Reflexes, e.g. increased diminished		
Communication	Normal ☐ Record best level of communication, e.g. single words, signs, gesture		
Behaviour‡	Normal ☐ Describe, e.g. hand flapping—consider video of unusual behaviour		

* Use free text/line-drawings supplemented by clinical photographs to describe any unusual features.

† OFC, Occipital–frontal circumference. Centiles are for chronological age, but you can also look at them for height age, for instance for a child 4 years old, but with a height age of 2 years, you can determine whether the head is normal for age or proportionate for height age.

‡ See 'Behavioural pattern profile (Shalev and Hall 2004)' in this Appendix for more detailed assessment of behaviour.

Embryonic fetal development (overview)

For an overview of embryonic fetal development, see Figure A16.

Age (days)	Length (mm)	Stage * (Streeter)	Gross appearance	CNS	Eye	Ear	Face
4		III	Blastocyst				
8	1	IV	Embryo, Trophoblast, Endometrium				
12	2	V	Ectoderm, Amniotic sac, Endoderm, Yolk sac				
19	1	IX	Ant. head fold, Body stalk, Heart	Enlargement of anterior neural plate			
23	2	X Early somites	Foregut, Allantois	Partial fusion neural folds	Optic evagination	Otic placode	Mandible Hyoid arches
28	4	XII 21–29 somites		Closure neural tube Rhombencephalon, mesen, prosen, Ganglia V VII VIII X	Optic cup	Otic invagination	Fusion, mand. arches
34	7	XIV		Cerebellar plate Cervical and mesencephalic flexures	Lens invagination	Otic vesicle	Olfactory placodes
38	11	XVI		Dorsal pontine flexure Basal lamina Cerebral evagination Neural hypophysis	Lens detached Pig-mented retina	Endolymphatic sac Ext. auditory meatus Tubotympanic recess	Nasal swellings
45	17	XVIII		Olfactory evagination Cerebral hemisphere	Lens fibres Migration of retinal cells Hyaloid vessels		Choana, 1° palate
51	22	XX		Optic nerve to brain	Corneal body Mesoderm No lumen in optic stalk		
56	26	XXII			Eyelids	Spiral cochlear duct Tragus	

* The embryonic ages for Streeter's stages XII–XXII have been altered in accordance with the human data from Iffy, L. *et al.* (1967). *Acta anat.* **66**,178.

Age (days)	Limbs	Heart	Gut, abdomen	Lung	Urogenital	Other
4						Early blastocyst with inner cell mass and cavitation (58 cells) lying free within the uterine cavity
8						Implantation Trophoblast invasion Embryonic disc with endoblast and ectoblast
12			Yolk sac			Early amnion sac. Extraembryonic mesoblast, angioblast Chorionic gonadotropin
19		Merging mesoblast anterior to prechordal plate	Stomatodeum Cloaca		Allantois	Primitive streak Hensen's node Notochord Prechordal plate Blood cells in yolk sac
23		Single heart tube Propulsion	Foregut		Mesonephric ridge	Yolk sac larger than amnion sac
28	Arm bud	Ventric outpouching Gelatinous reticulum	Rupture stomatodeum Evagination of thyroid, liver and dorsal pancreas	Lung bud	Mesonephric duct enters cloaca	Rathke's pouch Migration of myotomes from somites
34	Leg bud	Auric. outpouching Septum primum	Pharyngeal pouches yield parathyroids, lat. thyroid, thymus Stomach broadens	Bronchi	Ureteral evag. Urorect sept. Germ cells Gonadal ridge Coelom, Epithelium	
38	Hand plate, Mesench. condens. Innervation	Fusion mid A-V canal Muscular vent. sept.	Intestinal loop into yolk stalk Caecum Gallbladder Hepatic ducts Spleen	Main lobes	Paramesonephric duct Gonad ingrowth of coelomic epithelium	Adrenal cortex (from coelomic epithelium) invaded by sympathetic cells=medulla Jugular lymph sacs
45	Finger rays, Elbow	Aorta Pulmonary artery Valves Membrane ventricular septum	Duodenal lumen obliterated Caecum rotates right Appendix	Tracheal cartil.	Fusion urorect. septum Open urogenital memb., anus Epith. cords in testicle	Early muscle
51	Clearing, central cartil.	Septum secundum			S-shaped vesicles in nephron blastema connect with collecting tubules from calyces	Superficial vascular plexus low on cranium
56	Tubular bones				A few large glomeruli Short secretory tubules Tunica albuginea Testicle, interstitial cells	Superficial vascular plexus at vertex

(Adapted from Smith 1982, by permission)

Figure A16 Embryonic fetal development.
This article was published in *Smith's Recognizable Patterns of Human Malformation*, Seventh Edition, Jones & Jones & del Campo, Copyright Elsevier 2013.

Age (weeks)	Length C-R (cm)	Length Tot (cm)	Weight (gm)	Gross appearance	CNS	Eye, ear	Face, mouth	Cardiovascular	Lung
7	2.8			(illustration)	Cerebral hemisphere; Infundibulum, Rathke's; Primitive cereb. cortex; Olfactory lobes; Dura and pia mater	Lens nearing final shape	Palatal swellings; Dental lamina. Epithel	Pulmonary vein into left atrium	Pleuroperitoneal canals close
8	3.7			(illustration)	Spinal cord histology	Eyelid; Ear canals	Nares plugged; Rathke's pouch detach; Sublingual gland	A–V bundle; Sinus venosus absorbed into auricle	Bronchioles
10	6.0				Cerebellum	Iris; Ciliary body; Eyelids fuse; Lacrimal glands; Spiral gland different	Lips; Nasal cartilage; Palate		Laryngeal cavity reopened
12	8.8			(illustration)	Corpora quadrigemina; Cerebellum prominent; Myelination begins	Retina layered; Eye axis forward	Tonsillar crypts; Cheeks	Accessory coats, blood vessels	Elastic fibres
16	14			(illustration)	Cord-cervical & lumbar enlarged; Cauda equina	Scala vestibuli; Cochlear duct; Scala tympani; Inner ear ossified	Palate complete; Enamel and dentine	Cardiac muscle condensed	Segmentation of bronchi complete
20				(illustration)	Typical layers in cerebral cortex; Cauda equina at first sacral level		Ossification of nose		Decrease in mesenchyme; Capillaries penetrate linings of tubules
24		32	800	(illustration)	Cerebral fissures and convolutions	Eyelids reopen; Retinal layers complete; Perceive light	Nares reopen; Calcification of tooth primordia		Change from cuboidal to flattened epithelium; Alveoli
28		38.5	1100	(illustration)	Cauda equina, at L–3; Myelination within brain	Auricular cartilage	Taste sense		Vascular components adequate for respiration
32		43.5	1600	Accumulation of fat					Number of alveoli still incomplete
36		47.5	2600			Lacrimal duct canalised	Rudimentary frontal maxillary sinuses	Closure of foramen ovale, ductus arteriosus, umbilical vessels, ductus venosus	
38		50	3200					Relative hypertrophy left ventricle	
First postnatal year +				(illustration)	Continuing organization of axonal networks; Cerebrocortical function motor co-ordination; Myelination continues until 2–3 years	Iris pigmented, 5 months; Mastoid air cells; Co-ordinate vision 3–5 months; Maximal vision by 5 years	Salivary gland ducts became canalized; Teeth begin to erupt 5–7 months; Relatively rapid growth of mandible and nose		Continue adding new alveoli

Age (weeks)	Gut	Urogenital	Skeletal muscle	Skeleton	Skin	Blood, thymus, lymph	Endocrine
7	Pancreas, dorsal and ventral fusion	Renal vesicles (illustration)	Differentiation forward final shape	Cartilaginous models of bones; Chondrocranium; Tail regression	Mammary gland		Parathyroid associated with thyroid; Sympathetic neuroblasts invade adrenal
8	Liver relatively large; Intestinal villi	Mullerian ducts fusing	Muscles well represented; Movement	Ossification centre; Sternum	Basal layer	Bone marrow; Thymus halves unite; Lymphoblasts around the lymph sacs	Thyroid follicles
10	Gut withdrawal from cord; Pancreatic alveoli; Anal canal	Ovary distinguishable; Testosterone; Renal excretion; Bladder sac; Mullerian tube into urogenital sinus; Vaginal sacs, prostate	Perineal muscles	Joints	Hair follicles; Melanocytes	Enucleated RBCs; Thymus yields reticulum and corpuscles; Thoracic duct; Lymph nodes: axillary iliac	Adrenalin; Noradrenalin
12	Gut muscle layers; Pancreatic islets; Bile	Seminal vesicle; Regression, genital ducts		Tail degenerated; Notochord degenerated	Corium, 3 layers; Scalp, body hair; Sebaceous glands; Nails beginning; Palm creases	Blood principally from bone marrow; Thymus—medullary and lymphoid	Testicle—Leydig cells; Thyroid—colloid in follicle; Anterior pituitary acidophilic granules; Ovary—prim. follicles
16	Omentum fusing with transverse colon, Sacs, desc. colon attach to body wall; Meconium; Gastric, intest. glands	Typical kidney; Mesonephros involuting; Uterus and vagina; Primary follicles	In-utero movement can be detected	Distinct bones	Dermal ridge pattern; Hand creases; Sweat glands; Keratinization; Scalp hair pattern		Anterior pituitary—basophilic granules
20		No further collecting tubules			Hair at eyebrow; Verix caseosa; Nail plates; Mammary budding	Blood formation decreasing liver	
24		Urine osmolarity continues to be relatively low		Only a few secondary epiphyseal centre's ossified in knee	Eccrine sweat; Lanugo hair prominent; Nails to toe tips		Testes—decrease in Leydig cells
28				Ossification of 2nd epiph. centres hamate, capitate, proximal humerus, femur; New ossif 2nd epiph. centres till 10–12 years; Ossif. of epiphyses lat, 16–18 yrs			Testes descend
32					Nails to fingertips		
36							
38						Haemoglobin 17–18g; Leukocytosis	
First postnatal year +					New hair gradual loss of lanugo hair	Transient (8 wk) erythroid hypoplasia; Haemoglobin 11–12 g; 75 gamma globulin produced by 6 weeks; Lymph nodes develop cortex, medulla	Transient estrinization of fetal zone; Adrenal—regression of fetal zone; Gonadotropin with feminization of ♀ 9–12 yr (on self); masc 10–14 yr (on self)

(Adapted from Smith 1982, by permission)

Figure A16 Continued

Family tree sheet and symbols

Usage of standardized pedigree nomenclature reduces the chances for incorrect interpretation of patient and family medical and genetic information (see Figures A17 and A18). It may also improve the quality of patient care provided by genetic professionals and facilitate communication between researchers involved with genetic family studies (Bennett et al. 1995).

Reference

Bennett RL, Steinhaus KA, Uhrich SB, et al. Recommendations for standardized human pedigree nomenclature. Pedigree Standardization Task Force of the National Society of Genetic Counselors. Am J Hum Genet 1995; **56**: 745–52.

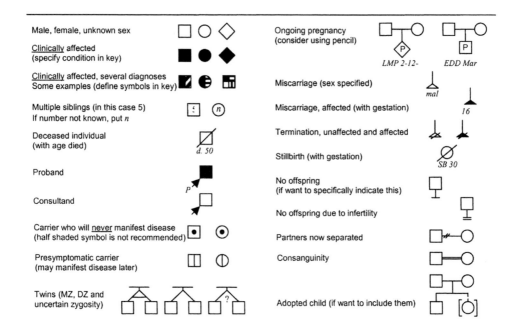

Figure A17 Recommended symbols for pedigree drawing.
Reproduced from *Journal of Genetic Counseling*, Recommendations for standardized human pedigree nomenclature, volume 4, issue 4, 1995, with permission of Springer and National Society of Genetic Counsellors.

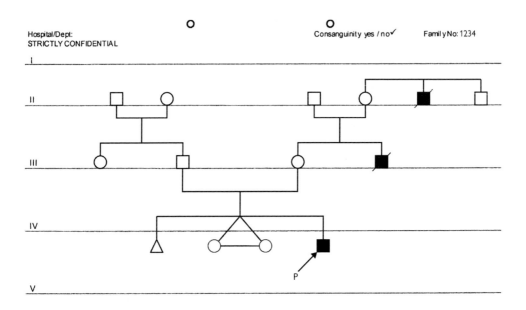

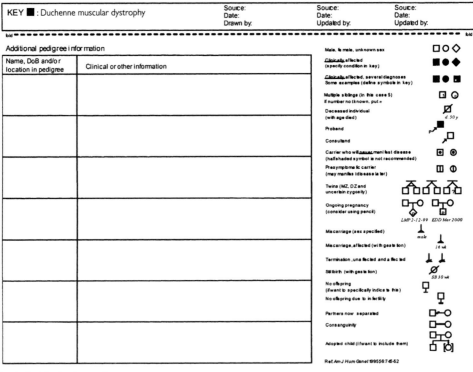

Sample sheet for drawing a pedigree.

Figure A18 Sample sheet for drawing a pedigree.
Reproduced from *Journal of Genetic Counseling*, Recommendations for standardized human pedigree nomenclature, volume 4, issue 4, 1995, with permission of Springer and National Society of Genetic Counsellors.

Haploid autosomal lengths of human chromosomes

Daniel (1979) studied interchange segment sizes and the sizes of chromosome imbalance arising from the different modes of meiotic segregation in a selected sample of reciprocal translocations (Rcp). The study population included spontaneous abortions and children born with chromosomal imbalance. He concluded that:

(1) the interchange segments were larger in the spontaneous abortion Rcp;

(2) all of the imbalances observed in full-term neonates plotted close to the origin and to the left of the line joining 4% trisomy to 2% monosomy;

(3) the imbalances observed in the neonates in each individual Rcp were of the smallest size possible arising by any segregation mode.

Haploid autosomal length (HAL)

To determine the amount of particular segmental imbalance as a fraction of the haploid autosomal length (HAL):

(1) measure the length of the entire chromosome using a millimetre ruler;

(2) measure the length of the chromosome segment involved in the imbalance using a millimetre ruler;

(3) determine the percentage of the length of that specific chromosome that would be involved in the imbalance, e.g. for the segment 4q13.3–qter, this represents 18% of the length of chromosome 4;

(4) from Table A11, determine the percentage of the total HAL, i.e. chromosome 4 represents 6.3% of HAL, 18% × 6.3% = 1.14%, hence the imbalance represents 1.14% of HAL which falls within the envelope of potentially viable imbalance (see Figure 5.1 in 'Autosomal reciprocal translocations—background', Chapter 5, 'Chromosomes', p.636).

Example

For the unbalanced karyotype 46,XX, der(20)t(14;20)(q24;q13.3), the segment 14q24–qter represents 33% of the length of chromosome 14, hence the imbalance represents 33% × 3.56% = 1.18% of HAL as a trisomy. In this rearrangement, there is no monosomy and so it falls within the triangle of potentially viable imbalance (see Figure 5.1 in 'Autosomal reciprocal translocations—background', Chapter 5, 'Chromosomes', p. 636).

References

Daniel A. Structural differences in reciprocal translocations. Potential for a model of risk in Rcp. *Hum Genet* 1979; **51**: 171–82.

Gardner RJM, Sutherland GR. *Chromosome abnormalities and genetic counseling*, Oxford monographs on medical genetics no. 31, 3rd edn. Oxford University Press, New York, 2004.

Table A11 Percentage of haploid autosomal length (HAL) that each autosome constitutes

Chromosome	% of HAL	Chromosome	% of HAL
1	8.44	12	4.66
2	8.02	13	3.74
3	6.83	14	3.56
4	6.30	15	3.46
5	6.08	16	3.36
6	5.90	17	3.25
7	5.36	18	2.93
8	4.93	19	2.67
9	4.80	20	2.56
10	4.59	21	1.90
11	4.61	22	2.04

Investigation of lethal metabolic disorder or skeletal dysplasia

Metabolic autopsy

A diagnosis is vitally important in order to be able to advise about recurrence risks and possibly to offer prenatal diagnosis in a subsequent pregnancy. If it has not been possible to make a diagnosis during life and there is a suspicion of an underlying metabolic disorder, the following samples taken immediately after death can substantially increase the chance of making a diagnosis and enable the diagnostic process to continue after death.

- Plasma: heparinized, separated, and deep frozen.
- Blood spots on Guthrie card for acylcarnitine.
- Urine in plain universal container: deep frozen.
- Blood in EDTA (ethylenedinitrilotetraacetate) for DNA extraction and storage.
- Skin for fibroblast culture taken into tissue culture medium and stored in a fridge at 4–8°C.
- Liver biopsy snap frozen for histochemistry/enzymology.
- Muscle snap frozen for histochemistry/enzymology/immunohistochemistry.
- Consider clinical photographs.
- Consider skeletal X-rays in a baby.

Investigation of the fetus and baby with a skeletal dysplasia

A diagnosis is vitally important in order to be able to advise about appropriate management and also recurrence risks.

- DNA storage, genomic analysis, WES/WGS as available. Cord blood, fetal blood sample, placental tissue, and skin biopsy can all be used. Many skeletal dysplasias have known mutations.
- Skin biopsy.
- Radiology: full skeletal survey.
- Clinical photography.
- Clinical measurements: length, span, OCF.

If the baby dies, it is possible to get most of the information required, even if a post-mortem examination is refused. If a post-mortem is performed, it should include bone histology.

Reference

Leonard JV, Morris AAM. Inborn errors of metabolism around the time of birth [review article]. *Lancet* 2000; **356**: 583–7.

ISCN nomenclature

For symbols and abbreviated terms used in the description of chromosomes and chromosomal abnormalities, see Table A12. For *in situ* hybridization symbols and abbreviations, see Table A13.

Table A12 Symbols and abbreviated terms used in the description of chromosomes and chromosomal abnormalities

add	mar
additional material of unknown origin	marker chromosome
46,XX,add(1)(p36)	47,XX,+mar
arrow (→)	mat
from–to, in detailed system	maternal origin
46,XX,add(1)(?::p36 → qter)	46,XX,der(5)t(1;5)(p36;q24)mat
brackets, square ([ ])	minus sign (–)
surround the absolute number of	loss
cells in each clone	45,XX, –21
45,X[20]/46,XX[10]	p
colon, single (:)	short arm of chromosome
break, in detailed system	46,XX,add(1)(p36)
46,XX,del(6)(qter → p21:)	parentheses
colon, double (::)	surround structurally altered chromosome
break and reunion, in detailed system	and breakpoints
46,XX,del(6)(qter → p11::p21lpter)	46,XX,der(5)t(1;5)(p36;q24)mat
comma (,)	pat
separates chromosome numbers, sex chromosomes,	paternal origin
and chromosome abnormalities	46,XX,der(5)t(1;5)(p36;q24)pat
45,XX,add(1)(p36),–21	plus sign (+)
decimal point (.)	gain
denotes subbands	47,XX,+21
46,XX,add(1)(p36.1)	q
del	long arm of chromosome
deletion	46,XX,der(5)t(1;5)(p36;q24)pat
46,XX,del(6)(qter → p21:)	question mark (?)
de novo	questionable identification of a chromosome or
designates a chromosome abnormality that	chromosome structure
has not been inherited	47,XX,+?21
46,XX,del(22)(q11.2q11.2)*de novo*	r
der	ring chromosome
derivative chromosome	46,X,r(X)
46,XX,der(5)t(1;5)(p36;q24)pat	rec
dic	recombinant chromosome
dicentric	46,XX,rec(4)dup(4q)inv(4)(p14q34)
46,X,dic(X)(p11)	s
dup	satellite
duplication	46,XX,12ps
46,XX,dup(5)(p13p23)	sce
fra	sister chromatid exchange
fragile site	Sce(9)(p11p23)
46,Y,fra(X)(q27.3)	semicolon (;)
h	separates altered chromosomes and breakpoints in
heterochromatin, constitutive	structural rearrangements involving more than one
46,XY,16qh+	chromosome
hsr	46,XX,t(1;5)(p36;q24)
homogeneously staining region	slant line (/)
46,XX,hsr(14)(q21)	separates clones
i	45,X/46,XX
isochromosome	t
46,X,i(X)(p10)	translocation
ins	46,XX,t(1;5)(p36;q24)
insertion	ter
46,XX,ins(5)(q12q22q34)	terminal (end of chromosome)
inv	46,XX,add(1)(?::p36 → qter)
inversion	upd
46,XX,inv(9)(p11q13)	uniparental disomy
	46,XX,upd(15)(mat)

Data from Mitelman F (ed.), *ISCN (2013): an international system for human cytogenetic nomenclature*, Karger, 2013.

Table A13 *In situ* hybridization: symbols and abbreviations

minus sign (–)
  absent from a specific chromosome
  46,XX.ish del(22)(q11.2q11.2)(D22S735–)
plus sign (+)
  present on a specific chromosome
  46,XX.ish del(22)(q11.2q11.2)(D22S735-,D22S422+)
multiplication sign (x)
  precedes the number of signals seen
  46,XX.ish 22q11.2(D22S735 x 2)
period (.)
  separates cytogenetic observations from results of *in situ* hybridization
  46,XX.ish del(22)(q11.2q11.2)(D22S735–)
semicolon (;)
  separates probes on different derivative chromosomes
  46,XX, t(1;5)(p36;q24).ish t(1;5)(D1S432+,D5S563–; D1S432–,D5S563)
FISH
  fluorescence *in situ* hybridization
ish
  in situ hybridization; when used without a prefix applies to chromosomes (usually metaphase or prometaphase) of
    dividing cells
  46,XX.ish del(22)(q11.2q11.2)(D22S735–)
nuc ish
  Nuclear or interphase *in situ* hybridization
  nuc ish 18cen(D18Z1 x 3)
wcp
  whole chromosome paint
  46,XX,r(9).ish r(9)(wcp9+)

Data from Mitelman F (ed.), *ISCN (2013): an international system for human cytogenetic nomenclature*, Karger, 2013.

Reference

Mitelman F (ed.). *ISCN (1995): an international system for human
  cytogenetic nomenclature*. Karger, Basel, 1995.

Karyotypes

For normal metaphase spread, normal male G-banded karyotype, normal female G-banded karyotype, and trisomy 21 G-banded karyotype, see Figures A19, A20, A21, and A22, respectively.

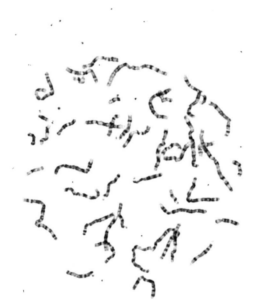

Figure A19 Normal metaphase spread.

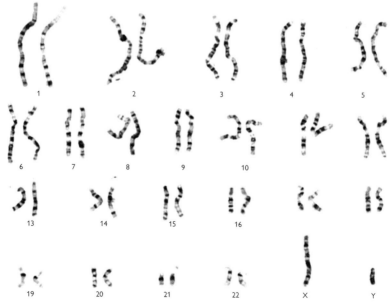

Figure A20 Normal male G-banded karyotype.

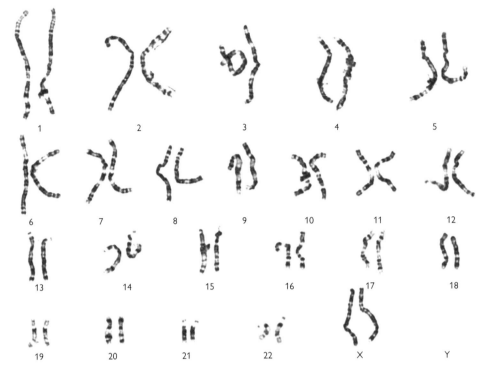

Figure A21 Normal female G-banded karyotype.

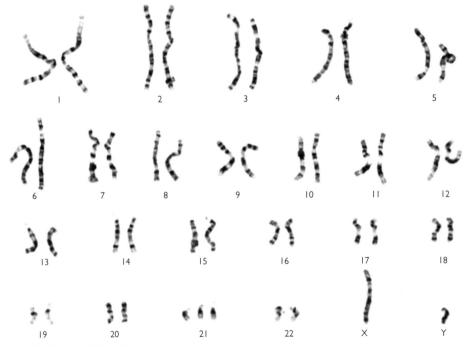

Figure A22 Trisomy 21 G-banded karyotype.

Normal range of aortic root dimensions

Nomograms standardly used to detect aortic dilatation by echocardiography in children and adults are based on M-mode data. Aortic root dilatation is overdiagnosed when two-dimensional echocardiographic data are compared with M-mode nomograms. This appendix provides nomograms devised for two-dimensional echocardiography. Figures A23 and A24 give nomograms for calculation of body surface area (BSA) in children and adults, respectively. Figures A25 and A26 then give 95% normal confidence limits for aortic root diameter at sinuses of Valsalva in relation to BSA in children and adults, respectively. Figure A26 gives normal echo values for aortic diameter as a function of BSA.

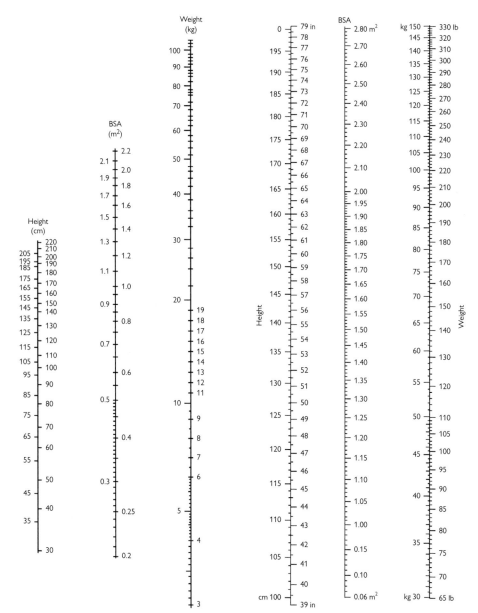

Figure A23 Nomogram for calculation of body surface area (BSA) in children. To use the nomogram, a ruler is aligned with the height and weight on the two lateral axes. The point at which the centre line is intersected gives the corresponding value for BSA.

Figure A24 Nomogram for calculation of body surface area (BSA) in adults. The point at which the centre line is intersected gives the corresponding value for BSA.

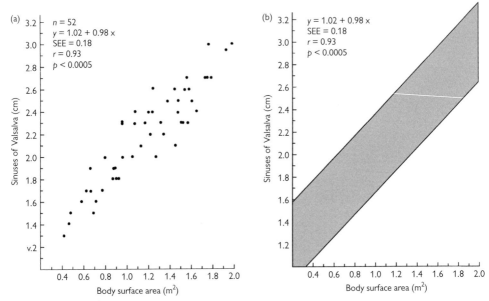

Figure A25 (a) Relation of body surface area (BSA) to aortic root diameter in normal infants and children. (b) The grey area represents the 95% confidence interval (CI) for aortic root diameter at sinuses of Valsalva in infants and children.
Reprinted from *American Journal of Cardiology*, volume 64, issue 8, Roman MJ, *et al.*, Two dimensional aortic root dimensions in normal children and adults, pp. 507–512, copyright 1989, with permission from Elsevier.

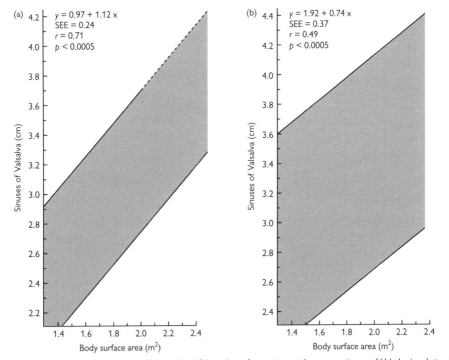

Figure A26 The grey area represents the 95% normal confidence limits for aortic root diameter at sinuses of Valsalva in relation to body surface area (BSA) in: (a) adults under 40 years of age; (b) adults 40 years of age and older.
Reprinted from *American Journal of Cardiology*, volume 64, issue 8, Roman MJ, *et al.*, Two dimensional aortic root dimensions in normal children and adults, pp. 507–512, copyright 1989, with permission from Elsevier.

References

Henry WL, Ware J, Gardin JM, Hepner SI, McKay J, Weiner M. Echocardiographic measurements in normal subjects. Growth-related changes that occur between infancy and early adulthood. *Circulation* 1978; **57**: 278–85.

Roman MJ, Devereux RB, Kramer-Fox R, O'Loughlin J. Two dimensional aortic root dimensions in normal children and adults. *Am J Cardiol* 1989; **64**: 507–12.

Paternity testing

In the UK, paternity testing for social or legal indications is not undertaken as part of health care but is available privately through several agencies (see list at end of article).

Typical testing methodology

A child inherits half of his/her DNA from each parent. DNA samples are analysed using polymerase chain reaction (PCR) and short tandem repeat (STR) profiling. Every STR marker in the child's pattern should be present in either the mother's or father's DNA. If, for example, 16 highly polymorphic STRs are used when a mother, alleged father, and child are tested, proof of paternity can be established with a minimum certainty of 99.99% or, alternatively, DNA analysis can prove non-paternity with 100% certainty. DNA from children is often collected as a mouth swab; samples from the mother and alleged father are collected as mouth swabs or blood samples.

There are commercial operations in most developed countries. Contact your molecular genetics lab for details of reputable centres.

Patterns of cancer

For cancer risks and non-cancerous manifestations for key cancer-predisposing genes and syndromes, see Table A14.

Expert advisers: Marc Tischkowitz, Reader and Honorary Consultant Physician in Medical Genetics, Department of Medical Genetics, University of Cambridge and East Anglian Medical Genetics Service, Cambridge, UK, Amy Taylor, Principal Genetic Counsellor, Cambridge University Hospital, Cambridge, UK, and David Greenberg, Principal Investigator, Research Institute at Nationwide Children's Hospital, Columbus, USA.

Table A14 Cancer risks and non-cancerous manifestations for key cancer-predisposing genes and syndromes. Lifetime percentage risks (%) or relative risks (RR) are given where available

	Skin	Breast	Colorectal	Gastric	Pancreas	Liver	Hepato-biliary tract	Small bowel	Prostate	Uterus
BRCA1		50–80%								
BRCA2	Melanoma?	50–80%			3–6%				15% by 65 years	
PALB2		33–58%			+					
RAD51C		?								
RAD51D										
MLH1/MSH2[a]	Sebaceous neoplasms 1–9%		50–80%	6–13%	?		1.4–4%	3–6%	+	25–60%
MSH6[a]	?		30–60%	?	?		?	?	?	50–80%
PMS2[a]	?		15–20%	?	?		?	?	?	5–35%
FAP	Sebaceous cysts		~100%	Fundic gland polyps	?	~1% hepatoblastoma	+	Duodenal polyps, duodenal cancer 4–12%		
MUTYH[b]	Sebaceous gland tumours		Polyposis, colorectal cancer 43–100%	Fundic gland polyps				Duodenal polyps, duodenal cancer 3–4%		
Peutz–Jeghers	Mucocutaneous pigmentation	30–60%	39%	29%	11–36%			13%		9%
Cowden	Melanoma 2–9%	70–95%	5–17%							17–40%
Juvenile polyposis syndrome			17–22%	Gastric polyps Cancer risk 21%						
TP53	Melanoma?	50–85%			RR 2–19					?
CDH1		55% lobular	?	50–80% Diffuse						
Gorlin	BCC 80% by 50 years									
RB1										

Cervix	Ovary	Lung	Para-thyroid	Thyroid	Adrenal	Eye	Brain/nervous system	Bone/soft tissue	Kidney	Uroth-elial	Testi-cular	Leukaemia/lymphoma
	30–50%											
	10–20%											
	?											
	~10%											
	~10%											
	4–12%				Adreno-cortical cancer		1–3% (CNS) Turcot syndrome			1–4%		
	?				?		?			?		
	?				?		?			?		
				Papillary thyroid 1–12%		CHRPE 50–80%	?	Osteomas, desmoids (Gardner syndrome)				
						CHRPE 5.5%	?					
10%	21% (sex cord tumors with annular tubules)	15%									Large cell calcifying Sertoli cell tumors	
									Renal cell carcinoma			
				20–50%					17–50%			
				Follicular type is over-represented								
	?	Bron-choalveolar		Non-medullary?	Adreno-cortical cancer +++ in children, + in adults		RR 19–60	RR 49–203 (bone sarcoma); RR 33–102 (soft tissue sarcoma)	Renal cell carcinoma?			Leukaemia, Hodgkin's and non-Hodgkin's lymphoma?
							Medullo-blastoma in children 5%	Jaw keratocysts				
		++				90% retino-blastoma	++	++				

Table A14 Continued

	Skin	Breast	Colorectal	Gastric	Pancreas	Liver	Hepato-bilary tract	Small bowel	Prostate	Uterus
MEN1				Gastri-noma	Insulinoma, glucagonoma, VIPoma			Gastrinoma		
MEN2	MEN2B mucosal neuromas									
HLRCC	Leiomyomas									Benign fibroids +++
NF1	Neurofibromas	8% by 50 years								
NF2	Neurofibromas									Benign fibroids +
DICER1										
BAP1	Melanoma									
CDKN2A	Melanoma 50–80%				++					
FLCN										
VHL					Neuro-endocrine tumours (5–17%), cysts					
SDHA										
SDHB				Gastro-intestinal stromal tumour?						
SDHC										
SDHD										

Cervix	Ovary	Lung	Parathyroid	Thyroid	Adrenal	Eye	Brain/nervous system	Bone/soft tissue	Kidney	Urothelial	Testicular	Leukaemia/lymphoma
		Carcinoid	100% hyperparathyroidism (non-malignant)	Thymic carcinoid	Adrenal tumours 20–40%, adrenocortical cancer 1%		Anterior pituitary 10–60%, meningioma 8%, ependymoma 1%					
			MEN2A parathyroid disease 20–30%	Medullary thyroid carcinoma 95–100%	Phaeochromocytoma 50%							
									Type II papillary 10–16%			
						Optic gliomas	Malignant peripheral nerve sheath tumours (10%)					Leukaemia, juvenile chronic myelogenous leukaemia
							Gliomas, brainstem/cerebellar astrocytoma					
						Posterior subcapsular cataracts	Bilateral vestibular schwannomas. Other schwannomas, meningiomas, ependymomas					
Cervical PNET, sarcoma botryoides	Sertoli–Leydig cell tumour of the ovary	Pleuropulmonary blastoma 10–20%		Multinodular goitre 80–100%		Intraocular medulloepithelioma	Pituitary blastoma	Embryonal rhabdomyosarcoma	Wilms +			
		Mesothelioma				Uveal melanoma			Renal cell carcinoma +			
		Lung cysts							Oncocytomas, renal cell cancer			
					Phaeochromocytoma (10–20%)	Retinal haemangioblastoma	Haemangioblastoma (56%), Endolymphatic sac tumours (10%)		Renal cell carcinoma (25%)		Epididymal tumours	
					Phaeochromocytoma +		Paragangliomas +					
				Thyroid?	Phaeochromocytoma 52% by 60 years		Paragangliomas 29% by 60 years (higher risk of malignancy)		Renal cell carcinoma 14% by 70 years			
					Phaeochromocytoma +		Paragangliomas +					
					Phaeochromocytoma 71% by 60 years		Paragangliomas 29% by 60 years		Renal cell carcinoma 8% by 70 years			

Table A14 Continued

		Skin	Breast	Colorectal	Gastric	Pancreas	Liver	Hepato-bilary tract	Small bowel	Prostate	Uterus
Carney triad					Gastro-intestinal stromal tumour				Oeso-phageal leiomyoma		
Carney Stratakis syndrome					Gastro-intestinal stromal tumour						
Carney complex			Myxomas								
MAX											
Hyper parathyroidism–jaw tumour syndrome											
Mean age of diagnosis for the UK (25th–75th quartiles)[c]	F	58 (49–74)	63 (52–75)	73 (66–83)	75 (70–85)	74 (67–83)					67 (59–76)
	M	60 (44–74)		71 (64–79)	72 (65–80)	70 (63–79)				73 (67–80)	
Lifetime UK population risk[c]	F (%)	1 in 56 (1.8)	1 in 8 (12.5)	1 in 19 (5)	1 in 120 (0.8)	1 in 74 (1.4)	1 in 215 (0.5)	1 in 1250 (0.08)	1 in 830 (0.12)		1 in 40 (2.5)
	M (%)	1 in 55 (1.8)	1 in 868 (0.1)	1 in 14 (7)	1 in 64 (1.6)	1 in 73 (1.4)	1 in 120 (0.8)			1 in 8 (12.5)	

Where the percentage risks are unknown, +/++/+++ are used for low, medium, and high increased risk.

? = association remains unproven.

[a] Risks for Lynch syndrome (heterozygous)—see main text for associated constitutional mismatch repair deficiency risks in biallelic mutation carriers.

[b] Risks for biallelic mutation carriers.

[c] General risks for each cancer site.

Main sources of information: Gene Reviews, http://www.ncbi.nlm.nih.gov/books/NBK1116/; CR-UK Cancer Stats (for population figures).

Additional useful tools: Familial Cancer Database, http://www.familialcancerdatabase.nl.

Cervix	Ovary	Lung	Para-thyroid	Thyroid	Adrenal	Eye	Brain/nervous system	Bone/soft tissue	Kidney	Uroth-elial	Testi-cular	Leukaemia/lymphoma
		Pulmonary chondroma			Adrenal cortical adenoma		Paragangliomas					
							Paragangliomas					
							Malignant psammomatous melanotic schwannoma					
					Phaeochromocytoma		Paragangliomas					
			Hyperparathyroidism 70% (in 10–15% caused by parathyroid carcinoma					Ossifying fibromas of the mandible or maxilla 30–40%	Renal cysts, hamartomas, Wilms tumour			
52 (37–68)	65 (55–76)						59 (48–74) brain		68 (60–79)			66 (57–82) leukaemia
		72 (65–80)					57 (46–71) brain		66 (59–76)			63 (55–78) leukaemia
1 in 134 (0.7)	1 in 70 (1.4)	1 in 18 (5.5)		1 in 90 (1.1)			Brain 1 in 150 (0.67)		1 in 90 (1.1)			Leukaemia
		1 in 14 (7)							1 in 56 (1.8)			1 in 110 (0.9%)

Radiological investigations including magnetic resonance imaging (MRI)

MRI

T1-weighted sequences typically demonstrate the cerebral anatomy well and are frequently used pre- and post-intravenous contrast medium (gadolinium DTPA (diethyltriaminepentaacetic acid)) to aid identification of pathology through typical patterns of vascular enhancement, in a similar fashion to computerized tomography (CT).

T2-weighted sequences are particularly useful for demonstrating oedema and for focal tumour detection, which both have increased signal and appear 'bright' on the images. T2-weighted sequences are limited in some situations by the fact that cerebrospinal fluid (CSF) also appears with increased signal and this may mask some subtle lesion (e.g. cortical tubers) close to fluid-filled regions such as the ventricles. In this situation, FLAIR (fluid-attenuated inversion recovery) sequences are helpful as they provide effective T2-weighting for oedema, tumours, and tuberous sclerosis (TSC) tubers, while suppressing the signal from fluid, making it appear dark.

Background radiation exposure

For effective radiation doses in adults, compared to background radiation exposure, please refer to the Radiological Society of North America, Inc at RadiologyInfo.org, http://www.radiologyinfo.org/en/pdf/safety-xray.pdf.

Skeletal dysplasia charts

For an approach to the radiological diagnosis of lethal and other skeletal dysplasias presenting at birth, see Table A15.

For the genetic basis and main radiological and clinical features of non-lethal skeletal dysplasias, see Table A16.

Table A15 An approach to the radiological diagnosis of lethal and other skeletal dysplasias presenting at birth

SKELETAL DYSPLASIAS PRESENTING AT BIRTH

DIAGNOSIS †	ALWAYS LETHAL *	LIMBS SHORT	LIMBS BENT/ANGULATED	LIMBS DISLOCATION	LIMBS FEMUR/TIBIA/FIBULA	LIMBS POLY-DACTYLY	SKULL OSSIFICATION	RIBS SHORT	RIBS BEADED/FRACTURED	SPINE PLATY-SPONDYLY	SPINE SOME ABSENT OSSIFICATION	PELVIS "TRIDENT" "SPIKEY"	BONE DENSITY ▲▼ + FRACTURE
ACHONDROPLASIA - HETERO:		rhizo.						+				+	
- HOMO:	+	rhizo.						+				+	
THANATOPHORIC I	+	++	+					++		++		+	
II	+	+	+				Clover leaf	+		+		+	
(Thanatophoric Variants)													
ACHONDROGENESIS I	+	++					▼	+	+		+		
II	+	++						+			+		
HYPOCHONDROGENESIS	+	+						+		+	+		
SPONDYLO-EPIPHYSEAL DYSPLASIA CONGENITA		(rhizo.)						+		+			
OSTEOGENESIS IMPERFECTA IIA	+	+	+				▼		+	+			▼ +
IIB	+	+	+						+				▼ +
IIC	+	+	+				▼		+				▼ +
III		(+)	(+)						+				▼ +
HYPOPHOSPHATASIA Lethal	+	+			Fib. ▼		▼		+	+	+		▼ +
Surviving			+										
CAMPOMELIC	+		+	+	Fib. ▼								
KYPHOMELIC		rhizo.	+										
DIASTROPHIC		+ (1st M.C. ++)		+						(+) (Scoliosis)			
METATROPIC		+			Dumb-bell			+		++			
KNIEST		+			Dumb-bell					(+)			
FIBROCHONDROGENESIS	+	+			Dumb-bell			++		++			
CHONDRODYSPLASIA PUNCTATA		rhizo. (+)											stippled ectopic calcification
OSTEOPETROSIS							▲						▲ +
PYCNODYSOSTOSIS							▲						▲ +
SHORT RIB SYNDROMES I Saldino-Noonan	+	+				+		++				+	
II Majewski	+	meso.			Oval Tibia	+		++					
III Verma-Naumoff	+	+				+		++				+	
Beemer	+	meso.				(+)		++					
Asphyxiating Thoracic (Jeune)		(+)				(+)		++				+	
Ellis van Creveld		meso.				+		++				+	
Atelosteogenesis I	+	rhizo.	+	+	Fib. ▼			+		+			
II	+	rhizo.		+	Fib. ▼								
III		rhizo.		+	(Fib. ▼)								
Boomerang / De La Chappelle	+	+	+		Fib. ▼			+		+	(+)	(+)	
Opsismodysplasia		+						+		+	+	+	
Schneckenbecken	+	+			Dumb-bell			+			+	+	
Dyssegmental Dysplasia I		+	+					+					
II	+	+	+					+					

All these findings should be easily observed by the non-specialist

† Grouped according to main radiographic features and (approximately) in descending order of frequency.

* Short limbs can be identified on ultrasound by 20 weeks gestation in the lethal conditions and a few non-lethal.

( ) In parenthesis – the finding may be present but mild, or absent.

▼ – indicates: 'reduced, short, hypoplastic or absent'.

▲ – indicates: 'increased, dense'.

Tissues should be stored from all these severe skeletal dysplasias to enable confirmatory genetic testing and/or prenatal diagnosis. Cryopreserved fibroblasts are suggested.

R. Wynne-Davies, C.M. Hall and J. Hurst for the Skeletal Dysplasia Group for Teaching and Research, Occasional publication no. 8c (2016) Edited by C.M. Hall, A.C. Offiah, M. Irving and S. Mansour. Reproduced with kind permission.

Table A16 Genetic basis and main radiological and clinical features of non-lethal skeletal dysplasias

DIAGNOSTIC GROUPS	MAIN RADIOLOGICAL FEATURES			MAIN ASSOCIATED ANOMALIES OR COMPLICATIONS	GENE (WHERE KNOWN)
	LIMBS		OSSIFICATION AND DENSITY		
	Deformity	Hands affected			
	Coxa vara / Malalignment				
1. SPONDYLOEPIPHYSEAL DISORDERS (1)					
Multiple epiphyseal dysplasia	(+) +	+ (V)	Delay		COMP, COL9A1/2/3, MATN3, DTDST (AR)
Stickler syndrome				Cleft palate, myopia, hearing **V**	COL2A1, COL11A1/2, COL9A1 (AR)
Chondrodysplasia punctata – mild/severe – Conradi		+ (V)	Punctate calcification	Cataract, cardiac, skin lesions	ARSE (XLR), PEX7/ DHAPAT/AGPS (AR), EBP (XLD)
2. SPONDYLOEPIPHYSEAL DISORDERS (2)					
Congenita	++		Delay at hips	Cleft palate, myopia	COL2A1
Tarda—X-linked AD/AR	+				SEDL
Progressive arthropathy	Contractures		Advanced	Contractures	WISP3
3. METAPHYSEAL and SPONDYLOMETAPHYSEAL					
MCD Schmidt	+				COL10A1
MCD McKusick	(+)	+ V		Blood **V**, hair **V**	RMRP
MCD Jansen	(+) +	+		Hypercalcaemia, hearing **V**, fractures	PTHR
MCD Shwachman	+		Delay	Pancreas **V**, blood **V**	SBDS
SMD Kozlowski					TRPV4
SMD Sutcliffe	+				(Strudwick COL2A1)
4. SHORT LIMBS, NORMAL TRUNK					
Achondroplasia	(+) Tib/fib	+ V		Spinal stenosis	FGFR3
Hypochondroplasia	Tib/fib	(+)			FGFR3
Dyschondrosteosis	Madelung	Wrist			SHOX
Acromesomelic	(+)	+ V	Hand advanced		GDF5 (CDMP1), NPR2, BMPR1B
Acrodysostosis		+ V	Hand advanced		PRKAR1A, PDE4D
Chondroectodermal (EVC)	+ knees	Polydac	Infant advanced	Cardiac, hair **V**	EVC1, EVC2
Asphyxiating thoracic (Jeune)		Polydac	Infant advanced	(Nephritis)	IFT80, DYNC2H1, TTC21B, WDR19/ NPHP13, NPHP12
5. SHORT LIMBS and TRUNK					
Pseudoachondroplasia	+	+ V	Delay at hips	(Severe joint laxity)	COMP
Diastrophic dysplasia	(+) Contractures	1st MC **V**	Delay/advanced	Cleft palate	DTDST
Metatropic dysplasia	+		Delay		TRPV4
Kniest dysplasia	(+)		Advanced	Cleft palate, myopia, hearing **V**	COL2A1
Dyggve–Melchior–Clausen			Delay	(Intellectual impairment)	DYM

Table A16 Continued

DIAGNOSTIC GROUPS	MAIN RADIOLOGICAL FEATURES				MAIN ASSOCIATED ANOMALIES OR COMPLICATIONS	GENE (WHERE KNOWN)
	LIMBS			OSSIFICATION AND DENSITY		
	Deformity		Hands affected			
	Coxa vara	Malalignment				
7. STORAGE DISORDERS						
Hurler (MPS I)	Valg	Contractures, hip dislocated	MC point		Intellectual impairment	*IDUA*
Hunter (MPS II)	Valg	Contractures	MC point		Intellectual impairment	*IDS*
Scheie (MPS IS)		Contractures				*IDUA*
Sanfilippo (MPS III)	Valg				Intellectual impairment	*SGSH(A)*, *NAGLU(B)*, *HGSNAT(C)*, *GNS9(D)*
Mannosidosis					Intellectual impairment	*MANBA*, *MAN2B1*
Maroteaux–Lamy (MPS VI)	Valg	Contractures	MC point			*ARSB*
Morquio (MPS IV)	Valg	++ knees	MC point	Hip advanced, then destroyed	Joint laxity, atlanto-axial instability	*GALNS* (type A), *GLB1* (type B)
Mucolipidoses	Valg	Contractures	MC point		Periosteal cloaking	*NEU1 (MLS 1)*, *GNPTAB (MLS 2/3)*, *GLB1 (GM1)*

+, feature present, increased, larger than normal; V, decreased, smaller, shorter than normal; ( ), the finding may or may not be present.

R. Wynne-Davies, C.M. Hall and J. Hurst for the Skeletal Dysplasia Group for Teaching and Research, Occasional publication no. 8c (2016) Edited by C.M. Hall, A.C. Offiah, M. Irving and S. Mansour. Reproduced with kind permission.

Staging of puberty

See 'Centile charts for height, weight, and occipital-frontal circumference (OFC)' in this appendix, pp. 815–822. The staging below is taken from Tanner (1962).

Girls: pubertal stages (98th–2nd centiles)

Breast development

Stage 1   Pre-adolescent: elevation of papilla only.

Stage 2   Breast bud stage: elevation of the breast and papilla as a small mound. Enlargement of areola diameter (8.2–13.8 years).

Stage 3   Further enlargement and elevation of the breast and areola, with no separation of their contours (9.7–14.3 years).

Stage 4   Projection of the areola and papilla to form a secondary mound above the level of the breast (10.5–15.7 years).

Pubic hair

Stage 1   Pre-adolescent: the vellus over the pubes is not further developed than that over the abdominal wall, i.e. no pubic hair.

Stage 2   Sparse growth of long slightly pigmented downy hair, straight or slightly curled, chiefly along labia (9.4–14.4 years).

Stage 3   Considerably darker, coarser, and more curled. The hair spreads sparsely over the junction of the pubes (10.2–15.2 years).

Stage 4   Hair now adult in type, but the area covered is still considerably smaller than in the adult. No spread to the medial surface of the thighs (11.2–16 years).

Stage 5   Adult in quantity and type.

Menarche

11–15 years (98th–2nd centiles); 10.3–15.7 years (99.6th–0.4th centile).

Republished with permission of Wiley, from *Growth at adolescence: with a general consideration of the effects of hereditary and environmental factors upon growth and maturation from birth to maturity*, Tanner JM, 1962; permission conveyed through Copyright Clearance Center, Inc.

Boys: pubertal stages (98th–2nd centiles)

Genital (penis) development

Stage 1   Pre-adolescent: testes, scrotum, and penis are of about the same size and proportion as in early childhood.

Stage 2   Enlargement of the scrotum and testes. Skin of the scrotum reddens and changes in texture. Little or no enlargement of the penis at this stage (9.8–14.2 years).

Stage 3   Enlargement of the penis, which occurs at first mainly in length; further growth of the testes and scrotum (11.1–14.3 years).

Stage 4   Increased size of the penis with growth and breadth and development of the glans. Testes and scrotum larger; scrotal skin darkened (12.1–15.9 years).

Stage 5   Genitalia adult in size and shape.

Pubic hair

Stage 1   Pre-adolescent: the vellus over the pubes is not further developed than that over the abdominal wall, i.e. no pubic hair.

Stage 2   Sparse growth of long, slightly pigmented downy hair, straight or slightly curled, chiefly at the base of the penis (10.3–14.2 years).

Stage 3   Considerably darker, coarser, and more curled. The hair spreads sparsely over the junction of the pubes (11.1–14.9 years).

Stage 4   Hair now adult in type, but the area covered is still considerably smaller than in the adult. No spread to the medial surface of the thighs (12.1–15.9 years).

Stage 5   Adult in quantity and type.

Republished with permission of Wiley, from *Growth at adolescence: with a general consideration of the effects of hereditary and environmental factors upon growth and maturation from birth to maturity*, Tanner JM, 1962; permission conveyed through Copyright Clearance Center, Inc.

References

Child Growth Foundation. *Boys four-in-one growth charts.* Harlow Printing Ltd, South Shields, 1996.

Child Growth Foundation. *Girls four-in-one growth charts.* Harlow Printing Ltd, South Shields, 1996.

Tanner JM. *Growth at adolescence*, 2nd edn. Blackwell Scientific, Oxford, 1962.

Surveillance for individuals at increased genetic risk of colorectal cancer

For a summary of recommendations for high- and moderate-risk family groups, see Tables A17 and A18. For a summary of recommendations for high-risk disease groups, see Table A19.

Expert adviser

Ian M Frayling, Consultant Genetic Pathologist, Cardiff & Vale University Health Board, Cardiff University, Institute of Medical Genetics, University Hospital of Wales, Cardiff, UK.

Table A17 Summary of recommendations for colorectal cancer screening and surveillance in high-risk family groups

Family history categories*	Lifetime risk of CRC death (without surveillance)	Screening procedure	Age at initial screen	Screening interval and procedure	Procedures/year/ 300 000
At-risk HNPCC (fulfils modified Amsterdam criteria,† or untested FDR of proven mutation carrier)	1 in 5 (male) 1 in 13 (female)	MMR gene testing of affected relative Colonoscopy ± OGD	Colonoscopy from age 25 years OGD from age 50 years	18–24 months colonoscopy (2-yearly OGD from age 50 years)	50
MMR gene carrier	1 in 2.5 (male) 1 in 6.5 (female)	Colonoscopy ± OGD			
At-risk FAP (member of FAP family with no mutation identified)	1 in 4	APC gene testing of affected relative Colonoscopy or alternating colonoscopy/flexible sigmoidoscopy	Puberty Flexible approach important, making allowance for variation in maturity	Annual colonoscopy or alternating colonoscopy/flexible sigmoidoscopy until aged 30 years Thereafter 3- to 5-yearly until 60 years Procto-colectomy or colectomy if +ve	2
Fulfils clinical FAP criteria, or proven APC mutation carrier opting for deferred surgery—prophylactic surgery normally strongly recommended	1 in 2	Colonoscopy or alternating colonoscopy/flexible sigmoidoscopy OGD with forward and side-viewing scope	Usually at diagnosis. Otherwise puberty Flexible approach important, making allowance for variation in maturity	Recommendation for procto-colectomy and pouch/colectomy before age 30 years Cancer risk increases dramatically age >30 years Twice-yearly colonoscopy or alternating colonoscopy/flexible sigmoidoscopy	1
FAP post-colectomy and IRA	1 in 15 (rectal cancer)	Flexible rectoscopy Forward and side-viewing OGD	After surgery OGD from age 30 years	Annual flexible rectoscopy 3-yearly forward and side-viewing OGD	3 (dependent on surgical practice)
FAP post-procto-colectomy and pouch	Negligible	DRE and pouch endoscopy Forward and side-viewing OGD	After surgery OGD from age 30 years	Annual exams alternating flexible/rigid pouch endoscopy 3-yearly forward and side-viewing OGD	3 (dependent on surgical practice)
MUTYH-associated polyposis (MAP)	1 in 2–2.5	Genetic testing Colonoscopy ± OGD	Colonoscopy from age 25 years OGD from age 30 years	Mutation carriers should be counselled about the available limited evidence Options include prophylactic colectomy and ileorectal anastomosis; or biennial colonoscopy surveillance 3- to 5-yearly gastro-duodenoscopy	4

(Continued)

Table A17 Continued

Family history categories*	Lifetime risk of CRC death (without surveillance)	Screening procedure	Age at initial screen	Screening interval and procedure	Procedures/year/ 300 000
One FDR with MSI-H colorectal cancer AND IHC shows loss of MSH2, MSH6, or PMS2 expression	1 in 5 (male) 1 in 13 (female) (likely overestimate)	Colonoscopy ± OGD	Colonoscopy from age 25 years OGD from age 50 years	2-yearly colonoscopy (with OGD aged >50 years)	<5, but variable, depending on extent of use of MSI and IHC tumour analysis
MLH1 loss and MSI specifically excluded (MLH1 loss in elderly patient with right-sided tumour is usually somatic epigenetic event)					
Peutz–Jeghers syndrome	1 in 6	Genetic testing of affected relative Colonoscopy ± OGD	Colonoscopy from age 25 years OGD from age 25 years Small bowel MRI/enteroclysis	2-yearly colonoscopy Consider colectomy and IRA for colonic cancer Small bowel VCE or MRI/enteroclysis 2- to 4-yearly OGD 2-yearly	3
Juvenile polyposis	1 in 6	Genetic testing of affected relative Colonoscopy ± OGD	Colonoscopy from age 15 years OGD from age 25 years	2-yearly colonoscopy and OGD. Extend interval aged >35 years	3

* The Amsterdam criteria for identifying HNPCC are: three or more relatives with colorectal cancer; one patient a first-degree relative of another; two generations with cancer; and one cancer diagnosed below the age of 50 or other HNPCC-related cancers, e.g. endometrial, ovarian, gastric, upper urothelial, and biliary tree.

† Clinical genetics referral and family assessment required, if not already in place or referral was not initiated by Clinical genetics.

FAP, familial adenomatosis polyposis; FDR, first-degree relative (sibling, parent, or child) with colorectal cancer; HNPCC, hereditary non-polyposis colorectal cancer; IHC, immunohistochemistry of tumour material from affected proband; MSI-H, microsatellite instability—high (two or more MSI markers show instability); OGD, oesophagogastroduodenoscopy; VCE, video capsule endoscopy.

Reproduced from *Gut*, Cairnes *et al.*, Guidelines for colorectal cancer screening and surveillance in moderate and high risk groups (update from 2002), 59(5), Table 2, page 683, Copyright 2010, with permission from BMJ Publishing Group Ltd.

Table A18 Summary of recommendations for colorectal cancer screening and surveillance in moderate-risk family groups

Moderate-risk family history categories	Lifetime risk of CRC death (without surveillance)#	Screening procedure	Age at initial screen (if older at presentation, instigate forthwith)	Screening procedure and interval	Procedures/year/300 000
†Colorectal cancer in three FDR in first-degree kinship*, none <50 years	~1 in 6–10	Colonoscopy	50 years	5-yearly colonoscopy to age 75 years	~18
†Colorectal cancer in two FDR in first-degree kinship*, mean age <60 years	~1 in 6–10	Colonoscopy	50 years	5-yearly colonoscopy to age 75 years	~60
‡Colorectal cancer in two FDR ≥60 years	~1 in 12	Colonoscopy	55 years	Once-only colonoscopy at age 55 years. If normal—no follow-up	12
‡Colorectal cancer in one FDR <50 years	~1 in 12	Colonoscopy	55 years	Once-only colonoscopy at age 55 years. If normal—no follow-up	10
All other family history of colorectal cancer	>1 in 12	None	N/A	N/A	None
Incident colorectal cancer case (age <50 years, or MMR prediction >10%), not fulfilling Lynch syndrome (LS) criteria	N/A	Tumour MSI and/or IHC analysis§. If no tumour testing available, consider genetics referral	N/A	Standard post-op follow-up, unless LS features on tumour analysis or a mutation identified, then LS surveillance applies	20

* Affected relatives who are first-degree relatives of each other AND at least one is a first-degree relative of the consultand. No affected relative <50 years old (otherwise high-risk criteria would apply). Combinations of three affected relatives in a first-degree kinship include: parent and aunt/uncle and/or grandparent; OR two siblings/one parent; OR two siblings/one parent. Combinations of two affected relatives in a first-degree kinship include a parent and grandparent, or >2 siblings, or >2 children, or child + sibling. Where both parents are affected, these count as being within the first-degree kinship.

† Clinical genetics referral recommended.

‡ Centres may vary, depending on capacity and referral agreements. Ideally, all such cases should be flagged systematically for future audit on a national scale.

§ Refer to clinical genetics if IHC loss or MSI-H.

Cancer Research UK (http://info.cancerresearchuk.org/cancerstats) and ISD Scotland (http://www.isdscotland.org/isd/183.html).

FDR, first-degree relative (sibling, parent, or child) with colorectal cancer; IHC, immunohistochemistry of tumour material from affected proband; MSI-H, microsatellite instability—high (two or more MSI markers show instability).

Reproduced from *Gut*, Cairnes et al., Guidelines for colorectal cancer screening and surveillance in moderate and high risk groups (update from 2002), 59(5), Table 3, page 683, Copyright 2010, with permission from BMJ Publishing Group Ltd.

Table A19 Summary of recommendations for colorectal cancer screening and surveillance in high-risk disease groups

High-risk disease groups		Screening procedure	Time of initial screen	Screening procedure and interval
Colorectal cancer		Consultation, CT, LFTs, and colonoscopy	Colonoscopy within 6 months of resection *only* if colon evaluation preop incomplete	CT liver scan within 2 years post-op. Colonoscopy 5-yearly until comorbidity outweighs
Colonic adenomas	Low risk 1–2 adenomas, both <1 cm	Colonoscopy	5 years or no surveillance	Cease follow-up after negative colonoscopy
	Intermediate risk 3–4 adenomas, OR at least one adenoma ≥1 cm	Colonoscopy	3 years	3-yearly until two consecutive negative colonoscopies, then no further surveillance
	High risk ≥5 adenomas or ≥3 with at least one ≥1 cm	Colonoscopy	1 year	Annual colonoscopy until out of this risk group, then interval colonoscopy as per intermediate risk group
	Piecemeal polypectomy	Colonoscopy or flexi-sig (depending on polyp location)	3 months—consider open surgical resection if incomplete healing of polypectomy scar	

Reproduced from *Gut*, Cairnes *et al.*, Guidelines for colorectal cancer screening and surveillance in moderate and high risk groups (update from 2002), 59(5), Table 4, Copyright 2010, with permission from BMJ Publishing Group Ltd.

Index

Note: Figures, tables, and boxes are indicated by 'f', 't' or 'b' following the page number, for example 46f would indicate a figure on page 45.